Meyler's Side Effects of Drugs

The International Encyclopedia of Adverse Drug Reactions and Interactions

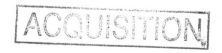

Complementary to this volume

Side Effects of Drugs Annuals 24–29 (1999–2006)
Edited by Jeffrey K. Aronson (Earlier annuals are no longer available in print)

Drugs During Pregnancy and Lactation, Second edition (2006)
Edited by Christof Schaefer et al.

The Law and Ethics of the Pharmaceutical Industry (2005)
By Graham Dukes

Introduction to Clinical Pharmacology, Fifth edition (2006)
By Marilyn Edmunds

Principles of Clinical Pharmacology, Second edition (2006)
Edited by Arthur Atkinson et al.

Writing Clinical Research Protocols (2006)
By E. De Renzo

A Pharmacology Primer (2003)
By Terry Kenakin

Publishing history of *Meyler's Side Effects of Drugs*

*Volume**	*Date of publication*	*Editors*
First published in Dutch	1951	L Meyler
First published in English	1952	L Meyler
First updating volume	1957	L Meyler
Second volume	1958	L Meyler
Third volume	1960	L Meyler
Fourth volume	1964	L Meyler
Fifth volume	1966	L Meyler, C Dalderup, W Van Dijl, and HGG Bouma
Sixth volume	1968	L Meyler and A Herxheimer
Seventh volume	1972	L Meyler and A Herxheimer
Eighth volume	1975	MNG Dukes
Ninth edition	1980	MNG Dukes
Tenth edition	1984	MNG Dukes
Eleventh edition	1988	MNG Dukes
Twelfth edition	1992	MNG Dukes
Thirteenth edition	1996	MNG Dukes
Fourteenth edition	2000	MNG Dukes & JK Aronson
Fifteenth edition	2006	JK Aronson

*The first eight volumes were updates; the ninth edition was the first encyclopedic version and updating continued with the Side Effects of Drugs Annual (SEDA) series.

At various times, full or shortened editions of volumes in the Side Effects series have appeared in French, Russian, Dutch, German, and Japanese.
The website of *Meyler's Side Effects of Drugs* can be viewed at:
   http://www.elsevier.com/locate/Meyler.

Meyler's Side Effects of Drugs

The International Encyclopedia of Adverse Drug Reactions and Interactions

Fifteenth edition

Editor

JK Aronson, MA, DPhil, MBChB, FRCP, FBPharmacol S
Oxford, United Kingdom

Honorary Editor

MNG Dukes, MA, DPhil, MB, FRCP
Oslo, Norway

ELSEVIER

AMSTERDAM • BOSTON • HEIDELBERG • LONDON • NEW YORK • OXFORD
PARIS • SAN DIEGO • SAN FRANCISCO • SINGAPORE • SYDNEY • TOKYO

Elsevier
Radarweg 29, PO Box 211, 1000 AE Amsterdam, The Netherlands

Fifteenth edition 2006
Reprinted 2007

British Library Cataloguing in Publication Data
A catalogue record for this book is available from the British Library

Library of Congress Cataloging-in-Publication Data
A catalog record for this book is available from the Library of Congress

ISBN: 978-0-444-50998-7 (Set)
ISBN: 978-0-444-52251-1 (Volume 1)
ISBN: 978-0-444-52252-8 (Volume 2)
ISBN: 978-0-444-52253-5 (Volume 3)
ISBN: 978-0-444-52254-2 (Volume 4)
ISBN: 978-0-444-52255-9 (Volume 5)
ISBN: 978-0-444-52256-6 (Volume 6)

For information on all Elsevier publications
visit our website at books.elsevier.com

Printed and bound in *Great Britain*

07 08 09 10 10 9 8 7 6 5 4 3 2

Contents

Contributors

In this list the main contributors to the Encyclopedia are identified according to the original chapter material to which they made the most contribution. Most have contributed the relevant chapters in one or more editions of the *Side Effects of Drugs Annuals* 23-27 and/or the 14th edition of *Meyler's Side Effects of Drugs*. A few have contributed individual monographs to this edition.

M. Allwood
Derby, United Kingdom
Intravenous infusions—solutions and emulsions

M. Andersen
Odense, Denmark
Antihistamines

M. Andrejak
Amiens, France
Drugs affecting blood coagulation, fibrinolysis, and hemostasis

J.K. Aronson
Oxford, United Kingdom
Antiepileptic drugs
Antiviral drugs
Positive inotropic drugs and drugs used in dysrhythmias

S. Arroyo
Milwaukee, Wisconsin, USA
Antiepileptic drugs

I. Aursnes
Oslo, Norway
Drugs that affect lipid metabolism

H. Bagheri
Toulouse, France
Radiological contrast agents

A.M. Baldacchino
London, United Kingdom
Opioid analgesics and narcotic antagonists

D. Battino
Milan, Italy
Antiepileptic drugs

Z. Baudoin
Zagreb, Croatia
General anesthetics and therapeutic gases

A.G.C. Bauer
Rotterdam, The Netherlands
Antihelminthic drugs
Dermatological drugs, topical agents, and cosmetics

M. Behrend
Deggendorf, Germany
Drugs acting on the immune system

T. Bicanic
London, United Kingdom
Antiprotozoal drugs

L. Biscarini
Perugia, Italy
Anti-inflammatory and antipyretic analgesics and drugs used in gout

J. Blaser
Zurich, Switzerland
Various antibacterial drugs

C. Bokemeyer
Tübingen, Germany
Cytostatic drugs

S. Borg
Stockholm, Sweden
Antidepressant drugs

J. Bousquet
Montpellier, France
Antihistamines

P.J. Bown
Redhill, Surrey, United Kingdom
Opioid analgesics and narcotic antagonists

C.N. Bradfield
Auckland, New Zealand
General anesthetics and therapeutic gases

C.C.E. Brodie-Meijer
Amstelveen, The Netherlands
Metal antagonists

P.W.G. Brown
Sheffield, United Kingdom
Radiological contrast agents

A. Buitenhuis
Amsterdam, The Netherlands
Sex hormones and related compounds, including hormonal contraceptives

H. Cardwell
Auckland, New Zealand
Local anesthetics

A. Carvajal
Valladolid, Spain
Antipsychotic drugs

R. Cathomas
Zurich, Switzerland
Drugs acting on the respiratory tract

A. Cerny
Zurich, Switzerland
Various antibacterial drugs

G. Chevrel
Lyon, France
Drugs acting on the immune system

C.C. Chiou
Bethesda, Maryland, USA
Antifungal drugs

N.H. Choulis
Attika, Greece
Metals
Miscellaneous drugs and materials, medical devices, and techniques not dealt with in other chapters

L.G. Cleland
Adelaide, Australia
Corticotrophins, corticosteroids, and prostaglandins

P. Coates
Adelaide, Australia
Miscellaneous hormones

J. Costa
Badalona, Spain
Corticotrophins, corticosteroids, and prostaglandins

P. Cottagnoud
Bern, Switzerland
Various antibacterial drugs

P.C. Cowen
Oxford, United Kingdom
Antidepressant drugs

S. Curran
Huddersfield, United Kingdom
Hypnosedatives and anxiolytics

H.C.S. Daly
Perth, Western Australia
Local anesthetics

A.C. De Groot
Hertogenbosch, The Netherlands
Dermatological drugs, topical agents, and cosmetics

M.D. De Jong
Amsterdam, The Netherlands
Antiviral drugs

A. Del Favero
Perugia, Italy
Anti-inflammatory and antipyretic analgesics and drugs used in gout

P. Demoly
Montpellier, France
Antihistamines

J. Descotes
Lyon, France
Drugs acting on the immune system

A.J. De Silva
Ragama, Sri Lanka
Snakebite antivenom

H.J. De Silva
Ragama, Sri Lanka
Gastrointestinal drugs

F.A. De Wolff
Leiden, The Netherlands
Metals

S. Dittmann
Berlin, Germany
Vaccines

M.N.G. Dukes
Oslo, Norway
Antiepileptic drugs
Antiviral drugs
Metals
Sex hormones and related compounds, including hormonal contraceptives

H.W. Eijkhout
Amsterdam, The Netherlands
Blood, blood components, plasma, and plasma products

E.H. Ellinwood
Durham, North Carolina, USA
Central nervous system stimulants and drugs that suppress appetite

C.J. Ellis
Birmingham, United Kingdom
Drugs used in tuberculosis and leprosy

P. Elsner
Jena, Germany
Dermatological drugs, topical agents, and cosmetics

T. Erikkson
Lund, Sweden
Thalidomide

E. Ernst
Exeter, United Kingdom
Treatments used in complementary and alternative medicine

M. Farré
Barcelona, Spain
Corticotrophins, corticosteroids, and prostaglandins

P.I. Folb
Cape Town, South Africa
Cytostatic drugs
Intravenous infusions—solutions and emulsions

J.A. Franklyn
Birmingham, United Kingdom
Thyroid hormones and antithyroid drugs

M.G. Franzosi
Milan, Italy
Beta-adrenoceptor antagonists and antianginal drugs

J. Fraser
Glasgow, Scotland
Cytostatic drugs

H.M.P. Freie
Maastricht, The Netherlands
Antipyretic analgesics

C. Fux
Bern, Switzerland
Various antibacterial drugs

P.J. Geerlings
Amsterdam, The Netherlands
Drugs of abuse

A.H. Ghodse
London, United Kingdom
Opioid analgesics and narcotic antagonists

P.L.F. Giangrande
Oxford, United Kingdom
Drugs affecting blood coagulation, fibrinolysis, and hemostasis

G. Gillespie
Perth, Australia
Local anaesthetics

G. Girish
Sheffield, United Kingdom
Radiological contrast agents

V. Gras-Champel
Amiens, France
Drugs affecting blood coagulation, fibrinolysis, and hemostasis

A.I. Green
Boston, Massachusetts, USA
Drugs of abuse

A.H. Groll
Münster, Germany
Antifungal drugs

H. Haak
Leiden, The Netherlands
Miscellaneous drugs and materials, medical devices, and techniques not dealt with in other chapters

F. Hackenberger
Bonn, Germany
Antiseptic drugs and disinfectants

J.T. Hartmann
Tübingen, Germany
Cytostatic drugs

K. Hartmann
Bern, Switzerland
Drugs acting on the respiratory tract

A. Havryk
Sydney, Australia
Drugs acting on the respiratory tract

E. Hedayati
Auckland, New Zealand
General anesthetics and therapeutic gases

E. Helsing
Oslo, Norway
Vitamins

R. Hoigné
Wabern, Switzerland
Various antibacterial drugs

A. Imhof
Seattle, Washington, USA
Various antibacterial drugs

L.L. Iversen
Oxford, United Kingdom
Cannbinoids

J. W. Jefferson
Madison, Wisconsin, USA
Lithium

D.J. Jeffries
London, United Kingdom
Antiviral drugs

M. Joerger
St Gallen, Switzerland
Drugs acting on the respiratory tract

G.D. Johnston
Belfast, Northern Ireland
Positive inotropic drugs and drugs used in dysrhythmias

P. Joubert
Pretoria, South Africa
Antihypertensive drugs

A.A.M. Kaddu
Entebbe, Uganda
Antihelminthic drugs

C. Koch
Copenhagen, Denmark
Blood, blood components, plasma, and plasma products

H. Kolve
Münster, Germany
Antifungal drugs

H.M.J. Krans
Hoogmade, The Netherlands
Insulin, glucagon, and oral hypoglycemic drugs

M. Krause
Scherzingen, Switzerland
Various antibacterial drugs

S. Krishna
London, United Kingdom
Antiprotozoal drugs

M. Kuhn
Chur, Switzerland
Drugs acting on the respiratory tract

R. Latini
Milan, Italy
Beta-adrenoceptor antagonists and antianginal drugs

T.H. Lee
Durham, North Carolina, USA
Central nervous system stimulants and drugs that
suppress appetite

P. Leuenberger
Lausanne, Switzerland
Drugs used in tuberculosis and leprosy

M. Leuwer
Liverpool, United Kingdom
Neuromuscular blocking agents and skeletal muscle
relaxants

G. Liceaga Cundin
Guipuzcoa, Spain
Drugs that affect autonomic functions or the
extrapyramidal system

P.O. Lim
Dundee, Scotland
Beta-adrenoceptor antagonists and antianginal drugs

H.-P. Lipp
Tübingen, Germany
Cytostatic drugs

C. Ludwig
Freiburg, Germany
Drugs acting on the immune system

T.M. MacDonald
Dundee, Scotland
Beta-adrenoceptor antagonists and antianginal drugs

G.T. McInnes
Glasgow, Scotland
Diuretics

I.R. McNicholl
San Francisco, California, USA
Antiviral drugs

P. Magee
Coventry, United Kingdom
Antiseptic drugs and disinfectants

A.P. Maggioni
Firenze, Italy
Beta-adrenoceptor antagonists and antianginal drugs

J.F. Martí Massó
Guipuzcoa, Spain
Drugs that affect autonomic functions or the
extrapyramidal system

L.H. Martín Arias
Valladolid, Spain
Antipsychotic drugs

M.M.H.M. Meinardi
Amsterdam, The Netherlands
Dermatological drugs, topical agents, and cosmetics

D.B. Menkes
Wrexham, United Kingdom
Hypnosedatives and anxiolytics

R.H.B. Meyboom
Utrecht, The Netherlands
Metal antagonists

T. Midtvedt
Stockholm, Sweden
Various antibacterial drugs

G. Mignot
Saint Paul, France
Gastrointestinal drugs

S.K. Morcos
Sheffield, United Kingdom
Radiological contrast agents

W.M.C. Mulder
Amsterdam, The Netherlands
Dermatological drugs, topical agents, and cosmetics

S. Musa
Wakefield, United Kingdom
Hypnosedatives and anxiolytics

K.A. Neftel
Bern, Switzerland
Various antibacterial drugs

A.N. Nicholson
Petersfield, United Kingdom
Antihistamines

L. Nicholson
Auckland, New Zealand
General anesthetics and therapeutic gases

I. Öhman
Stockholm, Sweden
Antidepressant drugs

H. Olsen
Oslo, Norway
Opioid analgesics and narcotic antagonists

I. Palmlund
London, United Kingdom
Diethylstilbestrol

J.N. Pande
New Delhi, India
Drugs used in tuberculosis and leprosy

J.K. Patel
Boston, Massachusetts, USA
Drugs of abuse

J.W. Paterson
Perth, Australia
Drugs acting on the respiratory tract

K. Peerlinck
Leuven, Belgium
Drugs affection blood coagulation, fibrinolysis, and
hemostasis

E. Perucca
Pavia, Italy
Antiepileptic drugs

E.H. Pi
Los Angeles, California, USA
Antipsychotic drugs

T. Planche
London, United Kingdom
Antiprotozoal drugs

B.C.P. Polak
Amsterdam, The Netherlands
Drugs used in ocular treatment

T.E. Ralston
Worcester, Massachusetts, USA
Drugs of abuse

P. Reiss
Amsterdam, The Netherlands
Antiviral drugs

H.D. Reuter
Köln, Germany
Vitamins

I. Ribeiro
London, United Kingdom
Antiprotozoal drugs

T.D. Robinson
Sydney, Australia
Drugs acting on the respiratory tract

Ch. Ruef
Zurich, Switzerland
Various antibacterial drugs

M. Schachter
London, United Kingdom
Drugs that affect autonomic functions or the
extrapyramidal system

A. Schaffner
Zurich, Switzerland
Various antibacterial drugs
Antifungal drugs

S. Schliemann-Willers
Jena, Germany
Dermatological drugs, topical agents, and cosmetics

M. Schneemann
Zürich, Switzerland
Antiprotozoal drugs

S.A. Schug
Perth, Australia
Local anesthetics

G. Screaton
Oxford, United Kingdom
Drugs acting on the immune system

J.P. Seale
Sydney, Australia
Drugs acting on the respiratory tract

R.P. Sequeira
Manama, Bahrain
Central nervous system stimulants and drugs that
suppress appetite

T.G. Short
Auckland, New Zealand
General anesthetics and therapeutic gases

D.A. Sica
Richmond, Virginia, USA
Diuretics

G.M. Simpson
Los Angeles, California, USA
Antipsychotic drugs

J.J. Sramek
Beverly Hills, California, USA
Antipsychotic drugs

A. Stanley
Birmingham, United Kingdom
Cytostatic drugs

K.J.D. Stannard
Perth, Australia
Local anesthetics

B. Sundaram
Sheffield, United Kingdom
Radiological contrast agents

J.A.M. Tafani
Toulouse, France
Radiological contrast agents

M.C. Thornton
Auckland, New Zealand
Local anesthetics

B.S. True
Campbelltown, South Australia
Corticotrophins, corticosteroids, and prostaglandins

C. Twelves
Glasgow, Scotland
Cytostatic drugs

W.G. Van Aken
Amsterdam, The Netherlands
Blood, blood components, plasma, and plasma products

C.J. Van Boxtel
Amsterdam, The Netherlands
Sex hormones and related compounds, including
hormonal contraceptives

G.B. Van der Voet
Leiden, The Netherlands
Metals

P.J.J. Van Genderen
Rotterdam, The Netherlands
Antihelminthic drugs

R. Verhaeghe
Leuven, Belgium
Drugs acting on the cerebral and peripheral circulations

J. Vermylen
Leuven, Belgium
Drugs affecting blood coagulation, fibrinolysis, and hemostasis

P. Vernazza
St Gallen, Switzerland
Antiviral drugs

T. Vial
Lyon, France
Drugs acting on the immune system

P. Vossebeld
Amsterdam, The Netherlands
Blood, blood components, plasma, and plasma products

G.M. Walsh
Aberdeen, United Kingdom
Antihistamines

T.J. Walsh
Bethesda, Maryland, USA
Antifungal drugs

R. Walter
Zurich, Switzerland
Antifungal drugs

D. Watson
Auckland, New Zealand
Local anesthetics

J. Weeke
Aarhus, Denmark
Thyroid hormones and antithyroid drugs

C.J.M. Whitty
London, United Kingdom
Antiprotozoal drugs

E.J. Wong
Boston, Massachusetts, USA
Drugs of abuse

C. Woodrow
London, United Kingdom
Antiprotozoal drugs

Y. Young
Auckland, New Zealand
General anesthetics and therapeutic gases

F. Zannad
Nancy, France
Antihypertensive drugs

J.-P. Zellweger
Lausanne, Switzerland
Drugs used in tuberculosis and leprosy

A. Zinkernagel
Zürich, Switzerland
Antiprotozoal drugs

M. Zoppi
Bern, Switzerland
Various antibacterial drugs

O. Zuzan
Hannover, Germany
Neuromuscular blocking agents and skeletal muscle relaxants

Foreword

My doctor is
A good doctor
He made me no
Iller than I was

Willem Hussem (The Netherlands) 1900–1974
Translation: Peter Raven

"*Primum non nocere*"—in the first place, do no harm—is often cited as one of the foundation stones of sound medical care, yet its origin is uncertain. Hippocrates? There are some who will tell you so;[1] but the phrase is not a part of the Hippocratic Oath, and the Father of Medicine wrote in any case in his native Greek.[2] It could be that the Latin phrase is from the Roman physician Galenius, while others attribute it to Scribonius Largus, physician to one of the later Caesars,[3] and there is a lot of reason to believe that it actually originated in 19th century England.[4] Hippocrates himself, in the first volume of his *Epidemics*, put it at all events better in context: "When dealing with diseases have two precepts in mind: to procure benefit and not to harm."[5] One must not become overly obsessed by the safety issue, but it is a necessary element in good medical care.

The ability to do good with the help of medicines has developed immensely within the last century, but with it has come the need to keep a watchful eye on the possibility of inflicting harm on the way. The challenge is to recognize at the earliest possible stage the adverse effects that a valuable drug may induce, and to find ways of containing them, so that risk never becomes disproportionate to benefit. The process of drug development will sometimes result in methods of treatment that are more specific to their purpose than were their predecessors and hence less likely to produce unwanted complications; yet the more novel a therapeutic advance the greater the possibility of its eliciting adverse effects of a type so unfamiliar that they are not specifically looked for and long remained unrecognized when they do occur. The entire process of keeping medicines safe today involves all those concerned with them, whether as researchers, manufacturers, regulators, prescribers, dispensers, or users, and it demands an effective and honest flow of information and thought between them.

For several decennia, concerned by its own errors in the past, the science of therapeutics put unbounded faith in the ability of well-planned clinical trials to arrive at the truth about the properties of medicines. Insofar as efficacy was concerned that was and remains a sound move, closing the door to charlatanism as well as to well-meant amateurism. Therapeutic trials with a new medicine were also able to delineate those adverse effects that occurred in a fair proportion of users. If serious, they would bar the drug from entry to the market altogether, while if transient and reasonably tolerable they would form the basis for warnings and precautions as well as the occasional contraindication. The problem lay with those adverse drug reactions that occurred rather less commonly or not at all in populations recruited for therapeutic trials, yet which could soon arise in the much broader spectrum of patients exposed to the drug once it was marketed across the world. The influence of race or climate might explain some of them; others might reflect interactions with foods, alcohol, or other drugs; yet others could only be explained, if at all, in terms of the particular susceptibility of certain individuals. Scattered across the globe, these effects might readily be overlooked, regarded as coincidental, or at worst dismissed contemptuously as "merely anecdotal".

The seriousness of the adverse effects issue became very apparent even as the reputation of controlled trials deservedly grew, and it touched on both newer and older drugs. The thalidomide calamity, involving several thousand cases of drug-induced phocomelia, was fortunately recognized by Widukind Lenz and others in the light of individual case reports within two years of the introduction of the product. On the other hand, generations elapsed between the patenting of aspirin in 1899 and the realization in 1965 that it might induce Reye's syndrome when used to treat fever in children. Such events, and many less spectacular, showed that, however vital well-controlled studies had become, there was good reason to remain alert for signals emerging from individual cases. Unanticipated events occurring during drug treatment might indeed reflect mere coincidence, but again they might not; and for many of the patients who suffered in consequence there was nothing in the least anecdotal about them.

Fortunately, the 1950s and 1960s of the 20th century saw the first positive reactions to the adverse reaction issue. Effective drug regulation emerged in one country after another. In 1952, Prof. Leo Meyler of The Netherlands produced his first "Side Effect of Drugs" to pull together data from the world literature. A number of national adverse reaction monitoring bureaux were established to gather data from the field and examine carefully reports of suspected side effects of medicines, creating the basis for the World Health Organization to establish its global reporting system. The pharmaceutical industry has increasingly realized its duty to collect and pass on the information that comes into its possession through its wide contacts with the health professions. Later years have seen the emergence, notably in Sweden and in Britain, of systems through which patients themselves can report possible adverse effects to the medicines they have taken. All these processes fit together in what the French language so appropriately terms "pharmacovigilance", with vigilance as the watchword for all concerned.

In this continuing development, the medical literature provides a resource with vast potential. The world is believed to have some 20 000 medical journals, of which a nuclear group of a thousand or so can be relied upon to publish reports and analyses of adverse effects—not only in the framework of formal investigations but also in letters, editorials, and reports of meetings large and small. Much of that information comprises not so much firm facts as emergent knowledge, based directly on experience in the field and calling urgently for attention. The book that Leo Meyler created has, in the course of fifteen editions and with the support of an ever-larger team of professionals, provided the means by which that attention can be mobilized. It has become the world's principal tool in bringing together, encyclopedically but critically, the evidence on the basis of which adverse drug effects and interactions can be recognized, discussed, and accommodated into medical practice. Together with its massive database and its complementary *Side Effects of Drugs Annuals*, it has evolved into a vital instrument in ensuring that drugs are used wisely and well and with due caution, in the light of all that is known about them.

There is nothing else like it, nor need there be; across the world, *Meyler* has become a pillar of responsible medical care.

M.N. Graham Dukes
Honorary Editor, *Meyler's Side Effects of Drugs*
Oslo, Norway

Notes

1. Lichtenhaeler C. Histoire de la Médicine, Fayard, Paris, 1978:117.
2. Smith CM. Origin and uses of *Primum non nocere*. J Clin Pharmacol 2005;45:371–7.
3. Albrecht H. Primum nil nocere. Die Zeit, 6 April, 2005.
4. Notably in a book by Inman T. *Foundation for a New Theory and Practice of Medicine*. London, 1860.
5. I am indebted to Jeffrey Aronson for his own translation of the Greek original from Hippocrates *Epidemics*, Book I, Section XI, which seems to convey the meaning of the original [ἀσκεῖν περὶ τὰ νοσημάτα δύο, ὠφελεῖν ἤ μὴ βλάπτειν] rather better than the published translations of his work.

Preface

This is a completely new edition of what has become the standard reference text in the field of adverse drug reactions and interactions since Leopold Meyler published his first review of the subject 55 years ago. Although we have retained the old title, *Meyler's Side Effects of Drugs*, the subtitle of this edition, *The Encyclopedia of Adverse Drug Reactions and Interactions*, reflects both modern terminology and the scope of the review. The structure of the book may have changed, but the *Encyclopedia* remains the most comprehensive reference source on adverse drug reactions and interactions and a major source of informed discussion about them.

Scope

The scope of the *Encyclopedia* remains wide. It covers not only the vast majority of prescription drugs, old and new, but also non-prescribed substances (such as anesthetics, antiseptics, lifestyle compounds, and drugs of abuse), herbal medicines, devices (such as blood glucose meters), and methods in alternative and complementary medicine. For this edition, entries on some substances that were regarded as obsolete, such as thalidomide and smallpox vaccine, have been rewritten and restored. Other compounds, such as diethylstilbestrol, although no longer in use, continue to cast their shadow and are included. Yet others, currently regarded as obsolete, have been retained, both for historical reasons and because one can never be sure when an old compound may once more become relevant or provide useful information in relation to another compound. Some drugs have been withdrawn from the market in some countries since the last edition of *Meyler* was published; rofecoxib, cisapride, phenylpropanolamine, and kava (see Piperaceae) are examples. Nevertheless, detailed monographs have been included on these substances because of the lessons that they can teach us and in some cases because of their relevance to other compounds in their classes that are still available; it is also not possible to predict whether these compounds will eventually reappear in some other form or for some new indication.

In the last 15 years there has been increasing emphasis on the use of high-quality evidence in therapeutic practice, principally as obtained from large, randomized clinical trials and from systematic reviews of the results of many such trials. However, while it has been possible to obtain useful information about the beneficial effects of interventions in this way, evidence about harms, including adverse drug reactions, has been more difficult to obtain. Even trials that yield good estimates of benefits are poor at providing evidence about harms for several reasons:

- benefits are usually single, whereas harms are usually multiple;
- the chance of any single form of harm is usually smaller than the chance of benefit and therefore more difficult to detect; however, multiple harms can accumulate and affect the benefit-to-harm balance;
- benefits are identifiable in advance, whereas harms are not or not always;

- the likely time-course of benefits can generally be predicted, while the time-course of harms often cannot and may be much delayed by comparison with the duration of a trial.

For all these reasons, larger and sometimes longer studies are needed to detect harms. In recent years attempts have been made to conduct systematic reviews of adverse reactions, but these have also been limited by several problems:

- harms are in general poorly collected in randomized trials and trials may not last long enough to detect them all;
- even when they are well collected, as is increasingly happening, they are often poorly reported;
- even when they are well reported in the body of a report, they may not be mentioned in titles and abstracts;
- even when they are well reported in the body of a report, they may be poorly indexed in large databases.

All this means that it is difficult to collect information on adverse drug reactions from randomized, controlled trials for systematic review. This can be seen from the evidence provided in Table 1, which shows the proportion of different types of information that have been used in the preparation of two volumes of the *Side Effects of Drugs Annual*, proportions that are likely be the same in this *Encyclopedia*.

Wherever possible, emphasis in this *Encyclopedia* has been placed on information that has come from systematic reviews and clinical trials of all kinds; this is reflected in new headings under which trial results are reported (observational studies, randomized studies, placebo-controlled studies). However, because many reports of adverse drug reactions (about 30%) are anecdotal, with evidence from one or just a few cases, many individual case studies (see below) have also been included. We need better methods to make use of the information that this large body of anecdotes provides.

Structure

The first major change that readers will notice is that the chapter structure of previous editions has given way to a monographic structure. That is because some of the information about individual drugs has previously been scattered over different chapters in the book; for example ciclosporin was previously covered in Chapter 37 and in scattered sections throughout Chapter 45; it is now dealt with in a single monograph. The monographs are arranged in alphabetical order, with cross-referencing as required. For example, if you turn to the monograph on cetirizine, you will be referred to the complementary general monograph on antihistamines, where much information that is relevant to cetirizine is given; the monograph on cetirizine itself contains information that is relevant only to cetirizine and not to other antihistamines. Within each monograph the material is arranged in the same way as in the *Side Effects of Drugs Annuals* (see "How to use this book").

Case Reports

A new feature, recognizable from the Annuals, but not incorporated into previous editions, is the inclusion of case reports of adverse effects. This feature reflects the fact that about 30% of all the literature that is reported and discussed in the Annuals derives from such reports (see Table 1). In some cases the only information about an adverse effect is contained in an anecdotal report; in other cases the report illustrates a variant form of the reaction. A case report also gives more immediacy to an adverse reaction, allowing the reader to appreciate more precisely the exact nature of the reported event.

Classification of Adverse Drug Reactions

Another new feature of this edition is the introduction of the DoTS method of classifying adverse drug reactions, based on the **Dose** at which they occur relative to the beneficial dose, the **Time-course** of the reaction, and individual **Susceptibility factors** (see "How to use this book"). This has been done for selected adverse effects, and I hope that as volumes of SEDA continue to be published and the *Encyclopedia's* electronic database is expanded, it will be possible to classify increasing numbers of adverse reactions in this way.

References

Because all the primary and secondary literature is thoroughly surveyed in the Annuals, the *Encyclopedia* has become increasingly compact relative to the amount of information available (even though it has increased in absolute size), with many unreferenced statements and cross-references to the Annuals, on the assumption that all the information would be readily available to the reader, although that may not always be the case. To restore all the reference material on which the *Encyclopedia* has been based as it has evolved over so many years would be a gargantuan task, but in this edition a major start has been made. Many references to original

material have been restored, and there is now hardly a statement that is not backed up by at least one reference to primary literature. In addition, almost all of the material that was published in Annuals 23 to 27 (SEDA-23 to SEDA-27) has been included, complete with citations. This has resulted in the inclusion of more than 40 000 references in this edition. Readers will still have to refer to earlier editions of the Annual (SEDA-1 to SEDA-22) and occasionally to earlier editions of *Meyler's Side Effects of Drugs* for more detailed descriptions, but now that the *Encyclopedia* is available electronically this will be repaired in future editions.

Methods and Contributors

I initially prepared the text of the *Encyclopedia* by combining text from the 14th edition of *Meyler's Side Effects of Drugs* and the five most recent annuals (SEDA-23 to SEDA-27). [Later literature is covered in SEDA-28 and the forthcoming SEDA-29.] I next restored missing references to the material and extended it where important information had not been included. The resulting monographs were then sent to experts for review, and their comments were incorporated into the finished monographs. I am grateful to all those, both authors of chapters in previous editions and Annuals and those who have reviewed the monographs for this edition, for their hard work and for making their expertise available.

Acknowledgements

This 15th edition of *Meyler's Side Effects of Drugs* was initiated and carefully planned with Joke Jaarsma at Elsevier, who has provided unstinting support during the production of several previous editions of *Meyler's Side Effects of Drugs* and the *Side Effects of Drugs Annuals*. Early discussions with Dieke van Wijnen at Elsevier about the structure of the text were invaluable. Professor Leufkens from the Faculty of Pharmacy at the University of Utrecht was instrumental in helping us to assemble the preliminary content for this edition; pharmacy students in his department entered the text

Table 1 Types of articles on adverse drug reactions published in 6576 papers in the world literature during 1999 and 2003 (as reviewed in SEDA-24 and SEDA-28)

Type of article	Number of descriptions* (%)
An anecdote or set of anecdotes (that is reported case histories)	2084 (29.9)
A major, randomized, controlled trial or observational study	1956 (28.1)
A minor, randomized, controlled trial or observational study or a non-randomized study (including case series)	1099 (15.8)
A major review, including non-systematic statistical analyses of published studies	951 (13.7)
A brief commentary (for example an editorial or a letter)	362 (5.19)
An experimental study (animal or in vitro)	263 (3.77)
A meta-analysis or other form of systematic review	172 (2.47)
Official statements (for example by Governmental organizations, the WHO, or manufacturers)	75 (1.07)
Total no. of descriptions*	6962
Total no. of articles	6576

* Some articles are described in more than one way

electronically into templates under the guidance of Joke Zwetsloot from Elsevier. Christine Ayorinde provided excellent assistance while I expanded and edited the material. The International Non-proprietary Names were checked by Renée Aronson. At Elsevier the references were then checked and collated by Liz Perill, who also copyedited the material, with Ed Stolting, and shepherded it through conversion to different electronic formats. Bill Todd created the indexes. Stephanie Diment oversaw the project and coordinated everyone's efforts.

The History of Meyler

The history of *Meyler's Side Effects of Drugs* goes back 55 years; a full account can be found at http://www.elsevier.com/locate/Meyler and the various volumes are listed before the title page of this set. When Leopold Meyler, a physician, experienced unwanted effects of drugs that were used to treat his tuberculosis, he discovered that there was no single text to which medical practitioners could turn for information about the adverse effects of drug therapy; Louis Lewin's text *Die Nebenwirkungen der Arzneimittel* ("The Untoward Effects of Drugs") of 1881 had long been out of print (SEDA-27, xxv–xxix). Meyler therefore surveyed the current literature, initially in Dutch as *Schadelijke Nevenwerkingen van Geneesmiddelen* (Van Gorcum, 1951), and then in English as *Side Effects of Drugs* (Elsevier, 1952). He followed up with what he called

surveys of unwanted effects of drugs. Each survey covered a period of two to four years and culminated in Volume VIII (1976), edited by Graham Dukes (SEDA-23, xxiii–xxvi), Meyler having died in 1973. By then the published literature was too extensive to be comfortably encompassed in a four-yearly cycle, and an annual cycle was started instead; the first *Side Effects of Drugs Annual* (SEDA-1) was published in 1977. The four-yearly review was replaced by a complementary critical encyclopaedic survey of the entire field; the first encyclopaedic edition of *Meyler's Side Effects of Drugs*, which appeared in 1980, was labelled the ninth edition.

Since then, *Meyler's Side Effects of Drugs* has been published every four years, providing an encyclopaedic survey of the entire field. Had the cycle been adhered to, the 15th edition would have been published in 2004, but over successive editions the quantity and nature of the information available in the text has changed. In the new millennium it was clear that for this edition a revolutionary approach was needed, and that has taken a little longer to achieve, with a great deal of effort from many different individuals.

We have come a long way since Meyler published his first account in a book of 192 pages. I think that he would have approved of this new *Encyclopedia*.

J. K. Aronson
Oxford, October 2005

How to use this book

In a departure from its previous structure, this edition of *Meyler's Side Effects of Drugs* is presented as individual drug monographs in alphabetical order. In many cases a general monograph (for example Antihistamines) is complemented by monographs about specific drugs (for example acrivastine, antazoline, etc.); in that case a cross-reference is given from the latter to the former.

Monograph Structure

Within each monograph the information is presented in sections as follows:

GENERAL INFORMATION

Includes, when necessary, notes on nomenclature, information about the results of observational studies, comparative studies, and placebo-controlled studies in relation to reports of adverse drug reactions, and a general summary of the major adverse effects.

ORGANS AND SYSTEMS

Cardiovascular (includes heart and blood vessels)
Respiratory
Ear, nose, throat
Nervous system (includes central and peripheral nervous systems)
Neuromuscular function
Sensory systems (includes eyes, ears, taste)
Psychological, psychiatric
Endocrine (includes hypothalamus, pituitary, thyroid, parathyroid, adrenal, pancreas, sex hormones)
Metabolism
Nutrition (includes effects on amino acids, essential fatty acids, vitamins, micronutrients)
Electrolyte balance (includes sodium, potassium)
Mineral balance (includes calcium, phosphate)
Metal metabolism (includes copper, iron, magnesium, zinc)
Acid–base balance
Fluid balance
Hematologic (includes blood, spleen, and lymphatics)
Mouth and teeth
Salivary glands
Gastrointestinal (includes esophagus, stomach, small bowel, large bowel)
Liver
Biliary tract
Pancreas
Urinary tract (includes kidneys, ureters, bladder, urethra)
Skin
Hair
Nails
Sweat glands
Serosae (includes pleura, pericardium, peritoneum)
Musculoskeletal (includes muscles, bones, joints)
Sexual function
Reproductive system (includes uterus, ovaries, breasts)
Immunologic (includes effects on the immune system and hypersensitivity reactions)
Autacoids

Infection risk
Body temperature
Multiorgan failure
Trauma
Death

LONG-TERM EFFECTS

Drug abuse
Drug misuse
Drug tolerance
Drug resistance
Drug dependence
Drug withdrawal
Genotoxicity
Mutagenicity
Tumorigenicity

SECOND-GENERATION EFFECTS

Fertility
Pregnancy
Teratogenicity
Fetotoxicity
Lactation

SUSCEPTIBILITY FACTORS (relates to features of the patient)

Genetic factors
Age
Sex
Physiological factors
Cardiac disease
Renal disease
Hepatic disease
Thyroid disease
Other features of the patient

DRUG ADMINISTRATION

Drug formulations
Drug additives
Drug contamination (includes infective agents)
Drug adulteration
Drug dosage regimens (includes frequency and duration of administration)
Drug administration route
Drug overdose

DRUG–DRUG INTERACTIONS
FOOD–DRUG INTERACTIONS
SMOKING
OTHER ENVIRONMENTAL INTERACTIONS
INTERFERENCE WITH DIAGNOSTIC TESTS
DIAGNOSIS OF ADVERSE DRUG REACTIONS
MANAGEMENT OF ADVERSE DRUG REACTIONS
MONITORING THERAPY

Classification of Adverse Drug Reactions

Selected major reactions are classified according to the DoTS system (BMJ 2003;327:1222–5). In this system adverse reactions are classified according to the **Dose** at which they usually occur relative to the beneficial dose, the **Time-course** over which they occur, and the **Susceptibility factors** that make them more likely, as follows:

1   **Relation to dose**

- *Toxic reactions* (reactions that occur at supratherapeutic doses)
- *Collateral reactions* (reactions that occur at standard therapeutic doses)
- *Hypersusceptibility reactions* (reactions that occur at subtherapeutic doses in susceptible patients)

2   **Time-course**

- *Time-independent reactions* (reactions that occur at any time during a course of therapy)
- *Time-dependent reactions*
    - Immediate reactions (reactions that occur only when a drug is administered too rapidly)
    - First-dose reactions (reactions that occur after the first dose of a course of treatment and not necessarily thereafter)
    - Early reactions (reactions that occur early in treatment then abate with continuing treatment)
    - Intermediate reactions (reactions that occur after some delay but with less risk during longer-term therapy, owing to the "healthy survivor" effect)
    - Late reactions (reactions the risk of which increases with continued or repeated exposure), including withdrawal reactions (reactions that occur when, after prolonged treatment, a drug is withdrawn or its effective dose is reduced)
    - Delayed reactions (reactions that occur some time after exposure, even if the drug is withdrawn before the reaction appears)

3   **Susceptibility factors**

- *Genetic*
- *Age*
- *Sex*
- *Physiological variation*
- *Exogenous factors* (for example drug–drug or food–drug interactions, smoking)
- *Diseases*

Drug Names And Spelling

Drugs are usually designated by their recommended or proposed International Non-proprietary Names (rINN or pINN); when these are not available, chemical names have been used. If a fixed combination has a generic combination name (for example co-trimoxazole for trimethoprim + sulfamethoxazole) that name has been used; in some cases brand names have been used.

Spelling

Where necessary, for indexing purposes, American spelling has been used, for example anemia rather than anaemia, estrogen rather than oestrogen.

Cross-references

The various editions of *Meyler's Side Effects of Drugs* are cited in the text as SED-l3, SED-14, etc.; the *Side Effects of Drugs Annuals* 1-22 are cited as SEDA-1, SEDA-2, etc. This edition includes most of the contents of SEDA-23 to SEDA-27. SEDA-28 and SEDA-29 are separate publications, which were prepared in parallel with the preparation of this edition.

Indexes

Index of drug names

An index of drug names provides a complete listing of all references to a drug for which adverse effects and/or drug interactions are described. The monograph on herbal medicines contains tabulated cross-indexes to the plants that are covered in separate monographs.

Index of adverse effects

This index is necessarily selective, since a particular adverse effect may be caused by very large numbers of compounds; the index is therefore mainly directed to adverse effects that are particularly serious or frequent, or are discussed in special detail; before assuming that a given drug does not have a particular adverse effect, consult the relevant monograph.

Alphabetical list of drug monographs

The number in parentheses after each heading is the number of the corresponding chapter in the Side Effects of Drug Annuals (SEDA-28 and later) in which the item is usually covered.

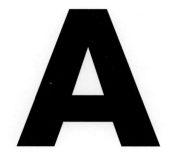

Abacavir

See also Nucleoside analogue reverse transcriptase inhibitors (NRTIs)

General Information

Abacavir is a guanidine analogue that inhibits HIV reverse transcriptase. In vitro, its potency is similar to that of zidovudine, protease inhibitors, and dual nucleoside combinations. There is evidence that abacavir is effective in reducing viral load and increasing the CD4 count in HIV-infected patients. Viral resistance is not rapidly selected for, but cross-resistance has been shown to other analogues of cytosine and guanidine (didanosine, lamivudine, and zalcitabine).

Abacavir has good oral systemic availability and penetrates the nervous system. It does not interfere with drugs that are metabolized by liver microsomal cytochrome P450 (1). It has no other significant drug interactions and can be administered without food restrictions.

Observational studies

The effects of abacavir have been evaluated in a study in over 13 000 adults who no longer responded to commercially available treatment regimens (2). By month 2 of treatment with abacavir, plasma HIV-1 RNA concentrations fell by at least half a log unit in 31% of patients, and in 5.6% of the patients HIV-1 RNA concentrations fell to under 400 copies/ml. Serious drug-related adverse events were reported by 7.7% of patients. The most common were nausea, skin rash, diarrhea, malaise or fatigue, and fever. About 4.6% of patients had a hypersensitivity reaction that was possibly drug-related.

General adverse effects

The adverse effects of abacavir that have been most often observed in clinical trials are fatigue, nausea and vomiting, abdominal pain, diarrhea, headache, rash, and dyspepsia (3,4). Allergic reactions lead to withdrawal of therapy in about 3% of patients (5). These can be severe, and anaphylaxis has been reported after rechallenge in a patient with an apparent allergic reaction to abacavir (6). It is wise to avoid rechallenge when allergy is suspected (7). In one study nausea and vomiting occurred in 38–57% of patients, headache in 27–41%, malaise and fatigue in 28%, diarrhea in 18–23%, and weakness in 29% (8). There was also one case of agranulocytosis accompanied by a skin rash.

Organs and Systems

Nervous system

Vertigo has been attributed to abacavir (9).

- A 44-year-old African-American developed vertigo, tinnitus in both ears, headache behind the eyes, and left ear pain and hearing loss soon after starting to take abacavir, lamivudine, and stavudine. There was left-sided nystagmus and vestibular tests showed evidence of vestibular impairment. An MRI scan was normal. All the antiretroviral drugs were withdrawn and he improved. When lamivudine and stavudine were restarted, with nevirapine, the vertigo did not recur.

Metabolism

While abacavir has been associated with hyperglycemia in individual cases (10), there were no significant effects on blood glucose concentration in clinical trials.

- A 47-year-old man, with normoglycemia and no family history of diabetes mellitus, who was taking highly active antiretroviral therapy, was given abacavir for treatment intensification. He became lethargic and hyperglycemic. Despite metformin and glibenclamide, the hyperglycemia continued. Abacavir was withdrawn, and within 2 weeks his blood glucose concentration returned to baseline and the hypoglycemic drugs were withdrawn.

This patient was also taking hydrochlorothiazide, but the time-course of onset and resolution were consistent with abacavir-induced hyperglycemia.

Immunologic

The risk of allergic reactions to abacavir may be as high as 10% (11). However, the incidence is more usually reported to be 3–5% (12,13). Allergic reactions usually occur within the first 28 days of therapy and rarely thereafter. They are characterized by non-specific complaints suggestive of an upper respiratory tract infection, fever, rash, nausea, and vomiting. Resolution of the symptoms occurs within days of withdrawal. Severe and even fatal reactions to readministration have been observed, and it has been suggested that rechallenge is contraindicated in any patients who have had an allergic reaction (7). However, it is safe to rechallenge patients who have stopped treatment because of other types of adverse reaction. Of 1201 patients treated in clinical trials, 219 interrupted abacavir therapy for reasons other than allergy; on reintroduction there were no cases of allergy or anaphylaxis (14).

The susceptibility factors associated with allergic reactions have been sought in an analysis of all protocols conducted by GlaxoSmithKline that involved abacavir exposure for at least 24 weeks with a quality-assured or validated clinical database by 30 June 2000 ($n = 5332$) (15). There were 197 allergic reactions (3.7%). The risks of allergic reactions were lower in black people (OR = 0.59; 95% CI = 0.38, 0.91) than in other ethnic groups, and in patients who had received previous therapy for HIV-1 infection with other antiretroviral agents (OR = 0.58; 95% CI = 0.44, 0.78) compared with those receiving therapy for the first time.

Genetic factors affecting the immune response to abacavir have been sought in patients who had taken abacavir for more than 6 weeks, 18 with hypersensitivity reactions and 167 without (16). HLA-B*5701 was present in 14 of the 18 patients with abacavir hypersensitivity, and in four of the 167 others (OR = 117; 95% CI = 29, 481). The combination of HLA-DR7 and

HLA-DQ3 was found in 13 of the 18 and five of the 167 (OR = 73; CI = 20, 268). HLA-B*5701, HLA-DR7, and HLA-DQ3 were present in combination in 13 of the 18 and none of the 167 (OR = 822; CI = 43, 15 675). Other MHC markers also present on the 57.1 ancestral haplotype to which these three markers belong confirmed the presence of haplotype-specific linkage disequilibrium, and mapped potential susceptibility loci to a region bounded by C4A6 and HLA-C. HLA-B*5701, HLA-DR7, and HLA-DQ3 had a positive predictive value for hypersensitivity of 100%, and a negative predictive value of 97%. The authors concluded that susceptibility to abacavir hypersensitivity is carried on the 57.1 ancestral haplotype and that withholding abacavir from those with HLA-B*5701, HLA-DR7, and HLA-DQ3 should reduce the prevalence of hypersensitivity from 9% to 2.5% without inappropriately denying abacavir to any patient.

In a retrospective case-control study of patients with allergic reactions, HLA-B57 was present in 39 of 84 patients compared with 4 of 113 controls (17). However, there were few women and other ethnic groups in the study, and so these findings relate largely to white men.

In a multicenter trial, 128 children were randomly assigned to zidovudine + lamivudine ($n = 36$), to zidovudine + abacavir ($n = 45$), or to lamivudine + abacavir ($n = 47$) (18). One child had an allergic reaction to abacavir and stopped taking it, as did three with possible reactions.

References

1. Ravitch JR, Bryant BJ, Reese MJ, et al. In vivo and in vitro studies of the potential for drug interactions involving the anti-retroviral 1592 in humans. 5th Conference on Retroviruses and Opportunistic Infections, Chicago, 1–5 February 1998: Abstract 634.
2. Kessler HA, Johnson J, Follansbee S, Sension MG, Mildvan D, Sepulveda GE, Bellos NC, Hetherington SV. Abacavir expanded access program for adult patients infected with human immunodeficiency virus type 1. Clin Infect Dis 2002;34(4):535–42.
3. Kumar PN, Sweet DE, McDowell JA, Symonds W, Lou Y, Hetherington S, LaFon S. Safety and pharmacokinetics of abacavir (1592U89) following oral administration of escalating single doses in human immunodeficiency virus type 1-infected adults. Antimicrob Agents Chemother 1999;43(3):603–8.
4. Vernazza PL, Katlama C, Clotet B, et al. Intensification of stable background (SBG) antiretroviral therapy (ART) with Ziagen (ABC,1592). 6th Conference on Retroviruses and Opportunistic Infections, Chicago, Jan 31–Feb 4 1999.
5. Staszewski S. Coming therapies: abacavir. Int J Clin Pract Suppl 1999;103:35–8.
6. Walensky RP, Goldberg JH, Daily JP. Anaphylaxis after rechallenge with abacavir. AIDS 1999;13(8):999–1000.
7. Escaut L, Liotier JY, Albengres E, Cheminot N, Vittecoq D. Abacavir rechallenge has to be avoided in case of hypersensitivity reaction. AIDS 1999;13(11):1419–20.
8. Tikhomirov V, Namek K, Hindes R. Agranulocytosis induced by abacavir. AIDS 1999;13(11):1420–1.
9. Fantry LE, Staecker H. Vertigo and abacavir. AIDS Patient Care STDS 2002;16(1):5–7.
10. Modest GA, Fuller J, Hetherington SV, Lenhard JM, Powell GS. Abacavir and diabetes. N Engl J Med 2001;344(2):142–4.
11. Katlama C, Fenske S, Gazzard B, Lazzarin A, Clumeck N, Mallolas J, Lafeuillade A, Mamet JP, Beauvais L; AZL30002 European study team. TRIZAL study: switching from successful HAART to Trizivir (abacavir–lamivudine–zidovudine combination tablet): 48 weeks efficacy, safety and adherence results. HIV Med 2003;4(2):79–86.
12. Hervey PS, Perry CM. Abacavir: a review of its clinical potential in patients with HIV infection. Drugs 2000;60(2):447–79.
13. Henry K, Wallace RJ, Bellman PC, Norris D, Fisher RL, Ross LL, Liao Q, Shaefer MS; TARGET Study Team. Twice-daily triple nucleoside intensification treatment with lamivudine–zidovudine plus abacavir sustains suppression of human immunodeficiency virus type 1: results of the TARGET Study. J Infect Dis 2001;183(4):571–8.
14. Loeliger AE, Steel H, McGuirk S, Powell WS, Hetherington SV. The abacavir hypersensitivity reaction and interruptions in therapy. AIDS 2001;15(10):1325–6.
15. Symonds W, Cutrell A, Edwards M, Steel H, Spreen B, Powell G, McGuirk S, Hetherington S. Risk factor analysis of hypersensitivity reactions to abacavir. Clin Ther 2002;24(4):565–73.
16. Mallal S, Nolan D, Witt C, Masel G, Martin AM, Moore C, Sayer D, Castley A, Mamotte C, Maxwell D, James I, Christiansen FT. Association between presence of HLA-B*5701, HLA-DR7, and HLA-DQ3 and hypersensitivity to HIV-1 reverse-transcriptase inhibitor abacavir. Lancet 2002;359(9308):727–32.
17. Hetherington S, Hughes AR, Mosteller M, Shortino D, Baker KL, Spreen W, Lai E, Davies K, Handley A, Dow DJ, Fling ME, Stocum M, Bowman C, Thurmond LM, Roses AD. Genetic variations in HLA-B region and hypersensitivity reactions to abacavir. Lancet 2002;359(9312):1121–2.
18. Paediatric European Network for Treatment of AIDS (PENTA). Comparison of dual nucleoside-analogue reverse-transcriptase inhibitor regimens with and without nelfinavir in children with HIV-1 who have not previously been treated: the PENTA 5 randomised trial. Lancet 2002;359(9308):733–40.

Abciximab

See also Monoclonal antibodies

General Information

Abciximab is a Fab fragment of the chimeric human-murine monoclonal antibody 7E3, which binds to the platelet glycoprotein IIb/IIIa receptor and inhibits platelet aggregation (1).

Abciximab is used for prevention of cardiac ischemic events in patients undergoing percutaneous coronary intervention and to prevent myocardial infarction in patients with unstable angina who do not respond to conventional treatment. It has also been used for thrombolysis in patients with peripheral arterial occlusive disease and arterial thrombosis (2).

Besides bleeding, other adverse reactions that have been associated with abciximab include back pain, hypotension, nausea, and chest pain (but with an incidence not significantly different from that observed with placebo).

Organs and Systems

Respiratory

Lung hemorrhage is a rare but potentially lethal complication of antithrombotic and antiplatelet therapy. The incidence of spontaneous pulmonary hemorrhage after the use of platelet glycoprotein IIb/IIIa inhibitors has been analysed from the medical records of 1020 consecutive patients who underwent coronary interventions (3). Diffuse pulmonary hemorrhage developed in seven patients, two of whom died and five of whom had activated clotting times greater than 250 seconds during the procedure. Activated partial thromboplastin time measured at the time of lung hemorrhage was raised in all cases (mean 85, range 69–95 seconds). All had a history of congestive heart failure, and had raised pulmonary capillary wedge pressures and/or left ventricular end-diastolic pressures at the time of the procedure. Six patients also had evidence of baseline radiographic abnormalities.

Nervous system

Seven patients undergoing neurointerventional procedures who received abciximab developed fatal intracerebral hemorrhages (4). The procedures included angioplasty and stent placement in the cervical internal carotid artery ($n = 4$), angioplasty of the intracranial carotid artery ($n = 1$), and angioplasty of the middle cerebral artery ($n = 2$). Aggressive antithrombotic treatment is used as adjuvant to angioplasty and/or stent placement to reduce the rate of ischemic and thrombotic complications associated with these procedures. Intravenous abciximab has a short life (10 minutes), but its inhibitory effect on platelets lasts for 48 hours. The exact cause of abciximab-associated intracerebral hemorrhage is unclear.

Hematologic

Bleeding

The primary risk associated with abciximab is bleeding. In the EPIC trial in high-risk angioplasty, 14% of patients who received a bolus of abciximab followed by an infusion had a major bleeding complication rate, versus 7% in the placebo group (5). The most marked excess of major bleeding episodes occurred at the site of vascular puncture, but there were also a substantial number of gastrointestinal haemorrhages. However, the therapeutic regimen used was not adjusted for body weight, and the risk of major bleeding was also related to the heparin dose per kg and not only to the use of abciximab (6).

In 7800 patients with chest pain and either ST segment depression or a positive troponin test, the addition of abciximab to unfractionated heparin or low molecular weight heparin in the treatment of acute coronary syndrome was not associated with any significant reduction in cardiac events, but a doubled risk of bleeding (7).

An analysis of data from the EPIC trial identified a series of factors that predicted vascular access site bleeding or the need for vascular access site surgery in abciximab-treated patients (8). They comprised larger vascular access sheath size, the presence of acute myocardial infarction at enrolment, female sex, higher baseline hematocrits, lower body weight, and a longer time spent in the catheterization laboratory.

It must be emphasized that patients in the EPIC trial received high-dose heparin and that vascular access site sheaths were left in place for 12–16 hours. In subsequent studies, the risk of vascular site bleeding was probably reduced by using lower doses of heparin and removing sheaths sooner. This was the case in the EPILOG trial in which heparin was withdrawn immediately after the coronary procedure and vascular sheaths were removed as soon as possible (9). The incidence of major bleeding in this study was not significantly higher with abciximab than with placebo. Nevertheless, the incidence of minor bleeding complications was significantly higher in the abciximab plus standard dose heparin group (but not in the abciximab plus low dose heparin group) compared with placebo. In the EPISTENT trial, all patients received low dose, body weight-adjusted heparin: Here the incidence of both major and minor bleeding complications was low and not significantly different between treatment groups (10).

It would therefore seem possible to reduce the incidence of bleeding complications when using abciximab during prophylactic coronary revascularization procedures. This is unfortunately not the case so far in the setting of primary angioplasty for myocardial infarction after intense anticoagulation (17% of major hemorrhagic complications versus 9.5 in placebo recipients) (11). The risk of serious bleeding complications is also increased in rescue situations when high doses of heparin have been used (12), but here it can be reduced by giving protamine to reverse heparin anticoagulation before abciximab therapy (13). There is also a high incidence of major bleeding in patients who receive abciximab during percutaneous coronary revascularization after unsuccessful thrombolytic therapy. It has been suggested that abciximab should not be administered within 18 hours after thrombolytic therapy (14).

It must be emphasized that very few episodes of abciximab-related bleeding are life-threatening and that in none of the trials with abciximab as well as with other glycoprotein IIb/IIIa antagonists has there been an excess of intracranial hemorrhage (15).

However, the bleeding risk in patients enrolled in trials may not be representative of the population actually being given abciximab. To clarify this, a review of adverse events in patients receiving glycoprotein IIb/IIIa inhibitors reported to the FDA has been undertaken (16,17). The FDA received 450 reports of deaths related to treatment with glycoprotein IIb/IIIa inhibitors between November 1, 1997 and December 31, 2000; these were reviewed and a standard rating system for assessing causation was applied to each event. Of the 450 deaths, 44% were considered to be definitely or probably attributable to glycoprotein IIb/IIIa inhibitors.

The mean age of patients who died was 69 years and 47% of the deaths were in women. All of the deaths that were deemed to be definitely or probably associated with glycoprotein IIb/IIIa inhibitors were associated with excessive bleeding, most often in the nervous system.

Thrombocytopenia

The other significant risk associated with abciximab is thrombocytopenia. Data pooled from three major trials showed that thrombocytopenia (under 100×10^9/l) was significantly more frequent in those who received a bolus dose of abciximab followed by an infusion than in placebo recipients (3.7 versus 2%). Severe thrombocytopenia (under 50×10^9/l) was also more frequent with abciximab (1.1 versus 0.5%) (18). Very acute and profound thrombocytopenia (under 20×10^9/l) within 24 hours after administration has been observed in 0.3–0.7% of patients treated with abciximab for the first time (15,18–20).

During postmarketing surveillance of the first 4000 patients treated with abciximab in France, 25 cases of thrombocytopenia (0.6%) were reported, with five severe cases (0.15%) and three acute profound forms (0.08%). In all cases reported, the role of heparin must be taken into account. The thrombocytopenia associated with abciximab differs with that associated with heparin by its rapid onset (within 24 hours), its reversal after platelet transfusion, and its possible association with hemorrhage but not with thrombosis.

Positive human anti-chimeric antibodies have been detected in 6% of patients (generally in low titers) but were not associated with hypersensitivity or allergic reactions. Preliminary data indicate that abciximab can be safety readministered, although a greater incidence of thrombocytopenia after administration has been reported with a lesser efficacy of platelet transfusion (12).

Thrombocytopenia due to abciximab usually occurs within 12–96 hours, but there has been a report of acute profound thrombocytopenia after 7 days (21).

- A 65-year-old woman with type 2 diabetes mellitus and coronary artery disease received a 0.25 mg/kg bolus of abciximab at the time of intervention followed by an infusion of 10 micrograms/minute for 12 hours. Her baseline platelet counts were 286×10^9/l before use, 385×10^9/l at 2 hours, and 296×10^9/l at 18 hours. On day 7 she developed petechiae over her legs and her platelet count was 1×10^9/l. Coagulation tests were normal and there was no evidence of heparin-induced thrombocytopenia. She received 10 units of single-donor platelets and recovered slowly over the next 4 days. The platelet count was 114×10^9/l on day 12.

In another case of profound thrombocytopenia after abciximab there was a delayed onset (6 days after therapy) (22). The authors speculated that preceding treatment with methylprednisolone may have delayed the onset of thrombocytopenia.The mechanism of severe thrombocytopenia associated with abciximab is unclear. Further administration should be avoided, but other glycoprotein IIb/IIIa inhibitors (eptifibatide and tirofiban)

have been successfully used in patients with history of abciximab-induced thrombocytopenia.

Thrombocytopenia after a second exposure to abciximab in nine patients showed that each had a strong immunoglobulin IgG antibody that recognized platelets sensitized with abciximab (23). Five patients also had IgM antibodies. Thrombocytopenia occurred four times as often as after the first exposure. The mechanism is not understood, but these findings suggest that it may be antibody-mediated. These antibodies were also found in 77 of 104 healthy patients, but in the patients the antibodies were specific for murine sequences in abciximab, causing the life-threatening thrombocytopenia.

Nine patients who developed profound thrombocytopenia after a second exposure to abciximab had an IgG antibody that recognized platelets sensitized with abciximab. In contrast, in 104 healthy subjects, in whom IgG antibodies reactive with abciximab-coated platelets were found in 77, the antibodies were specific for murine sequences in abciximab and were capable of causing life-threatening thrombocytopenia (23).

Ethylenediaminetetra-acetate can cause pseudothrombocytopenia by activating platelet agglutination, resulting in a spuriously low platelet count (SEDA-21, 250). Of 66 patients who received abciximab after coronary revascularization, 17 developed thrombocytopenia and 9 developed severe thrombocytopenia (24). However, of these 26 patients, 18 had pseudothrombocytopenia. True thrombocytopenia occurred at 4 hours after infusion whereas pseudothrombocytopenia occurred within the first 24 hours. The mechanism of pseudothrombocytopenia may be the effect of EDTA on the calcium-dependant glycoprotein IIb/IIIa complex, which frees the antigenic binding site on glycoprotein IIb available to IgM antibody. This increased antibody binding may cause platelet clumping and lead to false thrombocytopenia. True thrombocytopenia did not lead to hemorrhagic complications, but the patients required platelet transfusion.

Immunologic

Human antichimeric antibodies, specific to the murine epitope of Fab antibody fragments, have been observed in patients treated with abciximab. These antibodies are IgG antibodies and have so far not correlated with any adverse effects (12).

Because of its antigenic potential, there are theoretical concerns about the readministration of abciximab, and this has been studied in 1342 patients, who underwent percutaneous coronary interventions and received abciximab at least twice (25). There were no cases of anaphylaxis, and there were only five minor allergic reactions, none of which required termination of the infusion. There was clinically significant bleeding in 31 patients, including one with intracranial hemorrhage. There was thrombocytopenia (platelet count below 100×10^9/l) in 5% and profound thrombocytopenia (platelet count below 20×10^9/l) in 2%. In patients who received abciximab within 1 month of a previous treatment (n = 115), the risks of thrombocytopenia and profound thrombocytopenia were 17 and 12% respectively. Human chimeric antibody titers before readministration did not correlate with adverse outcomes or bleeding, but were associated with thrombocytopenia and profound thrombocytopenia.

An anaphylactic reaction to abciximab has been reported (26).

• An obese 46-year-old woman with prolonged angina pectoris underwent coronary angiography. She had no known drug allergies, but on administration of an iodinated contrast media she developed anaphylactic shock. After successful resuscitation angiography was completed and she was given aspirin, ticlopidine for a month, and metoprolol. Five months later she developed chest pain again, and angiography was repeated after pretreatment with prednisone and diphenhydramine and she was given abciximab. Within 5 minutes she had an anaphylactic reaction, requiring resuscitation.

This case shows that anaphylactic reactions to abciximab can occur even after pretreatment with prednisone and diphenhydramine for a known allergy to iodine.

Susceptibility Factors

Renal disease

The available data do not suggest an increased risk of bleeding with abciximab among patients with mild to moderate renal insufficiency (19), even though there is reduced platelet aggregation in renal insufficiency.

References

1. Ibbotson T, McGavin JK, Goa KL. Abciximab: an updated review of its therapeutic use in patients with ischaemic heart disease undergoing percutaneous coronary revascularisation. Drugs 2003;63(11):1121–63.
2. Schweizer J, Kirch W, Koch R, Muller A, Hellner G, Forkmann L. Use of abciximab and tirofiban in patients with peripheral arterial occlusive disease and arterial thrombosis. Angiology 2003;54(2):155–61.
3. Ali A, Hashem M, Rosman HS, Kazmouz G, Gardin JM, Schrieber TL. Use of platelet glycoprotein IIb/IIIa inhibitors and spontaneous pulmonary hemorrhage. J Invasive Cardiol 2003;15(4):186–8.
4. Qureshi AI, Saad M, Zaidat OO, Suarez JI, Alexander MJ, Fareed M, Suri K, Ali Z, Hopkins LN. Intracerebral hemorrhages associated with neurointerventional procedures using a combination of antithrombotic agents including abciximab. Stroke 2002;33(7):1916–19.
5. The EPIC Investigation. Use of a monoclonal antibody directed against the platelet glycoprotein IIb/IIIa receptor in high-risk coronary angioplasty. N Engl J Med 1994;330(14):956–61.
6. Aguirre FV, Topol EJ, Ferguson JJ, Anderson K, Blankenship JC, Heuser RR, Sigmon K, Taylor M, Gottlieb R, Hanovich G, et al. Bleeding complications with the chimeric antibody to platelet glycoprotein IIb/IIIa integrin in patients undergoing percutaneous coronary intervention. EPIC Investigators. Circulation 1995; 91(12):2882–90.
7. James S, Armstrong P, Califf R, Husted S, Kontny F, Niemminen M, Pfisterer M, Simoons ML, Wallentin L. Safety and efficacy of abciximab combined with dalteparin in treatment of acute coronary syndromes. Eur Heart J 2002;23(19):1538–45.
8. Blankenship JC, Hellkamp AS, Aguirre FV, Demko SL, Topol EJ, Califf RM. Vascular access site complications after percutaneous coronary intervention with abciximab in the Evaluation of c7E3 for the Prevention of Ischemic Complications (EPIC) trial. Am J Cardiol 1998;81(1):36–40.
9. The EPILOG Investigators. Platelet glycoprotein IIb/IIIa receptor blockade and low-dose heparin during percutaneous coronary revascularization. N Engl J Med 1997;336(24):1689–96.
10. The EPISTENT Investigators. Evaluation of Platelet IIb/IIIa Inhibitor for Stenting. Randomised placebo-controlled and balloon-angioplasty-controlled trial to assess safety of coronary stenting with use of platelet glycoprotein-IIb/IIIa blockade. Lancet 1998;352(9122): 87–92.
11. Brener SJ, Barr LA, Burchenal JE, Katz S, George BS, Jones AA, Cohen ED, Gainey PC, White HJ, Cheek HB, Moses JW, Moliterno DJ, Effron MB, Topol EJ. Randomized, placebo-controlled trial of platelet glycoprotein IIb/IIIa blockade with primary angioplasty for acute myocardial infarction. ReoPro and Primary PTCA Organization and Randomized Trial (RAPPORT) Investigators. Circulation 1998;98(8): 734–41.
12. Ferguson JJ, Kereiakes DJ, Adgey AA, Fox KA, Hillegass WB Jr, Pfisterer M, Vassanelli C. Safe use of platelet GP IIb/IIIa inhibitors. Am Heart J 1998;135(4):S77–89.
13. Kereiakes DJ, Broderick TM, Whang DD, Anderson L, Fye D. Partial reversal of heparin anticoagulation by intravenous protamine in abciximab-treated patients undergoing percutaneous intervention. Am J Cardiol 1997;80(5):633–4.
14. Kleiman NS. A risk-benefit assessment of abciximab in angioplasty. Drug Saf 1999;20(1):43–57.
15. Pinton P. Thrombopénies sous abciximab dans le traitement des syndromes coronariens aigus par angioplastie. [Abciximab-induced thrombopenia during treatment of acute coronary syndromes by angioplasty.] Ann Cardiol Angeiol (Paris) 1998;47(5):351–8.
16. Brown DL. Deaths associated with platelet glycoprotein IIb/IIIa inhibitor treatment. Heart 2003;89(5):535–7.
17. McLenachan JM. Who would I not give IIb/IIIa inhibitors to during percutaneous coronary intervention? Heart 2003;89(5):477–8.
18. Berkowitz SD, Harrington RA, Rund MM, Tcheng JE. Acute profound thrombocytopenia after C7E3 Fab (abciximab) therapy. Circulation 1997;95(4):809–13.
19. Foster RH, Wiseman LR. Abciximab. An updated review of its use in ischaemic heart disease. Drugs 1998;56(4):629–65.
20. Joseph T, Marco J, Gregorini L. Acute profound thrombocytopenia after abciximab therapy during coronary angioplasty. Clin Cardiol 1998;21(11):851–2.
21. Sharma S, Bhambi B, Nyitray W, Sharma G, Shambaugh S, Antonescu A, Shukla P, Denny E. Delayed profound thrombocytopenia presenting 7 days after use of abciximab (ReoPro). J Cardiovasc Pharmacol Ther 2002;7(1):21–4.
22. Schwarz S, Schwab S, Steiner HH, Hacke W. Secondary hemorrhage after intraventricular fibrinolysis: a cautionary note: a report of two cases. Neurosurgery 1998;42(3): 659–63.
23. Curtis BR, Swyers J, Divgi A, McFarland JG, Aster RH. Thrombocytopenia after second exposure to abciximab is caused by antibodies that recognize abciximab-coated platelets. Blood 2002;99(6):2054–9.

24. Schell DA, Ganti AK, Levitt R, Potti A. Thrombocytopenia associated with c7E3 Fab (abciximab). Ann Hematol 2002;81(2):76–9.
25. Dery JP, Braden GA, Lincoff AM, Kereiakes DJ, Browne K, Little T, George BS, Sane DC, Cines DB, Effron MB, Mascelli MA, Langrall MA, Damaraju L, Barnathan ES, Tcheng JE; ReoPro Readministration Registry Investigators. Final results of the ReoPro readministration registry. Am J Cardiol 2004;93(8):979–84.
26. Pharand C, Palisaitis DA, Hamel D. Potential anaphylactic shock with abciximab readministration. Pharmacotherapy 2002;22(3):380–3.

Abecarnil

General Information

Abecarnil is a partial agonist at the benzodiazepine-GABA receptor complex, and is used in generalized anxiety disorder. Its pharmacology suggests that it may be less likely to produce sedation and tolerance, but data thus far have not shown clear differences in its adverse effects from those of classical benzodiazepines, such as alprazolam, diazepam, and lorazepam. As expected, both acute adverse effects and tolerance are dose-related.

In a multicenter, double-blind trial, abecarnil (mean daily dose 12 mg), diazepam (mean daily dose 22 mg), or placebo were given in divided doses for 6 weeks to 310 patients with generalized anxiety disorder (1). Those who had improved at 6 weeks could volunteer to continue double-blind treatment for a total of 24 weeks. Slightly more patients who took diazepam (77%) and placebo (75%) completed the 6-week study than those who took abecarnil (66%). The major adverse events during abecarnil therapy were similar to those of diazepam, namely drowsiness, dizziness, fatigue, and difficulty in coordination. Abecarnil and diazepam both produced statistically significantly more symptom relief than placebo at 1 week, but at 6 weeks only diazepam was superior to placebo. In contrast to diazepam, abecarnil did not cause withdrawal symptoms. The absence of a placebo control makes it difficult to interpret the results of another study of the use of abecarnil and diazepam in alcohol withdrawal, which appeared to show comparable efficacy and adverse effects of the two drugs (2).

References

1. Rickels K, DeMartinis N, Aufdembrinke B. A double-blind, placebo-controlled trial of abecarnil and diazepam in the treatment of patients with generalized anxiety disorder. J Clin Psychopharmacol 2000;20(1):12–18.
2. Anton RF, Kranzler HR, McEvoy JP, Moak DH, Bianca R. A double-blind comparison of abecarnil and diazepam in the treatment of uncomplicated alcohol withdrawal. Psychopharmacology (Berl) 1997;131(2):123–9.

Abetimus

General Information

Abetimus is a selective immunomodulator for the treatment of systemic lupus erythematosus. It induces tolerance in B lymphocytes directed against double-stranded DNA by cross-linking surface antibodies. It also reduces serum double-stranded DNA antibodies and splenic double-stranded DNA antibody-producing cells in BXSB mice, giving improved renal function and histopathology, as well as prolonged survival (1).

In a phase-2, partly randomized, double-blind, placebo-controlled study of three different doses of abetimus in 58 patients, seven did not receive all doses because of adverse events (2). Five withdrew because of adverse events related to their lupus erythematosus: non-renal exacerbations ($n = 2$), hematuria and hypertension ($n = 1$), worsening rash ($n = 1$), and nephritis ($n = 1$). One patient withdrew because of cellulitis and another because of a localized *Herpes zoster* infection. None of the reported adverse events was considered to be definitely related to the drug.

Subsequently, La Jolla Pharmaceuticals terminated two previously established licensing agreements for abetimus (3). One of the agreements was with Leo Pharmaceutical Products of Denmark, which was licensed to market abetimus in Europe and the Middle East, and the other was with Abbott Laboratories. Abbott returned all rights to abetimus to La Jolla Pharmaceuticals in September 1999, based on the results of an analysis of a phase-2/phase-3 trial of abetimus in patients with systemic lupus erythematosus and a history of renal disease, which had been stopped in May 1999 because the primary end-point (the time to worsening of renal function) was much shorter than expected. A further analysis then showed that the number of exacerbations in responders treated with abetimus was less than half the number in the patients treated with placebo. Responders also had a significant reduction in the use of high-dose glucocorticoids and cyclophosphamide.

Another phase-3 placebo-controlled trial called PEARL (Program Enabling Antibody Reduction in Lupus) was conducted in the USA in 317 patients with lupus nephritis, who were treated with abetimus 100 mg/week. The trial was completed in December 2002 and preliminary results were reported in February 2003. However, in April 2003, La Jolla Pharmaceuticals ended the trial, in order to conserve resources for the continued development of the drug.

In September 2000, the US FDA granted orphan drug status to abetimus for the treatment of lupus nephritis; the EU did likewise in November 2001.

References

1. Coutts SM, Plunkett ML, Iverson GM, Barstad PA, Berner CM. Pharmacological intervention in antibody mediated disease. Lupus 1996;5(2):158–9.
2. Furie RA, Cash JM, Cronin ME, Katz RS, Weisman MH, Aranow C, Liebling MR, Hudson NP, Berner CM, Coutts S,

de Haan HA. Treatment of systemic lupus erythematosus with LJP 394. J Rheumatol 2001;28(2):257–65.

3. Anonymous. Abetimus: Abetimus sodium, LJP 394. BioDrugs 2003;17(3):212–15.

Acamprosate

General Information

Acamprosate (calcium acetylhomotaurinate) has been postulated to act by restoring the alcohol-induced neurotransmission imbalance of inhibition-excitation inputs believed to underlie alcohol dependence (1,2). The molecular structure of acamprosate explains its specificity toward the basic molecular mechanisms involved in the pathophysiology of alcohol dependence. A competitive interaction has been described between spermidine and acamprosate, suggesting a specific binding site for acamprosate on N-methyl-D-aspartate receptors (3).

To test the role of acamprosate as an aid in preventing relapse after detoxification, 296 alcohol-dependent patients entered a prospective, multicenter, randomized, double-blind, placebo-controlled study of acamprosate 666 mg tablets tds for 180 days (4). Unlike previous studies, acamprosate was prescribed from the start of alcohol withdrawal, rather than after the detoxification process. During the treatment period, 110 patients dropped out. The two treatment groups were balanced with regard to baseline values and reasons for discontinuation. There was no difference between the groups in the severity of withdrawal symptoms, as measured by the CIWA-Ar (Clinical Institute Withdrawal Assessment for Alcohol scale). Acamprosate given during withdrawal did not cause unwanted effects. The overall incidence of adverse events was similar in the two groups. The number of patients who presented at least one new adverse event (not present at baseline) during the course of the study was 99 with acamprosate and 94 with placebo. Nevertheless, there was a trend for gastrointestinal adverse events to be reported more often in the acamprosate-treated patients ($n = 61$) compared with placebo ($n = 46$). The individual adverse events that were reported more often with acamprosate were diarrhea, dyspepsia, constipation, and flatulence. Pruritus was reported by seven of those who took acamprosate and five of those who took placebo.

Organs and Systems

Gastrointestinal

Acamprosate can cause diarrhea and mild abdominal pain (5).

References

1. Littleton J. Acamprosate in alcohol dependence: how does it work? Addiction 1995;90(9):1179–88.
2. Zeise ML, Kasparov S, Capogna M, Zieglgansberger W. Acamprosate (calciumacetylhomotaurinate) decreases postsynaptic potentials in the rat neocortex: possible involvement of excitatory amino acid receptors. Eur J Pharmacol 1993;231(1):47–52.
3. Naassila M, Hammoumi S, Legrand E, Durbin P, Daoust M. Mechanism of action of acamprosate. Part I. Characterization of spermidine-sensitive acamprosate binding site in rat brain. Alcohol Clin Exp Res 1998;22(4):802–9.
4. Gual A, Lehert P. Acamprosate during and after acute alcohol withdrawal: a double-blind placebo-controlled study in Spain. Alcohol Alcohol 2001;36(5):413–18.
5. Graham R, Wodak AD, Whelan G. New pharmacotherapies for alcohol dependence. Med J Aust 2002;177(2):103–7.

Acebutolol

See also Beta-adrenoceptor antagonists

General Information

Acebutolol is a beta-adrenoceptor antagonist with membrane-stabilizing activity that is sometimes cited as being cardioselective but has considerable effects on bronchioles and peripheral blood vessels.

Organs and Systems

Respiratory

Bronchiolitis obliterans has been attributed to acebutolol (1).

Liver

Six cases of reversible hepatitis have been attributed to acebutolol (2).

Immunologic

Patients taking acebutolol relatively commonly develop antinuclear antibodies (3,4).

Drug Administration

Drug overdose

The membrane-stabilizing activity of beta-blockers can play a major role in toxicity. Of 208 deaths in subjects who had taken beta-blockers, 206 occurred with drugs that have membrane-stabilizing activity. This quinidine-like effect can be reversed by sodium bicarbonate, which is also used to counteract the cardiotoxic effects of cyclic antidepressants, which also have membrane-stabilizing activity.

- An overdose of acebutolol (6.4 mg) in a 48-year-old man caused cardiac arrest with ventricular tachycardia (5). An intravenous bolus of sodium bicarbonate 50 mmol produced sinus rhythm.

References

1. Camus P, Lombard JN, Perrichon M, Piard F, Guerin JC, Thivolet FB, Jeannin L. Bronchiolitis obliterans organising pneumonia in patients taking acebutolol or amiodarone. Thorax 1989;44(9):711–15.

2. Tanner LA, Bosco LA, Zimmerman HJ. Hepatic toxicity after acebutolol therapy. Ann Intern Med 1989;111(6):533–534.
3. Booth RJ, Bullock JY, Wilson JD. Antinuclear antibodies in patients on acebutolol. Br J Clin Pharmacol 1980;9(5):515–17.
4. Cody RJ Jr, Calabrese LH, Clough JD, Tarazi RC, Bravo EL. Development of antinuclear antibodies during acebutolol therapy. Clin Pharmacol Ther 1979;25(6):800–5.
5. Donovan KD, Gerace RV, Dreyer JF. Acebutolol-induced ventricular tachycardia reversed with sodium bicarbonate. J Toxicol Clin Toxicol 1999;37(4):481–4.

Acecainide

See also Antidysrhythmic drugs

General Information

Acecainide (*N*-acetylprocainamide) is the main metabolite of procainamide, and it has antidysrhythmic activity (1). However, in contrast to procainamide, which has Class Ib activity, the main action of acecainide is that of Class III.

Apart from the lupus-like syndrome, the adverse effects of acecainide are as common as those of procainamide. The commonest affect the gastrointestinal tract and the central nervous system. Anorexia, nausea, vomiting, diarrhea, and abdominal pain are common, as are insomnia, dizziness, light-headedness, tingling sensations, and blurred vision. Other reported unwanted effects include skin rashes, constipation, and reduced sexual function (2–5).

Organs and Systems

Cardiovascular

Acecainide prolongs the QT interval and can therefore cause ventricular dysrhythmias (6). The risk is increased in renal insufficiency, since acecainide is mainly eliminated unchanged via the kidneys.

Immunologic

The main advantage of acecainide over procainamide is the lower incidence of the lupus-like syndrome. Many fewer patients develop antinuclear antibodies during long-term treatment with acecainide than during long-term treatment with procainamide (7).

There are also reports of remission of lupus-like syndrome without recurrence in patients in whom acecainide has been used as a replacement for procainamide (8–10). Furthermore, patients in whom procainamide has previously caused a lupus-like syndrome have been reported not to suffer from the syndrome on subsequent long-term treatment with acecainide (8). However, one patient suffered mild arthralgia while taking acecainide, having had a more severe arthropathy while taking procainamide (8).

Susceptibility Factors

Renal disease

Because acecainide is eliminated mostly unchanged by renal excretion, with a half-life of about 7 hours, its clearance is reduced in patients with renal impairment, who are at increased risk of adverse effects. This means that elderly people, who generally have a degree of renal impairment, are also at increased risk.

Monitoring Drug Therapy

The target plasma concentration range of acecainide is 15–25 µg/ml. The adverse effects of acecainide increase in frequency at concentrations above 30 µg/ml (11).

References

1. Atkinson AJ Jr, Ruo TI, Piergies AA. Comparison of the pharmacokinetic and pharmacodynamic properties of procainamide and N-acetylprocainamide. Angiology 1988;39(7 Pt 2):655–67.
2. Roden DM, Reele SB, Higgins SB, Wilkinson GR, Smith RF, Oates JA, Woosley RL. Antiarrhythmic efficacy, pharmacokinetics and safety of N-acetylprocainamide in human subjects: comparison with procainamide. Am J Cardiol 1980;46(3):463–8.
3. Winkle RA, Jaillon P, Kates RE, Peters F. Clinical pharmacology and antiarrhythmic efficacy of N-acetylprocainamide. Am J Cardiol 1981;47(1):123–30.
4. Atkinson AJ Jr, Lertora JJ, Kushner W, Chao GC, Nevin MJ. Efficacy and safety of N-acetylprocainamide in long-term treatment of ventricular arrhythmias. Clin Pharmacol Ther 1983;33(5):565–76.
5. Domoto DT, Brown WW, Bruggensmith P. Removal of toxic levels of N-acetylprocainamide with continuous arteriovenous hemofiltration or continuous arteriovenous hemodiafiltration. Ann Intern Med 1987;106(4):550–2.
6. Piergies AA, Ruo TI, Jansyn EM, Belknap SM, Atkinson AJ Jr. Effect kinetics of N-acetylprocainamide-induced QT interval prolongation. Clin Pharmacol Ther 1987;42(1):107–12.
7. Lahita R, Kluger J, Drayer DE, Koffler D, Reidenberg MM. Antibodies to nuclear antigens in patients treated with procainamide or acetylprocainamide. N Engl J Med 1979;301(25):1382–5.
8. Kluger J, Leech S, Reidenberg MM, Lloyd V, Drayer DE. Long-term antiarrhythmic therapy with acetylprocainamide. Am J Cardiol 1981;48(6):1124–32.
9. Kluger J, Drayer DE, Reidenberg MM, Lahita R. Acetylprocainamide therapy in patients with previous procainamide-induced lupus syndrome. Ann Intern Med 1981;95(1):18–23.
10. Stec GP, Lertora JJ, Atkinson AJ Jr, Nevin MJ, Kushner W, Jones C, Schmid FR, Askenazi J. Remission of procainamide-induced lupus erythematosus with N-acetylprocainamide therapy. Ann Intern Med 1979;90(5):799–801.
11. Connolly SJ, Kates RE. Clinical pharmacokinetics of N-acetylprocainamide. Clin Pharmacokinet 1982;7(3):206–20.

Aceclofenac

See also Non-steroidal anti-inflammatory drugs

General Information

Despite claims that aceclofenac is a COX-2 selective inhibitor, experience shows that its adverse effects profile is similar to that of the non-selective NSAIDs.

Organs and Systems

Gastrointestinal

Symptoms of gastrointestinal intolerance in patients taking aceclofenac commonly require withdrawal, at a rate of 3–15% (SEDA-20, 91).

Liver

Acute hepatitis has been reported with aceclofenac (SEDA-21, 103).

Skin

Aceclofenac cream can cause erythema, itching, and a burning sensation in under 3% of patients (SEDA-20, 91). Aceclofenac can cause photosensitivity.

- After starting twice-daily topical application of a cream containing aceclofenac, a woman developed acute eczema affecting the sun-exposed areas of her legs (1).

Immunologic

A hypersensitivity reaction characterized by multiple purpuric lesions and reduced renal function has been described in an elderly patient (SEDA-18, 103), and there have been reports of hypersensitivity vasculitis (SEDA-20, 91) (SEDA-21, 103).

Reference

1. Goday Bujan JJ, Garcia Alvarez-Eire GM, Martinez W, del Pozo J, Fonseca E. Photoallergic contact dermatitis from aceclofenac. Contact Dermatitis 2001;45(3):170.

Acemetacin

See also Non-steroidal anti-inflammatory drugs

General Information

Acemetacin is an indometacin derivative with the same adverse effects profile (SEDA-6, 94). In an open multi-center study, 187 of 280 patients had adverse effects (57% gastrointestinal); treatment had to be stopped in 7% (1). The use of acemetacin is limited and there is no justification for claims that it has advantages over existing NSAIDs.

Reference

1. Heiter A, Tausch G, Eberl R. Ergebnisse einer Langstudie mit Acemetacin bei der Behandlung von Patienten mit chronischer Polyarthritis. [Results of a long-term study with acemetacin in the therapy of patients suffering from rheumatoid arthritis.] Arzneimittelforschung 1980;30(8A):460–3.

Acetylcholinesterase inhibitors

General Information

Cholinesterase inhibitors increase parasympathetic nervous system (cholinergic) activity indirectly by inhibiting acetylcholinesterase, thereby preventing the breakdown of acetylcholine. They are only effective in the presence of acetylcholine. They are listed in Table 1.

The cholinesterase inhibitors are used in the treatment of Alzheimer's disease (tacrine, 7-methoxytacrine, donepezil, metrifonate, and rivastigmine), the treatment and diagnosis of myasthenia gravis (distigmine, edrophonium, neostigmine, physostigmine, prostigmine, and pyridostigmine), and the treatment of atony of the intestine or bladder. In the eye, they increase the flow rate of aqueous humor across the trabeculum, reduce resistance to its flow, and consequently lower the intraocular pressure.

Use of acetylcholinesterase inhibitors in Alzheimer's disease

Of the acetylcholinesterase inhibitors, tacrine, methoxytacrine, metrifonate, donepezil hydrochloride, and rivastigmine are used in the treatment of Alzheimer's disease. In 12–30% of patients with Alzheimer's disease, tacrine causes an increase in hepatic transaminase activity. Abdominal adverse effects are very frequent, for example nausea, anorexia, diarrhea. The peripheral cholinomimetic effects of tacrine occur in a very high proportion of patients, probably the majority. The hepatic effects seem to be such that the use of these new (and in some cases still experimental) drugs would not be justified in

Table 1 Acetylcholinesterase inhibitors

Ambenonium
Diisopropyl fluorophosphate (Diflos)
Distigmine
Donepezil
Ecothiopate
Edrophonium
Eserine
Methoxytacrine
Metrifonate
Neostigmine
Physostigmine
Prostigmine
Pyridostigmine
Rivastigmine
Tacrine and 7-methoxytacrine

other-than-serious disease states, but they are reversible if the drug is withdrawn.

General adverse effects

The acetylcholinesterase inhibitors have the effects that one would expect to result from their promoting nicotinic and muscarinic cholinergic activity, including unwanted effects such as bradycardia, miosis, colic, and hypersalivation. Adverse reactions have been stated to be relatively more common with neostigmine than with some other drugs such as pyridostigmine or ambenonium, but it is doubtful whether the benefit to harm balance indeed differs, since neostigmine also tends to be more effective in certain patients. Ambenonium is relatively likely to cause headache. When neostigmine and pyridostigmine are used as bromide salts, bromide rashes can occur.

Local adverse effects

Acetylcholinesterase inhibitors as eye drops have more intense effects in myopic and young patients, causing aggravation of myopia, blurred vision, and periorbital pain, due to congestion of the iris and ciliary body. Anterior and posterior synechiae can develop. Allergic reactions have been reported as has epithelial toxicity. The acetylcholinesterase inhibitors can cause pseudopemphigoid reactions in the eyelids and occlusion of the lacrimal puncta (SED-12, 1198) (1). The danger that a miotic agent will produce retinal detachment is directly proportional to the capacity of the drug to produce spasm of the ciliary body. Retinal detachment has been reported after the use of cholinergic agents, but they can also be coincidental.

Systemic effects

The commonest effects of the acetylcholinesterase inhibitors are headache and periorbital pain. Signs of vagal stimulation can occur, with nausea, vomiting, sweating, hypersalivation, lacrimation, hypotension, bradycardia, bronchial constriction, respiratory failure, and nightmares. These reactions essentially occur during intensive treatment for acute closed-angle glaucoma, requiring frequent instillations of pilocarpine. Elderly people and young children are at particular risk.

Organs and Systems

Cardiovascular

With any acetylcholinesterase inhibitor, bradycardia can, with excessive dosage, proceed to dysrhythmias (SEDA-13, 114) and even asystole.

- A 67-year-old man underwent left upper lobectomy for a presumed malignancy 11 years after cardiac transplantation (2). He had had no cardiac symptoms since his transplant. Suxamethonium was used as a muscle relaxant and was reversed with glycopyrrolate 0.8 mg and neostigmine 4 mg. Within a few minutes, he developed asystole, which lasted for about 45 seconds. He subsequently made a full recovery.

The authors speculated that some degree of cardiac reinnervation may have occurred; they recommended that

this type of response should be anticipated in future anesthesia in such patients and that therapeutic measures, such as a beta-adrenoceptor agonist, should be available.

Another case of asystole has been reported with the very short-acting cholinesterase inhibitor edrophonium (3).

- A 49-year-old woman was given intravenous edrophonium chloride 2 mg as part of the investigation of an acute myopathy following gastrointestinal surgery. She had also received 60 mg of intravenous labetalol in the 14 hours before the edrophonium was given: presumably this was for a raised blood pressure, but that was not specified. Labetalol caused transient but severe bradycardia (heart rate about 20/minute). Immediately after the injection of edrophonium, she developed asystole, which was treated immediately with atropine and recovered in 10 seconds.

Such reactions are extremely rare, but in this case the risk was undoubtedly enhanced by previous beta-blockade.

With physostigmine, hypertension has been both demonstrated in animal experiments and observed in a series of patients after intravenous use in relatively high doses; it has also occurred during use of low doses of oral physostigmine in an elderly patient with Alzheimer's disease (SEDA-12, 125).

Nervous system

During a trial of oral physostigmine, myoclonus occurred in two patients with probable Alzheimer's disease (SEDA-12, 125).

Gastrointestinal

To reduce the incidence of residual paralysis after the administration of non-depolarizing neuromuscular blocking agents, some advocate the routine use of anticholinesterase drugs at the end of surgery. However, it has been suggested that this practice might increase the risk of postoperative nausea and vomiting. Clinical trials have produced contradictory results. A meta-analysis of the available data suggested that omitting routine neostigmine may reduce the incidence of emesis only when a large dose (2.5 mg) is used (4). With a smaller dose (1.5 mg), there was no difference. The incidence of clinically relevant residual paralysis was 1 in 30 in the control groups. There were no cases of residual curarization in the treatment groups when either edrophonium 500 µg/kg or neostigmine 1.5 mg was given in combination with atropine. Therefore, the question of whether or not routine anticholinesterase administration is beneficial for the patient is still open to debate. Other adverse effects of anticholinesterase drugs, such as bronchial hypersecretion or intestinal hypermotility, could increase morbidity, and we do not know whether all of these adverse effects are completely blocked by the concomitant use of a parasympatholytic agent (5). It should be taken into account that the incidence of residual curarization may be reduced as effectively by the use of neuromuscular transmission monitoring (6,7). Some believe that anticholinesterase drugs should be used to reverse residual neuromuscular block that produces clinical symptoms or is detected by neuromuscular transmission monitoring.

Musculoskeletal

Any acetylcholinesterase inhibitor can produce muscular fasciculation followed by voluntary muscle paralysis, and these muscular effects can serve as a valuable sign of approaching overdosage. Two patients, one with dystrophia myotonica and the other with progressive muscular dystrophy, presented with respiratory difficulties, necessitating prolonged mechanical ventilation. As these difficulties are as good as impossible to predict, short-acting neuromuscular blockers should preferably be used, thus avoiding the need for pharmacological reversal (8).

Immunologic

Severe urticaria and anaphylaxis associated with pyridostigmine (an unspecified dose) occurred in a 54-year-old woman with myasthenia gravis (9). Urticaria started almost immediately after introduction of the drug but was partially controlled by the antihistamine cetirizine. However, pyridostigmine was stopped after 2 months and the urticaria resolved completely. Rechallenge with oral pyridostigmine led to an anaphylactic reaction that was treated with subcutaneous adrenaline. There were no sequelae.

Second-Generation Effects

Teratogenicity

Microcephaly occurred in the child of a woman taking a high dose of pyridostigmine (10).

- A 24-year-old woman had suffered from myasthenia gravis from the unusually early age of 10 years. During her first pregnancy, pyridostigmine was her sole medication. Because of deterioration in her symptoms during the pregnancy, the dosage was increased until she was taking 1500–3000 mg/day, or 4–8 times the maximum recommended dose. This still did not produce much clinical improvement but was nevertheless continued throughout the pregnancy. She needed an emergency cesarean section at 36 weeks because of fetal bradycardia. The baby was microcephalic.

The authors failed to find any other cause for this abnormality and concluded that the excessive dose of pyridostigmine had been responsible for the fetal damage.

Fetotoxicity

Acetylcholinesterase inhibitors can probably be safely used in pregnancy when needed, provided the dosage is carefully regulated. Reversible muscle weakness in a newborn infant was attributed to relative overdosage of the mother with pyridostigmine bromide (11).

Susceptibility Factors

Age

Elderly people need to be treated with caution because of their greater susceptibility to the cardiovascular effects of the acetylcholinesterase inhibitors; this is particularly relevant to their use in Alzheimer's disease.

Other features of the patient

Special caution is recommended when acetylcholinesterase inhibitors are given to patients with inflammatory, infiltrative, or degenerative disease of the cardiac conducting system, patients taking digitalis, calcium channel blockers, or beta-blockers, and patients with myocardial ischemia. Appropriate resuscitative equipment should be readily available.

Neostigmine or other anticholinesterase inhibitors are regularly used in anesthesia to reverse neuromuscular block; however, in patients with neuromuscular disorders, this reversal can present unforeseen difficulties. All anticholinesterase inhibitors must be cautiously dosed if severe adverse reactions are to be avoided. When these drugs are given orally, administration should be suspended during periods of severe constipation, in light of one reported case in which neostigmine accumulated in the gastrointestinal tract of a child during a constipative phase and was thereafter rapidly absorbed, with fatal results (SED-12, 326). Anticholinesterase drugs are contraindicated in bronchial asthma.

Drug–Drug Interactions

Anticholinergic drugs

The effect of acetylcholinesterase inhibitors can be reduced by drugs with anticholinergic effects, such as antihistamines or neuroleptic drugs (12).

Suxamethonium

Acetylcholinesterase inhibitor eye drops or exposure to organophosphate insecticides can reduce the activity of plasma cholinesterase and pseudocholinesterase, creating a potentially fatal hazard for surgical patients receiving suxamethonium. During induction of general anesthesia, the presence of anticholinesterase activity in the serum can potentiate the effect of curare-like drugs, such as suxamethonium, used as muscle relaxants, with prolonged apnea after intubation and death. Such eye drops should be stopped 6 weeks before the operation. The importance of inquiring about the use of drugs cannot be overemphasized. Patients often do not regard eye drops as medications and omit this information from their medical history. Complaints of excessive sweating, intermittent diarrhea, muscle weakness, and fatigue over a long period may be due to the usage of ecothiopate eye drops (phospholine iodide 0.25%) for glaucoma and can disappear when the eye drops are withdrawn (13).

References

1. Friart A, Hermans L, De Valeriola Y. Unusual side-effect of a dobutamine stress echocardiography. Am J Noninvasive Cardiol 1993;7:63–4.
2. Bjerke RJ, Mangione MP. Asystole after intravenous neostigmine in a heart transplant recipient. Can J Anaesth 2001;48(3):305–7.
3. Okun MS, Charriez CM, Bhatti MT, Watson RT, Swift TR. Asystole induced by edrophonium following beta blockade. Neurology 2001;57(4):739.

4. Tramèr MR, Fuchs-Buder T. Omitting antagonism of neuromuscular block: effect on postoperative nausea and vomiting and risk of residual paralysis. A systematic review. Br J Anaesth 1999;82(3):379–86.

5. Bevan DR, Donati F, Kopman AF. Reversal of neuromuscular blockade. Anesthesiology 1992;77(4):785–805.

6. Mortensen R, Berg H, El-Mahdy A, Viby-Mogensen J. Perioperative monitoring of neuromuscular transmission using acceleromyography prevents residual neuromuscular block following pancuronium. Acta Anaesthesiol Scand 1995;39(6):797–801.

7. Shorten GD, Merk H, Sieber T. Perioperative train-of-four monitoring and residual curarization. Can J Anaesth 1995;42(8):711–15.

8. Buzello W, Krieg N, Schlickewei A. Hazards of neostigmine in patients with neuromuscular disorders. Report of two cases. Br J Anaesth 1982;54(5):529–34.

9. Castellano A, Cabrera M, Robledo T, Martinez-Cocera C, Cimarra M, Llamazares AA, Chamorro M. Anaphylaxis by pyridostigmine. Allergy 1998;53(11):1108–9.

10. Niesen CE, Shah NS. Pyridostigmine-induced microcephaly. Neurology 2000;54(9):1873–4.

11. Blackhall MI, Buckley GA, Roberts DV, Roberts JB, Thomas BH, Wilson A. Drug-induced neonatal myasthenia. J Obstet Gynaecol Br Commonw 1969;76(2):157–62.

12. Carnahan RM, Lund BC, Perry PJ, Chrischilles EA. The concurrent use of anticholinergics and cholinesterase inhibitors: rare event or common practice? J Am Geriatr Soc 2004;52(12):2082–7.

13. Alexander WD. Systemic side effects with eye drops. BMJ (Clin Res Ed) 1981;282(6273):1359.

Acetylcysteine

General Information

Acetylcysteine (*N*-acetylcysteine) is used as a mucolytic and to treat paracetamol overdose.

Acetylcysteine splits disulfide bonds in mucoproteins and thus lowers mucus viscosity, resulting in a larger volume of sputum. It is normally administered by inhalation as a nebulized solution or aerosol, although it can also be taken orally. Acetylcysteine is also an antioxidant and may protect the lung from free radicals generated by inflammatory cells activated by influenza virus infection. Treatment for 6 months with acetylcysteine 600 mg bd significantly reduced the frequency and severity of influenza-like episodes. Adverse effects were reported by 9% of patients who complained of dysuria, epigastric pain, nausea and vomiting, constipation or diarrhea, and flushing (SEDA-22, 195).

The place of mucolytic drugs in respiratory disease has recently been reviewed (1). The authors suggested that they have been inappropriately used in the past. As mucolytic agents do not improve lung function tests in COPD, the European Respiratory Society and the American Thoracic Society guidelines discourage their use in the treatment of COPD. Future trials should evaluate clinical symptoms and quality of life as well as lung function tests. Mucolytic agents should be evaluated earlier in the natural history of COPD, when mucus hypersecretion is the major feature and before lung function has deteriorated.

Acetylcysteine is used intravenously as an antidote for severe paracetamol poisoning, in which it acts as a thiol donor.

Oral acetylcysteine has been investigated for the treatment of cancer. Acetylcysteine 600 mg/day was compared with retinol 300 000 U/day, the combination, and a placebo in a total of 2191 patients treated for 2 years. Adverse effects were reported by 14% of those who took acetylcysteine, compared with 23% of those who took retinol and 25% of those who took the combination. The most common adverse effect attributed to acetylcysteine was dyspepsia. In healthy volunteers, higher doses of acetylcysteine, 600 mg taken two or three times daily for 4 weeks, caused more adverse effects: 25 and 61% of the volunteers, respectively, reported gastrointestinal adverse effects (SEDA-20, 184).

There has been a systematic review of published randomized studies of the use of *N*-acetylcysteine in chronic bronchitis (2). A total of 39 trials were considered, of which only nine were included in the meta-analysis. In all cases, oral *N*-acetylcysteine had been used in a dosage of 200–300 mg bd for 4–32 weeks. There were gastrointestinal adverse effects (dyspepsia, diarrhea, and heartburn) in 10% of 2011 patients, and 6.5% withdrew because of their symptoms. However, the rate of gastrointestinal adverse effects was higher in the placebo group (11% with a withdrawal rate of 7.1%). There was no exacerbation of chronic bronchitis in 49% of patients treated with acetylcysteine compared with 31% of placebo-treated patients, a relative benefit of 1.56 (95% CI = 1.37, 1.77). There was also symptom improvement with treatment: 61% reported improvement in symptoms with acetylcysteine compared with 35% with placebo.

Organs and Systems

Respiratory

Aerosol therapy with acetylcysteine can cause bronchoconstriction. In 31 ambulant asthmatics using 10% acetylcysteine solution, there was a mean reduction of 55% in the FEV_1 in 19 subjects. The addition of 0.05% isoprenaline reduced the number of patients who developed bronchoconstriction from 19 to 5 (SEDA-5, 170). In two placebo-controlled studies, involving over 700 patients, there was no difference in adverse effects between oral acetylcysteine and a placebo. There was, however, no improvement in FEV_1 in these studies (3).

Immunologic

Hypersensitivity reactions have been reported when acetylcysteine is given intravenously in paracetamol overdose. A generalized erythematous rash can develop, and itching, nausea, vomiting, dizziness, and severe breathlessness with bronchospasm and tachycardia have been reported (SEDA-5, 170). Angioedema with hypotension and bronchospasm have also been described (4). Wheal responses to high concentrations of acetylcysteine (20 mg/ml) were significantly greater in those who reacted to the drug. In two patients with a positive reaction the response could be inhibited by prior therapy with an antihistamine. As hypersensitivity reactions have been reported in up to

3% of patients receiving intravenous acetylcysteine for paracetamol overdose, physicians need to be prepared for these reactions (5). A pseudo-allergic reaction on the basis of histamine liberation, rather than an immunological etiology, is suggested as the mechanism (6,7).

Management guidelines for the treatment of anaphylactoid reactions to intravenous acetylcysteine have been developed. Patients who develop only flushing of the skin require no treatment. Urticaria should be treated with diphenhydramine and acetylcysteine infusion can be continued. If angioedema or respiratory distress occur, diphenhydramine should be given and the acetylcysteine infusion stopped; it can be restarted 1 hour after the administration of diphenhydramine if no symptoms are present (SEDA-22, 195).

Drug–Drug Interactions

Antibiotics

The 5% solution, for inhalation, almost completely inactivates penicillin and cephalosporins in vitro and reduces the activity of tetracycline.

References

1. Del Donno M, Olivieri D. Mucoactive drugs in the management of chronic obstructive pulmonary disease. Monaldi Arch Chest Dis 1998;53(6):714–19.
2. Stey C, Steurer J, Bachmann S, Medici TC, Tramer MR. The effect of oral N-acetylcysteine in chronic bronchitis: a quantitative systematic review. Eur Respir J 2000;16(2):253–62.
3. British Thoracic Society Research Committee. Oral N-acetylcysteine and exacerbation rates in patients with chronic bronchitis and severe airways obstruction. Thorax 1985;40(11):832–5.
4. Mant TG, Tempowski JH, Volans GN, Talbot JC. Adverse reactions to acetylcysteine and effects of overdose. BMJ (Clin Res Ed) 1984;289(6439):217–19.
5. Bonfiglio MF, Traeger SM, Hulisz DT, Martin BR. Anaphylactoid reaction to intravenous acetylcysteine associated with electrocardiographic abnormalities. Ann Pharmacother 1992;26(1):22–5.
6. Bateman DN, Woodhouse KW, Rawlins MD. Adverse reactions to N-acetylcysteine. Lancet 1984;2(8396):228.
7. Tenenbein M. Hypersensitivity-like reactions to N-acetylcysteine. Vet Hum Toxicol 1984;26(Suppl 2):3–5.

Acetylsalicylic acid

General Information

A century after its introduction, acetylsalicylic acid (aspirin) is by far the most commonly used analgesic, sharing its leading position with the relative newcomer paracetamol (acetaminophen), and notwithstanding the fact that other widely used compounds of their class, like ibuprofen and naproxen, have in recent years been introduced in over-the-counter versions. Both are also still being prescribed by physicians and are generally used for mild to moderate pain, fever associated with common everyday illnesses, and disorders ranging from head colds and influenza to toothache and headache. Their greatest use is by consumers who obtain them directly at the pharmacy, and in many countries outside pharmacies as well. Perhaps this wide availability and advertising via mass media lead to a lack of appreciation by the lay public that these are medicines with associated adverse effects. Both have at any rate been subject to misuse and excessive use, leading to such problems as chronic salicylate intoxication with aspirin, and severe hepatic damage after overdose with paracetamol. Both aspirin and paracetamol have featured in accidental overdosage (particularly in children) as well as intentional overdosage.

In an investigation of Canadian donors who had not admitted to drug intake, 6–7% of the blood samples taken were found to have detectable concentrations of acetylsalicylic acid and paracetamol (1). Such drugs would be potentially capable of causing untoward reactions in the recipients.

To offer some protection against misuse of analgesics, many countries have insisted on the use of packs containing total quantities less than the minimum toxic dose (albeit usually the one obtained for healthy young volunteers and thus disregarding the majority of the population), and supplied in child-resistant packaging. Most important, however, is the need to provide education for the lay public to respect such medicines in general for the good they can do, but more especially for the harm that can arise but which can be avoided. There is a definite role for the prescribing physician, as informing the patient seems to prevent adverse events (2).

The sale of paracetamol or aspirin in dosage forms in which they are combined with other active ingredients offers considerable risk to the consumer, since the product as sold may not be clearly identified as containing either of these two analgesics. Brand names sometimes obscure the actual composition of older formulations that contain one or both of these analgesics in combination with, for example, a pyrazolone derivative and/or a potentially addictive substance. For instance, in Germany, with the EC harmonization of the Drug Law of 1990, the manufacturers of drugs already marketed before 1978 had the opportunity of exchanging even the active principles without being obliged to undergo a new approval procedure or to abandon their brand name. Combination formulations are still being promoted and sold, and not exclusively in developing countries. Consequently, the patient who is so anxious to allay all his symptoms that he takes several medications concurrently may without knowing it take several doses of aspirin or paracetamol at the same time, perhaps sufficient to cause toxicity. It is essential that product labels clearly state their active ingredients by approved name together with the quantity per dosage form (3).

The antipyretic analgesics, with the non-steroidal anti-inflammatory drugs (NSAIDs), share a common mechanism of action, namely the inhibition of prostaglandin synthesis from arachidonic acid and their release. More precisely their mode of action is thought to result from inhibition of both the constitutive and the inducible isoenzymes (COX-1 and COX-2) of the cyclo-oxygenase pathway (4). However, aspirin and paracetamol are distinguishable from most of the NSAIDs by their ability to inhibit prostaglandin synthesis in the nervous system, and thus the hypothalamic center for body temperature regulation, rather than acting mainly in the periphery.

Endogenous pyrogens (and exogenous pyrogens that have their effects through the endogenous group) induce the hypothalamic vascular endothelium to produce prostaglandins, which activate the thermoregulatory neurons by increasing AMP concentrations. The capacity of the antipyretic analgesics to inhibit hypothalamic prostaglandin synthesis appears to be the basis of their antipyretic action. Neither aspirin nor paracetamol affects the synthesis or release of endogenous pyrogens and neither will lower body temperature if it is normal.

While aspirin significantly inhibits peripheral prostaglandin and thromboxane synthesis, paracetamol is less potent as a synthetase inhibitor than the NSAIDs, except in the brain, and paracetamol has only a weak anti-inflammatory action. It is simple to ascribe the analgesic activity of aspirin to its capacity to inhibit prostaglandin synthesis, with a consequent reduction in inflammatory edema and vasodilatation, since aspirin is most effective in the pain associated with inflammation or injury. However, such a peripheral effect cannot account for the analgesic activity of paracetamol, which is less well understood.

As a prostaglandin synthesis inhibitor, aspirin, like other NSAIDs, is associated with irritation of and damage to the gastrointestinal mucosa. In low doses it can also increase bleeding by inhibiting platelet aggregation; in high doses, prolongation of the prothrombin time will contribute to the bleeding tendency. Intensive treatment can also produce unwanted nervous system effects (salicylism).

Depending on the criteria used, the incidence of aspirin hypersensitivity is variously estimated as being as low as 1% or as high as 50%, the highest frequency being found in asthmatics. The condition is characterized by bronchospasm (asthma), urticaria, angioedema, and vasomotor rhinitis, each occurring alone or in combination, often leading to severe and even life-threatening reactions. There is no clear evidence of an association with tumors, apart from the possible peripheral contribution of aspirin to the development of urinary tract neoplasms in patients with analgesic nephropathy. Indeed, some authors have suggested a role for salicylates in reducing the incidence of colorectal tumors and breast tumors.

The following are absolute contraindications to the use of aspirin:

- children under 16;
- people with hypersensitivity to salicylates, NSAIDs, or tartrazine;
- people with peptic ulceration;
- people with known coagulopathies, including those induced as part of medical therapy.

The following are relative contraindications to the use of long-term analgesic doses of aspirin:

- gout, since normal analgesic doses impede the excretion of uric acid (high doses have a uricosuric effect); an additional problem in gout is that salicylates reduce the uricosuric effects of sulfinpyrazone and probenecid;
- variant angina; a daily dose of 4 g has been found to provoke attacks both at night-time and during the day (5,6), perhaps owing to direct triggering of coronary arterial spasm; blockade of the synthesis of PGI_z, which normally protects against vasoconstriction, could be involved;
- diabetes mellitus, in which aspirin can in theory interfere with the actions of insulin and glucagon sufficiently to derange control;
- some days before elective surgery (even in coronary artery bypass grafting) or delivery, especially if extradural anesthesia is used (7), although recent data seem reassuring (8); aspirin increases bleeding at dental extraction or perioperatively;
- in elderly people, who may develop gastrointestinal bleeding;
- anorectal inflammation (suppositories);
- pre-existing gastrointestinal disease, liver disease, hypoalbuminemia, hypovolemia, in the third trimester of pregnancy, perioperatively, or in patients with threatening abortion.

Assessing the benefit-to-harm balance of low-dose aspirin in preventing strokes and heart attacks

Although there is clear evidence of benefit of acetylsalicylic acid (aspirin) in secondary prevention of strokes and heart attacks, the question of whether aspirin should also be prescribed for primary prevention in asymptomatic people is still debatable. Trials in primary prevention have given contrasting results (9,10), and aspirin can cause major harms (for example severe gastrointestinal bleeding and hemorrhagic stroke).

Furthermore, despite evidence of the efficacy of aspirin in secondary prevention, its use in patients at high risk of strokes and heart attacks remains suboptimal (11). A possible explanation for this underuse may be concern about the relative benefit in relation to the potential risk for serious hemorrhagic events. Accurate evaluation of the benefits and harms of aspirin is therefore warranted.

Two meta-analyses have provided some information. The first examined the benefit and harms of aspirin in subjects without known cardiovascular or cerebrovascular disease (primary prevention) (12). The authors selected articles published between 1966 and 2000—five large controlled studies of primary prevention that lasted at least 1 year and nine studies of the effects of aspirin on gastrointestinal bleeding and hemorrhagic stroke. The five randomized, placebo-controlled trials included more than 50 000 patients and the meta-analysis showed that aspirin significantly reduced the risk of the combined outcome (confirmed non-fatal myocardial infarction or death from coronary heart disease) (OR = 0.72; 95% CI = 0.60, 0.87). However, aspirin increased the risk of major gastrointestinal bleeding (OR = 1.7; CI = 1.4, 2.1) significantly, while the small increase found for hemorrhagic stroke (OR = 1.4; CI = 0.9, 2.0) was not statistically significant. All-cause mortality was not significantly affected (OR = 0.93; CI = 0.84; 1.02). Most important was the finding that the net effect of aspirin improved with increasing risk of coronary heart disease. The meta-analysis showed that for 1000 patients with a 5% risk of coronary heart disease events over 5 years, aspirin would prevent 6–20 myocardial infarctions but would cause also 0–2 hemorrhagic strokes and 2–4 major gastrointestinal bleeds. For patients at lower risk (1% over 5 years), aspirin would prevent 1–4 myocardial infarctions but would still cause 0–2 hemorrhagic strokes and 2-4 major gastrointestinal bleeds.

Therefore when deciding to use aspirin in primary prophylaxis, one should take account of the relative utility of the different outcomes that are prevented or caused by aspirin.

The other meta-analysis (13) compared the benefits of aspirin in secondary prevention with the risk of gastrointestinal bleeding. An earlier analysis of this problem included patients at various levels of risk and doses of aspirin that would currently be regarded as too high (14), and may therefore have either under-represented the benefit or exaggerated the risk. In another analysis there was no difference in the risk of gastrointestinal bleeding across the whole range of doses used (15).

The meta-analysis reviewed all randomized, placebo-controlled, secondary prevention trials of at least 3-months duration published from 1970 to 2000. The dosage of aspirin was 50–325 mg/day. Six studies contributed 6300 patients to the analysis (3127 on aspirin and 3173 on placebo). Aspirin reduced all-cause mortality by 18%, the number of strokes by 20%, myocardial infarctions by 30%, and other vascular events by 30%. On the other hand, patients who took aspirin were 2.5 times more likely than those who took placebo to have gastrointestinal tract bleeds. The number of patients needed to be treated (NNT) to prevent one death from any cause was 67 and the NNT to cause one gastrointestinal bleeding event was 100. In other words 1.5 lives can be saved for every gastrointestinal bleed attributed to aspirin. Although the risk of gastrointestinal bleeding was increased by aspirin, the hemorrhagic events were manageable and led to no deaths. On the basis of these data we can conclude that the benefits–harm balance for low-dose aspirin in the secondary prevention of cardiovascular and cerebrovascular events is highly favorable. The same conclusions have been drawn from the systematic overview published by the Antithrombotic Trialists Collaboration Group, which analysed data from 287 studies involving 135 000 patients (16).

As far as primary prevention of cardiovascular events is concerned, it appears that aspirin can reduce heart attacks and strokes but increases gastrointestinal and intracranial bleeding. The decision to use aspirin in primary prevention should therefore take into account the fact that the net effect of aspirin improves with increasing risk of coronary heart disease as well as the values that patients attach to the main favorable and unfavorable outcomes.

Organs and Systems

Cardiovascular

Apart from rare reports of variant angina pectoris and vasculitis theoretically related to thromboxane, aspirin is not associated with adverse effects on the cardiovascular system (17,18), except an increase in circulating plasma volume after large doses.

Respiratory

The effect of aspirin on bronchial musculature is discussed in the section on Immunologic in this monograph.

Salicylates can cause pulmonary edema, particularly in the elderly, especially if they are or have been heavy smokers (19).

Chronic salicylate toxicity can cause pulmonary injury, leading to respiratory distress. Lung biopsy may show diffuse alveolar damage and fibrosis (20).

Nervous system

Salicylism is a reaction to very high circulating concentrations of salicylate, characterized by tinnitus, dizziness, confusion, and headache.

Encephalopathy secondary to hyperammonemia has been reported in those rare cases of liver failure that are associated with high doses of aspirin, and this also forms a major feature of Reye's syndrome (see the section on Liver in this monograph).

One case-control study showed no increased risk of intracerebral hemorrhage in patients using aspirin or other NSAIDs in low dosages as prophylaxis against thrombosis (21). However, intracerebral hemorrhage has been reported with aspirin, even in low doses, and in the SALT study (22) and the Physicians Health Study of 1989 (23) hemorrhagic stroke and associated deaths occurred with aspirin.

Sensory systems

Eyes
Well-documented acute myopia and increased ocular pressure attributed to aspirin has been described (24).

Ears
With the high concentrations achieved in attempted suicide, tinnitus and hearing loss, leading to deafness, develop within about 5 hours, usually with regression within 48 hours, but permanent damage can occur. Disturbed balance, often with vertigo, can develop, as well as nausea, usually with maintenance of consciousness, even without treatment. It has been postulated that in this state depolarization of the cochlear hair cells occurs, similar to the changes induced by pressure. Tinnitus is also a symptom of salicylism.

Metabolism

Aspirin lowers plasma glucose concentrations in C-peptide-positive diabetic subjects and in normoglycemic persons (25). This is of no clinical significance.

Fluid balance

NSAIDs can cause fluid retention, but this has rarely been reported with aspirin.

- Severe fluid retention, possibly due to impaired renal tubular secretion, has been reported in a 29-year-old woman taking aspirin (1.5 g/day for several days) for persistent headache (26). During rechallenge with aspirin (0.5 g tds for 3 days) a dynamic renal scintigram showed a substantial fall in tubular filtration. Withdrawal was followed by complete uneventful recovery.

Pulmonary edema is a feature of salicylate intoxication, but this patient was taking a therapeutic dosage.

Hematologic

Thrombocytopenia, agranulocytosis, neutropenia, aplastic anemia, and even pancytopenia have been reported in association with aspirin. The prospect for recovery from the latter is poor, mortality approaching 50%.

Hemolytic anemia can occur in patients with glucose-6-phosphate dehydrogenase deficiency or erythrocyte glutathione peroxidase deficiency (SED-9, 128) (27–29). Whether these reports have anything more than anecdotal value (SEDA-17, 97) is not known.

Simple iron deficiency caused by occult blood loss occurs with a frequency of 1%, and upper gastrointestinal bleeding resulting from regular aspirin ingestion is the reason for hospitalization in about 15 patients per 100 000 aspirin users per year. Aspirin causes bleeding of sufficient severity to lead to iron deficiency anemia in 10–15% of patients taking it continuously for chronic arthritis. Some individuals are particularly at risk because of pregnancy, age, inadequate diet, menorrhagia, gastrectomy, or malabsorption syndromes.

Macrocytic anemia associated with folate deficiency has been described in patients with rheumatoid arthritis (30) and also in patients who abuse analgesic mixtures containing aspirin (30).

Effects on coagulation

Aspirin in high doses for several days can reduce prothrombin concentrations and prolong the prothrombin time. This will contribute to bleeding problems initiated by other factors, including aspirin's local irritant effects on epithelial cells. It is therefore very risky to use aspirin in patients with bleeding disorders. The effect will contribute to increased blood loss at parturition, spontaneous abortion, or menorrhagia, and may be linked to persistent ocular hemorrhage, particularly in older people, with or without associated surgical intervention (31,32).

By virtue of its effects on both cyclo-oxygenase isoenzymes, aspirin inhibits platelet thromboxane A_2 formation. This effect in the platelet is irreversible and will persist for the lifetime of the platelet (that is up to 10 days), since the platelet cannot synthesize new cyclo-oxygenase. It is of clinical significance that the dose of aspirin necessary to inhibit platelet thromboxane A_2 (around 40 mg/day) is much lower than that needed to inactivate the subendothelial prostacyclin (PGI_2). Hence, platelet aggregation is inhibited, with some associated dilatation of coronary and cerebral arterioles, at doses that do not interfere with prostacyclin inhibition. It is important, in considering the dosage of aspirin for prophylaxis (see below), to appreciate that prostacyclin is a general inhibitor of platelet aggregation, while aspirin, as a cyclo-oxygenase inhibitor, affects aggregation from a limited number of stimuli, for example ADP, adrenaline, thromboxane A_2. It is also worth recalling that the vascular endothelium can synthesize new cyclo-oxygenase, so that any effect on prostacyclin synthesis is of limited duration only (SEDA-12, 74) (33).

Several long-term studies have been carried out since the 1980s to determine the prophylactic usefulness of these effects on clotting. It is now clear that aspirin in dosages of around 300 mg/day can be used successfully for secondary prophylaxis in patients with coronary artery disease, in order to reduce the incidence of severe myocardial infarction, and in patients with cerebrovascular disease to reduce the incidence of transient ischemic attacks and strokes. There is some suggestion that higher doses of aspirin may be required in women. A major drawback has been the high incidence of gastrointestinal adverse effects and particularly bleeding in aspirin-treated groups (5,6,10,34). In view of the age group involved, bleeding can have serious implications. In an attempt to avoid this high proportion of ill-effects and yet retain the benefits of prophylactic antithrombotic treatment, a few trials have been conducted using aspirin in a dose of 162 mg (ISIS-2) (35) and 75 mg (RISC) (36) in symptomatic coronary heart disease, with good evidence of efficacy. Two studies have been reported in patients with cerebrovascular events, namely the Dutch TIA trial with aspirin 30 versus 283 mg (21) and the SALT study with aspirin 75 mg (22). The former did not show any difference in efficacy between the 30 and 283 mg dose groups, but there was no placebo control. The latter study showed a significant reduction in thrombotic stroke. However, intracerebral hemorrhage has been reported with aspirin, even in low doses, and in this as well as in the Physicians Health Study of 1989 (23), hemorrhagic stroke and associated deaths occurred with aspirin. On the other hand, the incidence of serious gastrointestinal events was much lower than previously described.

As nearly all of the risks seem to be dose-related (SEDA-21, 96), there is a good prospect that an even lower daily dose of aspirin may offer advantages in antithrombotic prophylaxis without an increased risk of bleeding, but the results of further such studies are still awaited (9).

Relatively few patients developed a prolonged bleeding time while taking aspirin or other NSAIDs and only few had significant intraoperative blood loss. There is variation in the response of patients for unknown reasons and so the recommendation that NSAIDs should be withdrawn before elective surgery awaits confirmation (SEDA-19, 96).

Gastrointestinal

Gastric ulceration and hemorrhage
DoTS classification
  Dose-relation: collateral effect
  Time-course: intermediate
  Susceptibility factors: age (over 65); sex (women); disease (peptic ulceration)

The gastrointestinal adverse effects of aspirin and the other NSAIDs are the most common. While some argue against a causative relation between aspirin ingestion and chronic gastric ulceration, the current consensus favors such a relation, while admitting that other factors, such as *Helicobacter pylori*, are likely to play a part. Patients aged over 65 years and women are more at risk, as are those who take aspirin over prolonged periods in a daily dose of about 2 g or more.

However, there is no ambiguity about the association of aspirin with gastritis, gastric erosions, or extensions of existing peptic ulcers, all of which are demonstrable by endoscopy. Even after one or two doses, superficial erosions have been described in over 50% of healthy subjects. This association is now almost universally accepted as the standard basis for comparative testing of NSAIDs and other drugs (21,37–39). Whether it is of benefit to use other drugs concomitantly to prevent the effect of gastric acid on the mucosa, and thus reduce the risk of gastric ulceration, is discussed further in this monograph.

Dyspepsia, nausea, and vomiting occur in 2–6% of patients after aspirin ingestion. Patients with rheumatoid arthritis seem to be more sensitive, and the frequency of aspirin-induced dyspepsia in this group is 10–30% (SEDA-9, 129). However, these symptoms are generally poor predictors of the incidence of mucosal damage (SEDA-18, 90).

The bleeding that occurs is usually triggered by erosions and aggravated by the antithrombotic action of aspirin. While it is reported to occur in up to 100% of regular aspirin takers, bleeding tends to be asymptomatic in young adults, unless it is associated with peptic ulceration, but it is readily detectable by endoscopy and the presence of occult blood in the feces. Hematemesis and melena are less often seen, the odds ratio being 1.5–2.0 in an overview of 21 low-dose aspirin prevention studies (40). A degree of resultant iron deficiency anemia is common. Such events are more commonly seen in older people in whom there is a significant proportion of serious bleeding and even deaths. Major gastrointestinal bleeding has an incidence of 15 per 100 000 so-called heavy aspirin users. However, the interpretation of "heavy" and of quantities of aspirin actually taken is to a large extent subjective and very dependent on the questionable accuracy of patient reporting. The risk appears to be greater in women, smokers, and patients concurrently taking other NSAIDs, and is possibly affected by other factors not yet established (41). Gastrointestinal perforation can occur without prodromes. Aspirin increases the risk of major upper gastrointestinal bleeding and perforation two- to three-fold in a dose-related manner, but deaths are rare.

Incidence

Of the estimated annual 65 000 upper gastrointestinal emergency admissions in the UK, nearly 20% (including deaths in 3.4%) are attributable to the use of prostaglandin synthesis inhibitors (42). As might be expected with an inhibitor of prostaglandin synthesis, the cytoprotective effects of prostaglandin E and prostacyclin

(PGI_2) are reduced by aspirin, as is the inhibitory action on gastric acid secretion. This effect may be both direct, as is the case with aspirin released in the stomach (or the lower rectum in the case of aspirin suppositories), and indirect following absorption and distribution via the systemic circulation; attempts to reduce the problems by coating and buffering can therefore have only limited success. The indirect type of effect is shown by the fact that these adverse gastric effects can also be exerted by parenteral lysine acetylsalicylate (SEDA-10, 72). The local effects depend in part on the tablet particle size, solubility, and rate of gastric absorption, while the most important variable appears to be gastric pH. On the other hand, within-day changes in the pharmacokinetics of the analgesic compounds may be involved in the prevalence of gastrointestinal adverse effects.

The estimates of gastrointestinal complication rates from aspirin are generally derived from clinical trials (SEDA-21, 100). However, the applicability of the results of such trials to the general population may be debatable, as protocols for these studies often are designed precisely to avoid enrollment of patients who are at risk of complications. Indeed differences in benefit-to-harm balance have been found in trials using the same dose of aspirin (43,44). For this reason, a population-based historical cohort study on frequency of major complications of aspirin used for secondary stroke prevention may be of interest (45). The study identified 588 patients who had a first ischemic stroke, transient ischemic attack, or amaurosis fugax during the study period. Of these, 339 patients had taken aspirin for an average of 1.7 years. The mean age of patients who had taken aspirin was 74 years. Complications occurred within 30 days of initiation of treatment in one patient, between 30 days and 6 months in 10 patients, between 6 months and 1 year in seven patients, and between 1 year and 2 years in two patients. Estimated standardized morbidity ratio of gastrointestinal hemorrhage (determined on the basis of 10 observed events and 0.661 expected events, during 576 person-years of observation) was 15 (95% CI = 7, 28). The estimated standardized morbidity ratio of intracerebral hemorrhage (determined on the basis of only one event and 0.59 expected events) was 1.7 (CI = 0.04, 9.4). One patient had a fatal gastrointestinal hemorrhage. Unfortunately these complication rates must be considered estimates, because aspirin therapy was not consistently recorded. However, the rates of complications were similar to those observed in some randomized clinical trials. On the basis of these data and of those of a meta-analysis of 16 trials involving more than 95 000 patients (45), the overall benefits of aspirin, measured in terms of preventing myocardial infarction and ischemic stroke, clearly outweigh the risks.

Dose-relatedness

The question of whether the risk of gastrointestinal hemorrhage with long-term aspirin is related to dose within the usual therapeutic dosage range (SEDA-12, 100) (15,46) merits attention. In a meta-analysis of the incidence of gastrointestinal hemorrhage associated with long-term aspirin and the effect of dose in 24 randomized, controlled clinical trials including almost 66 000 patients exposed for an average duration of 28 months to a wide range of different doses of aspirin (50–1500 mg/day), gastrointestinal hemorrhage occurred in 2.47% of patients taking aspirin compared with 1.42% taking placebo (OR = 1.68; 95% CI = 1.51, 1.88). In patients taking low doses of aspirin (50–162.5 mg/day; n = 49 927), gastrointestinal hemorrhage occurred in 2.3% compared with 1.45% taking placebo (OR = 1.56; 95% CI = 1.40, 1.81). The pooled OR for gastrointestinal hemorrhage with low-dose aspirin was 1.59 (95% CI = 1.4, 1.81). A meta-regression to test for a linear relation between the daily dose of aspirin and the risk of gastrointestinal hemorrhage gave a pooled OR of 1.015 (95% CI = 0.998, 1.047) per 100 mg dose reduction. The reduction in the incidence of gastrointestinal hemorrhage was estimated to be 1.5% per 100 mg dose reduction, but this was not significant.

These data are in apparent contrast with others previously reported (SEDA-21, 100) (14), which showed that gastrointestinal hemorrhage was related to dose in the usual dosage range. Many reasons may explain these contrasting results, the most important being differences in the definition of the hemorrhagic events, in study design, in the population studied, and in the presence of accessory risk factors (47–49).

The recent trends toward the use of lower doses of aspirin have been driven by the belief that these offer a better safety profile while retaining equivalent therapeutic efficacy. Despite the large number of patients enrolled in randomized clinical trials and included in meta-analyses, there is no firm evidence that dose reduction significantly lowers the risk of gastrointestinal bleeding. Patients and doctors therefore need to consider the trade-off between the benefits and harms of long-term treatment with aspirin. Meanwhile, it seems wise to use the lowest dose of proven efficacy.

A systematic review of 17 epidemiological studies conducted between 1990 and 2001 has provided further data on this topic (50). The effect of aspirin dosage was investigated in five studies. There was a greater risk of gastrointestinal complications with aspirin in dosages over 300 mg/day than in dosages of 300 mg/day or less. However, users of low-dose aspirin still had a two-fold increased risk of such complications compared with non-users, with no clear evidence of a dose-response relation at dosages under 300 mg/day, confirming previous findings (15). The study also addressed the question of whether the aspirin formulation affects gastrotoxicity. The pooled relative risks of gastrointestinal complications in four studies were 2.4 (95%; CI = 1.9, 2.9) for enteric-coated aspirin, 5.3 (3.0, 9.2) for buffered formulations, and 2.6 (2.3, 2.9) for plain aspirin, compared with non-use. These data confirm those from previous studies (SEDA-21, 100) (15), which negate any protective effect of the most frequently used aspirin formulations. Furthermore, there were higher relative risks, compared with non-use, for gastrointestinal complications in patients who used aspirin regularly (RR = 3.2; CI = 2.6, 5.9) than in patients who used it occasionally (2.1; 1.7, 2.6), and

during the first month of use (4.4; 3.2, 6.1) compared with subsequent months (2.6; 2.1, 3.1).

Comparative studies
A comparative study of gastrointestinal blood loss after aspirin 972 mg qds for 4 days versus different doses of piroxicam (20 mg od, 5 mg qds, and 10 mg qds) showed that piroxicam did not increase fecal blood loss, whereas aspirin did. Gastroscopic evidence of irritation was also greater with aspirin (51).

In a randomized trial comparing ticlopidine (500 mg/day) with aspirin (1300 mg/day) for the prevention of stroke in high-risk patients, the incidence of bleeding was similar in both groups, although more patients treated with aspirin developed peptic ulceration or gastrointestinal hemorrhage (52).

Risk factors
A study of the risk factors for gastrointestinal perforation, a much less frequent event than bleeding, has confirmed that aspirin and other NSAIDs increase the risk of both upper and lower gastrointestinal perforation (OR 6.7, CI 3.1–14.5 for NSAIDs) (53). Gastrointestinal perforation has been associated with other factors, such as coffee consumption, a history of peptic ulcer, and smoking. The combination of NSAIDs, smoking, and alcohol increased the risk of gastrointestinal perforation (OR 10.7, CI 3.8–30) (SEDA-21, 97).

Associated effects
Aspirin can also play a role in esophageal bleeding, ulceration, or benign stricture, and it should be considered as a possible cause in patients, particularly the elderly, who present with any of these features. There have also been reports of rectal stricture in the elderly, associated with the use of aspirin suppositories. Effects on both these strictures emphasize the significance of a direct local action of aspirin as well as a systemic action and underlines the relevance of the involvement of oxygen-derived free radicals in the pathogenesis of mucosal lesions in the gastrointestinal tract (54–56).

A gastrocolic fistula developed in a 47-year-old woman taking aspirin and prednisone for rheumatoid arthritis (57). Other similar case reports have been published (58,59).

Long-term effects
The effects on the stomach of continued exposure to aspirin remain controversial. While in short-term use, gastric mucosal erosions may often be recurrent but transient and comparatively trivial lesions, with longer administration there seems to be an increased risk of progression to ulceration.

Prophylaxis
Intravenous administration, or the use of enteric-coated formulations or modified-release products all appear to reduce the risk both of bleeding and more particularly of erosions/ulceration. However, because of the indirect effect noted above, such formulations do not eliminate the risk, although they may reduce the incidence of

gastric or duodenal ulcer, as may buffered aspirin (60,61).

Considerable attention in recent years has been directed toward the efficacy of using synthetic forms of PGE_2, histamine H_2 receptor antagonists, proton pump inhibitors, or antacids, either to heal peptic ulcers associated with use of prostaglandin inhibitors or more significantly to act prophylactically to protect against ulceration or bleeding associated with aspirin or the NSAIDs. With the exception of PGE_2, there is no convincing evidence to justify their prophylactic use, as they do not reduce the risk of significant gastrointestinal events. In contrast, their soothing effect on gastrointestinal symptoms may ultimately result in more severe complications (62). Since all these agents carry their own potential risks, it is more than questionable whether administration to a patient with normal gastrointestinal mucosa is justified. Generally, use of prostaglandin inhibitors should be limited to the shortest possible duration, thereby minimizing, but not eliminating, the risk of gastrointestinal damage. Only high-risk patients should be eligible for prophylactic drug therapy. Well-known risk factors for the development of mucosal lesions of the gastrointestinal tract are age (over 75 years), a history of peptic ulcer, or gastrointestinal bleeding, and concomitant cardiac disease.

Liver

Aspirin can cause dose-related focal hepatic necrosis that is usually asymptomatic or anicteric. Much of the evidence for hepatotoxicity of aspirin and the salicylates has been shown in children (63,64), usually in patients with connective tissue disorders, taking relatively high long-term dosages for Still's disease, rheumatoid arthritis, or occasionally systemic lupus erythematosus. Rises in serum transaminases seem to be the most common feature (in up to 50% of patients) and are usually reversible on withdrawal, but they occasionally lead to fatal hepatic necrosis. Severe and even fatal metabolic encephalopathy can also occur, as in Reye's syndrome (see the section on Reye's syndrome in this monograph). One can easily overload the young patient's individual metabolic capacity. The co-existence of hypoalbuminemia may be a particular risk factor; in patients with hypoalbuminemia of 35 g/l or less, close monitoring of the aspartate transaminase is advisable, especially if the concentration of total serum salicylate is 1.1 mmol/l or higher (65). Plasma salicylate concentrations in serious cases have usually been in excess of 1.4 mmol/l and liver function tests return rapidly to normal when the drug is withdrawn. Finally, a very small number of cases of chronic active hepatitis have been attributed to aspirin (66).

Reye's syndrome

First defined as a distinct syndrome in 1963, Reye's syndrome came to be regarded some years later as an adverse effect of aspirin. In fact, the position is more complex, and the syndrome still cannot be assigned a specific cause. There is general agreement that the disorder presents a few days after the prodrome of a viral illness. Well over a dozen different viruses have so far been implicated, including influenza A and B, adenovirus, *Varicella*, and reovirus. Various other factors have also been incriminated, including aflatoxins, certain pesticides, and such antioxidants as butylated hydroxytoluene. Only in the case of aspirin have some epidemiological studies been conducted, and these appeared to show a close correlation with cases of Reye's syndrome. It was these studies that led to regulatory action against the promotion of salicylate use in children. However, doubt has been thrown on the clarity of the link, and it now seems increasingly likely that while there is some association with aspirin, the etiology is in fact multifactorial, including some genetic predisposition. Studies in Japan did not support the US findings, while studies in Thailand and Canada invoked other factors.

Two characteristic phenomena are present in Reye's syndrome.

1. Damage to mitochondrial structures, with pleomorphism, disorganization of matrix, proliferation of smooth endoplasmic reticulum, and an increase in peroxisomes; mitochondrial enzyme activity is severely reduced, but cytoplasmic enzymes are unaffected. The changes first appear in single cells, but may spread to all hepatocytes. Recovery may be complete by 5–7 days. While these changes are most evident in liver cells, similar effects have been seen in cerebral neurons and skeletal muscle. There appears to be a block in beta-oxidation of fatty acids (inhibition of oxidation of NAB-linked substrates). In vitro aspirin selectively inhibits mitochondrial oxidation of medium- and long-chain fatty acids.
2. An acute catabolic state with hypoglycemia, hyperammonemia, raised activities of serum aspartate transaminase and creatine phosphokinase, and increased urinary nitrogen and serum long chain dicarboxylic acid.

Despite our lack of understanding of the syndrome, the decision taken in many countries to advise against the use of salicylates in children under 12 made an impact, in terms of a falling incidence of Reye's syndrome (SEDA-16, 96; SEDA-17, 97).

Over the last 25 years, in the USA, the incidence of Reye's syndrome has fallen significantly—from the time that the advice was introduced up to 1999 there were 25 reported cases, but 15 were in adolescents aged 12–17 years, and 8% of cases occurred in patients aged 15 years or over (67). In the UK, in view of these findings, the Commission on Safety of Medicines (CSM) amended its original statement and advised that aspirin should be avoided in febrile illnesses or viral infections in patients aged under 16 years. However, the appropriateness of this decision has been challenged (68). This is because the incidence of Reye's syndrome is already low and is falling; furthermore, restricting the use of aspirin leaves paracetamol and ibuprofen as the only available therapeutic alternatives, and their safety is not absolutely guaranteed and might be even worse than that of aspirin.

Urinary tract

Aspirin is associated with a small but significant risk of hospitalization for acute renal insufficiency (SEDA-19, 95).

When aspirin is used by patients on sodium restriction or with congestive heart failure, there tends to be a reduction in the glomerular filtration rate, with preservation of normal renal plasma flow. Some renal tubular epithelial shedding can also occur.

Severe systemic disease involving the heart, liver, or kidneys seems to predispose the patient to the effects of aspirin and other NSAIDs on renal function (69).

Chronic renal disease

Renal papillary necrosis has been reported after long-term intake or abuse of aspirin and other NSAIDs (SEDA-11, 85) (SEDA-12, 79). The relation between long-term heavy exposure to analgesics and the risk of chronic renal disease has been the object of intensive toxicological and epidemiological research for many years (SEDA-24, 120) (70). Most of the earlier reports suggested that phenacetin-containing analgesics probably cause renal papillary necrosis and interstitial nephritis. In contrast, there was no convincing epidemiological evidence that non-phenacetin-containing analgesics (including paracetamol, aspirin, mixtures of the two, and NSAIDs) cause chronic renal disease. Moreover, findings from epidemiological studies should be interpreted with caution, because of a number of inherent limitations and potential biases in study design (71). Two methodologically sound studies have provided information on this topic.

The first was the largest cohort study conducted thus far to assess the risk of renal dysfunction associated with analgesic use (72). Details of analgesic use were obtained from 11 032 men without previous renal dysfunction participating in the Physicians' Health Study (PHS), which lasted 14 years. The main outcome measure was a raised creatinine concentration defined as 1.5 mg/dl (133 µmol/l) or higher and a reduced creatinine clearance of 55 ml/minute or less. In all, 460 men (4.2%) had a raised creatinine concentration and 1258 (11%) had a reduced creatinine clearance. Mean creatinine concentrations and creatinine clearances were similar among men who did not use analgesics and those who did. This was true for all categories of analgesics (paracetamol and paracetamol-containing mixtures, aspirin and aspirin-containing mixtures, and other NSAIDs) and for higher-risk groups, such as those aged 60 years or over or those with hypertension or diabetes.

These data are convincing, as the large size of the PHS cohort should make it possible to examine and detect even modest associations between analgesic use and a risk of renal disease. Furthermore, this study included more individuals who reported extensive use of analgesics than any prior case-control study. However, the study had some limitations, the most important being the fact that the cohort was composed of relatively healthy men, most of whom were white. These results cannot therefore be generalized to the entire population. However, the study clearly showed that there is not a strong association between chronic analgesic use and chronic renal dysfunction among a large cohort of men without a history of renal impairment.

The second study was a Swedish nationwide, population-based, case-control study of early-stage chronic renal insufficiency in men whose serum creatinine concentration exceeded 3.4 mg/dl (300 µmol/l) or women whose serum creatinine exceeded 2.8 mg/dl (250 µmol/l) (73). In all, 918 patients with newly diagnosed renal insufficiency and 980 controls were interviewed and completed questionnaires about their lifetime consumption of analgesics. Compared with controls, more patients with chronic renal insufficiency were regular users of aspirin (37 versus 19%) or paracetamol (25 versus 12%). Among subjects who did not use aspirin regularly, the regular use of paracetamol was associated with a risk of chronic renal insufficiency that was 2.5 times as high as that for non-users of paracetamol. The risk increased with increasing cumulative lifetime dose. Patients who took 500 g or more over a year (1.4 g/day) during periods of regular use had an increased odds ratio for chronic renal insufficiency (OR = 5.3; 95% CI = 1.8, 15). Among subjects who did not use paracetamol regularly, the regular use of aspirin was associated with a risk of chronic renal insufficiency that was 2.5 times as high as that for non-users of aspirin. The risk increased significantly with an increasing cumulative lifetime dose of aspirin. Among the patients with an average intake of 500 g or more of aspirin per year during periods of regular use, the risk of chronic renal insufficiency was increased about three-fold (OR = 3.3; CI = 1.4, 8.0). Among patients who used paracetamol in addition to aspirin, the risk of chronic renal insufficiency was increased about two-fold when regular aspirin users served as the reference group (OR = 2.2; CI = 1.4, 3.5) and non-significantly when regular paracetamol users were used as controls (OR = 1.6; CI = 0.9, 2.7). There was no relation between the use of other analgesics (propoxyphene, NSAIDs, codeine, and pyrazolones) and the risk of chronic renal insufficiency. Thus, the regular use of paracetamol, or aspirin, or both was associated dose-dependently with an increased risk of chronic renal insufficiency. The OR among regular users exceeded 1.0 for all types of chronic renal insufficiency, albeit not always significantly. These results are consistent with exacerbating effects of paracetamol and aspirin on chronic renal insufficiency, regardless of accompanying disease.

How can we explain the contrasting results of these two studies? A possible explanation lies in the different populations studied. In the PHS study, relatively healthy individuals were enrolled while in the Swedish study all the patients had pre-existing severe renal or systemic disease, suggesting that such disease has an important role in causing analgesic-associated chronic renal insufficiency. People without pre-existing disease who use analgesics may have only a small risk of end-stage renal disease.

Skin

Hypersensitivity reactions, such as urticaria and angioedema, are relatively common in subjects with aspirin hypersensitivity. Purpura, hemorrhagic vasculitis, erythema multiforme, Stevens–Johnson syndrome, and Lyell's syndrome have also been reported, but much less often. Fixed drug eruptions, probably hypersensitive in origin, are periodically described. In some patients they do not recur on rechallenge, that is the sensitivity disappears (74).

Musculoskeletal

There is evidence that salicylates together with at least some NSAIDs suppress proteoglycan biosynthesis independently of effects on prostaglandin synthesis (75). Thus, prolonged use of these agents can accentuate deterioration of articular cartilage in weight-bearing arthritic joints. If this is proved, the problem will be of greatest relevance to elderly people with osteoarthritis, a condition in which this use of prostaglandin inhibitors is questionable.

Immunologic

Aspirin hypersensitivity

Of adult asthmatics 2–20% have aspirin hypersensitivity (9). The mechanism is related to a deficiency in bronchodilator prostaglandins; prostaglandin inhibition may make arachidonic acid produce more leukotrienes with bronchoconstrictor activity. Oral challenge in asthmatic patients is an effective but potentially dangerous method for establishing the presence of aspirin hypersensitivity (63).

The term "aspirin allergy" is better avoided, in the absence of identification of a definite antigen–antibody reaction. This topic has been reviewed (SEDA-17, 94) (SEDA-18, 90).

Epidemiology
Aspirin hypersensitivity is relatively common in adults (about 20%). Estimates of the prevalence of aspirin-induced asthma vary from 3.3 to 44% in different reports (SEDA-5, 169), although it is often only demonstrable by challenge tests with spirometry, and only 4% have problems in practice. Patients with existing asthma and nasal polyps or chronic urticaria have a greater frequency of hypersensitivity (76), and women appear to be more susceptible than men, perhaps particularly during the child-bearing period of life (77). Acute intolerance to aspirin can develop even in patients who have taken the drug for some years without problems.

There is considerable cross-reactivity with other NSAIDs and the now widely banned food colorant tartrazine (78). Cross-sensitization between aspirin and tartrazine is common; for example, in one series 24% of aspirin-sensitive patients also reacted to tartrazine (SEDA-9, 76).

Mechanism
The current theory of the mechanism relates to the inhibition of cyclo-oxygenases (79) and a greater degree of interference with PGE_2 synthesis, allowing the bronchoconstrictor PGF_2 to predominate in susceptible individuals.

PGE_2 inhibition in macrophages may also unleash bronchial cytotoxic lymphocytes, generated by chronic viral infection, leading to destruction of virus-infected cells in the respiratory tract (80). When urticaria occurs, it may result from increased release of leukotrienes LTC_4, D_4, and E_4, which also induces bronchoconstriction, with a shunt of arachidonic acid toward lipoxygenation in aspirin-sensitive asthmatics (SEDA-18, 93). Aspirin-induced asthma patients show hyper-reactivity to inhaled metacholine and sulpyrine.

Features
The features of aspirin hypersensitivity include bronchospasm, acute and usually generalized urticaria, angioedema, severe rhinitis, and shock. These reactions can occur alone or in various combinations, developing within minutes or a few hours of aspirin ingestion, and lasting until elimination is complete. They can be life-threatening. The bronchospastic type of reaction predominates in adults, only the urticarial type being found in children. The frequency of recurrent urticaria is significantly greater in adults (3.8 versus 0.3%).

People with asthma may be particularly sensitive to acetylsalicylic acid, which may be given alone or as a constituent of a combination medicine. The association between aspirin sensitivity, nasal polyps, and rhinitis in asthma is well known.

Henoch–Schönlein purpura has been reported (81).

Life-threatening respiratory distress, facial edema, and lethargy occurred in a woman with a history of severe asthma and aspirin hypersensitivity (SEDA-22, 118).

Aspirin-sensitive subjects may have attacks induced by other NSAIDs (82).

Fish oil can also cause exacerbation of asthma in aspirin-sensitive patients (83).

Prophylaxis and treatment
Asthma induced by aspirin is often severe and resistant to treatment. Avoidance of aspirin and substances to which there is cross-sensitivity is the only satisfactory solution. Desensitization is not usually successful and repeated treatments are needed to maintain any effect (84,85).

Long-Term Effects

Tumorigenicity

Studies on the tumor-inducing effects of heavy use of analgesics, especially those that contain phenacetin, have given contrasting results (SEDA-21, 100) (86,87). There has been a case-control study of the role of habitual intake of aspirin on the occurrence of urothelial cancer and renal cell carcinoma (88). In previous studies there was a consistent association between phenacetin and renal cell carcinoma, but inconclusive results with respect to non-phenacetin analgesics. In 1024 patients with renal cell carcinoma and an equal number of matched controls, regular use of analgesics was a significant risk factor for renal cell carcinoma (OR = 1.6; CI = 1.4, 1.9). The risk was significantly increased by aspirin, NSAIDs, paracetamol, and phenacetin, and within each class of analgesic the risk increased with increasing exposure. Individuals in the highest exposure categories had about a 2.5-fold increase in risk relative to non-users or irregular users of analgesics. However, exclusive users of aspirin who took aspirin 325 mg/day or less for cardiovascular problems were not at an increased risk of renal cell carcinoma (OR = 0.9; CI = 0.6, 1.4).

Second-Generation Effects

Teratogenicity

It is perhaps surprising that aspirin, which is teratogenic in rodents, and which by virtue of its capacity to inhibit prostaglandin synthesis would be expected to affect the development of the renal and cardiovascular systems, has shown no evidence of teratogenesis in humans, despite very widespread use in pregnant women. Perhaps increased production of prostaglandins during pregnancy overrides the effects of aspirin in the usual dosages, and the intervention of placental metabolism protects the human fetus from exposure to aspirin. Whatever the explanation, there are very few reports in which aspirin can be implicated as a human teratogen and a few studies (89,90) have provided positive reassurance.

Fetotoxicity

Because aspirin is an antithrombotic agent and can promote bleeding, it should be avoided in the third trimester of pregnancy and at parturition (91). At parturition there is a second reason for avoiding aspirin, since its prostaglandin-inhibiting capacity could mean that it will delay parturition and induce early closure of the ductus arteriosus in the near-term fetus, as other NSAIDs do (92). However, its use in low doses in pregnancy may prevent retardation of fetal growth (93).

Susceptibility Factors

Age

In view of the association with Reye's syndrome, aspirin should be avoided in children aged under 16.

Drug Administration

Drug formulations

Although the use of enteric-coated aspirin can reduce its direct adverse effect on the stomach (SEDA-10, 72), it could in principle transfer these to some extent to the intestine; modified-release NSAIDs have sometimes caused intestinal perforation.

Enteric coating reduces the rate of absorption of aspirin. In cases of severe overdosage this can cause difficulties in diagnosis and treatment, since early plasma salicylate measurements are unreliable, maximum blood concentrations sometimes not being reached until 60 or 70 hours after overdose (94,95). Another complication of the use of enteric-coated aspirin is the risk of gastric outlet obstruction and the resulting accumulation of tablets because of subclinical pyloric stenosis.

Drug overdose

Acute poisoning

Acute salicylate poisoning is a major clinical hazard (96), although it is associated with low major morbidity and mortality, in contrast to chronic intoxication (SEDA-17,

98). It can cause alkalemia or acidemia, alkaluria or aciduria, hyperglycemia or hypoglycemia, and water and electrolyte imbalances. However, the usual picture is one of hypokalemia with metabolic acidosis and respiratory alkalosis. Effects on hearing have been referred to in the section on Sensory systems in this monograph. Nausea, vomiting, tinnitus, hyperpnea, hyperpyrexia, confusion, disorientation, dizziness, coma, and/or convulsions are common. They are expressions of the nervous system effects of the salicylates. Gastrointestinal hemorrhage is frequent.

Serum salicylate concentrations above 3.6 mmol/l are likely to be toxic, and concentrations of 5.4 mmol/l can easily prove fatal.

After ingestion, drug absorption can be prevented by induction of emesis, gastric lavage, and the administration of active charcoal; drug excretion is enhanced by administering intravenous alkalinizing solutions, hemoperfusion, and hemodialysis (97). Forced diuresis is dangerous and unnecessary.

Fluid and electrolyte management is the mainstay of therapy. The immediate aim must be to correct acidosis, hyperpyrexia, hypokalemia, and dehydration. In severe cases vitamin K_1 should be given to counteract hypoprothrombinemia.

Chronic poisoning

Chronic salicylate intoxication is commonly associated with chronic daily headaches, lethargy, confusion, or coma. Since headache is a feature, it can easily be misdiagnosed if the physician is not aware that aspirin has been over-used. Depression of mental status is usually present at the time of diagnosis, when the serum salicylate concentration is at a peak. The explanation of depression, manifested by irritability, lethargy, and unresponsiveness, occurring 1–3 days after the start of therapy for aspirin intoxication, lies in a persistently high concentration of salicylate in the central nervous system, while the serum salicylate concentration falls to non-toxic values. The delayed unresponsiveness associated with salicylate intoxication appears to be closely associated with the development of cerebral edema of uncertain cause. The encephalopathy that ensues appears to be directly related to increased intracranial pressure, a known effect of prostaglandin synthesis inhibitors; it responds to mannitol (98).

Drug–Drug Interactions

Alcohol

Although ethanol itself has no effect on bleeding time, it enhances the effect of aspirin when given simultaneously or up to at least 36 hours after aspirin ingestion (99). Ethanol also promotes gastric bleeding.

The FDA has announced its intention to require alcohol warnings on all over-the-counter pain medications that contain acetylsalicylic acid, salicylates, paracetamol, ibuprofen, ketoprofen, or naproxen. The proposed warnings are aimed at alerting consumers to the specific risks incurred from heavy alcohol consumption and its interaction with analgesics. For products that contain paracetamol, the warning indicates the risks of liver damage in those who drink more than three alcoholic beverages a day. For formulations that contain salicylates or the mentioned NSAIDs, three or more alcoholic beverages will increase the risk of stomach bleeding (100).

Anticoagulants

The effects on coagulation are additive if aspirin is used concurrently with anticoagulants. There are also other interaction mechanisms: the effect of the coumarins is temporarily increased by protein binding displacement, and if aspirin causes gastric hemorrhages, the latter may well be more severe when anticoagulants are being given.

Aspirin should therefore generally be avoided in patients adequately treated with anticoagulants. The most relevant information on hemorrhagic complications occurring during prophylaxis with antiplatelet drugs, whether used singly or in combination, has been provided by well-controlled prospective trials with aspirin (17), aspirin combined with dipyridamole (101), or aspirin compared with oral anticoagulants (102).

Antihypertensive drugs

An increase in mean supine blood pressure has been reported with aspirin (SEDA-19, 92). Aspirin may therefore interfere with antihypertensive pharmacotherapy, warranting caution, especially in the elderly.

Captopril

Aspirin is thought to reduce the antihypertensive effect of captopril (103).

Carbonic anhydrase inhibitors

In two children, aspirin potentiated the slight metabolic acidosis induced by carbonic anhydrase inhibitors (SEDA-9, 79) (104).

Glucocorticoids

The effects of aspirin on gastrointestinal mucosa will lead to additive effects if it is used concurrently with other drugs that have an irritant effect on the stomach, notably other NSAIDs or glucocorticoids (105,106).

Heparin

Risk factors for heparin-induced bleeding include concomitant use of aspirin (107).

Intrauterine contraceptive devices

The supposed mechanisms of action of intrauterine contraceptive devices (IUCDs) include a local inflammatory response and increased local production of prostaglandins that prevent sperm from fertilizing ova (108,109). As aspirin has both anti-inflammatory and antiprostaglandin properties, the contraceptive effectiveness of an IUCD can be reduced by the drug, although the effect on periodic bleeding may prevail.

Methotrexate

Aspirin displaces methotrexate from its binding sites and also inhibits its renal tubular elimination, so that the dosage of concurrently used methotrexate should be reduced (except once-a-week low-dose treatment in rheumatoid arthritis) (110).

Nitrates

Aspirin in low dosages (under 300 mg/day) is widely used in cardiovascular prophylaxis, but its use is accompanied by an increased risk of gastrointestinal bleeding (SEDA-21, 100). Of particular interest therefore are data from a retrospective case-control study showing that nitrate therapy may reduce the risk of aspirin-induced gastrointestinal bleeding (111). As nitrates are often used in the same population of patients, such data merit further confirmation from larger prospective studies.

NSAIDs

The effects of aspirin on gastrointestinal mucosa will lead to additive effects if it is used concurrently with other drugs that have an irritant effect on the stomach, notably other NSAIDs or glucocorticoids (105,106). Salicylates can be displaced from binding sites by some NSAIDs such as naproxen, or in turn displace others such as piroxicam.

Sodium valproate

Aspirin displaces sodium valproate from protein binding sites (112) and reduces its hepatic metabolism (113).

Streptokinase

Major hemorrhagic complications, including cerebral hemorrhage, can occur with aspirin (SEDA-23, 116) and the same is also true for thrombolytic therapy of acute ischemic stroke (114). A post hoc analysis of the Multicenter Acute Stroke Trial in Italy showed a negative interaction of aspirin and streptokinase in acute ischemic stroke (115). In 156 patients who received streptokinase plus aspirin and 157 patients treated with streptokinase alone, the combined regimen significantly increased early case fatality at days 3–10 (53 versus 30; OR = 2.5; CI = 1.2, 3.6). The excess in deaths was solely due to treatment and was not explained by the main prognostic predictors. Deaths in the combination group were mainly cerebral (42 versus 24; OR = 2.0; CI = 1.3, 3.7) and associated with hemorrhagic transformation (22 versus 11; OR = 2.2; CI = 1.0, 5.0). The data suggest that aspirin should be avoided when thrombolytic agents are used for acute ischemic stroke.

Uricosuric drugs

In low dosages (up to 2 g/day), aspirin reduces urate excretion and blocks the effects of probenecid and other uricosuric agents (116). However, in 11 patients with gout, aspirin 325 mg/day had no effect on the uricosuric action of probenecid (117). In higher dosages (over 5 g/day), salicylates increase urate excretion and inhibit the effects of spironolactone, but it is not clear that these phenomena are of importance.

Food-Drug Interactions

Food allergens

Aspirin seems to potentiate the effects of food allergens, but this is uncertain (SEDA-10, 72).

Interference with Diagnostic Tests

Thyroid function tests

Through competitive binding to thyroid-binding globulin, salicylates in high concentrations can displace thyroxine and triiodothyronine, thus interfering with the results of diagnostic thyroid function tests (118).

References

1. MacIntyre A, Gray JD, Gorelick M, Renton K. Salicylate and acetaminophen in donated blood. CMAJ 1986;135(3):215–16.
2. Wynne HA, Long A. Patient awareness of the adverse effects of non-steroidal anti-inflammatory drugs (NSAIDs). Br J Clin Pharmacol 1996;42(2):253–6.
3. National Drugs Advisory Board. Availability of aspirin and paracetamol. Annual Report 1987:24.
4. Mitchell JA, Akarasereenont P, Thiemermann C, Flower RJ, Vane JR. Selectivity of nonsteroidal antiinflammatory drugs as inhibitors of constitutive and inducible cyclooxygenase. Proc Natl Acad Sci USA 1993;90(24):11693–7.
5. Antiplatelet Trialists' Collaboration. Secondary prevention of vascular disease by prolonged antiplatelet treatment. BMJ (Clin Res Ed) 1988;296(6618):320–31.
6. Hennekens CH, Buring JE, Sandercock P, Collins R, Peto R. Aspirin and other antiplatelet agents in the secondary and primary prevention of cardiovascular disease. Circulation 1989;80(4):749–56.
7. Macdonald R. Aspirin and extradural blocks. Br J Anaesth 1991;66(1):1–3.
8. de Swiet M, Redman CW. Aspirin, extradural anaesthesia and the MRC Collaborative Low-dose Aspirin Study in Pregnancy (CLASP). Br J Anaesth 1992;69(1):109–10.
9. Steering Committee of the Physicians' Health Study Research Group. Final report on the aspirin component of the ongoing Physicians' Health Study. N Engl J Med 1989;321(3):129–35.
10. Peto R, Gray R, Collins R, Wheatley K, Hennekens C, Jamrozik K, Warlow C, Hafner B, Thompson E, Norton S, et al. Randomised trial of prophylactic daily aspirin in British male doctors. BMJ (Clin Res Ed) 1988;296(6618):313–16.
11. Stafford RS. Aspirin use is low among United States outpatients with coronary artery disease. Circulation 2000;101(10):1097–101.
12. Hayden M, Pignone M, Phillips C, Mulrow C. Aspirin for the primary prevention of cardiovascular events: a summary of the evidence for the U.S. Preventive Services Task Force. Ann Intern Med 2002;136(2):161–72.
13. Weisman SM, Graham DY. Evaluation of the benefits and risks of low-dose aspirin in the secondary prevention of cardiovascular and cerebrovascular events. Arch Intern Med 2002;162(19):2197–202.
14. Roderick PJ, Wilkes HC, Meade TW. The gastrointestinal toxicity of aspirin: an overview of randomised controlled trials. Br J Clin Pharmacol 1993;35(3):219–26.
15. Derry S, Loke YK. Risk of gastrointestinal haemorrhage with long term use of aspirin: meta-analysis. BMJ 2000;321(7270):1183–7.
16. Antithrombotic Trialists' Collaboration. Collaborative meta-analysis of randomised trials of antiplatelet therapy for prevention of death, myocardial infarction, and stroke in high risk patients. BMJ 2002;324(7329):71–86.
17. Aspirin Myocardial Infarction Study Research Group. A randomized, controlled trial of aspirin in persons recovered from myocardial infarction. JAMA 1980;243(7):661–9.
18. Habbab MA, Szwed SA, Haft JI. Is coronary arterial spasm part of the aspirin-induced asthma syndrome? Chest 1986;90(1):141–3.
19. Heffner JE, Sahn SA. Salicylate-induced pulmonary edema. Clinical features and prognosis. Ann Intern Med 1981;95(4):405–9.
20. Grabe DW, Manley HJ, Kim JS, McGoldrick MD, Bailie GR. Respiratory distress caused by salicylism confirmed by lung biopsy. Clin Drug Invest 1999;17:79–81.
21. The Dutch TIA Trial Study Group. A comparison of two doses of aspirin (30 mg vs. 283 mg a day) in patients after a transient ischemic attack or minor ischemic stroke. N Engl J Med 1991;325(18):1261–6.
22. The SALT Collaborative Group. Swedish Aspirin Low-Dose Trial (SALT) of 75 mg aspirin as secondary prophylaxis after cerebrovascular ischaemic events. Lancet 1991;338(8779):1345–9.
23. Final report on the aspirin component of the ongoing Physicians' Health Study. Steering Committee of the Physicians' Health Study Research Group. N Engl J Med 1989;321(3):129–35.
24. Rohr WD. Transitorische Myopisierung und Drucksteigerung als Medikamentennebenwirkung. [Transitory myopia and increased ocular pressure as side effects of drugs.] Fortschr Ophthalmol 1984;81(2):199–200.
25. Prince RL, Larkins RG, Alford FP. The effect of acetylsalicylic acid on plasma glucose and the response of glucose regulatory hormones to intravenous glucose and arginine in insulin treated diabetics and normal subjects. Metabolism 1981;30(3):293–8.
26. Manfredini R, Ricci L, Giganti M, La Cecilia O, Kuwornu Afi H, Chierici F, Gallerani M. An uncommon case of fluid retention simulating a congestive heart failure after aspirin consumption. Am J Med Sci 2000;320(1):72–4.
27. Necheles TF, Steinberg MH, Cameron D. Erythrocyte glutathione-peroxidase deficiency. Br J Haematol 1970;19(5):605–12.
28. Meloni T, Forteleoni G, Ogana A, Franca V. Aspirin-induced acute haemolytic anaemia in glucose-6-phosphate dehydrogenase-deficient children with systemic arthritis. Acta Haematol 1989;81(4):208–9.
29. Levy M, Heyman A. Hematological adverse effects of analgesic anti-inflammatory drugs. Hematol Rev 1990;4:177.
30. Williams JO, Mengel CE, Sullivan LW, Haq AS. Megaloblastic anemia associated with chronic ingestion of an analgesic. N Engl J Med 1969;280(6):312–13.
31. Kingham JD, Chen MC, Levy MH. Macular hemorrhage in the aging eye: the effects of anticoagulants. N Engl J Med 1988;318(17):1126–7.
32. Werblin TP, Peiffer RL. Persistent hemorrhage after extracapsular surgery associated with excessive aspirin ingestion. Am J Ophthalmol 1987;104(4):426.
33. Hanley SP, Bevan J, Cockbill SR, Heptinstall S. Differential inhibition by low-dose aspirin of human venous prostacyclin synthesis and platelet thromboxane synthesis. Lancet 1981;1(8227):969–71.

34. The Canadian Cooperative Study Group. A randomized trial of aspirin and sulfinpyrazone in threatened stroke. N Engl J Med 1978;299(2):53–9.

35. ISIS-2 (Second International Study of Infarct Survival) Collaborative Group. Randomised trial of intravenous streptokinase, oral aspirin, both, or neither among 17,187 cases of suspected acute myocardial infarction: ISIS-2. Lancet 1988;2(8607):349–60.

36. The RISC Group. Risk of myocardial infarction and death during treatment with low dose aspirin and intravenous heparin in men with unstable coronary artery disease. Lancet 1990;336(8719):827–30.

37. Blower AL, Brooks A, Fenn GC, Hill A, Pearce MY, Morant S, Bardhan KD. Emergency admissions for upper gastrointestinal disease and their relation to NSAID use. Aliment Pharmacol Ther 1997;11(2):283–91.

38. Piper DW, McIntosh JH, Ariotti DE, Fenton BH, MacLennan R. Analgesic ingestion and chronic peptic ulcer. Gastroenterology 1981;80(3):427–32.

39. Petroski D. Endoscopic comparison of various aspirin preparations-gastric mucosal adaptability to aspirin restudied. Curr Ther Res 1989;45:945.

40. Szabo S. Pathogenesis of gastric mucosal injury. S Afr Med J 1988;74(Suppl):35.

41. Faulkner G, Prichard P, Somerville K, Langman MJ. Aspirin and bleeding peptic ulcers in the elderly. BMJ 1988;297(6659):1311–13.

42. Freeland GR, Northington RS, Hedrich DA, Walker BR. Hepatic safety of two analgesics used over the counter: ibuprofen and aspirin. Clin Pharmacol Ther 1988;43(5):473–9.

43. Hansson L, Zanchetti A, Carruthers SG, Dahlof B, Elmfeldt D, Julius S, Menard J, Rahn KH, Wedel H, Westerling S. Effects of intensive blood-pressure lowering and low-dose aspirin in patients with hypertension: principal results of the Hypertension Optimal Treatment (HOT) randomised trial. HOT Study Group. Lancet 1998;351(9118):1755–62.

44. Meade TW, Brennan PJ, Wilkes HC, Zuhrie SR. Thrombosis prevention trial: randomised trial of low-intensity oral anticoagulation with warfarin and low-dose aspirin in the primary prevention of ischaemic heart disease in men at increased risk. The Medical Research Council's General Practice Research Framework. Lancet 1998;351(9098):233–41.

45. Petty GW, Brown RD Jr, Whisnant JP, Sicks JD, O'Fallon WM, Wiebers DO. Frequency of major complications of aspirin, warfarin, and intravenous heparin for secondary stroke prevention. A population-based study. Ann Intern Med 1999;130(1):14–22.

46. Sorensen HT, Mellemkjaer L, Blot WJ, Nielsen GL, Steffensen FH, McLaughlin JK, Olsen JH. Risk of upper gastrointestinal bleeding associated with use of low-dose aspirin. Am J Gastroenterol 2000;95(9):2218–24.

47. Tramèr MR, Moore RA, Reynolds DJ, McQuay HJ. Quantitative estimation of rare adverse events which follow a biological progression: a new model applied to chronic NSAID use. Pain 2000;85(1–2):169–82.

48. Weil J, Langman MJ, Wainwright P, Lawson DH, Rawlins M, Logan RF, Brown TP, Vessey MP, Murphy M, Colin-Jones DG. Peptic ulcer bleeding: accessory risk factors and interactions with non-steroidal anti-inflammatory drugs. Gut 2000;46(1):27–31.

49. Tramèr MR. Aspirin, like all other drugs, is a poison. BMJ 2000;321(7270):1170–1.

50. Garcia Rodriguez LA, Hernandez-Diaz S, de Abajo FJ. Association between aspirin and upper gastrointestinal complications: systematic review of epidemiologic studies. Br J Clin Pharmacol 2001;52(5):563–71.

51. Bianchine JR, Procter RR, Thomas FB. Piroxicam, aspirin, and gastrointestinal blood loss. Clin Pharmacol Ther 1982;32(2):247–52.

52. Hass WK, Easton JD, Adams HP Jr, Pryse-Phillips W, Molony BA, Anderson S, Kamm B. A randomized trial comparing ticlopidine hydrochloride with aspirin for the prevention of stroke in high-risk patients. Ticlopidine Aspirin Stroke Study Group. N Engl J Med 1989;321(8):501–7.

53. Lanas A, Serrano P, Bajador E, Esteva F, Benito R, Sainz R. Evidence of aspirin use in both upper and lower gastrointestinal perforation. Gastroenterology 1997;112(3):683–9.

54. Bonavina L, DeMeester TR, McChesney L, Schwizer W, Albertucci M, Bailey RT. Drug-induced esophageal strictures. Ann Surg 1987;206(2):173–83.

55. Schreiber JB, Covington JA. Aspirin-induced esophageal hemorrhage. JAMA 1988;259(11):1647–8.

56. Barrier CH, Hirschowitz BI. Controversies in the detection and management of nonsteroidal antiinflammatory drug-induced side effects of the upper gastrointestinal tract. Arthritis Rheum 1989;32(7):926–32.

57. Suazo-Barahona J, Gallegos J, Carmona-Sanchez R, Martinez R, Robles-Diaz G. Nonsteroidal anti-inflammatory drugs and gastrocolic fistula. J Clin Gastroenterol 1998;26(4):343–5.

58. Gutnik SH, Willmott D, Ziebarth J. Gastrocolic fistula-secondary to aspirin abuse. S D J Med 1993;46(10):358–60.

59. Levine MS, Kelly MR, Laufer I, Rubesin SE, Herlinger H. Gastrocolic fistulas: the increasing role of aspirin. Radiology 1993;187(2):359–61.

60. Mielants H, Verbruggen G, Schelstraete K, Veys EM. Salicylate-induced gastrointestinal bleeding: comparison between soluble buffered, enteric-coated, and intravenous administration. J Rheumatol 1979;6(2):210–18.

61. Malfertheiner P, Stanescu A, Rogatti W, Ditschuneit H. Effects of microencapsulated vs. enteric-coated acetylsalicylic acid on gastric and duodenal mucosa: an endoscopic study. J Clin Gastroenterol 1988;10(3):269–72.

62. Singh G, Ramey DR, Morfeld D, Shi H, Hatoum HT, Fries JF. Gastrointestinal tract complications of nonsteroidal anti-inflammatory drug treatment in rheumatoid arthritis. A prospective observational cohort study. Arch Intern Med 1996;156(14):1530–6.

63. Ward MR. Reye's syndrome: an update. Nurse Pract 1997;22(12):45–6, 49–50, 52–3.

64. Food and Drug Administration, HHS. Labeling for oral and rectal over-the-couter drug products containing aspirin and nonaspirin salicylates; Reye's Syndrome warning. Final rule. Fed Regist 2003;68(74):18861–9.

65. Zimmerman HJ. Effects of aspirin and acetaminophen on the liver. Arch Intern Med 1981;141(3 Spec No):333–42.

66. Gitlin N. Salicylate hepatotoxicity: the potential role of hypoalbuminemia. J Clin Gastroenterol 1980;2(3):281–5.

67. Belay ED, Bresee JS, Holman RC, Khan AS, Shahriari A, Schonberger LB. Reye's syndrome in the United States from 1981 through 1997. N Engl J Med 1999;340(18):1377–82.

68. Langford NJ. Aspirin and Reye's syndrome: is the response appropriate? J Clin Pharm Ther 2002;27(3):157–60.

69. Plotz PH, Kimberly RP. Acute effects of aspirin and acetaminophen on renal function. Arch Intern Med 1981;141(3 Spec No):343–8.

70. Delzell E, Shapiro S. A review of epidemiologic studies of nonnarcotic analgesics and chronic renal disease. Medicine (Baltimore) 1998;77(2):102–21.

71. McLaughlin JK, Lipworth L, Chow WH, Blot WJ. Analgesic use and chronic renal failure: a critical review of the epidemiologic literature. Kidney Int 1998;54(3):679–86.

72. Rexrode KM, Buring JE, Glynn RJ, Stampfer MJ, Youngman LD, Gaziano JM. Analgesic use and renal function in men. JAMA 2001;286(3):315–21.

73. Fored CM, Ejerblad E, Lindblad P, Fryzek JP, Dickman PW, Signorello LB, Lipworth L, Elinder CG, Blot WJ, McLaughlin JK, Zack MM, Nyren O. Acetaminophen, aspirin, and chronic renal failure. N Engl J Med 2001;345(25):1801–8.

74. Kanwar AJ, Belhaj MS, Bharija SC, Mohammed M. Drugs causing fixed eruptions. J Dermatol 1984;11(4):383–5.

75. Brandt KD, Palmoski MJ. Effects of salicylates and other nonsteroidal anti-inflammatory drugs on articular cartilage. Am J Med 1984;77(1A):65–9.

76. Oates JA, FitzGerald GA, Branch RA, Jackson EK, Knapp HR, Roberts LJ 2nd. Clinical implications of prostaglandin and thromboxane A2 formation (1). N Engl J Med 1988;319(11):689–98.

77. Settipane RA, Constantine HP, Settipane GA. Aspirin intolerance and recurrent urticaria in normal adults and children. Epidemiology and review. Allergy 1980;35(2):149–54.

78. Farr RS, Spector SL, Wangaard CH. Evaluation of aspirin and tartrazine idiosyncrasy. J Allergy Clin Immunol 1979;64(6 pt 2):667–8.

79. Szczeklik A. The cyclooxygenase theory of aspirin-induced asthma. Eur Respir J 1990;3(5):588–93.

80. Szczeklik A. Aspirin-induced asthma: pathogenesis and clinical presentation. Allergy Proc 1992;13(4):163–73.

81. Sola Alberich R, Jammoul A, Masana L. Henoch-Schonlein purpura associated with acetylsalicylic acid. Ann Intern Med 1997;126(8):665.

82. Martelli NA. Bronchial and intravenous provocation tests with indomethacin in aspirin-sensitive asthmatics. Am Rev Respir Dis 1979;120(5):1073–9.

83. Ritter JM, Taylor GW. Fish oil in asthma. Thorax 1988;43(2):81–3.

84. Anonymous. Aspirin sensitivity in asthmatics. BMJ 1980;281(6246):958–9.

85. Pleskow WW, Stevenson DD, Mathison DA, Simon RA, Schatz M, Zeiger RS. Aspirin desensitization in aspirin-sensitive asthmatic patients: clinical manifestations and characterization of the refractory period. J Allergy Clin Immunol 1982;69(1 Pt 1):11–19.

86. Dubach UC, Rosner B, Pfister E. Epidemiologic study of abuse of analgesics containing phenacetin. Renal morbidity and mortality (1968-1979). N Engl J Med 1983;308(7):357–62.

87. Dubach UC, Rosner B, Sturmer T. An epidemiologic study of abuse of analgesic drugs. Effects of phenacetin and salicylate on mortality and cardiovascular morbidity (1968 to 1987). N Engl J Med 1991;324(3):155–60.

88. Gago-Dominguez M, Yuan JM, Castelao JE, Ross RK, Yu MC. Regular use of analgesics is a risk factor for renal cell carcinoma. Br J Cancer 1999;81(3):542–8.

89. Slone D, Siskind V, Heinonen OP, Monson RR, Kaufman DW, Shapiro S. Aspirin and congenital malformations. Lancet 1976;1(7974):1373–5.

90. Werler MM, Mitchell AA, Shapiro S. The relation of aspirin use during the first trimester of pregnancy to congenital cardiac defects. N Engl J Med 1989;321(24):1639–42.

91. Rumack CM, Guggenheim MA, Rumack BH, Peterson RG, Johnson ML, Braithwaite WR. Neonatal intracranial hemorrhage and maternal use of aspirin. Obstet Gynecol 1981;58(Suppl 5):S52–6.

92. Shapiro S, Siskind V, Monson RR, Heinonen OP, Kaufman DW, Slone D. Perinatal mortality and birth-weight in relation to aspirin taken during pregnancy. Lancet 1976;1(7974):1375–6.

93. Uzan S, Beaufils M, Breart G, Bazin B, Capitant C, Paris J. Prevention of fetal growth retardation with low-dose aspirin: findings of the EPREDA trial. Lancet 1991;337(8755):1427–31.

94. Anonymous. Poisoning with enteric-coated aspirin. Lancet 1981;2(8238):130.

95. Pierce RP, Gazewood J, Blake RL Jr. Salicylate poisoning from enteric-coated aspirin. Delayed absorption may complicate management. Postgrad Med 1991;89(5):61–4.

96. Temple AR. Acute and chronic effects of aspirin toxicity and their treatment. Arch Intern Med 1981;141(3 Spec No):364–9.

97. Meredith TJ, Vale JA. Non-narcotic analgesics. Problems of overdosage. Drugs 1986;32(Suppl 4):177–205.

98. Dove DJ, Jones T. Delayed coma associated with salicylate intoxication. J Pediatr 1982;100(3):493–6.

99. Deykin D, Janson P, McMahon L. Ethanol potentiation of aspirin-induced prolongation of the bleeding time. N Engl J Med 1982;306(14):852–4.

100. Anonymous. Alcohol warning on over-the-counter pain medications. WHO Drug Inf 1998;12:16.

101. Diener HC, Cunha L, Forbes C, Sivenius J, Smets P, Lowenthal A; European Stroke Prevention Study. 2. Dipyridamole and acetylsalicylic acid in the secondary prevention of stroke. J Neurol Sci 1996;143(1-2):1–13.

102. Enquete de prevention secondaire de l'infarctus du Myocarde' Research Group. A controlled comparison of aspirin and oral anticoagulants in prevention of death after myocardial infarction. N Engl J Med 1982; 307(12):701–8.

103. Moore TJ, Crantz FR, Hollenberg NK, Koletsky RJ, Leboff MS, Swartz SL, Levine L, Podolsky S, Dluhy RG, Williams GH. Contribution of prostaglandins to the antihypertensive action of captopril in essential hypertension. Hypertension 1981;3(2):168–73.

104. Cowan RA, Hartnell GG, Lowdell CP, Baird IM, Leak AM. Metabolic acidosis induced by carbonic anhydrase inhibitors and salicylates in patients with normal renal function. BMJ (Clin Res Ed) 1984;289(6441):347–8.

105. Brooks PM, Day RO. Nonsteroidal antiinflammatory drugs—differences and similarities. N Engl J Med 1991;324(24):1716–25.

106. McInnes GT, Brodie MJ. Drug interactions that matter. A critical reappraisal. Drugs 1988;36(1):83–110.

107. Levine MN, Raskob G, Landefeld S, Kearon C. Hemorrhagic complications of anticoagulant treatment. Chest 1998;114(Suppl 5):S511–23.

108. World Health Organization (WHO). Mechanism of action, safety and efficacy of intrauterine devices. In: Technical Report Series. Geneva: WHO, 1987;753:91.

109. Croxatto HB, Ortiz ME, Valdez E. IUD mechanisms of action. In: Bardin CW, Mishell DR, editors. Proceedings from the 4th International Conference on IUDs. Boston: Butterworth-Heinemann, 1994:44.

110. Offerhaus L. Drug interactions at excretory mechanisms. Pharmacol Ther 1981;15(1):69–78.

111. Lanas A, Bajador E, Serrano P, Arroyo M, Fuentes J, Santolaria S. Effects of nitrate and prophylactic aspirin on upper gastrointestinal bleeding: a retrospective case-control study. J Int Med Res 1998;26(3):120–8.

112. Orr JM, Abbott FS, Farrell K, Ferguson S, Sheppard I, Godolphin W. Interaction between valproic acid and aspirin in epileptic children: serum protein binding and metabolic effects. Clin Pharmacol Ther 1982;31(5):642–9.

113. Abbott FS, Kassam J, Orr JM, Farrell K. The effect of aspirin on valporic acid metabolism. Clin Pharmacol Ther 1986;40(1):94–100.

114. Multicentre Acute Stroke Trial—Italy (MAST-I) Group. Randomised controlled trial of streptokinase, aspirin, and combination of both in treatment of acute ischaemic stroke. Lancet 1995;346(8989):1509–14.

115. Ciccone A, Motto C, Aritzu E, Piana A, Candelise L. Negative interaction of aspirin and streptokinase in acute ischemic stroke: further analysis of the Multicenter Acute Stroke Trial—Italy. Cerebrovasc Dis 2000;10(1):61–4.

116. Akyol SM, Thompson M, Kerr DN. Renal function after prolonged consumption of aspirin. BMJ (Clin Res Ed) 1982;284(6316):631–2.

117. Harris M, Bryant LR, Danaher P, Alloway J. Effect of low dose daily aspirin on serum urate levels and urinary excretion in patients receiving probenecid for gouty arthritis. J Rheumatol 2000;27(12):2873–6.

118. Samuels MH, Pillote K, Ashex D, Nelson JC. Variable effects of nonsteroidal antiinflammatory agents on thyroid test results. J Clin Endocrinol Metab 2003;88(12): 5710–5716.

Aciclovir

General Information

Aciclovir is an acyclic purine nucleoside. Its antiviral activity depends upon intracellular phosphorylation to its triphosphate derivative. Because of its higher affinity for viral thymidine kinase, aciclovir is phosphorylated at a much higher rate by the viral enzyme. Thus, it is almost exclusively active in infected cells, fulfilling one of the selectivity principles of antiviral drugs. In addition, aciclovir triphosphate serves as a better substrate for viral than for host cell DNA polymerase and thereby causes preferential termination of viral DNA synthesis (1).

Aciclovir is active against *Herpes simplex* virus type 1 (HSV-1), HSV-2, *Varicella zoster* virus (VZV), *Herpesvirus simiae*, and to a lesser degree Epstein–Barr virus (EBV). Resistant strains of HSV can arise owing to the emergence of thymidine kinase-deficient mutants. Other forms of resistance patterns are less common (2,3).

Aciclovir is used topically or systemically, orally or intravenously. Its therapeutic potential is most impressive in active parenchymal or systemic HSV infections. The latency stage of the viral infection is not affected. Since the blood–brain barrier is well penetrated, aciclovir is the treatment of choice for HSV encephalitis.

Very few adverse effects, generally of minor importance, have been reported (4). In immunosuppressed patients abnormal liver function, encephalopathy, and myelosuppression have been observed; however, it is unclear at present whether these adverse effects are related to the drug itself or to the underlying disorder (5–7).

Comparative studies

The effects of aciclovir and valaciclovir for anogenital herpes have been studied in HIV-infected individuals in two controlled trials (8). In the first study, 1062 patients with CD4+ counts over 100×10^6/l received valaciclovir or aciclovir for 1 year and were assessed monthly. In the second study, 467 patients were treated episodically for at least 5 days with valaciclovir or aciclovir and were assessed daily. Valaciclovir was as effective as aciclovir for suppression and episodic treatment of herpesvirus infections. Hazard ratios for the time to recurrence with valaciclovir 500 mg bd and 1000 mg od compared with aciclovir were 0.73 (95% CI = 0.50, 1.06) and 1.31 (0.94, 1.82). Valaciclovir 1000 mg bd and aciclovir had similar effects on the duration of infective episodes (HR = 0.92; CI = 0.75, 1.14). The most common adverse events, which occurred at similar rates with all regimens, were diarrhea, headache, infections, rashes, nausea, rhinitis, pharyngitis, abdominal pain, fever, depression, and cough.

Organs and Systems

Nervous system

Neurotoxicity secondary to aciclovir is rare and is associated with high plasma concentrations (SEDA-18, 299), such as result from impaired renal function (9). Although the risk is greatest with intravenous administration, neurotoxicity has previously been noted with oral use.

Symptoms of neurotoxicity, which usually appear within the first 24–72 hours of administration, include tremor, myoclonus, confusion, lethargy, agitation, hallucinations, dysarthria, asterixis, ataxia, hemiparesthesia, and seizures. While aciclovir-induced neurotoxicity is most prevalent with intravenous administration, it has also been reported after oral use in patients with terminal renal insufficiency on hemodialysis.

Neurotoxicity possibly secondary to the topical use of aciclovir has also been described (10).

- A 59-year-old woman on hemodialysis was treated with oral aciclovir 200 mg/day for ophthalmic Herpes zoster. After a few days, an ophthalmic aciclovir cream was started (one application every 6 hours) because of ipsilateral *Herpes* keratitis. After 1 week of combined oral and topical treatment, she became confused, with dysarthria and audiovisual hallucinations. Aciclovir was withdrawn and hemodialysis was initiated. Complete resolution of symptoms was achieved after three hemodialysis sessions in 3 days. Aciclovir plasma concentrations before hemodialysis were high (45 μmol/l) and fell rapidly during hemodialysis.

There is no conclusive evidence for the contribution of the topically administered aciclovir to the high plasma concentrations and subsequent neurotoxicity in this case. However, the authors argued that the existence of high aciclovir plasma concentrations, in spite of careful adjustment of the oral dosage, pointed to significant topical absorption of the drug, especially since the absorption of aciclovir through the skin and mucous membranes may be unpredictable.

Coma has been attributed to oral aciclovir (11).

- A 73-year-old man with acute respiratory failure, presumed to be secondary to amiodarone toxicity, developed sepsis and acute renal insufficiency, and required intermittent hemodialysis. Following a *Herpes simplex* labialis infection he was treated with oral aciclovir (400 mg tds). The next day he became sleepy, disoriented, and agitated. Over the next 48 hours his neurological condition deteriorated and he responded to pain only, had uncoordinated eye movements, tremors, facial and jaw myoclonus, increased reflexes, and hypertonia. After 7 days of aciclovir he became unresponsive and comatose. Aciclovir was withdrawn and hemodialysis carried out more frequently. His neurological status improved over a period of 4 days. Trough plasma concentrations of aciclovir were well above the upper limit of the usual target range.

This appears to be the first case of coma attributable to oral aciclovir. The fact that the patient was receiving oral rather than intravenous aciclovir and was on regular hemodialysis made neurotoxicity unlikely, and this emphasizes the need to be wary of this potentially serious complication in seriously ill elderly patients.

Sensory systems

Local application of 3% ophthalmic ointment can cause mild transient stinging. Diffuse, superficial, punctate, non-progressive keratopathy can develop. This quickly resolves after withdrawal (12,13).

Psychological, psychiatric

One report described reversible psychiatric adverse effects in three dialysis patients receiving intravenous aciclovir (8–10 mg/kg/day) (14).

Hematologic

Neutropenia and thrombocytopenia occurred in an 8-year-old boy who was treated with aciclovir 200 mg bd for 5 months for "chronic cold sores" (15). After withdrawal of aciclovir, the absolute neutrophil and platelet counts normalized within days. There was no recurrence of oral herpes lesions during the ensuing month.

Urinary tract

Renal impairment has been associated with the use of intravenous aciclovir. Transient increases in serum creatinine and urea have been observed in 14% of patients treated with bolus injections (16). These are related to crystal formation in the lower renal tubules when the solubility of aciclovir in urine is exceeded. Slow (1-hour) intravenous infusion and adequate hydration are therefore mandatory. Bolus doses are to be avoided. Dosage modifications for patients with renal insufficiency are based on creatinine clearance (4).

- Crystalluria due to aciclovir occurred within 24 hours of the start of therapy with 500 mg 8-hourly in a 4-year-old African-American boy (17). Slow intravenous infusion over 1–2 hours and volume repletion avoids the problem.

Renal toxicity has not been described in infants treated with intravenous aciclovir, 5–10 mg/kg every 8 hours for 5–10 days (18) or in children receiving aciclovir 500 mg/m^2 intravenously (19) or orally (4).

Skin

Skin reactions to aciclovir are mostly mild and transitory, including pruritus, pain, rashes, contact dermatitis, and photoallergic contact dermatitis. However, serious reactions occasionally occur (20). Antiviral drugs that have been implicated include topical aciclovir, cidofovir, idoxuridine, imiquimod, lamivudine, penciclovir, podophyllin, podophyllotoxin, trifluridine, tromantadine, vidarabine, intralesional and ophthalmic solutions of interferon, intravitreal injections of fomivirsen and foscarnet, and intraocular implants of ganciclovir. Patch-testing in these cases only rarely caused positive reactions to the antiviral drug.

A case of possible aciclovir-induced Stevens–Johnson syndrome has been reported in an HIV-positive patient with mycobacterial disease (21). However, Stevens–Johnson syndrome is associated with *Herpes simplex* infection and can be prevented by aciclovir (22).

Immunologic

Although allergy to aciclovir is unusual, it can occur; in one case it resulted in a skin rash (23).

- A 38-year-old woman of African descent, with a history of atopy and mild asthma, developed a periumbilical, erythematous, maculopapular rash and generalized pruritus after starting aciclovir. The reaction resolved within a few days after withdrawal, recurred when famciclovir was used, and again resolved when famciclovir was withdrawn. She was successfully stabilized on suppressive therapy after a graded challenge with aciclovir four times a day for 5 days.

Cross-reactivity between aciclovir and famciclovir is unusual. Aciclovir desensitization may be a novel method of treating patients with aciclovir allergy.

Contact sensitization to aciclovir is rare, but frequent application to inflamed skin in relapsing *Herpes simplex* may increase the risk of allergy. Severe contact dermatitis in a teenager has been reported.

- A 16-year-old girl with an 11-year history of frequent cold sores developed an erythematous rash and severe contact dermatitis during oral and topical aciclovir therapy (24). Patch tests showed contact sensitization to aciclovir and to the related compound ganciclovir.
- In a 44-year-old woman who used topical aciclovir for genital herpes, aciclovir contact allergy was associated with a systemic contact allergic reaction with an erythematous vesiculobullous eruption in the labial and perioral skin and a rash on the upper trunk and extremities (25). Patch tests were positive to aciclovir, valaciclovir, and ganciclovir, but not to famciclovir.

Pre-existing vesicular edematous cheilitis (probably due to contact allergy to the protecting lip salve) was aggravated after application of Zovirax cream (26). Patch tests to the lip salve were positive, but in addition there were positive photopatch tests to Zovirax cream, but not to its separate constituents.

Second-Generation Effects

Pregnancy

Animal data suggest that aciclovir is probably safe in pregnancy. There are no reports of teratogenicity in humans, and a report of 312 pregnant women exposed to aciclovir showed no increase in the number of birth defects compared with the numbers expected in the general population (27). However, data from larger numbers of human pregnancies are not available to draw reliable conclusions about the safety of aciclovir in pregnancy.

Drug Administration

Drug administration route

Local necrosis and inflammation can occur due to extravasation of the drug at the site of injection (28).

Various local adverse effects of aciclovir eye-drops have been reported, including pruritus, burning sensations, and irritative or allergic conjunctivitis. Persistent superficial punctate keratitis, delayed epithelial healing, and epithelial dysplasia can develop (29).

References

1. Wagstaff AJ, Faulds D, Goa KL. Aciclovir. A reappraisal of its antiviral activity, pharmacokinetic properties and therapeutic efficacy. Drugs 1994;47(1):153–205.
2. Erlich KS, Mills J, Chatis P, Mertz GJ, Busch DF, Follansbee SE, Grant RM, Crumpacker CS. Acyclovir-resistant *Herpes simplex* virus infections in patients with the acquired immunodeficiency syndrome. N Engl J Med 1989;320(5):293–6.
3. Sacks SL, Wanklin RJ, Reece DE, Hicks KA, Tyler KL, Coen DM. Progressive esophagitis from acyclovir-resistant *Herpes simplex*. Clinical roles for DNA polymerase mutants and viral heterogeneity? Ann Intern Med 1989;111(11):893–9.
4. Drucker JL, Tucker WE, Szczech M Jr. Safety studies of acyclovir: preclinical and clinical. In: Baker DA, editor. Acyclovir Therapy for Herpesvirus Infections. New York: Marcel Dekker, 1990:15.
5. Wade JC, Meyers JD. Neurologic symptoms associated with parenteral acyclovir treatment after marrow transplantation. Ann Intern Med 1983;98(6):921–5.
6. Wade JC, Hintz M, McGuffin R, Springmeyer SC, Connor JD, Meyers JD. Treatment of cytomegalovirus pneumonia with high-dose acyclovir. Am J Med 1982;73(1A):249–56.
7. Straus SE, Smith HA, Brickman C, de Miranda P, McLaren C, Keeney RE. Acyclovir for chronic mucocutaneous *Herpes simplex* virus infection in immunosuppressed patients. Ann Intern Med 1982;96(3):270–7.
8. Conant MA, Schacker TW, Murphy RL, Gold J, Crutchfield LT, Crooks RJ, Acebes LO, Aiuti F, Akil B, Anderson J, Melville RL, Ballesteros Martin J, Berry A, Weiner M, Black F, Anderson PL, Bockman W, Borelli S, Bradbeer CS, Braffman M, Brandon W, Clark R, Wisniewski T, Bruun JN, Burdge D, Caputo RM, Chateauvert M, LaLonde R, Chiodo F, et al.; International Valaciclovir HSV Study Group. Valaciclovir versus aciclovir for *Herpes simplex* virus infection in HIV-infected individuals: two randomized trials. Int J STD AIDS 2002;13(1):12–21.
9. Ernst ME, Franey RJ. Acyclovir- and ganciclovir-induced neurotoxicity. Ann Pharmacother 1998;32(1):111–13.
10. Gomez Campdera FJ, Verde E, Vozmediano MC, Valderrabano F. More about acyclovir neurotoxicity in patients on haemodialysis. Nephron 1998;78(2):228–9.
11. Rajan GR, Cobb JP, Reiss CK. Acyclovir induced coma in the intensive care unit. Anaesth Intensive Care 2000;28(3):305–7.
12. McGill J, Tormey P. Use of acyclovir in herpetic ocular infection. Am J Med 1982;73(1A):286–9.
13. Richards DM, Carmine AA, Brogden RN, Heel RC, Speight TM, Avery GS. Acyclovir. A review of its pharmacodynamic properties and therapeutic efficacy. Drugs 1983;26(5):378–438.
14. Tomson CR, Goodship TH, Rodger RS. Psychiatric side-effects of acyclovir in patients with chronic renal failure. Lancet 1985;2(8451):385–6.
15. Grella M, Ofosu JR, Klein BL. Prolonged oral acyclovir administration associated with neutropenia and thrombocytopenia. Am J Emerg Med 1998;16(4):396–8.
16. Brigden D, Rosling AE, Woods NC. Renal function after acyclovir intravenous injection. Am J Med 1982;73(1A):182–5.
17. Blossom AP, Cleary JD, Daley WP. Acyclovir-induced crystalluria. Ann Pharmacother 2002;36(3):526.
18. Yeager AS. Use of acyclovir in premature and term neonates. Am J Med 1982;73(1A):205–9.
19. Blanshard C, Benhamou Y, Dohin E, Lernestedt JO, Gazzard BG, Katlama C. Treatment of AIDS-associated gastrointestinal cytomegalovirus infection with foscarnet and ganciclovir: a randomized comparison. J Infect Dis 1995;172(3):622–8.
20. Holdiness MR. Contact dermatitis from topical antiviral drugs. Contact Dermatitis 2001;44(5):265–9.
21. Fazal BA, Turett GS, Justman JE, Hall G, Telzak EE. Stevens–Johnson syndrome induced by treatment with acyclovir. Clin Infect Dis 1995;21(4):1038–9.
22. Cheriyan S, Patterson R. Recurrent Stevens–Johnson syndrome secondary to *Herpes simplex*: a follow up on a successful management program. Allergy Asthma Proc 1996;17(2):71–3.
23. Kawsar M, Parkin JM, Forster G. Graded challenge in an aciclovir allergic patient. Sex Transm Infect 2001;77(3):204–5.
24. Wollenberg A, Baldauf C, Rueff F, Przybilla B. Allergic contact dermatitis and exanthematous drug eruption following aciclovir-cross reaction with ganciclovir. Allergo J 2000;9:96–9.
25. Lammintausta K, Makela L, Kalimo K. Rapid systemic valaciclovir reaction subsequent to aciclovir contact allergy. Contact Dermatitis 2001;45(3):181.
26. Rodriguez WJ, Bui RH, Connor JD, Kim HW, Brandt CD, Parrott RH, Burch B, Mace J. Environmental exposure of primary care personnel to ribavirin aerosol when supervising treatment of infants with respiratory syncytial virus infections. Antimicrob Agents Chemother 1987;31(7):1143–6.
27. Andrews EB, Yankaskas BC, Cordero JF, Schoeffler K, Hampp S. Acyclovir in pregnancy registry: six years' experience. The Acyclovir in Pregnancy Registry Advisory Committee. Obstet Gynecol 1992;79(1):7–13.
28. Sylvester RK, Ogden WB, Draxler CA, Lewis FB. Vesicular eruption. A local complication of concentrated acyclovir infusions. JAMA 1986;255(3):385–6.
29. Ohashi Y. Treatment of herpetic keratitis with acyclovir: benefits and problems. Ophthalmologica 1997;211(Suppl 1):29–32.

Acipimox

General Information

Acipimox (*S*-methylpyrazine-2-carboxylic acid 4-oxide) is structurally related to nicotinic acid. There were flushing and gastrointestinal disturbances in 7137 patients, of whom 15% stopped taking the drug because of adverse effects; there were no adverse effects on blood glucose or uric acid (1). Of 32 patients with hypertriglyceridemia, excessive hypertriglyceridemia, and combined hyper-lipidemia, acipimox had to be withdrawn in 10 cases, because of adverse effects or absence of clinical response (2). The other 22 completed 6 months of treatment with no adverse effects. The authors claimed that acipimox is much better tolerated than nicotinic acid; it has fewer adverse effects and can therefore be used as a second-line drug.

Organs and Systems

Metabolism

In an open study, blood glucose was on average slightly lowered in 3009 type II diabetics given acipimox for at least 2 months (3).

References

1. Ganzer BM. Langzeitstudie zu acipimox. Pharmazie 1990;135:31.
2. Yeshurun D, Hamood H, Morad N, Naschitz J. [Acipimox (Olbetam) as a secondary hypolipemic agent in combined hypertriglyceridemia and hyperlipidemia.] Harefuah 2000;138(8):650–3, 710.
3. Lavezzari M, Milanesi G, Oggioni E, Pamparana F. Results of a phase IV study carried out with acipimox in type II diabetic patients with concomitant hyperlipoproteinaemia. J Int Med Res 1989;17(4):373–80.

Acivicin

See also Cytostatic and immunosuppressant drugs

General Information

Acivicin is a cytostatic antibiotic, a glutamine analogue, which is a potent inhibitor of l-asparagine synthetase and other l-glutamine amidotransferases and has its cytotoxic action by blocking nucleotide biosynthesis.

Besides myelotoxicity, acivicin is neurotoxic, and can cause lethargy and auditory and visual hallucinations. Some patients have nystagmus, incontinence, and severe depression (1,2).

References

1. Willson JK, Knuiman MW, Skeel RT, Wolter JM, Pandya KJ, Falkson G, Chang YC. Phase II clinical trial of acivicin in advanced breast cancer: an Eastern Cooperative Oncology Group Study. Cancer Treat Rep 1986;70(10):1237–8.
2. Booth BW, Korzun AH, Weiss RB, Ellison RR, Budman D, Khojasteh A, Wood W. Phase II trial of acivicin in advanced breast carcinoma: a Cancer and Leukemia Group B Study. Cancer Treat Rep 1986;70(10):1247–8.

Acoraceae

See also Herbal medicines

General Information

Acorus calamus was originally classified as a member of the arum family (Araceae), but is now designated as belonging to its own family, the Acoraceae, of which it is the only member.

Acorus calamus

Acorus calamus (calamus root, sweet flag, rat root, sweet sedge, flag root, sweet calomel, sweet myrtle, sweet cane, sweet rush, beewort, muskrat root, pine root) contains several active constituents called "asar-ones." The basic structure is 2,4,5-trimethoxy-1-propenyl-benzene, which is related to the hallucinogen 3,4-methylenedioxyphenylisopropylamine (MDA). The amounts of the asarones in calamus rhizomes vary considerably with the botanical variety. For example, there are high concentrations in triploid calamus from Eastern Europe but none detectable in the diploid North American variety.

Acorus calamus has been used as a hallucinogen since ancient times and it has several uses in folk medicine. It may have been one of the constituents of the Holy Oil that God commanded Moses to make (Exodus 30) and is mentioned by ancient writers on medicine, such as Hippocrates, Theophrastus, Dioscorides, and Celsus (http://www.a1b2c3.com/drugs/var002.htm). Walt Whitman's 39 "Calamus poems" are to be found in his well-known collection "Leaves of Grass."

Acorus calamus has in vitro antiproliferative and immunosuppressive actions (1).

Acorus calamus contains beta-asarone [(Z)-1,2,4-trimethoxy-5-prop-1-enyl-benzene], which is carcinogenic (2). Commercial calamus preparations have mutagenic effects in bacteria (3), while calamus oil (Jammu variety) is carcinogenic in rats.

References

1. Mehrotra S, Mishra KP, Maurya R, Srimal RC, Yadav VS, Pandey R, Singh VK. Anticellular and immunosuppressive properties of ethanolic extract of *Acorus calamus* rhizome. Int Immunopharmacol 2003;3(1):53–61.
2. Bertea CM, Azzolin CM, Bossi S, Doglia G, Maffei ME. Identification of an EcoRI restriction site for a rapid and precise determination of beta-asarone-free *Acorus calamus* cytotypes. Phytochemistry 2005;66(5):507–14.

3. Sivaswamy SN, Balachandran B, Balanehru S, Sivaramakrishnan VM. Mutagenic activity of south Indian food items. Indian J Exp Biol 1991;29(8):730–7.

Acrisorcin

See also Disinfectants and antiseptics

General Information

Acrisorcin (aminoacridine 4-hexylresorcinolate) has been used for induction of abortion in mid-trimester pregnancies. Abortion was produced when a 0.1% solution of acrisorcin was introduced into the extra-amniotic space in 23 women. All patients aborted after a mean induction-delivery interval of 59 hours (SEDA-11, 474) (1).

Reference

1. Lewis BV, Pybus A, Stilwell JH. The oxytocic effect of acridine dyes and their use in terminating mid-trimester pregnancies. J Obstet Gynaecol Br Commonw 1971;78(9):838–42.

Acrivastine

See also Antihistamines

General Information

Acrivastine is a second-generation antihistamine that has not been the subject of recent studies; earlier work was insufficient to substantiate statements that it was non-sedating.

Organs and Systems

Nervous system

Five of thirty-five patients taking acrivastine reported drowsiness compared with none in the placebo group (SEDA-14, 135). In another study acrivastine 8 mg did not impair nervous system function (SEDA-21, 172). The usual dose is 8 mg tds, which is effective in treating seasonal allergic rhinitis and has been stated to be without sedative effects (1). However, acrivastine does have a small but significant additive effect with alcohol at a dose of 8 mg (2).

References

1. Gibbs TG, Irander K, Salo OP. Acrivastine in seasonal allergic rhinitis: two randomized crossover studies to evaluate efficacy and safety. J Int Med Res 1988;16(6):413–19.
2. Cohen AF, Hamilton MJ, Peck AW. The effects of acrivastine (BW825C), diphenhydramine and terfenadine in combination with alcohol on human CNS performance. Eur J Clin Pharmacol 1987;32(3):279–88.

Acrylic bone cement

General Information

Local biocompatibility

Although polymerized polymethylmethacrylate is a biocompatible material, it is not biocompatible during the brief time it takes to set, during which it releases 130 calories/gram and can cause a rise in temperature up to 120°C. This temperature rise can be reduced by various techniques, although the thermal tolerance of the tissues affected is low (56°C and 72°C for coagulation of body proteins and bone collagen respectively). This is the main factor that is responsible for bone necrosis associated with acrylic bone cement. To avoid this, sucrose crystals have been added to acrylic cement. The mixture has a lower polymerization temperature and greater porosity, allowing for better ingrowth of bone into the cement pores (1); however, the resultant lower mechanical resistance limits its use (2,3). The same can be achieved by adding tricalcium phosphate, which lowers the reaction temperature. The non-polymerized monomer is cytotoxic (4), which can cause histopathological changes in soft tissues and bones.

Regional damage

Regional damage from methylmethacrylate is generally the result of poor surgical technique, whereby the cement inadvertently reaches other tissues and structures. For example, leaking methylmethacrylate cement during fixation of the acetabular cup in a total hip replacement can cause sciatic nerve compression and result in severe lasting leg pain (5).

Organs and Systems

Cardiovascular

Cardiovascular reactions to acrylic bone cement are a common complication in bone surgery. It is believed that cementation activates an adrenocortical response, increasing the blood pressure during general anesthesia (6,7); during spinal anesthesia this response is suppressed and the blood pressure falls. The mechanism is thought to be by a direct effect on the blood pressure through the kallikrein–kinin system, since aprotinin (Trasylol), an inhibitor of kallikrein, prevents the fall in arterial pressure if it is given during the application of acrylic bone cement (8).

Some investigators suggested that implantation of acrylic bone cement into the femur increases plasma histamine, which, especially in elderly patients with pre-existing cardiac diseases and/or hypovolemia, can cause serious, sometimes fatal, cardiovascular complications (9).

Respiratory

Since adverse effects in humans develop within 2–5 minutes of fixation, with features of pulmonary insufficiency, direct pulmonary damage has been postulated, with the cardiovascular effects being a consequence of hypoxemia (10–12). This has been demonstrated by lactase dehydrogenase isomer determinations, fractions 3 and 4 being significantly raised. These isozymes are released as a result of pulmonary mitochondrial injury caused by hypoxia. Methylmethacrylate monomer vapour can irritate the respiratory tract, eyes, and skin.

Immunologic

Methylmethacrylate is essentially an immunologically inert implant material, but it induces an inflammatory mononuclear cell migration (13,14). Both cemented and cementless prostheses cause a foreign-body-type host response. A new connective tissue capsule is formed around the artificial joint, which is coarser than normal. The reaction is partly granulomatous, with a tendency to necrosis and loosening of the prosthesis. After an initial necrotic phase of 2–3 weeks repair follows, leading to stabilization within 2 years.

Sensitization can occur in patients, surgeons, and dentists and is occasionally reported (15). As most surgical gloves do not provide a reliable barrier, additional gloves are recommended. Contact dermatitis, dizziness, and nausea and vomiting occur. Ethylene oxide present in acrylic bone cement can cause acute allergic reactions in sensitized patients (16).

Infection risk

Addition of materials (for example antimicrobial drugs or radio-opaque contrast materials) to acrylic bone cement can cause mechanical weakness due to loss of homogeneity and greater water resorption. Antimicrobial drugs have been added to combat the problem of microbial adherence. However, this can lead to a considerable dead biofilm mass on the polymethylmethacrylate surface, promoting late infections by providing a surface attractive to other strains of bacteria (17).

References

1. Rijke AM, Rieger MR, McLaughlin RE, McCoy S. Porous acrylic cement. J Biomed Mater Res 1977;11(3):373–94.
2. Feith R. Arcrylic cement. Ned Tijdschr Geneeskd 1978;122:64.
3. Rijke AM. Bijwerkingen van methylmethacrylaat-botcement. [Side effects of methylmethacrylate bone cement.] Ned Tijdschr Geneeskd 1980;124(6):180–3.
4. Fediukovich LV, Egorova AB. Genotoksicheskii effekt akrilatov. [Genotoxic effect of acrylates.] Gig Sanit 1991;(12):62–4.
5. Oleksak M, Edge AJ. Compression of the sciatic nerve by methylmethacrylate cement after total hip replacement. J Bone Joint Surg Br 1992;74(5):729–30.
6. Svartling N, Lehtinen AM, Tarkkanen L. The effect of anaesthesia on changes in blood pressure and plasma cortisol levels induced by cementation with methylmethacrylate. Acta Anaesthesiol Scand 1986;30(3):247–52.
7. Esemenli BT, Toker K, Lawrence R. Hypotension associated with methylmethacrylate in partial hip arthroplasties. The role of femoral canal size. Orthop Rev 1991;20(7):619–23.
8. Arac SS, Ercan ZS, Turker RK. Prevention by aprotinin of the hypotension due to acrylic cement implantation into the bone. Curr Ther Res 1980;28:554.
9. Tryba M, Linde I, Voshage G, Zenz M. Histaminfreisetzung und kardiovaskulare Reaktionen nach Implantation von Knochenzement bei totalem Huftgelenkersatz. [Histamine release and cardiovascular reactions to implantation of bone cement during total hip replacement.] Anaesthesist 1991;40(1):25–32.
10. Saint-Maurice C, Migne J, Maurin JP, Vedrine Y, Raud J, Lamas JP. Accidents consécutifs au scellement des prothéses articulaires. [Complications following cementing of joint prosthesis.] Ann Anesthesiol Fr 1977;18(7-8):647–54.
11. Shirai K. [Untoward effect of monomeric methylmethacrylate cement on the respiratory system during surgery.] Masui 1975;24(9):886–90.
12. Pickering CA, Bainbridge D, Birtwistle IH, Griffiths DL. Occupational asthma due to methyl methacrylate in an orthopaedic theatre sister. BMJ (Clin Res Ed) 1986;292(6532):1362–3.
13. Santavirta S, Konttinen YT, Bergroth V, Gronblad M. Lack of immune response to methyl methacrylate in lymphocyte cultures. Acta Orthop Scand 1991;62(1):29–32.
14. Santavirta S, Gristina A, Konttinen YT. Cemented versus cementless hip arthroplasty. A review of prosthetic biocompatibility. Acta Orthop Scand 1992;63(2):225–32.
15. Donaghy M, Rushworth G, Jacobs JM. Generalized peripheral neuropathy in a dental technician exposed to methyl methacrylate monomer. Neurology 1991;41(7):1112–16.
16. Rumpf KW, Rieger J, Jansen J, Scherer M, Seubert S, Seubert A, Sellin HJ. Quincke's edema in a dialysis patient after administration of acrylic bone cement: possible role of ethylene oxide allergy. Arch Orthop Trauma Surg 1986;105(4):250–2.
17. Chang CC, Merritt K. Microbial adherence on poly(methyl methacrylate) (PMMA) surfaces. J Biomed Mater Res 1992;26(2):197–207.

Activated charcoal

General Information

Activated charcoal is a standard therapy for gut decontamination after self-poisoning. It has two uses. If given within an hour or two after acute self-poisoning it can adsorb the drug and prevent it from being absorbed; in this case a single dose of activated charcoal 50 g is sufficient. However, some drugs are secreted into the gut after absorption and can be adsorbed by charcoal, preventing re-absorption; in this case repeated doses of activated charcoal 50 g 6-hourly can be used.

In a randomized study in 401 patients who had taken an overdose of oleander seeds, which contain cardiac glycosides, activated charcoal 50 g every 6 hours for 3 days was compared with sterile water. There were fewer deaths in the treatment group, 2.5% versus 8% (1). There were no important adverse effects.

Organs and Systems

Respiratory

Pulmonary aspiration is an ever-present risk of using charcoal, especially in semi-conscious patients (2). Povidone, which is used as a suspending agent of charcoal, can cause pneumonitis, which can lead to respiratory failure and death.

Electrolyte balance

Hyponatremic dehydration has been described when charcoal was combined with sorbitol to treat theophylline overdose in a child (SED-12, 951) (3).

Gastrointestinal

- Esophageal laceration with charcoal mediastinum has been reported in a 19-year-old woman who underwent multiple attempts at orogastric lavage with isotonic saline followed by 50 g of activated charcoal and sorbitol via the orogastric tube for a drug overdose (4). She recovered after surgical intervention.

Two formulations of activated charcoal 50 g (Carbomix, made into a slurry with 400 ml of tap water, and Actidose-Aqua, which came as a 240 ml suspension) have been compared in a prospective, randomized, single-blind study in 97 patients (5). The mean total dose of Carbomix (26.5 g) was significantly higher than the mean total dose of Actidose-Aqua (19.5 g); the reasons for this difference were not stated. The rates of vomiting did not differ between patients who received Carbomix (6%) or Actidose-Aqua (8%), and were low compared with previous reports (13%).

Though usually innocuous, activated charcoal can in large or multiple doses, such as may be needed in severe poisoning, cause intestinal obstruction (3,6). Pseudo-obstruction can also occur if drugs that inhibit intestinal motility are given at the same time, and sometimes it is not clear which process has occurred (SED-12, 951) (SEDA-17, 426) (6).

References

1. de Silva HA, Fonseka MM, Pathmeswaran A, Alahakone DG, Ratnatilake GA, Gunatilake SB, Ranasinha CD, Lalloo DG, Aronson JK, de Silva HJ. Multiple-dose activated charcoal for treatment of yellow oleander poisoning: a single-blind, randomised, placebo-controlled trial. Lancet 2003;361(9373):1935-8.
2. Menzies DG, Busuttil A, Prescott LF. Fatal pulmonary aspiration of oral activated charcoal. BMJ 1988;297(6646): 459-60.
3. Watson WA, Cremer KF, Chapman JA. Gastrointestinal obstruction associated with multiple-dose activated charcoal. J Emerg Med 1986;4(5):401-7.
4. Caravati EM, Knight HH, Linscott MS Jr, Stringham JC. Esophageal laceration and charcoal mediastinum complicating gastric lavage. J Emerg Med 2001;20(3):273-6.
5. Boyd R, Hanson J. Prospective single blinded randomised controlled trial of two orally administered activated charcoal preparations. J Accid Emerg Med 1999;16(1):24-5.
6. Atkinson SW, Young Y, Trotter GA. Treatment with activated charcoal complicated by gastrointestinal obstruction requiring surgery. BMJ 1992;305(6853):563.

Adefovir

General Information

Adefovir is an adenine analogue reverse transcriptase inhibitor. While it has activity against both HIV and hepatitis B, its use in HIV infection is limited by nephrotoxicity due to the high doses needed (1). The dose used for treatment of hepatitis B is about one-tenth that needed to treat HIV infection, so patients with hepatitis B must have co-infection with HIV ruled out before treatment is started.

Organs and Systems

Liver

In 35 patients co-infected with hepatitis B virus and HIV given adefovir 10 mg/day plus lamivudine 150 mg bd as part of treatment for hepatitis B and followed for 48 weeks, common adverse effects included raised transaminases, particularly alanine transaminase, increased serum creatinine, and increased blood glucose (2). Concerns about the study include the small number of patients and the lack of a comparison group.

Urinary tract

Adefovir is nephrotoxic, particularly at high doses, and the possible mechanism has been investigated in a 39-year-old man, who had severe acute tubular degenerative changes mainly affecting the proximal tubule; the mitochondria were significantly enlarged, possibly as a result of depletion of mitochondrial DNA (3).

References

1. Danta M, Dusheiko G. Adefovir dipivoxil: review of a novel acyclic nucleoside analogue. Int J Clin Pract 2004;58(9): 877-86.
2. Benhamou Y, Bochet M, Thibault V, Calvez V, Fievet MH, Vig P, Gibbs CS, Brosgart C, Fry J, Namini H, Katlama C, Poynard T. Safety and efficacy of adefovir dipivoxil in patients co-infected with HIV-1 and lamivudine-resistant hepatitis B virus: an open-label pilot study. Lancet 2001;358(9283):718-23.
3. Tanji N, Tanji K, Kambham N, Markowitz GS, Bell A, D'agati VD. Adefovir nephrotoxicity: possible role of mitochondrial DNA depletion. Hum Pathol 2001;32(7):734-40.

Ademetionine

General Information

Ademetionine (S-adenosylmethionine) has anti-inflammatory and analgesic effects in animals. Convincing evidence of these effects in man is still lacking. In trials in osteoarthritis, as presented at a symposium organized by the manufacturers (and thus open to selection bias), ademetionine was well tolerated

(1). In a large, uncontrolled, short-term Phase IV trial, adverse effects (moderate or severe) were reported by 21% of the patients, with withdrawal in 5.2%. Adverse effects were mainly gastrointestinal (nausea, stomach-ache, heartburn, diarrhea), CNS symptoms (headache, dizziness, sleep disturbances, fatigue), and skin rashes.

Reference

1. di Padova C. S-adenosylmethionine in the treatment of osteoarthritis. Review of the clinical studies. Am J Med 1987;83(5A):60–5.

Adenosine and adenosine triphosphate (ATP)

See also Antidysrhythmic drugs

General Information

Adenosine and adenosine triphosphate (ATP), its phosphorylated derivative, have been used to treat acute paroxysmal supraventricular tachycardias and adenosine has also been used in the diagnosis of narrow-and broad-complex tachycardias (SEDA-16, 176).

Several reviews of the clinical pharmacology, actions, therapeutic uses, and adverse reactions and interactions of adenosine and ATP have appeared (1–4). After intravenous administration adenosine enters cells, disappearing from the blood with a half-life of less than 10 seconds; intracellularly it is phosphorylated to cyclic AMP. Its mechanism of action as an antidysrhythmic drug is not known, but it may act by an effect at adenosine receptors on the cell membrane. Its electrophysiological effects are to prolong AV nodal conduction time by prolonging the AH interval, without an effect on the HV interval. The pharmacological and adverse effects of adenosine triphosphate are similar to those of adenosine.

Although adenosine and ATP very commonly cause adverse effects, they are generally mild and usually transient, because adenosine is rapidly eliminated from the blood (with a half-life of less than 10 seconds). Adverse effects have been reported in 81% of patients given adenosine and 94% of patients given ATP (5). Exercise reduces the non-cardiac adverse effects and the incidence of major dysrhythmias (6). Reducing the duration of adenosine infusion from 6 to 4 minutes reduced the incidence of chest discomfort and ischemic ST segment changes, but had no impact on non-cardiac effects (7).

Several studies have reported the efficacy and safety of adenosine and ATP in the treatment of tachycardias in children (8–11).

In 18 children with aortic valve disease or Kawasaki disease, adenosine stress myocardial perfusion imaging was associated with the usual adverse effects, most commonly flushing and dyspnea (12).

Exercise reduces both non-cardiac adverse effects and dysrhythmias in patients who are given adenosine for diagnostic purposes in myocardial perfusion imaging (SEDA-21, 197). This has been confirmed in two studies. In the first of these, 793 patients were given an intravenous infusion of adenosine 140 micrograms/kg/minute while exercising for 6 minutes or for a similar time without exercise (13). The rate of hypotension and dysrhythmias was significantly less in those who exercised (14 of 507) than in those who did not exercise (16 of 286). Overall reactions were more common in women than in men (5.7 versus 1.8%). All the adverse effects were transient and no specific therapy was required. The authors attributed the difference to the increase in sympathetic tone during exercise, which would have partly counteracted the hypotension and the negative chronotropic and negative dromotropic effects of adenosine. However, there was a major difference between the two groups, in that those who did not take exercise were considered unfit for exercise, which may have been associated with an increased risk of adverse effects. Nevertheless, the authors discarded that possibility, because the frequency of adverse reactions in those who did not take exercise was similar to frequencies that have previously been reported.

In the second study 19 patients received an intravenous infusion of adenosine 140 micrograms/kg/minute for 4 minutes during exercise or for 6 minutes without exercise; the patients undertook both protocols (14). Again, there were fewer adverse effects in those who took exercise, but only hypotension, chest pain, and headache were significantly different; there was a reduction in the frequency of flushing, which was almost significant. In addition, adverse effects were experienced for longer and the severity was greater in those who did not take exercise.

Organs and Systems

Cardiovascular

The most common cardiac effects are atrioventricular block, sinus bradycardia, and ventricular extra beats. Occasionally serious dysrhythmias occur (SEDA-17, 219), including ventricular fibrillation (15). ATP can cause transient atrial fibrillation (16). Chest pain occurs in 30–50% of patients and dyspnea and chest discomfort in 35–55%. Chest pain can occur in patients with and without coronary artery disease, and the symptoms are not always typical of cardiac pain.

Myocardial ischemia
Adenosine can cause cardiac ischemia by activating adenosine A1 receptors in the heart. However, in a double-blind, placebo-controlled, crossover study in eight healthy volunteers, adenosine 100 μg/kg/minute did not alter ischemic pain in an exercising arm (17). Otherwise, the usual adverse effects were noted, including facial flushing and mild chest tightness.

Hypotension
When adenosine (70 micrograms/kg/minute) was given by intravenous infusion to 45 patients with acute myocardial infarction preceding balloon angioplasty, one patient developed persisting hypotension in conjunction with a large inferolateral myocardial infarction (18). Transient hypotension in three other patients resolved with a reduction in dosage. There were no cases of atrioventricular block.

Symptomatic hypotension has occasionally been reported in patients with myocardial infarction who have been given adenosine (SEDA-20, 174).

An infusion of adenosine, 25 micrograms/kg, in 15 women undergoing anesthesia for major gynecological procedures was effective in maintaining hemodynamic stability during operation in addition to conventional anesthesia (19). It caused a significantly greater fall in systolic blood pressure and increase in heart rate than remifentanil in a comparable group. In four cases ephedrine was required for hypotension that was refractory to intravenous fluids or a temporary reduction in the infusion rate of adenosine. Two patients also required atropine for prolonged bradycardia.

Cardiac dysrhythmias

In patients with ischemic heart disease adenosine can prolong the QT_c interval and can increase the frequency of ventricular extra beats when there is myocardial scarring. It also causes increased release of catecholamines, and this may be the mechanism whereby it causes dysrhythmias in susceptible patients. If a dysrhythmia occurs, theophylline or one of its derivatives may be beneficial (20).

Of 100 patients who received intravenous adenosine in hospital (mean dose 7.8 mg) two had a dysrhythmia other than that for which they were being treated (21).

- A 53-year-old man with a dilated cardiomyopathy was given adenosine 6 mg for a regular broad-complex tachycardia; the dysrhythmia resolved but was followed by prolonged asystole and cyanosis for about 15 seconds.
- A 64-year-old woman with atrial fibrillation was given adenosine 12 mg; she developed a non-sustained polymorphous ventricular tachycardia followed by sustained ventricular fibrillation requiring DC shock.

In the whole series, about 40% of the patients received adenosine unnecessarily, having atrial fibrillation or atrial flutter, and the authors suggested that misuse of this sort resulted in unnecessary expense and increased risks of adverse effects. Most of this misuse was attributed to misdiagnosis by house officers who thought that rapid atrial fibrillation was a paroxysmal supraventricular tachycardia. Very few thought that adenosine would be likely to terminate atrial fibrillation.

Adenosine is contraindicated in patients with aberrant conduction pathways, because it can cause cardiac dysrhythmias. Supraventricular dysrhythmias occurred in three children with Wolff–Parkinson–White syndrome who were given intravenous adenosine (22).

There have been reports of cardiac dysrhythmias in patients given either an intravenous infusion of adenosine or a single bolus dose.

- A 38-year-old man was given intravenous adenosine 6 mg for a narrow-complex tachycardia (20). Within about 1 minute his heart rate fell from 230/minute to bradycardia and then asystole. Cardiopulmonary resuscitation was ineffective. At autopsy there was a 75% occlusion of one of the coronary arteries (unspecified).

The cause of the dysrhythmia in response to adenosine was not clear. He was not known to be taking other drugs

(for example dipyridamole) that might have potentiated the action of adenosine.

- A 56-year-old man was given adenosine 12 mg for a narrow-complex tachycardia on four occasions, and on each occasion developed transient atrial fibrillation for a few minutes thereafter. He had a concealed left-sided accessory pathway, which was successfully ablated (23).
- An 86-year-old woman was given adenosine 12 mg intravenously for sustained supraventricular tachycardia, which terminated but was followed by atrial fibrillation and paroxysmal ventricular tachycardia (24). Cardioversion was unsuccessful, but normal sinus rhythm was obtained with procainamide. This followed an anteroseptal myocardial infarction.
- A 75-year-old man who had had coronary bypass surgery was given an intravenous infusion of adenosine for stress testing (25). After 1 minute he developed a three-beat run of wide-complex tachycardia, followed by a 20-second run of a regular wide-complex tachycardia at a rate of 115/minute. There was left bundle branch block, and the tachycardia ended spontaneously. Adenosine infusion was continued and some ventricular extra beats with the same configuration occurred. In this case there was impaired perfusion of the left ventricle.
- In a 60-year-old woman with atrial flutter with 2:1 block and a ventricular rate of 130/minute, the ventricular rate increased paradoxically to 260/minute with 1:1 conduction after intravenous administration of adenosine 6 mg; it responded to intravenous amiodarone 300 mg (26).
- A 52-year-old woman with a wide-complex tachycardia was given adenosine 6, 12, and another 12 mg as intravenous bolus doses; immediately after the third dose she developed ventricular fibrillation (27). She recovered with cardioversion.

In the last case the authors did not discuss the possibility that the presence of digoxin (serum concentration 1.8 ng/ml) may have contributed; the risk of cardiac dysrhythmias after electrical cardioversion is increased in the presence of digoxin (SEDA-8, 174), and the same might be true of chemical cardioversion.

In a prospective study of 187 episodes of tachycardia in 127 unselected patients adenosine was given in an average dose of 9.7 mg (28). In 108 cases, adenosine induced transient ventricular extra beats or non-sustained ventricular tachycardia after successful termination of supraventricular tachycardia; more than half had a right bundle branch block morphology that suggested that the dysrhythmias had originated from the inferior left ventricular septum.

Heart block

The frequency of atrioventricular block has been studied in 600 patients who underwent stress testing with intravenous adenosine 140 micrograms/kg/minute for 6 minutes (29). The patients were young (under 49 years old; $n = 75$), middle-aged (50–65 years; $n = 214$), old (66–75 years; $n = 195$), or very old (over 75 years; $n = 116$). The respective frequencies of first-degree atrioventricular block were 15, 9.3, 14, and 17% (overall

Table 1 The incidence of atrioventricular block with adenosine

Type of block	Baseline PR interval over 200 ms ($n = 43$)	Baseline PR interval under 200 ms ($n = 557$)
Further prolongation of PR interval	49%	10%
Second-degree block	37%	8%
Third-degree block	14%	1%

average 13%), of second-degree block 15, 7.0, 8.7, and 16% (overall average 10%), and of third-degree block 2.7, 2.3, 1.0, and 2.6% (overall average 2.0%). The differences with age were not statistically significant. All types of atrioventricular block were of short duration, were well tolerated, and did not require withdrawal of adenosine or specific treatment.

In four out of nine patients with heart transplants second-degree or third-degree atrioventricular block occurred during the administration of adenosine 140 micrograms/kg/minute over 6 minutes (30). In two patients the infusion had to be interrupted because of severe discomfort and chest pain.

The incidence of atrioventricular block has been reported in 600 consecutive patients who underwent stress myocardial perfusion imaging with adenosine (140 micrograms/kg/minute for 6 minutes), and of whom 43 had first-degree heart block before adenosine and 557 had a baseline PR interval less than 200 ms (Table 1) (31). The heart block in all cases was of short duration, was not associated with any specific symptoms, and in no case required specific treatment. The risk of atrioventricular block during adenosine infusion was not increased by the presence of other drugs that might have caused atrioventricular block (digitalis, beta-blockers, diltiazem, verapamil).

Respiratory

Adenosine can cause bronchoconstriction with asthma (32), and a history of bronchoconstriction is a contraindication to intravenous adenosine.

In 94 patients with chronic obstructive pulmonary disease who were given adenosine in an initial dosage of 50 micrograms/kg/minute, increasing to 140 micrograms/kg/minute if adverse effects did not occur, there was only a slight and insignificant fall in FEV_1 at the highest dose of adenosine (33). However, four patients had a fall in FEV_1 of 20% or more, although without shortness of breath or evidence of bronchospasm; in these the dosage of adenosine was reduced to 100 micrograms/kg/minute. Two other patients had shortness of breath with no fall in FEV_1 or bronchospasm, and the dosage was reduced to 100 micrograms/kg/minute. There was no difference in the fall in FEV_1 between patients who had a history of asthma and those who did not. Other adverse effects included light-headedness ($n = 26$), dyspnea ($n = 17$), headache ($n = 14$), flushing ($n = 8$), hypotension ($n = 7$), chest pain ($n = 6$), and nausea ($n = 2$). In a subsequent study in 117 patients, two had symptomatic bronchospasm during adenosine infusion. In two other patients in whom bronchospasm was present before

treatment, bronchospasm did not develop when adenosine was infused at the highest dosage.

In another study, 63 of 122 patients had breathlessness during cardiac stress testing with adenosine but none had associated bronchospasm (34). Pre-test lung function did not predict the risk of breathlessness and neither chronic obstructive airways disease nor smoking increased the risk. The authors concluded that breathlessness during adenosine stress testing is not due to bronchospasm.

Nervous system

Adenosine has been used intrathecally to treat pain, but can itself cause backache (SEDA-23, 197) (35). In a placebo-controlled study in 40 healthy volunteers, who were given intrathecal adenosine 2 mg in 2 ml of saline, 13 had a mild headache, nine had mild to moderate backache, and one had mild aching in the thigh, compared with none of those who were given saline alone (36). No headaches or leg aches occurred later than 6 hours after the injection, but the backaches occurred at 6–24 hours; there were no later symptoms.

In a randomized, double-blind study of two doses of intrathecal adenosine in 35 volunteers with experimental hypersensitivity induced by capsaicin, intrathecal adenosine 0.5 or 2 mg in 2 ml of saline, but not saline alone, equally reduced areas of allodynia and hyperalgesia from capsaicin (37). There were adverse effects in 1, 2, and 6 of the volunteers who received saline, 0.5 mg, and 2.0 mg of adenosine respectively. The adverse effects were headache, backache, and leg or groin ache. Intravenous aminophylline 5 mg/kg, given 2 hours after the adenosine, did not reverse the effects of adenosine.

Of 12 healthy volunteers given an intrathecal injection of adenosine (500–2000 micrograms) one volunteer had transient lumbar pain lasting 30 minutes after an injection of 2000 micrograms (38). There were no adverse effects at lower doses.

Adenosine can cause increased intracranial pressure (39).

Gastrointestinal

Adenosine can cause transient epigastric pain mimicking that of peptic ulceration (40).

Immunologic

- An anaphylactic reaction has been reported in a 75-year-old woman who was given adenosine 12 mg for a supraventricular tachycardia. She developed bronchospasm and profound inspiratory stridor, her arterial blood pressure fell to 50/30 mmHg from an arterial systolic pressure of 70 mmHg, and she recovered with appropriate treatment (41).

Death

Two cases of sudden death have been reported soon after the administration of adenosine for presumed supraventricular tachycardia, which turned out to be atrial fibrillation (42). The authors thought that both patients may have been unable to cope with the sudden momentary loss of cardiac function that would have occurred immediately after the administration of adenosine; in one case, a patient with chronic lung disease, bronchospasm may have contributed.

Drug Administration

Drug administration route

The standard regimen for stress testing with intravenous adenosine is 140 micrograms/kg/minute for 6 minutes. However, in 599 patients a 3-minute infusion was associated with a lower frequency of some adverse effects (specifically flushing, headache, neck pain, and atrioventricular block) and had similar sensitivity in the diagnosis of coronary artery disease (43).

Intracoronary adenosine has been compared with intravenous adenosine for the measure of fractional flow reserve in 52 patients with coronary artery lesions (44). The intravenous dose was 140 micrograms/kg/minute and the intracoronary bolus dose was 15–20 micrograms to the right coronary artery and 18–24 micrograms to the left coronary artery. The two routes of administration were equally effective in measuring hyperemic flow, and adverse effects were limited to two patients who received intravenous adenosine; one patient had severe nausea and one patient with asthma had an episode of bronchospasm.

The use of intrathecal adenosine in patients with chronic neuropathic pain (35,45) has been briefly reviewed (46).

Drug–Drug Interactions

General

Adenosine does not interact with digoxin, disopyramide, flecainide, or quinidine.

Ciclosporin

Endogenous plasma adenosine concentrations were measured in 14 kidney transplant recipients taking ciclosporin and compared with five transplant recipients not taking ciclosporin, two taking sirolimus (FK506), six patients with chronic renal insufficiency, and ten controls (47). Plasma adenosine concentrations were significantly higher in those taking ciclosporin and sirolimus and in the patients taking ciclosporin the plasma adenosine concentrations correlated with serum ciclosporin concentrations. An in vitro study showed that ciclosporin inhibited the uptake of adenosine by erythrocytes. The authors concluded that since adenosine is immunosuppressant, the raised concentrations of adenosine in patients taking ciclosporin might contribute to the immunosuppressive action of ciclosporin. A further mechanism of the increase in adenosine concentration was possibly increased tissue release secondary to ciclosporin-induced vasoconstriction. The relevance of these results to the use of therapeutic intravenous adenosine in patients already taking ciclosporin is not clear.

Dipyridamole

Dipyridamole inhibits the uptake of adenosine by cells and so increases its effects; this causes a large reduction in the effective dose of adenosine (48).

Sirolimus

In two kidney transplant recipients taking sirolimus (FK506), plasma adenosine concentrations were significantly increased (47). The relevance of these results to the use of therapeutic intravenous adenosine in patients already taking sirolimus is not clear.

Xanthines

Antagonists at adenosine receptors should inhibit the action of adenosine, and indeed theophylline increases the dose of adenosine needed for conversion of supraventricular tachycardia (49).

Diagnosis of Adverse Drug Reactions

In 34 patients given midazolam or placebo in a double-blind study, midazolam significantly reduced patients' experiences of palpitation and chest pain but had no effects on other adverse events (50). These effects were probably due to amnesia rather than a true reduction in the incidence of adverse events, and it is uncertain that the benefit to harm ratio is worth while. However, the authors suggested that midazolam might be useful in patients who have previously had unpleasant adverse reactions to adenosine.

References

1. Camm AJ, Garratt CJ. Adenosine and supraventricular tachycardia. N Engl J Med 1991;325(23):1621–9.
2. Harper KJ. Adenosine in the acute treatment of PSVT. Drug Ther 1992;March:53–72.
3. Rankin AC, Brooks R, Ruskin JN, McGovern BA. Adenosine and the treatment of supraventricular tachycardia. Am J Med 1992;92(6):655–64.
4. Hori M, Kitakaze M. Adenosine, the heart, and coronary circulation. Hypertension 1991;18(5):565–74.
5. Rankin AC, Oldroyd KG, Chong E, Dow JW, Rae AP, Cobbe SM. Adenosine or adenosine triphosphate for supraventricular tachycardias? Comparative double-blind randomized study in patients with spontaneous or inducible arrhythmias. Am Heart J 1990;119(2 Pt 1):316–23.
6. Pennell DJ, Mavrogeni SI, Forbat SM, Karwatowski SP, Underwood SR. Adenosine combined with dynamic exercise for myocardial perfusion imaging. J Am Coll Cardiol 1995;25(6):1300–9.
7. O'Keefe JH Jr, Bateman TM, Handlin LR, Barnhart CS. Four- versus 6-minute infusion protocol for adenosine thallium-201 single photon emission computed tomography imaging. Am Heart J 1995;129(3):482–7.
8. Dimitriu AG, Nistor N, Russu G, Cristogel F, Streanga V, Varlam L. Value of intravenous ATP in the diagnosis and treatment of tachyarrhythmias in children. Rev Med Chir Soc Med Nat Iasi 1998;102(3–4):100–2.
9. Pfammatter JP, Bauersfeld U. Safety issues in the treatment of paediatric supraventricular tachycardias. Drug Saf 1998;18(5):345–56.
10. Sherwood MC, Lau KC, Sholler GF. Adenosine in the management of supraventricular tachycardia in children. J Paediatr Child Health 1998;34(1):53–6.
11. Bakshi F, Barzilay Z, Paret G. Adenosine in the diagnosis and treatment of narrow complex tachycardia in the pediatric intensive care unit. Heart Lung 1998;27(1):47–50.

12. Prabhu AS, Singh TP, Morrow WR, Muzik O, Di Carli MF. Safety and efficacy of intravenous adenosine for pharmacologic stress testing in children with aortic valve disease or Kawasaki disease. Am J Cardiol 1999;83(2):284–6.

13. Thomas GS, Prill NV, Majmundar H, Fabrizi RR, Thomas JJ, Hayashida C, Kothapalli S, Payne JL, Payne MM, Miyamoto MI. Treadmill exercise during adenosine infusion is safe, results in fewer adverse reactions, and improves myocardial perfusion image quality. J Nucl Cardiol 2000;7(5):439–46.

14. Elliott MD, Holly TA, Leonard SM, Hendel RC. Impact of an abbreviated adenosine protocol incorporating adjunctive treadmill exercise on adverse effects and image quality in patients undergoing stress myocardial perfusion imaging. J Nucl Cardiol 2000;7(6):584–9.

15. Mulla N, Karpawich PP. Ventricular fibrillation following adenosine therapy for supraventricular tachycardia in a neonate with concealed Wolff–Parkinson–White syndrome treated with digoxin. Pediatr Emerg Care 1995;11(4):238–9.

16. Strickberger SA, Man KC, Daoud EG, Goyal R, Brinkman K, Knight BP, Weiss R, Bahu M, Morady F. Adenosine-induced atrial arrhythmia: a prospective analysis. Ann Intern Med 1997;127(6):417–22.

17. Rae CP, Mansfield MD, Dryden C, Kinsella J. Analgesic effect of adenosine on ischaemic pain in human volunteers. Br J Anaesth 1999;82(3):427–8.

18. Garratt KN, Holmes DR Jr, Molina-Viamonte V, Reeder GS, Hodge DO, Bailey KR, Lobl JK, Laudon DA, Gibbons RJ. Intravenous adenosine and lidocaine in patients with acute myocardial infarction. Am Heart J 1998;136(2):196–204.

19. Zarate E, Sa Rego MM, White PF, Duffy L, Shearer VE, Griffin JD, Whitten CW. Comparison of adenosine and remifentanil infusions as adjuvants to desflurane anesthesia. Anesthesiology 1999;90(4):956–63.

20. Christopher M, Key CB, Persse DE. Refractory asystole and death following the prehospital administration of adenosine. Prehosp Emerg Care 2000;4(2):196–8.

21. Knight BP, Zivin A, Souza J, Goyal R, Man KC, Strickberger A, Morady F. Use of adenosine in patients hospitalized in a university medical center. Am J Med 1998;105(4):275–80.

22. Jaeggi E, Chiu C, Hamilton R, Gilljam T, Gow R. Adenosine-induced atrial pro-arrhythmia in children. Can J Cardiol 1999;15(2):169–72.

23. Israel C, Klingenheben T, Gronefeld G, Hohnloser SH. Adenosine-induced atrial fibrillation. J Cardiovasc Electrophysiol 2000;11(7):825.

24. Kaplan IV, Kaplan AV, Fisher JD. Adenosine induced atrial fibrillation precipitating polymorphic ventricular tachycardia. Pacing Clin Electrophysiol 2000;23(1):140–1.

25. Misra D, Van Tosh A, Schweitzer P. Adenosine induced monomorphic ventricular tachycardia. Pacing Clin Electrophysiol 2000;23(6):1044–6.

26. Ruiz Ruiz MJ, Rivero Guerrero JA, Barrera Cordero A, de Teresa E. Empeoramiento de la taquicardia Supraventricular tras la administracion de adenosina: un efecto paradojico. [Worsening of supraventricular tachycardia after intravenous after adenosine administration: a paradoxical effect.] Med Clin (Barc) 2001;117(7):276.

27. Parham WA, Mehdirad AA, Biermann KM, Fredman CS. Case report: adenosine induced ventricular fibrillation in a patient with stable ventricular tachycardia. J Interv Card Electrophysiol 2001;5(1):71–4.

28. Tan HL, Spekhorst HH, Peters RJ, Wilde AA. Adenosine induced ventricular arrhythmias in the emergency room. Pacing Clin Electrophysiol 2001;24(4 Pt 1):450–5.

29. Alkoutami GS, Reeves WC, Movahed A. The frequency of atrioventricular block during adenosine stress testing in young, middle-aged, young-old, and old-old adults. Am J Geriatr Cardiol 2001;10(3):159–61.

30. Toft J, Mortensen J, Hesse B. Risk of atrioventricular block during adenosine pharmacologic stress testing in heart transplant recipients. Am J Cardiol 1998;82(5):696–7.

31. Alkoutami GS, Reeves WC, Movahed A. The safety of adenosine pharmacologic stress testing in patients with first-degree atrioventricular block in the presence and absence of atrioventricular blocking medications. J Nucl Cardiol 1999;6(5):495–7.

32. Ng WH, Polosa R, Church MK. Adenosine bronchoconstriction in asthma: investigations into its possible mechanism of action. Br J Clin Pharmacol 1990;30(Suppl 1): S89–98.

33. Johnston DL, Scanlon PD, Hodge DO, Glynn RB, Hung JC, Gibbons RJ. Pulmonary function monitoring during adenosine myocardial perfusion scintigraphy in patients with chronic obstructive pulmonary disease. Mayo Clin Proc 1999;74(4):339–46.

34. Balan KK, Critchley M. Is the dyspnea during adenosine cardiac stress test caused by bronchospasm? Am Heart J 2001;142(1):142–5.

35. Belfrage M, Segerdahl M, Arner S, Sollevi A. The safety and efficacy of intrathecal adenosine in patients with chronic neuropathic pain. Anesth Analg 1999;89(1):136–42.

36. Eisenach JC, Hood DD, Curry R. Phase I safety assessment of intrathecal injection of an American formulation of adenosine in humans. Anesthesiology 2002;96(1):24–8.

37. Eisenach JC, Curry R, Hood DD. Dose response of intrathecal adenosine in experimental pain and allodynia. Anesthesiology 2002;97(4):938–42.

38. Rane K, Segerdahl M, Goiny M, Sollevi A. Intrathecal adenosine administration: a phase 1 clinical safety study in healthy volunteers, with additional evaluation of its influence on sensory thresholds and experimental pain. Anesthesiology 1998;89(5):1108–15.

39. Clarke KW, Brear SG, Hanley SP. Rise in intracranial pressure with intravenous adenosine. Lancet 1992; 339(8786):188–9.

40. Watt AH, Lewis DJ, Horne JJ, Smith PM. Reproduction of epigastric pain of duodenal ulceration by adenosine. BMJ (Clin Res Ed) 1987;294(6563):10–12.

41. Shaw AD, Boscoe MJ. Anaphylactic reaction following intravenous adenosine. Anaesthesia 1999;54(6):608.

42. Haynes BE. Two deaths after prehospital use of adenosine. J Emerg Med 2001;21(2):151–4.

43. Treuth MG, Reyes GA, He ZX, Cwajg E, Mahmarian JJ, Verani MS. Tolerance and diagnostic accuracy of an abbreviated adenosine infusion for myocardial scintigraphy: a randomized, prospective study. J Nucl Cardiol 2001;8(5):548–54.

44. Jeremias A, Whitbourn RJ, Filardo SD, Fitzgerald PJ, Cohen DJ, Tuzcu EM, Anderson WD, Abizaid AA, Mintz GS, Yeung AC, Kern MJ, Yock PG. Adequacy of intracoronary versus intravenous adenosine-induced maximal coronary hyperemia for fractional flow reserve measurements. Am Heart J 2000;140(4):651–7.

45. Sjolund KF, Segerdahl M, Sollevi A. Adenosine reduces secondary hyperalgesia in two human models of cutaneous inflammatory pain. Anesth Analg 1999;88(3):605–10.

46. Kopf A, Ruf W. Novel drugs for neuropathic pain. Curr Opin Anaesthesiol 2000;13:577–83.

47. Guieu R, Dussol B, Devaux C, Sampol J, Brunet P, Rochat H, Bechis G, Berland YF. Interactions between cyclosporine A and adenosine in kidney transplant recipients. Kidney Int 1998;53(1):200–4.

48. Watt AH, Bernard MS, Webster J, Passani SL, Stephens MR, Routledge PA. Intravenous adenosine in the treatment of supraventricular tachycardia: a dose-ranging study and interaction with dipyridamole. Br J Clin Pharmacol 1986;21(2):227–30.

49. diMarco JP, Sellers TD, Lerman BB, Greenberg ML, Berne RM, Belardinelli L. Diagnostic and therapeutic use of adenosine in patients with supraventricular tachyarrhythmias. J Am Coll Cardiol 1985;6(2):417–25.
50. Hourigan C, Safih S, Rogers I, Jacobs I, Lockney A. Randomized controlled trial of midazolam premedication to reduce the subjective adverse effects of adenosine. Emerg Med (Fremantle) 2001;13(1):51–6.

Adiphenine

General Information

Adiphenine, in the doses generally used (up to 60 mg/day), is of disputed value. It may have a non-specific relaxant action on the gastrointestinal muscle and some local anesthetic effect on the buccal mucosa. The evidence on its effects is meager and it seems like an anticholinergic drug that has been promoted in doses that are often too low to result in either a useful therapeutic effect or in adverse effects.

Adrenaline

See also Anticholinergic drugs

General Information

Note on nomenclature

Although epinephrine is the recommended International Non-proprietary Name (rINN), there are good reasons why the name adrenaline should be preferred, based on usage, history, etymology, and, most importantly, risk of clinical errors (1).

Adrenaline is a catecholamine with agonist effects at both α- and β-adrenoceptors.

The use of adrenaline is largely limited to subcutaneous administration for the immediate relief of anaphylactic shock. Intramuscular doses of 0.1 ml of a 1:1000 solution are often given repeatedly, up to a maximum of some 2 ml in 5 minutes. Although the sensitivity of individuals to adrenaline varies considerably, the adverse reactions to such doses are generally limited to mild cardiovascular effects.

Intravenous administration of adrenaline for treatment of systemic anaphylactic shock should be undertaken with extreme caution, even in patients without a history of cardiovascular disease. At all times the patient must be monitored and emergency treatment should be available. Even the infiltration of low doses of adrenaline for local hemostasis can be attended by these risks; one patient developed ventricular tachycardia and severe hypertension after receiving 3.75 mg locally for this purpose (SEDA-17, 160), and the value of this treatment is in any case today regarded as dubious (SEDA-17, 161).

Subcutaneous adrenaline has been used to prevent the immediate adverse effects of snake antivenom, although evidence of its efficacy is scanty (2). A large clinical trial is under way in Sri Lanka.

Adrenaline was at one time a component of asthma sprays, and dilated cardiomyopathy was described after many years of use (3).

Adrenaline has been largely abandoned as an adjuvant to local anesthetics, although in a 1:80 000 concentration it is still sometimes used in dental and in epidural anesthesia.

Dipivefrin

Dipivefrin (dipivalyl epinephrine) is a prodrug of adrenaline, used topically in the treatment of glaucoma. Its potential advantages include a longer duration of action, increased local availability, greater potency, greater stability, and fewer adverse effects. The effect on pupil size is insignificant, no objective sight-threatening effects are observed, and central visual acuity and visual fields are not affected after application of a 0.1% solution of dipivefrine. However, minor sporadic and transient burning or stinging sensations can occur.

Organs and Systems

Cardiovascular

When the limits of tolerance are approached, there may be palpitation, extra beats, and a rise in blood pressure. In sensitive individuals or at high doses, ventricular fibrillation, subarachnoid hemorrhage, and even hemiplegia have been known to occur. Adrenaline can occasionally cause pulmonary edema (4,5). It is possible that in at least some of these cases the drug has been inadvertently injected intravenously.

Ventricular dysrhythmias have been reported in a case of adrenaline overdose (6).

- A 5-year-old boy was given subcutaneous adrenaline 1:1000 after a severe allergic reaction to a bee sting. Inadvertently, 10 times the correct dose was given. He developed extra beats and two brief runs of ventricular tachycardia, but recovered fully after about 20 minutes. Creatine kinase activity, both total and the MB fraction, was slightly raised in this patient (total 603 IU/l, MB fraction 161 IU/l; upper limits of the local reference range 243 and 15 IU/l), suggesting cardiac damage.

Life-threatening torsade de pointes has been observed when an epidural anesthetic was given using 20 ml of bupivacaine containing only 1:200 000 adrenaline (7).

When adrenaline 0.4 ml of a 1 mg/ml solution was inadvertently injected into the penile skin of a 12-hour-old neonate the skin blanched and the error was immediately understood (8). After repeated doses of phentolamine (total 0.65 mg) the skin regained its normal color. There were no sequelae.

Adrenaline is occasionally used as a hemostatic agent, with rare complications. However, they do occur, as noted in a report from Lyon (9).

- A 64-year-old man with diabetes and hypertension bled from a site in the lower rectum. A local injection of adrenaline 0.2 mg successfully stopped the hemorrhage, but very soon after he became hypotensive, with rapid atrial fibrillation (ventricular rate not given), the first time he had experienced this. He reverted spontaneously to sinus rhythm within 24 hours.

The authors suggested that if this type of procedure is contemplated in elderly patients with cardiovascular disease an anesthetist should be present to monitor cardiovascular status; it may in any case be wiser to avoid adrenaline altogether in favor of other means of hemostasis.

A more unusual site of adrenaline injection has been described in a Canadian report (10).

- A 79-year-old woman developed pituitary apoplexy in an adenomatous gland and was being prepared for *trans*-sphenoidal hypophysectomy. Topical adrenaline (1:1000) was applied to both nostrils and then 1.5 ml of 1% lidocaine containing 1:100 000 adrenaline was injected into the nasal mucosa. The blood pressure immediately rose from 100/50 to 230/148 mmHg and the pulse rate from 48 to 140/minute. Although she was treated immediately with esmolol and intravenous glyceryl trinitrate, resulting in normalization of her blood pressure, subsequent investigations showed that she had had a painless myocardial infarction. She made a full recovery after pituitary surgery.

The authors suggested that if adrenaline is to be used in such cases, even lower concentrations might be advisable. This is reasonable, although one also wonders in this case whether her blood pressure may have been lowered too rapidly.

Sensory systems

Melanic conjunctivocorneal pigmentation has been reported with an incidence of 30% with adrenaline (11,12).

Cystoid macular edema has been reported to occur in 2.8% of the patients receiving adrenaline especially in aphakic or pseudophakic eyes (13). Cystoid macular edema has also been seen after the use of dipivefrine, but in the classic case described in 1982 pretreatment with timolol maleate may have predisposed the eye to this complication (14).

Central retinal vein thrombosis occurred in a 75-year-old man 20 minutes after the ipsilateral insertion of a 1% adrenaline-soaked cotton wool stick (15). Unfortunately, his visual acuity did not improve.

Metabolism

Lactic acidosis has been observed, persisting for some hours after deliberate intravenous misuse of 20 mg adrenaline by an addict (SED-12, 308). Six of 19 patients who were given adrenaline for hypotension after undergoing cardiopulmonary bypass developed lactic acidosis, though the ultimate outcome was favorable (SEDA-22, 154).

Mouth and teeth

Facial swelling due to drug-induced sialadenosis was repeatedly observed in one patient who controlled her asthma symptoms with an adrenaline inhaler (SEDA-14, 119).

Susceptibility Factors

Cardiovascular

In susceptible individuals, an attack of angina pectoris can be precipitated by adrenaline, and in any form of cardiac disease caution is indicated; at one time an attempt was made to use high doses of adrenaline for the early treatment of ventricular fibrillation, but its pharmacological effects swing the balance against its use, the immediate survival rate actually being reduced.

Hyperthyroidism

Patients with hyperthyroidism are unduly sensitive to the effects of adrenaline (SEDA-14, 179).

Drug Administration

Drug administration route

While the absorption of adrenaline from a subcutaneous injection in healthy subjects is variable (and sometimes very slow) absorption from an inhaled dose is rapid and reliable (16). The main adverse effect from the inhaled route, for example in a dose of 3–4.5 mg, is gastrointestinal discomfort, with nausea and sometimes vomiting; this seems to be a local effect since it does not occur with injections. However, both forms produce mild tremor and palpitation in some individuals.

Since adrenaline is so short acting, the metabolic and other adrenergic effects which it can produce are unlikely to be elicited unless a depot formulation is used; in the latter event, hyperglycemia may occur.

Drug–Drug Interactions

Beta-adrenoceptor antagonists

Small quantities of adrenaline, such as are present as an additive in local anesthetic formulations, can be dangerously potentiated by beta-adrenoceptor blockers; propranolol should be discontinued at least 3 days in advance of administering such products for local anesthesia. A combined infusion of adrenaline and propranolol has been used for diagnosing insulin resistance, but it can evoke cardiac dysrhythmias, even in patients without signs of coronary disease (17).

Halothane

Halothane and some other anesthetics sensitize patients to the risk of adrenaline-induced ventricular dysrhythmias and acute pulmonary edema, especially if hypoxia is present (18,19).

Hyaluronidase

Adrenaline is physically incompatible with hyaluronidase (20).

Monoamine oxidase inhibitors

Monoamine oxidase inhibitors have been said to potentiate the hypertensive effects of adrenaline, but there is no good clinical evidence of such an interaction (21). Nevertheless, care should be taken when contemplating the use of adrenaline in patients taking a monoamine oxidase inhibitor.

Sodium novobiocin

Adrenaline is physically incompatible with sodium novobiocin (20).

Sodium warfarin

Adrenaline is physically incompatible with sodium warfarin (20).

Tricyclic antidepressants

Tricyclic antidepressants inhibit the uptake of catecholamines, such as adrenaline, into sympathetic neurons and can enhance the cardiovascular effects, so that even the small amounts of adrenaline present as additives in some local anesthetics can have a marked effect on the cardiovascular system.

References

1. Aronson JK. "Where name and image meet"—the argument for "adrenaline". BMJ 2000;320(7233):506–9.
2. Nuchpraryoon I, Garner P. Interventions for preventing reactions to snake antivenom. Cochrane Database Syst Rev 2000:(2):CD002153. http://www.update-software.com/abstracts/ab002153.htm.
3. Stewart MJ, Fraser DM, Boon N. Dilated cardiomyopathy associated with chronic overuse of an adrenaline inhaler. Br Heart J 1992;68(2):221–2.
4. Worthen M, Placik B, Argano B, MacCanon DM, Luisada AA. On the mechanism of epinephrine-induced pulmonary edema. Jpn Heart J 1969;10(2):133–41.
5. Ersoz N, Finestone SC. Adrenaline-induced pulmonary oedema and its treatment. A report of two cases. Br J Anaesth 1971;43(7):709–12.
6. Davis CO, Wax PM. Prehospital epinephrine overdose in a child resulting in ventricular dysrhythmias and myocardial ischemia. Pediatr Emerg Care 1999;15(2):116–18.
7. Jackman WM, Friday KJ, Anderson JL, Aliot EM, Clark M, Lazzara R. The long QT syndromes: a critical review, new clinical observations and a unifying hypothesis. Prog Cardiovasc Dis 1988;31(2):115–72.
8. Adams MC, McLaughlin KP, Rink RC. Inadvertent concentrated epinephrine injection at newborn circumcision: effect and treatment. J Urol 2000;163(2):592.
9. Galoo E, Godon P, Potier V, Vergeau B. Fibrillation auriculaire compliquant une hémostase endoscopique rectale par injection d' adrénaline. [Atrial fibrillation following a rectal endoscopic injection using epiphedrine solution.] Gastroenterol Clin Biol 2002;26(1):99–100.
10. Chelliah YR, Manninen PH. Hazards of epinephrine in transsphenoidal pituitary surgery. J Neurosurg Anesthesiol 2002;14(1):43–6.
11. Macho MS, Vicente MC, Salorio MS. Depositos pigmentarios conjunctivales producidos por epinefrina. [Conjunctival pigmentary deposits produced by epinephrine.] Arch Soc Esp Oftalmol 1973;33:537.
12. Zolog N, Leibovici M. La "mélanose" conjonctivale par épinéphrine. [Conjunctival melanosis caused by epinephrine.] Bull Mem Soc Fr Ophtalmol 1973;86(0):198–200.
13. Larricart P. Les affections retiniennes. [Retinal diseases.] Bull Soc Ophtalmol Fr 1985;Spec No:193–211.
14. Mehelas TJ, Kollarits CR, Martin WG. Cystoid macular edema presumably induced by dipivefrin hydrochloride (Propine). Am J Ophthalmol 1982;94(5):682.
15. Maaranen TH, Mantyjarvi MI. Central retinal artery occlusion after a local anesthetic with adrenaline on nasal mucosa. J Neuroophthalmol 2000;20(4):234–5.
16. Heilborn H, Hjemdahl P, Daleskog M, Adamsson U. Comparison of subcutaneous injection and high-dose inhalation of epinephrine—implications for self-treatment to prevent anaphylaxis. J Allergy Clin Immunol 1986;78(6):1174–9.
17. Lampman RM, Santinga JT, Bassett DR, Savage PJ. Cardiac arrhythmias during epinephrine–propranolol infusions for measurement of in vivo insulin resistance. Diabetes 1981;30(7):618–20.
18. Mattig W, Radam R. Todesfall nach Adrenalinanwendung unter Halothannarkose. Dtsch Gesundheitsw 1977;32:953.
19. Woldorf NM, Pastore PN. Extreme epinephrine sensitivity with a general anesthesia. Arch Otolaryngol 1972;96(3):272–7.
20. Griffin JP, D'Arcy PF. A Manual of Adverse Drug Interactions. 2nd ed. Bristol: John Wright and Sons Ltd, 1985.
21. Yagiela JA. Adverse drug interactions in dental practice: interactions associated with vasoconstrictors. Part V of a series. J Am Dent Assoc 1999;130(5):701–9.

Adrenoceptor agonists

See also Individual agents

General Information

Adrenoceptor agonists evoke physiological responses similar to those produced by stimulation of adrenergic nerves or the physiological release of adrenaline (see Table 1). For many of these responses it is currently possible to conclude that only an alpha-adrenoceptor or a beta-adrenoceptor is involved, and in some cases one can distinguish a $beta_1$ from a $beta_2$ response. In some cases, however, the distinction is not clear: most adrenoceptor agonists, however specific to a particular receptor type they are claimed to be, will for example on occasion stimulate central nervous functions, resulting in nervousness, insomnia, tremors, dizziness, or headache. In some organ systems both alpha-adrenoceptors and beta-adrenoceptors are present; thus, the nature of the response produced will depend either on the concentrations achieved or on other factors; whether, for example, the uterus contracts or relaxes in response to an adrenergic drug depends in part on the hormonal balance in the system at that moment.

Alpha-adrenoceptor agonists, such as clonidine, are little used nowadays in the treatment of hypertension or migraine. Clonidine is used epidurally, in combination with opioids, neostigmine, and anesthetic and analgesic agents, to produce segmental analgesia, particularly for postoperative relief of pain after obstetrical and surgical

Table 1 Adrenoceptors and the effects of agonists

Organs and systems	Receptor	Response to an agonist
Cardiovascular		
Heart		
Sinoatrial node	β_1	Increased heart rate
Atria	β_1	Increased contractility and conduction velocity
Atrioventricular node and conduction system	β_1	Increased conduction velocity and automaticity
Ventricles	β_1	Increased contractility, conduction velocity, automaticity, rate of idiopathic pacemakers
Blood vessels		
Coronary	α, β_2	Constriction
Skin, mucosa	α	Constriction
Skeletal muscle	α or β_2	Constriction or dilatation
Cerebral	α	Slight constriction
Pulmonary	α or β_2	Constriction or dilatation
Abdominal viscera	α or β_2	Constriction or dilatation
Salivary glands	α	Constriction
Respiratory		
Bronchial muscle	β_2	Relaxation
Bronchial glands	α_1, β_2	Decreased or increased secretion
Nervous system		
Cerebral function	Various	Stimulation
Eyes		
Radial muscle, iris	α	Contraction (mydriasis)
Ciliary muscle	β	Relaxation for far vision (slight)
Hematologic		
Spleen capsule	α	Contraction
Salivary glands	α_1	Potassium and water secretion
	β	Amylase secretion
Gastrointestinal		
Motility and tone	α_1, β_1, β_2	Decrease (usually)
Sphincters	α	Contraction (usually)
Secretion of various substances	Various	Inhibition
Liver		
Glycogenolysis and gluconeogenesis	α_1, β_2	Stimulation
Gallbladder		
Bile ducts	β_2	Relaxation
Urinary tract		
Ureter; tone, motility	β_2	Relaxation (usually)
Bladder; detrusor	β	Relaxation (usually)
Trigone, sphincter	α	Contraction
Renal vessels	α_1, β_1, β_2	Primary contraction
Skin		
Pilomotor muscles	α	Contraction
Sweat glands	α	Slight local secretion
Musculoskeletal		
Muscle glycogenolysis	β	Stimulation
Sexual function		
Uterus	α, β_2	Variable effect[a]
Male sex function	α_1	Ejaculation

[a] Response depends inter alia on hormonal status.

procedures. Apraclonidine is available for the short-term reduction of intraocular pressure.

The drugs that were developed some 40 years ago as general beta-adrenoceptor agonists have largely fallen into disuse with the development of more selective beta$_1$-adrenoceptor agonists (for use in cardiac failure) and beta$_2$-adrenoceptor agonists (for use in airways disease and threatened premature labor).

Beta$_3$-adrenoceptor agonists

Stimulation of beta-adrenoceptors on the cell surface of adipocytes promotes lipolysis and energy expenditure. These receptors are neither beta$_1$-adrenoceptors nor beta$_2$-adrenoceptors, and they have been termed atypical or beta$_3$-adrenoceptors. Some atypical agonists (BRL 26830 A, BRL 35135, CL 316243, and D 7114) have been developed and assessed for their ability to stimulate these receptors and hence to induce weight loss. The BRL compounds appear to exaggerate physiological tremor, presumably through an effect on beta$_2$-adrenoceptors; the two other compounds are said to be more selective.

Ajmaline and its derivatives

See also Antidysrhythmic drugs

General Information

Ajmaline and its derivatives, prajmalium bitartrate (rINN; *N*-propylajmaline), lorajmine (rINN; chloroacetylajmaline), detajmium bitartrate (rINN), and diethylaminohydroxypropylajmaline, are *Rauwolfia* alkaloids. Their use is restricted by serious adverse effects, such as neutropenia and cardiac dysrhythmias, which have been reviewed (1). Other adverse effects include dizziness, headache, and a sensation of warmth after intravenous injection.

Organs and Systems

Cardiovascular

Ajmaline occasionally causes cardiac dysrhythmias (SEDA-17, 219). Of 1995 patients who were given ajmaline 1 mg/kg intravenously during an electrophysiological study, 63 developed a supraventricular tachydysrhythmia (atrial flutter, fibrillation, or tachycardia), and seven an atrioventricular re-entrant tachycardia (2). Those most at risk were older patients, those with underlying cardiac disease, and those with a history of dysrhythmias or sinus node dysfunction.

Two cases of torsade de pointes have been reported in association with prolongation of the QT interval (3). Polymorphous ventricular tachycardia has been reported in three cases (4–6).

- A 13-year-old boy with Brugada syndrome (right bundle branch block with persistent ST segment elevation) was given an injection of ajmaline 1 mg/kg and developed greater ST segment elevation and more marked right bundle branch block morphology (7). This was followed by short runs of non-sustained polymorphic ventricular tachycardia, gradually increasing until monomorphic ventricular tachycardia occurred. The dysrhythmia eventually resolved without further treatment.

It is unwise to give antidysrhythmic drugs to patients with Brugada syndrome.

Nervous system

Neurological effects have occasionally been reported in patients taking ajmaline derivatives; they include confusion and cranial nerve palsies (8,9).

Hematologic

Neutropenia is a relatively common and important adverse effect of ajmaline (10). Of the three main mechanisms that cause neutropenia (immune, toxic, and autoimmune) two have been associated with ajmaline: immune and autoimmune neutropenia.

Liver

Ajmaline can cause hepatitis or cholestasis. Cholestasis has been reported in association with neutropenia (11) and with fever and eosinophilia (12). Although acute liver damage due to ajmaline is usually reversible, there has been a report of persistent jaundice due to long-lasting cholestasis (13).

Immunologic

Hypersensitivity to ajmaline is rare, but there has been a report of an immune interstitial nephritis in association with fever (14).

Drug Administration

Drug overdose

In overdosage ajmaline can cause heart block and dysrhythmias, hypotension, malaise, vertigo, respiratory depression, and coma (15). In one series of 38 cases there were nine deaths (24%) (16). Treatment of overdosage includes the intravenous administration of molar sodium lactate for dysrhythmias, conduction disturbances, and circulatory failure; a pacemaker may be required.

- After an overdose of detajmium bitartrate in a dose of 18 mg/kg, a 36-year-old woman developed ventricular flutter, which responded to treatment with lidocaine, defibrillation, glucagon, noradrenaline, and sodium chloride (17). Hypokalemia responded to intravenous potassium chloride.
- A 57-year-old man took ajmaline 1000 mg with suicidal intent (18). He was unconscious and hypotensive and had serious disturbances in cardiac conduction. His serum and urine ajmaline concentrations were high. Although only 4% of the ingested dose was excreted following forced diuresis, all evidence of toxicity disappeared within 21 hours.

Various types of cardiac dysrhythmia have previously been reported after overdosage of ajmaline (SEDA-2, 162).

References

1. Schwartz JB, Keefe D, Harrison DC. Adverse effects of antiarrhythmic drugs. Drugs 1981;21(1):23–45.
2. Brembilla-Perrot B, Terrier de la Chaise A. Provocation of supraventricular tachycardias by an intravenous class I antiarrhythmic drug. Int J Cardiol 1992;34(2):189–98.
3. Haverkamp W, Monnig G, Kirchhof P, Eckardt L, Borggrefe M, Breithardt G. Torsade de pointes induced by ajmaline. Z Kardiol 2001;90(8):586–90.
4. Kaul U, Mohan JC, Narula J, Nath CS, Bhatia ML. Ajmaline-induced torsade de pointes. Cardiology 1985;72(3):140–3.
5. Kolar J, Humhal J, Karetova D, Novak M. "Torsade de pointes" po mezokainu a ajmalinu u nemocne s intermitertni sinokomorovou blokadou. Priznivy recebny vliv vysokych davek izoprenalinu. [Torsade de pointes after mesocaine and ajmaline in a patient with intermittent atrioventricular block. Favorable therapeutic effect of high doses of isoprenaline.] Cas Lek Cesk 1987;126(48):1503–7.

6. Schmitt C, Brachmann J, Schols W, Beyer T, Kubler W. Proarrhythmischer Effekt von Ajmalin bei idiopathischer ventrikulärer Tachykardie. [Proarrhythmic effect of ajmaline in idiopathic ventricular tachycardia.] Dtsch Med Wochenschr 1989;114(3):99–102.

7. Pinar Bermudez E, Garcia-Alberola A, Martinez Sanchez J, Sanchez Munoz JJ, Valdes Chavarri M. Spontaneous sustained monomorphic ventricular tachycardia after administration of ajmaline in a patient with Brugada syndrome. Pacing Clin Electrophysiol 2000;23(3):407–9.

8. Aquaro G, Marra S, Paolillo V, Pavia M. Complicanze neurologiche in corso di terapia con 17-MDCAA. [Neurological complications during therapy with 17 MDCAA.] G Ital Cardiol 1977;7(3):304–8.

9. Lessing JB, Copperman IJ. Severe cerebral confusion produced by prajmalium bitartrate. BMJ 1977;2(6088):675.

10. Brna TG Jr. Agranulocytosis from antiarrhythmic agents. What to watch for when a medication is first prescribed. Postgrad Med 1991;89(1):181–8.

11. Offenstadt G, Boisante L, Onimus R, Amstutz P. Agranulocytose et hepatite cholestatique au cours d'un traitement par l'ajmaline. [Agranulocytosis and cholestatic hepatitis during treatment with ajmaline.] Ann Med Interne (Paris) 1976;127(8–9):622–7.

12. Buscher HP, Talke H, Rademacher HP, Gessner U, Oehlert W, Gerok W. Intrahepatische Cholestase durch N-Propyl-Ajmalin. [Intrahepatic cholestasis due to N-propyl ajmaline.] Dtsch Med Wochenschr 1976;101(18):699–703.

13. Chammartin F, Levillain P, Silvain C, Chauvin C, Beauchant M. Hepatite prolongée a l'ajmaline—description d'un cas et revue de la litterature. [Prolonged hepatitis due to ajmaline—description of a case and review of the literature.] Schweiz Rundsch Med Prax 1989;78(20):582–4.

14. Dupond JL, Herve P, Saint-Hillier Y, Guyon B, Colas JM, Perol C, Leconte des Floris R. Anurie recidivant a 3 reprises; complication exceptionelle d'un traitement antiarythmique. J Med Besancon 1975;11:231.

15. Tempe JD, Jaeger A, Beissel J, Burg E, Mantz JM. Intoxications aigués par trois drogues cardiotropes: l'ajmaline, la chloroquine, la digitaline. J Med Strasbourg (Eur Med) 1976;7:569.

16. Conso F, Bismuth C, Riboulet G, Efthymiou ML. Intoxication aiguë par l'ajmaline. [Acute poisoning by ajmaline.] Therapie 1979;34(4):529–30.

17. Mobis A, Minz DH. Suizidale Tachmalcor-Intoxikation–Ein Fallbericht. [Suicidal Tachmalcor poisoning—a case report.] Anaesthesiol Reanim 1999;24(4):109–10.

18. Almog C, Maidan A, Pik A, Schlesinger Z. Acute intoxication with ajmaline. Isr J Med Sci 1979;15(7):570–2.

Alatrofloxacin and trovafloxacin

See also Fluoroquinolones

General Information

Alatrofloxacin is a fluoronaphthyridone that is hydrolysed to the active moiety, trovafloxacin, after intravenous administration. This fourth-generation broad-spectrum fluoroquinolone has activity against Gram-positive, Gram-negative, anerobic, and atypical respiratory pathogens. Because it has significant hepatotoxicity, the list of appropriate indications for trovafloxacin has been restricted.

In a multicenter, double-blind, randomized comparison of trovafloxacin 200 mg and clarithromycin 500 mg bd in 176 subjects with acute exacerbations of chronic bronchitis, the most common adverse effects of trovafloxacin were nausea (5%), dizziness (5%), vomiting (3%), and constipation (3%) (1). Because trovafloxacin is hepatotoxic, the list of appropriate indications has been limited to patients who have at least one of several specified infections, such as nosocomial pneumonia or complicated intra-abdominal infections that are serious and life- or limb-threatening in the physician's judgement.

Trovafloxacin may down-regulate cytokine mRNA transcription in human peripheral blood mononuclear cells stimulated with lipopolysaccharide or lipoteichoic acid (2). Likewise, trovafloxacin inhibited *Salmonella typhimurium*-induced production of TNFα, HIV-1 replication, and reactivation of latent HIV-1 in promonocytic U1 cells at concentrations comparable to the plasma and tissue concentrations achieved by therapeutic dosages (3).

Organs and Systems

Cardiovascular

Phlebitis can occur during parenteral administration of trovafloxacin. High concentrations of trovafloxacin (2 mg/ml) significantly reduced intracellular ATP content in cultured endothelial cells and reduced concentrations of ADP, GTP, and GDP (4). These in vitro data suggest that high doses of trovafloxacin are not compatible with maintenance of endothelial cell function and may explain the occurrence of phlebitis. Commercial formulations should be diluted and given into large veins.

Nervous system

Alatrofloxacin can cause seizures (5).

- A 37-year-old Asian man received several antibiotics (including intravenous ceftazidime, gentamicin, meropenem, metronidazole, and vancomycin) postoperatively. After 3 weeks he was given alatrofloxacin 75 mg in 25 ml of dextrose 5% (1.875 mg/ml) and developed generalized clonus. On rechallenge, infusing at half the initial rate, the seizure recurred. A CT scan of the brain was normal.

Seizures are rare but have occurred during treatment with other fluoroquinolones. This is the first report of a case of seizures associated with slow infusion of alatrofloxacin. However, as of 21 June 2000, the manufacturers had received 53 reports of seizures through worldwide postmarketing surveillance. In rat hippocampus slices, trovafloxacin had significant convulsive potential; the underlying mechanism is hitherto incompletely understood.

Trovafloxacin has been associated with diffuse weakness due to a demyelinating polyneuropathy in a patient without an underlying neurological disorder (6).

Hematologic

Alatrofloxacin has been associated with severe leukopenia (7).

- A 79-year-old white man was treated with intravenous alatrofloxacin mesylate 200 mg bd for 5 days. His leukocyte count fell from 10.9×10^9/l to 2.2×10^9/l; the hemoglobin did not change. Alatrofloxacin was withdrawn, and 3 days later the leukocyte count had increased to 11.5×10^9/l.

The mechanism of trovafloxacin-induced leukopenia is unknown. Nevertheless, since quinolones exert their antibacterial effect by inhibiting bacterial DNA gyrase and since similar topoisomerases are involved in the organization and function of mammalian DNA, it is possible that trovafloxacin acts by modulating bone marrow stem-cell DNA production.

Alatrofloxacin has been associated with severe thrombocytopenia (8).

- A 54-year-old woman was given alatrofloxacin 300 mg intravenously qds and on day 4 developed epistaxis. Her platelet count was 7×10^9/l, with normal hemoglobin and white blood cell counts. Direct antiglobulin testing showed coating of erythrocytes with polyspecific immunoproteins, and platelet-associated antibody testing was positive for IgM and IgG antibodies. Alatrofloxacin was withdrawn and azithromycin was given instead. She was given methylprednisolone 125 mg intravenously bd and the platelet count fell to 2×10^9/l and then rose, reaching 60×10^9/l on day 8.

During clinical trials, thrombocytopenia occurred in under 1% of more than 7000 patients who received alatrofloxacin or trovafloxacin.

Liver

More than 100 cases of hepatotoxicity associated with trovafloxacin have been reported to the FDA.

- A 19-year-old woman developed severe acute hepatitis and peripheral eosinophilia during oral trovafloxacin therapy for recurrent sinusitis (9). Liver biopsy showed extensive centrilobular hepatocyte necrosis, probably causing veno-occlusive disease. Clinical and laboratory abnormalities resolved completely after prolonged treatment with steroids.
- A 66-year-old man had taken trovafloxacin 100 mg/day for 4 weeks for refractory chronic sinusitis (10). For several years he had also taken allopurinol, doxepin, hydrochlorothiazide, losartan, metoprolol, and nabumetone. He developed nausea, vomiting, malaise, and abdominal distension. His white cell count was 8000×10^9/l with 16% eosinophils; his serum aspartate transaminase was 537 IU/l, alanine transaminase 841 IU/l, direct bilirubin 17 μmol/l; total bilirubin 27 μmol/l, alkaline phosphatase 111 IU/l; blood urea nitrogen 5 μmol/l; and creatinine 190 μmol/l. Tests for hepatitis A, B, and C were negative. A biopsy of the liver showed centrilobular and focal periportal necrosis and eosinophilic infiltration; the sinusoids were dilated and contained lymphocytes and eosinophils; many hepatocytes were undergoing mitosis. After withdrawal of trovafloxacin and treatment with prednisone, his hepatic and renal function returned to normal, and the eosinophilia gradually resolved.

Skin

The photosensitizing potential of trovafloxacin 200 mg od has been compared with that of ciprofloxacin 500 mg bd,

lomefloxacin 400 mg od, and placebo in 48 healthy men (aged 19–45 years) (11). Trovafloxacin had significantly less photosensitizing potential than either ciprofloxacin or lomefloxacin. Photosensitivity seemed to be induced only by wavelengths in the UVA region, was maximal at 24 hours, and had a short-term effect.

Musculoskeletal

Trovafloxacin inhibited growth and extracellular matrix mineralization in MC3T3-E1 osteoblast-like cell cultures (12). The IC_{50} was 0.5 μg/ml, which is below clinically achievable serum concentrations. The authors suggested that the clinical relevance of this observation to bone healing in orthopedic patients should be evaluated.

Second-Generation Effects

Teratogenicity

In an ex vivo study, trovafloxacin crossed the human placenta by simple diffusion and neither accumulated in the media nor bound to tissues or accumulated in the placenta (13). This implies that it should have no effects on the fetus if given during pregnancy.

Susceptibility Factors

Age

The pharmacokinetics of a single intravenous dose of alatrofloxacin have been determined in six infants aged 3–12 months and in 14 children aged 2–12 years (14). The peak trovafloxacin concentration at the end of the infusion was 4.3 μg/ml; the volume of distribution at steady state was 1.6 l/kg, clearance 2.5 ml/min/kg, and the half-life 9.8 hours, with no age-related differences. Less than 5% of the administered dose was excreted in the urine over 24 hours.

Other features of the patient

The pharmacokinetics of trovafloxacin after the administration of alatrofloxacin were not substantially altered in seven critically ill patients (three men, four women) with APACHE II scores of 27 (range 15–32) and normal or mildly impaired hepatic function (15).

Monitoring Therapy

In 17 patients aged over 18 years with severe acute community-acquired pneumonia trovafloxacin concentrations were persistently high in the sputum, bronchial secretions, bronchoalveolar lavage fluid, and epithelial lining fluid, with no significant difference between these compartments (16). The authors proposed that measurement of sputum concentrations could be used to monitor the outcome of treatment.

References

1. Sokol WN Jr, Sullivan JG, Acampora MD, Busman TA, Notario GF. A prospective, double-blind, multicenter study comparing clarithromycin extended-release with

trovafloxacin in patients with community-acquired pneumonia. Clin Ther 2002;24(4):605–15.

2. Purswani M, Eckert S, Arora H, Johann-Liang R, Noel GJ. The effect of three broad-spectrum antimicrobials on mononuclear cell responses to encapsulated bacteria: evidence for down-regulation of cytokine mRNA transcription by trovafloxacin. J Antimicrob Chemother 2000;46(6): 921–9.

3. Gollapudi S, Gupta S, Thadepalli H. Salmonella typhimurium-induced reactivation of latent HIV-1 in promonocytic U1 cells is inhibited by trovafloxacin. Int J Mol Med 2000;5(6):615–18.

4. Armbruster C, Robibaro B, Griesmacher A, Vorbach H. Endothelial cell compatibility of trovafloxacin and levofloxacin for intravenous use. J Antimicrob Chemother 2000;45(4):533–5.

5. Melvani S, Speed BR. Alatrofloxacin-induced seizures during slow intravenous infusion. Ann Pharmacother 2000;34(9):1017–19.

6. Murray CK, Wortmann GW. Trovafloxacin-induced weakness due to a demyelinating polyneuropathy. South Med J 2000;93(5):514–15.

7. Mitropoulos FA, Angood PB, Rabinovici R. Trovafloxacin-associated leukopenia. Ann Pharmacother 2001;35(1):41–4.

8. Gales BJ, Sulak LB. Severe thrombocytopenia associated with alatrofloxacin. Ann Pharmacother 2000;34(3):330–4.

9. Lazarczyk DA, Goldstein NS, Gordon SC. Trovafloxacin hepatotoxicity. Dig Dis Sci 2001;46(4):925–6.

10. Chen HJ, Bloch KJ, Maclean JA. Acute eosinophilic hepatitis from trovafloxacin. N Engl J Med 2000;342(5):359–60.

11. Ferguson J, McEwen J, Al-Ajmi H, Purkins L, Colman PJ, Willavize SA. A comparison of the photosensitizing potential of trovafloxacin with that of other quinolones in healthy subjects. J Antimicrob Chemother 2000;45(4):503–9.

12. Holtom PD, Pavkovic SA, Bravos PD, Patzakis MJ, Shepherd LE, Frenkel B. Inhibitory effects of the quinolone antibiotics trovafloxacin, ciprofloxacin, and levofloxacin on osteoblastic cells in vitro. J Orthop Res 2000;18(5):721–7.

13. Casey B, Bawdon RE. Ex vivo human placental transfer of trovafloxacin. Infect Dis Obstet Gynecol 2000;8(5–6):228–9.

14. Bradley JS, Kearns GL, Reed MD, Capparelli EV, Vincent J. Pharmacokinetics of a fluoronaphthyridone, trovafloxacin (CP 99,219), in infants and children following administration of a single intravenous dose of alatrofloxacin. Antimicrob Agents Chemother 2000;44(5):1195–9.

15. Olsen KM, Rebuck JA, Weidenbach T, Fish DN. Pharmacokinetics of intravenous trovafloxacin in critically ill adults. Pharmacotherapy 2000;20(4):400–4.

16. Peleman RA, Van De Velde V, Germonpre PR, Fleurinck C, Rosseel MT, Pauwels RA. Trovafloxacin concentrations in airway fluids of patients with severe community-acquired pneumonia. Antimicrob Agents Chemother 2000;44(1):178–80.

Albendazole

See also Benzimidazoles

General Information

Albendazole, a benzimidazole derivative closely related to mebendazole (qv), is used in the treatment of helminth infections, such as gastrointestinal roundworms, hydatid disease, neurocysticercosis, larva migrans cutanea, and strongyloidiasis (1). Provided that an adequate concentration is attained within the cyst, it is scolicidal. In high doses given for prolonged periods or cyclically, it is effective in echinococcosis, in which it is given in a dosage of 10 mg/kg/day for 4 weeks, repeated in six cycles with 2-week rest periods between each cycle, although even with this high dose only about one-third of patients enjoy a complete cure, some 70% having a partial response. Albendazole is also active against *Pneumocystis jiroveci*, and is effective in prophylaxis and treatment in immuno-suppressed mice (2). In hydatid disease a combination of albendazole and praziquantel is effective when either agent has failed when used alone (SED-12, 707) (3).

Observational studies

Ankylostomiasis

Albendazole has been used in the treatment of human hookworm and trichuriasis. In a mass-treatment report from Western Australia 295 individuals in a remote rural area were treated with albendazole 400 mg/day for 5 days because of possible *Giardia lamblia* and hookworm infections (4). The 37% prevalence of *Giardia* fell to 12% between days 6 and 9, but rose again to 28% between days 18 and 30. The effect on hookworms (*Ankylostoma duodenale*) was more pronounced and more sustained with a reduction of the pretreatment prevalence of hookworm infections from 76% before treatment to 0% after 3–4 weeks. The tolerability of the drug was judged to be excellent by 89%, good by 1%, and moderately good by 1%, while 9% gave no response. Adverse effects were reported by five individuals and consisted of mild abdominal pain ($n = 2$), mild or moderate diarrhea ($n = 2$), moderate fever ($n = 1$), and weakness ($n = 1$).

Ascariasis

The efficacy of 2 years of mass chemotherapy against ascariasis has been evaluated in Iran (5). A single dose of albendazole 400 mg was given at 3-month intervals for 2 years to every person, except children under 2 years of age and pregnant women. After 2 years of treatment the prevalences, based on 2667 post-treatment samples, had fallen (Table 1). There were no adverse effects of mass treatment with albendazole.

Echinococcosis

Hydatid disease is a common zoonosis caused by the larval cysts of *Echinococcus granulosus*. Hydatid cysts most commonly form in the liver, but can occur in any organ. The management and operative complications in 70 patients with hydatid disease aged 10–78 years have been studied retrospectively to assess the impact of albendazole and praziquantel compared with surgery (6). In all,

Table 1 Changes in prevalences of helminthic infections in patients treated with albendazole

Helminth	Number (%) of positive tests before treatment ($n = 3098$)	Number (%) of positive tests after treatment ($n = 2667$)
Ascaris lumbricoides	1198 (39%)	196 (7.4%)
Trichuris trichiura	22 (0.7%)	5 (0.2%)
Hymenolepis nana	63 (2%)	49 (1.8%)

39 patients received albendazole and praziquantel in combination and 19 received albendazole alone; none was treated with praziquantel alone. The combined use of albendazole and praziquantel preoperatively significantly reduced the number of cysts that contained viable protoscolices. During the 12-year follow-up period an initial 3 months of drug treatment (albendazole throughout and praziquantel for 2 weeks), re-assessment, followed by either surgery or continuation with chemotherapy was found to be a rational treatment algorithm. In 11 patients albendazole, given for a median of 3 months at a dose of 400 mg bd, had adverse effects: five patients developed nausea and six had abnormal liver function tests. Therapy was withdrawn in two patients owing to altered liver function.

The efficacy of albendazole emulsion has been studied in 212 patients with hydatid disease of the liver, aged 4–82 years (7). Two regimens of albendazole were given for a variable period (3 months to more than 1 year); 67 adults received albendazole 10 mg/kg/day and 145 adults received 12.5 mg/kg/day. The overall cure rate was 75%. In the follow-up study the recurrence rate was 10%. The highest cure rate was observed in those who received albendazole 12.5 mg/kg/day for 9 months. At the start of therapy about 15% of the patients had mild pruritus, rash, and transient gastric pain, which resolved without specific therapy. Two patients had alopecia. There were frequent rises in serum transaminase activities in both groups but not to above 30–50 IU/l, except in six patients, who had values above 200 IU/l. In two patients albendazole was withdrawn because of vomiting. In one patient who took 12.5 mg/kg/day severe adverse effects, such as anorexia, jaundice, anemia, edema, and hypoproteinemia, developed, necessitating withdrawal. Reintroduction of albendazole 10 mg/kg/day was uneventful.

The use of albendazole and mebendazole in patients with hydatidosis has been evaluated in 448 patients with *E. granulosis* hydatid cysts who received continuous treatment with albendazole 10–12 mg/kg/day for 3–6 months daily orally in a total dose of (323 patients) twice or mebendazole 50 mg/kg/day (8). At the end of treatment, 82% of the cysts treated with albendazole and 56% of the cysts treated with mebendazole showed degenerative changes. During long-term follow-up 25% of these cysts showed relapse, which took place within 2 years in 78% of cases. Further treatment with albendazole induced degenerative changes in over 90% of the relapsed cysts, without induction of more frequent or more severe adverse effects, as observed during the first treatment period. Adverse effects during the first treatment period consisted of raised transaminases with albendazole (67 of 323 patients) and mebendazole (16 of 125 patients), and abdominal pain in 12 and 11% respectively. With both drugs, occasional patients experienced headache, abdominal distension, vertigo, urticaria, jaundice, thrombocytopenia, fever, or dyspepsia, but most of these are known manifestations of *Echinococcus* infection. Six of 323 patients taking albendazole withdrew because of adverse effects compared with eight of 125 patients taking mebendazole. It appears that albendazole is more effective than mebendazole in the treatment of hydatid cysts caused by *E. granulosis* and that both the intensity and frequency of the usually mild adverse effects are comparable.

Filariasis

Treatment of patients with high *Loa loa* microfilaraemia is sometimes complicated by an encephalopathy, suggested to be related to a rapid killing of large number of *L. loa* microfilariae. If the *L. loa* microfilarial count could be reduced more slowly, before ivermectin is distributed, ivermectin-related encephalopathy might be prevented. In 125 patients with *L. loa* microfilariasis the effect of albendazole (800 mg/day for three consecutive days) or multivitamin tablets on *L. loa* microfilarial load and the occurrence of encephalopathy were studied (9). *L. loa* microfilarial loads were followed for 9 months. There was no significant change in the overall microfilarial loads among those treated with albendazole, although the loads in patients with more than 8000 microfilariae/ml tended to fall more progressively during the first 3 months of follow-up. There were no cases of encephalopathy. The main adverse effects reported were itching (in eight patients taking albendazole and seven taking multivitamins), abdominal pain (two taking albendazole), and diarrhea (one taking albendazole, two taking multivitamins); overall analysis showed no significant difference in these events between the groups. Albendazole was associated with modest but significantly raised plasma transaminase activities.

Neurocysticercosis

In a report on the use of albendazole 15 mg/kg/day in two divided doses for 14 days in the treatment of persistent neurocysticercosis (10), adverse reactions were monitored in 43 patients with seizures and a solitary cysticercal cyst, who had not been treated before. In all patients CT scans confirmed the presence of a solitary cyst less than 2 cm in diameter. Antiepileptic treatment was continued. In seven patients dexamethasone 8 mg/day in four divided doses was given for the first 5–7 days after the start of treatment. Follow-up CT scans at 4–10 weeks after the start of treatment showed responses in 20 patients, with complete disappearance in seven patients and a reduction to 50% of the pretreatment size in the other 13. There were adverse effects in 15 patients, with a maximum on the fifth day after the start of treatment. Six patients had severe headaches, 11 had partial seizures, and 2 had epileptic seizures and severe postictal hemiparesis that persisted for a week or more. Because of these serious adverse effects treatment was discontinued in seven patients and dexamethasone was added in those patients who were not already taking it, although its use proved questionable. Adverse effects were seen in three of seven patients who took prophylactic steroid therapy and in 12 of 36 patients who did not.

Albendazole was effective in neurocysticercosis in an optimal dosage of 15 mg/kg/day divided in two doses every 12 hours for 8 days (11). It was generally well tolerated, although several patients had adverse reactions during the first few days after the start of treatment, consisting of headache, vomiting, and exacerbation of neurological symptoms caused by an inflammatory reaction to antigens from degenerating cysts, necessitating the concomitant use of glucocorticoids. In very large cysticerci, or cysticerci located in risky areas like the brainstem, these reactions may rarely be life-threatening.

Protozoal infections

The efficacy of albendazole 800 mg bd for 14 days for persistent diarrhea due to cryptosporidiosis ($n = 10$), isosporiasis ($n = 54$), or microsporidiosis ($n = 23$) has been studied in 153 HIV-positive patients (12). Albendazole reduced the burden of protozoal infection and promoted mucosal recovery in 87 patients who had a complete clinical response. Two patients reported nausea and vomiting. One patient developed leukopenia (1.9×10^9/l) after treatment and four patients developed thrombocytopenia ($51–98 \times 10^9$/l).

Toxocariasis

The efficacy of albendazole plus prednisolone has been studied in five patients aged 11–72 years with ocular toxocariasis (13). All had uveitis and retinochoroidal granulomas. Their symptoms had persisted for a mean of 14 months (range 3 days to 24 months). The adults were treated with albendazole 800 mg bd for 2 weeks plus prednisolone starting at 1.5 mg/kg/day tapering over 3 months. The children were treated with 400 mg bd for 2 weeks plus prednisolone 1.0 mg/kg/day. All tolerated the therapy well without adverse effects. In particular, there were no significant hypersensitivity reactions to dying *Toxocara* larvae. The uveitis resolved in all cases and there were no relapses. After treatment, all the granulomas had disappeared, leaving heavily pigmented chorioretinal scars without loss of vision.

Comparative studies

The use of albendazole and mebendazole in patients with hydatidosis has been evaluated in 448 patients with *E. granulosis* hydatid cysts who received continuous treatment with albendazole 10–12 mg/kg/day for 3–6 months daily orally in a total dose of (323 patients) twice or mebendazole 50 mg/kg/day (8). At the end of treatment, 82% of the cysts treated with albendazole and 56% of the cysts treated with mebendazole showed degenerative changes. During long-term follow-up 25% of these cysts showed relapse, which took place within 2 years in 78% of cases. Further treatment with albendazole induced degenerative changes in over 90% of the relapsed cysts, without induction of more frequent or more severe adverse effects, as observed during the first treatment period. Adverse effects during the first treatment period consisted of raised transaminases with albendazole (67 of 323 patients) and mebendazole (16 of 125 patients), and abdominal pain in 12 and 11% respectively. Headache occurred in eight patients taking albendazole and three taking mebendazole, abdominal distension in seven and five patients, vertigo in five and one, urticaria in five and three, jaundice in one and one, thrombocytopenia in two and none, fever in three and none, dyspepsia in two and four, and tachycardia in two and none. Six of 323 patients taking albendazole withdrew because of adverse effects compared with eight of 125 patients taking mebendazole. It appears that albendazole is more effective than mebendazole in the treatment of hydatid cysts caused by *E. granulosis* and that both the intensity and frequency of the usually mild adverse effects are comparable.

In a randomized trial in Mexico (14) 622 children with *Trichuris* were randomized to either albendazole 400 mg/day for 3 days, one dose of albendazole 400 mg, or one dose of pyrantel 11 mg/kg. The aim was to study efficacy and the effects on growth. After three courses at 1 year the level of infection with *Trichuris* was reduced by 99% in the 3-day albendazole treatment group, by 87% in the single-dose albendazole treatment group, and by 67% in the pyrantel group. There were no significant differences in the increases in height, weight, or arm circumference, but contrary to expectations there was a lower increase in the thickness of the triceps skin fold in those given 3-day courses of albendazole. This was only found in the patients with lower pretreatment *Trichuris* stool egg counts. These findings suggest that although elimination of *Trichuris* may promote growth in children, albendazole in a dose of 1200 mg/kg every 4 months may have an independent negative effect on growth. In an accompanying commentary (15) it was concluded that the suggestion that relatively high doses of albendazole may affect growth deserves study, but that this possible effect must be weighed against the negative effect of prolonged helminthic infestation on children's health, growth, and cognitive function. However, it is unlikely that high-dose treatment will be standard in mass-treatment campaigns, and these results should not deter the use of single-dose albendazole in mass-treatment programs in high-risk populations.

In 110 children with ascariasis or trichuriasis the efficacy of a single dose of albendazole 400 mg has been compared with that of nitazoxanide 100 mg bd for 3 days in children aged 1–3 years and 200 mg bd for 3 days in children aged 4–11 years (16). Nitazoxanide cured 89 and 89% of the cases of ascariasis and trichuriasis respectively. Albendazole cured 91 and 58% of the cases of ascariasis and trichuriasis respectively. Abdominal pain ($n = 9$), nausea ($n = 1$), diarrhea ($n = 2$), and headache ($n = 1$) were reported as mild adverse effects in 105 patients who took nitazoxanide, and abdominal pain ($n = 1$), nausea ($n = 1$), and vomiting ($n = 1$) were reported as adverse effects in 54 patients who took albendazole. All the adverse events were mild and transient and drug withdrawal was not necessary.

Placebo-controlled studies

Albendazole has been used in the treatment and prophylaxis of microsporidiosis in patients with AIDS. In a small, double-blind, placebo-controlled trial from France (17) the efficacy and safety of treatment with albendazole was studied in four patients treated with albendazole 400 mg bd for 3 weeks and in four patients treated with placebo. Microsporidia were cleared in all patients given albendazole but in none of those given placebo. Afterwards all eight patients were again randomized to receive either maintenance treatment with albendazole 400 mg bd or no treatment for the next 12 months; none of the three patients taking maintenance treatment had a recurrence, while three of the five who took no maintenance therapy developed a recurrence. During the double-blind part of the trial there were no serious adverse effects in the patients who took albendazole, although two complained of headache, one of abdominal pain, one had raised transaminase activities, and one had thrombocytopenia. However, half the patients were also taking anti-HIV triple therapy, which makes it difficult to assess these abnormalities. The authors concluded that the adverse effects were not serious and did not hinder maintenance therapy. The tentative conclusion derived from these findings is that albendazole may be useful in the treatment of microsporidiosis, which in patients with AIDS often leads to debilitating chronic diarrhea and is difficult to treat.

Use in non-infective conditions

The efficacy of albendazole has been evaluated in a few patients with either hepatocellular carcinoma ($n = 1$) or colorectal cancer and hepatic metastases refractory to other forms of treatment ($n = 8$) (18). Apart from hematological and biochemical indices, the tumor markers carcinoembryonic antigen (CEA) and alpha-fetoprotein (AFP) were measured to monitor treatment efficacy. One other patient with a neuroendocrine cancer and a mesothelioma was treated on a compassionate basis and only monitored for adverse effects. Albendazole was given orally in a dose of 10 mg/kg/day in two divided doses for 28 days. Albendazole reduced CEA in two patients and in the other five patients with measurable tumor markers, serum CEA or AFP was stabilized in three. In the seven patients who completed this pilot study, albendazole was well tolerated and there were no significant changes in any hematological, kidney, or liver function tests. However, three patients were withdrawn because of severe neutropenia, which resulted in the death of one. Neutropenia was more frequent than is usually experienced in the treatment of hydatid disease. The authors speculated that this may relate to reduced metabolism in patients with liver cancer or liver metastases, leading to the passage of unmetabolized drug into the circulation.

General adverse effects

As with other antihelminthic drugs, the general adverse effects of albendazole can reflect the destruction of the parasite rather than a direct action of the drug; pyrexia is likely to be seen, even in the absence of other problems. Albendazole was well tolerated in 30-day courses of 10–14 mg/kg/day separated by 2-week intervals.

Its adverse effects are similar to those of mebendazole and are possibly more common because of better and more reliable absorption.

The direct adverse effects of albendazole are few and usually minor, and consist of gastrointestinal upsets, dizziness, rash, and alopecia, which usually do not require drug withdrawal. Early pyrexia and neutropenia can also occur. Cyst rupture can also occur, as with mebendazole. About 15% of patients treated with albendazole at higher doses develop raised serum transaminases, necessitating careful monitoring and sometimes withdrawal of treatment after prolonged use. Careful monitoring of leukocyte and platelet counts is also indicated. The possibility of teratogenicity and embryotoxicity from animal studies suggests that the drug should be avoided in pregnancy.

Organs and Systems

Nervous system

Used in the treatment of neurocysticercosis, albendazole (like praziquantel) can cause a CSF syndrome characterized by fever, headaches, meningism, and exacerbation of some or many of the neurological signs of the disease; it is thought to be due to a local reaction to dying and dead larvae and can be attenuated by prednisone (SED-12, 707) (19,20).

Since neurocysticercosis is a neurological infection, it is not surprising that when treating it with any drug some of the neurological reactions to that drug (or to the death of the parasite) are particularly pronounced. For example, with a dose of 1.5 mg/kg continued for some time in cases of neurocysticercosis, a majority of patients initially develop intolerance in the form of headache, vomiting, fever, and occasionally diplopia and meningeal irritation (21). Even shorter and less intensive treatment has produced similar effects. However, all of these symptoms are probably due to the death of the parasite, and if therapy is continued they usually disappear within a few days. Nevertheless, they can be alarming and demand treatment. Data from large studies mention somnolence and even transient hemiparesis as incidental adverse effects.

Very rarely, in cases of neurocysticercosis, the reaction of the nervous system to the death of the parasite is extremely violent. In one case cerebral edema resulted in permanent neurological damage (22), while other patients have suffered hydrocephalus or acute intracranial hypertension requiring treatment, for example with glucocorticoids or mannitol (23).

Albendazole has sometimes aggravated extrapyramidal disorders or precipitated seizures in patients with prior epileptic symptoms. The risk of intracranial hypertension has led some to suggest that glucocorticoids should be given preventively when using albendazole in neurocysticercosis (24); however, dexamethasone can interact with albendazole, increasing its plasma concentrations (25), and it is not clear whether this might produce new problems.

Encephalopathy is an adverse event related to the treatment of *L. loa* with diethylcarbamazine or ivermectin, and it has also been related to albendazole (11).

- A 55-year-old woman from Cameroon took oral albendazole 200 mg bd for a symptomatic *L. loa* infection with microfilaremia of 152 microfilariae/ml and a *Mansonella perstans* infection of 133 microfilariae/ml. Three days after the start of therapy she developed an encephalopathy. Albendazole was withdrawn and she recovered without any specific treatment within the next 16 hours. On day 4, the *L. loa* microfilarial count was 29 microfilariae/ml.

The clinical presentation, the interval after starting treatment, the evolution of the episode, and the results of cerebral spinal fluid analysis and electroencephalography in this case were similar to those seen in cases of encephalopathy following treatment of *L. loa* with ivermectin or diethylcarbamazine. However, pretreatment filaremia was relatively low and *L. loa* microfilariae were not detectable in the cerebral spinal fluid. Thus, pre-existing conditions might increase the susceptibility to encephalopathy.

Sensory systems

An allergic conjunctivitis was seen in cases of industrial occupational skin reactions to albendazole (26).

Hematologic

There have been various reports of bone marrow depression. In one study (27) two of 20 patients had a reversible drop in leukocyte count. Pancytopenia, reversible on withdrawal, has been documented in an elderly woman (28). Even with high doses neutropenia occurs in under 1% of cases. In the older literature an occasional hematological death was reported.

A megakaryocytic thrombocytopenia attributed to albendazole has been reported (29).

- A 25-year-old woman who had been taking albendazole 13 mg/kg/day for 5 months for hepatic and pulmonary echinococcosis developed fatigue, bleeding gums, and prolonged menstrual bleeding. She had ecchymoses and petechiae over her legs, marked thrombocytopenia ($10 \times 10^9/l$), a mild iron deficiency anemia, and a normal leukocyte count. There was no antiplatelet immunoglobulin. A bone marrow aspiration showed absent megakaryocytes with normal granulocytes and mild erythroid hyperplasia. A cytogenetic study of the bone marrow showed normal karyotype and immunophenotype. The albendazole was withdrawn and oral iron given. At follow-up 2 months later all laboratory abnormalities had resolved.

Gastrointestinal

With a single oral dose of albendazole 400 mg, there is usually little more in the way of adverse effects than mild gastrointestinal disturbances (notably epigastric pain or dry mouth), occurring only in about 6% of patients in some large series; a few patients have abdominal pain. With higher doses, irritation of the central nervous system can lead to nausea and vomiting.

Diarrhea occurs in a few patients taking albendazole and is usually mild. However, a typical case of pseudomembranous colitis has been documented, although the patient also had AIDS and intestinal microsporidiosis and had taken a number of other drugs; the complication responded to vancomycin (30).

Liver

Even in single low doses a transient increase in transaminase activities has been repeatedly reported, generally affecting up to 13–20% of patients taking albendazole (SEDA-18, 315) (31). At the higher doses some evidence of moderate hepatitis has been claimed to be present in almost all patients, but in one series with high doses of albendazole or mebendazole for echinococcosis only 17% had a (generally slight) increase in serum transaminases, and a fair number of these had pre-existent liver disorders (32). Like various other adverse effects, the increase in transaminases may be attributable to the breakdown of liver cysts; it is almost always reversible and is usually not a reason for withdrawal; it does not become more marked during long-term treatment. A very occasional individual develops jaundice (33) or some other manifestation of hepatitis (34).

Skin

A generalized rash has sometimes been seen in patients taking albendazole (SEDA-15, 334), and skin complications (including urticaria and contact dermatitis) are a potential problem in employees in the pharmaceutical industry if they undergo heavy exposure to the drug (26).

- A 38-year-old woman with cough, eosinophilia, and pulmonary infiltrates due to visceral larva migrans from *Toxocara canis* infection took albendazole 600 mg for 8 weeks and developed slight transient skin eruptions (35).

Stevens–Johnson syndrome was reported in a man who took albendazole 400 mg/day for toxocariasis (36).

Hair

There are various well-documented reports of reversible alopecia in patients taking albendazole (SEDA-17, 358) (SEDA-22, 324), which in one study occurred in 2% of cases (SEDA-18, 315) and in another study in one case of 20 (SED-13, 913) (27).

- Severe alopecia has been described in an almost 3-year-old child who took albendazole 400 mg/d for 3 days; 2 months later alopecia developed and resolved within 1 month (37).
- When one woman took 400 mg bd for 10 months for hydatid disease, she lost much of her hair; no other likely cause could be identified, and her hair growth recovered when the drug was stopped (38).

Oddly, however, a fair proportion of patients when specifically questioned seem to remark that their hair growth has actually improved during treatment (SED-13, 913) (27).

Musculoskeletal

Myalgia and arthralgia can occur in patients taking albendazole (39). However, these symptoms are often features of the disease being treated.

Second-Generation Effects

Teratogenicity

It has been emphasized that albendazole is teratogenic in animals and should not be used in pregnancy (40).

Drug–Drug Interactions

Antiepileptic drugs

The pharmacological interactions of the antiepileptic drugs phenytoin, carbamazepine, and phenobarbital with albendazole have been studied in 32 adults with active intraparenchymatous neurocysticercosis (41):

- nine patients took phenytoin 3–4 mg/kg/day;
- nine patients took carbamazepine 10–20 mg/kg/day;
- five patients took phenobarbital 1.5–4.5 mg/kg/day;
- nine patients took no antiepileptic drugs.

All were treated with albendazole 7.5 mg/kg every 12 hours on 8 consecutive days. Phenytoin, carbamazepine, and phenobarbital all induced the oxidative metabolism of albendazole to a similar extent in a non-enantioselective manner. In consequence, there was a significant reduction in the plasma concentration of the active metabolite of albendazole, albendazole sulfoxide.

Cimetidine

The poor intestinal absorption of albendazole, which may be enhanced by a fatty meal, contributes to difficulties in predicting its therapeutic response in echinococcosis. The effect of cimetidine co-administration on the systemic availability of albendazole has been studied in six healthy men (42). After an overnight fast, a single oral dose of albendazole (10 mg/kg) was administered on an empty stomach with water, a fatty meal, grapefruit juice, or grapefruit juice plus cimetidine. The systemic availability of albendazole was reduced by cimetidine. There were no adverse events. These results are consistent with presystemic metabolism of albendazole by CYP3A4.

References

1. Venkatesan P. Albendazole. J Antimicrob Chemother 1998;41(2):145–7.
2. Bartlett MS, Edlind TD, Lee CH, Dean R, Queener SF, Shaw MM, Smith JW. Albendazole inhibits *Pneumocystis carinii* proliferation in inoculated immunosuppressed mice. Antimicrob Agents Chemother 1994;38(8):1834–7.
3. Cook GC. Tropical medicine. Postgrad Med J 1991;67(791):798–822.
4. Reynoldson JA, Behnke JM, Gracey M, Horton RJ, Spargo R, Hopkins RM, Constantine CC, Gilbert F, Stead C, Hobbs RP, Thompson RC. Efficacy of albendazole against *Giardia* and hookworm in a remote Aboriginal community in the north of Western Australia. Acta Trop 1998;71(1):27–44.
5. Fallah M, Mirarab A, Jamalian F, Ghaderi A. Evaluation of two years of mass chemotherapy against ascariasis in Hamadan, Islamic Republic of Iran. Bull World Health Organ 2002;80(5):399–402.
6. Ayles HM, Corbett EL, Taylor I, Cowie AG, Bligh J, Walmsley K, Bryceson AD. A combined medical and surgical approach to hydatid disease: 12 years' experience at the Hospital for Tropical Diseases, London. Ann R Coll Surg Engl 2002;84(2):100–5.
7. Chai J, Menghebat, Jiao W, Sun D, Liang B, Shi J, Fu C, Li X, Mao Y, Wang X, Dolikun, Guliber, Wang Y, Gao F, Xiao S. Clinical efficacy of albendazole emulsion in treatment of 212 cases of liver cystic hydatidosis. Chin Med J (Engl) 2002;115(12):1809–13.
8. Franchi C, Di Vico B, Teggi A. Long-term evaluation of patients with hydatidosis treated with benzimidazole carbamates. Clin Infect Dis 1999;29(2):304–9.
9. Tsague-Dongmo L, Kamgno J, Pion SD, Moyou-Somo R, Boussinesq M. Effects of a 3-day regimen of albendazole (800 mg daily) on *Loa loa* microfilaraemia. Ann Trop Med Parasitol 2002;96(7):707–15.
10. Rajshekhar V. Incidence and significance of adverse effects of albendazole therapy in patients with a persistent solitary cysticercus granuloma. Acta Neurol Scand 1998;98(2):121–3.
11. Sotelo J, Jung H. Pharmacokinetic optimisation of the treatment of neurocysticercosis. Clin Pharmacokinet 1998;34(6):503–15.
12. Zulu I, Veitch A, Sianongo S, McPhail G, Feakins R, Farthing MJ, Kelly P. Albendazole chemotherapy for AIDS-related diarrhoea in Zambia—clinical, parasitological and mucosal responses. Aliment Pharmacol Ther 2002;16(3):595–601.
13. Barisani-Asenbauer T, Maca SM, Hauff W, Kaminski SL, Domanovits H, Theyer I, Auer H. Treatment of ocular toxocariasis with albendazole. J Ocul Pharmacol Ther 2001;17(3):287–94.
14. Forrester JE, Bailar JC 3rd, Esrey SA, Jose MV, Castillejos BT, Ocampo G. Randomised trial of albendazole and pyrantel in symptomless trichuriasis in children. Lancet 1998;352(9134):1103–8.
15. Winstanley P. Albendazole for mass treatment of asymptomatic trichuris infections. Lancet 1998;352(9134):1080–1.
16. Juan JO, Lopez Chegne N, Gargala G, Favennec L. Comparative clinical studies of nitazoxanide, albendazole and praziquantel in the treatment of ascariasis, trichuriasis and hymenolepiasis in children from Peru. Trans R Soc Trop Med Hyg 2002;96(2):193–6.
17. Molina JM, Chastang C, Goguel J, Michiels JF, Sarfati C, Desportes-Livage I, Horton J, Derouin F, Modai J. Albendazole for treatment and prophylaxis of microsporidiosis due to *Encephalitozoon intestinalis* in patients with AIDS: a randomized double-blind controlled trial. J Infect Dis 1998;177(5):1373–7.
18. Morris DL, Jourdan JL, Pourgholami MH. Pilot study of albendazole in patients with advanced malignancy. Effect on serum tumor markers/high incidence of neutropenia. Oncology 2001;61(1):42–6.
19. Teggi A, Lastilla MG, De Rosa F. Therapy of human hydatid disease with mebendazole and albendazole. Antimicrob Agents Chemother 1993;37(8):1679–84.
20. Desser KB, Baden M. Allergic reaction to pyrvinium pamoate. Am J Dis Child 1969;117(5):589.
21. Escobedo F, Penagos P, Rodriguez J, Sotelo J. Albendazole therapy for neurocysticercosis. Arch Intern Med 1987;147(4):738–41.
22. Noboa C. Albendazole therapy for giant subarachnoid cysticerci. Arch Neurol 1993;50(4):347–8.
23. Garcia HH, Gilman RH, Horton J, Martinez M, Herrera G, Altamirano J, Cuba JM, Rios-Saavedra N, Verastegui M, Boero J, Gonzalez AE. Albendazole therapy for neurocysticercosis: a prospective double-blind trial comparing 7 versus 14 days of treatment. Cysticercosis Working Group in Peru. Neurology 1997;48(5):1421–7.
24. Del Brutto OH. Clues to prevent cerebrovascular hazards of cysticidal drug therapy. Stroke 1997;28(5):1088.
25. Takayanagui OM, Lanchote VL, Marques MP, Bonato PS. Therapy for neurocysticercosis: pharmacokinetic interaction of albendazole sulfoxide with dexamethasone. Ther Drug Monit 1997;19(1):51–5.
26. Macedo NA, Pineyro MI, Carmona C. Contact urticaria and contact dermatitis from albendazole. Contact Dermatitis 1991;25(1):73–5.
27. Steiger U, Cotting J, Reichen J. Albendazole treatment of echinococcosis in humans: effects on microsomal metabolism and drug tolerance. Clin Pharmacol Ther 1990;47(3):347–53.
28. Fernandez FJ, Rodriguez-Vidigal FF, Ledesma V, Cabanillas Y, Vagace JM. Aplastic anemia during treatment with albendazole. Am J Hematol 1996;53(1):53–4.
29. Yildiz BO, Haznedaroglu IC, Coplu L. Albendazole-induced amegakaryocytic thrombocytopenic purpura. Ann Pharmacother 1998;32(7–8):842.
30. Shah V, Marino C, Altice FL. Albendazole-induced pseudomembranous colitis. Am J Gastroenterol 1996;91(7):1453–4.
31. Horton RJ. Albendazole in treatment of human cystic echinococcosis: 12 years of experience. Acta Trop 1997;64(1–2):79–93.

32. Teggi A, Lastilla MG, Grossi G, Franchi C, De Rosa F. Increase of serum glutamic-oxaloacetic and glutamic-pyruvic transaminases in patients with hydatid cysts treated with mebendazole and albendazole. Mediterr J Infect Parasit Dis 1995;10:85–90.

33. Choudhuri G, Prasad RN. Jaundice due to albendazole. Indian J Gastroenterol 1988;7(4):245–6.

34. Luchi S, Vincenti A, Messina F, Parenti M, Scasso A, Campatelli A. Albendazole treatment of human hydatid tissue. Scand J Infect Dis 1997;29(2):165–7.

35. Inoue K, Inoue Y, Arai T, Nawa Y, Kashiwa Y, Yamamoto S, Sakatani M. Chronic eosinophilic pneumonia due to visceral larva migrans. Intern Med 2002;41(6):478–82.

36. Dewerdt S, Machet L, Jan-Lamy V, Lorette G, Therizol-Ferly M, Vaillant L. Stevens–Johnson syndrome after albendazole. Acta Dermatol Venereol 1997;77(5):411.

37. Herdy R. Alopecia associated to albendazole: a case report. An Bras Dermatol 2000;75:715–19.

38. Al Karawi M, Kasawy MI, Mohamed AL. Hair loss as a complication of albendazole therapy. Saudi Med J 1988;9:530.

39. Supali T, Ismid IS, Ruckert P, Fischer P. Treatment of *Brugia timori* and *Wuchereria bancrofti* infections in Indonesia using DEC or a combination of DEC and albendazole: adverse reactions and short-term effects on microfilariae. Trop Med Int Health 2002;7(10):894–901.

40. Bialek R, Knobloch J. Parasitare Infektionen in der Schwangerschaft und konnatale Parasitosen. II. Teil: Helmintheninfektionen. [Parasitic infections in pregnancy and congenital parasitoses. II. Helminth infections.] Z Geburtshilfe Neonatol 1999;203(3):128–33.

41. Lanchote VL, Garcia FS, Dreossi SA, Takayanagui OM. Pharmacokinetic interaction between albendazole sulfoxide enantiomers and antiepileptic drugs in patients with neurocysticercosis. Ther Drug Monit 2002;24(3):338–45.

42. Nagy J, Schipper HG, Koopmans RP, Butter JJ, Van Boxtel CJ, Kager PA. Effect of grapefruit juice or cimetidine coadministration on albendazole bioavailability. Am J Trop Med Hyg 2002;66(3):260–3.

Albumin

General Information

Adverse reactions to human serum albumin are uncommon and usually mild, such as itching and urticaria. Serious reactions are rare. A patient who has reacted violently to albumin on one occasion may tolerate it well on another after being given an antihistamine such as diphenhydramine (1). Aggregates present in protein preparations may be the cause of some reactions. Another postulated cause may be the presence of antibodies against genetic variants of human albumin (2). Hypotensive reactions due to the presence of a prekallikrein activator in some batches of formulations can occur.

Albumin has been used to prevent the ovarian hyperstimulation syndrome (OHSS) associated with ovulation stimulation. In 98 women albumin had no positive effect on OHSS (3). Because of adverse effects, such as exacerbation of ascites in OHSS, nausea, vomiting, febrile reactions, allergic reactions, anaphylaxis, and the risk of pathogen transmission, albumin should not be used to prevent OHSS.

Adverse events during plasma exchanges in 28 adults with Guillain–Barré syndrome have been described in a study of 28 French and Swiss intensive care units (4). The study was based on 220 patients allocated either to plasma exchange or not. A total of 105 patients underwent 390 plasma exchanges (55 received albumin in 208 sessions as replacement fluid and 50 received fresh plasma in 182 sessions). Altogether, 253 adverse incidents were recorded, and in 15 patients plasma exchange had to be discontinued because of severe intolerance, which included bradycardia ($n = 3$), intercurrent complications (mainly infections), and technical difficulties. Fresh frozen plasma was associated with significantly more adverse incidents than albumin. The occurrence of adverse events was related to the preplasma exchange hemoglobin. Age, sex, previous history, neurological severity, and the need for mechanical ventilation did not modify the risk of adverse effects. The possibility that some of the events described in this series were attributable to the underlying disease rather than to the plasma exchange was not ruled out.

Organs and Systems

Cardiovascular

Albumin infusions can increase capillary permeability (5) and albumin infusion during resuscitation can result in hypervolemia, due to overfilling of the circulation (6).

It has been postulated that cardiac pump function can be reduced by binding of free calcium to albumin (6).

Metabolism

Acute normovolemic hemodilution to a hematocrit of 22% was performed in a prospective randomized study in 20 patients undergoing gynecological surgery (7). In one group 35% of the blood volume was replaced by 5% albumin while the other group received 6% hydroxyethyl starch solutions containing chloride concentrations of 150 and 15 mmol/l. Neither solution contained bicarbonate or citrate. After acute normovolemic hemodilution the blood volume remained constant in both groups. The plasma albumin concentration fell after hemodilution with hydroxyethyl starch and increased after hemodilution with albumin. There was a slight metabolic acidosis with hyperchloremia and a concomitant fall in anion gap in both groups. The acidosis, which was attributed to hyperchloremia and dilution of bicarbonate in the extracellular volume, was considered to be of no clinical relevance. The authors proposed that acidosis during acute normovolemic hemodilution can be avoided when the composition of electrolytes in colloid solutions is more physiological, as in lactate-buffered solutions.

Hematologic

Albumin can inhibit platelet aggregation (6). In addition, coagulation defects can result from dilution after albumin administration (6).

Liver

Intravenous albumin formulations contain a significant amount of ammonium, with concentrations up to 800 µmol/l (8). The concentration of ammonium seems to be batch dependent and related to storage time, the highest concentration being in the oldest formulations. Ammonium is probably liberated from protein and/or amino acids during storage, enhanced in the presence of oxygen. Although this might potentially contribute to deterioration of hepatic encephalopathy in patients receiving this treatment, that was not shown in this small study.

Immunologic

Immunological reactions to human serum albumin tend to be non-IgE-mediated anaphylactic reactions (0.011% of cases treated), about a third of which are life-threatening (9). A case in which the mechanism seemed to be IgE-mediated anaphylaxis against native albumin has been reported (10).

A meta-analysis of 193 albumin-treated women versus 185 controls showed a significant reduction of severe OHSS after administration of human albumin; two cases of urticaria and one case of an anaphylactic reaction were reported (11).

Death

In July 1998, The Cochrane Injuries Group Albumin Reviewers published a meta-analysis comparing the use of albumin with the use of crystalloids or no treatment in critically ill patients (12). The review was based on 30 randomized, controlled studies, involving a total of 1419 patients with hypovolemia due to trauma, surgery, burns, or hypoalbuminemia. There was excess mortality in the albumin group of about 6%, and the authors concluded that albumin should not be used outside rigorously conducted randomized controlled trials. The review elicited numerous mostly critical comments. For example, it was commented that a meta-analysis is not exact and that in this specific studythe study had conflated three separate indications that were not comparable (5).

An Expert Working Party of the Committee on Safety of Medicines was set up to examine these findings and to advise on any necessary regulatory action. The Working Party concluded that there is insufficient evidence of harm to warrant withdrawal of albumin products from the market and that the effect of albumin on mortality can only be discovered by conducting large, purpose-designed, randomized, controlled trials (13). It was recommended that a number of changes be made to the product information for human albumin. Specifically, the Expert Working Party recommended that the indication for human albumin solutions should be focused on the use of albumin to replace lost fluids, rather than the underlying illness that resulted in hypovolemia, and that albumin deficiency in itself was not an appropriate indication. The product information should contain warnings about the risks of hypervolemia and cardiovascular overload and emphasize that hemodynamic monitoring in patients who receive albumin should be undertaken to avoid these complications. A warning that special care should be taken when administering albumin in pathological states that affect capillary integrity should also be included.

However, the validity of these findings has been questioned, because some papers chosen for meta-analysis by the Cochrane group were suggested to have been incorrectly included (14,15). The results obtained from the meta-analysis have also been challenged by another meta-analysis of albumin administration in critically ill patients, which showed no increased risk in mortality (16). This illustrates the need for high-quality, randomized, controlled trials to generate definitive evidence.

Second-Generation Effects

Pregnancy

Hypovolemic shock due to acute blood loss during delivery is one of the major causes of maternal mortality. It has been suggested that albumin may increase the risk of death, and crystalloids have been suggested to be the volume expanders of choice (17).

Drug Administration

Drug contamination

Aluminium

Contamination of albumin solutions with aluminium and consequent toxic effects have been described (18). Analysis of albumin from 20 suppliers showed aluminium contents varying from 1.03 to 1301 µmol/l depending on the batch and the manufacturer (19). Aluminium overloading is especially likely to occur in patients with impaired renal function who receive large volumes of albumin, leading to osteodystrophy and encephalopathy (20).

The source of contamination is the fractionation apparatus and can be located to containers, filters, and final product containers. The increase in aluminium content over the shelf-life period is due to the fact that the glass vial releases aluminium ions. This process is catalysed by the residual citrate content of albumin formulations and depends on the storage temperature as well as on the relation of the inner glass surface to the amount of liquid. For 10 ml bottles, stability of the aluminium content below 200 ng/ml cannot be guaranteed for the shelf life, irrespective of storage conditions.

In 50 ml and 100 ml bottles stored at temperatures below 8°C, the increase in aluminium content is sufficiently slowed down, so that it does not rise beyond 200 ng/ml within the 3-year shelf life. However, at storage temperatures exceeding 8°C, the aluminium content can increase beyond 200 ng/ml. According to stability studies, this threshold value is not passed before 12 months of storage at these higher temperatures.

An Austrian manufacturer of human albumin 20 and 25% voluntarily recalled the products because the pharmacopoeial specification for aluminium (200 ng/ml or less) for treatment of premature infants and dialysis patients cannot be guaranteed over the whole shelf life of 3 years when stored at temperatures above 8°C (21).

The Paul Ehrlich Institut of Germany recalled certain batches of human albumin products (Human Albumin 20%, Human Albumin 20% Immuno, Human Albumin Immuno 20%, Human Albumin 25% Immuno), including batches that had exceeded 12 months of shelf life (22). This action was taken after quality assurance tests had shown that the aluminium content of these batches had exceeded the maximum acceptable concentration of 200 ng/ml.

Infections

The transmission of viral infections via albumin can be eliminated through pasteurization, and albumin treated in this way has an unblemished safety record in this regard, although there is little information on the safety of albumin with respect to hepatitis A and parvovirus (5). The production process excludes transmission of viruses such as hepatitis B and C and HIV (6). There have been no cases of HIV transmission attributed to this type of product, although many batches are known in retrospect to have been derived from HIV-contaminated pools (23).

Drug–Drug Interactions

ACE inhibitors

In a child with chronic renal insufficiency perioperative hypotension occurred after plasma volume expansion using 4% albumin (24). The fall in blood pressure was attributed to the combination of a low concentration of prekallikrein-activating factor in albumin and the use of an angiotensin-converting enzyme (ACE) inhibitor. When ACE is inhibited, the half-life of bradykinin is significantly prolonged and the concomitant administration of prekallikrein activator is likely to cause significant prolonged hypotension. To prevent this, the authors suggested withdrawing ACE inhibitors 24 hours before surgery or alternatively avoiding albumin in patients taking ACE inhibitors.

Furosemide

In children with the nephrotic syndrome, albumin in combination with furosemide carries a risk of thrombotic complications. In 12 children although antithrombin and alpha-2 macroglobulin fell, which is in accordance with a thrombotic tendency, there were no thrombotic complications (25). Furthermore, there was a fall in fibrinogen concentration, which is not consistent with a thrombotic tendency.

References

1. Edelman BB, Straughn MA, Getz P, Schwartz E. Uneventful plasma exchange with albumin replacement in a patient with a previous anaphylactoid reaction to albumin. Transfusion 1985;25(5):435–6.
2. Naylor DH, Anhorn CA, Laschinger C, Males F, Chodirker WB. Antigenic differences between normal human albumin and a genetic variant. Transfusion 1982;22(2):128–33.
3. Ben-Chetrit A, Eldar-Geva T, Gal M, Huerta M, Mimon T, Algur N, Diamant YZ, Margalioth EJ. The questionable use of albumin for the prevention of ovarian hyperstimulation syndrome in an IVF programme: a randomized placebo-controlled trial. Hum Reprod 2001;16(9):1880–4.
4. Bouget J, Chevret S, Chastang C, Raphael JC. Plasma exchange morbidity in Guillain-Barré syndrome: results from the French prospective, randomized, multicenter study. The French Cooperative Group. Crit Care Med 1993;21(5):651–8.
5. Drummond GB, Ludlam CA. Is albumin harmful? Br J Haematol 1999;106(2):266–9.
6. Tjoeng MM, Bartelink AK, Thijs LG. Exploding the albumin myth. Pharm World Sci 1999;21(1):17–20.
7. Rehm M, Orth V, Scheingraber S, Kreimeier U, Brechtelsbauer H, Finsterer U. Acid-base changes caused by 5% albumin versus 6% hydroxyethyl starch solution in patients undergoing acute normovolemic hemodilution: a randomized prospective study. Anesthesiology 2000;93(5):1174–83.
8. Chamuleau RA, Jorning GG, Korse FG, Roos PJ. Ammonium in intravenous albumin preparations. Lancet 1993;342(8879):1110–11.
9. Ring J, Messmer K. Incidence and severity of anaphylactoid reactions to colloid volume substitutes. Lancet 1977;1(8009):466–9.
10. Stafford CT, Lobel SA, Fruge BC, Moffitt JE, Hoff RG, Fadel HE. Anaphylaxis to human serum albumin. Ann Allergy 1988;61(2):85–8.
11. Aboulghar M, Evers JH, Al-Inany H. Intravenous albumin for preventing severe ovarian hyperstimulation syndrome: a Cochrane review. Hum Reprod 2002;17(12):3027–32.
12. Roberts I, Berger A. Human albumin administration in critically ill patients: systematic review of randomised controlled trials. Cochrane Injuries Group Albumin Reviewers. BMJ 1998;317(7153):235–40.
13. Anonymous. Albumin (human)—review of safety: conclusions. WHO Pharm Newslett 1999;7/8:1.
14. Waller C. Albumin and hypovolaemia. Lancet 2002;359(9325):2278.
15. Horsey P. Albumin and hypovolaemia: is the Cochrane evidence to be trusted? Lancet 2002;359(9300):70–2.
16. Dubois MJ, Vincent JL. Use of albumin in the intensive care unit. Curr Opin Crit Care 2002;8(4):299–301.
17. Hofmeyr GJ, Mohlala BK. Hypovolaemic shock. Best Pract Res Clin Obstet Gynaecol 2001;15(4):645–62.
18. el Habib R, Eygonnet JP. Aluminium bone disease. BMJ (Clin Res Ed) 1987;295(6610):1415–16.
19. Maharaj D, Fell GS, Boyce BF, Ng JP, Smith GD, Boulton-Jones JM, Cumming RL, Davidson JF. Aluminium bone disease in patients receiving plasma exchange with contaminated albumin. BMJ (Clin Res Ed) 1987;295(6600):693–6.
20. Anonymous. Encephalopathy. Encephalopathy 1992;92.
21. Anonymous. Albumin (human) batches withdrawn: increase in aluminium levels. WHO Newsletter 1998;9/10:1.
22. Anonymous. Albumin (human) batches withdrawn: increase in aluminium levels. WHO Newsletter 1999;1/2:1.
23. Cuthbertson B, Rennie JG, Aw D, Reid KG. Safety of albumin preparations manufactured from plasma not tested for HIV antibody. Lancet 1987;2(8549):41.
24. Fong SY, Hansen TG. Perioperative hypotension following plasma volume expansion with albumin in an angiotensin-converting enzyme inhibited infant. Br J Anaesth 2000;84(4):537–8.
25. Bircan Z, Katar S, Batum S, Yavuz Yilmaz A, Comert S, Vitrinel A. The effect of albumin and furosemide therapy on hemostatic parameters in nephrotic children. Int Pediatr 2001;16:235–7.

Alclofenac

See also Non-steroidal anti-inflammatory drugs

General Information

While the pattern of alclofenac toxicity resembles that of other NSAIDs, the frequency of adverse effects differs widely. Allergic reactions have been reported more frequently and skin rashes have been particularly common. Hypersensitivity reactions, including anaphylactic shock, severe generalized vasculitis, hepatotoxicity, and nephrotoxicity, have been observed. Alclofenac has therefore been withdrawn in several countries (1). Blood dyscrasias and neurological symptoms are rare.

Reference

1. Morison WL, Baughman RD, Day RM, Forbes PD, Hoenigsmann H, Krueger GG, Lebwohl M, Lew R, Naldi L, Parrish JA, Piepkorn M, Stern RS, Weinstein GD, Whitmore SE. Consensus workshop on the toxic effects of long-term PUVA therapy. Arch Dermatol 1998;134(5):595–8.

Alcuronium

See also Neuromuscular blocking drugs

General Information

Alcuronium is a synthetic derivative of toxiferine, an alkaloid of calabash curare, and is a non-depolarizing relaxant with properties and adverse effects similar to those of D-tubocurarine. It is about twice as potent as D-tubocurarine, 0.15–0.25 mg/kg usually being adequate for abdominal relaxation, and has a similar onset time and a slightly shorter duration of action. It is bound to albumin (40%), and requirements for alcuronium are less if the plasma albumin levels are low, as may occur in hepatic disease.

Like D-tubocurarine, alcuronium does not undergo biotransformation. Excretion occurs mainly in the urine (80–85%), but, as with D-tubocurarine, some is also excreted in the bile (15–20%) (1). Persistent relaxation has been reported in renal insufficiency (2) and the drug is relatively contraindicated in this condition.

Organs and Systems

Cardiovascular

Tachycardia, hypotension, and a fall in total peripheral resistance all occur to an extent similar to that seen with D-tubocurarine, according to most studies (3–6). Others have reported that these effects are short-lived (7). Doses of 0.2 mg/kg or more may be associated with the more extreme cardiovascular effects. Blockade of cardiac muscarinic receptors (8), histamine release, and, possibly, some ganglionic blockade (although it has a very low

ganglion-blocking activity in animals) (8) may all play a role in the production of the cardiovascular effects of alcuronium.

Nervous system

Two patients in intensive care treated with infusions of large amounts of alcuronium developed fixed dilated pupils. Within 6–24 hours after stopping the infusion the pupils became normally reactive again (9).

This is a very important and dangerous adverse effect, since the presence of fixed dilated pupils may lead to the mistaken diagnosis of brain death in coma patients if other neurological diagnostic procedures are not carried out.

Immunologic

Histamine release and anaphylactoid reactions occur with alcuronium (10–12). The precise incidence is not clear. Erythema is said to occur much less frequently than after D-tubocurarine (3). A retrospective study in Australia (13) showed that 37% of serious anaphylactoid reactions reported there were associated with alcuronium; alcuronium, however, at that time accounted for almost 50% of the total muscle relaxant consumption in Australia, and if this is taken into account the likelihood of a serious reaction is less than with D-tubocurarine, as others have also concluded (14). Clinical features reported range from erythema to severe hypotension and tachycardia (15) and bronchospasm (16,17). In a large prospective surveillance study (SEDA-15, 125) (SED-12, 473) involving over 1400 patients given alcuronium (initial dose 0.25 + 0.09 mg/kg), there were adverse reactions in almost 18% of the patients, with moderate hypotension (20–50% fall) in 13%, severe hypotension in 0.8%, and bronchospasm in 0.1%.

Second-Generation Effects

Fetotoxicity

Placental transfer (SEDA-6, 130) (18), occurs and is increased if alcuronium is rapidly injected (19). No complications attributable to neuromuscular block were seen in the newborn.

Susceptibility Factors

Hepatic disease

In liver cancer in children, resistance to alcuronium has been reported (SEDA-13, 104) (20).

Other features of the patient

In patients with burns, dosage requirements are increased (21).

Drug–Drug Interactions

Penicillamine

Penicillamine-induced myasthenia gravis (SED-10, 415) was probably the cause of extremely prolonged apnea occurring in two patients given alcuronium (SEDA-12, 111) (22,23). Patients receiving penicillamine should be treated as if they had no myasthenia; if a muscle relaxant is required, they should be given a test dose (of about one-tenth the usual dose), with monitoring of the response, before a full dose is administered.

References

1. Raaflaub J, Frey P. Pharmakokinetik von Diallylnortoxiferin beim Menschen. [Pharmacokinetics of diallyl-nor-toxiferine in man.] Arzneimittelforschung 1972;22(1):73–8.
2. Havill JH, Mee AD, Wallace MR, Chin LS, Rothwell RP. Prolonged curarisation in the presence of renal impairment. Anaesth Intensive Care 1978;6(3):234–8.
3. Pandit SK, Dundee JW, Stevenson HM. A clinical comparison of pancuronium with tubocurarine and alcuronium in major cardiothoracic surgery. Anesth Analg 1971;50(6):926–35.
4. Coleman AJ, Downing JW, Leary WP, Moyes DG, Styles M. The immediate cardiovascular effects of pancuronium, alcuronium and tubocurarine in man. Anaesthesia 1972;27(4):415–22.
5. Baraka A. A comparative study between diallylnortoxiferine and tubocurarine. Br J Anaesth 1967;39(8):624–8.
6. Brandli FR. Pancuronium und Alcuronium: Ein klinischer Vergleich. [Pancuronium and alcuronium: a clinical comparison.] Prakt Anaesth 1976;11:239.
7. Tammisto T, Welling I. The effect of alcuronium and tubocurarine on blood pressure and heart rate: a clinical comparison. Br J Anaesth 1969;41(4):317–22.
8. Hughes R, Chapple DJ. Effects on non-depolarizing neuromuscular blocking agents on peripheral autonomic mechanisms in cats. Br J Anaesth 1976;48(2):59–68.
9. Rao U, Milligan KR. Fixed dilated pupils associated with alcuronium infusions. Anaesthesia 1993;48(10):917.
10. Chan CS, Yeung ML. Anaphylactic reaction to alcuronium. Case report. Br J Anaesth 1972;44(1):103–5.
11. Rowley RW. Hypersensitivity reaction to diallyl nortoxiferine (Alloferine). Anaesth Intensive Care 1975;3:74.
12. Fisher MM, Hallowes RC, Wilson RM. Anaphylaxis to alcuronium. Anaesth Intensive Care 1978;6(2):125–8.
13. Fisher MM, Munro I. Life-threatening anaphylactoid reactions to muscle relaxants. Anesth Analg 1983;62(6):559–64.
14. Galletly DC, Treuren BC. Anaphylactoid reactions during anaesthesia. Seven years' experience of intradermal testing. Anaesthesia 1985;40(4):329–33.
15. Panning B, Peest D, Kirchner E, Schedel I. Anaphylaktoider Schock nach Alloferin. [Anaphylactoid shock following Alloferin.] Anaesthesist 1985;34(4):211–12.
16. Fadel R, Herpin-Richard N, Rassemont R, Salomon J, David B, Laurent M, Henocq E. Choc anaphylactique à la diallylnortoxiferine: étude clinique et immunologique. [Anaphylactic shock from diallylnortoxiferine. Clinical and immunological studies.] Ann Fr Anesth Réanim 1982;1(5):531–4.
17. Plotz J, Schreiber W. Vergleichende Untersuchung von Atracurium und Alcuronium zur Intubation älterer Patienten in Halothannarkose. [Comparative study of atracurium and alcuronium for the intubation of older patients in halothane anesthesia.] Anaesthesist 1984;33(11):548–51.
18. Ho PC, Stephens ID, Triggs EJ. Caesarean section and placental transfer of alcuronium. Anaesth Intensive Care 1981;9(2):113–18.
19. Thomas J, Climie CR, Mather LE. The placental transfer of alcuronium. A preliminary report. Br J Anaesth 1969;41(4):297–302.
20. Brown TC, Gregory M, Bell B, Campbell PC. Liver tumours and muscle relaxants. Electromyographic studies in children. Anaesthesia 1987;42(12):1284–6.
21. Sarubin J. Erhöhter Bedarf an Alloferin bei Verbrennungspatienten. [Increased requirement of alcuronium in burned patients.] Anaesthesist 1982;31(8):392–5.
22. Fried MJ, Protheroe DT. D-penicillamine induced myasthenia gravis. Its relevance for the anaesthetist. Br J Anaesth 1986;58(10):1191–3.
23. Blanloeil Y, Baron D, Gazeau MF, Nicolas F. Curarisation prolongée au cours d'un syndrôme myasthénique induit par la D-pénicillamine. [Prolonged neuromuscular blockade during D-penicillamine-induced myasthenia.] Anesth Analg (Paris) 1980;37(7–8):441–3.

Aldesleukin

General Information

Aldesleukin (interleukin-2, celmoleukin, proleukin, teceleukin) is produced by activated T lymphocytes and has pleiotropic immunological effects, including the proliferation of T lymphocytes. Non-glycosylated recombinant aldesleukin has been approved for the treatment of metastatic renal cell carcinoma (1) and is also being investigated in other malignant neoplasms. Low-dose aldesleukin is a relatively safe treatment of HIV infection (SEDA-20, 334).

The adverse effects of aldesleukin include fever, chills, malaise, skin rash, nausea, vomiting (often resistant to antiemetics), diarrhea, fluid retention, myalgia, insomnia, disorientation, life-threatening hypotension, and the capillary leak syndrome (which can be preceded by weight gain) (SEDA-15, 491) (2).

In early trials, aldesleukin was given with lymphokine-activated killer (LAK) cells or tumor-infiltrating lymphocytes. However, later data showed that the addition of LAK cells does not improve the therapeutic response in renal cell carcinoma and can produce more pulmonary toxicity and hypotension (1). Compared with aldesleukin or interferon alfa alone, the combination of aldesleukin plus interferon alfa produces a significantly longer event-free survival without effect on the overall survival, but induces substantial toxicity with severe and resistant hypotension (3). The optimal safe and effective dose and schedule of administration of aldesleukin is not yet well defined, and a variety of regimens have been tested, with doses of 600 000 units/kg by intermittent bolus intravenous infusion or 18 106 units/m² by continuous subcutaneous or intravenous infusion.

Considerable efforts have been made to limit the toxic effects of aldesleukin, which are dose- and schedule-dependent (4). Low-dose aldesleukin, continuous infusion, and/or subcutaneous administration are preferred by various investigators, because of their reluctance to use conventional high-dose or bolus dose administration. Such regimens were considered as effective and safe for outpatients (5,6).

A thorough analysis of 255 patients from seven phase II trials treated with the currently recommended high dose of aldesleukin for metastatic renal cell carcinoma has been presented (7). Although severe toxicity, generally attributable to the capillary leak syndrome, was found in most patients, the problems receded promptly after withdrawal of treatment. Deaths related to aldesleukin-induced toxicity were reported in 4% of patients, and were caused by myocardial infarction, respiratory failure, gastrointestinal toxicity, or sepsis.

Use in patients with HIV infection

The use, benefits, and adverse effects of aldesleukin in HIV-infected patients have been extensively reviewed (8). Aldesleukin significantly increased the $CD4^+$ cell count without an increase in viral load. However, many questions remain unanswered. In particular, it is still not known whether immunological improvements translate into clinical benefit. Regardless of how aldesleukin is administered—intravenously, subcutaneously, or as polyethylene glycol-modified (pegylated) aldesleukin—adverse effects are generally not treatment-limiting. As the duration of adverse effects was shorter with the subcutaneous route, these patients may be treated as outpatients (9).

In two randomized, controlled studies (44 patients given subcutaneous aldesleukin, 58 given a modified-release polyethylene glycol-modified formulation, 27 given continuous intravenous aldesleukin, and 50 controls), aldesleukin was well tolerated and a minority of patients required drug withdrawal because of adverse events (10,11). The overall adverse effects profile of both routes of administration was very similar, but was substantially less severe than previously described with high-dose aldesleukin. It consisted mostly of fatigue, nasal/sinus congestion, fever above 38°C, headache, gastrointestinal disorders, stomatitis, somnolence, and mood change. Increased bilirubin and alanine transaminase activities were more frequent than in the control group. None of the patients developed the capillary leak syndrome or significant hypertension, but cardiomyopathy, attempted suicide, ulcerative colitis, and exacerbation of hepatitis B were identified in one patient each among 85 patients treated with aldesleukin (10). Erythema and injection site reactions were observed in 66–69% of patients who received subcutaneous aldesleukin, and skin biopsies showed a perivascular infiltrate with lymphocytes and some eosinophils.

Use in patients with metastatic melanoma

In an analysis of data from 270 patients with metastatic melanoma in eight clinical trials, high-dose aldesleukin (8.4–9.8 MU/kg during each cycle) produced an overall objective response rate of 16%, with 17 complete responses and 26 partial responses (12). Although the response rate was low, there was a durable response for at least 24 months in 10 of 17 complete responders. Adverse effects were primarily the same as those previously described in patients with metastatic renal cell carcinoma, and severe hypotension (64%) was the most frequent. Six patients died from bacterial sepsis, but none was taking prophylactic antibiotics.

In a randomized trial, 102 patients with metastatic melanoma had more frequent treatment-related adverse effects, particularly hematological suppression in patients

treated with tamoxifen, cisplatin, and dacarbazine followed by interferon alfa and aldesleukin, than in patients treated with chemotherapy alone, but there was no increase in survival (13).

General adverse effects

The frequencies of severe adverse effects of aldesleukin (7) are listed in Table 1 and the most frequent reasons for withdrawal of high-dose intravenous aldesleukin in Table 2.

Table 1 The frequencies of severe adverse effects of aldesleukin

General symptoms	
Fever and chills	24%
Weakness	4%
Edema	2%
Sepsis	6%
Cardiovascular	
Hypotension	74%
Supraventricular dysrhythmias	3%
Myocardial damage (angina, infarction)	4%
Respiratory	
Dyspnea	17%
Adult respiratory distress syndrome	<1%
Respiratory failure	2%
Nervous system	
Coma, seizures	4%
Psychiatric	
Behavioral changes	28%
Hematologic	
Thrombocytopenia	21%
Anemia	18%
Gastrointestinal	
Nausea and vomiting	25%
Diarrhea	22%
Stomatitis	4%
Gastrointestinal bleeding	4%
Intestinal perforation	<1%
Liver	
Hyperbilirubinemia	21%
Raised transaminases	10%
Raised alkaline phosphatase	9%
Urinary tract	
Oliguria or anuria	46%
Raised blood urea nitrogen	16%
Raised serum creatinine	14%
Acidosis	6%
Skin	
Pruritus and erythema	4%
Musculoskeletal	
Arthralgia	1%
Myalgia	1%
Death	4%

Table 2 The most frequent reasons for withdrawal of high-dose intravenous aldesleukin

Constitutional symptoms	17%
Cardiovascular	
Hypotension	19%
Atrial dysrhythmias	10%
Respiratory	
Pulmonary toxicity	12%
Nervous system	
Disorientation	10%
Hematologic	
Thrombocytopenia	7%
Gastrointestinal	
Nausea or vomiting	4%
Diarrhea	6%
Liver	
Hyperbilirubinemia	5%
Urinary tract	
Oliguria	9%
Raised creatinine concentration	13%

High-dose aldesleukin is associated with a wide range of adverse effects, and practical guidelines for their avoidance and management have been detailed (14). Constitutional symptoms (malaise, fever, chills and asthenia) are universal in patients treated with high-dose aldesleukin (4). Although they are usually suppressed by paracetamol (acetaminophen), indometacin, or pethidine, they are one of the major reasons for stopping treatment. Myalgia and arthralgia are sometimes associated with the flu-like symptoms.

A wide range of aldesleukin-induced adverse effects is associated with the capillary leak syndrome, which is characterized by an increase in vascular permeability with subsequent leakage of fluids and proteins into the extravascular space (4). This results in a third–space clinical syndrome, generalized or peripheral edema, weight gain, cardiovascular and pulmonary complications with hypotension, pericardial, and pleural effusions, ascites, oliguria, and prerenal azotemia. Symptoms usually resolve in a few days after aldesleukin withdrawal. Studies on the mechanism have raised a number of hypotheses, such as damage to the endothelial cells, release of secondary cytokines, and activation of the complement cascade (15).

Denileukin diftitox

Denileukin diftitox is a fusion protein formed by binding human aldesleukin to the cytotoxic A chain of diphtheria toxin. This product binds to the aldesleukin receptor and inhibits protein synthesis, resulting in cell death. It has been approved for treatment of persistent or recurrent cutaneous T cell lymphoma and is being evaluated in patients with severe psoriasis.

In 71 patients with cutaneous T cell lymphomas randomized to denileukin diftitox 9 or 18 μg/kg/day, flu-like and gastrointestinal symptoms were observed in 92%

(16). About 60% had an acute hypersensitivity reaction, with dyspnea, back pain, hypotension, and chest pain or tightness within 24 hours of infusion. A vascular leak syndrome, as defined by the presence of at least two of edema, hypoalbuminemia, and hypotension, occurred in 25%.

A dose-escalation study in 35 patients with psoriasis confirmed that constitutional symptoms in response to denileukin diftitox were dose-related and less frequent at lower doses (below 5 micrograms/kg/day) (17). There was only one case of mild vascular leak syndrome. Skin reactions compatible with delayed hypersensitivity reactions were noted in three patients, including one case of exfoliative dermatitis.

The more severe adverse effects of denileukin diftitox consisted of acute hypersensitivity reactions during or within 24 hours of infusion in 69% of patients, and a vascular leak syndrome in 27% of patients, which was severe in 6%. In contrast to acute hypersensitivity reactions, the vascular leak syndrome was typically delayed and occurred within the first 2 weeks of infusion (18). Whether this was due to a direct action of denileukin diftitox or to tumor lysis syndrome is unknown.

Organs and Systems

Cardiovascular

Hemodynamic and cardiac complications are the major limitations of high-dose aldesleukin and have been described in both adults (19,20) and children (21). Significant hypotension requiring meticulous maintenance therapy with intravenous fluids or low-dose vasopressors was observed in most patients (22). The clinical findings were very similar to the hemodynamic pattern seen in early septic shock. Aldesleukin-induced increases in plasma nitrate and nitrite concentrations correlated with the severity of hypotension (23).

Among other cardiovascular complications, cardiac dysrhythmias were reported in 6–10% of patients, angina pectoris or documented myocardial infarction in 3–4%, and mortality due to myocardial infarction in 1–2% (4). Severe myocardial dysfunction, myocarditis, and cardiomyopathy have been seldom reported (SED-13, 1103) (SEDA-20, 334) (SEDA-22, 406).

The cardiopulmonary toxicity of high-dose intravenous bolus aldesleukin has been analysed in 199 metastatic melanoma or renal cell carcinoma patients without underlying cardiac disease (24). Cardiovascular events occurred within hours after starting infusion, persisted throughout aldesleukin therapy, and normalized within 1–3 days after treatment withdrawal. Hypotension was the most frequent adverse effect (53% of treatment courses) and resolved promptly with vasopressor treatment. Unexpectedly, the response to treatment was significantly better in patients with melanoma who had hypotension. There were cardiac dysrhythmias in 9% of patients; they mostly consisted of easily manageable atrial fibrillation or supraventricular tachycardia. Further courses of aldesleukin in 11 of these patients produced recurrent dysrhythmias in only two, and long-term treatment of dysrhythmias was never required. High-degree atrioventricular block and repetitive episodes of ventricular tachycardia were each observed once. Although 11% of patients had raised creatine kinase activity before or during treatment, only 2.5% had a documented rise in the MB isoenzyme fraction.

At-risk patients include those with pre-existing cardiac disease, whereas age, performance status, and sex are not significantly associated with cardiopulmonary toxicity. In view of this risk, it is reasonable to monitor cardiac function and creatine kinase activity closely in all patients, or to exclude those with significant underlying coronary or cardiorespiratory disease. Pretreatment cardiac screening has greatly reduced the incidence of myocardial infarction, ischemia, and related dysrhythmias, and two-dimensional and Doppler echocardiography was suggested to be helpful to anticipate cardiovascular toxicity (25). A reduction in systemic vascular resistance, stroke work index, and left ventricular ejection fraction are usually involved in the pathophysiology of cardiac dysfunction. Clinical, electrocardiographic, and radionuclide ventriculography monitoring in 22 patients undergoing a 5-day continuous intravenous infusion of aldesleukin for various cancers showed that reversible left ventricular dysfunction accounted for most of the observed hemodynamic changes (26). Indeed, significant coronary disease was usually not observed in patients undergoing cardiac catheterization, which argues for direct myocardial damage (24). In isolated reports, clinical and histological findings of eosinophilic, lymphocytic, or mixed lymphocytic–eosinophilic myocarditis also suggested an immune-mediated drug reaction (SED-13, 1103) (SEDA-22, 406).

Aldesleukin-induced cardiac eosinophilic infiltration has been reported (27).

- After 25 days of treatment with continuous aldesleukin infusion (up to 150 000 units/kg/day) for stage IV Hodgkin's disease, a 26-year-old woman had increased fatigue, tachycardia, hypotension, and hypothermia. Echocardiography showed bilateral intraventricular masses. Her maximal absolute eosinophil count was $11.4 \times 10^9/l$ and the platelet count was $17 \times 10^9/l$. Despite aldesleukin withdrawal, her condition deteriorated and she died. Postmortem examination showed biventricular thrombi and prominent eosinophilic infiltration of the endomyocardium.

Of 10 subsequent patients who received prolonged infusions of aldesleukin and were monitored by echocardiography, one developed asymptomatic changes in cardiac function, with features suggestive of early thrombus formation and a reduced ejection fraction during weeks 6–8. The maximal absolute eosinophil count was $5 \times 10^9/l$. These abnormalities resolved on aldesleukin withdrawal.

Conjugates of aldesleukin with polyethylene glycol produce less cardiovascular toxicity (SEDA-20, 333).

Respiratory

Dose-related cough has been reported as the most frequent adverse effect of inhaled aldesleukin (28).

Among 199 patients with metastatic melanoma or renal cell carcinoma treated with high-dose intravenous bolus aldesleukin, there was severe respiratory distress in 3.2% of treatment courses, but intubation was required in only one (24). This is far less common than earlier estimates

that 10–30% of patients develop respiratory distress severe enough to warrant mechanical ventilation in 5–20% of cases (4). The improvement may be related to the current strict selection criteria for the evaluation of pulmonary function, limited fluid management strategy, prophylactic antibiotics, and prompt withdrawal of treatment in patients presenting with shortness of breath, rales, or persistent hypoxemia.

Pulmonary features of the adverse effects of aldesleukin include lung opacities, diffuse pulmonary interstitial edema, pleural effusions, alveolar edema, and hypoxemia, with full and rapid recovery after treatment withdrawal (29,30).

Aldesleukin-induced increase in lung capillary permeability or direct cardiac dysfunction is thought to be a likely mechanism of this adverse effect, and a localized vascular leak syndrome, attributed to activation of eosinophils in the lung and subsequent deposition of the eosinophil major basic protein, has also been suggested, as reported in a 49-year-old woman with breast cancer (31).

There is no significant association between pre-existing clinical dysfunction and radiological interstitial edema (30). Very severe adult respiratory distress syndrome requiring double lung transplantation has been reported in one patient (32).

Nervous system

Severe pain resulting from a previously asymptomatic thoracic spine metastasis has been attributed to aldesleukin in a 64-year-old man with metastatic renal cell carcinoma (33).

Fatal acute leukoencephalopathy with brain perivascular foci demyelination (34) and delayed progressive cognitive dysfunction (35) have been reported in isolated cases.

The neurotoxicity of aldesleukin is usually dose-related and can be treatment-limiting (36).

Sensory systems

Transient episodes of amaurosis or scotomata, both of which recurred after aldesleukin rechallenge, have been described (37). Three other patients had visual phenomena, including diplopia, scotomata, and palinopsia during treatment, which resolved on withdrawal of aldesleukin (38).

Psychological, psychiatric

Aldesleukin can cause moderate impairment of cognitive function, with disorientation, confusion, hallucinations, sleep disturbances, and sometimes severe behavioral changes requiring transient neuroleptic drug administration (39–41). Some of the cognitive deficits mimicked those observed in dementias, such as Alzheimer's disease. Several studies have also shown increased latency and reduced amplitude of event-related evoked potentials in patients with cognitive impairment (41,42). Other infrequent adverse effects included paranoid delusions, hallucinations, loss of interest, sleep disturbances or drowsiness, reduced energy, fatigue, anorexia, and malaise. Coma and seizures were exceptionally noted.

Symptoms occurred within 1 week of treatment and complete recovery was usually noted after aldesleukin withdrawal.

In 10 patients with advanced tumors, low-dose subcutaneous aldesleukin produced significant psychological changes; increased depression scores, psychasthenia, and conversion hysteria were the most common findings (43).

The short-term occurrence of depressive symptoms has been investigated by using the Montgomery and Asberg Depression Rating Scale (MADRS) before and after 3 and 5 days of treatment in 48 patients without a previous psychiatric history and treated for renal cell carcinoma or melanoma with aldesleukin alone ($n = 20$), aldesleukin plus interferon alfa-2b ($n = 6$), or interferon alfa-2b alone ($n = 22$) (44). On day 5, patients in the aldesleukin groups had significantly higher MADRS scores, whereas there were no significant changes in the patients who received interferon alfa-2b alone. Eight of 26 patients given aldesleukin and only three of 22 given interferon alfa-2b alone had severe depressive symptoms. Depressive symptoms occurred as early as the second day of aldesleukin treatment and were more severe in the patients who received both cytokines. Early detection of mood changes can be useful in pinpointing patients at risk of subsequent severe neuropsychiatric complications.

Neuropsychiatric symptoms are less frequent with subcutaneous aldesleukin (4). No predictive or predisposing factors have been clearly identified. Whether a direct effect of aldesleukin on neuronal tissues, an increased vascular brain permeability with a subsequent increased brain water content, or an aldesleukin-induced release of neuroendocrine hormones (beta-endorphin, ACTH, or cortisol), accounted for these effects, is unknown. A possible immune-mediated cerebral vasculitis has also been reported in one patient (SEDA-20, 334).

Endocrine

Various hormonal and metabolic effects of aldesleukin are temporally related to hypotension. Transient serum rises in ACTH, cortisol, beta-endorphin, adrenaline and noradrenaline have been found, whereas there were no significant changes in the plasma concentrations of several other hormones (4).

An acute episode of adrenal insufficiency secondary to adrenal hemorrhage occurred in one patient receiving aldesleukin (45).

Thyroid

Since the first reports of hypothyroidism, a number of studies have reported the occurrence of thyroid dysfunction in patients receiving aldesleukin alone or in combination with LAK cells, interferon alfa, interferon gamma, or tumor necrosis factor alfa (SED-13, 1104) (46). Symptoms were usually observed after 2–4 months of treatment (47–49), and mostly consisted of moderate hypothyroidism, which resolved after immunotherapy withdrawal or thyroxine treatment (49,50). Patients treated with aldesleukin plus interferon alfa more commonly developed biphasic thyroiditis with subsequent hypothyroidism or hyperthyroidism (50–53).

The possibility of a positive correlation between the development of thyroid dysfunction and the probability of a favorable tumor response has been debated (47,49,54). The incidence of thyroid dysfunction did not correlate with the dose or the underlying disease, but increased with treatment duration (46). In a large survey of 281 cancer patients receiving low-dose (72 000 IU/kg) or high-dose (720 000 IU/kg) aldesleukin, up to 41% of previously euthyroid cancer patients developed thyroid dysfunction (55). Combined immunotherapy was also associated with more frequent thyroid disorders. Aldesleukin plus interferon alfa produced thyroid dysfunction in 20–91% of patients (46), and the incidence of laboratory thyroid dysfunction reached 100% in patients given five or six cycles of both cytokines (51). Aldesleukin plus interferon alfa also tended to be a risk factor for the development of biphasic thyroiditis (49).

Female sex and the presence of antithyroid antibodies correlated significantly with the development of thyroid disease (49,56). This, together with the findings of strong expression of HLA-DR antigens on thyrocytes or the presence of mononuclear cell infiltrates on histological examination of the thyroid, makes an autoimmune phenomenon likely (49,52). However, a possible direct effect of immunotherapy on thyroid hormonal function has also been suggested in patients who had no detectable thyroid antibodies. There was a significant decrease in TSH concentration, while thyroid autoantibodies were not significantly raised (57).

Metabolism

Reversible insulin-dependent diabetes mellitus has been described in a predisposed patient (SEDA-20, 334).

Aldesleukin can cause lipid disorders. Recurrent and marked hypocholesterolemia with reduced high- and low-density lipoproteins, and slight increases in plasma triglycerides have been observed after high-dose aldesleukin (SEDA-21, 375) (4).

Nutrition

Severe, but reversible hypovitaminosis C was noted in patients receiving high-dose aldesleukin plus LAK cells (58).

Hematologic

Hematological adverse effects of aldesleukin typically included transient anemia, thrombocytopenia, eosinophilia, neutropenia, extreme lymphopenia, and rebound lymphocytosis (4,59). Transient suppression of hemopoiesis by secondary cytokines, peripheral platelet destruction, and increased endothelium margination of lymphocytes are possible mechanisms.

Hematological toxicity was analysed in 199 patients treated with a high-dose intravenous bolus aldesleukin regimen for metastatic melanoma or renal cell carcinoma (60). Anemia requiring transfusions was noted in 14% of all treatment courses and severe thrombocytopenia occurred in 2.2%, with three patients suffering from serious hemorrhages. Severe leukopenia was infrequent and not associated with infectious episodes. Early transient lymphopenia (93% reduction) was followed by rebound lymphocytosis up to 198% above baseline values. Except for severe thrombocytopenia, treatment withdrawal was not required in this study. Other investigators found that reductions in platelet count correlated with a significant increase in ex vivo platelet functional activity, but there were no episodes of bleeding or thrombosis (61).

Aldesleukin can produce sustained eosinophilia, possibly mediated by interleukin-5 or GM-CSF, but this was not associated with allergic reactions (62).

In 42 patients with advanced cancer treated with aldesleukin and lymphokine-activated killer cells from autologous lymphocytes, there were reduced numbers of circulating erythroid and granulocyte/macrophage progenitors, with recovery after withdrawal (63). Patients developed severe anemia (partly due to phlebotomy, cytopheresis, and hemodilution), thrombocytopenia, lymphopenia, and eosinophilia, with mild neutropenia and rebound lymphocytosis after treatment was stopped.

The severity of hematological disorders was not affected by previous chemotherapy for metastatic melanoma or renal cell carcinoma and there was no correlation with response to treatment (60). However, others have found that moderate to severe dose-related thrombocytopenia occurred particularly in patients previously treated with cytotoxic agents (64). Subcutaneous low-dose aldesleukin therapy reduced the frequency and intensity of hematological toxicity, and the combination of aldesleukin plus interferon alfa produced either moderate additional toxicity or no significant enhancement (65).

Most patients develop significant, but promptly reversible coagulation disorders with prolongation of the partial thromboplastin time (the most frequent effect), hypoprothrombinemia, and reduced functional concentrations of several clotting factors II, IX, X, XI, and XII (60,66,67). No clear mechanism of aldesleukin-induced coagulopathy has been identified, and the efficacy of prophylactic vitamin K has been disputed (67). Other data suggest that aldesleukin may activate the coagulation and fibrinolytic system (64,68), but the clinical relevance of these findings is not clear.

A mean splenic index increase of 64% was found on computed tomography after a mean of 66 days of aldesleukin treatment for non-hematological malignancies (69). Splenomegaly persisted after an average of 215 days after the completion of aldesleukin treatment and was not associated with tumor progression.

Mouth and teeth

Oral effects of aldesleukin include xerostomia with reversible salivary gland hypofunction, a burning sensation in the mouth, taste disorders, mucosal atrophy, mucositis, glossitis, and ulcerative lesions (70,71).

Gastrointestinal

Minor gastrointestinal adverse effects, that is anorexia, nausea, vomiting, and diarrhea, were noted in about 80% of patients (4).

Incidental case reports included symptomatic exacerbation of Crohn's disease (72) and transient painful swelling of the appendix (SEDA-21, 376).

Severe and sometimes fatal intestinal complications have been described in 1.3–7% of patients receiving aldesleukin alone or in combination with LAK cells or interferon alfa, including intestinal ischemia, bowel ulceration or perforation, and colosplenic fistula (73–75). It has been suggested that severe diarrhea may be an indicator of subsequent colonic ischemia (75).

Liver

Mild liver dysfunction, hypophosphatemia, and hypomagnesmia are the most common laboratory abnormalities caused by aldesleukin (76,77). About 20% of patients develop mild to severe intrahepatic cholestasis with reversible and dose-dependent rises in bilirubin and alkaline phosphatase while serum transaminases were only slightly increased (4,78). Recurrence of cholestasis after aldesleukin rechallenge was not always observed (79). The mechanism of aldesleukin-induced intrahepatic cholestasis is unknown, but it might be mediated by activation of Kupfer cells and the subsequent release of cytokines (SEDA-20, 335). Focal fatty infiltrates of the liver mimicking metastases were also reported in a patient receiving both aldesleukin and a short course of interferon alfa (80).

Biliary tract

Gall-bladder changes have been reported in patients given aldesleukin and should be promptly recognized to avoid unnecessary intervention in symptomatic patients (SED-13, 1105) (81). Further systematic ultrasonographic examination in 25 HIV-infected patients treated with low-dose aldesleukin (6–18 MU/day) confirmed that most patients had gall-bladder wall thickening (80%), abnormal echo texture (64%), and intramural fluid (52%) or pericholecystic fluid (20%) (82). The frequency and severity of ultrasonographic abnormalities correlated with a higher dose of aldesleukin, as did complaints of right upper quadrant pain (24%). Although these findings mimicked those observed with acute cholecystitis, clinical symptoms and ultrasonographic abnormalities rapidly reversed after aldesleukin withdrawal or between two cycles.

Aldesleukin-induced cholecystopathy has been described in patients with cancer and was fully investigated in seven of 29 HIV-infected patients (81). Right upper quadrant abdominal pain and gallbladder wall thickening at sonography developed after 4–5 days of treatment and spontaneously resolved after withdrawal or dosage reduction. Similar symptoms recurred after renewed administration of aldesleukin. Although suggestive of acalculous cholecystitis, surgery is not required because this disorder is usually benign.

Pancreas

Acute pancreatitis has been described after high-dose bolus aldesleukin therapy (83).

Urinary tract

The renal toxicity associated with aldesleukin is dose-related. It manifests as uremia, oliguria, fluid retention, and pronounced renal tubular sodium reabsorption (77). No evidence of tubular dysfunction has been found. There is reduced renal plasma flow associated with reduced renal prostaglandin synthesis and increased plasma renin activity, which may explain the mechanism (84).

Oliguria or anuria, and increased serum creatinine concentrations occurred in over 90% of patients receiving high-dose aldesleukin (4).

Proteinuria, ranging in degree from traces to a frank, but reversible nephrotic syndrome (85,86), was sometimes observed, and a possible role of contaminants has been discussed (87).

In 199 patients with metastatic melanoma or renal cell carcinoma with high-dose intravenous bolus aldesleukin, severe oliguria, hypotension, and weight gain were frequent, and raised serum creatinine concentrations (mean peak 2.7 mg/dl) were the cause of treatment withdrawal in 13% of cycles (88). There were also various changes on urinalysis. The highest creatinine concentrations were found in patients with renal carcinoma and in elderly, male, or nephrectomized patients. There was no evidence of any long-term renal defect, and renal dysfunction was therefore not considered to be a treatment-limiting factor provided that patients were carefully managed for hypotension or oliguria.

It has been suggested that low-to-intermediate doses of aldesleukin alone or associated with interferon alfa may be safer under outpatient conditions (5). Patients over 60 years of age and individuals with previously raised serum creatinine concentrations have been thought to be likely to have longer-lasting and more severe renal impairment, but neither previous nephrectomy nor the interval between nephrectomy and initiation of aldesleukin therapy were associated with a higher risk of renal insufficiency (4).

A prerenal mechanism secondary to the vascular leak syndrome is commonly involved in the pathophysiology of acute renal insufficiency. In addition it has been suggested that a direct intrinsic intrarenal effect of aldesleukin with a higher than expected reduction in glomerular filtration rate or tubular dysfunction (85,89) is involved. Several isolated cases of acute interstitial or tubulointerstitial nephritis with predominant T lymphocyte infiltration of the kidneys (90–92) and the exacerbation of a subclinical IgA glomerulonephritis (93) suggested altered cell-mediated immunity.

Risk factors for renal dysfunction have been analysed in 72 patients with metastatic renal cell cancer treated with high-dose aldesleukin (18 MU/m²/day), interferon alfa (5 MU/m²/day), and lymphokine-activated killer lymphocytes (94). There was some type of renal dysfunction in 97%, of whom 69% developed renal toxicity of grade 2 (creatinine 260–525 µmol/l) or grade 3 (creatinine 525–1050 µmol/l). Although renal function commonly resolved between successive treatment courses, six patients had a persistently raised creatinine concentration (more than 20% above baseline). Among the various potential risk factors, a multivariate analysis showed that the significant risk factors for severe renal dysfunction were male sex, pre-treatment hypertension, and sepsis during treatment.

Skin

Cutaneous reactions to aldesleukin generally comprise pruritus, flushing, mild to moderate erythematous macular and desquamative eruptions, while generalized erythroderma or photosensitivity have occasionally been observed (95). The severity was not dose-dependent and did not correlate with other systemic reactions. Histological and immunopathological examination of the skin showed mild infiltrates of activated T helper lymphocytes and increased expression of HLA-DR and intercellular adhesion molecule-1 on keratinocytes and endothelial cells, and a possible role of interferon gamma has been suggested (96–98). Other adverse effects included erosions in surgical scars, multiple superficial cutaneous ulcers, and telogen effluvium (95).

Injection site reactions have been noted after subcutaneous aldesleukin (SEDA-21, 376). Localized lobular panniculitis after subcutaneous injections was further exacerbated by intravenous aldesleukin in one patient (99).

An unusually high incidence of skin erythema (70–85%) was noted in patients who received aldesleukin after autologous bone marrow transplantation. Histological examination showed features of cutaneous graft-versus-host disease or T cell epidermal infiltrates, but cutaneous toxicity was not reproduced in patients receiving low-dose aldesleukin (100,101).

The potential role of localized vertebral palliative radiotherapy before aldesleukin treatment was denied, since the area of cutaneous toxicity was broader than the irradiated field.

Aldesleukin given alone or aldesleukin plus interferon alfa produced a high incidence of vitiligo in patients with metastatic melanoma, irrespective of whether or not they had received chemotherapy (102–104). A possible correlation between aldesleukin-induced vitiligo and a favorable tumor response was found (102) but has also been disputed (103).

Some isolated reports have given rise to the suggestion that aldesleukin can exacerbate cutaneous reactions compatible with an immune-mediated phenomenon (105). Case reports included recurrence of quiescent pemphigus vulgaris, fatal dermatitis exfoliativa compatible with pemphigus vulgaris, exacerbation of localized or widespread psoriasis, acute reactivation of eczema, rapid progression of scleroderma with myositis, and leukocytoclastic vasculitis (SED-13, 1106) (SEDA-20, 335) (SEDA-21, 376).

Immunostimulation due to aldesleukin may have also played a role in the occurrence or unmasking of erythema nodosum, linear IgA bullous dermatosis, and life-threatening extensive bullous skin eruption or toxic epidermal necrolysis (SED-13, 1106) (SEDA-21, 376) (106).

Because aldesleukin stimulates T cells, it has been suggested to have favored the development of successive episodes of multifocal fixed drug eruption in response to chemically unrelated drugs (paracetamol, ondansetron, and tropisetron) in a 43-year-old patient (107).

Musculoskeletal

Joint or muscle pains have sometimes been reported in patients receiving aldesleukin, as has shoulder arthralgia with normal radiography and scintigraphic imaging consistent with bilateral synovitis (4,108).

Rare reports have suggested that aldesleukin can reactivate or cause rheumatoid arthritis (109) or cause necrotizing myositis with positive antinuclear antibodies (SEDA-20, 335).

Interstitial edema and local fluid retention resulting from increased vascular permeability has been suggested to cause unilateral or bilateral carpal tunnel syndrome with sensorimotor median neuropathy (SEDA-20, 334) (110).

Sexual function

A reversible reduction in testosterone concentrations has been observed in men who have received aldesleukin (4).

Immunologic

Aldesleukin was thought to be the triggering factor in the occurrence of sarcoidosis in a 36-year-old patient with AIDS stabilized for a long time by highly active antiretroviral therapy (111).

There have been very few reports of angioedema in patients receiving aldesleukin (112).

Interleukin antibodies

Recombinant aldesleukin-binding antibodies were detected in the half of 205 patients with metastatic cancer but there were neutralizing antibodies in only 7% (113). No significant difference in incidence was found between subcutaneous and continuous intravenous administration. In another study, none of the patients receiving aldesleukin alone developed neutralizing antibodies, whereas 18% of patients treated with aldesleukin and interferon alfa-2b had antibodies (114). Whatsoever, the clinical relevance of recombinant aldesleukin-neutralizing antibodies has not been accurately evaluated and a loss of response was apparently documented in only one patient (115).

Autoimmune disorders

Aldesleukin sometimes causes acute exacerbation of latent autoimmune disease, as has been further exemplified by the following description, which also included the first report of aldesleukin-induced myasthenia gravis (116).

- A 64-year-old man with non-insulin-dependent diabetes was given 14 large doses of aldesleukin (600 000 IU/kg every 8 hours) for metastatic renal cell carcinoma. One week after the completion of the first cycle he had a reversible episode of hyperosmolar, non-ketotic hyperglycemia, and insulin was started. A second cycle 3 months later was associated with hypotension, mild weakness of the right shoulder, and increased activity of creatine kinase (CK)-MB fraction. After four doses of the third cycle he again had hypotension and a raised CK-MB fraction. Two weeks later, he developed typical features of myasthenia gravis and required mechanical ventilation. Acetylcholine receptor antibodies were found and there was an inflammatory primary myositis on muscle biopsy. He gradually recovered with prednisone, pyridostigmine, and daily insulin.

In this case, which was marked by three autoimmune complications (insulin-dependent diabetes mellitus, myositis, and myasthenia gravis) in a single patient, a retrospective analysis of the patient's serum before aldesleukin therapy showed the presence of antibodies against glutamic acid decarboxylase, insulin, islet cell antigen, and striated muscle, but was negative for acetylcholine receptor antibodies. Immune stimulation by aldesleukin was

therefore thought to have caused broken tolerance to self-antigens and enhanced latent autoimmunity.

Infection risk

Clinically relevant infectious complications occurred with an incidence of 10–40% after intravenous aldesleukin (4). A retrospective study showed a 13% incidence of confirmed bacterial infections during 935 treatment courses of high-dose aldesleukin; opportunistic infections were not more frequent (117). The most commonly isolated pathogens were *Staphylococcus aureus*, *Staphylococcus epidermidis*, and *Escherichia coli*. Documented infections affected mostly the catheter site or the urinary tract. Infections were usually noted during the first (68%) or second (21%) course of aldesleukin therapy, that is 4–9 days and 13–18 days after the start of treatment. Bacterial sepsis was mostly related to the use of central venous catheters and fatal septic shock was rarely recorded. There was also an increased incidence of infectious complications in patients receiving subcutaneous aldesleukin plus interferon alfa (118), but these findings were not confirmed in patients who received subcutaneous aldesleukin alone (119,120). Previous colonization of the skin with *S. aureus* and skin desquamation increased the risk of nosocomial bacteremia (117). Age, underlying tumor, source, dose and duration of intravenous aldesleukin, or the concomitant use of LAK cells were not risks factors, and severe neutropenia was not associated with bacteremia. The prophylactic use of antibiotics and systematic screening led to a significant reduction in the frequency of infections, from 22 to 7% of patients over 3 years (117).

The mechanism of these complications is not fully understood. A reduction in neutrophil chemotaxis, superoxide production, and/or neutrophil Fc receptor expression have been suggested to be involved. Impaired cell-mediated or humoral immune responses have also been shown after high-dose aldesleukin, but the clinical consequences of these findings are unknown.

Long-Term Effects

Tumorigenicity

Isolated case reports have described relapses of acute myeloid leukemia or the proliferation of leukemic blasts cells with phenotypic changes in a patient with acute myelocytic leukemia; a high percentage of blasts expressed the CD25 antigen in both reports (121,122). A reversible increase in peripheral monoclonal B cell lymphocyte count in a patient with B cell lymphocytic lymphoma and Hodgkin's disease in a woman receiving aldesleukin for metastatic melanoma were also documented in single reports.

Drug–Drug Interactions

General

The potential of aldesleukin to participate in drug interactions has been investigated in 18 patients who underwent surgical resection of hepatic metastases (123). Compared with seven control patients who did not receive aldesleukin before surgery, six patients who received 9 or 12 MU/m^2 from days 7–3 before hepatectomy had a significant fall in the activities of total cytochromes and several mono-oxygenases. No such effect was found in five patients treated with 3 or 6 MU/m^2 before hepatectomy. This suggests that high-dose aldesleukin might cause drug interactions by inhibiting hepatic drug metabolism.

Contrast media

More frequent allergic reactions to iodinated and non-ionic contrast media injection were observed when radiological examination was performed within a period ranging from 2 to 6 weeks up to 2 years after withdrawal of aldesleukin in patients who had previously tolerated contrast media well (124,125). These reactions usually appeared within 1–4 hours after contrast media injection, but delayed reactions up to 24 hours were sometimes noted. The most frequent symptoms were diarrhea, vomiting, influenza-like symptoms, skin rash, pruritus, and facial edema, and rarely included hypotension, dyspnea, and oliguria. The overall incidence was 5–15%, but as high as 28% of patients receiving aldesleukin via arterial infusion (126). This incidence is therefore about 3–4 times higher than in the general population undergoing contrast media examination. "Recall" reactions to aldesleukin have been suggested as an explanation, since these complications more closely resemble immediate adverse effects to aldesleukin than typical contrast media reactions. Putative enhancement of the immune response to iodine-containing contrast media after aldesleukin has also been suggested.

Cytotoxic drugs

An unexpected high incidence of type I allergic reactions to cisplatin and dacarbazine has been observed, several hours after administration to patients on a combination of aldesleukin and interferon alfa (127). The reactions occurred at least after the first cycle and increased in incidence thereafter, suggesting that immunotherapy can sensitize patients to several chemotherapeutic agents.

In a phase III trial in 190 patients with metastatic melanoma, sequential chemotherapy with dacarbazine, cisplatin, and vinblastine plus interferon alfa and aldesleukin modestly increased the response rates and produced considerably more frequent and severe adverse effects than chemotherapy alone (128). In particular, severe episodes of anemia and thrombocytopenia that required blood or platelet transfusions were 2–6 times more frequent in the chemotherapy group.

Morphine

Acute encephalopathy with typical signs of morphine intoxication occurred in a patient taking aldesleukin (129).

Non-steroid anti-inflammatory agents

Non-steroidal anti-inflammatory agents used to reduce fever and other aldesleukin adverse effects can theoretically potentiate aldesleukin nephrotoxicity by inhibiting prostaglandin synthesis. However this effect was deemed unlikely by several authors (85).

References

1. Law TM, Motzer RJ, Mazumdar M, Sell KW, Walther PJ, O'Connell M, Khan A, Vlamis V, Vogelzang NJ, Bajorin DF. Phase III randomized trial of interleukin-2 with or without lymphokine-activated killer cells in the treatment of patients with advanced renal cell carcinoma. Cancer 1995;76(5):824–32.
2. Javadpour N, Lalehzarian M. A phase I-II study of high-dose recombinant human interleukin-2 in disseminated renal-cell carcinoma. Semin Surg Oncol 1988;4(3):207–9.
3. Negrier S, Escudier B, Lasset C, Douillard JY, Savary J, Chevreau C, Ravaud A, Mercatello A, Peny J, Mousseau M, Philip T, Tursz T. Recombinant human interleukin-2, recombinant human interferon alfa-2a, or both in metastatic renal-cell carcinoma. Groupe Francais d'Immunotherapie. N Engl J Med 1998;338(18):1272–8.
4. Vial T, Descotes J. Clinical toxicity of interleukin-2. Drug Saf 1992;7(6):417–33.
5. Schomburg A, Kirchner H, Atzpodien J. Renal, metabolic, and hemodynamic side-effects of interleukin-2 and/or interferon alpha: evidence of a risk/benefit advantage of subcutaneous therapy. J Cancer Res Clin Oncol 1993;119(12):745–55.
6. Stadler WM, Vogelzang NJ. Low-dose interleukin-2 in the treatment of metastatic renal-cell carcinoma. Semin Oncol 1995;22(1):67–73.
7. Fyfe G, Fisher RI, Rosenberg SA, Sznol M, Parkinson DR, Louie AC. Results of treatment of 255 patients with metastatic renal cell carcinoma who received high-dose recombinant interleukin-2 therapy. J Clin Oncol 1995;13(3):688–96.
8. Piscitelli SC, Bhat N, Pau A. A risk-benefit assessment of interleukin-2 as an adjunct to antiviral therapy in HIV infection. Drug Saf 2000;22(1):19–31.
9. Levy Y, Capitant C, Houhou S, Carriere I, Viard JP, Goujard C, Gastaut JA, Oksenhendler E, Boumsell L, Gomard E, Rabian C, Weiss L, Guillet JG, Delfraissy JF, Aboulker JP, Seligmann M. Comparison of subcutaneous and intravenous interleukin-2 in asymptomatic HIV-1 infection: a randomised controlled trial. ANRS 048 study group. Lancet 1999;353(9168):1923–9.
10. Carr A, Emery S, Lloyd A, Hoy J, Garsia R, French M, Stewart G, Fyfe G, Cooper DA. Outpatient continuous intravenous interleukin-2 or subcutaneous, polyethylene glycol-modified interleukin-2 in human immunodeficiency virus-infected patients: a randomized, controlled, multicenter study. Australian IL-2 Study Group. J Infect Dis 1998;178(4):992–9.
11. Hengge UR, Goos M, Esser S, Exner V, Dotterer H, Wiehler H, Borchard C, Muller K, Beckmann A, Eppner MT, Berger A, Fiedler M. Randomized, controlled phase II trial of subcutaneous interleukin-2 in combination with highly active antiretroviral therapy (HAART) in HIV patients. AIDS 1998;12(17):F225–34.
12. Atkins MB, Lotze MT, Dutcher JP, Fisher RI, Weiss G, Margolin K, Abrams J, Sznol M, Parkinson D, Hawkins M, Paradise C, Kunkel L, Rosenberg SA. High-dose recombinant interleukin 2 therapy for patients with metastatic melanoma: analysis of 270 patients treated between 1985 and 1993. J Clin Oncol 1999;17(7):2105–16.
13. Rosenberg SA, Yang JC, Schwartzentruber DJ, Hwu P, Marincola FM, Topalian SL, Seipp CA, Einhorn JH, White DE, Steinberg SM. Prospective randomized trial of the treatment of patients with metastatic melanoma using chemotherapy with cisplatin, dacarbazine, and tamoxifen alone or in combination with interleukin-2 and interferon alfa-2b. J Clin Oncol 1999;17(3):968–75.

14. Schwartzentruber DJ. Guidelines for the safe administration of high-dose interleukin-2. J Immunother 2001;24(4):287–93.

15. Baluna R, Vitetta ES. Vascular leak syndrome: a side effect of immunotherapy. Immunopharmacology 1997;37(2–3):117–32.

16. Olsen E, Duvic M, Frankel A, Kim Y, Martin A, Vonderheid E, Jegasothy B, Wood G, Gordon M, Heald P, Oseroff A, Pinter-Brown L, Bowen G, Kuzel T, Fivenson D, Foss F, Glode M, Molina A, Knobler E, Stewart S, Cooper K, Stevens S, Craig F, Reuben J, Bacha P, Nichols J. Pivotal phase III trial of two dose levels of denileukin diftitox for the treatment of cutaneous T cell lymphoma. J Clin Oncol 2001;19(2):376–88.

17. Martin A, Gutierrez E, Muglia J, McDonald CJ, Guzzo C, Gottlieb A, Pappert A, Garland WT, Bagel J, Bacha P. A multicenter dose-escalation trial with denileukin diftitox (ONTAK, DAB(389)IL-2) in patients with severe psoriasis. J Am Acad Dermatol 2001;45(6):871–81.

18. Railan D, Fivenson DP, Wittenberg G. Capillary leak syndrome in a patient treated with interleukin 2 fusion toxin for cutaneous T cell lymphoma. J Am Acad Dermatol 2000;43(2 Pt 1):323–4.

19. Sosman JA, Kohler PC, Hank JA, Moore KH, Bechhofer R, Storer B, Sondel PM. Repetitive weekly cycles of interleukin-2. II. Clinical and immunologic effects of dose, schedule, and addition of indomethacin. J Natl Cancer Inst 1988;80(18):1451–61.

20. Richards JM, Barker E, Latta J, Ramming K, Vogelzang NJ. Phase I study of weekly 24-hour infusions of recombinant human interleukin-2. J Natl Cancer Inst 1988;80(16):1325–8.

21. Nasr S, McKolanis J, Pais R, Findley H, Hnath R, Waldrep K, Ragab AH. A phase I study of interleukin-2 in children with cancer and evaluation of clinical and immunologic status during therapy. A Pediatric Oncology Group Study. Cancer 1989;64(4):783–8.

22. Groeger JS, Bajorin D, Reichman B, Kopec I, Atiq O, Pierri MK. Haemodynamic effects of recombinant interleukin-2 administered by constant infusion. Eur J Cancer 1991;27(12):1613–16.

23. Citterio G, Pellegatta F, Lucca GD, Fragasso G, Scaglietti U, Pini D, Fortis C, Tresoldi M, Rugarli C. Plasma nitrate plus nitrite changes during continuous intravenous infusion interleukin 2. Br J Cancer 1996;74(8):1297–301.

24. White RL Jr, Schwartzentruber DJ, Guleria A, MacFarlane MP, White DE, Tucker E, Rosenberg SA. Cardiopulmonary toxicity of treatment with high dose interleukin-2 in 199 consecutive patients with metastatic melanoma or renal cell carcinoma. Cancer 1994;74(12):3212–22.

25. Citterio G, Fragasso G, Rossetti E, Di Lucca G, Bucci E, Foppoli M, Guerrieri R, Matteucci P, Polastri D, Scaglietti U, Tresoldi M, Chierchia SL, Rugarli C. Isolated left ventricular filling abnormalities may predict interleukin-2-induced cardiovascular toxicity. J Immunother Emphasis Tumor Immunol 1996;19(2):134–41.

26. Fragasso G, Tresoldi M, Benti R, Vidal M, Marcatti M, Borri A, Besana C, Gerundini PP, Rugarli C, Chierchia S. Impaired left ventricular filling rate induced by treatment with recombinant interleukin 2 for advanced cancer. Br Heart J 1994;71(2):166–9.

27. Junghans RP, Manning W, Safar M, Quist W. Biventricular cardiac thrombosis during interleukin-2 infusion. N Engl J Med 2001;344(11):859–60.

28. Huland E, Heinzer H, Huland H. Treatment of pulmonary metastatic renal-cell carcinoma in 116 patients using inhaled interleukin-2 (IL-2). Anticancer Res 1999;19(4A):2679–83.

29. Davis SD, Berkmen YM, Wang JC. Interleukin-2 therapy for advanced renal cell carcinoma: radiographic evaluation of response and complications. Radiology 1990;177(1):127–31.

30. Saxon RR, Klein JS, Bar MH, Blanc P, Gamsu G, Webb WR, Aronson FR. Pathogenesis of pulmonary edema during interleukin-2 therapy: correlation of chest radiographic and clinical findings in 54 patients. Am J Roentgenol 1991;156(2):281–5.

31. O'Hearn DJ, Leiferman KM, Askin F, Georas SN. Pulmonary infiltrates after cytokine therapy for stem cell transplantation. Massive deposition of eosinophil major basic protein detected by immunohistochemistry. Am J Respir Crit Care Med 1999;160(4):1361–5.

32. Brichon PY, Barnoud D, Pison C, Perez I, Guignier M. Double lung transplantation for adult respiratory distress syndrome after recombinant interleukin 2. Chest 1993;104(2):609–10.

33. Trufflandier N, Gille O, Palussiere J, Prie L, Pointillart V, Ravaud A. Symptomatic neurological epidural metastasis with interleukin-2 therapy in metastatic renal cell carcinoma. Tumori 2002;88(4):338–40.

34. Vecht CJ, Keohane C, Menon RS, Punt CJ, Stoter G. Acute fatal leukoencephalopathy after interleukin-2 therapy. N Engl J Med 1990;323(16):1146–7.

35. Meyers CA, Yung WK. Delayed neurotoxicity of intraventricular interleukin-2: a case report. J Neurooncol 1993;15(3):265–7.

36. Buter J, de Vries EG, Sleijfer DT, Willemse PH, Mulder NH. Neuropsychiatric symptoms during treatment with interleukin-2. Lancet 1993;341(8845):628.

37. Bernard JT, Ameriso S, Kempf RA, Rosen P, Mitchell MS, Fisher M. Transient focal neurologic deficits complicating interleukin-2 therapy. Neurology 1990;40(1):154–5.

38. Friedman DI, Hu EH, Sadun AA. Neuro-ophthalmic complications of interleukin 2 therapy. Arch Ophthalmol 1991;109(12):1679–80.

39. Denicoff KD, Rubinow DR, Papa MZ, Simpson C, Seipp CA, Lotze MT, Chang AE, Rosenstein D, Rosenberg SA. The neuropsychiatric effects of treatment with interleukin-2 and lymphokine-activated killer cells. Ann Intern Med 1987;107(3):293–300.

40. Caraceni A, Martini C, Belli F, Mascheroni L, Rivoltini L, Arienti F, Cascinelli N. Neuropsychological and neurophysiological assessment of the central effects of interleukin-2 administration. Eur J Cancer 1993;29A(9):1266–9.

41. Walker LG, Wesnes KP, Heys SD, Walker MB, Lolley J, Eremin O. The cognitive effects of recombinant interleukin-2 (rIL-2) therapy: a controlled clinical trial using computerised assessments. Eur J Cancer 1996;32A(13):2275–83.

42. Pace A, Pietrangeli A, Bove L, Rosselli M, Lopez M, Jandolo B. Neurotoxicity of antitumoral IL-2 therapy: evoked cognitive potentials and brain mapping. Ital J Neurol Sci 1994;15(7):341–6.

43. Pizzi C, Caraglia M, Cianciulli M, Fabbrocini A, Libroia A, Matano E, Contegiacomo A, Del Prete S, Abbruzzese A, Martignetti A, Tagliaferri P, Bianco AR. Low-dose recombinant IL-2 induces psychological changes: monitoring by Minnesota Multiphasic Personality Inventory (MMPI). Anticancer Res 2002;22(2A):727–32.

44. Capuron L, Ravaud A, Dantzer R. Early depressive symptoms in cancer patients receiving interleukin 2 and/or interferon alfa-2b therapy. J Clin Oncol 2000;18(10):2143–51.

45. VanderMolen LA, Smith JW 2nd, Longo DL, Steis RG, Kremers P, Sznol M. Adrenal insufficiency and interleukin-2 therapy. Ann Intern Med 1989;111(2):185.

46. Vial T, Descotes J. Immune-mediated side-effects of cytokines in humans. Toxicology 1995;105(1):31–57.

47. Kruit WH, Bolhuis RL, Goey SH, Jansen RL, Eggermont AM, Batchelor D, Schmitz PI, Stoter G. Interleukin-2-induced thyroid dysfunction is correlated with treatment duration but not with tumor response. J Clin Oncol 1993;11(5):921–4.

48. Preziati D, La Rosa L, Covini G, Marcelli R, Rescalli S, Persani L, Del Ninno E, Meroni PL, Colombo M, Beck-Peccoz P. Autoimmunity and thyroid function in patients with chronic active hepatitis treated with recombinant interferon alpha-2a. Eur J Endocrinol 1995;132(5):587–93.

49. Vialettes B, Guillerand MA, Viens P, Stoppa AM, Baume D, Sauvan R, Pasquier J, San Marco M, Olive D, Maraninchi D. Incidence rate and risk factors for thyroid dysfunction during recombinant interleukin-2 therapy in advanced malignancies. Acta Endocrinol (Copenh) 1993;129(1):31–8.

50. Schwartzentruber DJ, White DE, Zweig MH, Weintraub BD, Rosenberg SA. Thyroid dysfunction associated with immunotherapy for patients with cancer. Cancer 1991;68(11):2384–90.

51. Jacobs EL, Clare-Salzler MJ, Chopra IJ, Figlin RA. Thyroid function abnormalities associated with the chronic outpatient administration of recombinant interleukin-2 and recombinant interferon-alpha. J Immunother 1991;10(6):448–55.

52. Pichert G, Jost LM, Zobeli L, Odermatt B, Pedia G, Stahel RA. Thyroiditis after treatment with interleukin-2 and interferon alpha-2a. Br J Cancer 1990;62(1):100–4.

53. Reid I, Sharpe I, McDevitt J, Maxwell W, Emmons R, Tanner WA, Monson JR. Thyroid dysfunction can predict response to immunotherapy with interleukin-2 and interferon-2 alpha. Br J Cancer 1991;64(5):915–18.

54. Weijl NI, Van der Harst D, Brand A, Kooy Y, Van Luxemburg S, Schroder J, Lentjes E, Van Rood JJ, Cleton FJ, Osanto S. Hypothyroidism during immunotherapy with interleukin-2 is associated with antithyroid antibodies and response to treatment. J Clin Oncol 1993;11(7):1376–83.

55. Krouse RS, Royal RE, Heywood G, Weintraub BD, White DE, Steinberg SM, Rosenberg SA, Schwartzentruber DJ. Thyroid dysfunction in 281 patients with metastatic melanoma or renal carcinoma treated with interleukin-2 alone. J Immunother Emphasis Tumor Immunol 1995;18(4):272–8.

56. Kung AW, Lai CL, Wong KL, Tam CF. Thyroid functions in patients treated with interleukin-2 and lymphokine-activated killer cells. Q J Med 1992;82(297):33–42.

57. Monig H, Hauschild A, Lange S, Folsch UR. Suppressed thyroid-stimulating hormone secretion in patients treated with interleukin-2 and interferon-alpha 2b for metastatic melanoma. Clin Investig 1994;72(12):975–8.

58. Marcus SL, Dutcher JP, Paietta E, Ciobanu N, Strauman J, Wiernik PH, Hutner SH, Frank O, Baker H. Severe hypovitaminosis C occurring as the result of adoptive immunotherapy with high-dose interleukin 2 and lymphokine-activated killer cells. Cancer Res 1987;47(15):4208–12.

59. Aulitzky WE, Tilg H, Vogel W, Aulitzky W, Berger M, Gastl G, Herold M, Huber C. Acute hematologic effects of interferon alpha, interferon gamma, tumor necrosis factor alpha and interleukin 2. Ann Hematol 1991;62(1):25–31.

60. MacFarlane MP, Yang JC, Guleria AS, White RL Jr, Seipp CA, Einhorn JH, White DE, Rosenberg SA. The hematologic toxicity of interleukin-2 in patients with metastatic melanoma and renal cell carcinoma. Cancer 1995;75(4):1030–7.

61. Oleksowicz L, Zuckerman D, Mrowiec Z, Puszkin E, Dutcher JP. Effects of interleukin-2 administration on platelet function in cancer patients. Am J Hematol 1994;45(3):224–31.

62. Macdonald D, Gordon AA, Kajitani H, Enokihara H, Barrett AJ. Interleukin-2 treatment-associated eosinophilia is mediated by interleukin-5 production. Br J Haematol 1990;76(2):168–73.

63. Ettinghausen SE, Moore JG, White DE, Platanias L, Young NS, Rosenberg SA. Hematologic effects of immunotherapy with lymphokine-activated killer cells and recombinant interleukin-2 in cancer patients. Blood 1987;69(6):1654–60.

64. Fleischmann JD, Shingleton WB, Gallagher C, Ratnoff OD, Chahine A. Fibrinolysis, thrombocytopenia, and coagulation abnormalities complicating high-dose interleukin-2 immunotherapy. J Lab Clin Med 1991;117(1):76–82.

65. Schomburg A, Kirchner H, Atzpodien J. Hematotoxicity of interleukin-2 in man: clinical effects and comparison of various treatment regimens. Acta Haematol 1993;89(3):119–31.

66. Birchfield GR, Rodgers GM, Girodias KW, Ward JH, Samlowski WE. Hypoprothrombinemia associated with interleukin-2 therapy: correction with vitamin K. J Immunother 1992;11(1):71–5.

67. Oleksowicz L, Strack M, Dutcher JP, Sussman I, Caliendo G, Sparano J, Wiernik PH. A distinct coagulopathy associated with interleukin-2 therapy. Br J Haematol 1994;88(4):892–4.

68. Baars JW, de Boer JP, Wagstaff J, Roem D, Eerenberg-Belmer AJ, Nauta J, Pinedo HM, Hack CE. Interleukin-2 induces activation of coagulation and fibrinolysis: resemblance to the changes seen during experimental endotoxaemia. Br J Haematol 1992;82(2):295–301.

69. Ratcliffe MA, Roditi G, Adamson DJ. Interleukin-2 and splenic enlargement. J Natl Cancer Inst 1992;84(10):810–11.

70. Marmary Y, Shiloni E, Katz J. Oral changes in interleukin-2 treated patients: a preliminary report. J Oral Pathol Med 1992;21(5):230–1.

71. Nagler A, Nagler R, Ackerstein A, Levi S, Marmary Y. Major salivary gland dysfunction in patients with hematological malignancies receiving interleukin-2-based immunotherapy post-autologous blood stem cell transplantation (ABSCT). Bone Marrow Transplant 1997;20(7):575–80.

72. Sparano JA, Brandt LJ, Dutcher JP, DuBois JS, Atkins MB. Symptomatic exacerbation of Crohn disease after treatment with high-dose interleukin-2. Ann Intern Med 1993;118(8):617–18.

73. Post AB, Falk GW, Bukowski RM. Acute colonic pseudo-obstruction associated with interleukin-2 therapy. Am J Gastroenterol 1991;86(10):1539–41.

74. Rahman R, Bernstein Z, Vaickus L, Penetrante R, Arbuck S, Kopec I, Vesper D, Douglass HO Jr, Foon KA. Unusual gastrointestinal complications of interleukin-2 therapy. J Immunother 1991;10(3):221–5.

75. Sparano JA, Dutcher JP, Kaleya R, Caliendo G, Fiorito J, Mitsudo S, Shechner R, Boley SJ, Gucalp R, Ciobanu N, et al. Colonic ischemia complicating immunotherapy with interleukin-2 and interferon-alpha. Cancer 1991;68(7):1538–44.

76. Sondel PM, Kohler PC, Hank JA, Moore KH, Rosenthal NS, Sosman JA, Bechhofer R, Storer B. Clinical and immunological effects of recombinant interleukin 2 given by repetitive weekly cycles to patients with cancer. Cancer Res 1988;48(9):2561–7.

77. Webb DE, Austin HA 3rd, Belldegrun A, Vaughan E, Linehan WM, Rosenberg SA. Metabolic and renal effects of interleukin-2 immunotherapy for metastatic cancer. Clin Nephrol 1988;30(3):141–5.

78. Fisher B, Keenan AM, Garra BS, Steinberg SM, White DE, DiBisceglie AM, Hoofnagle JH, Yolles P, Rosenberg SA, Lotze MT. Interleukin-2 induces profound

reversible cholestasis: a detailed analysis in treated cancer patients. J Clin Oncol 1989;7(12):1852–62.

79. Punt CJ, Henzen-Logmans SC, Bolhuis RL, Stoter G. Hyperbilirubinaemia in patients treated with recombinant human interleukin-2 (rIL-2). Br J Cancer 1990;61(3):491.

80. Lilenbaum RC, Lilenbaum AM, Hryniuk WM. Interleukin 2-induced focal fatty infiltrate of the liver that mimics metastases. J Natl Cancer Inst 1995;87(8):609–10.

81. Powell FC, Spooner KM, Shawker TH, Premkumar A, Thakore KN, Vogel SE, Kovacs JA, Masur H, Feuerstein IM. Symptomatic interleukin-2-induced chole-cystopathy in patients with HIV infection. Am J Roentgenol 1994;163(1):117–21.

82. Premkumar A, Walworth CM, Vogel S, Daryanani KD, Venzon DJ, Kovacs JA, Feuerstein IM. Prospective sono-graphic evaluation of interleukin-2-induced changes in the gallbladder. Radiology 1998;206(2):393–6.

83. Birchfield GR, Ward JH, Redman BG, Flaherty L, Samlowski WE. Acute pancreatitis associated with high-dose interleukin-2 immunotherapy for malignant mela-noma. West J Med 1990;152(6):714–16.

84. Christiansen NP, Skubitz KM, Nath K, Ochoa A, Kennedy BJ. Nephrotoxicity of continuous intravenous infusion of recombinant interleukin-2. Am J Med 1988;84(6):1072–5.

85. Shalmi CL, Dutcher JP, Feinfeld DA, Chun KJ, Saleemi KR, Freeman LM, Lynn RI, Wiernik PH. Acute renal dysfunction during interleukin-2 treatment: sugges-tion of an intrinsic renal lesion. J Clin Oncol 1990;8(11):1839–46.

86. Hisanaga S, Kawagoe H, Yamamoto Y, Kuroki N, Fujimoto S, Tanaka K, Kurokawa M. Nephrotic syndrome associated with recombinant interleukin-2. Nephron 1990;54(3):277–8.

87. Heslan JM, Branellec AI, Lang P, Lagrue G. Recombinant interleukin-2-induced proteinuria: fact or artifact? Nephron 1991;57(3):373–4.

88. Guleria AS, Yang JC, Topalian SL, Weber JS, Parkinson DR, MacFarlane MP, White RL, Steinberg SM, White DE, Einhorn JH, et al. Renal dys-function associated with the administration of high-dose interleukin-2 in 199 consecutive patients with metastatic melanoma or renal carcinoma. J Clin Oncol 1994;12(12):2714–22.

89. Heys SD, Eremin O, Franks CR, Broom J, Whiting PH. Lithium clearance measurements during recombinant interleukin 2 treatment: tubular dysfunction in man. Ren Fail 1993;15(2):195–201.

90. Diekman MJ, Vlasveld LT, Krediet RT, Rankin EM, Arisz L. Acute interstitial nephritis during continuous intravenous administration of low-dose interleukin-2. Nephron 1992;60(1):122–3.

91. Feinfeld DA, D'Agati V, Dutcher JP, Werfel SB, Lynn RI, Wiernik PH. Interstitial nephritis in a patient receiving adoptive immunotherapy with recombinant interleukin-2 and lymphokine-activated killer cells. Am J Nephrol 1991;11(6):489–92.

92. Vlasveld LT, van de Wiel-van Kemenade E, de Boer AJ, Sein JJ, Gallee MP, Krediet RT, Mellief CJ, Rankin EM, Hekman A, Figdor CG. Possible role for cytotoxic lym-phocytes in the pathogenesis of acute interstitial nephritis after recombinant interleukin-2 treatment for renal cell cancer. Cancer Immunol Immunother 1993;36(3):210–13.

93. Chan TM, Cheng IK, Wong KL, Chan KW, Lai CL. Crescentic IgA glomerulonephritis following interleukin-2 therapy for hepatocellular carcinoma of the liver. Am J Nephrol 1991;11(6):493–6.

94. Kruit WH, Schmitz PI, Stoter G. The role of possible risk factors for acute and late renal dysfunction after high-

dose interleukin-2, interferon alpha and lymphokine-acti-vated killer cells. Cancer Immunol Immunother 1999; 48(6):331–5.

95. Asnis LA, Gaspari AA. Cutaneous reactions to recombi-nant cytokine therapy. J Am Acad Dermatol 1995;33(3):393–410.

96. Blessing K, Park KG, Heys SD, King G, Eremin O. Immunopathological changes in the skin following recombinant interleukin-2 treatment. J Pathol 1992; 167(3):313–19.

97. Dummer R, Miller K, Eilles C, Burg G. The skin: an immunoreactive target organ during interleukin-2 admin-istration? Dermatologica 1991;183(2):95–9.

98. Wolkenstein P, Chosidow O, Wechsler J, Guillaume JC, Lescs MC, Brandely M, Avril MF, Revuz J. Cutaneous side effects associated with interleukin 2 administration for metastatic melanoma. J Am Acad Dermatol 1993;28(1):66–70.

99. Baars JW, Coenen JL, Wagstaff J, van der Valk P, Pinedo HM. Lobular panniculitis after subcutaneous administration of interleukin-2 (IL-2), and its exacerbation during intravenous therapy with IL-2. Br J Cancer 1992;66(4):698–9.

100. Costello R, Blaise D, Jacquemier J, Monges G, Stoppa AM, Viens P, Olive D, Bouabdallah M, Brandely, Gastaut JA. Induction of cutaneous "graft-versus-host like" reaction by recombinant IL-2 after autologous bone marrow transplantation. Bone Marrow Transplant 1995;16(1):199–200.

101. Massumoto C, Benyunes MC, Sale G, Beauchamp M, York A, Thompson JA, Buckner CD, Fefer A. Close simulation of acute graft-versus-host disease by interleu-kin-2 administered after autologous bone marrow trans-plantation for hematologic malignancy. Bone Marrow Transplant 1996;17(3):351–6.

102. Richards JM, Gilewski TA, Ramming K, Mitchel B, Doane LL, Vogelzang NJ. Effective chemotherapy for melanoma after treatment with interleukin-2. Cancer 1992;69(2):427–9.

103. Wolkenstein P, Revuz J, Guillaume JC, Avril MF, Chosidow O. Autoimmune disorders and interleukin-2 therapy: a step toward "unanswered questions". Arch Dermatol 1995;131(5):615–16.

104. Scheibenbogen C, Hunstein W, Keilholz U. Vitiligo-like lesions following immunotherapy with IFN alpha and IL-2 in melanoma patients. Eur J Cancer 1994;30A(8):1209–11.

105. Gustafsson LL, Eriksson LS, Dahl ML, Eleborg L, Ericzon BG, Nyberg A. Cyclophosphamide-induced acute liver failure requiring transplantation in a patient with genetically deficient debrisoquine metabolism: a cau-sal relationship? J. Intern Med 1996;240(5):311–14.

106. Segura Huerta AA, Tordera P, Cercos AC, Yuste AL, Lopez-Tendero P, Reynes G. Toxic epidermal necrolysis associated with interleukin-2. Ann Pharmacother 2002;36(7–8):1171–4.

107. Bernand S, Scheidegger EP, Dummer R, Burg G. Multifocal fixed drug eruption to paracetamol, tropisetron and ondansetron induced by interleukin 2. Dermatology 2000;201(2):148–50.

108. Baron NW, Davis LP, Flaherty LE, Muz J, Valdivieso M, Kling GA. Scintigraphic findings in patients with shoulder pain caused by interleukin-2. Am J Roentgenol 1990;154(2):327–30.

109. Massarotti EM, Liu NY, Mier J, Atkins MB. Chronic inflammatory arthritis after treatment with high-dose interleukin-2 for malignancy. Am J Med 1992;92(6):693–7.

110. Heys SD, Mills KL, Eremin O. Bilateral carpal tunnel syndrome associated with interleukin 2 therapy. Postgrad Med J 1992;68(801):587–8.

111. Blanche P, Gombert B, Rollot F, Salmon D, Sicard D. Sarcoidosis in a patient with acquired immunodeficiency syndrome treated with interleukin-2. Clin Infect Dis 2000;31(6):1493–4.

112. Baars JW, Wagstaff J, Hack CE, Wolbink GJ, Eerenberg-Belmer AJ, Pinedo HM. Angioneurotic oedema and urticaria during therapy with interleukin-2 (IL-2). Ann Oncol 1992;3(3):243–4.

113. Scharenberg JGM, Stam AGM, von Blomberg BME, et al. The development of anti-interleukin-2 (IL-2) antibodies in patient treated with recombinant IL-2 does not interfere with clinical responsiveness. Proc Am Assoc Cancer Res 1993;34:464.

114. Atzpodien J, Hanninen EL, Kirchner H, Knuver-Hopf J, Poliwoda H. Human antibodies to recombinant interleukin-2 in patients with hypernephroma. J Interfer Res 1994;14:177–8.

115. Kirchner H, Korfer A, Evers P, Szamel MM, Knuver-Hopf J, Mohr H, Franks CR, Pohl U, Resch K, Hadam M, et al. The development of neutralizing antibodies in a patient receiving subcutaneous recombinant and natural interleukin-2. Cancer 1991;67(7):1862–4.

116. Fraenkel PG, Rutkove SB, Matheson JK, Fowkes M, Cannon ME, Patti ME, Atkins MB, Gollob JA. Induction of myasthenia gravis, myositis, and insulin-dependent diabetes mellitus by high-dose interleukin-2 in a patient with renal cell cancer. J Immunother 2002;25(4):373–8.

117. Pockaj BA, Topalian SL, Steinberg SM, White DE, Rosenberg SA. Infectious complications associated with interleukin-2 administration: a retrospective review of 935 treatment courses. J Clin Oncol 1993;11(1):136–47.

118. Jones AL, Cropley I, O'Brien ME, Lorentzos A, Moore J, Jameson B, Gore ME. Infectious complications of subcutaneous interleukin-2 and interferon-alpha. Lancet 1992;339(8786):181–2.

119. Buter J, de Vries EG, Sleijfer DT, Willemse PH, Mulder NH. Infection after subcutaneous interleukin-2. Lancet 1992;339(8792):552.

120. Schomburg AG, Kirchner HH, Atzpodien J. Cytokines and infection in cancer patients. Lancet 1992;339(8800):1061.

121. Macdonald D, Jiang YZ, Swirsky D, Vulliamy T, Morilla R, Bungey J, Barrett AJ. Acute myeloid leukaemia relapsing following interleukin-2 treatment expresses the alpha chain of the interleukin-2 receptor. Br J Haematol 1991;77(1):43–9.

122. Spiekermann K, O'Brien S, Estey E. Relapse of acute myelogenous leukemia during low dose interleukin-2 (IL-2) therapy. Phenotypic evolution associated with strong expression of the IL-2 receptor alpha chain. Cancer 1995;75(7):1594–7.

123. Elkahwaji J, Robin MA, Berson A, Tinel M, Letteron P, Labbe G, Beaune P, Elias D, Rougier P, Escudier B, Duvillard P, Pessayre D. Decrease in hepatic cytochrome P450 after interleukin-2 immunotherapy. Biochem Pharmacol 1999;57(8):951–4.

124. Choyke PL, Miller DL, Lotze MT, Whiteis JM, Ebbitt B, Rosenberg SA. Delayed reactions to contrast media after interleukin-2 immunotherapy. Radiology 1992;183(1):111–14.

125. Shulman KL, Thompson JA, Benyunes MC, Winter TC, Fefer A. Adverse reactions to intravenous contrast media in patients treated with interleukin-2. J Immunother 1993;13(3):208–12.

126. Zukiwski AA, David CL, Coan J, Wallace S, Gutterman JU, Mavligit GM. Increased incidence of hypersensitivity to iodine-containing radiographic contrast media after interleukin-2 administration. Cancer 1990;65(7):1521–4.

127. Heywood GR, Rosenberg SA, Weber JS. Hypersensitivity reactions to chemotherapy agents in patients receiving chemoimmunotherapy with high-dose interleukin 2. J Natl Cancer Inst 1995;87(12):915–22.

128. Eton O, Legha SS, Bedikian AY, Lee JJ, Buzaid AC, Hodges C, Ring SE, Papadopoulos NE, Plager C, East MJ, Zhan F, Benjamin RS. Sequential biochemotherapy versus chemotherapy for metastatic melanoma: results from a phase III randomized trial. J Clin Oncol 2002;20(8):2045–52.

129. Bortolussi R, Fabiani F, Savron F, Testa V, Lazzarini R, Sorio R, De Conno F, Caraceni A. Acute morphine intoxication during high-dose recombinant interleukin-2 treatment for metastatic renal cell cancer. Eur J Cancer 1994;30A(12):1905–7.

Aldose reductase inhibitors

General Information

Aldose reductase inhibitors (SEDA-19, 397) (SEDA-20, 399) (SEDA-21, 447) (SEDA-22, 477) have been developed for the treatment of secondary complications in diabetes (1,2). They include alrestatin, benurestat, epalrestat, fidarestat, imirestat, lidorestat, minalrestat, ponalrestat, ranirestat, risarestat, sorbinil, tolrestat, zenarestat, and zopolrestat (all rINNs).

The aldose reductase inhibitors inhibit or reduce secondary complications induced by diabetes, specifically in tissues in which glucose uptake is not insulin-dependent (probably neural tissue, the lens, and glomeruli). Many of them (including alrestatin, imirestat, ponalrestat, and sorbinil) have been used in clinical trials, but have been withdrawn because of adverse effects or lack of effect (2). Their main adverse effects include fever, nausea, diarrhea, increases in liver enzymes, skin rashes, including toxic epidermal necrolysis and Stevens–Johnson syndrome, marked thrombocytopenia, lymphadenopathy, splenomegaly, and adult respiratory distress syndrome.

Tolrestat was withdrawn because of deaths from fatal hepatic necrosis (3) and poor efficacy in clinical trials. Sorbinil was withdrawn because of hypersensitivity reactions in more than 10% of patients.

Organs and Systems

Gastrointestinal

Nausea, vomiting, abdominal fullness, and diarrhea are reported with aldose reductase inhibitors (1).

References

1. Tsai SC, Burnakis TG. Aldose reductase inhibitors: an update. Ann Pharmacother 1993;27(6):751–4.
2. Krans HM. Recent clinical experience with aldose reductase inhibitors. Diabet Med 1993;10(Suppl 2):S44–8.
3. Foppiano M, Lombardo G. Worldwide pharmacovigilance systems and tolrestat withdrawal. Lancet 1997;349(9049):399–400.

Alemtuzumab

See also Monoclonal antibodies

General Information

Alemtuzumab (campath-1H) is a humanized monoclonal antibody specific for the CDw52 antigen, present on cell membranes of lymphocytes and monocytes. It has been used for treatment of patients with rheumatoid arthritis and vasculitis, is being investigated for the treatment of chronic lymphocytic leukemia, and has been used to deplete circulating lymphocytes in patients with multiple sclerosis (1). In 2001, alemtuzumab was approved in Europe for the treatment of chronic B cell lymphocytic leukemia that had been treated previously with alkylating agents and was refractory to fludarabine (2). It has also been used for induction of immunosuppression/tolerance in liver transplant recipients (3,4) and kidney/pancreas transplant recipients (5).

The major adverse effects (fever, nausea, skin rash, and hypotension) may well be related to the release of cytokines as a consequence of lysis of the target lymphocytes (6). Of four patients treated with alemtuzumab, three developed antibodies against it, but without affecting the plasma concentrations and without obvious clinical consequences. Other adverse effects have included mild renal impairment and transient thrombocytopenia.

Organs and Systems

Respiratory

Of 22 patients, median age 61 years, who had received a median of three previous types of therapy for mycosis fungoides or Sézary syndrome and were given alemtuzumab in increasing doses (from 3 to 30 mg three times a week for 12 weeks), 11 had no infectious complications, one had fatal pulmonary aspergillosis 2.5 months after the end of treatment, and another contracted fatal *Mycobacterium* pneumonia 10 months after the end of treatment (7).

Endocrine

Nine of 27 patients with multiple sclerosis developed antibodies against the thyrotropin receptor and carbimazole-responsive autoimmune hyperthyroidism after a 5-day pulse of alemtuzumab, a finding that was not reported in patients treated for other disorders (1).

Hematologic

In 50 patients with advanced, low-grade, non-Hodgkin's lymphoma alemtuzumab produced marked lymphopenia and neutropenia, which were the probable cause of frequent severe infections (8). Seven patients developed opportunistic infections and nine had bacterial septicemia; three patients died from infectious complications. Severe resistant autoimmune thrombocytopenia has also been noted in one patient, but the evidence that alemtuzumab was involved was limited (9).

Immunologic

Reactivation of cytomegalovirus is a frequent complication during treatment with alemtuzumab in patients with chronic lymphocytic leukemia (10), and other organisms are occasionally described.

- A 52-year-old man with B cell chronic lymphocytic leukemia had weight loss and a steadily rising blood lymphocyte count (11). He received alemtuzumab as first-line treatment as part of a clinical trial. After 12 weeks the leukemia completely remitted. Three years later he received chlorambucil for progressive disease and had a partial remission. After another 2 years his chemotherapy regimen was change to fludarabine and cyclophosphamide. After a further year his disease became rapidly progressive, with anemia, splenomegaly, and lymphadenopathy. Alemtuzumab was reintroduced and standard prophylaxis treatment was started with co-trimoxazole, valaciclovir, and fluconazole. After 8 weeks he developed fever up to 39°C. There was no evidence of bacterial or viral infection. His general condition worsened rapidly and he showed signs of acute hepatitis, renal insufficiency, disseminated intravascular coagulation, and finally respiratory failure. He died 14 days after the start of the fever. Adenovirus 5 was recovered from the lung, spleen, liver, and blood.

Among 18 patients with chronic lymphocytic leukemia, one with a long-lasting lymphocytopenia died 3 months after treatment, owing to progressive multifocal leukoencephalopathy; papovavirus was isolated from the cerebrospinal fluid (12).

References

1. Coles AJ, Wing M, Smith S, Coraddu F, Greer S, Taylor C, Weetman A, Hale G, Chatterjee VK, Waldmann H, Compston A. Pulsed monoclonal antibody treatment and autoimmune thyroid disease in multiple sclerosis. Lancet 1999;354(9191):1691–5.
2. Robak T. Alemtuzumab in the treatment of chronic lymphocytic leukemia. BioDrugs 2005;19(1):9–22.
3. Calne RY. Prope tolerance with alemtuzumab. Liver Transpl 2005;11(3):361–3.
4. Marcos A, Eghtesad B, Fung JJ, Fontes P, Patel K, Devera M, Marsh W, Gayowski T, Demetris AJ, Gray EA, Flynn B, Zeevi A, Murase N, Starzl TE. Use of alemtuzumab and tacrolimus monotherapy for cadaveric liver transplantation: with particular reference to hepatitis C virus Transplantation 2004;78(7):966–71.
5. Keven K, Basu A, Tan HP, Thai N, Khan A, Marcos A, Starzl TE, Shapiro R. Cytomegalovirus prophylaxis using oral ganciclovir or valganciclovir in kidney and pancreas-kidney transplantation under antibody preconditioning. Transplant Proc 2004;36(10):3107–12.
6. Watts RA, Isaacs JD, Hale G, Hazleman BL, Waldmann H. CAMPATH-1H in inflammatory arthritis. Clin Exp Rheumatol 1993;11(Suppl 8):S165–7.
7. Lundin J, Hagberg H, Repp R, Cavallin-Stahl E, Freden S, Juliusson G, Rosenblad E, Tjonnfjord G, Wiklund T, Osterborg A. Phase 2 study of alemtuzumab (anti-CD52 monoclonal antibody) in patients with advanced mycosis fungoides/Sezary syndrome. Blood 2003;101(11):4267–72.

8. Lundin J, Osterborg A, Brittinger G, Crowther D, Dombret H, Engert A, Epenetos A, Gisselbrecht C, Huhn D, Jaeger U, Thomas J, Marcus R, Nissen N, Poynton C, Rankin E, Stahel R, Uppenkamp M, Willemze R, Mellstedt H. CAMPATH-1H monoclonal antibody in therapy for previously treated low-grade non-Hodgkin's lymphomas: a phase II multicenter study. European Study Group of CAMPATH-1H Treatment in Low-Grade Non-Hodgkin's Lymphoma. J Clin Oncol 1998;16(10):3257–63.
9. Otton SH, Turner DL, Frewin R, Davies SV, Johnson SA. Autoimmune thrombocytopenia after treatment with Campath 1H in a patient with chronic lymphocytic leukaemia. Br J Haematol 1999;106(1):261–2.
10. Laurenti L, Piccioni P, Cattani P, Cingolani A, Efremov D, Chiusolo P, Tarnani M, Fadda G, Sica S, Leone G. Cytomegalovirus reactivation during alemtuzumab therapy for chronic lymphocytic leukemia: incidence and treatment with oral ganciclovir. Haematologica 2004;89(10):1248–52.
11. Cavalli-Bjorkman N, Osby E, Lundin J, Kalin M, Osterborg A, Gruber A. Fatal adenovirus infection during alemtuzumab (anti-CD52 monoclonal antibody) treatment of a patient with fludarabine-refractory B cell chronic lymphocytic leukemia. Med Oncol 2002;19(4):277–80.
12. Uppenkamp M, Engert A, Diehl V, Bunjes D, Huhn D, Brittinger G. Monoclonal antibody therapy with CAMPATH-1H in patients with relapsed high- and low-grade non-Hodgkin's lymphomas: a multicenter phase I/II study. Ann Hematol 2002;81(1):26–32.

Alfadolone and alfaxolone

See also General anesthetics

General Information

Alfadolone and alfaxolone are two steroid anesthetics that were used in combination. However, the mixture has been withdrawn because of safety considerations regarding the solvent used, polyethoxylated castor oil (Cremophor EL), which can cause non-IgE-mediated anaphylactic (anaphylactoid) reactions (SED-10, 189) (1).

Reference

1. Anonymous. Glaxo discontinues Althesin. Scrip 1984;882:17.

Alfentanil

General Information

Alfentanil is a potent short-acting opioid used in anesthesia. Beside its effects on opioid receptors, there is some evidence that it may affect acetylcholine, since intrathecal neostigmine produced a dose-dependent increase in the effect of alfentanil (SEDA-22, 3). Its rapid onset and short duration of action make alfentanil suitable for use in day care, although it is important to treat adverse effects before discharge.

Alfentanil is an ideal analgesic for focused and ambulatory interventions. In a prospective, uncontrolled study in three consecutive groups of outpatients undergoing shock-wave lithotripsy, group 1 (152 patients) had an induction dose of a combination of propofol 0.8 mg/kg and alfentanil 8 µg/kg; in group 2 (78 patients) and group 3 (250 patients), the induction dose was reduced by 20% (1). For all three groups the maintenance dose was a mixture of propofol 0.25 mg/kg and alfentanil 5 µg/kg given via a PCA device with a lock-out time of 5 minutes. In groups 1 and 2 the lithotripter was equipped with a standard electromagnetic shock-wave emitter (the EMSE 200), while in group 3 an upgraded EMSE F150 was used. Analgesic consumption was lower in the patients treated with the EMSE 150; groups 2 and 3, with a 20% reduction in induction dose, did not compensate by using more PCA. Groups 2 and 3 also had a significant reduction in the incidence of oxygen desaturation. The intravenous administration of a mixture of alfentanil and propofol, using the updated EMSE F150 device as in group 3, was therefore considered to be safe and reliable, with good patient tolerance and rapid recovery.

In a non-comparative study of 24 consecutive outpatients undergoing extracorporeal shock-wave lithotripsy, alfentanil (initial dose 15 µg/kg followed by 0.38 µg/kg/minute) and propofol (initial dose 1 mg/kg followed by 59 µg/kg/minute) were used for sedation (2). Both alfentanil and propofol were effective and safe, provided respiratory and cardiovascular parameters were routinely monitored.

Organs and Systems

Cardiovascular

When alfentanil 30 µg/kg was given to six healthy volunteers there were no clinical changes in respiratory or cardiovascular function (SEDA-16, 78).

Bradycardia often occurs with the combination of a potent short-acting opioid with suxamethonium during induction of anesthesia, and alfentanil has been reported to have caused sinus arrest in three patients (SEDA-17, 79) (3).

In one study alfentanil was particularly likely to cause hemodynamic instability and myocardial ischemia; however, drug interactions or the dosage regimen may have been responsible (4).

Respiratory

Significant respiratory depression occurs after alfentanil in doses in excess of 1000 µg and delayed-onset respiratory depression has been reported. Used as a general anesthetic for urgent cesarean section, alfentanil can cause marked neonatal respiratory depression, which is reversible with naloxone (SEDA-16, 78).

- A 35-year-old man developed recurrent respiratory depression after being given alfentanil 0.0125 mg/kg for vitreoretinal surgery (5). General anesthesia was induced with a combination of propofol, rocuronium, and alfentanil, subsequent inhalation of isoflurane, and three additional doses of alfentanil (total 0.04 mg/kg over 2 hours). The pulse oxygen saturation fluctuated and was as low as 89% 180 minutes after extubation.

The severity of respiratory depression with alfentanil has been assessed in 49 patients undergoing abdominal hysterectomy under general anesthetic, who were randomly allocated to three groups (6). Group 1 did not receive alfentanil during surgery, group 2 received alfentanil 30 μg/kg, and group 3 received a bolus dose of alfentanil 10–20 μg/kg and an alfentanil infusion increasing in increments of 0.25–0.5 mg/kg/minute. In this randomized double-blind study alfentanil had respiratory depressant effects (measured by plethysmography and pulse oximetry), in one patient in group 1 and three each in groups 2 and 3, but there were no cases of clear-cut recurrent respiratory depression.

Nervous system

Increased intracranial pressure in normal pressure hydrocephalus patients has been described (SEDA-17, 79). An acute dystonic reaction has been reported in an untreated patient with Parkinson's disease (SEDA-16, 78).

Simultaneous scalp and depth electrode recordings were performed on five patients with complex partial epilepsy who underwent alfentanil anesthesia induction before depth electrode removal (7). Five equal bolus doses of alfentanil 100 μg were given to each patient at 60-second intervals (total dose 500 μg). Epileptiform activity was increased in three of the five, but without clinical evidence of seizure activity.

Gastrointestinal

Alfentanil is associated with a high incidence of nausea and vomiting. Droperidol can reduce emetic symptoms but moclobemide does not (SEDA-17, 79).

- A 30-year-old woman with multiple body injuries required five general anesthetics in under 7 days for reconstructive surgery and dressing changes. In order to avoid further general anesthesia she was given a target-controlled infusion of alfentanil in 50 ml of 0.9% sodium chloride (a total dose of 5 mg over 35 minutes). There was one self-limiting episode of nausea with no vomiting. Oxygen saturation was 93–98% on air. There were no episodes of hypotension, cardiac dysrhythmias, or sedation (8).

Musculoskeletal

Muscular rigidity involving many muscle groups has been described with alfentanil (SEDA-12, 62).

Immunologic

A possible hypersensitivity reaction to alfentanil was reported in an atopic 13-year-old girl who developed life-threatening bronchospasm and confluent urticarial wheals (9).

Second-Generation Effects

Fetotoxicity

Alfentanil 10 μg/kg in normal parturients does not reduce Apgar scores, but a higher dose (15–30 μg/kg) is recommended for attenuation of the "stress" response in nonpregnant patients. In a randomized, placebo-controlled, double-blind study alfentanil was used in 40 patients in a dose of 10 μg/kg 1 minute before induction of anesthesia in 40 uncomplicated cesarean deliveries to determine whether it would reduce the maternal stress response after tracheal intubation without subsequent neonatal depression (10). There was a small but significant improvement in maternal hemodynamic stability in the alfentanil group at the expense of early but transient neonatal depression.

Susceptibility Factors

Age

Care is needed when alfentanil is used in the elderly, in whom the elimination of alfentanil is slower (11).

Other features of the patient

Recovery times were shorter in smokers than in non-smokers (12).

Alfentanil is 90% protein bound, and variability in protein binding can affect its actions. In 10 patients who received standardized anesthesia and alfentanil to a target concentration of 150 ng/ml for postoperative analgesia interindividual variation in plasma protein binding explained at least 39% of the interindividual variability in alfentanil requirements (13). There was a high incidence of adverse effects: seven patients had emesis and five had urinary retention.

Drug–Drug Interactions

Benzodiazepines

Muscle rigidity after high-dose opioid can be reduced by the benzodiazepines midazolam and diazepam (SEDA-19, 82).

Diltiazem

Diltiazem reduces the elimination of alfentanil and prolongs the time to tracheal extubation (SEDA-21, 86); erythromycin may do the same (14).

Fluconazole

There has been a double-blind randomized control study of the effect of the antifungal drug fluconazole 400 mg on the pharmacokinetics and pharmacodynamics of intravenous alfentanil (15). Fluconazole given either orally or intravenously 1 hour before alfentanil 20 μg/kg intravenously caused a significant doubling of the half-life, by inhibition of CYP3A4, which metabolizes alfentanil. Intravenous and oral fluconazole both increased alfentanil-induced respiratory depression by reducing the respiratory rate by 10–15% compared with alfentanil alone. Alfentanil should therefore be given cautiously to patients taking fluconazole and the authors suggested that such patients require 60% less alfentanil for maintenance of analgesia, irrespective of the mode of administration of the antifungal drug.

Ketamine

Eight healthy men participated in a 2-day study in which alfentanil was given to a constant plasma concentration of

50 ng/ml followed by the addition of ketamine at escalating plasma concentrations of 50, 100, and 200 ng/ml (16). The resting hypoventilation induced by alfentanil was antagonized by ketamine 200 ng/ml, but not 50 ng/ml.

Reserpine

The combination of reserpine with alfentanil is reported to cause ventricular dysrhythmias (SEDA-17, 79).

Tranylcypromine

There is no interaction of alfentanil with the monoamine oxidase inhibitor tranylcypromine (SEDA-17, 79).

References

1. Tailly GG, Marcelo JB, Schneider IA, Byttebier G, Daems K. Patient-controlled analgesia during SWL treatments. J Endourol 2001;15(5):465–71.
2. Nociti JR, Zuccolotto SN, Cagnolatl CA, Oliveira ACM, Bastos MM. Propofol and alfentanil sedation for extracorporeal shock wave lithotripsy. Rev Bras Anestesiol 2002;1:74–8.
3. Ananthanarayan C. Sinus arrest after alfentanil and suxamethonium. Anaesthesia 1989;44(7):614.
4. Nathan HJ. Narcotics and myocardial performance in patients with coronary artery disease. Can J Anaesth 1988;35(3Pt 1):209–13.
5. Calenda E, Muraine M. Recurrent respiratory depression after low doses of alfentanil. Eur J Anaesthesiol 1999;16(3):206.
6. Snijdelaar DG, Katz J, Clairoux M, Sandler AN. Respiratory effects of intraoperative alfentanil infusion in post-abdominal hysterectomy patients: a comparison of high versus low dose. Acute Pain 2000;3:131–9.
7. Ross J, Kearse LA Jr, Barlow MK, Houghton KJ, Cosgrove GR. Alfentanil-induced epileptiform activity: a simultaneous surface and depth electroencephalographic study in complex partial epilepsy. Epilepsia 2001;42(2):220–5.
8. Gallagher G, Rae CP, Watson S, Kinsella J. Target-controlled alfentanil analgesia for dressing change following extensive reconstructive surgery for trauma. J Pain Symptom Manage 2001;21(1):1–2.
9. Coventry DM, Stone P. Hypersensitivity reactions to alfentanil? Anaesthesia 1988;43(10):887–8.
10. Gin T, Ngan-Kee WD, Siu YK, Stuart JC, Tan PE, Lam KK. Alfentanil given immediately before the induction of anesthesia for elective cesarean delivery. Anesth Analg 2000;90(5):1167–72.
11. Kent AP, Dodson ME, Bower S. The pharmacokinetics and clinical effects of a low dose of alfentanil in elderly patients. Acta Anaesthesiol Belg 1988;39(1):25–33.
12. Dechene JP. Alfentanil as an adjunct to thiopentone and nitrous oxide in short surgical procedures. Can Anaesth Soc J 1985;32(4):346–50.
13. van den Nieuwenhuyzen MC, Engbers FH, Burm AG, Vletter AA, van Kleef JW, Bovill JG. Target-controlled infusion of alfentanil for postoperative analgesia: contribution of plasma protein binding to intra-patient and inter-patient variability. Br J Anaesth 1999;82(4):580–5.
14. Ahonen J, Olkkola KT, Salmenpera M, Hynynen M, Neuvonen PJ. Effect of diltiazem on midazolam and alfentanil disposition in patients undergoing coronary artery bypass grafting. Anesthesiology 1996;85(6):1246–52.
15. Palkama VJ, Isohanni MH, Neuvonen PJ, Olkkola KT. The effect of intravenous and oral fluconazole on the pharmacokinetics and pharmacodynamics of intravenous alfentanil. Anesth Analg 1998;87(1):190–4.
16. Persson J, Scheinin H, Hellstrom G, Bjorkman S, Gotharson E, Gustafsson LL. Ketamine antagonises alfentanil-induced hypoventilation in healthy male volunteers. Acta Anaesthesiol Scand 1999;43(7):744–52.

Alfuzosin

See also Alpha-adrenoceptor antagonists

General Information

Alfuzosin is a uroselective $alpha_1$-adrenoceptor antagonist used to relieve the symptoms of prostatic hyperplasia (1). Its safety has been investigated in a large prospective 3-year open trial in 3228 patients with benign prostatic hyperplasia. There were no unexpected adverse effects. Only 4.2% of the patients dropped out owing to adverse effects.

In a large database of 7093 patients with lower urinary tract symptoms related to benign prostatic hyperplasia treated for up to 3 years with alfuzosin in general practice, adverse events were reported in a very complex and uninformative way (2). In another paper, the same authors reported on a subcohort of 2829 patients, with special focus on effects on quality of life. Adverse events occurred in 15% of the patients, 1.7% died during the study, and 5.2% had serious effects, which the authors did not detail, but which they stated were not related to treatment. Most adverse effects occurred during the first 3 months of treatment (3). In another database of 3095 Spanish patients taking alfuzosin 5 mg bd for 60 days, adverse events were reported in 3.3% of the patients, and led to drug withdrawal in 1.6%; postural hypotension occurred in 1.8% (4).

Organs and Systems

Nervous system

Dizziness, headache, postural hypertension, and other symptoms familiar from the older alpha-blockers occur primarily during the first 2 weeks of treatment with alfuzosin (1).

Liver

Hepatitis potentially related to alfuzosin has been reported (5).

- A 63-year-old man, who had taken amiloride and alfuzosin for 9 months for hypertension and benign prostatic hyperplasia, became jaundiced. His aspartate transaminase was 3013 IU/l, alanine transaminase 2711 IU/l, alkaline phosphatase 500 IU/l, and total bilirubin 415 µmol/l. Viral causes, autoimmune hepatitis, and biliary obstruction were excluded. After withdrawal of alfuzosin, his liver function tests gradually returned to normal within 6 months.

Immunologic

Dermatomyositis has been attributed to alfuzosin.

- A 75-year-old man, who had taken alfuzosin for 1 year, developed muscle pain and weakness over 4 days, accompanied by tenderness and swelling of the deltoid muscles (6). There was erythema, with rash, periungual purpura, and erythematous plaques over the finger joints. Serum CK, LDH, and transaminase activities were raised and ANA was positive. An MRI scan showed findings consistent with inflammation of muscle and a biopsy confirmed the diagnosis of dermatomyositis. Three days after drug withdrawal there was no improvement, so prednisone was started and he recovered within a few days. The temporal relation in this case was weak.

- Dermatomyositis, with typical clinical effects, biochemical tests, electromyography, and muscle biopsy, occurred in a 75-year-old man who had taken alfuzosin for 1 year (7). There was no malignancy and he recovered fully after alfuzosin withdrawal (timing not given).

References

1. McKeage K, Plosker GL. Alfuzosin: a review of the therapeutic use of the prolonged-release formulation given once daily in the management of benign prostatic hyperplasia. Drugs 2002;62(4):633–53.
2. Lukacs B, Grange JC, Comet D, McCarthy C. History of 7,093 patients with lower urinary tract symptoms related to benign prostatic hyperplasia treated with alfuzosin in general practice up to 3 years. Eur Urol 2000;37(2):183–90.
3. Lukacs B, Grange JC, Comet D. One-year follow-up of 2829 patients with moderate to severe lower urinary tract symptoms treated with alfuzosin in general practice according to IPSS and a health-related quality-of-life questionnaire. BPM Group in General Practice. Urology 2000;55(4):540–6.
4. Sanchez-Chapado M, Guil M, Alfaro V, Badiella L, Fernandez-Hernando N. Safety and efficacy of sustained-release alfuzosin on lower urinary tract symptoms suggestive of benign prostatic hyperplasia in 3,095 Spanish patients evaluated during general practice. Eur Urol 2000;37(4):421–7.
5. Zabala S, Thomson C, Valdearcos S, Gascon A, Pina MA. Alfuzosin-induced hepatotoxicity. J Clin Pharm Ther 2000;25(1):73–4.
6. Vela-Casasempere P, Borras-Blasco J, Navarro-Ruiz A. Alfuzosin-associated dermatomyositis. Br J Rheumatol 1998;37(10):1135–6.
7. Schmutz J-L, Barbaud A, Trechot PH. Alfuzosine, inducteur de dermatomyosite. [Alfuzosine-induced dermatomyositis.] Ann Dermatol Venereol 2000;127(4):449.

Algae

General Information

Algae are members of the kingdom Protista. They include Bacillariophyta (unicellular diatoms), Charophyta (freshwater stoneworts), Chrysophyta (photosynthetic, unicellular organisms), Cyanobacteria (photosynthetic bacteria), Dinophyta (dinoflagellates), and the various types of seaweeds.

There are three major groups of seaweeds: the green algae (Chlorophyta), the brown algae (Phaeophyta), and the red algae (Rhodophyta).

Kelp is a general name for seaweed preparations obtained from different species of Phaeophyta (such as

Ascophyllum nodosum, *Fucus vesiculosus*, *Fucus serratus*, *Laminaria* species, and *Macrocystis pyrifera*). As kelp contains iodine, it occasionally produces hyperthyroidism (1), hypothyroidism, or extrathyroidal reactions, such as skin eruptions. It can also contain contaminants such as arsenic, and bone marrow depression and autoimmune thrombocytopenia have been described in consequence (2).

Anaphylaxis to *Laminaria* has been described (3–5).

Laminaria has been used to induce abortion and can cause uterine rupture especially in primipara.

- A 32-year-old woman in her 25th week of gestation was hospitalized for endouterine fetal death (6). She had had two previous cesarean sections. Cervical dilatation was induced with a Hagar dilator and laminaria tents, and sudden spontaneous and strong contractions led to uterine rupture.

References

1. de Smet PA, Stricker BH, Wilderink F, Wiersinga WM. Hyperthyreoïdie tijdens het gebruik van kelptabletten. [Hyperthyroidism during treatment with kelp tablets.] Ned Tijdschr Geneeskd 1990;134(21):1058–9.
2. Pye KG, Kelsey SM, House IM, Newland AC. Severe dyserythropoiesis and autoimmune thrombocytopenia associated with ingestion of kelp supplements. Lancet 1992;339(8808):1540.
3. Knowles SR, Djordjevic K, Binkley K, Weber EA. Allergic anaphylaxis to *Laminaria*. Allergy 2002;57(4):370.
4. Cole DS, Bruck LR. Anaphylaxis after *Laminaria* insertion. Obstet Gynecol 2000;95(6 Pt 2):1025.
5. Nguyen MT, Hoffman DR. Anaphylaxis to *Laminaria*. J Allergy Clin Immunol 1995;95(1 Pt 1):138–9.
6. Menaldo G, Alemanno MG, Brizzolara M, Campogrande M. La *Laminaria* nell'induzione d'aborto al 2no trimestre. Caso di rottura d'utero. [*Laminaria* in induction of abortion in the 2d trimester. Case of uterine rupture.] Minerva Ginecol 1981;33(6):599–601.

Alimemazine

See also Neuroleptic drugs

General Information

Alimemazine is a phenothiazine derivative with sedative antihistaminic and antimuscarinic effects.

Organs and Systems

Nervous system

Neuroleptic malignant syndrome has been reported with alimemazine (1).

- A 4-year-old girl with damage in the basal ganglia who was receiving increasing doses of alimemazine for sedative purposes developed neuroleptic malignant syndrome. The alimemazine was withdrawn and she received dantrolene and supportive measures, including ventilation under sedation and paralysis with midazolam and vecuronium. As her symptoms were unchanged, she was given increasing doses of bromocriptine and improved. A few days after bromocriptine withdrawal, the neuroleptic malignant syndrome recurred and was complicated by cardiorespiratory arrest.

Reference

1. van Maldegem BT, Smit LM, Touw DJ, Gemke RJ. Neuroleptic malignant syndrome in a 4-year-old girl associated with alimemazine. Eur J Pediatr 2002;161(5):259–61.

Aliphatic alcohols

See also Disinfectants and antiseptics

General Information

The lower aliphatic alcohols (ethanol, isopropanol, 2-propanol, *N*-propanol, and 1-propanol) are widely used for skin antisepsis. In appropriate concentrations, these alcohols are bactericidal to most of the common pathogenic bacteria, but some rare species survive and can grow, especially since these alcohols are inactive against dried spores.

Seven cases of gaseous edema were observed in the former German Democratic Republic (GDR) after intramuscular injections following rubbing of the skin with ethanol (SEDA-11, 474); this led to a national recommendation that alcohols should not be used to cleanse the skin before intramuscular injection, injection of vasoconstrictors, injections in patients with disturbed peripheral circulation, or before lumbar, paraneural, or intra-articular injection and puncture (SEDA-11, 474) (1).

Organs and Systems

Cardiovascular

Skin disinfection before insertion of peripheral infusion catheters is standard practice. Ethanol 70% has been compared with 2% iodine dissolved in 70% ethanol in a prospective, randomized trial in 109 patients who were given infusions of prednisone and theophylline (2). Phlebitis occurred six times in the ethanol group and 12 times in the iodine group. The relative risk reduction of 53% failed to reach significance, but the power of the study was only 0.55, so there was a 45% chance of missing a true difference. As vast numbers of catheters are inserted each year, a small difference in phlebitis rate could save many patients discomfort.

Skin

Skin reactions to ethanol are extremely rare, although allergic contact dermatitis due to lower aliphatic alcohols has been described (SEDA-11, 474) (3). However, in premature infants of very low birth weight, second-degree and third-degree chemical skin burns were reported after the use of isopropanol, either for conduction in electrocardiography, for the preparation of the umbilical stump for arterial catheterization, or for cleansing before herniotomy (SEDA-11, 474) (4,5). Possible causes are hypoperfusion of the skin by local pressure and general hypoperfusion derived from hypoxia, hypothermia, and acidosis. Immediate drying of the skin of small premature infants after antisepsis with alcoholic formulations and carefully avoiding that the alcohol is absorbed by the diapers is recommended.

Drug Administration

Drug administration route

When it is not possible to perform surgical treatment for omphalocele, application of ethanol is probably the safest method. However, dosage and frequency of application should be as limited, since absorption and intoxication can occur (SEDA-11, 474) (6).

References

1. Spengler W. Stellungnahme der Hauptabteilung Hygiene und Staatlichen Hygieninspektion im Ministerium für Gesundheitswesen zur Diskussion über die Hautdesinfektion vor Injektionen und Punktionen. Med Aktuell 1977;3:51.
2. de Vries JH, van Dorp WT, van Barneveld PW. A randomized trial of alcohol 70% versus alcoholic iodine 2% in skin disinfection before insertion of peripheral infusion catheters. J Hosp Infect 1997;36(4):317–20.
3. Ludwig E, Hausen BM. Sensitivity to isopropyl alcohol. Contact Dermatitis 1977;3(5):240–4.
4. Schick JB, Milstein JM. Burn hazard of isopropyl alcohol in the neonate. Pediatrics 1981;68(4):587–8.
5. Klein BR, Leape LL. Skin burn from Freon preparation. Surgery 1976;79(1):122.
6. Schroder CH, Severijnen RS, Monnens LA. Vergiftiging door desinfectans bij conservatieve behandeling van twee patiënten met omfalokele. [Poisoning by disinfectants in the conservative treatment of 2 patients with omphalocele.] Tijdschr Kindergeneeskd 1985;53(2):76–9.

Alizapride

General Information

Alizapride is a substituted benzamide related to some neuroleptic drugs. In one study alizapride, in doses that were less effective than normal doses of metoclopramide, was equally likely to cause extrapyramidal effects and more likely to cause hypotension (SED-12, 939) (SEDA-17, 413).

In another study, doses of 5 mg/kg (but not less) caused diarrhea and orthostatic hypotension (SEDA-9, 311); the incidence of diarrhea may well be higher than with metoclopramide (1). Other recorded effects include a sensation of bodily heat and trismus (SEDA-10, 323).

Drug–Drug Interactions

Diazepam

Alizapride increases the absorption rate of concurrently administered diazepam (2).

References

1. Moreno I, Rosell R, Abad-Esteve A, Barnadas A, Carles J, Ribelles N. Randomized trial for the control of acute vomiting in cisplatin-treated patients: high-dose metoclopramide with dexamethasone and lorazepam as adjuncts versus high-dose alizapride plus dexamethasone and lorazepam. Study of the incidence of delayed emesis. Oncology 1991;48(5):397–402.
2. McGeown MG. Renal disease associated with drugs. In: D'Arcy PF, Griffin JP, editors. Iatrogenic Diseases. 3rd ed. Oxford-New York-Tokyo: Oxford University Press, 1986:790.

Alkylating cytostatic agents — nitrosoureas

See also Cytostatic and immunosuppressant drugs

General Information

Alkylating cytostatic drugs include (all rINNs):

- Nitrosoureas: carmustine, lomustine, nimustine, streptozocin
- *N*-lost derivatives: chlormethine, cyclophosphamide, estramustine
- Others: busulfan, chlorambucil, dacarbazine, ifosfamide, melphalan, mitobronitol, mitomycin, procarbazine, thiotepa, temozolomide, treosulfan.

The first two groups (apart from cyclophosphamide) are covered in this monograph.

Nitrosoureas

Carmustine (BCNU) is used to treat myeloma, lymphomas, breast cancer, and brain tumors, Topical carmustine has been used to treat mycosis fungoides (1).

Lomustine (CCNU) is used to treat lymphomas and some solid tumors, particularly brain tumors, often in combination with procarbazine and vincristine (2).

Nimustine (ACNU) is used to treat malignant glioma (3).

Streptozocin (streptozotocin) is produced by *Streptomyces achromogenes*. It is used to treat metastatic islet cell carcinoma of the pancreas, but because of its high nephrotoxic and emetogenic potential should be reserved for patients with symptomatic or progressive disease.

N-lost derivatives

Chlormethine (mechlorethamine, mustine, nitrogen mustard) is mainly used topically in the early stages of mycosis fungoides (4).

Cyclophosphamide (see separate monograph) is used in the treatment of various solid tumors, and as an immunosuppressant in conditions such as Wegener's granulomatosis and in conditioning regimens for bone marrow transplantation.

Estramustine is a conjugated derivative of estradiol and chlormethine, mainly used to treat prostate cancer (5,6).

Organs and Systems

Respiratory

Carmustine pulmonary toxicity is well documented. Eight patients developed interstitial pulmonary fibrosis 12–17 years after exposure to carmustine in a total dose of carmustine of 770–1410 mg/m^2 (7).

Lung fibrosis has been described in a long-term follow up 13–17 years after treatment of 31 children given carmustine for brain tumors; 6 died, and of 8 still available for study, 6 had upper zone fibrotic changes of their lungs on X-ray (8).

Sensory systems

A 2.7% ocular complication rate in 112 patients treated with a cumulative dose of carmustine 370 mg/m^2 for intracranial tumors has been recorded (9).

Eye pain and blindness due to retinal and optic nerve damage are recognized hazards of intracarotid carmustine therapy reference. They are thought to be due, at least in part, to the ethanol content of the diluent. Nimustine (ACNU) is water-soluble and ethanol-free. In a study of 30 patients with malignant gliomas, 123 infusions of nimustine and 53 of carmustine were administered (10). Eye pain was experienced during all carmustine infusions but not with nimustine, and one patient developed unilateral blindness after carmustine. In another study, carmustine was administered in solution with 5% dextrose in water (11). All the patients experienced ipsilateral orbital pain and scleral erythema, suggesting that carmustine itself contributes to the toxicity. Seven additional patients were treated wearing an ocular compression device to decrease blood flow and had not experienced any ocular complications.

Mineral balance

A patient with androgen-independent prostate cancer developed hypocalcemia during treatment with estramustine (12). The total serum calcium concentrations before and after the initiation of estramustine were 2.1 and 1.1 mmol/l respectively. This prompted a retrospective survey of hypocalcemia in 135 consecutive patients taking estramustine; 20% were affected. The authors speculated that estramustine may cause hypocalcemia by inhibiting mobilization of calcium and the action of parathyroid hormone on the skeleton.

Hematologic

Of 91 patients treated with topical carmustine, three developed reversible bone marrow depression (13).

Urinary tract

Nephrotoxicity can rarely occur with lomustine, and all cases have been associated with cumulative doses of greater than 1500 mg/m^2 (14).

Skin

Local adverse effects of topical carmustine include tender erythema, superficial denudation or bullae, contact allergy, pigment alterations, and patchy telangiectasia (1).

Reproductive system

Gynecomastia severe enough to necessitate withdrawal of therapy was the main adverse effect of estramustine 560 mg/day for more than 1 year in prostatic carcinoma (15).

Breast pain with vaginal bleeding and diarrhea were dose-limiting when estramustine 840 mg/day was given for breast cancer (16).

Immunologic

Topical carmustine can cause hypersensitivity reactions, and three previous cases have been supplemented by a fourth (17).

- A 67-year-old woman used topical carmustine for a stage-I cutaneous T cell lymphoma. A second course was started after 6 months and resulted in severe erosive inflammation at the site of treatment. Patch tests with carmustine 0.1, 0.5, and 1% in water all gave positive results; 22 controls were tested with 0.1% carmustine and lomustine and were all negative.

The most common adverse effect of chlormethine is an allergic contact dermatitis (18). Neither reducing the concentration of drug applied nor shortening the time of contact appreciably reduces the frequency of this adverse effect, which occurs in 30–80% of patients, although in one study of 203 patients with mycosis fungoides the use of chlormethine ointment was associated with contact hypersensitivity in under 10% of cases (4). In an open, prospective study in 39 patients with cutaneous T cell lymphomas or parapsoriasis, chlormethine was applied topically and then washed off after 1 hour (19). There was cutaneous intolerance in 19 patients, six of whom had an allergic contact dermatitis after a mean period of 9.3 weeks, while the other 13 developed irritant contact dermatitis after a longer period. Cutaneous intolerance did not differ significantly according to the number of applications per week or the extent of body area treated. Comparison with published studies showed no significant difference in the number of cases of cutaneous intolerance after short-term application, although their occurrence was delayed. Therapeutic response was decreased appreciably by short-term application as compared with results in the literature.

Long-Term Effects

Tumorigenicity

Chlormethine can act as a tumor promotor. In most cases squamous cell carcinomas and basal cell carcinomas have been reported. Two cases of small malignant melanoma, 3 mm in diameter, have been reported in patients with mycosis fungoides stage 1a, with latency intervals of 18 and 10 months after withdrawal of local application, which had been conducted for 18 months and almost 3 years respectively (20).

Second-Generation Effects

Fertility

In 21 boys treated with carmustine or lomustine alone or in combination with procarbazine and vincristine for brain tumors, there were 20 cases of persistent testicular damage (21). From assessment of testicular size it was thought that most those affected would remain infertile. This supports the idea that germinal epithelium is more susceptible than Leydig cells to cytostatic-induced damage.

References

1. Zackheim HS. Topical carmustine (BCNU) in the treatment of mycosis fungoides. Dermatol Ther 2003;16(4):299–302.
2. Prados MD, Seiferheld W, Sandler HM, Buckner JC, Phillips T, Schultz C, Urtasun R, Davis R, Gutin P, Cascino TL, Greenberg HS, Curran WJ Jr. Phase III randomized study of radiotherapy plus procarbazine, lomustine, and vincristine with or without BUdR for treatment of anaplastic astrocytoma: final report of RTOG 9404. Int J Radiat Oncol Biol Phys 2004;58(4):1147–52.
3. Weller M, Muller B, Koch R, Bamberg M, Krauseneck P; Neuro-Oncology Working Group of the German Cancer Society. Neuro-Oncology Working Group 01 trial of nimustine plus teniposide versus nimustine plus cytarabine chemotherapy in addition to involved-field radiotherapy in the first-line treatment of malignant glioma. J Clin Oncol 2003;21(17):3276–84.
4. Kim YH, Martinez G, Varghese A, Hoppe RT. Topical nitrogen mustard in the management of mycosis fungoides: update of the Stanford experience. Arch Dermatol 2003;139(2):165–73.
5. Kimura M, Sasagawa T, Tomita Y, Katagiri A, Morishita H, Saito T, Tanikawa T, Kawasaki T, Saito K, Nishiyama T, Kasahara T, Hara N, Takahashi K. [Intermittent oral hormonal chemotherapy using estramustine phosphate and etoposide for the treatment of hormone-refractory prostate cancer.] Hinyokika Kiyo 2003;49(12):709–14.
6. Eastham JA, Kelly WK, Grossfeld GD, Small EJ; Cancer and Leukemia Group B. Cancer and Leukemia Group B (CALGB) 90203: a randomized phase 3 study of radical prostatectomy alone versus estramustine and docetaxel before radical prostatectomy for patients with high-risk localized disease. Urology 2003;62(Suppl 1):55–62.
7. Hasleton PS, O'Driscoll BR, Lynch P, Webster A, Kalra SJ, Gattamaneini HR, Woodcock AA, Poulter LW. Late BCNU lung: a light and ultrastructural study on the delayed effect of BCNU on the lung parenchyma. J Pathol 1991;164(1):31–6.
8. O'Driscoll BR, Hasleton PS, Taylor PM, Poulter LW, Gattameneni HR, Woodcock AA. Active lung fibrosis up to 17 years after chemotherapy with carmustine (BCNU) in childhood. N Engl J Med 1990;323(6):378–82.
9. Elsas T, Watne K, Fostad K, Hager B. Ocular complications after intracarotid BCNU for intracranial tumors. Acta Ophthalmol (Copenh) 1989;67(1):83–6.
10. Papavero L, Loew F, Jaksche H. Intracarotid infusion of ACNU and BCNU as adjuvant therapy of malignant gliomas. Clinical aspects and critical considerations. Acta Neurochir (Wien) 1987;85(3–4):128–37.
11. Johnson DW, Parkinson D, Wolpert SM, Kasdon DL, Kwan ES, Laucella M, Anderson ML. Intracarotid chemotherapy with 1,3-bis-(2-chloroethyl)-1-nitrosourea (BCNU) in 5% dextrose in water in the treatment of malignant glioma. Neurosurgery 1987;20(4):577–83.

12. Park DS, Vassilopoulou Sellin R, Tu S. Estramustine-related hypocalcemia in patients with prostate carcinoma and osteoblastic metastases. Urology 2001;58(1):105.

13. Zackheim HS, Epstein EH Jr, McNutt NS, Grekin DA, Crain WR. Topical carmustine (BCNU) for mycosis fungoides and related disorders: a 10-year experience. J Am Acad Dermatol 1983;9(3):363–74.

14. Ellis ME, Weiss RB, Kuperminc M. Nephrotoxicity of lomustine. A case report and literature review. Cancer Chemother Pharmacol 1985;15(2):174–5.

15. Asakawa M, Wada S, Hayahara N, Yayumoto R, Kishimoto T, Maekawa M, Morikawa Y, Kawakita J, Umeda M, Horii A, et al. [Clinical study of estramustine phosphate disodium (Estracyt) on prostatic cancer—results of long-term therapy for 38 patients with prostatic cancer.] Hinyokika Kiyo 1990;36(11):1361–9.

16. Wada T, Morikawa E, Houjou T, Kadota K, Mori N, Matsunami N, Watatani M, Yasutomi M. [Clinical evaluation of estramustine phosphate in the treatment of patients with advanced breast cancers.] Gan To Kagaku Ryoho 1990;17(9):1901–4.

17. Thomson KF, Sheehan-Dare RA, Wilkinson SM. Allergic contact dermatitis from topical carmustine. Contact Dermatitis 2000;42(2):112.

18. Goday JJ, Aguirre A, Raton JA, Diaz-Perez JL. Local bullous reaction to topical mechlorethamine (mustine). Contact Dermatitis 1990;22(5):306–7.

19. Foulc P, Evrard V, Dalac S, Guillot B, Delaunay M, Verret JL, Dreno B. Evaluation of a 1-h exposure time to mechlorethamine in patients undergoing topical treatment. Br J Dermatol 2002;147(5):926–30.

20. Amichai B, Grunwald MH, Goldstein J, Finkelstein E, Halevy S. Small malignant melanoma in patients with mycosis fungoides. J Eur Acad Dermatol Venereol 1998;11(2):155–7.

21. Clayton PE, Shalet SM, Price DA, Campbell RH. Testicular damage after chemotherapy for childhood brain tumors. J Pediatr 1988;112(6):922–6.

Alkylating cytostatic agents — *N*-lost derivatives

See also Cytostatic and immunosuppressant drugs

General Information

The *N*-lost cytostatic drugs are alkylating agents that include chlormethine (mechlorethamine, mustine, nitrogen mustard), cyclophosphamide, and estramustine (all rINNs). Chlormethine is mainly used topically in the early stages of mycosis fungoides (1). Estramustine is a conjugated derivative of estradiol and chlormethine, mainly used to treat prostate cancer (2).

Organs and Systems

Mineral balance

A patient with androgen-independent prostate cancer developed hypocalcemia during treatment with estramustine (3). The total serum calcium concentrations before and after the initiation of estramustine were 2.1 and 1.1 mmol/l respectively. This prompted a retrospective survey of hypocalcemia in 135 consecutive patients taking estramustine; 20% were affected. The authors speculated that estramustine may cause hypocalcemia by inhibiting mobilization of calcium and the action of parathyroid hormone on the skeleton.

Reproductive system

Gynecomastia severe enough to necessitate withdrawal of therapy was the main adverse effect of estramustine 560 mg/day for more than 1 year in prostatic carcinoma (4).

Breast pain with vaginal bleeding and diarrhea were dose-limiting when estramustine 840 mg/day was given for breast cancer (5).

Immunologic

The most common adverse effect of chlormethine is an allergic contact dermatitis (6). Neither reducing the concentration of drug applied nor shortening the time of contact appreciably reduces the frequency of this adverse effect, which occurs in 30–80% of patients, although in one study of 203 patients with mycosis fungoides, the use of chlormethine ointment was associated with contact hypersensitivity in under 10% of cases (1). In an open, prospective study in 39 patients with cutaneous T cell lymphomas or parapsoriasis, chlormethine was applied topically and then washed off after 1 hour (7). There was cutaneous intolerance in 19 patients, six of whom had an allergic contact dermatitis after a mean period of 9.3 weeks, while the other 13 developed irritant contact dermatitis after a longer period. Cutaneous intolerance did not differ significantly according to the number of applications per week or the extent of body area treated. Comparison with published studies showed no significant difference in the number of cases of cutaneous intolerance after short-term application, although their occurrence was delayed. Therapeutic response was decreased appreciably by short-term application as compared with results in the literature.

Long-Term Effects

Tumorigenicity

Chlormethine can act as a tumor promotor. In most cases squamous cell carcinomas and basal cell carcinomas have been reported. Two cases of small malignant melanoma, 3 mm in diameter, have been reported in patients with mycosis fungoides stage 1a, with latency intervals of 18 and 10 months after withdrawal of local application, which had been conducted for 18 months and almost 3 years respectively (8).

References

1. Kim YH, Martinez G, Varghese A, Hoppe RT. Topical nitrogen mustard in the management of mycosis fungoides: update of the Stanford experience. Arch Dermatol 2003;139(2):165–73.

2. Eastham JA, Kelly WK, Grossfeld GD, Small EJ; Cancer and Leukemia Group B. Cancer and Leukemia Group B

(CALGB) 90203: a randomized phase 3 study of radical prostatectomy alone versus estramustine and docetaxel before radical prostatectomy for patients with high-risk localized disease. Urology 2003;62(Suppl 1):55–62.

3. Park DS, Vassilopoulou Sellin R, Tu S. Estramustine-related hypocalcemia in patients with prostate carcinoma and osteoblastic metastases. Urology 2001;58(1):105.

4. Asakawa M, Wada S, Hayahara N, Yayumoto R, Kishimoto T, Maekawa M, Morikawa Y, Kawakita J, Umeda M, Horii A, et al. [Clinical study of estramustine phosphate disodium (Estracyt) on prostatic cancer—results of long-term therapy for 38 patients with prostatic cancer.] Hinyokika Kiyo 1990;36(11):1361–9.

5. Wada T, Morikawa E, Houjou T, Kadota K, Mori N, Matsunami N, Watatani M, Yasutomi M. [Clinical evaluation of estramustine phosphate in the treatment of patients with advanced breast cancers.] Gan To Kagaku Ryoho 1990;17(9):1901–4.

6. Goday JJ, Aguirre A, Raton JA, Diaz-Perez JL. Local bullous reaction to topical mechlorethamine (mustine). Contact Dermatitis 1990;22(5):306–7.

7. Foulc P, Evrard V, Dalac S, Guillot B, Delaunay M, Verret JL, Dreno B. Evaluation of a 1-h exposure time to mechlorethamine in patients undergoing topical treatment. Br J Dermatol 2002;147(5):926–30.

8. Amichai B, Grunwald MH, Goldstein J, Finkelstein E, Halevy S. Small malignant melanoma in patients with mycosis fungoides. J Eur Acad Dermatol Venereol 1998;11(2):155–7.

Allopurinol

General Information

Allopurinol is an inhibitor of xanthine oxidase, used to lower serum uric acid concentrations in the long-term treatment of gout and in the prevention of acute gout in people who are susceptible to hyperuricemia. Allopurinol is itself metabolized to its active metabolite, oxipurinol, by xanthine oxidase.

Comparisons with antimonials in leishmaniasis

Allopurinol has an antileishmanial effect in vitro and in animals, its effect being strongly increased by the addition of antimonial compounds. Allopurinol alone as well as in combination with meglumine antimoniate has been used in clinical studies. In a small study in patients with leishmaniasis and HIV infection, clinical and parasitological cure was achieved in four of five cases treated for 4 weeks, but in only one of the six treated for 3 weeks (1).

Allopurinol and meglumine antimoniate (Glucantime) have been evaluated in a randomized controlled trial in 150 patients with cutaneous leishmaniasis (2). They received oral allopurinol (15 mg/kg/day) for 3 weeks or intramuscular meglumine antimoniate (30 mg/kg/day, corresponding to 8 mg/kg/day of pentavalent antimony, for 2 weeks), or combined therapy. There were a few adverse effects in those who used allopurinol: nausea, heartburn ($n = 3$), and mild increases in transaminases ($n = 2$). These symptoms subsided on drug withdrawal.

In an open study, 72 patients each received meglumine antimoniate (60 mg/kg/day) or allopurinol (20 mg/kg/day) plus low-dose meglumine antimoniate (30 mg/kg/day) for 20 days, and each was followed for 30 days after the end of treatment (3). Only six patients in the combined treatment group complained of mild abdominal pain and nausea; however, one patient who received meglumine antimoniate developed a skin eruption. Generalized muscle pain and weakness occurred in four patients.

Organs and Systems

Nervous system

Apart from headache and vertigo, adverse effects of allopurinol involving the nervous system are rare. Transient peripheral neuropathy has been reported (SEDA-18, 107).

Seizures, which were unresponsive to standard anticonvulsive therapy, disappeared when allopurinol was withdrawn in a patient with a primary neurological disorder (4).

In contrast, occasional reports that allopurinol may have an anticonvulsive effect prompted its use in therapy-resistant epileptic patients. Withdrawal in one of these patients precipitated a convulsive status epilepticus (SEDA-16, 114).

- A 60-year-old man developed aseptic meningitis after taking allopurinol on two separate occasions (5).

Sensory systems

Allopurinol can reportedly cause cataracts (6), but in one study there was no evidence to confirm this risk (SEDA-15, 104).

Hematologic

Eosinophilia and leukocytosis are part of a general hypersensitivity reaction to allopurinol. Leukopenia and neutropenia are sometimes associated with allopurinol. Patients taking cytostatic therapy are more susceptible to bone marrow depression if they take allopurinol as well (SED-9, 155); however, this has not been confirmed in other reports (7). Agranulocytosis is extremely rare.

Cases of aplastic anemia, some in patients with renal insufficiency, have been reported (SEDA-13, 84) (8–10), confirming the need to reduce the dose of allopurinol in patients with renal insufficiency and to monitor toxicity (SEDA-16, 114).

Liver

Hepatitis can be part of a generalized hypersensitivity reaction. Hepatotoxicity ranges from mild granulomatous hepatitis to severe hepatocellular necrosis (SED-5, 155) (SEDA-4, 70). Renal impairment seems to be a prerequisite for a severe hepatic reaction.

Urinary tract

Vasculitis due to a general hypersensitivity reaction can cause renal insufficiency and oliguria. Histological findings are vasculitis and tubular necrosis with fibrinoid deposits. Acute renal insufficiency due to xanthine crystals in the kidney tubules during antineoplastic chemotherapy has been reported (11).

Since allopurinol blocks xanthine conversion to uric acid, urinary xanthine excretion is increased, creating a risk of xanthine crystal formation in the urinary system or even in muscles; this can result in nephrolithiasis (12). It is still an open question whether a predisposition to renal disease or renal disease itself is required to precipitate these adverse effects. It is also not known whether increased excretion of orotic acid, due to an interaction of allopurinol with pyrimidine formation, has any consequences for these adverse effects or for its role in reducing glucose tolerance.

Granulomatous interstitial nephritis (SEDA-12, 94) and two cases of interstitial cystitis have been described during long-term treatment with allopurinol (SEDA-21, 108).

Skin

Skin reactions have a general incidence of 10%, are more common in patients with renal disorders and in those taking thiazide diuretics, and are closely correlated with persistently high serum concentrations of oxipurinol (13). The positive association of severe skin reactions with HLA haplotypes AW33 and B17 suggests a genetic predisposition to these reactions (14).

Rash, urticaria, erythematous eruptions, papulovesicular reactions, and pruritus may be the only signs of hypersensitivity or may be part of a generalized reaction.

Dangerous reactions such as exfoliative dermatitis and Lyell's syndrome rarely develop (SEDA-5, 108).

Unusual skin lesions with a benign lymphocyte infiltration have been documented (SEDA-14, 96). Toxic pustuloderma can be added to the list (SEDA-18, 108).

An allopurinol-induced fixed drug eruption was successfully treated by desensitization (SEDA-21, 108).

Allopurinol can uncover latent lichen planus (15).

Musculoskeletal

Myositis and rhabdomyolysis have been attributed to allopurinol (16).

- A 73-year-old woman with chronic renal insufficiency developed generalized muscular weakness and pain 6 days after starting to take allopurinol 200 mg/day. Her serum creatine kinase activity was increased and the diagnosis was rhabdomyolysis, attributed to severe myositis. The serum concentration of oxipurinol was also high. The muscle weakness resolved in 7 weeks with intermittent hemodiafiltration.

Fever, myalgia, and arthralgia have been reported in a patient taking captopril and allopurinol (17).

Acute gout can be exacerbated at the beginning of allopurinol treatment unless the drug is combined with colchicine or an anti-inflammatory drug (18).

Immunologic

Hypersensitivity reactions to allopurinol occur in about 10–15% of patients. Desensitization with both oral and intravenous allopurinol has been successful (SEDA-17, 114). In the allopurinol hypersensitivity syndrome, the skin is most prominently involved (19). Symptoms develop after 2–5 weeks of treatment. Hepatic involvement is present in 40% and renal involvement in 45%; 25% of patients have combined renal and hepatic lesions. The hypersensitivity syndrome has been estimated to occur in 1 in 1000 hospitalized patients. A major complication is an extensive cutaneous staphylococcal infection with septicemia and endocarditis. Gastrointestinal hemorrhage, disseminated intravascular coagulation, adult respiratory distress syndrome, cerebral vasculitis, and peripheral axonal neuropathy have also been described (SEDA-21, 109). Death occurs in 20–30% of patients with severe hypersensitivity syndrome.

One report has presented evidence of a possible association between severe drug-induced erythema multiforme and reactivation of infection with human herpesvirus 6. The reactivation is thought to have contributed in some way to the development of allopurinol hypersensitivity reactions (20).

Allopurinol has been associated, albeit rarely, with pANCA (antineutrophil cytoplasmic antibodies with a peripheral pattern) positivity. A generalized cutaneous vasculitis has been associated with the presence in the serum of pANCA and antimyeloperoxidase antibodies (21). A skin biopsy of a lesion showed leukocytoclastic vasculitis with eosinophilic infiltration. Allopurinol was withdrawn and the symptoms resolved completely. The possible drug causes of ANCA-positive vasculitis with high titers of antimyeloperoxidase antibodies in 30 new patients have been reviewed (22). The findings illustrate that this type of vasculitis is a predominantly drug-induced disorder. Only 12 of the 30 cases were not related to a drug. Allopurinol was implicated in two of the other 18 cases.

Treatment of the allopurinol hypersensitivity syndrome includes drug withdrawal and the administration of systemic corticosteroids (prednisone 40–200 mg/day) for several months. Desensitization strategies allow some patients to resume allopurinol therapy later without any further problem (23–25). The standard desensitization protocol consists of an initial allopurinol dosage of 50 µg/day, increasing every 3 days to a target of 50–100 mg/day. The interval between dosage increases can be extended to 5 days or more in elderly patients with multiple co-morbidity. Using this protocol, desensitization was successful in 25 out of 32 patients (78%); 28 patients completed the desensitization protocol and 21 did so without requiring deviation from the standard dosage schedule and without adverse effects. During the follow-up for 902 patient-months, seven of the 28 patients had recurrent skin eruptions after completing the desensitization protocol and after rechallenge with allopurinol. Desensitization to allopurinol is not recommended for all patients, but it can be useful in selected patients who have had a pruritic maculopapular eruption during treatment with allopurinol and who cannot be treated with other drugs.

Susceptibility Factors

Renal disease

Renal impairment and diuretic therapy predispose to an increased frequency of adverse effects. The exact mechanisms have still to be elucidated. The active metabolite, oxipurinol or alloxanthine, accumulates in renal insufficiency and also in patients taking a low protein diet (13).

Drug–Drug Interactions

Aluminium hydroxide

When aluminium hydroxide is given with allopurinol, the serum uric acid concentration can increase, probably because the antacid reduces the absorption of allopurinol (SEDA-13, 84).

Ampicillin

Concomitant administration of allopurinol with ampicillin may increase the incidence of adverse skin reactions. In one study, these occurred in 22% of patients taking the combination (26). However, this interaction was not confirmed in a later investigation (27).

Ciclosporin

Two well-documented reports have described a marked increase in ciclosporin serum concentrations when allopurinol was co-administered (SEDA-18, 108).

Cytostatic drugs

The risk of bone marrow depression by cytostatic drugs is potentiated by allopurinol, which also appears to potentiate the therapeutic effect of purine cytostatic drugs, since it competitively inhibits their metabolic breakdown. Studies in animals suggest that this reaction occurs only with oral mercaptopurine (28), although there is older evidence that the toxicity of cyclophosphamide and other cytostatic drugs can be increased by allopurinol (SED-9, 156). The danger of combining allopurinol with azathioprine has been confirmed by cases of bone marrow suppression, particularly in patients with impaired renal function (SEDA-16, 114).

Thiazides

Thiazides enhance the excretion of orotic acid, which is already increased during allopurinol treatment, but the implications for the frequency of adverse effects are not known.

References

1. Laguna F, Lopez-Velez R, Soriano V, Montilla P, Alvar J, Gonzalez-Lahoz JM. Assessment of allopurinol plus meglumine antimoniate in the treatment of visceral leishmaniasis in patients infected with HIV. J Infect 1994;28(3):255–9.
2. Esfandiarpour I, Alavi A. Evaluating the efficacy of allopurinol and meglumine antimoniate (Glucantime) in the treatment of cutaneous leishmaniasis. Int J Dermatol 2002;41(8):521–4.
3. Momeni AZ, Reiszadae MR, Aminjavaheri M. Treatment of cutaneous leishmaniasis with a combination of allopurinol and low-dose meglumine antimoniate. Int J Dermatol 2002;41(7):441–3.
4. Weiss EB, Forman P, Rosenthal IM. Allopurinol-induced arteritis in partial HGPRTase deficiency. Atypical seizure manifestation. Arch Intern Med 1978;138(11):1743–4.
5. Greenberg LE, Nguyen T, Miller SM. Suspected allopurinol-induced aseptic meningitis. Pharmacotherapy 2001;21(8):1007–9.
6. Lerman S, Megaw J, Fraunfelder FT. Further studies on allopurinol therapy and human cataractogenesis. Am J Ophthalmol 1984;97(2):205–9.
7. Boston Collaborative Drug Surveillance Program. Allopurinol and cytotoxic drugs. Interaction in relation to bone marrow depression. JAMA 1974;227(9):1036–40.
8. Stolbach L, Begg C, Bennett JM, Silverstein M, Falkson G, Harris DT, Glick J. Evaluation of bone marrow toxic reaction in patients treated with allopurinol. JAMA 1982;247(3):334–6.
9. Ohno I, Ishida Y, Hosoya T, Kobayashi M, Sakai O. [Allopurinol induced aplastic anemia in a patient with chronic renal failure.] Ryumachi 1990;30(4):281–6.
10. Okafuji K, Shinohara K. [Aplastic anemia probably induced by allopurinol in a patient with renal insufficiency.] Rinsho Ketsueki 1990;31(1):85–8.
11. Gomez GA, Stutzman L, Chu TM. Xanthine nephropathy during chemotherapy in deficiency of hypoxanthine-guanine phosphoribosyltransferase. Arch Intern Med 1978;138(6):1017–19.
12. Stote RM, Smith LH, Dubb JW, Moyer TP, Alexander F, Roth JL. Oxypurinol nephrolithiasis in regional enteritis secondary to allopurinol therapy. Ann Intern Med 1980;92(3):384–5.
13. Hande KR, Noone RM, Stone WJ. Severe allopurinol toxicity. Description and guidelines for prevention in patients with renal insufficiency. Am J Med 1984;76(1):47–56.
14. Chan SH, Tan T. HLA and allopurinol drug eruption. Dermatologica 1989;179(1):32–3.
15. Chau NY, Reade PC, Rich AM, Hay KD. Allopurinol-amplified lichenoid reactions of the oral mucosa. Oral Surg Oral Med Oral Pathol 1984;58(4):397–400.
16. Terawaki H, Suzuki T, Yoshimura K, Hasegawa T, Takase H, Nemoto T, Hosoya T. [A case of allopurinol-induced muscular damage in a chronic renal failure patient.] Nippon Jinzo Gakkai Shi 2002;44(1):50–3.
17. Samanta A, Burden AC. Fever, myalgia, and arthralgia in a patient on captopril and allopurinol. Lancet 1984;1(8378):679.
18. Kot TV, Day RO, Brooks PM. Preventing acute gout when starting allopurinol therapy. Colchicine or NSAIDs? Med J Aust 1993;159(3):182–4.
19. Lupton GP, Odom RB. The allopurinol hypersensitivity syndrome. J Am Acad Dermatol 1979;1(4):365–74.
20. Suzuki Y, Inagi R, Aono T, Yamanishi K, Shiohara T. Human herpesvirus 6 infection as a risk factor for the development of severe drug-induced hypersensitivity syndrome. Arch Dermatol 1998;134(9):1108–12.
21. Choi HK, Merkel PA, Niles JL. ANCA-positive vasculitis associated with allopurinol therapy. Clin Exp Rheumatol 1998;16(6):743–4.
22. Choi HK, Merkel PA, Walker AM, Niles JL. Drug-associated antineutrophil cytoplasmic antibody-positive vasculitis: prevalence among patients with high titers of antimyeloperoxidase antibodies. Arthritis Rheum 2000;43(2):405–13.
23. Tanna SB, Barnes JF, Seth SK. Desensitization to allopurinol in a patient with previous failed desensitization. Ann Pharmacother 1999;33(11):1180–3.
24. Vazquez-Mellado J, Guzman Vazquez S, Cazarin Barrientos J, Gomez Rios V, Burgos-Vargas R. Desensitisation to allopurinol after allopurinol hypersensitivity syndrome with renal involvement in gout. J Clin Rheumatol 2000;6:266–8.

25. Fam AG, Dunne SM, Iazzetta J, Paton TW. Efficacy and safety of desensitization to allopurinol following cutaneous reactions. Arthritis Rheum 2001;44(1):231–8.

26. Boston Collaborative Drug Surveillance Program. Excess of amphicillin rashes associated with allopurinol or hyperuricemia. A report from the Boston Collaborative Drug Surveillance Program, Boston University Medical Center. N Engl J Med 1972;286(10):505–7.

27. Sonntag MR, Zoppi M, Fritschy D, Maibach R, Stocker F, Sollberger J, Buchli W, Hess T, Hoigne R. Exantheme unter haufig angewandten Antibiotika and antibakteriellen Chemotherapeutika (Penicilline, speziell Aminopenicilline, Cephalosporine und Cotrimoxazol) sowie Allopurinol. [Exanthema during frequent use of antibiotics and antibacterial drugs (penicillin, especially aminopenicillin, cephalosporin and cotrimoxazole) as well as allopurinol. Results of The Berne Comprehensive Hospital Drug Monitoring Program.] Schweiz Med Wochenschr 1986;116(5):142–5.

28. Zimm S, Narang PK, Ricardi R, et al. The effect of allopurinol on the pharmacokinetics of oral and parenteral (i.v.) 6-mercaptopurine Proc Am Assoc Cancer Res 1982;23:210.

Almitrine

General Information

Almitrine is a respiratory stimulant that improves hypoxemia in about 80% of patients with severe chronic obstructive pulmonary disease (SEDA-17, 212). Oral almitrine bimesilate (100 mg/day) increased PaO_2 in patients with severe chronic obstructive pulmonary disease without altering mean pulmonary artery pressure (1). Adverse effects were rarely observed and it was concluded that long-term treatment was safe. In other studies, respiratory, digestive, and neurological symptoms have been noted but were often pre-existent (2,3).

Organs and Systems

Gastrointestinal

Mild gastrointestinal symptoms have sometimes occurred (nausea, accelerated intestinal transit) but they regress spontaneously or after symptomatic treatment (2,3).

References

1. Weitzenblum E, Schrijen F, Apprill M, Prefaut C, Yernault JC. One year treatment with almitrine improves hypoxaemia but does not increase pulmonary artery pressure in COPD patients. Eur Respir J 1991;4(10):1215–22.

2. Ansquer JC, Bertrand A, Blaive B, Charpin J, Chretien J, Decroix G, Kalb JC, Lissac J, Michel FB, Morere P, et al. Intérêt thérapeutique et acceptabilié du Vectarion 50 mg comprimés enrobés (bismésilate d'almitrine) à la dose de 100 mg/jour. Etude des resultats gazometriques, cliniques et biologiques en traitement prolonge pendant 1 an. [Therapeutic importance and tolerance of coated 50 mg Vectarion tablets (almitrine bismesylate) at a dosage of 100 mg/day. Study of blood gas, clinical and biological

results after a year of long-term treatment.] Rev Mal Respir 1985;2(Suppl 1):S61–7.

3. Grassi V, Bottino G, Blasi A, Grassi C. Première expérience clinique italienne du bismésilate d'almitrine. [The first Italian clinical experience with almitrine bismesylate.] Rev Mal Respir 1985;2(Suppl 1):S53–60.

Aloeaceae

See also Herbal medicines

General Information

The family of Aloeaceae contains the single genus *Aloe*.

Aloe capensis and *Aloe vera*

Aloe capensis and *Aloe vera* (*Aloe barbadensis*) (Barbados aloe, burn plant, Curacao aloe, elephant's gall, first-aid plant, Hsiang dan, lily of the desert) contain several active constituents called aloins, including barbaloin, isobarbaloin, and aloe-emodin. Laxative anthranoid derivatives occur primarily in various laxative herbs (such as aloe, cascara sagrada, medicinal rhubarb, and senna) in the form of free anthraquinones, anthrones, dianthrones, and/or O- and C-glycosides derived from these substances. They produce harmless discoloration of the urine. Depending on intrinsic activity and dose, they can also produce abdominal discomfort and cramps, nausea, violent purgation, and dehydration. They can be distributed into breast milk, but not always in sufficient amounts to affect the suckling infant. Long-term use can result in electrolyte disturbances and in atony and dilatation of the colon. Several anthranoid derivatives (notably the aglycones aloe-emodin, chrysophanol, emodin, and physicon) are genotoxic in bacterial and/or mammalian test systems (SEDA-12, 409).

Aloe species contain laxative anthranoid derivatives, the main active ingredient being isobarbaloin. Large doses are claimed to cause nephritis and use during pregnancy is discouraged, since intestinal irritation might lead to pelvic congestion.

Aloes have been used on the skin to reduce the pain and swelling of burns, improve the symptoms of genital herpes and other skin conditions such as psoriasis, and to help heal wounds and frostbite. Aloe has been used orally to treat arthritis, asthma, diabetes, pruritus, peptic ulcers, and constipation. It may be effective in inflammatory bowel disease (1). It may reduce blood glucose in diabetes mellitus and blood lipid concentrations in hyperlipidemia (2).

Adverse effects

Aloe can reportedly cause muscle weakness, cardiac dysrhythmias, peripheral edema, bloody diarrhea, weight loss, stomach cramps, itching, redness, rash, pruritus, and a red coloration of the urine.

Liver

Hepatitis in a 57-year-old woman was linked to the ingestion of *A. vera*; the hepatitis resolved completely after withdrawal (3).

Gastrointestinal

- Melanosis coli occurred in a 39-year-old liver transplant patient who took an over-the-counter product containing aloe, rheum, and frangula (4). The typical brownish pigmentation of the colonic mucosa developed over 10 months. The medication was withdrawn and follow-up colonoscopy 1 year later showed normal looking mucosa. However, a sessile polypoid lesion was found in the transverse colon. Histology showed tubulovillous adenoma with extensive low-grade dysplasia.

Skin

Four patients had severe burning sensations after the application of *A. vera* to skin that had been subjected to chemical peel or dermabrasion (5).

Aloes can cause contact sensitivity (6,7).

Urinary tract

Acute renal insufficiency been attributed to *A. capensis*.

- A 47-year-old South African man developed acute oliguric renal insufficiency and liver dysfunction after taking an herbal medicine prescribed by a traditional healer to "clean his stomach" (8). After withdrawal of the remedy and dialysis he recovered slowly, but his creatinine concentration did not fully normalize. Analysis of the remedy showed that it consisted of *A. capensis* (*Aloe ferox* Miller), which contains the nephrotoxic compounds aloesin and aloesin A.

The authors also mentioned that 35% of all cases of acute renal insufficiency in Africa are due to traditional remedies.

Drug interactions

Massive intraoperative bleeding in a 35-year-old woman has been attributed to an interaction of preoperative *A. vera* tablets and sevoflurane, since both may inhibit platelet function (9).

References

1. Langmead L, Feakins RM, Goldthorpe S, Holt H, Tsironi E, De Silva A, Jewell DP, Rampton DS. Randomized, double-blind, placebo-controlled trial of oral *Aloe vera* gel for active ulcerative colitis. Aliment Pharmacol Ther 2004;19(7):739–47.
2. Vogler BK, Ernst E. Aloe vera: a systematic review of its clinical effectiveness. Br J Gen Pract 1999;49(447):823–8.
3. Rabe C, Musch A, Schirmacher P, Kruis W, Hoffmann R. Acute hepatitis induced by an *Aloe vera* preparation: a case report. World J Gastroenterol 2005;11(2):303–4.
4. Willems M, van Buuren HR, de Krijger R. Anthranoid self-medication causing rapid development of melanosis coli. Neth J Med 2003;61(1):22–4.
5. Hunter D, Frumkin A. Adverse reactions to vitamin E and *Aloe vera* preparations after dermabrasion and chemical peel. Cutis 1991;47(3):193–6.
6. Shoji A. Contact dermatitis to *Aloe arborescens*. Contact Dermatitis 1982;8(3):164–7.
7. Morrow DM, Rapaport MJ, Strick RA. Hypersensitivity to aloe. Arch Dermatol 1980;116(9):1064–5.
8. Luyckx VA, Ballantine R, Claeys M, Cuyckens F, Van den Heuvel H, Cimanga RK, Vlietinck AJ, De Broe ME, Katz IJ. Herbal remedy-associated acute renal failure secondary to Cape aloes. Am J Kidney Dis 2002;39(3):E13.

9. Lee A, Chui PT, Aun CS, Gin T, Lau AS. Possible interaction between sevoflurane and *Aloe vera*. Ann Pharmacother 2004;38(10):1651–4.

Alpha₁-antitrypsin

General Information

Alpha₁-antitrypsin neutralizes the activity of neutrophil elastase and is used to treat patients with homozygous deficiency of Alpha₁-antitrypsin (1). Adverse effects occur only rarely (2).

Organs and Systems

Cardiovascular

Chest pain and cyanosis occurred in 14 patients but the symptoms seemed to be related to the presence of sucrose in the product (1).

Immunologic

An acute allergic reaction to alpha₁-protease inhibitor has been reported (3).

References

1. Clark JA, Gross TP. Pain and cyanosis associated with alpha₁-proteinase inhibitor. Am J Med 1992;92(6):621–6.
2. Vogelmeier C, Kirlath I, Warrington S, Banik N, Ulbrich E, Du Bois RM. The intrapulmonary half-life and safety of aerosolized alpha₁-protease inhibitor in normal volunteers. Am J Respir Crit Care Med 1997;155(2):536–41.
3. Meyer FJ, Wencker M, Teschler H, Steveling H, Sennekamp J, Costabel U, Konietzko N. Acute allergic reaction and demonstration of specific IgE antibodies against alpha-1-protease inhibitor. Eur Respir J 1998;12(4):996–7.

Alpha-adrenoceptor antagonists

See also Individual agents

General Information

The postsynaptic alpha-adrenoceptor antagonists, indoramin, prazosin, and related quinazoline derivatives, block alpha₁-adrenoceptor-mediated vasoconstriction of peripheral blood vessels (both arterial and venous) and are effectively peripheral vasodilators (1,2). Qualitatively and quantitatively common adverse effects are generally similar, although indoramin has additional effects on other neurotransmitter systems and therefore tends to be considered separately. Their use in benign prostatic hyperplasia has been reviewed (3,4).

Several recent articles have reviewed the pharmacology, pharmacokinetics, mode of action, use, efficacy, and adverse effects of the selective alpha₁-adrenoceptor blockers doxazosin, prazosin, and terazosin in benign prostatic hyperplasia (5).

The frequencies and the profile of adverse effects of five major classes of antihypertensive agents have been assessed in an unselected group of 2586 chronically drug-treated hypertensive patients (6). This was accompanied by a questionnaire-based survey among patients attending a general practitioner. The percentage of patients who reported adverse effects spontaneously, on general inquiry, and on specific questioning were 16, 24, and 62% respectively. With alpha-blockers the figures were 15, 25, and 50%. The percentage of patients in whom discontinuation was due to adverse effects was 6.8% with alpha-blockers. Alpha-blockers were associated with less fatigue, cold extremities, sexual urge, and insomnia, and more bouts of palpitation than other antihypertensive drugs (RR = 2.5; CI = 1.2, 5.4). The authors did not find a significant effect of age on the pattern of adverse effects. Women reported more effects and effects that were less related to the pharmacological treatment.

The first-dose effect (profound postural hypotension and reflex tachycardia) is a well-recognized complication of the first dose of prazosin and related agents. This phenomenon is dose-related and can usually be avoided by using a low initial dosage taken at bedtime. During long-term treatment, orthostatic hypotension and dizziness is reported by about 10% of patients.

References

1. Grimm RH Jr. Alpha 1-antagonists in the treatment of hypertension. Hypertension 1989;13(5 Suppl):I131–6.
2. Luther RR. New perspectives on selective alpha 1 blockade. Am J Hypertens 1989;2(9):729–35.
3. Beduschi MC, Beduschi R, Oesterling JE. Alpha-blockade therapy for benign prostatic hyperplasia: from a nonselective to a more selective alpha1A-adrenergic antagonist. Urology 1998;51(6):861–72.
4. Narayan P, Man In't Veld AJ. Clinical pharmacology of modern antihypertensive agents and their interaction with alpha-adrenoceptor antagonists. Br J Urol 1998;81(Suppl 1):6–16.
5. Akduman B, Crawford ED. Terazosin, doxazosin, and prazosin: current clinical experience. Urology 2001;58(6 Suppl 1):49–54.
6. Olsen H, Klemetsrud T, Stokke HP, Tretli S, Westheim A. Adverse drug reactions in current antihypertensive therapy: a general practice survey of 2586 patients in Norway. Blood Press 1999;8(2):94–101.

Alpha-glucosidase inhibitors

General Information

Alpha-glucosidase inhibitors are competitive inhibitors of 1α-glucosidases, enzymes that are located in the brush border of epithelial cells, mainly in the upper half of the small intestine. The enzymes degrade complex carbohydrates into monosaccharides, which are absorbed. The alpha-glucosidase inhibitors bind reversibly in a dose-dependent manner to the oligosaccharide binding site of these enzymes and delay the degradation of polysaccharides and starch to glucose. They slow down food digestion in the gut, reducing peak blood glucose concentrations after meals. They also prevent reactive hypoglycemia, as can be seen after gastric operations, in dumping syndrome, and in idiopathic forms. When carbohydrates appear in the colon, bacterial fermentation can occur, leading to gastrointestinal adverse effects, of which flatulence and loose stools are the most frequent. During long-term treatment the colonic bacterial mass can increase. In elderly patients acarbose increases insulin sensitivity but not insulin release (1). Acarbose may reduce the incidence of colon cancer, the risk of which is 30% higher in people with diabetes than in the non-diabetic population (2).

The alpha-glucosidase inhibitors (polyhexose mimickers) in use are acarbose (rINN) (2–4), miglitol (rINN) (5–7), and voglibose (rINN), which is 20 times more potent (8).

Acarbose is not well absorbed and is mostly excreted in the feces. Miglitol is well absorbed from the gut and is almost completely excreted unchanged in the urine (9).

Observational studies

In a 2-year study of the tolerability and safety of acarbose in 2035 patients the incidence of adverse effects was 7.5% and of withdrawals 2.5% (10). Of 1907 patients, 444 (23%) reported one or more adverse events. In 143 patients the physician considered that there was a probable or possible relation between the adverse event (all gastrointestinal) and acarbose. There were 77 deaths, but none was considered to be related to acarbose; 52 stopped taking acarbose because of an adverse event and 45 were considered to be related to acarbose. Laboratory analyses were all within the reference ranges. HbA_{1c} fell by 1.92%.

The addition of metformin to acarbose in 49 patients produced a synergistic effect (11).

Of 1027 patients, 283 used acarbose as the treatment of choice (12). In 250 cases the physician was not sure of the benefit; 124 of these patients took acarbose and 126 patients took placebo besides regular therapy. In those taking acarbose HbA_{1c} fell. The adverse effects were bloating, flatulence, abdominal cramps, and diarrhea; there were moderate increases in serum transaminases.

Comparative studies

Voglibose and acarbose have been compared in 32 patients insufficiently treated by diet in an open crossover study (13). The metabolic results were identical. There were fewer adverse reactions in those who took voglibose. There was increased flatulence with acarbose in 96% and with voglibose in 57%; abdominal distension was reported in 17 and 10% respectively.

In an open study in 57 patients acarbose and gliclazide had the same effects on HbA_{1c}, blood glucose, and lipids, but the ratio of HDL to LDL cholesterol increased with acarbose (14). Acarbose caused flatulence in 30% and diarrhea in 3% and gliclazide caused at least one mild attack of hypoglycemia in 10%.

Placebo-controlled studies

The effect of adding acarbose (maximum 100 mg tds) or placebo to insulin (15) or metformin (16) has been investigated in 1946 patients with type 2 diabetes. The results were comparable with the results of the UK Prospective

Diabetes Study (17). After 3 years, 39% were still using acarbose compared with 58% using placebo. The main reasons for stopping were flatulence (30 versus 12%) or diarrhea (16 versus 8%). After 3 years the HbA_{1c} concentration was 0.5% lower (median 8.1 versus 8.6%). Acarbose was equally effective when added to diet, sulfonylurea, metformin, or insulin.

When acarbose or placebo was given to patients with type 1 diabetes taking insulin, acarbose reduced postprandial blood glucose but there was no difference in HbA_{1c}; the only adverse effects were gastrointestinal (18).

In a double-blind, placebo-controlled study in 74 patients for 2 years, acarbose 100 mg tds, after a stepwise increase in dosage over 5 weeks, improved HbA_{1c} (-1.71%) more than placebo (19). Two patients taking acarbose withdrew with drug-related adverse effects.

In a randomized, double-blind, placebo-controlled, crossover study 12 healthy subjects took acarbose 100 mg or voglibose 0.3 mg tds (20). Postprandial glucose, the rise in plasma immunoreactive insulin, and urinary immunoreactive C-peptide were higher with acarbose than voglibose. The flatus score was higher with acarbose than voglibose, but the stool score was not different and was higher than with placebo. Voglibose before the evening meal may improve nocturnal hypoglycemia during intensive insulin therapy (21).

Acarbose reduced insulin resistance in 192 patients over 65 years of age (mean age 70) in a double-blind, placebo-controlled study (22). HbA_{1c} was significantly but modestly reduced. The most frequent adverse effect was flatulence, which caused 12 patients (9 taking acarbose and 3 taking placebo) to withdraw.

In a multicenter, double-blind, placebo-controlled study, 81 patients, in whom treatment with metformin was inadequate, received extra acarbose or placebo during 24 weeks after a 4-week run-in period to establish the optimal dose of acarbose (23). HbA_{1c} was reduced by 1.02% and fasting blood glucose by 1.13 mmol/l. Gastrointestinal adverse effects were more common in the acarbose group.

In a placebo-controlled study of 154 patients taking glibenclamide or metformin, miglitol (starting at 25 mg tds and increasing to 50 or 100 mg tds for 24 weeks) caused more meteorism, flatulence, and diarrhea (24). When miglitol was added to metformin, HbA_{1c} improved and there was weight loss. In another study in 318 patients, more of the patients taking miglitol only or miglitol plus metformin withdrew because of flatulence and diarrhea than in the other groups (25).

The effects of miglitol 25 or 50 mg tds have been compared with placebo and various doses of glibenclamide in 411 patients aged over 60 years (mean 68 years) with mild type 2 diabetes insufficiently controlled by diet for 56 weeks (26). HbA_{1c} fell after 1 year by 0.92% (glibenclamide), 0.49% (miglitol 25 mg), and 0.40% (miglitol 50 mg). Gastrointestinal events were most common in patients taking miglitol. Most (88%) of the hypoglycemic events were minor and occurred in the patients taking glibenclamide. Mean body weight increased continuously and significantly in those taking glibenclamide. In the other groups weight fell by more than 1 kg. The rate of withdrawal was the same in all groups; withdrawal was mostly occasioned by cardiovascular effects in those

taking glibenclamide and by hyperglycemia, flatulence, or diarrhea in those taking miglitol.

When patients with inadequately controlled type 2 diabetes used glibenclamide plus metformin, miglitol, or placebo for 24 weeks in addition to their earlier therapy, fasting blood glucose concentrations improved with miglitol (24). Flatulence and diarrhea were significantly more common with miglitol. No patient stopped taking miglitol because of adverse effects.

General adverse effects

Acarbose and miglitol have been reviewed (13,27,28). Their major adverse effects are flatulence, abdominal discomfort, diarrhea, and bloating, particularly at the start of therapy, which sometimes prevent further use. They should not be given to patients with intestinal obstruction, malabsorption, inflammatory bowel disease, or hepatic impairment.

Organs and Systems

Sensory systems

Acarbose can cause altered taste sensation (29).

Metabolism

When acarbose is combined with insulin, the greatest effects are seen with regimens that involve only once- or twice-daily administration. The alpha-glucosidase inhibitors seem to be less effective when they are combined with intensive insulin therapy (30). In combination with insulin or oral hypoglycemic drugs the frequency of hypoglycemic episodes can increase; sucrose or higher carbohydrates are reported to be less effective, which can be understood from the mechanism of action.

Extreme weight loss has been attributed to acarbose (31).

- A 47-year-old woman weighing 59 kg took acarbose 50 mg tds. Her blood glucose improved but she lost about 1 kg/month. She had a sore tongue without oral ulcers and no evidence of malabsorption. Later she developed general weakness and iron deficiency anemia but no other evidence of malabsorption. After she had lost 7 kg in 5 months, acarbose was withdrawn. Her complaints disappeared, her weight normalized, and she had no signs of iron deficiency anemia, even without iron therapy.

Extreme weight loss due to acarbose is rare. In this case the mechanism was unclear.

In 36 Japanese patients who were relatively lean but had excess abdominal fat, glibenclamide and voglibose caused loss of weight and abdominal fat (32). The loss of abdominal fat was related to glycemic control. The ratio of subcutaneous to abdominal fat shifted toward subcutaneous fat only in those who took voglibose. Both voglibose and glibenclamide improved insulin sensitivity and the acute response to insulin.

Gastrointestinal

Abdominal pain and diarrhea with malabsorption have been described in patients taking acarbose, which can also cause carbohydrate malabsorption (33).

A review of miglitol included data on adverse effects in 3585 patients in well-designed clinical trials (34). Only the adverse effects in the gastrointestinal tract occurred with a significantly greater incidence with miglitol 50 or 100 mg tds. The adverse effects were the same as with other drugs in this class: flatulence, diarrhea, dyspepsia, and abdominal pain. There were no differences with monotherapy or combination therapy or in relation to age or ethnicity. There were more episodes of hypoglycemia when miglitol was combined with insulin but not with oral agents. The incidence of cardiovascular events was the same as with placebo.

Long-term acarbose had a good effect on late dumping syndrome in six patients with type 2 diabetes; one patient complained of increased flatulence (35).

Although acarbose often causes abdominal complaints, dietary manipulation has not been used to reduce the complaints (36).

In 120 patients with type 1 diabetes, acarbose lowered postprandial glucose but did not reduce HbA_{1c} (17). Four patients taking acarbose withdrew because of gastrointestinal effects, which improved after withdrawal. One of the placebo group withdrew because of gastrointestinal problems and one other patient taking acarbose withdrew with a Bell's palsy, which was not considered to be related to acarbose.

Ileus has also been reported with acarbose (37–40).

Paralytic ileus with intestinal pneumatosis cystoides has been reported (39).

- An 87-year-old woman, who took acarbose, glibenclamide, and mannitol (for constipation), developed abdominal distention and loss of appetite. An X-ray showed distention of the small intestine, with pockets of small gas bubbles in the submucosal space. When her drugs were withdrawn, her symptoms subsided and the radiological evidence of ileus disappeared by 5 days. Although she had an atonic bladder, there were no signs of neuropathy. She was also hypothyroid, which could have contributed.

Acarbose may also have caused pneumatosis cystoides intestinalis in a 55-year-old woman with pemphigus vulgaris (41).

Most cases of ileus with acarbose have been reported in Japan.

- A 73-year-old man with diabetic gangrene who had used insulin and acarbose 300 mg/day for 15 months developed ileus with abdominal pain and vomiting after he took PL granules (containing salicylamide, paracetamol, anhydrous caffeine, and promethazine methylene disalicylate) for a common cold (40). The ileus subsided after acarbose and the other drugs were withdrawn.

Although the ileus in this case was not clearly related to the use of acarbose, the combination of acarbose, which can cause ileus, with the other drugs that the patient was taking, may have caused it. The anticholinergic effect of promethazine methylene disalicylate may have contributed.

Lymphocytic colitis activated by acarbose has been reported (42).

- A 52-year-old man developed watery diarrhea 6–8 times a day 2 weeks after he had started to take acarbose 100 mg. In 3 weeks he lost 3 kg. Duodenal biopsies were normal; colon biopsies showed a large increase in intraepithelial lymphocytes. The mononuclear cells expressed CD-25, and HLA-DR antigen was increased in epithelial cells. Within 4 days of acarbose withdrawal the diarrhea had disappeared, and biopsies 4 months later showed that CD-25 expression in the cells of the lamina propria was improved and HLA-DR was no longer expressed by the epithelial cells. On rechallenge the diarrhea recurred within 3 days. Biopsies showed pronounced HLA-DR in the epithelial cells and CD-25 expression in some mononuclear cells in the lamina propria.

Non-digestable sugar substitutes and alpha-glucosidase inhibitors should probably not be used in combination.

Liver

Liver damage with raised liver enzymes has been described (16,43). Four case of liver damage by acarbose have been described in women aged 52–57, three established (44) and one probable (45). All had signs of liver impairment within 2–8 months after starting to take acarbose and the changes subsidized within a month after withdrawal. The first patient was given acarbose again; her liver enzymes increased after 3 days and normalized within 10 days after withdrawal. The second and third patients had liver biopsies, which confirmed hepatic changes.

- A 45-year-old man took acarbose 50 mg tds for a year and developed an aspartate transaminase of 62 U/l and an alanine transaminase of 127 /l, with negative serology; 3 months later the alanine transaminase was 153 U/l. After withdrawal of acarbose his liver enzymes normalized (46).
- A 54-year-old woman had fatigue and dark urine after taking acarbose 50 mg tds for 5 months (46). Her aspartate transaminase was 2436 U/l, alanine transaminase 2556 U/l, γ-glutamyl transpeptidase 601 U/l, and alkaline phosphatase 174 U/l; serology was negative and she had a normal liver and gall bladder on ultrasound. Her liver enzymes normalized 5 months after withdrawal.
- A 58-year-old man taking gliclazide 80 mg/day, atenolol 100 mg/day, and pravastatin 10 mg/day started to take acarbose 150 mg/day and benazepril 10 mg/day (47). After 2 weeks he developed weakness and myalgia and 1 week later his alanine transaminase was 22 times higher and aspartate transaminase 9 times higher than the upper limits of the reference ranges. Benazepril and pravastatin were withdrawn and his hypoglycemic therapy was changed to insulin. No viral or other antibodies related to liver disease were found. He improved and was given glibenclamide and acarbose instead of insulin. His enzymes increased 3 weeks later without subjective signs and he had an eosinophilia. A liver biopsy showed intralobular and periportal necrosis of liver cells and mononuclear infiltrates. Acarbose was withdrawn and he improved.
- A 57-year-old woman developed hepatitis 2 months after starting to take acarbose 100 mg tds (48). No other causes of hepatitis were found. Liver function tests normalized 3 months after withdrawal. Acarbose was reintroduced 3 years later and she again developed acute hepatitis. Liver function tests became normal 2 months after withdrawal.

- A 74-year-old woman who had used acarbose for 3 months developed progressive weakness and jaundice (49). Her bilirubin was 152 μmol/l (direct bilirubin 96 μmol/l). All of her liver enzymes were substantially raised. All other investigations were normal, except that she was positive for hepatitis C antigen. After withdrawal of acarbose everything became normal within 1 month.
- A 73-year-old woman who had taken acarbose 450 mg/day for 3 months became very tired and icteric (50). Her total bilirubin was 427 μmol/l (direct bilirubin 335 μmol/l) and her liver enzymes were very high. Liver biopsy showed cholestasis and cytolysis without eosinophils. Acarbose was continued for 3 days and her condition did not change. When the acarbose was withdrawn she improved rapidly.
- Another patient taking acarbose also had a serum alanine transaminase three times the upper limit of the reference range, but she had positive serology for hepatitis A (16).

Comparable reports have prompted a questionnaire investigation of 770 patients with type 2 diabetes at the start of acarbose therapy (51). Patients with one or more susceptibility factors for liver damage underwent ultrasonography and autoantibody assays. There was silent liver disease in 13% and 20 patients had a fatty liver without hepatic disease. In 15% of these patients there were slight reversible changes in transaminase activity after acarbose. This supports the supposition that severe hepatotoxic reactions to acarbose are idiosyncratic.

However, in a double-blind study in 100 patients with compensated non-alcoholic liver cirrhosis and type 2 diabetes, acarbose for 28 weeks did not alter liver function (52). The number of hypoglycemic episodes was reduced.

Skin

Erythema multiforme has been attributed to acarbose (53).

- A skin biopsy from a 58-year-old man showed necrosis of keratinocytes with lymphocytic and eosinophilic infiltration. Liver enzymes were normal. After withdrawal the rash disappeared. After 3 weeks, rechallenge with acarbose 50 mg caused the skin changes to reappear.

Second-Generation Effects

Pregnancy

In six women with gestational diabetes, acarbose 50 mg before meals normalized fasting and postprandial glucose concentrations (54). The pregnancies were uneventful and the neonates were healthy. Internal discomfort persisted during the whole pregnancy.

Drug–Drug Interactions

Colestyramine

Acarbose increases bowel motility, which reduces the effect of colestyramine.

Digoxin

Acarbose can reduce plasma concentrations of digoxin by impairing its absorption.

- An 82-year-old man with type 2 diabetes, taking digoxin and voglibose 0.9 mg/day, had digoxin serum concentrations in the target range (55). He was given acarbose 300 mg/day instead of voglibose and his digoxin concentrations fell from 0.8–2.0 ng/ml to 0.2–0.4 ng/ml. One month after restarting voglibose the digoxin concentrations were again in the target range.
- A 69-year-old woman with diabetes mellitus and heart failure repeatedly had unusual subtherapeutic plasma digoxin concentrations (56). When acarbose was withdrawn the plasma digoxin concentration rose.

In a randomized, crossover study in healthy men, acarbose 100–200 mg reduced the AUC and C_{max} of digoxin and prolonged its t_{max}, consistent with reduced absorption (57). However, in another study acarbose 50 mg tds for 12 days had no significant effect on the pharmacokinetics of a single oral dose of digoxin 0.75 mg (58).

In one study there was no interaction of voglibose with digoxin (59).

Glibenclamide

In a placebo-controlled study in six patients with type 2 diabetes, acarbose 300 mg/day for 7 days had no significant effect on the pharmacokinetics of a single dose of glibenclamide 5 mg (60).

Miglitol did not reduce the t_{max} or C_{max} of glibenclamide, but the 9-hour AUC was significantly reduced (61).

In a double-blind, crossover study in 12 healthy men, voglibose 5 mg tds for 8 days had no significant effect on the pharmacokinetics of a single dose of glibenclamide 1.75 mg (62).

Metformin

Acarbose reduces the absorption of metformin (63), as does miglitol (61).

Thioctic acid

In 24 healthy volunteers thioctic acid 600 mg orally had no significant effect on the actions of acarbose 50 mg and acarbose did not alter the pharmacokinetics of thioctic acid (64).

Warfarin

Acarbose may increase the availability of warfarin (65). However, neither miglitol (66) nor voglibose (67) has any effect.

References

1. Meneilly GS, Ryan EA, Radziuk J, Lau DC, Yale JF, Morais J, Chiasson JL, Rabasa-Lhoret R, Maheux P, Tessier D, Wolever T, Josse RG, Elahi D. Effect of acarbose on insulin sensitivity in elderly patients with diabetes. Diabetes Care 2000;23(8):1162–7.
2. Laube H. Acarbose: an update of its therapeutic use in diabetes treatment. Clin Drug Invest 2002;22:141–56.

3. Coniff R, Krol A. Acarbose: a review of US clinical experience. Clin Ther 1997;19(1):16–26.
4. Sels JP, Verdonk HE, Wolffenbuttel BH. Effects of acarbose (Glucobay) in persons with type 1 diabetes: a multicentre study. Diabetes Res Clin Pract 1998;41(2):139–45.
5. Johnston PS, Feig PU, Coniff RF, Krol A, Davidson JA, Haffner SM. Long-term titrated-dose alpha-glucosidase inhibition in non-insulin-requiring Hispanic NIDDM patients. Diabetes Care 1998;21(3):409–15.
6. Johnston PS, Feig PU, Coniff RF, Krol A, Kelley DE, Mooradian AD. Chronic treatment of African-American type 2 diabetic patients with alpha-glucosidase inhibition. Diabetes Care 1998;21(3):416–22.
7. Mitrakou A, Tountas N, Raptis AE, Bauer RJ, Schulz H, Raptis SA. Long-term effectiveness of a new alpha-glucosidase inhibitor (BAY m1099—miglitol) in insulin-treated type 2 diabetes mellitus. Diabet Med 1998;15(8):657–60.
8. Matsumoto K, Yano M, Miyake S, Ueki Y, Yamaguchi Y, Akazawa S, Tominaga Y. Effects of voglibose on glycemic excursions, insulin secretion, and insulin sensitivity in non-insulin-treated NIDDM patients. Diabetes Care 1998;21(2):256–60.
9. Clissold SP, Edwards C. Acarbose. A preliminary review of its pharmacodynamic and pharmacokinetic properties, and therapeutic potential. Drugs 1988;35(3):214–43.
10. Mertes G. Efficacy and safety of acarbose in the treatment of type 2 diabetes: data from a 2-year surveillance study. Diabetes Res Clin Pract 1998;40(1):63–70.
11. Hanefeld M, Bar K. Efficacy and safety of combined treatment of type 2 diabetes with acarbose and metformin. Diabetes Stoffwechsel 1998;7:186–90.
12. Scorpiglione N, Belfiglio M, Carinci F, Cavaliere D, De Curtis A, Franciosi M, Mari E, Sacco M, Tognoni G, Nicolucci A. The effectiveness, safety and epidemiology of the use of acarbose in the treatment of patients with type II diabetes mellitus. A model of medicine-based evidence. Eur J Clin Pharmacol 1999;55(4):239–49.
13. Vichayanrat A, Ploybutr S, Tunlakit M, Watanakejorn P. Efficacy and safety of voglibose in comparison with acarbose in type 2 diabetic patients. Diabetes Res Clin Pract 2002;55(2):99–103.
14. Salman S, Salman F, Satman I, Yilmaz Y, Ozer E, Sengul A, Demirel HO, Karsidag K, Dinccag N, Yilmaz MT. Comparison of acarbose and gliclazide as first-line agents in patients with type 2 diabetes. Curr Med Res Opin 2001;16(4):296–306.
15. Kelley DE, Bidot P, Freedman Z, Haag B, Podlecki D, Rendell M, Schimel D, Weiss S, Taylor T, Krol A, Magner J. Efficacy and safety of acarbose in insulin-treated patients with type 2 diabetes. Diabetes Care 1998;21(12):2056–61.
16. Rosenstock J, Brown A, Fischer J, Jain A, Littlejohn T, Nadeau D, Sussman A, Taylor T, Krol A, Magner J. Efficacy and safety of acarbose in metformin-treated patients with type 2 diabetes. Diabetes Care 1998;21(12):2050–5.
17. Holman RR, Cull CA, Turner RC. A randomized double-blind trial of acarbose in type 2 diabetes shows improved glycemic control over 3 years (U.K. Prospective Diabetes Study 44) Diabetes Care 1999;22(6):960–4.
18. Riccardi G, Giacco R, Parillo M, Turco S, Rivellese AA, Ventura MR, Contadini S, Marra G, Monteduro M, Santeusanio F, Brunetti P, Librenti MC, Pontiroli AE, Vedani P, Pozza G, Bergamini L, Bianchi C. Efficacy and safety of acarbose in the treatment of Type 1 diabetes mellitus: a placebo-controlled, double-blind, multicentre study. Diabet Med 1999;16(3):228–32.
19. Hasche H, Mertes G, Bruns C, Englert R, Genthner P, Heim D, Heyen P, Mahla G, Schmidt C, Schulze-Schleppinghof B, Steger-Johannsen G. Effects of acarbose treatment in type 2 diabetic patients under dietary training: a multicentre, double-blind, placebo-controlled, 2-year study. Diabetes Nutr Metab 1999;12(4):277–85.
20. Kageyama S, Nakamichi N, Sekino H, Fujita H, Nakano S. Comparison of the effects of acarbose and voglibose on plasma glucose, endogenous insulin sparing, and gastrointestinal adverse events in obese subjects: a randomized, placebo-controlled, double-blind, three-way crossover study. Curr Ther Res Clin Exp 2000;61:630–45.
21. Taira M, Takasu N, Komiya I, Taira T, Tanaka H. Voglibose administration before the evening meal improves nocturnal hypoglycemia in insulin-dependent diabetic patients with intensive insulin therapy. Metabolism 2000;49(4):440–3.
22. Josse RG, Chiasson JL, Ryan EA, Lau DC, Ross SA, Yale JF, Leiter LA, Maheux P, Tessier D, Wolever TM, Gerstein H, Rodger NW, Dornan JM, Murphy LJ, Rabasa-Lhoret R, Meneilly GS. Acarbose in the treatment of elderly patients with type 2 diabetes. Diabetes Res Clin Pract 2003;59(1):37–42.
23. Phillips P, Karrasch J, Scott R, Wilson D, Moses R. Acarbose improves glycemic control in overweight type 2 diabetic patients insufficiently treated with metformin. Diabetes Care 2003;26(2):269–73.
24. Standl E, Schernthaner G, Rybka J, Hanefeld M, Raptis SA, Naditch L. Improved glycaemic control with miglitol in inadequately-controlled type 2 diabetics. Diabetes Res Clin Pract 2001;51(3):205–13.
25. Chiasson JL, Naditch L; Miglitol Canadian University Investigator Group. The synergistic effect of miglitol plus metformin combination therapy in the treatment of type 2 diabetes. Diabetes Care 2001;24(6):989–94.
26. Johnston PS, Lebovitz HE, Coniff RF, Simonson DC, Raskin P, Munera CL. Advantages of alpha-glucosidase inhibition as monotherapy in elderly type 2 diabetic patients. J Clin Endocrinol Metab 1998;83(5):1515–22.
27. Lebovitz HE. Alpha-glucosidase inhibitors as agents in the treatment of diabetes. Diabetes Rev 1998;6:132–45.
28. Johnston PS, Coniff RF, Hoogwerf BJ, Santiago JV, Pi-Sunyer FX, Krol A. Effects of the carbohydrase inhibitor miglitol in sulfonylurea-treated NIDDM patients. Diabetes Care 1994;17(1):20–9.
29. Ruiz M, Matrone A, Alvari-as J, Burlando G, Jadzinsky M, Tesone P, Joge A, Bueno R, Castelli F, Fuente G, Gallego L, Garcia A, Del Hoyo N, Garcia S, Gianaula C, Maggiolo S, Marcello S, Mainetti H, Ortensi G, Righi S, Salzberg S, Traversa M, Vasta A, Vasquez V, Lemme L, Wendik A. Estudio multicentrico para determinar la eficacia y tolerancia de acarbose (Bay g 5421) en pacientes DMNID. Prensa Med Argent 1996;83:392–8.
30. Liebl A, Renner R, Hepp KD. Acarbose bei insulinbehandelten Diabetikern. Ein kritischer Überblick. Akt Endokrinol 1993;14:42–7.
31. Yoo WH, Park TS, Baek HS. Marked weight loss in a type 2 diabetic patient treated with acarbose. Diabetes Care 1999;22(4):645–6.
32. Takami K, Takeda N, Nakashima K, Takami R, Hayashi M, Ozeki S, Yamada A, Kokubo Y, Sato M, Kawachi S, Sasaki A, Yasuda K. Effects of dietary treatment alone or diet with voglibose or glyburide on abdominal adipose tissue and metabolic abnormalities in patients with newly diagnosed type 2 diabetes. Diabetes Care 2002;25(4):658–62.
33. Sobajima H, Mori M, Niwa T, Muramatsu M, Sugimoto Y, Kato K, Naruse S, Kondo T, Hayakawa T. Carbohydrate malabsorption following acarbose administration. Diabet Med 1998;15(5):393–7.
34. Scott LJ, Spencer CM. Miglitol: a review of its therapeutic potential in type 2 diabetes mellitus Drugs 2000;59(3):521–49.
35. Hasegawa T, Yoneda M, Nakamura K, Ohnishi K, Harada H, Kyouda T, Yoshida Y, Makino I. Long-term

effect of alpha-glucosidase inhibitor on late dumping syndrome. J Gastroenterol Hepatol 1998;13(12):1201–6.

36. Lindstrom J, Tuomilehto J, Spengler M. Acarbose treatment does not change the habitual diet of patients with type 2 diabetes mellitus. The Finnish Acargbos Study Group. Diabet Med 2000;17(1):20–5.

37. Nishii Y, Aizawa T, Hashizume K. Ileus: a rare side effect of acarbose. Diabetes Care 1996;19(9):1033.

38. Odawara M, Bannai C, Saitoh T, Kawakami Y, Yamashita K. Potentially lethal ileus associated with acarbose treatment for NIDDM. Diabetes Care 1997;20(7):1210–11.

39. Azami Y. Paralytic ileus accompanied by pneumatosis cystoides intestinalis after acarbose treatment in an elderly diabetic patient with a history of heavy intake of maltitol. Intern Med 2000;39(10):826–9.

40. Oba K, Kudo R, Yano M, Watanabe K, Ajiro Y, Okazaki K, Suzuki T, Nakano H, Metori S. Ileus after administration of cold remedy in an elderly diabetic patient treated with acarbose. J Nippon Med Sch 2001;68(1):61–4.

41. Maeda A, Yokoi S, Kunou T, Murata T. [A case of pneumatosis cystoides intestinalis assumed to be induced by acarbose administration for diabetes mellitus and pemphigus vulgaris.] Nippon Shokakibyo Gakkai Zasshi 2002;99(11):1345–9.

42. Piche T, Raimondi V, Schneider S, Hebuterne X, Rampal P. Acarbose and lymphocytic colitis. Lancet 2000;356(9237):1246.

43. Carrascosa M, Pascual F, Aresti S. Acarbose-induced acute severe hepatotoxicity. Lancet 1997;349(9053):698–9.

44. Fujimoto Y, Ohhira M, Miyokawa N, Kitamori S, Kohgo Y. Acarbose-induced hepatic injury. Lancet 1998;351(9099):340.

45. Diaz-Gutierrez FL, Ladero JM, Diaz-Rubio M. Acarbose-induced acute hepatitis. Am J Gastroenterol 1998;93(3):481.

46. Andrade RJ, Lucena M, Vega JL, Torres M, Salmeron FJ, Bellot V, Garcia-Escano MD, Moreno P. Acarbose-associated hepatotoxicity. Diabetes Care 1998;21(11):2029–30.

47. Mennecier D, Zafrani ES, Dhumeaux D, Mallat A. Hépatite aiguë induite par l'acarbose. [Acarbose-induced acute hepatitis.] Gastroenterol Clin Biol 1999;23(12):1398–9.

48. de la Vega J, Crespo M, Escudero JM, Sanchez L, Rivas LL. Hepatitis aguda por acarbosa. Descripcion de 2 episodios en una misma paciente. [Acarbose-induced acute hepatitis. Report of two events in the same patient.] Gastroenterol Hepatol 2000;23(6):282–4.

49. Madonia S, Pietrosi G, Pagliaro L. Acarbose-induced liver injury in an anti-hepatitis C virus positive patient. Dig Liver Dis 2001;33(7):615–16.

50. Fernandez AB, Gacia AM, Fabuel AT, Merino AB. Hepatitis aguda inducida por acarbosa. Med Clin 2001;117:317–18.

51. Gentile S, Turco S, Guarino G, Sasso FC, Torella R. Aminotransferase activity and acarbose treatment in patients with type 2 diabetes. Diabetes Care 1999;22(7):1217–18.

52. Gentile S, Turco S, Guarino G, Oliviero B, Annunziata S, Cozzolino D, Sasso FC, Turco A, Salvatore T, Torella R. Effect of treatment with acarbose and insulin in patients with non-insulin-dependent diabetes mellitus associated with non-alcoholic liver cirrhosis. Diabetes Obes Metab 2001;3(1):33–40.

53. Kono T, Hayami M, Kobayashi H, Ishii M, Taniguchi S. Acarbose-induced generalised erythema multiforme. Lancet 1999;354(9176):396–7.

54. Zarate A, Ochoa R, Hernandez M, Basurto L. Eficacia de la acarbosa para controlar el deterioro de la tolerancia a la glucosa durante la gestacion. [Effectiveness of acarbose in the control of glucose tolerance worsening in pregnancy.] Ginecol Obstet Mex 2000;68:42–5.

55. Nagai Y, Hayakawa T, Abe T, Nomura G. Are there different effects of acarbose and voglibose on serum levels of

56. Serrano JS, Jimenez CM, Serrano MI, Balboa B. A possible interaction of potential clinical interest between digoxin and acarbose. Clin Pharmacol Ther 1996;60(5):589–92.

57. Miura T, Ueno K, Tanaka K, Sugiura Y, Mizutani M, Takatsu F, Takano Y, Shibakawa M. Impairment of absorption of digoxin by acarbose. J Clin Pharmacol 1998;38(7):654–7.

58. Cohen E, Almog S, Staruvin D, Garty M. Do therapeutic doses of acarbose alter the pharmacokinetics of digoxin? Isr Med Assoc J 2002;4(10):772–5.

59. Kusumoto M, Ueno K, Fujimura Y, Kameda T, Mashimo K, Takeda K, Tatami R, Shibakawa M. Lack of kinetic interaction between digoxin and voglibose. Eur J Clin Pharmacol 1999;55(1):79–80.

60. Gerard J, Lefebvre PJ, Luyckx AS. Glibenclamide pharmacokinetics in acarbose-treated type 2 diabetics. Eur J Clin Pharmacol 1984;27(2):233–6.

61. Scheen AJ, Lefebvre PJ. Potential pharmacokinetics interference between alpha-glucosidase inhibitors and other oral antidiabetic agents. Diabetes Care 2002;25(1):247–8.

62. Kleist P, Ehrlich A, Suzuki Y, Timmer W, Wetzelsberger N, Lucker PW, Fuder H. Concomitant administration of the alpha-glucosidase inhibitor voglibose (AO-128) does not alter the pharmacokinetics of glibenclamide. Eur J Clin Pharmacol 1997;53(2):149–52.

63. Dachman AH. New contraindication to intravascular iodinated contrast material. Radiology 1995;197(2):545.

64. Gleiter CH, Schreeb KH, Freudenthaler S, Thomas M, Elze M, Fieger-Buschges H, Potthast H, Schneider E, Schug BS, Blume HH, Hermann R. Lack of interaction between thioctic acid, glibenclamide and acarbose. Br J Clin Pharmacol 1999;48(6):819–25.

65. Morreale AP, Janetzky K. Probable interaction of warfarin and acarbose. Am J Health Syst Pharm 1997;54(13):1551–2.

66. Schall R, Muller FO, Hundt HK, Duursema L, Groenewoud G, Middle MV. Study of the effect of miglitol on the pharmacokinetics and pharmacodynamics of warfarin in healthy males. Arzneimittelforschung 1996;46(1):41–6.

67. Fuder H, Kleist P, Birkel M, Ehrlich A, Emeklibas S, Maslak W, Stridde E, Wetzelsberger N, Wieckhorst G, Lucker PW. The alpha-glucosidase inhibitor voglibose (AO-128) does not change pharmacodynamics or pharmacokinetics of warfarin. Eur J Clin Pharmacol 1997;53(2):153–7.

Alphaprodine

General Information

Alphaprodine is a synthetic opioid that is rapidly absorbed after oral submucosal injection (1). It is used in pediatric dentistry, but it has been withdrawn from the market on a number of occasions because of concerns about its safety. Problems include hypoxia, reduced respiratory rate, and generalized venodilatation with local cyanosis.

Reference

1. Currie WR, Biery KA, Campbell RL, Mourino AP. Narcotic sedation: an evaluation of cardiopulmonary parameters and behavior modification in pediatric dental patients. J Pedod 1988;12(3):230–49.

Alpidem

General Information

Alpidem, like zolpidem, is an imidazopyridine, chemically distinct from the benzodiazepines. It binds selectively to a subset of benzodiazepine receptors (1), which may account for its apparently milder withdrawal effects and a relative dominance of anxiolytic over sedative and cognitive effects (2). Its effects are reversed by flumazenil (3). Alpidem was withdrawn in 1953 in France, the only country in which it was marketed, because of hepatotoxicity (4).

References

1. Lader M. Psychiatric disorders. In: Speight T, Holford N, editors. Avery's Drug Treatment, 4th ed. Auckland: ADIS International Press, 1997:1437.
2. Lader M. Clinical pharmacology of anxiolytic drugs: past, present and future. In: Biggio G, Sanna E, Costa E, editors. GABA-A Receptors and Anxiety. From Neurobiology to Treatment. New York: Raven Press, 1995:135.
3. Zivkovic B, Morel E, Joly D, Perrault G, Sanger DJ, Lloyd KG. Pharmacological and behavioral profile of alpidem as an anxiolytic. Pharmacopsychiatry 1990;23(Suppl 3):108–13.
4. Cassano GB, Petracca A, Borghi C, Chiroli S, Didoni G, Garreau M. A randomized, double-blind study of alpidem vs placebo in the prevention and treatment of benzodiazepine withdrawal syndrome. Eur Psychiatry 1996;11(2):93–9.

Alprazolam

See also Benzodiazepines

General Information

Alprazolam, a triazolobenzodiazepine, has been marketed as an anxiolytic with additional antidepressant properties; an analogue, adinazolam, also has partial antidepressant activity (1) and is useful in panic disorder. Like other benzodiazepines, alprazolam is effective in acute and generalized anxiety; its efficacy in panic disorder (2,3), premenstrual syndrome (4), and chronic pain (5) is complicated by high rates of adverse effects (6). On the other hand, low-dose alprazolam (1.4 mg/day) is useful and well tolerated in the treatment of anxiety associated with schizophrenia (SEDA-19, 34).

The value of the Saskatchewan data files in an acute adverse event signalling scheme has been evaluated using two benzodiazepines (7). The first 20 000 patients taking lorazepam and the first 8525 patients taking alprazolam were followed for 12 months after the initial prescription. The most frequent adverse drug reactions associated with these benzodiazepines were drowsiness, depression, impaired intellectual function and memory, lethargy, impaired coordination, dizziness, nausea and/or vomiting, skin rashes, and respiratory disturbance. Sleep disorders, depression, dizziness and/or vertigo, respiratory depression, gastrointestinal disorders, and inflammatory skin conditions occurred significantly more often during the first 30 days after the initial prescription than during the next 6 months.

Organs and Systems

Cardiovascular

Alprazolam has been associated with hypotension (8).

- A 76-year-old woman, who had a history of hypertension, valvular heart disease (mitral regurgitation) with chronic atrial fibrillation, chronic obstructive airways disease, diverticular disease of the sigmoid colon, and generalized anxiety disorder, developed severe hypotension with a tachycardia after taking alprazolam for 7 days. She also had severe weakness, depressed mood, and impaired gait and balance, without clinical features of neuromuscular disease.

Psychological, psychiatric

Rapid and sometimes serious mood swings to mania or depression, and other adverse effects, including enuresis, aggression, impaired memory, sedation, and ataxia, can occur in patients with panic disorder treated with alprazolam (SEDA-19, 34)(SEDA-20, 31).

Disinhibition has been reported as a major problem with alprazolam, particularly in patients with borderline personality disorder (9). Several case reports have suggested that alprazolam can cause behavioral disinhibition (10), in common with other benzodiazepines that are occasionally used for recreational or criminal purposes (11). In one study, covering the period January 1989 to June 1990, the medical records of 323 psychiatric inpatients treated with alprazolam, clonazepam, or no benzodiazepine were reviewed (12). The frequencies of behavioral disturbances were not significantly different in the different groups, suggesting that alprazolam does not have unique disinhibitory activity and that disinhibition with benzodiazepines may not be an important clinical problem in all psychiatric populations. The study design did not allow the establishment of a relation between the prescription of the benzodiazepine and worsening behaviors, and the findings need to be interpreted conservatively, because it was a retrospective review of a heterogeneous population.

Agoraphobia/panic disorder occurred in 31 patients, 15 of whom had originally been treated with alprazolam and 16 with placebo, had been previously followed during an 8-week treatment period, and had alprazolam-induced memory impairment (13). These patients were reviewed 3.5 years after treatment to determine whether the memory impairment persisted. Those who had used alprazolam performed as well as those who had taken placebo on the memory task and other objective tests. The performances in both groups were similar to pretreatment values. However, there were differences in subjective ratings: those who had used alprazolam rated themselves as less attentive and clear-headed and more incompetent and clumsy. Memory impairment found while patients were taking alprazolam did not persist 3.5 years later.

Abrupt withdrawal of alprazolam after prolonged treatment of panic disorder is associated with panic attacks.

- A 77-year-old married woman with panic attacks did not experience them while she took alprazolam 0.5 mg bd for 5 months; however, the attacks recurred after an increase in dose to 0.5 mg qds (14).

The authors suggested that the duration of action of alprazolam is too brief to prevent rebound anxiety with administration four times a day, but this explanation is highly speculative. This case illustrates the potential severity of alprazolam rebound and how its long-term use can exacerbate the symptoms for which it was originally administered.

Endocrine

Alprazolam can alter dehydroepiandrosterone and cortisol concentrations. Of 38 healthy volunteers who received a single intravenous dose of alprazolam 2 mg over 2 minutes (phase I), 15 of 25 young men (aged 22–35 years) and all 13 elderly men (aged 65–75 years) responded to alprazolam and agreed to participate in a crossover study of placebo and alprazolam infusion to plateau for 9 hours (15). Plasma samples at 0, 1, 4, and 7 hours were assayed for steroid concentrations. Alprazolam produced:

(a) significant increases in dehydroepiandrosterone concentrations at 7 hours in both the young and elderly men;
(b) significant reductions in cortisol concentrations;
(c) no change in dehydroepiandrosterone-S concentrations.

The results suggest that alprazolam modulates peripheral concentrations of dehydroepiandrosterone and that dehydroepiandrosterone and/or dehydroepiandrosterone-S may have an in vivo role in modulating GABA receptor-mediated responses.

Skin

Alprazolam, which is lipid-soluble, can cause photosensitivity after a long duration of administration.

- A 65-year-old man developed pruritic erythema on sun-exposed areas (photosensitivity) due to alprazolam (16). A photopatch test was negative, but an oral photo-challenge test with UVA irradiation was positive after he had taken alprazolam for 17 days.

Long-Term Effects

Drug dependence

Dependence on alprazolam and withdrawal symptoms appear to present greater problems than with other benzodiazepines (SED-12, 98).

Drug withdrawal

Withdrawal symptoms have been described with alprazolam.

- A woman with paranoid schizophrenia developed catatonia 5 days after the abrupt withdrawal of olanzapine and alprazolam (17). The catatonic symptoms included mutism, prostration, waxy flexibility, oculogyric movements, and an inability to swallow. Her symptoms disappeared after administration of alprazolam and haloperidol, and there was no recurrence.
- A 39-year-old woman had withdrawal symptoms after her dose of alprazolam was reduced (18). Cognitive symptoms made it almost impossible for her to stop taking alprazolam or to continue psychotherapeutic treatment. The medication was stopped by means of a behavioral experiment, in which both patient and therapist were unaware of the way in which the medication was reduced, after which continuation of treatment became possible.

Pharmacological strategies for withdrawing alprazolam, by switching to a longer-acting agent, have been proposed (19).

Drug Administration

Drug overdose

The effects of alprazolam overdose have been reported (20,21).

- A 28-year-old African-American man took alprazolam 12 mg. He denied using alcohol, other prescription medications, over-the-counter medications, or illicit drugs. He denied any suicidal intent. He stated that he had taken this large dose because his usual dose of 1–2 mg had failed to relieve his anxiety. He was drowsy and his heart rate was 58/minute. He had marked first-degree atrioventricular block, with a PR interval of 500 ms.
- A 30-year-old woman, with a history of depression, was found dead after taking an unknown quantity of alprazolam, tramadol, and alcohol. At autopsy, only slight decomposition and diffuse visceral congestion were observed. Blood concentrations of alprazolam, alcohol, and tramadol were 0.21 mg/l, 1.29 g/kg, and 38 mg/l respectively.

Drug–Drug Interactions

Alcohol

In common with other benzodiazepines, alprazolam produces additional impairment of performance when it is taken together with alcohol (22). The combination can also produce behavioral disturbance and aggression (11,23).

Alosetron

In an open, randomized, crossover study in 12 healthy men and women, alosetron 1 mg bd did not affect the pharmacokinetics of a single oral dose of alprazolam 1 mg (24).

Dextropropoxyphene

Inhibition of alprazolam metabolism by dextropropoxyphene has been reported (25).

Grapefruit juice

There have been two studies of the effects of repeated ingestion of grapefruit juice on the pharmacokinetics and pharmacodynamics of both single and multiple oral doses of alprazolam in a total of 19 subjects (26). Grapefruit juice altered neither the steady-state plasma concentration of alprazolam nor its clinical effects.

Ketoconazole

In a double-blind, crossover, pharmacokinetic and pharmacodynamic study of the interaction of ketoconazole with alprazolam and triazolam, two CYP3A4 substrate drugs with different kinetic profiles, impaired clearance by ketoconazole had more profound clinical consequences for triazolam than for alprazolam (27).

Miocamycin

Hydroxylation of miocamycin metabolites is mainly performed by CYP3A4. Some macrolide antibiotics cause drug interactions that result in altered metabolism of concomitantly administered drugs by the formation of a metabolic intermediate complex with CYP450 or competitive inhibition of CYP450 (28). The resulting interactions can cause rhabdomyolysis (associated with the coadministration of some statins, for example lovastatin or simvastatin), hypoprothrombinemia (associated with warfarin), excessive sedation (associated with certain benzodiazepines, for example alprazolam, diazepam, midazolam, or triazolam), ataxia (associated with carbamazepine), and ergotism (associated with ergotamine).

Moclobemide

- A 44-year-old man developed the serotonin syndrome after taking moclobemide and alprazolam for 1 year (29). The symptoms developed after 4 days of extreme heat, which was thought to have contributed.

Nefazodone

Nefazodone is a weak inhibitor of CYP2D6 but a potent inhibitor of CYP3A4 and it increases plasma concentrations of drugs that are substrates of CYP3A4, such as alprazolam, astemizole, carbamazepine, ciclosporin, cisapride, terfenadine, and triazolam.

Oral contraceptives

Oral contraceptives alter the metabolism of some benzodiazepines that undergo oxidation (alprazolam, chlordiazepoxide, and diazepam) or nitroreduction (nitrazepam) (30). Oral contraceptives inhibit enzyme activity and reduce the clearances of these drugs. There is nevertheless no evidence that this interaction is of clinical importance. It should be noted that for other benzodiazepines that undergo oxidative metabolism, such as bromazepam or clotiazepam, no change has ever been found in oral contraceptive users. Some other benzodiazepines are metabolized by glucuronic acid conjugation. The clearance of temazepam was increased when oral contraceptives were administered concomitantly, but the clearances of lorazepam and oxazepam were not (31). Again, it is unlikely that this is an interaction of clinical importance.

Ritonavir

The inhibitory effect of ritonavir (a viral protease inhibitor) on the metabolism of alprazolam, a CYP3A-mediated reaction, has been investigated in a double-blind study (32). Ten subjects took alprazolam 1.0 mg plus either low-dose ritonavir (four doses of 200 mg) or placebo. Ritonavir reduced alprazolam clearance by 60%, prolonged its half-life, and magnified its benzodiazepine agonist effects, such as sedation and impairment of performance.

Sertraline

Sertraline (50–150 mg/day) had no effects on alprazolam metabolism in a randomized, double-blind, placebo-controlled study in 10 healthy volunteers (33).

Troleandomycin

Troleandomycin inhibits the metabolism of ecabapide and alprazolam by inhibition of CYP3A4 (34,35).

Venlafaxine

The effects of venlafaxine on the pharmacokinetics of alprazolam have been investigated in 16 healthy volunteers. Steady-state venlafaxine 75 mg bd did not inhibit CYP3A4 metabolism of a single dose of alprazolam 2 mg (36).

References

1. Ansseau M, Devoitille JM, Papart P, Vanbrabant E, Mantanus H, Timsit-Berthier M. Comparison of adinazolam, amitriptyline, and diazepam in endogenous depressive inpatients exhibiting DST nonsuppression or abnormal contingent negative variation. J Clin Psychopharmacol 1991;11(3):160–5.
2. Andersch S, Rosenberg NK, Kullingsjo H, Ottosson JO, Bech P, Bruun-Hansen J, Hanson L, Lorentzen K, Mellergard M, Rasmussen S, et al. Efficacy and safety of alprazolam, imipramine and placebo in treating panic disorder. A Scandinavian multicenter study. Acta Psychiatr Scand 1991;365(Suppl):18–27.
3. O'Sullivan GH, Noshirvani H, Basoglu M, Marks IM, Swinson R, Kuch K, Kirby M. Safety and side-effects of alprazolam. Controlled study in agoraphobia with panic disorder. Br J Psychiatry 1994;165(2):79–86.
4. Mortola JF. A risk-benefit appraisal of drugs used in the management of premenstrual syndrome. Drug Saf 1994;10(2):160–9.
5. Reddy S, Patt RB. The benzodiazepines as adjuvant analgesics. J Pain Symptom Manage 1994;9(8):510–14.
6. Verster JC, Volkerts ER. Clinical pharmacology, clinical efficacy, and behavioral toxicity of alprazolam: a review of the literature. CNS Drug Rev 2004;10(1):45–76.
7. Rawson NS, Rawson MJ. Acute adverse event signalling scheme using the Saskatchewan Administrative health care utilization datafiles: results for two benzodiazepines. Can J Clin Pharmacol 1999;6(3):159–66.
8. Ranieri P, Franzoni S, Trabucchi M. Alprazolam and hypotension. Int J Geriatr Psychiatry 1999;14(5):401–2.
9. Gardner DL, Cowdry RW. Alprazolam-induced dyscontrol in borderline personality disorder. Am J Psychiatry 1985;142(1):98–100.
10. Cowdry RW, Gardner DL. Pharmacotherapy of borderline personality disorder. Alprazolam, carbamazepine, trifluoperazine, and tranylcypromine. Arch Gen Psychiatry 1988;45(2):111–19.

11. Michel L, Lang JP. Benzodiazepines et passage à l'acte criminel. [Benzodiazepines and forensic aspects.] Encephale 2003;29(6):479–85.

12. Rothschild AJ, Shindul-Rothschild, Viguera A, Murray M, Brewster S. Comparison of the frequency of behavioral disinhibition on alprazolam, clonazepam, or no benzodiazepine in hospitalized psychiatric patients. J Clin Psychopharmacol 2000;20(1):7–11.

13. Kilic C, Curran HV, Noshirvani H, Marks IM, Basoglu M. Long-term effects of alprazolam on memory: a 3.5 year follow-up of agoraphobia/panic patients. Psychol Med 1999;29(1):225–31.

14. Bashir A, Swartz C. Alprazolam-induced panic disorder. J Am Board Fam Pract 2002;15(1):69–72.

15. Kroboth PD, Salek FS, Stone RA, Bertz RJ, Kroboth FJ 3rd. Alprazolam increases dehydroepiandrosterone concentrations. J Clin Psychopharmacol 1999;19(2):114–24.

16. Watanabe Y, Kawada A, Ohnishi Y, Tajima S, Ishibashi A. Photosensitivity due to alprazolam with positive oral photo-challenge test after 17 days administration. J Am Acad Dermatol 1999;40(5 Pt 2):832–3.

17. Roberge C, Mosquet B, Hamel F, Crete P, Starace J. Catatonie après sevrage d'un traitement par olanzapine et alprostadil. [Catatonia after olanzapine and alprazolam withdrawal.] J Clin Pharm 2001;20:163–5.

18. Meesters Y, Van Velzen CJM, Horwitz EH. Een cognitief aspect bij de afbouw van alprazolum. [A cognitive aspect related to the withdrawal of alprazolam; a case study.] Tijdschr Psychiatrie 2002;44:199–203

19. Rosenbaum JF. Switching patients from alprazolam to clonazepam. Hosp Community Psychiatry 1990;41(12):1302.

20. Mullins ME. First-degree atrioventricular block in alprazolam overdose reversed by flumazenil. J Pharm Pharmacol 1999;51(3):367–70.

21. Michaud K, Augsburger M, Romain N, Giroud C, Mangin P. Fatal overdose of tramadol and alprazolam. Forensic Sci Int 1999;105(3):185–9.

22. Linnoila M, Stapleton JM, Lister R, Moss H, Lane E, Granger A, Eckardt MJ. Effects of single doses of alprazolam and diazepam, alone and in combination with ethanol, on psychomotor and cognitive performance and on autonomic nervous system reactivity in healthy volunteers. Eur J Clin Pharmacol 1990;39(1):21–8.

23. Bond AJ, Silveira JC. The combination of alprazolam and alcohol on behavioral aggression. J Stud Alcohol 1993;11(Suppl):30–9.

24. D'Souza DL, Levasseur LM, Nezamis J, Robbins DK, Simms L, Koch KM. Effect of alosetron on the pharmacokinetics of alprazolam. J Clin Pharmacol 2001;41(4):452–4.

25. Hansen BS, Dam M, Brandt J, Hvidberg EF, Angelo H, Christensen JM, Lous P. Influence of dextropropoxyphene on steady state serum levels and protein binding of three anti-epileptic drugs in man. Acta Neurol Scand 1980;61(6):357–67.

26. Yasui N, Kondo T, Furukori H, Kaneko S, Ohkubo T, Uno T, Osanai T, Sugawara K, Otani K. Effects of repeated ingestion of grapefruit juice on the single and multiple oral-dose pharmacokinetics and pharmacodynamics of alprazolam. Psychopharmacology (Berl) 2000;150(2):185–90.

27. Greenblatt DJ, Wright CE, von Moltke LL, Harmatz JS, Ehrenberg BL, Harrel LM, Corbett K, Counihan M, Tobias S, Shader RI. Ketoconazole inhibition of triazolam and alprazolam clearance: differential kinetic and dynamic consequences. Clin Pharmacol Ther 1998;64(3):237–47.

28. Rubinstein E. Comparative safety of the different macrolides. Int J Antimicrob Agents 2001;18(Suppl 1):S71–6.

29. Butzkueven H. A case of serotonin syndrome induced by moclobemide during an extreme heatwave. Aust NZ J Med 1997;27(5):603–4.

30. Jochemsen R, van der Graaff M, Boeijinga JK, Breimer DD. Influence of sex, menstrual cycle and oral contraception on the disposition of nitrazepam. Br J Clin Pharmacol 1982;13(3):319–24.

31. Patwardhan RV, Mitchell MC, Johnson RF, Schenker S. Differential effects of oral contraceptive steroids on the metabolism of benzodiazepines. Hepatology 1983;3(2):248–53.

32. Greenblatt DJ, von Moltke LL, Harmatz JS, Durol AL, Daily JP, Graf JA, Mertzanis P, Hoffman JL, Shader RI. Alprazolam-ritonavir interaction: implications for product labeling. Clin Pharmacol Ther 2000;67(4):335–41.

33. Hassan PC, Sproule BA, Naranjo CA, Herrmann N. Dose-response evaluation of the interaction between sertraline and alprazolam in vivo. J Clin Psychopharmacol 2000;20(2):150–8.

34. Juurlink DN, Ito S. Comment: clarithromycin–digoxin interaction. Ann Pharmacother 1999;33(12):1375–6.

35. Piquette RK. Torsade de pointes induced by cisapride/clarithromycin interaction. Ann Pharmacother 1999;33(1):22–6.

36. Amchin J, Zarycranski W, Taylor KP, Albano D, Klockowski PM. Effect of venlafaxine on the pharmacokinetics of alprazolam. Psychopharmacol Bull 1998;34(2):211–19.

Alprostadil

See also Prostaglandins

General Information

Alprostadil is PGE_1 available for exogenous administration. Alprostadil is widely used in neonates with cyanotic congenital heart disease to maintain the patency of the ductus arteriosus. Reported adverse effects include fever, apnea, flushing, bradycardia, and hyperostosis. Continuous chronic infusion of alprostadil via a portable pump and neuromuscular electrical stimulation help to improve the quality of life in patients with severe chronic heart failure waiting for a donor heart, as both treatments can be performed at home.

Of 15 neonates with hypoplastic left heart syndrome (nine boys and six girls; median weight 3123 g) included in a cardiac transplant program between January 1993 and August 1996, who received continuous perfusion of alprostadil from the time of diagnosis of the cardiomyopathy, 13 received transplants and 6 died in the operating room (1). All had short-term adverse effects from the continuous perfusion of alprostadil, including slight fever and irritability. However, none had apneic pauses. Cortical hyperostosis occurred in 13 and antral hyperplasia in 12, but in all transplanted cases regression of the antral hyperplasia was seen after 6 months and regression of the cortical hyperostosis was seen after 12 months.

Organs and Systems

Cardiovascular

Moderate or severe phlebitis can occur at the site of venepuncture in some patients who receive alprostadil by infusion. It is sometimes severe enough to necessitate withdrawal of therapy. The frequency and severity of phlebitis has been investigated in 18 men, mean age 63 (range 47–78) years, with peripheral vascular disease who received a 2-hour infusion twice daily (2). Although it is usual to dissolve 60 micrograms of alprostadil in 500 ml of fluid to avoid phlebitis, in this study 200 ml was used to prevent volume overload. The solution was neutralized to pH 7.4 with 4 ml of 7% sodium bicarbonate. Two patients had grade 0, four grade 1, 11 grade 2, and one grade 3 phlebitis (by Dinley's criteria (3)). Age correlated negatively with the severity of phlebitis. Usually, alprostadil infusion therapy is stopped when phlebitis reaches grade 4 or more, but there were no such cases in this study.

Hematologic

Investigators from the Department of Pediatrics in Johns Hopkins Hospital, after seeing a neonate who had marked leukocytosis temporally related to alprostadil, conducted a retrospective study of neonatal leukocytosis induced by alprostadil in 45 neonates (4). They concluded that alprostadil infusion is a predictable cause of leukocytosis in neonates with congenital heart disease. Alprostadil-induced leukocytosis was especially prominent in three patients with splenic disorders associated with the heterotaxy syndrome. Many of the other adverse effects of alprostadil, including respiratory depression, hypotension, fever, and lethargy, were also associated with sepsis. The authors considered that it is reasonable to look for sepsis in infants receiving alprostadil, but that it is equally reasonable to withdraw empirical therapy once infection has been ruled out. Leukocytosis associated with alprostadil infusion has not been previously reported and is not listed in the alprostadil package insert.

Skin

Penile shaft lichen sclerosus has been reported in a 63-year-old man in association with alprostadil intracavernous injection for erectile dysfunction (5). The authors suggested that the lichen sclerosus had been caused by (1) an isomorphic response to the trauma of repeated needle injection; (2) a local cutaneous response to alprostadil-induced collagen synthesis or alprostadil-induced fibroblast production of IL-6, with secondary paracrine/autocrine-induced collagen synthesis by improper skin exposure by direct injection to the skin or by retrograde flow of alprostadil through the needle puncture tract; or (3) a random occurrence of separate events.

A neonate with transposition of the great vessels developed urticaria during treatment with alprostadil (6). While flushing and peripheral edema are well recognized, urticaria has not been described before.

Allergic contact dermatitis has been attributed to latanoprost (7).

- An 85-year-old man with glaucoma developed tearing, red eyes, and pruritic, edematous, eczematous eyelids. Treatment for presumed ocular rosacea and seborrhea with oral tetracyclines, topical glucocorticoids, and metronidazole gel was unhelpful. He was using topical carboxymethylcellulose sodium 1%, propylmethylcellulose 0.3%, polyvinyl alcohol 1.4%, latanoprost, and levobunolol. Patch-testing with a standard 64-antigen patch elicited a strong reaction only to balsam of Peru. However, repeated open application of levobunolol and latanoprost for 4 days elicited a strong positive reaction to latanoprost.

Musculoskeletal

Alprostadil infusion can produce bone cortical hyperostosis. Periosteal changes have been described in 15 neonates after the administration of alprostadil for more than 1 week (8). Serum alkaline phosphatase activity was significantly raised. The long bones and clavicles were most commonly involved and symmetrically affected. The scapula was involved in two cases and the ribs in seven. The involvement of clavicles has not been previously reported.

Hypertrophic osteoarthropathy has been reported in a woman with severe chronic heart failure who was referred for cardiac rehabilitation (9).

- A 56-year-old woman with muscle weakness and severe chronic heart failure (NYHA Class III) caused by aortic coarctation received an intravenous infusion of alprostadil 5 nanograms/kg/minute. Although her hemodynamics improved, her muscle weakness and exercise intolerance persisted. Neuromuscular electrical stimulation of both thigh muscles was begun. However, during simultaneous continuous intravenous infusion of alprostadil, she developed pain in her knees and elbows. The overlying skin was warm and dusky red and the subcutaneous tissues were swollen. The discomfort was aggravated by motion. There were signs of non-inflammatory synovial effusions and X-rays showed symmetric bilateral periosteal bone deposition in the distal humerus and synovial effusions in both knees. The bone scintigram showed increased bilateral symmetrical tracer uptake in both knees, ankles, wrists, and carpal bones, and increased radionuclide uptake in periarticular regions. Secondary hypertrophic osteoarthropathy caused by continuous intravenous infusion of alprostadil was diagnosed. The dosage of alprostadil was reduced to 2.5 nanograms/kg/minute, and the signs of osteoarthropathy disappeared within 5 days.

Sexual function

Intracavernosal alprostadil was effective and well tolerated in the treatment of erectile dysfunction, according to the results of a 6-month study (funded by Pharmacia & Upjohn) in 848 men (mean age 52 years) with at least a 4-month history of erectile dysfunction (10). This is provided that the individual dose is established by titration and patients receive training in injection techniques and periodic supervision during treatment. An initial dose was established for each patient and the patients then administered the alprostadil themselves at home. Of 727 evaluable patients, 682 (94%) had at least one erectile response after the injection of alprostadil, and 88% of injections lead to a satisfactory sexual response. The most commonly reported adverse event was penile pain, reported by 44% of patients, but only after 8% of injections. In just over half of the patients who had penile pain, the condition was reported as mild.

Prolonged erection, penile fibrosis, and priapism occurred in 8, 4, and 0.9% of patients respectively. Treatment was withdrawn because of medical events in 4% of patients, and drug-related events accounted for treatment withdrawal in 2% of patients.

There is a high dropout rate from self-injection therapy for erectile dysfunction. Of 86 patients aged 36–76 years who had been using home treatment for at least 3 months, 17 had discontinued treatment (11). The patients were evaluated by interview and clinical examination. Patients still in the program used one injection every 2 weeks, and those who had given up treatment had used one injection in 3 weeks. They were in the program for 39 and 16 months respectively, and had used a mean of 50 versus 12 injections respectively. There was no difference in the number of injections that produced unsatisfactory penile rigidity, prolonged erections, hematomas at the injection site, corporeal fibrosis, secondary penile deviation, or mean estimated duration of a drug-induced erection. Patient satisfaction, estimated partner satisfaction, increase in self-esteem, and negligible effort in performing injections were all significantly better for those still in the program. The authors commented that the reasons for dropout from self-injection therapy were not based on objective adverse effects and discomfort. Patients who leave the program are less motivated, less satisfied with the quality of drug-induced sexuality, consider the effort of giving the injections to be substantial, and have not achieved improved self-esteem.

There has been a report of a long-term follow-up program for treatment of erectile dysfunction in 32 patients who used alprostadil for a minimum of 5 years under standardized protocol conditions (12). All the patients had organic erectile dysfunction, and their mean age was 59 years. The period of observation was on average 75 months, and the mean dose of alprostadil was 14 µg. In all, 6799 injections were registered. The average number of injections was 213 per patient, 2.8 injections per month per patient. As regards adverse effects, hematomas occurred in 1.9% of the patients and there were five cases of prolonged erection (0.07%) caused by unauthorized redosing. Three patients developed reversible penile nodules. In 10 patients, the initial dosage had to be increased. Five patients dropped out after 5 years, none of them because of treatment complications.

The impact of treatment with transurethral alprostadil for erectile dysfunction on the quality of life of 249 men and their partners has been evaluated (13). The men had organic erectile dysfunction of more than 3 months' duration and self-administered transurethral alprostadil in an open, dose-escalating, outpatient study. Patients with a sufficient response ($n = 159$) were randomly assigned double-blind to either active medication or placebo for 3 months at home. Drug-related urogenital pain was reported by 12% of patients during outpatient dosing. However, this pain was usually mild, and only five patients (2%) discontinued treatment. One patient reported minor urethral bleeding/spotting. The transurethral administration of alprostadil was associated with minimal or no discomfort in 83–88% of patients. In the outpatient study, dizziness occurred in one patient and hypotension in one patient. During home treatment, drug-related urogenital pain was reported by 11 patients (14%), minor urethral bleeding/spotting by one (1.3%), and dizziness by 2 (2.6%). One patient reported prolonged erections on two occasions during home treatment, each lasting less than 5 hours.

The incidence of priapism after intracorporeal administration of alprostadil is 1%. Priapism after medicated urethral system for erection (MUSE) has been reported (14).

- A 57-year-old man with erectile impotence, who had previously been treated with intracorporeal injections of papaverine and alprostadil, resulting in recurrent episodes of priapism necessitating aspiration, decided to try intraurethral alprostadil (MUSE). The dose needed to achieve a full erection in the clinic was titrated to 1 µg, but after 5 months this was found to be inadequate unless supplemented by a hot bath before MUSE administration. The patient stated that with MUSE alone the erection lasted for 5–10 minutes but on the two previous occasions when he had had a hot bath for 20 minutes and then used MUSE, the erection had lasted 3–4 hours. However, on the third occasion, priapism lasted 20 hours and necessitated corporeal aspiration for detumescence.

Immunologic

When latanoprost was applied for 4 months to the eyes in 14 patients, there was an increase in HLA-DR expression (15). Since HLA-DR is a marker of ocular surface inflammation, these results suggested a subclinical inflammatory reaction to latanoprost. However, the clinical significance of HLA-DR expression is not clear.

References

1. Caballero S, Torre I, Arias B, Blanco D, Zabala JI, Sanchez Luna M. Efectos secundarios de la prostaglandina E1 en el manejo del sindrome de corazon izquierdo hipoplastico en espera de trasplante cardiaco. [Secondary effects of prostaglandin E1 on the management of hypoplastic left heart syndrome while waiting for heart transplantation.] An Esp Pediatr 1998;48(5):505–9.
2. Fujita M, Hatori N, Shimizu M, Yoshizu H, Segawa D, Kimura T, Iizuka Y, Tanaka S. Neutralization of prostaglandin E1 intravenous solution reduces infusion phlebitis. Angiology 2000;51(9):719–23.
3. Lewis GB, Hecker JF. Infusion thrombophlebitis. Br J Anaesth 1985;57(2):220–33.
4. Arav-Boger R, Baggett HC, Spevak PJ, Willoughby RE. Leukocytosis caused by prostaglandin E1 in neonates. J Pediatr 2001;138(2):263–5.
5. English JC 3rd, King DH, Foley JP. Penile shaft hypopigmentation: lichen sclerosus occurring after the initiation of alprostadil intracavernous injections for erectile dysfunction. J Am Acad Dermatol 1998;39(5 Pt 1):801–3.
6. Carter EL, Garzon MC. Neonatal urticaria due to prostaglandin E1. Pediatr Dermatol 2000;17(1):58–61.
7. Jerstad KM, Warshaw E. Allergic contact dermatitis to latanoprost. Am J Contact Dermat 2002;13(1):39–41.
8. Nadroo AM, Shringari S, Garg M, al-Sowailem AM. Prostaglandin induced cortical hyperostosis in neonates with cyanotic heart disease. J Perinat Med 2000;28(6):447–52.
9. Crevenna R, Quittan M, Hulsmann M, Wiesinger GF, Keilani MY, Kainberger F, Leitha T, Fialka-Moser V, Pacher R. Hypertrophic osteoarthropathy caused by PGE1

in a patient with congestive heart failure during cardiac rehabilitation. Wien Klin Wochenschr 2002;114(3):115–18.

10. Alvarez E, Andrianne R, Arvis G, Boezaart F, Buvat J, Czyzyk A, et al. The long-term safety of alprostadil (prostaglandin-E1) in patients with erectile dysfunction. The European Alprostadil Study Group. Br J Urol 1998;82(4):538–43.

11. Lehmann K, Casella R, Blochlinger A, Gasser TC. Reasons for discontinuing intracavernous injection therapy with prostaglandin E1 (alprostadil). Urology 1999;53(2):397–400.

12. Hauck EW, Altinkilic BM, Schroeder-Printzen I, Rudnick J, Weidner W. Prostaglandin E1 long-term self-injection programme for treatment of erectile dysfunction—a follow-up of at least 5 years. Andrologia 1999;31(Suppl 1):99–103.

13. Williams G, Abbou CC, Amar ET, Desvaux P, Flam TA, Lycklama a Nijeholt GA, Lynch SF, Morgan RJ, Muller SC, Porst H, Pryor JP, Ryan P, Witzsch UK, Hall MM, Place VA, Spivack AP, Todd LK, Gesundheit N. The effect of transurethral alprostadil on the quality of life of men with erectile dysfunction, and their partners. MUSE Study Group. Br J Urol 1998;82(6):847–54.

14. Bettocchi C, Ashford L, Pryor JP, Ralph DJ. Priapism after transurethral alprostadil. Br J Urol 1998;81(6):926.

15. Guglielminetti E, Barabino S, Monaco M, Mantero S, Rolando M. HLA-DR expression in conjunctival cells after latanoprost. J Ocul Pharmacol Ther 2002;18(1):1–9.

Aluminium

General Information

Aluminium is a metallic element (symbol Al; atomic no. 13), a light, silver-colored, malleable metal.

Aluminium is the most abundant of all metals and is obtained from bauxite ores by the production of alumina, which is then smelted to produce aluminium. Its abundance is demonstrated by the vast number of minerals and precious stones that contain aluminium, which include: albite, analcime, anorthite, beryl, chabazite, cimolite, dumortierite, epidote, euclase, feldspar, fuller's earth, glauconite, halloysite, harmotome, iolite, jadeite, kaolinite, kyanite, lazurite, leucite, margarite, melilite, montmorillonite, muscovite, natrolite, nepheline, noselite, penninite, phillipsite, piedmontite, pinite, prehnite, saponite, sapphirine, scapolite, scolecite, sillimanite, sodalite, spessartite, spodumene, staurolite, topaz, and vesuvianite (all of which contain salts or pure crystals of aluminium silicate); alunite (hydrous aluminium sulfate); cryolite (sodium aluminium fluoride); diaspore, gibbsite, and laterite (aluminium hydroxide); lazulite, sphaerite, turquoise, variscite, and wavellite (aluminium phosphate); scorodite and synadelphite (aluminium arsenate); and gmelinite (aluminium zeolite).

Note on nomenclature

Aluminium was first named (although not isolated) by Sir Humphry Davy, who originally called it alumium (1808) because it was found in alum, a name that had been extant since at least the 14th century. He later called it aluminum (1812), but others soon changed it to aluminium, in order to harmonize it with the many other elements whose names end in "ium" and because "aluminum" was thought not to have a particularly classical sound. For many years, both "aluminium" and "aluminum" were used in the USA, until the American Chemical Society adopted the form "aluminum" in 1925. However, "aluminium" is the official name recognized by the International Union of Pure and Applied Chemistry (IUPAC) and is the form that is used here.

Sources of exposure

Aluminium is widely used in medicine, pharmacy, food technology, and cosmetics. It is also a popular metal for making everyday objects, including kitchen utensils and other devices associated with food preparation. There is also some exposure, although generally limited, from the environment. Toxic effects of aluminium have been seen in patients treated with total parenteral nutrition contaminated with aluminium (1); high concentrations of aluminium have been detected in some intravenously administered solutions, such as human serum albumin (2) and in artificial breast milk substitutes. Exceptionally, a metallic aluminium object can become lodged in the body and give rise to aluminium toxicity (SEDA-20, 207). Additive intake from multiple medical and/or non-medical sources can prove excessive, and it can be important to recognize the many circumstances in which exposure occurs. Aluminium absorbed into the system is excreted in the bile, generally without obvious consequences (SEDA-12, 316).

Hyperaluminemia has been described in premature infants receiving prolonged intravenous alimentation, and in recipients of plasmapheresis receiving large volumes of replacement albumin solutions, which contain high concentrations of aluminium (3–4).

Many aluminium salts, including aluminium hydroxide gel, aluminium carbonate, aluminium glycinate, and aluminosilicate, are used therapeutically, and the absorption rate depends on the chemical species. Aluminium citrate is well absorbed (5), but aluminium hydroxide gel antacid is poorly absorbed (0.003%) (6). Aluminium glycinate is well absorbed and excreted in the urine. Poorly absorbed aluminium-containing formulations should be preferred for those who have poor renal function particularly elderly people.

Sucralfate is a basic aluminium salt of sucrose octasulfate.

Medical uses

The external medical uses of aluminium are many; water-soluble compounds such as alum have long been used as mild external antiseptic, astringent, antihydrotic, or styptic agents, and more recently in deodorants and antiperspirants. Metallic aluminium is also used in some wound dressings.

Internal use in medicine can exploit the alkaline nature and adsorptive capacities of aluminium compounds (as in antacid mixtures, antidiarrheal drugs, and vaccines). Aluminium is found in medications for antacid therapy and phosphate depletion; alternatives are under investigation (7). Patients on dialysis take large amounts of oral aluminium hydroxide as a means of reducing serum phosphate. Sucralfate is used to treat peptic ulceration and gastritis.

Aluminium is used as a vaccine adjuvant (8).

General adverse effects

Topical aluminium can occasionally cause skin irritation in sensitive individuals.

The systemic availability of aluminium is normally very low, because the gastrointestinal tract, skin, and lungs are excellent barriers to its entry; furthermore, the small amounts that pass these barriers are efficiently eliminated by the kidneys. However, problems can arise if the natural protective barriers are bypassed or if there is impaired renal function. Significant systemic effects are rare unless there is a high degree of absorption.

- Acute aluminium toxicity in one reported case followed the introduction of aluminium sulfate (alum) into the urinary tract to treat hemorrhagic cystitis; there was apparently both increased absorption, due to the mucosal lesion of the bladder wall, and an increased susceptibility due to pre-existing renal insufficiency (SED-13, 585).

Aluminium is toxic in patients on chronic hemodialysis and peritoneal dialysis and in those taking oral aluminium-containing medications. Aspects of aluminium safety (9) and metabolism (10) have been reviewed. The association between aluminium in drinking water and Alzheimer's disease continues to be discussed and remains controversial (11).

Although aluminium adjuvants have proven to be safe over six decades, adverse effects, such as erythema, subcutaneous nodules, and contact hypersensitivity, sometimes occur (12). The aluminium body burden has been estimated in infants during the first year of life for a standard immunization schedule compared with breast milk and formula diets (13). The calculated body burden of aluminium from immunization exceeds that from dietary sources, but is still below the minimal risk level equivalent curve during the brief period after injection.

Organs and Systems

Respiratory

Specific chemical exposures and exposure assessment methods relating to studies in the alumina and primary aluminium industry have been reviewed (14). In aluminium smelting, exposure to fluorides, coal tar pitch volatiles, and sulfur dioxide has tended to abate in recent years, but there is insufficient information about other exposures. Published epidemiological studies and quantitative exposure data for bauxite mining and alumina refining are virtually non-existent. Determination of possible exposure–response relations for this part of the industry through improved exposure assessment methods should be the focus of future studies.

Dental technicians are potentially exposed to various occupational dusts and chemicals and pulmonary granulomatosis has been reported (15).

- A dental laboratory technician developed progressive exertional dyspnea and cough associated with pulmonary granulomatosis. Lung function studies showed a restrictive pattern with a low diffusion capacity. A high-resolution CT scan showed micronodules in both lungs, corresponding to non-caseating foreign body granulomas at histological examination. Mineralogical studies showed the presence of silica, silicates, and aluminium. The lymphocytic transformation test was positive for beryllium with the bronchoalveolar lavage.

Combined histological, mineralogical, and immunological studies led to a diagnosis of pneumoconiosis, most likely related to occupational exposure to beryllium and aluminium.

The role of aluminium in the development of occupational asthma has never been convincingly substantiated. Occupational asthma has been attributed to aluminium welding (16).

- A 32-year-old man working in a leather plant performed electric arc welding on mild steel, using manual metal arc and inert gas metal arc techniques. About once a month he welded aluminium pieces using a manual arc process with a flux-coated electrode. After 4 years of intermittent exposure to these various welding processes, he developed chest tightness and wheezing that occurred specifically on days when he was welding aluminium. His asthmatic symptoms started 1–4 hours after the end of exposure to aluminium and persisted for several hours. He never had myalgia, chills, or fever. He was treated with inhaled budesonide (400 micrograms/day) and salbutamol when necessary. Inhalation challenges combined with exposure assessment provided evidence that aluminium can cause asthmatic reactions.

A syndrome known as "pot-room asthma" occurs in around 2% of new aluminium smelters each year, with a wide range of incidences around the world (17).

- In 1529 men in two smelting factories, work-related respiratory symptoms were reported significantly more often among the ingot mill, anode, and pot-room groups in factory A after adjusting for age and smoking, while in factory B, ingot employees were more likely to report work-related wheeze and pot-room employees were more likely to report work-related rhinitis (18). Symptoms tended to increase with increasing time in the pot-rooms, but were more likely to occur in new employees in the ingot mill and anode process groups.

Nervous system

The toxicology of aluminium in the brain has been reviewed (19,20).

Since 1976, aluminium has been known to be a cause of encephalopathy, a potentially fatal condition occurring primarily in patients on chronic dialysis (21). Difficulties in speech, disturbances of consciousness, and ataxia can be followed by psychotic episodes, personality changes, myoclonic jerks, electroencephalographic abnormalities, convulsions, and dementia. Accumulation of aluminium can be demonstrated in the gray matter of the brain and in other tissues. If not too advanced, the condition can recede after reduction of aluminium intake and use of deferoxamine.

- Intravesical irrigation with 1% alum for hemorrhagic cystitis resulted in sufficient absorption to produce encephalopathic symptoms in a teenage girl (22).

An identical condition can occur in aluminium plant workers and miners, and can be reproduced in animal experiments. However, some clinically similar encephalopathies do occur spontaneously (or possibly as a result of uremia) in children where no link with aluminium exposure can be found.

There have been reports that the use of surgical aluminium-containing bone cement can cause epileptic seizures as well as encephalopathy, at least when the cement is in direct contact with the cerebrospinal fluid, as can happen in neurosurgery (23,24) (SEDA-21, 232). In this connection it should be noted that such bone cements can produce high circulating concentrations of aluminium. One French study in six patients (25) noted mean plasma aluminium concentrations of up to 9.2 ng/ml, while up to 176 ng/ml was present in the postauricular cerebrospinal fluid (SEDA-22, 242). This aspect of aluminium cement merits further study.

Aluminium-containing antacids have been suggested to be the cause of idiopathic Parkinson's disease in a study of 200 patients and 200 age- and sex-matched controls. There was a significantly higher incidence of ulcers (diagnosed by X-ray or surgery) in the patients with Parkinson's disease compared with controls (14 versus 4%) (26,27). The ulcers typically preceded the diagnosis of Parkinson's disease by 10–20 years. Parkinson's disease occurs worldwide, suggesting perhaps that some ubiquitous toxin plays a role in its pathogenesis. Aluminium absorption resulting in raised blood concentrations has been detected in babies given "Infant Gaviscon" (which is based on aluminium alginate and is not in fact recommended by the manufacturers in the very young) and in adults given aluminium sucrose sulfate, though without apparent ill-effect.

Acute neurotoxic adverse effects of aluminium have been attributed to aluminium-containing surgical cement.

- A 52-year-old woman had a resection of an acoustic neuroma (28). Bone reconstruction was performed with an aluminium-containing cement and 6 weeks later she had loss of consciousness, myoclonic jerks, and persistent tonic-clonic seizures, effects resembling those of dialysis encephalopathy. She died 6 months later with septic complications. Light microscopy and electron microscopy of the brain showed pathognomonic aluminium-containing intracytoplasmic argyrophilic inclusions in the choroid plexus epithelia, neurons, and cortical glia. These changes are characteristic of dialysis-associated encephalopathy. Atomic absorption spectrometry showed an increase in the mean aluminium concentration in the cortex and subcortex, up to 9.3 µg/g (reference range under 2 µg/g); a laser microprobe showed increased aluminium in subcellular structures.

This case shows again the extraordinary neurotoxic potency of aluminium, which was initiated by about 30 mg and apparently caused by direct access of aluminium to the brain parenchyma via cerebrospinal fluid leakage.

Aluminium and Alzheimer's disease

The association between aluminium in drinking water and Alzheimer's disease continues to be discussed and remains controversial (11,29,30). The theory has been advanced that aluminium may be linked to the etiology of Alzheimer's disease (31), one suggestion being that the mechanism is the inhibition of tetrahydrobiopterin synthesis in the temporal cortex. This hypothesis has led to much debate (32–34), and more knowledge is accumulating regarding possible mechanisms of neurotoxicity (35).

One study has suggested that researchers looking for a connection between aluminium and Alzheimer's disease may have ignored the most important source of aluminium for the average person—foodstuffs that contain aluminium additives (36). The results implied that aluminium, added to such foods as anticaking agents, emulsifiers, thickeners, leaveners, and stabilizers, may have long-term adverse effects on health. However, the small sample size hampers any definitive conclusions, the odds ratios were very unstable, and the study had limited statistical power to rule out random errors.

The relation between different chemical forms of aluminium in drinking water and Alzheimer's disease has been studied in 68 patients with Alzheimer's disease, diagnosed according to recognized criteria and paired for age and sex with non-demented controls (37). Aluminium speciation was assessed using established standard analytical protocols along with quality control procedures (total aluminium, total dissolved aluminium, monomeric organic aluminium, monomeric inorganic aluminium, polymeric aluminium, Al^{3+}, AlOH, AlF, $AlH_3SiO_4^{2+}$, $AlSO_4$). The results suggested a possible association between monomeric aluminium exposition and Alzheimer's disease. In contrast to the results of earlier studies, this association was observed in a geographical environment characterized by low aluminium concentrations and a high pH.

However, others have suggested that the theory that aluminium plays a role in the pathogenesis of Alzheimer's disease has been largely discarded, as our understanding of the pathogenic mechanisms of Alzheimer's disease has advanced (38).

Sensory systems

Tissue lesions can be caused by local deposition of aluminium, for example in the eye (39)

- A 76-year-old man with a history of multiple melanomas noticed a gradually enlarging pigmented mass in his right eye. He had had successful pneumatic cryopexy of a retinal tear in the temporal region of the right eye 4 years before with no reported complications. Slit lamp examination showed a 4×2 mm elevated darkly pigmented conjunctival mass surrounding the insertion site of the lateral rectus. An excisional biopsy showed multiple foci of fine, jet-black, granular pigmentation in a perivascular distribution, with additional deposition throughout the conjunctival stroma. There were no melanocyte abnormalities or cellular atypia. Energy dispersive analysis of X-rays showed spectral peaks corresponding to heavy aluminium deposition with trace amounts of silicone.

Aluminium is often incorporated in cryoprobe tips for ophthalmic use, providing a possible source of local deposition. Other possibilities include a metallic foreign body and occupational exposure.

Mineral balance

The ability of aluminium gels to bind phosphate can result in clinical significant hypophosphatemia, which usually presents as myalgia, weakness, and bone pain, but can have more extreme consequences; one report described rickets with hypercalciuria after prolonged use, though the subject was an immobilized boy with spastic quadriplegia which can itself have affected the skeleton (40). Even relatively small doses of commonly used aluminium-containing liquid antacids (90–120 ml/day) can lead to adverse effects on calcium and phosphorus metabolism. During long-term therapy, a considerable loss of calcium may occur, resulting in skeletal demineralization (41). Collagen synthesis and matrix mineralization can be so seriously affected that a vitamin D-resistant osteomalacia develops (42). The adverse effects of aluminium overload on the bones respond to reduction in aluminium exposure, whether this has resulted from oral intake or use of aluminium in dialysis (43).

Metal metabolism

Severe copper deficiency has followed the intake of a gel containing bismuth, aluminium, magnesium, and sodium in a patient with pyloric stenosis (44).

Hematologic

Aluminium overload in uremic patients can lead to a microcytic hypochromic anemia (45). The mechanism is unknown, but it appears to involve inhibition of heme synthesis, either by inhibition of enzyme activity or by interference with the incorporation or utilization of iron. Exposure for 3 months is sufficient to reduce hematological values and cause significant increases in serum and urinary aluminium (46). The anemia can be reversed by lowering the aluminium intake or by chelation therapy with deferoxamine.

Gastrointestinal

Aluminium hydroxide can cause constipation, or even intestinal obstruction. Severe bowel dysfunction developed in 25 of 945 patients receiving long-term hemodialysis during 10 years (47). There was colonic perforation in 12 patients, six of whom died with peritonitis. In 10 other patients there was prolonged, severe, adynamic ileus that progressed to colonic pseudo-obstruction in eight. All had regularly taken aluminium hydroxide gel and had had chronic constipation before presentation.

Large doses of aluminium can be associated with fecal impaction and the development of intestinal obstruction in uremic patients (48). Impacted tablets have in some cases caused obstruction (SEDA-16, 417).

Aluminium hydroxide can have an aggravating effect on *Helicobacter pylori*-associated gastritis in patients with duodenal ulceration (49).

Liver

The histology and metal content of the liver have been studied in a patient with Wilson's disease (50). Copper and aluminium contents of the biopsied liver were measured simultaneously by neutron activation analysis. The copper content was markedly increased (814 µg/g dry weight) and there was an extremely high aluminium content (479 µg/g). On the other hand, macroscopically and histologically there was no evidence of cirrhosis, although there was mild fibrosis or inflammation of the liver. It is likely that toxic metals, such as aluminium, copper, and manganese, might be implicated in the pathogenesis of Wilson's disease.

Animal experiments suggest that aluminium may play a role in the pathogenesis of parenteral nutrition-induced hepatobiliary dysfunction (51).

Urinary tract

A patient who grossly overused an antacid containing aluminium and magnesium developed nephrolithiasis and bilateral ureteric obstruction as well as asymptomatic hypophosphatemia (SEDA-16, 417).

Irrigation of the urinary bladder with alum successfully controls vesical hematuria, but it can cause bladder spasm (52).

Skin

Aluminium causes histological changes at injection sites, and these stain with hematoxylin and eosin (53). Of four patients studied, one had a sclerosing lipogranuloma-like reaction with unlined cystic spaces containing crystalline material. Another presented as a large symptomatic subcutaneous swelling, which microscopically showed diffuse and widespread involvement of the subcutaneous tissues by a lymphoid infiltrate with prominent lymphoid follicles.

Contact allergy to topically applied aluminium compounds is rare but skin sensitization has been described (54). In one case the use of a cream for acne and hyperpigmentation was followed by dermatitis, and patch tests were positive to both aluminium sulfate and aluminium chloride. A more typical antecedent of sensitization is the injection of aluminium-adsorbed vaccines, and such patients may present with a granulomatous nodule at the site. Mixed contact sensitivity to nickel and aluminium has been reported to respond to antihistamine therapy (55).

Persistent skin lesions occurred in three patients after the administration of aluminium hydroxide-containing vaccines.

- A 19-year-old woman presented with multiple itchy nodules on the outer aspects of the upper arms at the sites of previous vaccine injections (56). There were several nodules, ranging from a few millimeters to 1 cm in diameter, some with overlying hyperpigmented skin. She had been receiving hyposensitization vaccines to treat recurrent extrinsic asthma and rhinitis for the previous 4 years. A skin biopsy showed a normal epidermis and upper dermis. There were multifocal unencapsulated granulomatous infiltrates in the deep dermis and subcutaneous tissues, disrupting the normal architecture of the latter. The infiltrate was predominantly composed of histiocytes with foreign body giant cells. There were also fibroblasts, fibrosis, and perivascular lymphocytes and plasma cells, with a few eosinophils. There was a granular basophilic material within the cytoplasm of some histiocytes. However, patch tests with aluminium chloride, nickel sulfate, and potassium dichromate were all negative. She was treated with potent topical corticosteroids and oral antihistamines, with some relief, but the nodules persisted 2 years later.

- A 37-year-old woman with a 5-year history of multiple itchy nodules on the outer aspects of the upper parts of the arms at sites of previous vaccine injections had been receiving hyposensitization vaccines to treat recurrent extrinsic asthma and rhinitis for 10 years (56). Physical examination and a biopsy of one of the nodules were identical to those of the previous case. Patch tests with aluminium chloride were negative. Symptomatic relief was obtained with topical corticosteroids and oral antihistamines. The nodules persisted for at least 3 years.

- A 52-year-old woman, allergic to wasp venom, was hyposensitized with a vaccine containing wasp venom precipitated on aluminium hydroxide (57). Each subcutaneous injection of the extract was followed by cooling of the acute local reaction at the injection site for about 1 hour. As soon as 24 hours after the second maintenance dose, she developed tender, erythematous, ill-demarcated, indurated plaques at the injection sites on both the lateral thighs. The lesions resolved spontaneously after several weeks, leaving residual hyperpigmentation and subcutaneous atrophy. They reappeared with each treatment, even after the vaccine was changed to a lyophilized, aluminium-free extract. No further lesions occurred when the injection sites were not cooled, even though the aluminium hydroxide vaccine was continued. Patch tests with the vaccine, aluminium hydroxide, human albumin, phenol, and aluminium chloride hexahydrate were all negative. A biopsy of the skin lesions showed lobular panniculitis, with lipocyte necrosis and a mixed cellular infiltrate of neutrophils, lymphocytes, and histiocytes. Ultrasound examination of the atrophic areas showed significantly thinner subcutaneous tissue than in the normal contralateral skin. Rechallenge with an ice pack alone on the upper arm caused a similar skin lesion to appear within 24 hours.

Various mechanisms were postulated to explain these persistent lesions, such as a non-allergic direct toxic effect of aluminium and a delayed hypersensitivity reaction to aluminium.

Four cases have been reported of persistent subcutaneous nodules at sites of hepatitis B vaccination due to aluminium sensitization (58). Symptoms included pruritic, sore, erythematous, and in two cases hyperpigmented, subcutaneous nodules, persisting for 8 months to 2 years. All the patients were positive for aluminium salts in patch tests, while immunization against hepatitis B was successful.

Musculoskeletal

Macrophagic myofasciitis has been reported in relation to immunization with an aluminium-based vaccine (59).

- A 5-year-old boy with chronic intestinal pseudo-obstruction required nighttime parenteral nutrition.

He had abnormal pupillary reflexes and urinary retention, suggesting diffuse dysautonomia. A 3-year-old child had developed delay and hypotonia. Both children had received age-appropriate immunizations. Quadriceps muscle biopsies showed the typical patchy, cohesive, centripetal infiltration of alpha-1-antitrypsin+, alpha-antichymotrypsin+, CD68+, PAS+, CD1a−, S-100−, factor XIII− granular macrophages with adjacent atrophy of myofibers, dilated blood vessels, and mild endomysial and perimysial fibrosis. There was no myonecrosis and no discrete granulomas. There was a single aluminium peak on energy dispersive X-ray microanalysis. Most infectious causes leading to macrophage activation were ruled out, thus implicating aluminium. Both patients improved gradually with time.

Heavy chronic use of antacids containing aluminium and magnesium hydroxide can cause serious skeletal impairment (60).

- A 39-year-old female pharmacist who self-medicated with high doses of a potent antacid containing aluminium and magnesium hydroxide for peptic ulcer disease consumed over 18 kg of elemental aluminium and 15 kg of elemental magnesium over 8 years. This resulted in severe osteomalacia, due to profound phosphate depletion. Bone biopsy showed stainable aluminium deposits along 28% of the total bone surface, which is a unique observation in a patient with normal renal function. Treatment included withdrawing the antacid and supplementation with phosphate, calcium, and vitamin D. This produced marked subjective and objective improvement, including a striking increase in her bone mineral density over the next 2 years.

Osteomalacia due to aluminium-containing antacids has been associated with stainable bone aluminium in patients with normal renal function (61).

- A 39-year-old woman who took high doses of aluminium and magnesium hydroxide for peptic ulcer disease (over 18 kg of elemental aluminium and 15 kg of elemental magnesium over 8 years) developed severe osteomalacia due to profound phosphate depletion (60). Bone biopsy showed stainable aluminium deposits along 28% of the total bone surface, a unique observation in a patient with normal renal function. Treatment included withdrawal of the antacid and supplementation with phosphate, calcium, and vitamin D. Her bone mineral density increased over the next 2 years.

Unexpected persistent aluminium-related bone disease occurred after renal transplantation following earlier use of aluminium hydroxide (62).

- A 59-year-old man presented with end-stage renal insufficiency. While on hemodialysis he had used aluminium hydroxide as a phosphate binder but then used calcium lactate instead after total parathyroidectomy. Oral vitamin D was discontinued after the parathyroidectomy. However, after he had received a renal transplant he developed aluminium-related bone disease and was treated with infusions of deferoxamine.

This is the first report of worsening aluminium-related bone disease after renal transplantation.

Hyperparathyroidism and aluminium hydroxide lead to aluminium-related bone disease; however, total parathyroidectomy does not lead to failure of aluminium mobilization after renal transplantation. This man had satisfactory graft function, and the aluminium excretion that was achieved by deferoxamine suggests that the renal transplant was not the limiting factor for the mobilization of aluminium. The most likely explanation was that he developed adynamic bone through a combination of vitamin D deficiency, hypoparathyroidism, and aluminium deposition. Vitamin D supplementation failed to prevent the osteodystrophy on its own. When aluminium chelation therapy was used, bone healing occurred and his symptoms improved.

Immunologic

Aluminium has a non-specific immunosuppressive action, which results in a lower incidence of transplant rejection in patients with high aluminium concentrations in the tissues; in the first instance one might consider this a reason for seeking to maintain a particularly high aluminium concentration in transplant patients. However, there are good reasons not to do so. Firstly, should infection occur, this immunosuppressive effect can lead to increased risk and higher mortality; work in dialysis patients has confirmed that an increased aluminium load raises the risk of infections (63). Secondly, after transplantations there already is a high aluminium concentration because of mobilization of aluminium from the storage pool. Aluminium loading before transplantation should therefore be avoided and excessive concentrations countered (64).

Aluminium salts are currently the only widely used adjuvants in human vaccines (65). Developments in the understanding of the structure, composition, and preparation of immunostimulating complexes (ISCOMs) have been reviewed and compared.

Susceptibility Factors

Renal disease

In many patients with severe renal disease there is a double risk: they are exposed to aluminium as a part of their treatment (in agents given for the control of serum phosphate concentrations, in aluminium-containing dialysis fluids and, in one case, in the form of bladder irrigation with alum) (66), and at the same time they have a reduced ability to eliminate it. Aluminium-containing phosphate binders are especially risky if used in combination with an alkalinizing citrate solution (Shohl's solution) (67,68); due to the formation of an aluminium citrate complex in the gastrointestinal tract, aluminium is absorbed more readily. In addition, aluminium citrate complex has a synergistic inhibitory action on bone growth and thus exacerbates aluminium-associated osteomalacia in chronic renal failure. Children with impaired renal function may be particularly susceptible to aluminium intoxication solely from oral aluminium loading (69).

When aluminium is used as a phosphate binder in patients on renal dialysis, absorption and accumulation can occur. Phosphate depletion accompanied by increased bone resorption and hypercalciuria (with a risk of osteomalacia) can result (70). Low phosphate diets exacerbate this risk. Concurrent use of oral citrate solutions may increase absorption of aluminium from aluminium hydroxide, resulting in high blood concentrations, especially when renal function is impaired (71).

Encephalopathy due to high serum aluminium concentrations has been reported in acute renal insufficiency (SEDA-17, 273) (72). Unsuspected intake of citrate from other sources has apparently promoted the occurrence of aluminium encephalopathy in renal insufficiency (73). Most reported instances of encephalopathy after alum irrigation have occurred in patients with compromised renal function.

- A 70-year-old man with advanced obstructive nephropathy began to hemorrhage from the bladder after decompression with a Foley catheter (74). He developed an encephalopathy after continuous irrigation with 1% alum for 2 days, associated with raised serum aluminium concentrations. Repeated treatment with deferoxamine and hemodialysis removed some aluminium, but he succumbed to bronchopneumonia. At autopsy his brain aluminium content was not excessive.

Prolonged exposure to aluminium in patients with chronic renal insufficiency can be involved in the pathogenesis of uremic pruritus, and increased calcium phosphate production seems to be an additional predisposing factor (75); certainly the incidence and intensity of pruritus in these uremic patients have been found to be related to the circulating concentrations of aluminium.

Slow accumulation of aluminium during long-term hemodialysis can cause osteomalacia (76), bone and joint pain and muscular weakness (77), iron-resistant microcytic anemia (78), and neurological disorders (79).

In 33 patients on hemodialysis, who were exposed to moderately high serum aluminium concentrations for less than 4 months, even moderately high aluminium concentrations produced significant hematological alterations and depletion of body iron stores before clinical manifestations were evident (80).

In all patients with chronic renal insufficiency, strict supervision of total aluminium intake is vital. The administration of aluminium should be stopped as soon as the serum concentration exceeds 150 µg/ml or at the appearance of the first symptoms of encephalopathy (81). According to current recommendations, dialysate solutions should contain less than 10 µg/l of aluminium (82). There is some controversy about the view that aluminium-containing medications used to control serum phosphate concentrations in uremic subjects should be replaced by calcium-containing phosphate binders (83). Another approach used to reduce the toxic risks of aluminium hydroxide may be to tailor doses to the phosphate concentration in serum, that is individualizing aluminium gel therapy (SED-12, 515).

Drug Administration

Drug overdose

Of 195 patients hospitalized after aluminium phosphide poisoning (84), 115 died. Death was related to the dose but not to the time between ingestion and arrival at the hospital. The non-survivors had more severe hypotension and metabolic acidosis than the survivors, who had more severe vomiting. Aluminium phosphide is highly toxic, with a fatal dose as low as 1.5 g. The dominant clinical feature in such cases is severe hypotension, and severe gastrointestinal derangement and cardiorespiratory failure can occur within a day of exposure (85).

Drug–Drug Interactions

Citrate

Citrate is included in many effervescent or dispersible tablets, and increased absorption of aluminium from the gastrointestinal tract has been reported (86–88).

Deferoxamine

Although deferoxamine is effective in treating aluminium overload, case reports have shown that it can induce an exacerbation of aluminium encephalopathy (89), possibly due to increased aluminium concentrations in the cerebrospinal fluid (90,91). During treatment with deferoxamine, plasma aluminium concentrations should be monitored, as concentrations exceeding 800–1000 µmol/l can exacerbate encephalopathy.

Diflunisal

Aluminium reduced the systemic availability of diflunisal by about 40% in healthy volunteers (92).

Prednisone

In five healthy volunteers and 12 patients with chronic active liver disease, antacids containing aluminium hydroxide and magnesium hydroxide significantly reduced the C_{max} and AUC of prednisone when administered with antacids. The systemic availability was reduced by up to 43% (93).

Silicon

Aluminium has a close chemical affinity with silicon, which may have a role in protecting against aluminium toxicity (94). Serum aluminium and silicon concentrations were measured in hemodialysis patients from four different centers. Although there was no relation across all centers combined, in one center there was a reciprocal relation in patients on home hemodialysis (who did not require reverse osmosis). Median (range) aluminium concentrations were higher, 2.2 (0.4–9.6) µmol/l when serum silicon was less than 150 µmol/l, and lower, 1.1 (0.2–2.8) µmol/l when serum silicon was greater than 150 µmol/l. In patients treated by hemodialysis without reverse osmosis, high serum silicon concentrations were associated with lower serum aluminium concentrations. Further work is needed to confirm a preventive role for silicon in the accumulation and subsequent toxicity of aluminium in dialysis patients.

Tetracyclines

The laboratory finding that aluminium hydroxide binds a variety of drugs, thus forming poorly absorbable salts or complexes, has led to a general rule of thumb that other drugs should not be taken within 1–2 hours of aluminium compounds. In most cases such interactions are clinically insignificant, but caution is advisable. The absorption of tetracyclines under these conditions can be reduced by as much as 90% (95).

References

1. Klein GL. Aluminum in parenteral products: medical perspective on large and small volume parenterals. J Parenter Sci Technol 1989;43(3):120–4.
2. Milliner DS, Shinaberger JH, Shuman P, Coburn JW. Inadvertent aluminum administration during plasma exchange due to aluminum contamination of albumin-replacement solutions. N Engl J Med 1985;312(3):165–7.
3. Sedman AB, Klein GL, Merritt RJ, Miller NL, Weber KO, Gill WL, Anand H, Alfrey AC. Evidence of aluminum loading in infants receiving intravenous therapy. N Engl J Med 1985;312(21):1337–43.
4. Monteagudo F, Wood L, Jacobs P, Folb P, Cassidy M. Aluminium loading during therapeutic plasma exchange. J Clin Apher 1987;3(3):161–3.
5. Fairweather-Tait S, Hickson K, McGaw B, Reid M. Orange juice enhances aluminium absorption from antacid preparation. Eur J Clin Nutr 1994;48(1):71–3.
6. Meshitsuka S, Inoue M. Urinary excretion of aluminum from antacid ingestion and estimation of its apparent biological half-time. Trace Elem Electrolytes 1998;15:132–5.
7. Burke SK. Renagel: reducing serum phosphorus in haemodialysis patients. Hosp Med 2000;61(9):622–7.
8. White JL, Hem SL. Characterization of aluminium-containing adjuvants. Dev Biol (Basel) 2000;103:217–28.
9. Hemstreet BA. Use of sucralfate in renal failure. Ann Pharmacother 2001;35(3):360–4.
10. Yokel RA, McNamara PJ. Aluminium toxicokinetics: an updated minireview. Pharmacol Toxicol 2001;88(4):159–67.
11. Flaten TP. Aluminium as a risk factor in Alzheimer's disease, with emphasis on drinking water. Brain Res Bull 2001;55(2):187–96.
12. Baylor NW, Egan W, Richman P. Aluminum salts in vaccines—US perspective. Vaccine 2002;20(Suppl 3):S18–23.
13. Keith LS, Jones DE, Chou CH. Aluminum toxicokinetics regarding infant diet and vaccinations. Vaccine 2002;20(Suppl 3):S13–17.
14. Benke G, Abramson M, Sim M. Exposures in the alumina and primary aluminium industry: an historical review. Ann Occup Hyg 1998;42(3):173–89.
15. Brancaleone P, Weynand B, De Vuyst P, Stanescu D, Pieters T. Lung granulomatosis in a dental technician. Am J Ind Med 1998;34(6):628–31.
16. Vandenplas O, Delwiche JP, Vanbilsen ML, Joly J, Roosels D. Occupational asthma caused by aluminium welding. Eur Respir J 1998;11(5):1182–4.
17. Abramson MJ, Wlodarczyk JH, Saunders NA, Hensley MJ. Does aluminum smelting cause lung disease? Am Rev Respir Dis 1989;139(4):1042–57.
18. Fritschi L, Beach J, Sim M, Abramson M, Benke G, Musk AW, de Klerk N, McNeil J. Respiratory symptoms and lung function in two prebake aluminum smelters. Am J Ind Med 1999;35(5):491–8.
19. Yokel RA. The toxicology of aluminum in the brain: a review. Neurotoxicology 2000;21(5):813–28.
20. Yokel RA. Brain uptake, retention, and efflux of aluminum and manganese. Environ Health Perspect 2002;110(Suppl 5):699–704.
21. Hoang-Xuan K, Perrotte P, Dubas F, Philippon J, Poisson FM. Myoclonic encephalopathy after exposure to aluminum. Lancet 1996;347(9005):910–11.

22. Kanwar VS, Jenkins JJ 3rd, Mandrell BN, Furman WL. Aluminum toxicity following intravesical alum irrigation for hemorrhagic cystitis. Med Pediatr Oncol 1996;27(1):64–7.

23. Hantson P, Mahieu P, Gersdorff M, Sindic C, Lauwerys R. Fatal encephalopathy after otoneurosurgery procedure with an aluminum-containing biomaterial. J Toxicol Clin Toxicol 1995;33(6):645–8.

24. Various authors Research issues in aluminium toxicity. J Toxicol Environ Health (Special Issue) 1996;48:527–686.

25. Guillard O, Pineau A, Fauconneau B, Chobaut JC, Desaulty A, Angot A, Le Borgne E, Furon O. Biological levels of aluminium after use of aluminium-containing bone cement in post-otoneurosurgery. J Trace Elem Med Biol 1997;11(1):53–6.

26. Altschuler E. Aluminum-containing antacids as a cause of idiopathic Parkinson's disease. Med Hypotheses 1999;53(1):22–3.

27. Strang RR. The association of gastro-duodenal ulceration and Parkinson's disease. Med J Aust 1965;310:842–3.

28. Reusche E, Pilz P, Oberascher G, Lindner B, Egensperger R, Gloeckner K, Trinka E, Iglseder B. Subacute fatal aluminum encephalopathy after reconstructive otoneurosurgery: a case report. Hum Pathol 2001; 32(10):1136–40.

29. Campbell A. The potential role of aluminium in Alzheimer's disease. Nephrol Dial Transplant 2002;17(Suppl 2):17–20.

30. Rondeau V. A review of epidemiologic studies on aluminum and silica in relation to Alzheimer's disease and associated disorders. Rev Environ Health 2002;17(2):107–21.

31. Martyn CN, Barker DJ, Osmond C, Harris EC, Edwardson JA, Lacey RF. Geographical relation between Alzheimer's disease and aluminum in drinking water. Lancet 1989;1(8629):59–62.

32. Kawachi I, Pearce N. Aluminium in the drinking water—is it safe? Aust J Public Health 1991;15(2):84–7.

33. Exley C. A molecular mechanism of aluminium-induced Alzheimer's disease? J Inorg Biochem 1999;76(2):133–40.

34. Sjogren B, Ljunggren KG, Basun H, Frech W, Nennesmo I. Reappraisal of aluminosis and dementia. Lancet 1999;354(9189):1559.

35. Yokel RA, Allen DD, Ackley DC. The distribution of aluminum into and out of the brain. J Inorg Biochem 1999;76(2):127–32.

36. Rogers MA, Simon DG. A preliminary study of dietary aluminium intake and risk of Alzheimer's disease. Age Ageing 1999;28(2):205–9.

37. Gauthier E, Fortier I, Courchesne F, Pepin P, Mortimer J, Gauvreau D. Aluminum forms in drinking water and risk of Alzheimer's disease. Environ Res 2000;84(3):234–46.

38. Munoz DG, Feldman H. Causes of Alzheimer's disease. CMAJ 2000;162(1):65–72.

39. Linebarger EJ, Kikkawa DO, Floyd B, Granet D, Booth M. Conjunctival aluminum deposition following pneumatic cryopexy. Arch Ophthalmol 1999;117(5):692–3.

40. Foldes J, Balena R, Ho A, Parfitt AM, Kleerekoper M. Hypophosphatemic rickets with hypocalciuria following long-term treatment with aluminum-containing antacid. Bone 1991;12(2):67–71.

41. Spencer H, Kramer L. Antacid-induced calcium loss. Arch Intern Med 1983;143(4):657–9.

42. Goodman WG. Bone disease and aluminum: pathogenic considerations. Am J Kidney Dis 1985;6(5):330–5.

43. Moriniere P, Cohen-Solal M, Belbrik S, Boudailliez B, Marie A, Westeel PF, Renaud H, Fievet P, Lalau JD, Sebert JL, et al. Disappearance of aluminic bone disease in a long term asymptomatic dialysis population restricting Al(OH)$_3$ intake: emergence of an idiopathic adynamic bone disease not related to aluminum. Nephron 1989;53(2):93–101.

44. van Kalmthout PM, Engels LG, Bakker HH, Burghouts JT. Severe copper deficiency due to excessive use of an antacid combined with pyloric stenosis. Dig Dis Sci 1982;27(9):859–61.

45. Shah NR, Oberkircher OR, Lobel JS. Aluminum-induced microcytosis in a child with moderate renal insufficiency. Am J Pediatr Hematol Oncol 1990;12(1):77–9.

46. Lin JL, Kou MT, Leu ML. Effect of long-term low-dose aluminum-containing agents on hemoglobin synthesis in patients with chronic renal insufficiency. Nephron 1996;74(1):33–8.

47. Adams PL, Rutsky EA, Rostand SG, Han SY. Lower gastrointestinal tract dysfunction in patients receiving long-term hemodialysis. Arch Intern Med 1982;142(2):303–6.

48. Salmon R, Aubert P, David R, Guedon J. Peritonite stercorale. Complication rare du traitement par les gels d'alumine chez les insuffisants renaux en dialyse chronique. [Stercoral peritonitis. Unusual complication of treatment by aluminum gels in patients with renal insufficiency under long-term hemodialysis.] Med Chir Dig 1979;8(4):329–31.

49. Meining A, Bosseckert H, Caspary WF, Nauert C, Stolte M. H2-receptor antagonists and antacids have an aggravating effect on *Helicobacter pylori* gastritis in duodenal ulcer patients. Aliment Pharmacol Ther 1997;11(4):729–34.

50. Yasui M, Kohmoto J, Ota K, Shinmen K, Tanaka H, Nogami H. [A case of neurologic type of Wilson's disease with increased aluminum in liver: comparative study with histological findings to metal contents in the liver.] No To Shinkei 1998;50(8):767–72.

51. Klein GL, Heyman MB, Lee TC, Miller NL, Marathe G, Gourley WK, Alfrey AC. Aluminum-associated hepatobiliary dysfunction in rats: relationships to dosage and duration of exposure. Pediatr Res 1988;23(3):275–8.

52. Praveen BV, Sankaranarayanan A, Vaidyanathan S. A comparative study of intravesical instillation of 15(s) 15-methyl PGF2-alpha and alum in the management of persistent hematuria of vesical origin. Int J Clin Pharmacol Ther Toxicol 1992;30(1):7–12.

53. Culora GA, Ramsay AD, Theaker JM. Aluminium and injection site reactions. J Clin Pathol 1996;49(10):844–7.

54. Bajaj AK, Gupta SC, Pandey RK, Misra K, Rastogi S, Chatterji AK. Aluminium contact sensitivity. Contact Dermatitis 1997;37(6):307–8.

55. Helgesen AL, Austad J. Contact urticaria from aluminium and nickel in the same patient. Contact Dermatitis 1997;37(6):303–4.

56. Nagore E, Martinez-Escribano JA, Tato A, Sabater V, Vilata JJ. Subcutaneous nodules following treatment with aluminium-containing allergen extracts. Eur J Dermatol 2001;11(2):138–40.

57. Mooser G, Gall H, Weber L, Peter RU. Cold panniculitis—an unusual differential diagnosis from aluminium allergy in a patient hyposensitized with aluminium-precipitated antigen extract. Contact Dermatitis 2001;44(6):368.

58. Skowron F, Grezard P, Berard F, Balme B, Perrot H. Persistent nodules at sites of hepatitis B vaccination due to aluminium sensitization. Contact Dermatitis 1998; 39(3):135–6.

59. Lacson AG, D'Cruz CA, Gilbert-Barness E, Sharer L, Jacinto S, Cuenca R. Aluminum phagocytosis in quadriceps muscle following vaccination in children: relationship to macrophagic myofasciitis. Pediatr Dev Pathol 2002;5(2):151–8.

60. Woodson GC. An interesting case of osteomalacia due to antacid use associated with stainable bone aluminum in a patient with normal renal function. Bone 1998;22(6):695–8.

61. Neumann L, Jensen BG. Osteomalacia from Al and Mg antacids. Report of a case of bilateral hip fracture. Acta Orthop Scand 1989;60(3):361–2.

62. Nicholas JC, Dawes PT, Davies SJ, Freemont AJ. Persisting aluminium-related bone disease after cadaveric renal transplantation. Nephrol Dial Transplant 1999;14(1):202–4.

63. Sulkova S, Valek A. Aluminium elimination in patients receiving regular dialysis treatment for chronic renal failure. Trace Elem Med 1991;8(Suppl 1):26–30.

64. Winterberg B, Korte R, Lison AE. Clinical impact of aluminium load in kidney transplant recipients. Trace Elem Med 1991;8(Suppl 1):46–8.

65. Sjolander A, Cox JC, Barr IG. ISCOMs: an adjuvant with multiple functions. J Leukoc Biol 1998;64(6):713–23.

66. Murphy CP, Cox RL, Harden EA, Stevens DA, Heye MM, Herzig RH. Encephalopathy and seizures induced by intravesical alum irrigations. Bone Marrow Transplant 1992;10(4):383–5.

67. Bakir AA, Hryhorczuk DO, Ahmed S, Hessl SM, Levy PS, Spengler R, Dunea G. Hyperaluminemia in renal failure: the influence of age and citrate intake. Clin Nephrol 1989;31(1):40–4.

68. Hewitt CD, Poole CL, Westervelt FB Jr, Savory J, Wills MR. Risks of simultaneous therapy with oral aluminium and citrate compounds. Lancet 1988;2(8615):849.

69. Freunlich M. The spectrum of aluminium toxicity in pediatrics. Int J Pediatr 1988;3:41.

70. Pivnick EK, Kerr NC, Kaufman RA, Jones DP, Chesney RW. Rickets secondary to phosphate depletion. A sequela of antacid use in infancy. Clin Pediatr (Phila) 1995;34(2):73–8.

71. Kirschbaum BB, Schoolwerth AC. Hyperaluminaemia associated with oral citrate and aluminium hydroxide. Hum Toxicol 1989;8(1):45–7.

72. Moreno A, Dominguez P, Dominguez C, Ballabriga A. High serum aluminium levels and acute reversible encephalopathy in a 4-year-old boy with acute renal failure. Eur J Pediatr 1991;150(7):513–14.

73. Sherrard DJ. Aluminum—much ado about something. N Engl J Med 1991;324(8):558–9.

74. Phelps KR, Naylor K, Brien TP, Wilbur H, Haqqie SS. Encephalopathy after bladder irrigation with alum: case report and literature review. Am J Med Sci 1999;318(3):181–5.

75. Friga V, Linos A, Linos DA. Is aluminum toxicity responsible for uremic pruritus in chronic hemodialysis patients? Nephron 1997;75(1):48–53.

76. Andress DL, Maloney NA, Coburn JW, Endres DB, Sherrard DJ. Osteomalacia and aplastic bone disease in aluminum-related osteodystrophy. J Clin Endocrinol Metab 1987;65(1):11–16.

77. Netter P, Kessler M, Burnel D, Hutin MF, Delones S, Benoit J, Gaucher A. Aluminum in the joint tissues of chronic renal failure patients treated with regular hemodialysis and aluminum compounds. J Rheumatol 1984;11(1):66–70.

78. Bia MJ, Cooper K, Schnall S, Duffy T, Hendler E, Malluche H, Solomon L. Aluminum induced anemia: pathogenesis and treatment in patients on chronic hemodialysis. Kidney Int 1989;36(5):852–8.

79. Alfrey AC, Mishell JM, Burks J, Contiguglia SR, Rudolph H, Lewin E, Holmes JH. Syndrome of dyspraxia and multifocal seizures associated with chronic hemodialysis. Trans Am Soc Artif Intern Organs 1972;18:257–61,266–7.

80. Gonzalez-Revalderia J, Casares M, de Paula M, Pascual T, Giner V, Miravalles E. Biochemical and hematological changes in low-level aluminum intoxication. Clin Chem Lab Med 2000;38(3):221–5.

81. Rottembourg J, Jaudon MC, Legrain M, Galli A. Les gels d'alumine chez les insuffisants rénaux chroniques. [Aluminum gels in chronic kidney failure patients. A potential risk of encephalopathy and osteopathy.] Ann Med Interne (Paris) 1980;131(2):71–4.

82. Sideman S, Manor D. The dialysis dementia syndrome and aluminum intoxication. Nephron 1982;31(1):1–10.

83. Arieff AI. Aluminum and the pathogenesis of dialysis encephalopathy. Am J Kidney Dis 1985;6(5):317–21.

84. Singh S, Singh D, Wig N, Jit I, Sharma BK. Aluminum phosphide ingestion—a clinico-pathologic study. J Toxicol Clin Toxicol 1996;34(6):703–6.

85. Andersen TS, Holm JW, Andersen TS. Forgiftning med muldvarpegasningsmidlet aluminiumfosfid. [Poisoning with aluminum phospholipide used as a poison against moles.] Ugeskr Laeger 1996;158(38):5308–9.

86. Dorhout Mees EJ, Basci A. Citric acid in calcium effervescent tablets may favour aluminium intoxication. Nephron 1991;59(2):322.

87. Main J, Ward MK. Potentiation of aluminium absorption by effervescent analgesic tablets in a haemodialysis patient. BMJ 1992;304(6843):1686.

88. Domingo JL, Gomez M, Llobet JM, Richart C. Effect of ascorbic acid on gastrointestinal aluminium absorption. Lancet 1991;338(8780):1467.

89. Campistol JM, Cases A, Botey A, Revert A. Acute aluminum encephalopathy in an uremic patient. Nephron 1989;51(1):103–6.

90. Ellenberg R, King AL, Sica DA, Posner M, Savory J. Cerebrospinal fluid aluminum levels following deferoxamine. Am J Kidney Dis 1990;16(2):157–9.

91. Warady BA, Ford DM, Gaston CE, Sedman AB, Huffer WE, Lum GM. Aluminum intoxication in a child: treatment with intraperitoneal desferrioxamine. Pediatrics 1986;78(4):651–5.

92. Verbeeck R, Tjandramaga TB, Mullie A, Verbesselt R, de Schepper PJ. Effect of aluminum hydroxide on diflunisal absorption. Br J Clin Pharmacol 1979;7(5):519–22.

93. Uribe M, Casian C, Rojas S, Sierra JG, Go VL. Decreased bioavailability of prednisone due to antacids in patients with chronic active liver disease and in healthy volunteers. Gastroenterology 1981;80(4):661–5.

94. Parry R, Plowman D, Delves HT, Roberts NB, Birchall JD, Bellia JP, Davenport A, Ahmad R, Fahal I, Altmann P. Silicon and aluminium interactions in haemodialysis patients. Nephrol Dial Transplant 1998;13(7):1759–62.

95. Gugler R, Allgayer H. Effects of antacids on the clinical pharmacokinetics of drugs. An update. Clin Pharmacokinet 1990;18(3):210–19.

Amantadine

General Information

Amantadine is a symmetrical C10 tricyclic amine with an unusual structure (1-adamantanamine hydrochloride). It interferes with virus uncoating (1) by blocking the M2 ion channel, which is needed to affect a pH change that helps to initiate the uncoating process. Most consistent antiviral activity has been observed against influenza A virus, but amantadine has little or no activity against influenza B virus (2). However, influenza A virus can become rapidly resistant to amantadine in vitro (3). Amantadine also promotes the release of dopamine from nerve endings, but may also delay its reuptake into synaptic vesicles.

Doses of 100–200 mg/day are often used and are usually well tolerated. The best-documented adverse reactions are nausea, psychotic episodes (mania, hallucinations, agitation, confusion), restless legs, and convulsions. Minor adverse reactions often resemble those caused by anticholinergic agents, for example blurred vision, dryness of the mouth, insomnia, lethargy, and rash. In rare cases, photosensitization has been described. Oral or aerosol administration can be accompanied by gastrointestinal or minor neurological symptoms, such as insomnia, light-headedness, concentration difficulties, nervousness, dizziness, and headache in individuals taking 200 mg/day (4). These symptoms disappear on withdrawal. More severe but rare complications include convulsions and coma (5,6). Local nasal adverse effects of the aerosolized form can mimic the symptoms of upper respiratory tract infection. In Parkinson's disease, in which doses of 200 mg/day or more have been used, minor adverse effects resembling those caused by anticholinergic agents (for example blurred vision, dry mouth, as well as livedo reticularis, rash, and photosensitization, can occur (SED-13, 874) (7,8).

Organs and Systems

Cardiovascular

Reversible congestive cardiac failure has been attributed to amantadine (9).

Nervous system

Insomnia is common with amantadine (10).
Myoclonus, especially vocal, can occur (11).

- A 48-year-old woman with a 17-year history of Parkinson's disease developed a sensorimotor peripheral neuropathy after taking amantadine 300 mg/day for 8 years (12). She had livedo reticularis after only 1 year of treatment and this had become increasingly extensive. Attempts to withdraw the drug resulted in worsening Parkinsonian symptoms. However, after the neuropathy had been diagnosed, amantadine was withdrawn, with improvement of the neurological symptoms within 6 weeks and complete resolution after 6 months. However, the livedo reticularis was still present 18 months after withdrawal.

This is the first description of peripheral neuropathy in these circumstances, but it suggests that chronic livedo reticularis may be a forerunner of more severe problems.

Three Japanese women aged 78–87 years who had taken amantadine 100–200 mg/day for 1 month to 5 years, in two cases together with co-careldopa, developed multifocal myoclonus and two were confused (13). Amantadine concentrations were high in the two patients in whom they were measured, at over 3000 ng/ml; a concentration over 1000 ng/ml is regarded as toxic. Amantadine was withdrawn and the myoclonus disappeared within 1–2 weeks and did not recur. Cortical myoclonus has also been described with levodopa and bromocriptine, but the mechanism is not known.

Sensory systems

Rarely, amantadine causes visual impairment due to corneal abrasions, local edema, and superficial keratitis (14).

Psychological, psychiatric

The risk of mental complications seems to increase substantially if doses of 200 mg or more are given (15). Amantadine can cause mania and is contraindicated in patients with bipolar affective disorder (16).

- While taking amantadine, an elderly man developed the Othello syndrome, a severe delusion of marital infidelity, as described in Shakespeare's plays *Othello* and *A Winter's Tale*; it abated with drug withdrawal (SEDA-17, 170).
- Amantadine and phenylpropanolamine may have caused intense recurrent déjà vu experiences in a healthy 39-year-old within 24 hours of starting both drugs for influenza (17).

Fluid balance

Resistant edema of the ankles in the absence of cardiac disease has repeatedly been described and well documented by rechallenge (18).

Skin

Livedo reticularis has been stated to occur in as many as 90% of patients; it is very common in female patients especially those with antiphospholipid antibodies (19).

Long-Term Effects

Drug withdrawal

On withdrawal of amantadine after long-term therapy, acute delirium with confusion, disorientation, agitation, and paranoia occurred in three patients (20). Reintroduction of the drug returned the patients to the baseline status.

In four patients, amantadine withdrawal was associated with delirium and confusion (21). The patients, three of them women, were aged 70–83 years and all but one were considered to have early dementia. Amantadine exposure was 1–5 years and the symptoms occurred within a week of drug withdrawal. In all cases they were reversed by reintroduction. The mechanism of the withdrawal reaction is unknown, but it should obviously be borne in mind, especially in elderly patients with long exposure to the drug and with already impaired cognitive function.

Neuroleptic malignant syndrome can occur on withdrawal of amantadine (22,23).

Susceptibility Factors

Renal disease

In a case of end-stage renal insufficiency, amantadine caused coma, though drug plasma concentrations were not greatly increased (SEDA-18, 160).

References

1. Bukrinskaya AG, Vorkunova NK, Narmanbetova RA. Rimantadine hydrochloride blocks the second step of influenza virus uncoating. Arch Virol 1980;66(3):275–82.

2. Oxford JS, Galbraith A. Antiviral activity of amantadine: a review of laboratory and clinical data. Pharmacol Ther 1980;11(1):181–262.

3. Heider H, Adamczyk B, Presber HW, Schroeder C, Feldblum R, Indulen MK. Occurrence of amantadine- and rimantadine-resistant influenza A virus strains during the 1980 epidemic. Acta Virol 1981;25(6):395–400.

4. Van Voris LP, Newell PM. Antivirals for the chemoprophylaxis and treatment of influenza. Semin Respir Infect 1992;7(1):61–70.

5. Bryson YJ, Monahan C, Pollack M, Shields WD. A prospective double-blind study of side effects associated with the administration of amantadine for influenza A virus prophylaxis. J Infect Dis 1980;141(5):543–7.

6. Ing TS, Daugirdas JT, Soung LS, Klawans HL, Mahurkar SD, Hayashi JA, Geis WP, Hano JE. Toxic effects of amantadine in patients with renal failure. Can Med Assoc J 1979;120(6):695–8.

7. Silver DE, Sahs AL. Livedo reticularis in Parkinson's disease patients treated with amantadine hydrochloride. Neurology 1972;22(7):665–9.

8. van den Berg WH, van Ketel WG. Photosensitization by amantadine (Symmetrel). Contact Dermatitis 1983;9(2):165.

9. Vale JA, Maclean KS. Amantadine-induced heart-failure. Lancet 1977;1(8010):548.

10. Huete B, Varona L. Insomnio durante el tratamiento con amantadina. [Insomnia during treatment with amantadine.] Rev Neurol 1997;25(148):2062.

11. Pfeiffer RF. Amantadine-induced "vocal" myoclonus. Mov Disord 1996;11(1):104–6.

12. Shulman LM, Minagar A, Sharma K, Weiner WJ. Amantadine-induced peripheral neuropathy. Neurology 1999;53(8):1862–5.

13. Matsunaga K, Uozumi T, Qingrui L, Hashimoto T, Tsuji S. Amantadine-induced cortical myoclonus. Neurology 2001;56(2):279–80.

14. Nogaki H, Morimatsu M. Superficial punctate keratitis and corneal abrasion due to amantadine hydrochloride. J Neurol 1993;240(6):388–9.

15. Hunter KR. Treatment of parkinsonsim. Prescr J 1976;16:101.

16. Rego MD, Giller EL Jr. Mania secondary to amantadine treatment of neuroleptic-induced hyperprolactinemia. J Clin Psychiatry 1989;50(4):143–4.

17. Taiminen T, Jaaskelainen SK. Intense and recurrent deja vu experiences related to amantadine and phenylpropanolamine in a healthy male. J Clin Neurosci 2001;8(5):460–2.

18. New Approvals/Indications. Pediatric indications for metaproterenol. Drug Ther 1992;Feb 22 and 38.

19. Paulson GW, Brandt JT. Amantadine, livedo reticularis, and antiphospholipid antibodies. Clin Neuropharmacol 1995;18(5):466–7.

20. Factor SA, Molho ES, Brown DL. Acute delirium after withdrawal of amantadine in Parkinson's disease. Neurology 1998;50(5):1456–8.

21. Sommer BR, Wise LC, Kraemer HC. Is dopamine administration possibly a risk factor for delirium? Crit Care Med 2002;30(7):1508–11.

22. Ito T, Shibata K, Watanabe A, Akabane J. Neuroleptic malignant syndrome following withdrawal of amantadine in a patient with influenza A encephalopathy. Eur J Pediatr 2001;160(6):401.

23. Simpson DM, Davis GC. Case report of neuroleptic malignant syndrome associated with withdrawal from amantadine. Am J Psychiatry 1984;141(6):796–7.

Amaranthaceae

See also Herbal medicines

General Information

The genera in the family of Amaranthaceae (Table 1) include cotton flower and rockwort.

Pfaffia paniculata and ginseng

Ginseng is an ambiguous vernacular term that can refer to *Panax* species such as *Panax ginseng* (Asian ginseng) and *Panax quinquefolius* (American ginseng), *Eleutherococcus senticosus* (Siberian ginseng), and *Pfaffia paniculata* (Brazilian ginseng). See ginseng in the monograph on Araliaceae.

Adverse effects
Respiratory

Asthma occurred in a patient who had been exposed to *Pfaffia paniculata* root powder used in the manufacturing of Brazil ginseng capsules (1). Airway hyper-reactivity was confirmed by a positive bronchial challenge to methacholine and sensitivity to the dust was confirmed by immediate skin test reactivity, a positive bronchial challenge (immediate response), and the presence of a specific IgE to an aqueous extract detected by ELISA. The bronchial response was inhibited by sodium cromoglicate. Unexposed subjects did not react to this ginseng extract with any of the tests referred to above. The same study performed with Korean ginseng (*Panax ginseng*) was negative.

Table 1 The genera of Amaranthaceae

Achyranthes (chaff flower)
Aerva (aerva)
Alternanthera (joyweed)
Amaranthus (pigweed)
Blutaparon (blutaparon)
Celosia (cock's comb)
Chamissoa (chamissoa)
Charpentiera (papala)
Cyathula (cyathula)
Froelichia (snake cotton)
Gomphrena (globe amaranth)
Gossypianthus (cotton flower)
Guilleminea (matweed)
Hermbstaedtia (hermbstaedtia)
Iresine (bloodleaf)
Lithophila (lithophila)
Nototrichium (rockwort)
Pfaffia (pfaffia)
Philoxerus (philoxerus)
Tidestromia (honeysweet)

Reference

1. Subiza J, Subiza JL, Escribano PM, Hinojosa M, Garcia R, Jerez M, Subiza E. Occupational asthma caused by Brazil ginseng dust. J Allergy Clin Immunol 1991;88(5):731–6.

Amfebutamone (bupropion)

See also Antidepressants, second-generation

General Information

Amfebutamone is an amphetamine-like drug. It is structurally and pharmacologically distinct from other antidepressants, and apparently enhances both dopamine and noradrenaline function in the brain (SEDA-8, 18) (SEDA-10, 20).

Amfebutamone is used to encourage smoking cessation and in some countries as an antidepressant. In some respects its adverse effects profile is similar to that of the SSRIs: insomnia, agitation, tremor, and nausea are most often reported.

Randomized controlled trials have shown that amfebutamone is less likely to cause sexual dysfunction than SSRIs (1,2), unlike SSRIs, which gives it an important advantage in some patients.

Amfebutamone has been used as an antidepressant for many years in the USA and Canada and is now licensed in Europe for smoking cessation. There has been concern about the number of serious adverse reactions associated with amfebutamone, with particular emphasis on the risk of seizures. Deaths have also been reported from myocarditis and liver failure (3). A problem in determining the role of amfebutamone in these adverse effects is that it is prescribed for heavy smokers who are at risk of serious co-morbid disorders, particularly cardiovascular and respiratory disease. However, it has been clear for some time that the use of amfebutamone is associated with an increased risk of seizures, though this is less with the modified-release formulation (SEDA-23, 20).

Organs and Systems

Cardiovascular

The UK Committee on Safety of Medicines has received over 200 reports of chest pain in patients taking amfebutamone, and a case of myocardial infarction has been reported.

- A 43-year-old man who had smoked up to 20 cigarettes daily for several years and had a family history of heart disease was given amfebutamone and stopped smoking after reaching the recommended dose (300 mg/day) (4). Three days later he developed central chest and arm pain and 1 day later stopped taking amfebutamone. Three days after this he developed classical symptoms of acute inferoposterolateral myocardial infarction. He was treated with thrombolytic therapy and discharged taking secondary prevention therapy.

It is difficult to know how far amfebutamone might have contributed to this acute cardiac event. However, continuing vigilance and case-control studies are warranted.

Nervous system

The main concern with the use of amfebutamone is that in higher dosages it is associated with a risk of seizures (0.4%). Early in 1986, advertising began to appear in advance of the expected release of amfebutamone in the USA. Abruptly, in March, distribution was halted because of reports of seizures in patients with bulimia. Although the risk is greater than that seen with SSRIs (about 0.1%), data have suggested that amfebutamone has approximately the same seizure potential as the tricyclic compounds (SEDA-8, 30). However, a higher seizure risk for amfebutamone than for tricyclic antidepressants has been reported in patients taking amfebutamone in doses over 450 mg/day (SEDA 17, 21). Furthermore, the manufacturers have noted an increased risk of seizures in patients taking over 600 mg/day in combination with lithium or antipsychotic drugs (SEDA-10, 20).

Of 279 patients who presented to a hospital emergency service between 1994 and 1998 with a first tonic-clonic seizure, 17 (6.1%) had seizures that were thought to be drug-related (5). The most common drug-induced causes were cocaine intoxication (6/17) and benzodiazepine withdrawal (5/17) followed by amfebutamone use (4/17). While one amfebutamone-associated seizure occurred in a 26-year-old woman without any other risk factors, the three other patients (all women) had additional risk factors, such as concomitant treatment with antidepressants that also lower seizure threshold and a history of bulimia nervosa. These results suggest that amfebutamone is not an infrequent cause of de novo seizures. However, because of the time frame of the study, many of the patients would have been taking standard-release amfebutamone. It would be of interest to repeat the study now that modified-release amfebutamone is available.

Amfebutamone lowers the seizure threshold and can cause paresthesia (6).

- A 38-year-old woman who was taking olanzapine 10 mg/day and lamotrigine 200 mg/day for a schizoaffective disorder started to take amfebutamone for a depressive mood swing. After 4 weeks the dose of amfebutamone was increased to 300 mg/day, at which point she complained of a twitching pain on the left side of her face. There was hypesthesia of two branches of the left trigeminal nerve, the ophthalmic and maxillary branches, and a reduced left corneal reflex. The amfebutamone was withdrawn and the neurological signs and symptoms disappeared within 8 days. Four weeks later, because of persisting depression, the amfebutamone was reintroduced; at a dosage of 300 mg/day identical neurological symptoms recurred.

The reason for this unusual reaction is not clear. Amfebutamone may potentiate dopamine neurotransmission, and dopamine D_2 receptors modulate trigeminal nerve function (7).

Amfebutamone has been reported to mimic transient ischemic attacks (8).

- A 67-year-old man with a strong history of ischemic heart disease, who had been smoking 20 cigarettes a day for many years, started to take amfebutamone (100 mg tds) as an aid to smoking cessation. One week later he had episodes of disorientation, a tingling sensation over his body, and roaring sounds in his ears. MRI scanning and angiography showed evidence of previous strokes. His current episodes were ascribed to transient ischemic attacks. He had stopped taking amfebutamone while in hospital and then restarted it 2 days after discharge, when the same symptoms recurred. He then stopped taking amfebutamone completely and over the next 9 months had no further neurological episodes.

It is possible that these symptoms were entirely due to amfebutamone, but more probably the amfebutamone interacted in some way with the patient's established cerebrovascular disease.

Acute dystonia is a recognized complication of treatment with antipsychotic drugs and it can also occur with SSRIs and the anxiolytic drug buspirone.

- A 44-year-old man took amfebutamone 300 mg/day and buspirone 45 mg/day for depression (9). Over 2–3 weeks he developed increasing neck stiffness, with tightening and spasm of the jaw muscles and pain in the left temporomandibular joint. He stopped taking his medications, and all his symptoms resolved over the next 3 weeks. Rechallenge with buspirone (45 mg/day) failed to reproduce the dystonic symptoms. The buspirone was withdrawn and amfebutamone 150 mg/day was started; the dystonic symptoms did not recur. However, 24 hours after the dose of amfebutamone was increased to 300 mg/day there was a return of neck stiffness and jaw spasm.

Amfebutamone has dopaminergic properties, which seem to have played a part in this dystonia. Whether the effect was initiated by concomitant buspirone therapy is unclear, but subsequently amfebutamone alone was sufficient to produce the dystonic symptoms.

Cases of visual hallucinations and tinnitus have been reported in patients taking amfebutamone (SEDA-17, 21).

Psychological, psychiatric

Amfebutamone potentiates dopamine neurotransmission and at higher doses can cause toxic delirium and psychosis, particularly in patients with a history of psychosis and those taking other dopaminergic medications (SEDA-8, 31).

- A 79-year-old man developed a paranoid psychosis with auditory hallucinations during treatment with amfebutamone (100 mg tds) (10). The symptoms remitted with reduction of the dose of amfebutamone and the introduction of haloperidol 5 mg/day.

Paranoid ideas and hallucinations can occur during the course of a severe depressive episode, but in this case the patient's mood was gradually improving, so a link with amfebutamone seems more likely. It seems prudent to dose amfebutamone conservatively in elderly patients.

In an open trial, two of 16 patients became psychotic and were withdrawn from the study (11). A more detailed report of this adverse effect described four of 13 patients who became psychotic during a trial of amfebutamone; three had a history of psychosis, but none had previously had this response to other antidepressants (12). The usual dosage range of amfebutamone is 300–750 mg/day, and the psychotic symptoms occurred at dosages of 300–500 mg/day. In two cases psychotic symptoms were absent at lower dosages, but in one case the dose was therapeutically inadequate.

Other reports of psychotic reactions and a manic syndrome associated with amfebutamone have appeared (SEDA-16, 10) (SEDA-17, 21). In two of these cases a possible drug interaction with fluoxetine, with inhibition of the metabolism of amfebutamone, could not be excluded.

Hematologic

Eosinophilia reportedly developed in a 72-year-old woman shortly after she was given amfebutamone. The eosinophil count fell rapidly after all medications (including glibenclamide and tolmetin) were withdrawn (13).

Skin

Adverse skin reactions, such as rash, urticaria, and pruritus, have been reported in 1–4% of patients taking amfebutamone (14).

Immunologic

Two cases of serum sickness-like reactions have been reported in association with amfebutamone when used as an aid to smoking cessation (15,16). Both patients developed localized swellings of the fingers and hands, urticaria, and arthralgia. In both cases treatment with antihistamines and corticosteroids produced rapid relief of symptoms.

In three other patients (two women, one man) a serum sickness-like reaction developed 6–21 days after the start of amfebutamone treatment (14). The symptoms, arthralgia, pruritus, and tongue swelling, abated within 2 weeks of treatment with oral corticosteroids. Serum sickness reactions to drugs are rare, and it will be important to find out whether amfebutamone carries an increased risk of this unusual reaction.

Death

Amfebutamone has been linked to 41 deaths (17). From the reports of suspected adverse events received by the Netherlands Pharmacovigilance Foundation, it appears that more than half concerned patients at risk of smoking-related diseases. In 15 cases there had been simultaneous use of amfebutamone with another antidepressant (10 patients), theophylline (1 patient), or insulin (4 patients). These combinations may lead to an increase in the risk of seizures. Furthermore, two patients reported having taken antiepileptic drugs, despite the fact that amfebutamone is contraindicated in patients with seizure disorders. These results suggest that the guidelines described in the product information are not being adhered to in some cases.

Drug Administration

Drug formulations

A modified-release formulation of amfebutamone has been marketed (18). There are insufficient data yet on the risk of seizures with higher doses of the modified-release formulation, but preliminary indications suggest that it is likely to be lower than that seen with the immediate-release formulation (18).

Drug overdose

Seizure is a significant risk in amfebutamone overdose.

- An 18-year-old man attempted suicide by taking amfebutamone 7.5 g (50×150 mg tablets) (19). On assessment 90 minutes later he was agitated and aggressive, with a resting pulse of 160 beats/minute and a blood pressure of 142/63 mmHg. He quickly developed a persistently low blood pressure (65/40 mmHg), followed by three generalized tonic-clonic seizures, which were controlled by diazepam. He was ventilated and a metabolic acidosis was corrected with sodium bicarbonate. Despite this, his blood pressure remained persistently low (70/40 mmHg) with a sinus tachycardia (150 beats/minute). Dopamine was ineffective and adrenaline was required. After 24 hours he was extubated and made a full recovery over the next 3 days.
- A 14-year-old boy took 1.5–3.0 g of amfebutamone and had a persistent tachycardia, seizures, and brief agitation and aggression (20). He also had visual hallucinations, disorientation, and confusion but recovered about 24 hours after ingestion.

These cases show that overdose of amfebutamone can be serious.

Drug–Drug Interactions

SSRIs

Amfebutamone is sometimes used to augment the action of other antidepressant drugs, but there are few data on the pharmacokinetic effects of this strategy. In an open study in 19 consecutive patients (7 men and 12 women), amfebutamone (150 mg/day for 8 weeks) did not alter plasma concentrations of paroxetine or fluoxetine (21). Plasma concentrations of venlafaxine increased, but concentrations of its active metabolite, O-desmethylvenlafaxine, fell. Overall tolerability was good and there was a significant reduction in depression rating scales. Sexual function, particularly orgasmic function in women, improved. These data suggest that adding amfebutamone to SSRI treatment does not alter plasma concentrations of SSRIs. The addition of amfebutamone to venlafaxine seems unlikely to cause pharmacokinetic problems in practice, because the increase in plasma concentration of the parent compound was offset by a reduction in the concentration of its major active metabolite. However, there is scope for an interaction of venlafaxine with amfebutamone and the effects in individual patients might be hard to predict. This study also supports clinical suggestions that the addition of amfebutamone to SSRI treatment can enhance antidepressant efficacy and improve sexual function. However, controlled trials are needed to confirm this view.

References

1. Coleman CC, Cunningham LA, Foster VJ, Batey SR, Donahue RM, Houser TL, Ascher JA. Sexual dysfunction associated with the treatment of depression: a placebo-controlled comparison of bupropion sustained release and sertraline treatment Ann Clin Psychiatry 1999;11(4):205–15.
2. Croft H, Settle E, Jr. Houser T, Batey SR, Donahue RM, Ascher JA. A placebo-controlled comparison of the antidepressant efficacy and effects on sexual functioning of sustained-release bupropion and sertraline. Clin Ther 1999;21(4):643–58.
3. Wooltorton E. Bupropion (Zyban, Wellbutrin SR): reports of deaths, seizures, serum sickness. CMAJ 2002;166(1):68.
4. Patterson RN, Herity NA. Acute myocardial infarction following bupropion (Zyban). Q J Med 2002;95(1):58–9.
5. Pesola GR, Avasarala J. Bupropion seizure proportion among new-onset generalized seizures and drug related seizures presenting to an emergency department. J Emerg Med 2002;22(3):235–9.
6. Amann B, Hummel B, Rall-Autenrieth H, Walden J, Grunze H. Bupropion-induced isolated impairment of sensory trigeminal nerve function. Int Clin Psychopharmacol 2000;15(2):115–16.
7. Peterfreund RA, Kosofsky BE, Fink JS. Cellular localization of dopamine D2 receptor messenger RNA in the rat trigeminal ganglion. Anesth Analg 1995;81(6):1181–5.
8. Humma LM, Swims MP. Bupropion mimics a transient ischemic attack. Ann Pharmacother 1999;33(3):305–7.
9. Detweiler MB, Harpold GJ. Bupropion-induced acute dystonia. Ann Pharmacother 2002;36(2):251–4.
10. Howard WT, Warnock JK. Bupropion-induced psychosis. Am J Psychiatry 1999;156(12):2017–18.
11. Dufresne R, Becker R, Blitzer R, et al. Safety and efficacy of bupropion. Drug Dev Res 1985;6:39.
12. Golden RN, James SP, Sherer MA, Rudorfer MV, Sack DA, Potter WZ. Psychoses associated with bupropion treatment. Am J Psychiatry 1985;142(12):1459–62.
13. Malesker MA, Soori GS, Malone PM, Mahowald JA, Housel GJ. Eosinophilia associated with bupropion. Ann Pharmacother 1995;29(9):867–9.
14. McCollom RA, Elbe DH, Ritchie AH. Bupropion-induced serum sickness-like reaction. Ann Pharmacother 2000;34(4):471–3.
15. Peloso PM, Baillie C. Serum sickness-like reaction with bupropion. JAMA 1999;282(19):1817.
16. Tripathi A, Greenberger PA. Bupropion hydrochloride induced serum sickness-like reaction. Ann Allergy Asthma Immunol 1999;83(2):165–6.
17. Bhattacharjee C, Smith M, Todd F, Gillespie M. Bupropion overdose: a potential problem with the new "miracle" anti-smoking drug. Int J Clin Pract 2001;55(3):221–2.
18. Settle EC, Jr. Bupropion sustained release: side effect profile. J Clin Psychiatry 1998;59(Suppl 4):32–6.
19. Ayers S, Tobias JD. Bupropion overdose in an adolescent. Pediatr Emerg Care 2001;17(2):104–6.
20. Carvajal Garcia-Pando A, Garcia del Pozo J, Sanchez AS, Velasco MA, Rueda de Castro AM, Lucena MI. Hepatotoxicity associated with the new antidepressants. J Clin Psychiatry 2002;63(2):135–7.
21. Kennedy SH, McCann SM, Masellis M, McIntyre RS, Raskin J, McKay G, Baker GB. Combining bupropion SR with venlafaxine, paroxetine, or fluoxetine: a preliminary report on pharmacokinetic, therapeutic, and sexual dysfunction effects. J Clin Psychiatry 2002;63(3):181–6.

Amfepramone (diethylpropion)

See also Anorectic drugs

General Information

Reports on the frequency of adverse reactions to amfepramone are not entirely consistent. The number of adverse effects reported by patients taking amfepramone closely paralleled the number in those taking placebo in one study in 90 obese individuals. In another 16-week controlled study in 95 subjects who took amfepramone 25 mg tds, the main adverse effect was nervousness. In 121 obese patients who took a shorter-acting form for an average of 4.4 months, adverse effects occurred in under 9%. They were nausea, vertigo in two patients, and nervousness and palpitation in another two; treatment was discontinued in three cases because of nausea, insomnia, and paresthesia (1). With long-acting amfepramone in a double-blind 16-week crossover study in 102 Austrian patients, adverse effects included nervousness, tension, nausea, dizziness, light-headedness, and dry mouth [SED-9, 14]. The main unwanted effects in a double-blind trial of modified-release amfepramone (Tenuate Dospan) in 50 pregnant women were euphoria, sweating, irritability, and palpitation. Nervousness and insomnia were reported in another controlled study in 75 pregnant women [SEDA-8, 17]. In neither of the last two studies were the adverse reactions serious enough to justify withdrawal.

Organs and Systems

Nervous system

Altogether the effects of amfepramone on the central nervous system are much less common than those of dexamphetamine; for example, 78 patients who had to stop treatment with amphetamine and benzfetamine were able to continue therapy with amfepramone. Even insomnia is uncommon if the drug is taken early in the day.

Long-Term Effects

Drug dependence

There have been some reports of addiction and psychotic manifestations with amfepramone (2) but these are much less frequent than are those associated with amphetamine or phenmetrazole.

Drug–Drug Interactions

Diazepam

In a comparative study using a fixed combination of amfepramone 75 mg plus diazepam 10 mg the adverse effects were milder than those found with other anorexigenic drugs [SED-9, 14]. However, there were mild

adverse effects (dry mouth, nervousness, and depression) in about half of the patients.

References

1. Matthews PA. Diethylpropion in the treatment of obese patients seen in general practice. Curr Ther Res Clin Exp 1975;17(4):340–6.
2. Willis JHP. The natural history of anorectic drug abuse. In: Garattini S, Samanin R, editors. Central Mechanisms of Anorectic Drugs. New York: Raven Press, 1978:367.

Amikacin

See also Aminoglycoside antibiotics

General Information

Amikacin is a semisynthetic derivative of kanamycin with similar pharmacokinetic properties and dosages. It is resistant to many of the bacterial R factor-mediated enzymes that inactivate kanamycin and gentamicin. Noteworthy is its effect against *Pseudomonas aeruginosa* and against most Gram-negative aerobes that are resistant to gentamicin and tobramycin. There are strains of *Staphylococcus aureus* that inactivate amikacin by phosphorylation and adenylation. Ticarcillin or azlocillin plus amikacin is considered one of the most efficacious empiric antibiotic combinations in febrile granulocytopenia in patients with cancer. On a weight basis amikacin is less active than gentamicin, and so the usual dose is 10–20 mg/kg/day. Wherever possible, peak concentrations of 40 µg/ml and troughs of 10 µg/ml should not be exceeded during twice-daily dosing.

Organs and Systems

Respiratory

Amikacin may have been the causative agent in an apneic episode in an infant on peritoneal dialysis (1).

Sensory systems

- A 43-year-old man, who was receiving hemodialysis through a permanent catheter developed severe irreversible sensorineural hearing loss after using an amikacin–heparin lock for 16 weeks (2). He suddenly developed a high-frequency sensorineural hearing loss of 40 decibels. His condition progressed over 1 week, despite immediate withdrawal of the amikacin–heparin lock, and he developed severe irreversible hearing loss below 80 decibels for both high and low frequencies.

Retinal toxicity can occur when aminoglycosides are given intravitreally for endophthalmitis.

- Preretinal hemorrhages developed in a 58-year old man who was treated with two intravitreal injections of amikacin (0.4 mg) and cefazolin (2.25 mg) 48 hours apart for postoperative endophthalmitis following routine extracapsular cataract extraction (3).

- Macular toxicity followed the use of intravitreal amikacin 0.2 mg for postoperative endophthalmitis in a 69-year-old white woman (4).

Ototoxicity was observed in three of 195 patients who received amikacin (15 mg/kg/day) with either cefepime (2 g bd) or ceftazidime (2 g tds) (5). Two patients had severe loss of hearing, which persisted after drug withdrawal and resulted in permanent disability. The other had mild ototoxicity that required no action and resolved spontaneously.

Urinary tract

After administration of the recommended doses of amikacin for 10 days, renal damage probably occurs in less than 10% of cases. Limited data support the view that amikacin is less nephrotoxic than other aminoglycosides, possibly because of lower binding affinity to proximal tubular cells or reduced potential to cause phospholipidosis (SEDA-20, 236). In several prospective randomized studies the liability of amikacin to cause nephrotoxicity was no greater than that of gentamicin or tobramycin (6–8). In a prospective study there was significantly lower nephrotoxicity with amikacin 15 mg/kg/day (4% toxicity) compared with netilmicin 7 mg/kg/day (12%) (9). As with other aminoglycosides, renal toxicity is reversible in most cases (10).

Nephrotoxicity occurred in five of 195 patients who received amikacin (15 mg/kg/day) with either cefepime (2 g bd) or ceftazidime (2 g tds) (5). In two patients the deterioration in renal function was mild and resolved without withdrawal of amikacin. In the three other patients, renal insufficiency necessitated drug withdrawal; two of these patients recovered, but one died with sepsis, and renal function was still abnormal at the time of death.

Long-Term Effects

Drug tolerance

In Spain, an epidemic strain of *Acinetobacter baumannii* with resistance to amikacin was isolated in eight different hospitals (11).

Susceptibility Factors

In an open study in eight young healthy Japanese women, the pharmacokinetics of amikacin were affected by the phase of the menstrual cycle (12). In patients with hematological malignancies, bodyweight, renal function, acute myeloblastic leukemia, and hypoalbuminemia were the most important co-variates for the interindividual variability in amikacin pharmacokinetics (13).

Drug Administration

Drug formulations

The pharmacokinetics and toxicity of liposomal amikacin have been investigated in a patient treated for advanced pulmonary multidrug-resistant tuberculosis (14). The serum concentrations of amikacin obtained with the liposomal formulation were considerably greater than those obtained with the conventional formulation. Liposomal amikacin was well tolerated and led to clinical improvement, but the patient's sputum remained smear- and culture-positive during the treatment period and for 9 months.

Drug administration route

Amikacin has been tested for compatibility with a chlorhexidine-bearing central venous catheter, the ARROWg+ard Blue Plus, and did not cause a substantial increase in chlorhexidine delivery (15). The amount of amikacin sulfate that was delivered was slightly less than the amount in the infusion solution (92%), but this was considered acceptable.

Drug–Drug Interactions

Penicillins

Amikacin may be inactivated by penicillins. This inactivation occurs not only with a mixture of the agents in solution but also in vivo, particularly in patients with renal insufficiency. Amikacin offers, at least in vitro, the advantage of being much less inactivated than tobramycin or gentamicin (16).

References

1. Cano F, Morales M, Delucchi A. Amykacin-related apneic episode in an infant on peritoneal dialysis. Pediatr Nephrol 2000;14(4):357.
2. Saxena AK, Panhotra BR, Naguib M. Sudden irreversible sensory-neural hearing loss in a patient with diabetes receiving amikacin as an antibiotic–heparin lock. Pharmacotherapy 2002;22(1):105–8.
3. Kumar A, Dada T. Preretinal haemorrhages: an unusual manifestation of intravitreal amikacin toxicity. Aust NZ J Ophthalmol 1999;27(6):435–6.
4. Galloway G, Ramsay A, Jordan K, Vivian A. Macular infarction after intravitreal amikacin: mounting evidence against amikacin. Br J Ophthalmol 2002;86(3):359–60.
5. Erman M, Akova M, Akan H, Korten V, Ferhanoglu B, Koksal I, Cetinkaya Y, Uzun O, Unal S; Febrile Neutropenia Study Group of Turkey. Comparison of cefepime and ceftazidime in combination with amikacin in the empirical treatment of high-risk patients with febrile neutropenia: a prospective, randomized, multicenter study. Scand J Infect Dis 2001;33(11):827–31.
6. Plaut ME, Schentag JJ, Jusko WJ. Aminoglycoside nephrotoxicity: comparative assessment in critically ill patients. J Med 1979;10(4):257–66.
7. Smith CR, Baughman KL, Edwards CQ, Rogers JF, Lietman PS. Controlled comparison of amikacin and gentamicin. N Engl J Med 1977;296(7):349–53.
8. Feld R, Valdivieso M, Bodey GP, Rodriguez V. Comparison of amikacin and tobramycin in the treatment of infection in patients with cancer. J Infect Dis 1977;135(1):61–6.
9. Noone M, Pomeroy L, Sage R, Noone P. Prospective study of amikacin versus netilmicin in the treatment of severe infection in hospitalized patients. Am J Med 1989;86(6 Pt 2):809–13.

10. Lane AZ, Wright GE, Blair DC. Ototoxicity and nephrotoxicity of amikacin: an overview of phase II and phase III experience in the United States. Am J Med 1977;62(6):911–18.
11. Vila J, Ruiz J, Navia M, Becerril B, Garcia I, Perea S, Lopez-Hernandez I, Alamo I, Ballester F, Planes AM, Martinez-Beltran J, de Anta TJ. Spread of amikacin resistance in Acinetobacter baumannii strains isolated in Spain due to an epidemic strain. J Clin Microbiol 1999;37(3):758–61.
12. Matsuki S, Kotegawa T, Tsutsumi K, Nakamura K, Nakano S. Pharmacokinetic changes of theophylline and amikacin through the menstrual cycle in healthy women. J Clin Pharmacol 1999;39(12):1256–62.
13. Romano S, Fdez de Gatta MM, Calvo MV, Caballero D, Dominguez-Gil A, Lanao JM. Population pharmacokinetics of amikacin in patients with haematological malignancies. J Antimicrob Chemother 1999;44(2):235–42.
14. Whitehead TC, Lovering AM, Cropley IM, Wade P, Davidson RN. Kinetics and toxicity of liposomal and conventional amikacin in a patient with multidrug-resistant tuberculosis. Eur J Clin Microbiol Infect Dis 1998;17(11):794–7.
15. Xu QA, Zhang Y, Trissel LA, Gilbert DL. Adequacy of a new chlorhexidine-bearing polyurethane central venous catheter for administration of 82 selected parenteral drugs. Ann Pharmacother 2000;34(10):1109–16.
16. Meyer RD. Amikacin. Ann Intern Med 1981;95(3):328–32.

Amiloride

See also Diuretics

General Information

Amiloride is a potassium-sparing diuretic that acts in the distal convoluted tubule independently of the action of aldosterone, inhibiting sodium channels. It is a relatively safe drug with few reported adverse effects.

Patients with congenital nephrogenic diabetes insipidus are often treated with a combination of a thiazide and a potassium-sparing diuretic, without consensus on the preferred potassium-sparing diuretic. A Japanese adult was systematically studied to determine the renal effects of hydrochlorothiazide plus amiloride and hydrochlorothiazide plus triamterene (1). The combination with amiloride was superior to that with triamterene in preventing excessive urinary potassium loss, hypokalemia, and metabolic alkalosis. These results suggest that amiloride is the preferred add-on therapy to hydrochlorothiazide in nephrogenic diabetes insipidus.

Organs and Systems

Cardiovascular

An isolated report (2) suggests that amiloride may have prodysrhythmic potential in a small proportion of patients with inducible sustained ventricular tachycardia.

Electrolyte balance

Amiloride has a specific effect on sodium flux in the renal tubules; severe hyponatremia has been reported with the combination of a thiazide diuretic and amiloride.

As a potassium-sparing diuretic, amiloride can cause hyperkalemia (3), even in patients who are taking a potassium-wasting diuretic (4). This effect can be enhanced by concomitant therapy with ACE inhibitors or angiotensin-II receptor antagonists. In five patients with diabetes mellitus over 50 years of age who were taking an ACE inhibitor the serum potassium rose markedly 8–18 days after the addition of amiloride (5). All but one had some degree of renal impairment. In four cases potassium concentrations were between 9.4 and 11 mmol/l.

Skin

Rashes with diarrhea and eosinophilia have been reported (6).

Immunologic

Sweden's National Adverse Reaction Monitoring System called the attention of physicians to a case in which a 73-year-old woman developed anaphylactic shock after taking only a single tablet of Moduretic (7). The National System had received three other reports on anaphylactic reactions to this combination, and by 1988 the WHO center in Uppsala had received eight others from other countries. Except for mild skin reactions, hypersensitivity reactions to hydrochlorothiazide alone are highly unusual and not of this type.

Drug–Drug Interactions

ACE inhibitors

Co-administration of potassium-sparing diuretics with ACE inhibitors can cause severe hyperkalemia (SED-14, 674). In a retrospective study, five patients developed extreme hyperkalemia (9.4–11 mmol/l) within 8–18 days of starting combination therapy with co-amilozide (amiloride + hydrochlorothiazide) and an ACE inhibitor (5).

Amphotericin

Amiloride is a therapeutic option in reducing potassium losses in patients receiving amphotericin. When it was given to 19 oncology patients with marked amphotericin-induced potassium depletion mean serum potassium concentrations increased in the 5 days before and after administration (from 3.4 to 3.9 mmol/l) (8). There was also a trend toward reduced potassium supplementation (48 versus 29 mmol/day). Adverse reactions were limited to hyperkalemia in two patients who took amiloride 20 mg/day and a high potassium intake.

Carbenoxolone

Amiloride inhibits the ulcer-healing properties of carbenoxolone (9).

Lithium

Although amiloride may reduce the renal clearance of lithium, it appears to be free of the troublesome interaction with lithium that complicates the use of thiazides and loop diuretics.

Pentamidine

Pentamidine is structurally similar to amiloride and can cause severe hyperkalemia if co-prescribed with potassium-sparing diuretics (10). This is a particularly important interaction in patients with AIDS.

Trimethoprim

Trimethoprim (SED-14, 675) is structurally similar to amiloride and can cause severe hyperkalemia if co-prescribed with potassium-sparing diuretics (10). This is a particularly important interaction in patients with AIDS.

Interference with Diagnostic Tests

Creatinine clearance

Amiloride does not alter renal function (11), but it does block the tubular secretion of creatinine, leading to falsely high measurements of creatinine clearance; inulin clearance is not affected similarly (6).

References

1. Konoshita T, Kuroda M, Kawane T, Koni I, Miyamori I, Tofuku Y, Mabuchi H, Takeda R. Treatment of congenital nephrogenic diabetes insipidus with hydrochlorothiazide and amiloride in an adult patient. Horm Res 2004;61(2):63–7.
2. Duff HJ, Mitchell LB, Kavanagh KM, Manyari DE, Gillis AM, Wyse DG. Amiloride. Antiarrhythmic and electrophysiologic actions in patients with inducible sustained ventricular tachycardia. Circulation 1989;79(6):1257–63.
3. Maddox RW, Arnold WS, Dewell WM Jr. Extreme hyperkalemia associated with amiloride. South Med J 1985;78(3):365.
4. Jaffey L, Martin A. Malignant hyperkalaemia after amiloride/hydrochlorothiazide treatment. Lancet 1981;1(8232):1272.
5. Chiu TF, Bullard MJ, Chen JC, Liaw SJ, Ng CJ. Rapid life-threatening hyperkalemia after addition of amiloride HCl/hydrochlorothiazide to angiotensin-converting enzyme inhibitor therapy. Ann Emerg Med 1997;30(5):612–15.
6. Vidt DG. Mechanism of action, pharmacokinetics, adverse effects, and therapeutic uses of amiloride hydrochloride, a new potassium-sparing diuretic. Pharmacotherapy 1981;1(3):179–87.
7. Anonymous. Moduretic-anaphylactic shock. Uppsala: WHO Collaborating Centre for Adverse Drug Reaction Monitoring, Adv React Newslett 1988;(3–4).
8. Bearden DT, Muncey LA. The effect of amiloride on amphotericin B-induced hypokalaemia. J Antimicrob Chemother 2001;48(1):109–11.
9. Reed PI, Lewis SI, Vincent-Brown A, Holdstock DJ, Gribble RJ, Murgatroyd RE, Baron JH. The influence of amiloride on the therapeutic and metabolic effects of carbenoxolone in patients with gastric ulcer. A double-blind controlled trial. Scand J Gastroenterol Suppl 1980;65:51–7.
10. Perazella MA. Drug-induced hyperkalemia: old culprits and new offenders. Am J Med 2000;109(4):307–14.
11. Maronde RF, Milgrom M, Vlachakis ND, Chan L. Response of thiazide-induced hypokalemia to amiloride. JAMA 1983;249(2):237–41.

Amineptine

See also Tricyclic antidepressants

General Information

Amineptine is a tricyclic antidepressant that selectively reduces the dopamine reuptake without affecting the uptake of noradrenaline or serotonin (5-HT) (1). In vivo, it increases striatal homovanillic acid concentrations without affecting the concentrations of other metabolites of dopamine, 3,4,dihydroxyphenylacetic acid (DOPAC) and 3-methoxytyramine. However, high doses of amineptine reduced the extracellular DOPAC concentration in the nucleus accumbens but not in the striatum. Long-term treatment with amineptine causes down-regulation of beta-adrenoceptors.

Amineptine has a seven-membered carbon side-chain and is reported to have more stimulant and fewer sedative effects than other tricyclic compounds, possibly owing to differential actions on dopaminergic rather than serotonergic mechanisms. Amineptine appears to have an unusual propensity for causing hepatocellular damage, which may limit its clinical use (2).

Amineptine increases the release and reduces the re-uptake of dopamine, and it is therefore not surprising that an amphetamine-like drug dependence has been reported (3–5). A withdrawal syndrome occurs and can be improved by clonidine (SEDA-16, 8).

Organs and Systems

Liver

Of all the tricyclic antidepressants, amineptine appears to be the most likely to cause liver damage. More than 26 cases of toxic hepatitis have been reported in France (6). In most cases, hepatitis occurred within the usual dosage range and recurred on rechallenge. However, in several instances it was reported after overdosage. There are other reports of hepatotoxicity associated with amineptine (7,8).

Skin

Amineptine has been reported (9) to cause particularly active acne, occurring beyond the usual distribution on the body and beyond the usual age, especially in women. The remedy recommended is withdrawal of amineptine.

A rosacea-like eruption on the face of a 76-year-old woman was associated with amineptine; the association was confirmed by re-challenge (10).

Long-Term Effects

Drug dependence

Dependence on amineptine in a patient also taking midazolam has been reported (11).

References

1. Garattini S. Pharmacology of amineptine, an antidepressant agent acting on the dopaminergic system: a review. Int Clin Psychopharmacol 1997;12(Suppl 3):S15–19.
2. Lefebure B, Castot A, Danan G, Elmalem J, Jean-Pastor MJ, Efthymiou ML. Hépatites aux antidépresseurs. [Hepatitis from antidepressants. Evaluation of cases from French Assoc Drug Surveillance Centers Techn Committee.] Thérapie 1984;39(5):509–16.
3. Ginestet D, Cazas O, Branciard M. Deux cas de dependance à l'amineptine. [2 cases of amineptine dependence.] Encephale 1984;10(4):189–91.
4. Castot A, Benzaken C, Wagniart F, Efthymiou ML. Surconsommation d'amineptine. [Amineptin abuse. Analysis of 155 cases. An evaluation of the official cooperative survey of Regional Centers of Pharmacovigilance.] Therapie 1990;45(5):399–405.
5. Bertschy G, Luxembourger I, Bizouard P, Vandel S, Allers G, Volmat R. Dépendance à l'amineptine. [Amineptin dependence. Detection of patients at risk. Report 8 Cases.] Encephale 1990;16(5):405–9.
6. Andrieu J, Doll J, Coffinier C. Hépatitis due à l'amineptine: quatre observations. [Hepatitis due to amineptin. 4 Cases.] Gastroenterol Clin Biol 1982;6(11):915–18.
7. Lazaros GA, Stavrinos C, Papatheodoridis GV, Delladetsima JK, Toliopoulos A, Tassopoulos NC. Amineptine induced liver injury. Report of two cases and brief review of the literature. Hepatogastroenterology 1996;43(10):1015–19.
8. Lonardo A, Grisendi A, Mazzone E. One more case of hepatic injury due to amineptine. Ital J Gastroenterol Hepatol 1997;29(6):580–1.
9. Thioly-Bensoussan D, Charpentier A, Triller R, Thioly F, Blanchet P, Tricoire N, Noury JY, Grupper C. Acne iatrogène à l'amineptine (Survector): à propos de 8 cases. [Iatrogenic acne caused by amineptin (Survector). Report of 8 cases.] Ann Dermatol Venereol 1988;115(11):1177–80.
10. Jeanmougin M, Civatte J, Cavelier-Balloy B. Toxidermie rosacéiforme à l'amineptine (Survector). [Rosaceous Drug Eruption Caused by Amineptin (Survector).] Ann Dermatol Venereol 1988;115(11):1185–6.
11. Perera I, Lim L. Amineptine and midazolam dependence. Singapore Med J 1998;39(3):129–31.

Aminocaproic acid

General Information

During normal fibrinolysis, inactive circulating plasminogen binds to fibrin through an active site that binds lysine. The bound plasminogen is then converted to plasmin by activators (such as tissue plasminogen activator, t-PA) and converted to plasmin, which breaks down the fibrin. Aminocaproic acid (ε-aminocaproic acid, EACA, 6-aminohexanoic acid, Amicar) and tranexamic acid (Cyklokapron) are structural analogues of lysine, which bind irreversibly to the lysine-binding sites on plasminogen, inhibiting binding to fibrin and thus the whole process of fibrinolysis (1,2). These agents inhibit the natural degradation of fibrin and so stabilize clots.

Aminocaproic acid was the first such agent to be used widely, but it has largely been superseded in clinical practice by tranexamic acid, which is about 10 times more potent. *Para*-aminomethylbenzoic acid (PAMBA) is similar to aminocaproic acid, but is about three times more active in inhibiting plasminogen activators (3). However, it is no longer used despite the fact that it is well tolerated.

Uses

Antifibrinolytic agents are of benefit in the treatment of primary menorrhagia (4–7), recurrent epistaxis (8), oral bleeding in patients with congenital and acquired coagulation disorders (9,10), hemorrhage associated with thrombolytic therapy, and to reduce blood loss associated with surgery (especially cardiac surgery, joint replacement, and orthotopic liver transplantation) (11–14). Antifibrinolytic therapy can be of value in other conditions as well (15–21). It is effective in the bleeding diathesis that can accompany acute promyelocytic leukemia (22,23), but it does not improve outcome after subarachnoid hemorrhage (24).

General adverse effects

Some adverse effects are associated with all antifibrinolytic agents, reflecting their effect on clot stability. Dissolution of extravascular blood clots may be resistant to physiological fibrinolysis. These drugs should not to be used to treat hematuria due to blood loss from the upper urinary tract, as this can provoke painful clot retention and even renal insufficiency associated with bilateral ureteric obstruction (25–31).

Well-controlled studies on aminocaproic acid in a limited number of patients showed no serious adverse effects. Minor unwanted effects have been reported in 10–20% of patients and include headache, nasal congestion, conjunctival suffusion, nausea, vomiting, diarrhea, and transient hypotension (32). Skin rashes have also been associated with aminocaproic acid, including maculopapular and morbilliform eruptions. Rarer dermatological reactions reported include purpuric rashes (33), bullous eruptions (34), and contact dermatitis with positive patch tests (35–37). Treatment with a high dose (the maximum daily dose is 36 g/day) can result in an osmotic diuresis (38).

Miscellaneous adverse reactions attributed by the authors of single case reports have included a psychotic reaction (39), convulsions after intravenous administration of aminocaproic acid in a 60-year-old man treated for bleeding esophageal varices (40), and renal insufficiency due to glomerular capillary thrombosis (31).

Aminocaproic acid used during cardiopulmonary bypass reduced mediastinal blood losses by about one-third, while transfusion requirements were unchanged (41). In one series of over 950 patients, not a single thromboembolic complication could be ascribed to aminocaproic acid. However, a few cases of muscle necrosis and rhabdomyolysis with renal insufficiency have been reported with aminocaproic acid (42,43).

Organs and Systems

Cardiovascular

Aminocaproic acid has been reported to cause acute right heart failure (44).

Acid–base balance

Metabolic acidosis associated with a high anion gap has been reported after the administration of aminocaproic acid to a woman with renal insufficiency (45).

Hematologic

Inhibition of plasminogen by tranexamic acid and aminocaproic acid could theoretically facilitate the development of thrombosis, but whether it actually does so has been the subject of contradictory reports. Episodes of venous and arterial thrombosis have been reported in association with treatment using either tranexamic acid or aminocaproic acid. These include thrombosis at unusual sites such as mesenteric thrombosis (46), aorta (47), retinal artery occlusion (48), and intracranial arterial thrombosis (49–51), as well as deep vein thrombosis in the legs (52).

- Massive pulmonary thromboembolism was reported in a 62-year-old woman seven days after treatment with high doses for subarachnoid hemorrhage (53).

Caution should also be taken in the administration of antifibrinolytic agents in disseminated intravascular coagulation (54).

Prophylactic use of histamine H_1 and H_2 receptor antagonists, aminocaproic acid, and hyposensitization have all been proposed as means of preventing idiosyncratic reactions to radiological contrast media. Aminocaproic acid was formerly used prophylactically in France, but carried a risk of massive intravascular coagulation (SEDA-17, 536).

Skin

- A 70-year-old man taking aminocaproic acid developed dermatitis with eosinophilia and positive patch tests on days 2 and 4 (55).

Musculoskeletal

Myopathy has occasionally been reported in association with aminocaproic acid therapy in both adults and children (42,56–64).

- Myonecrosis developed in a 22-year-old man who presented with dark smoky urine and calf tenderness, with progressive weakness and difficulty in walking, after treatment with aminocaproic acid for several weeks for traumatic hematuria; after withdrawal he recovered over 3 weeks (61).

A review of published cases confirmed that this complication is very rare and is usually associated with the administration of high doses for several weeks (43). The myopathy is often painful, and associated with raised creatine kinase activity and even myoglobinuria. Full resolution can be expected once the drug is withdrawn.

Susceptibility Factors

Renal disease

Two different case reports have dealt with previously unreported adverse effects of aminocaproic acid in patients with renal insufficiency.

- A patient with underlying chronic renal insufficiency, who underwent coronary bypass artery grafting and was treated with intravenous aminocaproic acid, developed hyperkalemia (6.7 mmol/l) (65). There was no other obvious cause for the acute increase in serum potassium.

The authors suggested that the structural similarity between aminocaproic acid and lysine and arginine underlies the mechanism of hyperkalemia; intravenous arginine can cause hyperkalemia (66,67). Furthermore, aminocaproic acid infusion in anephric dogs caused a rapid rise in serum potassium (68).

References

1. Astedt B. Clinical pharmacology of tranexamic acid. Scand J Gastroenterol Suppl 1987;137:22–5.
2. Hoylaerts M, Lijnen HR, Collen D. Studies on the mechanism of the antifibrinolytic action of tranexamic acid. Biochim Biophys Acta 1981;673(1):75–85.
3. Westlund LE, Lunden R, Wallen P. Effect of EACA, PAMBA, AMCA and AMBOCA on fibrinolysis induced by streptokinase, urokinase and tissue activator. Haemostasis 1982;11(4):235–41.
4. Nilsson L, Rybo G. Treatment of menorrhagia with an antifibrinolytic agent, tranexamic acid (AMCA): a double-blind invetsigation. Acta Obstet Gynecol Scand 1967;46:572–80.
5. Vermylen J, Verhaegen-Declercq ML, Verstraete M, Fierens F. A double blind study of the effect of tranexamic acid in essential menorrhagia. Thromb Diath Haemorrh 1968;20(3):583–7.
6. Callender ST, Warner GT, Cope E. Treatment of menorrhagia with tranexamic acid. A double-blind trial. BMJ 1970;4(729):214–16.
7. Prentice A. Fortnightly review. Medical management of menorrhagia. BMJ 1999;319(7221):1343–5.
8. Petruson B. A double-blind study to evaluate the effect in epistaxis with oral administration of the antifibrinolytic drug tranexamic acid (Cyklokapron). Acta Otolaryngol 1974;317(Suppl):57–61.
9. Forbes CD, Barr RD, Reid G, Thomson C, Prentice CR, McNicol GP, Douglas AS. Tranexamic acid in control of haemorrhage after dental extraction in haemophilia and Christmas disease. BMJ 1972;2(809):311–13.
10. Sindet-Pedersen S, Ramstrom G, Bernvil S, Blomback M. Hemostatic effect of tranexamic acid mouthwash in anticoagulant-treated patients undergoing oral surgery. N Engl J Med 1989;320(13):840–3.
11. Jordan D, Delphin E, Rose E. Prophylactic epsilon-aminocaproic acid (EACA) administration minimizes blood replacement therapy during cardiac surgery. Anesth Analg 1995;80(4):827–9.
12. Boylan JF, Klinck JR, Sandler AN, Arellano R, Greig PD, Nierenberg H, Roger SL, Glynn MF. Tranexamic acid reduces blood loss, transfusion requirements, and coagulation factor use in primary orthotopic liver transplantation. Anesthesiology 1996;85(5):1043–8.
13. Benoni G, Fredin H. Fibrinolytic inhibition with tranexamic acid reduces blood loss and blood transfusion after knee arthroplasty: a prospective, randomised, double-blind study of 86 patients. J Bone Joint Surg Br 1996;78(3):434–40.
14. Jansen AJ, Andreica S, Claeys M, D'Haese J, Camu F, Jochmans K. Use of tranexamic acid for an effective blood conservation strategy after total knee arthroplasty. Br J Anaesth 1999;83(4):596–601.

15. Gardner FH, Helmer RE 3rd. Aminocaproic acid. Use in control of hemorrhage in patients with amegakaryocytic thrombocytopenia. JAMA 1980;243(1):35–7.

16. Bartholomew JR, Salgia R, Bell WR. Control of bleeding in patients with immune and nonimmune thrombocytopenia with aminocaproic acid. Arch Intern Med 1989;149(9):1959–61.

17. von Holstein CC, Eriksson SB, Kallen R. Tranexamic acid as an aid to reducing blood transfusion requirements in gastric and duodenal bleeding. BMJ (Clin Res Ed) 1987;294(6563):7–10.

18. Henry DA, O'Connell DL. Effects of fibrinolytic inhibitors on mortality from upper gastrointestinal haemorrhage. BMJ 1989;298(6681):1142–6.

19. Jerndal T, Frisen M. Tranexamic acid (AMCA) and late hyphaema. A double blind study in cataract surgery. Acta Ophthalmol (Copenh) 1976;54(4):417–29.

20. Varnek L, Dalsgaard C, Hansen A, Klie F. The effect of tranexamic acid on secondary haemorrhage after traumatic hyphaema. Acta Ophthalmol (Copenh) 1980;58(5):787–93.

21. Uusitalo RJ, Ranta-Kemppainen L, Tarkkanen A. Management of traumatic hyphema in children. An analysis of 340 cases. Arch Ophthalmol 1988;106(9):1207–9.

22. Schwartz BS, Williams EC, Conlan MG, Mosher DF. Epsilon-aminocaproic acid in the treatment of patients with acute promyelocytic leukemia and acquired alpha-2-plasmin inhibitor deficiency. Ann Intern Med 1986;105(6):873–7.

23. Avvisati G, ten Cate JW, Buller HR, Mandelli F. Tranexamic acid for control of haemorrhage in acute promyelocytic leukaemia. Lancet 1989;2(8655):122–4.

24. Roos Y. Antifibrinolytic treatment in subarachnoid hemorrhage: a randomized placebo-controlled trial. STAR Study Group. Neurology 2000;54(1):77–82.

25. van Itterbeek H, Vermylen J, Verstraete M. High obstruction of urine flow as a complication of the treatment with fibrinolysis inhibitors of haematuria in haemophiliacs. Acta Haematol 1968;39(4):237–42.

26. Stark SN, White JG, Lange RL Jr, Krivit W. Epsilon amino caproic acid therapy as a cause of intrarenal obstruction in haematuria of haemophiliacs. Scand J Haematol 1965;79:99–107.

27. Coggins JT, Allen TD. Insoluble fibrin clots within the urinary tract as a consequence of epsilon aminocaprioic acid therapy. J Urol 1972;107(4):647–9.

28. Albronda T, Gokemeyer JD, van Haeflen TW. Transient acute renal failure due to tranexaminic acid therapy for diffuse intravascular coagulation. Neth J Med 1991;39(1–2):127–8.

29. Fernandez Lucas M, Liano F, Navarro JF, Sastre JL, Quereda C, Ortuno J. Acute renal failure secondary to antifibrinolytic therapy. Nephron 1995;69(4):478–9.

30. Wymenga LF, van der Boon WJ. Obstruction of the renal pelvis due to an insoluble blood clot after epsilon-aminocaproic acid therapy: resolution with intraureteral streptokinase instillations. J Urol 1998;159(2):490–2.

31. Charytan C, Purtilo D. Glomerular capillary thrombosis and acute renal failure after epsilon-amino caproic acid therapy. N Engl J Med 1969;280(20):1102–4.

32. McNicol GP, Fletcher AP, Alkjaersig N, et al. The use of epsilon-aminocaproic acid, a potent inhibitor of fibrinolytic activity, in the management of postoperative hematuria. J Urol 1961;86:829.

33. Chakrabarti A, Collett KA. Purpuric rash due to epsilon-aminocaproic acid. BMJ 1980;281(6234):197–8.

34. Brooke CP, Spiers EM, Omura EF. Noninflammatory bullae associated with epsilon-aminocaproic acid infusion. J Am Acad Dermatol 1992;27(5 Pt 2):880–2.

35. Tanaka M, Niizeki H, Miyakawa S. Contact dermatitis from epsilon-aminocaproic acid. Contact Dermatitis 1993;28(2):124.

36. Gonzalez Gutierrez ML, Esteban Lopez MI, Ruiz Ruiz MD. Positivity of patch tests in cutaneous reaction to aminocaproic acid: two case reports. Allergy 1995;50(9):745–6.

37. Miyamoto H, Okajima M. Allergic contact dermatitis from epsilon-aminocaproic acid. Contact Dermatitis 2000;42(1):50.

38. Lee P, Pompeius R. Antifibrinolytisk behandling och forcerad osmotisk diures efter transuretral prostataresektion. [Antifibrinolytic treatment and forced osmotic diuresis after transurethral prostatectomy.] Nord Med 1970;84(51):1624–6.

39. Wysenbeek AJ, Sella A, Vardi M, Yeshurun D. Acute delirious state after epsilon-aminocaproic acid. Lancet 1978;1(8057):221.

40. Rabinovici R, Heyman A, Kluger Y, Shinar E. Convulsions induced by aminocaproic acid infusion. DICP 1989;23(10):780–1.

41. Barrons RW, Jahr JS. A review of post-cardiopulmonary bypass bleeding, aminocaproic acid, tranexamic acid, and aprotinin. Am J Ther 1996;3(12):821–38.

42. Biswas CK, Milligan DA, Agte SD, Kenward DH, Tilley PJ. Acute renal failure and myopathy after treatment with aminocaproic acid. BMJ 1980;281(6233):115–16.

43. Seymour BD, Rubinger M. Rhabdomyolysis induced by epsilon-aminocaproic acid. Ann Pharmacother 1997;31(1):56–8.

44. Johansson SA. Acute right heart failure during treatment with epsilon amino caproic acid (E-ACA). Acta Med Scand 1967;182(3):331–4.

45. Budris WA, Roxe DM, Duvel JM. High anion gap metabolic acidosis associated with aminocaproic acid. Ann Pharmacother 1999;33(3):308–11.

46. Razis PA, Coulson IH, Gould TR, Findley IL. Acquired C1 esterase inhibitor deficiency. Anaesthesia 1986;41(8):838–40.

47. Hocker JR, Saving KL. Fatal aortic thrombosis in a neonate during infusion of epsilon-aminocaproic acid. J Pediatr Surg 1995;30(10):1490–2.

48. Parsons MR, Merritt DR, Ramsay RC. Retinal artery occlusion associated with tranexamic acid therapy. Am J Ophthalmol 1988;105(6):688–9.

49. Davies D, Howell DA. Tranexamic acid and arterial thrombosis. Lancet 1977;1(8001):49.

50. Agnelli G, Gresele P, De Cunto M, Gallai V, Nenci GG. Tranexamic acid, intrauterine contraceptive devices and fatal cerebral arterial thrombosis. Case report. Br J Obstet Gynaecol 1982;89(8):681–2.

51. Humbert P, Gutknecht J, Mallet H, Dupond JL, Leconte des Floris R. Acide tranéxamique et thrombose du sinus longitudinal supérieur. [Tranexamic acid and thrombosis of the superior longitudinal sinus.] Therapie 1987;42(1):65–6.

52. Endo Y, Nishimura S, Miura A. Deep-vein thrombosis induced by tranexamic acid in idiopathic thrombocytopenic purpura. JAMA 1988;259(24):3561–2.

53. Woo KS, Tse LK, Woo JL, Vallance-Owen J. Massive pulmonary thromboembolism after antifibrinolytic therapy. Ann Emerg Med 1989;18(1):116–17.

54. Giles AR. Disseminated intravascular coagulation. Edinburgh: Churchill Livingstone, 1994.

55. Villarreal O. Systemic dermatitis with eosinophilia due to epsilon-aminocaproic acid. Contact Dermatitis 1999;40(2):114.

56. Brodkin HM. Myoglobinuria following epsilon-aminocaproic acid (EACA) therapy. Case report. J Neurosurg 1980;53(5):690–2.

57. Frank MM, Sergent JS, Kane MA, Alling DW. Epsilon aminocaproic acid therapy of hereditary angioneurotic edema. A double-blind study. N Engl J Med 1972;286(15):808–12.

58. Korsan-Bengtsen K, Ysander L, Blohme G, Tibblin E. Extensive muscle necrosis after long-term treatment with aminocaproic acid (EACA) in a case of hereditary periodic edema. Acta Med Scand 1969;185(4):341–6.

59. Rizza RA, Sclonick S, Conley CL. Myoglobinuria following aminocaproic acid administration. JAMA 1976;236(16):1845–6.

60. Kennard C, Swash M, Henson RA. Myopathy due to epsilon amino-caproic acid. Muscle Nerve 1980;3(3):202–6.

61. Johnstone BR, Syme RR. Myonecrosis complicating epsilon aminocaproic acid treatment of traumatic haematuria. Br J Urol 1987;60(1):81–2.

62. MacKay AR, Sang U H, Weinstein PR. Myopathy associated with epsilon-aminocaproic acid (EACA) therapy. Report of two cases. J Neurosurg 1978;49(4):597–601.

63. Lane RJ, McLelland NJ, Martin AM, Mastaglia FL. Epsilon aminocaproic acid (EACA) myopathy. Postgrad Med J 1979;55(642):282–5.

64. Winter SS, Chaffee S, Kahler SG, Graham ML. Epsilon-aminocaproic acid-associated myopathy in a child. J Pediatr Hematol Oncol 1995;17(1):53–5.

65. Perazella MA, Biswas P. Acute hyperkalemia associated with intravenous epsilon-aminocaproic acid therapy. Am J Kidney Dis 1999;33(4):782–5.

66. Hertz P, Richardson JA. Arginine-induced hyperkalemia in renal failure patients. Arch Intern Med 1972;130(5):778–80.

67. Bushinsky DA, Gennari FJ. Life-threatening hyperkalemia induced by arginine. Ann Intern Med 1978;89(5 Pt 1):632–4.

68. Carroll HJ, Tice DA. The effects of epsilon amino-caproic acid upon potassium metabolism in the dog. Metabolism 1966;15(5):449–57.

Aminoglycoside antibiotics

See also Individual agents

General Information

Eleven aminoglycosides have been, or are still, important in medical practice: amikacin (rINN), gentamicin (pINN), isepamicin (rINN), kanamycin (rINN), neomycin (rINN), netilmicin (rINN), paromomycin (rINN), sisomicin (rINN), streptomycin (rINN) and dihydrostreptomycin (rINN), and tobramycin (rINN). The following aminoglycosides are also covered in separate monographs: amikacin, gentamicin, isepamicin, kanamycin, and tobramycin.

Being chemically similar, the aminoglycosides have many features in common, in particular their mechanism of antibacterial action, a broad antibacterial spectrum, partial or complete cross-resistance, bactericidal action in a slightly alkaline environment, poor absorption from the gastrointestinal tract, elimination by glomerular filtration, nephrotoxicity, ototoxicity, a potential to cause neuromuscular blockade, and partial or complete cross-allergy (1). Aminoglycosides have a moderate capacity for diffusion into bone tissue (2).

The aminoglycosides have probably more than one mechanism of action on bacterial cells. They cause misreading of the RNA code and/or inhibition of the polymerization of amino acids.

All the aminoglycosides have similar patterns of adverse reactions, although there are important differences with regard to their frequency and severity (Table 1).

Strategies for minimizing aminoglycoside toxicity include early bedside detection of cochlear and vestibular dysfunction, which should lead to prompt withdrawal, use of short periods of treatment, dosing intervals of at least 12 hours, monitoring of serum concentrations, and awareness of relative contraindications, such as renal or hepatic dysfunction, old age, hearing impairment, and previous recent aminoglycoside exposure (3).

Observational studies

In an open, randomized, comparative study of the efficacy, safety, and tolerance of two different antibiotic regimens in the treatment of severe community-acquired or nosocomial pneumonia, 84 patients were analysed (4). Half were treated with co-amoxiclav (amoxicillin 2 g and clavulanic acid 200 mg) every 8 hours plus a single-dose of 3–6 mg/kg of an aminoglycoside (netilmicin or gentamicin), and half with piperacillin 4 g and tazobactam 500 mg every 8 hours. The patients were treated for between 48 hours and 21 days. Clinical cure was achieved in 65% of patients with co-amoxiclav/aminoglycoside and in 81% of patients with piperacillin/tazobactam. Cure or improvement was observed in 84 and 90% respectively. Treatment failures were recorded in 14 versus 7%. One patient in each group relapsed. There was only one fatal outcome in the piperacillin/tazobactam group compared with six in the co-amoxiclav/aminoglycoside group. The adverse event rate was non-significantly lower in the

Table 1 Relative adverse effects of aminoglycoside antibiotics on eighth nerve function, the nervous system, and neuromuscular function

Aminoglycoside[1]	Usual parenteral dose (mg/kg/day)[2]	Site of adverse effect[3]			
		Vestibular function	Cochlear function	Nervous system	Neuromuscular function
Amikacin	10–15	+	++	++	+
Gentamicin	3–6	++	++	++	+
Kanamycin	10–20	+	+++	++	+
Netilmicin	3–6	+	+	++	+
Sisomicin	2–4	++	++	++	+
Streptomycin	10–20	+++	+	+	++
Dihydrostreptomycin	10–20	+	+++	+++	++
Tobramycin	3–6	++	++	++	+

[1] Neomycin and paromomycin: only accidental absorption after topical or gastrointestinal use.
[2] In general, older patients require lower doses. Low doses are required during therapy of infectious endocarditis when an aminoglycoside is given with a penicillin. Monitoring serum concentrations should be considered, particularly when using dosing regimens that involve more than one dose a day and high doses for several days.
[3] The number of signs (+) indicates the relative clinical importance of each reaction.

piperacillin/tazobactam group. In one patient given piperacillin/tazobactam, there were raised transaminases. In the co-amoxiclav/aminoglycoside group, acute renal insufficiency developed in two patients and possibly drug-related fever in one. Bacteriological efficacy was comparable (92% versus 96%). The authors concluded that piperacillin/tazobactam is highly efficacious in the treatment of severe pneumonia in hospitalized patients and compares favorably with the combination of co-amoxiclav plus an aminoglycoside.

General adverse effects

The main adverse reactions of aminoglycosides consist of kidney damage (often presenting as non-oliguric renal insufficiency) and ototoxicity, including vestibular and/or cochlear dysfunction. Neuromuscular transmission can be inhibited. Hypersensitivity reactions are most frequent after topical use, which should be avoided. Anaphylactic reactions can occur. Tumor-inducing effects have not been reported.

Pharmacoeconomics

The pharmacoeconomic impact of adverse effects of antimicrobial drugs is enormous. Antibacterial drug reactions account for about 25% of adverse drug reactions. The adverse effects profile of an antimicrobial agent can contribute significantly to its overall direct costs (monitoring costs, prolonged hospitalization due to complications or treatment failures) and indirect costs (quality of life, loss of productivity, time spent by families and patients receiving medical care). In one study an adverse event in a hospitalized patient was associated on average with an excess of 1.9 days in the length of stay, extra costs of $US2262 (1990–93 values), and an almost two-fold increase in the risk of death. In the outpatient setting, adverse drug reactions result in 2–6% of hospitalizations, and most of them were thought to be avoidable if appropriate interventions had been taken. In a review, economic aspects of antibacterial therapy with aminoglycosides have been summarized and critically evaluated (5).

Organs and Systems

Cardiovascular

Anecdotal reports refer to tachycardia, electrocardiographic changes, hypotension, and even cardiac arrest (6). In practice, effects on the cardiovascular system are unlikely to be of any significance.

Respiratory

Severe respiratory depression due to neuromuscular blockade has been observed (7). Bronchospasm can occur as part of a hypersensitivity reaction.

Neuromuscular function

The aminoglycosides have a curare-like action, which can be antagonized by calcium ions and acetylcholinesterase inhibitors (8). The mechanisms include reduced release of acetylcholine prejunctionally and an interaction with the postjunctional acetylcholine receptor-channel complex. While neomycin interacts with the open state of the receptor, streptomycin blocks the receptor (9).

Aminoglycoside-induced neuromuscular blockade can be clinically relevant in patients with respiratory acidosis, in myasthenia gravis, and in other neuromuscular diseases. Severe illness, the simultaneous use of anesthetics, for example in the immediate postoperative phase, and application of the antibiotic to serosal surfaces are predisposing factors (10).

With regard to this effect, neomycin is the most potent member of the group. Several deaths and cases of severe respiratory depression due to neomycin have been reported (11). Severe clinical manifestations are rare in patients treated with aminoglycosides that are administered in low doses, such as gentamicin, netilmicin, and tobramycin. In some cases the paralysis was reversed by prostigmine.

Sensory systems

Eyes

Collagen corneal shields pre-soaked with antibiotics are used as a means of delivering drug to the cornea and anterior chamber of the eye. Gentamicin damages the primate retina, particularly by macular infarction, and amikacin can have a similar effect; a subconjunctival injection of tobramycin causes macular infarction (SEDA-19, 245). This potentially devastating consequence suggests that care must be exercised when contemplating instillation of aminoglycosides directly into the eye. Allergic contact dermatitis causing conjunctivitis and blepharitis has been reported with topical ophthalmic tobramycin (12).

Ears

Ototoxicity is a major adverse effect of aminoglycoside antibiotics (13). They all affect both vestibular and cochlear function, but different members of the family have different relative effects (Table 1).

Differences between different aminoglycosides
Ototoxicity due to amikacin is primarily cochlear; however, in comparisons with equipotent dosages, ototoxicity was of the same order as that caused by gentamicin (14–16).

In 40 patients tobramycin had little effect on audiometric thresholds, but produced a change in the amplitude of the distortion products, currently considered an objective method for rapidly evaluating the functional status of the cochlea (17). In one case, tobramycin caused bilateral high-frequency vestibular toxicity, which subsequently showed clinical and objective evidence of functional recovery (18).

In a quantitative assessment of vestibular hair cells and Scarpa's ganglion cells in 17 temporal bones from 10 individuals with aminoglycoside ototoxicity, streptomycin caused a significant loss of both type I and type II hair cells in all five vestibular sense organs (19). The vestibular ototoxic effects of kanamycin appeared to be similar to those of streptomycin, whereas neomycin did not cause loss of vestibular hair cells. There was no significant loss of Scarpa's ganglion cells.

Incidence

The incidence of ototoxicity due to aminoglycosides varies in different studies, depending on the type of patients treated, the methods used to monitor cochlear and vestibular function, and the aminoglycoside used (20). Clinically recognizable hearing loss and vestibular damage occur in about 2–4% of patients, but pure-tone audiometry, particularly at high frequencies, and electronystagmography show hearing loss and/or vestibular damage in up to 26 and 10% respectively, despite careful dosage adjustment (21). In patients with *Pseudomonas* endocarditis receiving prolonged high-dose gentamicin, auditory toxicity was found in 44% (22,23).

A review of nearly 10000 adults suggested rates of 14% for amikacin, 8.6% for gentamicin, and 2.4% for netilmicin. Aminoglycoside toxicity is markedly lower in infants and children, with an incidence of 0–2%. A long duration of treatment and repeated courses or high cumulative doses appear to be critical for ototoxicity, which occurs in high frequency hearing beyond the range of normal speech.

There is a discrepancy between clinical observations, in which very few patients receiving aminoglycosides actually complain of hearing loss, and the reported incidences of ototoxicity in studies of audiometric thresholds. A major reason for this discrepancy relates to the fact that aminoglycosides cause high-frequency hearing loss well before they affect the speech frequency range in which they can be detected by the patient (21).

Gentamicin also damages the vestibular apparatus at a rate of 1.4–3.7%, resulting in vertigo and impaired balance. This effect is reversible in only about 50% from 1 week to 6 months after administration.

In a retrospective study in 81 men and 29 women, hearing loss of 15 decibels at two or more frequencies, or at least 20 decibels at at least one frequency, was found in 18% of patients treated with aminoglycosides (amikacin, kanamycin, and/or streptomycin) (24). In those treated with kanamycin the rate was 16%. Age, sex, treatment duration, total aminoglycoside dose, and first serum creatinine concentration were not associated with hearing loss.

Dose-relatedness

Hearing loss was attributed to repeated exposure to aminoglycosides in 12 of 70 patients with cystic fibrosis (one child) (25). There was a non-linear relation between the number of courses of therapy and the incidence of hearing loss. The severity of loss was not related to the number of courses. Assuming that the risk of hearing loss was independent of each course, the preliminary estimate of the risk was less than 2 per 100 courses.

Presentation

Clinically, cochlear ototoxicity is more frequent and easier to detect than vestibular toxicity; combined defects are relatively rare. Symptoms of cochlear damage include tinnitus, hearing loss, pressure, and sometimes pain in the ear. The manifestations of vestibular toxicity are dizziness, vertigo, ataxia, and nystagmus. These are often overlooked in severely ill, bed-ridden patients.

Symptoms of ototoxicity can occur within 3–5 days of starting treatment, but most patients with severe damage have received prolonged courses of aminoglycosides. In some cases, hearing loss progresses after the administration of the causative drug has been interrupted. The ototoxicity is reversible in only about 50% of patients. Permanent deafness is often seen in patients with delayed onset of symptoms, progressive deterioration after withdrawal of treatment, and hearing loss of over 25 db (21).

There are interesting differences in the toxicity patterns of aminoglycosides in animals. Gentamicin and tobramycin affect the cochlear and vestibular systems to a similar extent, while amikacin, kanamycin, and neomycin preferentially damage the cochlear and streptomycin the vestibular system. Netilmicin appears to be the least toxic (26,27).

In man, differences in the ototoxic risks of the currently used aminoglycosides are difficult to evaluate (20). There have been no prospective comparisons of more than two drugs using the same criteria in similar patient populations. However, several controlled comparisons of two aminoglycosides are available and provide some information. A survey of 24 such trials showed the following mean frequencies of ototoxicity: gentamicin 7.7%, tobramycin 9.7%, amikacin 13.8%, netilmicin 2.3% (28). There was also a lower incidence of netilmicin-induced inner ear damage compared with tobramycin in two studies (29,30).

Of 20 patients with Dandy's syndrome, 15 had previously been treated with aminoglycosides (13 with gentamicin and 2 with streptomycin), of whom 10 had symptoms of pre-existing chronic nephrosis or transitory renal insufficiency. In all 13 patients who had gentamicin, peripheral vestibular function was destroyed or severely damaged, whereas there was no hearing loss (31).

Mechanism

The mechanism of ototoxicity by aminoglycosides is still not fully clarified. Most of the experimental data have been gained in the guinea-pig model, which seems to resemble man.

Animal studies

Traditionally, toxic damage is considered to be the consequence of drug accumulation in the inner ear fluids (32,33). After a period of reversible functional impairment, destruction of outer hair cells occurs in the basilar turn of the cochlear duct and proceeds to the apex. Similar changes are found in the hair cells of the vestibular system. Gentamicin was detected in the outer hair cells in the cochlea of animals receiving non-ototoxic doses of the drug and continued to increase for several days after withdrawal (34). This was followed by a third and very much slower phase of elimination (estimated half-life 6 months), and in the absence of ototoxicity gentamicin could still be detected in the outer hair cells 11 months after treatment. This may explain why patients who receive several courses of aminoglycosides in a year may be more susceptible to ototoxicity, and suggests that the cumulative dose (and by implication the duration of therapy) is the more important determinant of cochlear damage. However, it has been questioned whether ototoxicity correlates with plasma perilymph or whole-tissue concentrations of aminoglycosides (33).

The effects of aminoglycosides on the medial efferent system have been assessed in awake guinea-pigs (35,36). The ensemble background activity and its suppression by contralateral acoustic stimulation was used as a tool to study the medial efferent system. A single intramuscular dose of gentamicin 150 mg/kg reduced or abolished the suppressive effect produced by activation of the olivoco-chlear system by contralateral low-level broadband noise stimulation. This effect was dose-dependent and could be demonstrated ipsilaterally on the compound action poten-tial, otoacoustic emissions, and ensemble background activity of the eighth nerve. Long-term gentamicin treat-ment (60 mg/kg for 10 days) had no effect, at least before the development of ototoxicity. Single-dose intramuscular netilmicin 150 mg/kg displayed blocking properties similar to gentamicin, although less pronounced, while amikacin 750 mg/kg and neomycin 150 mg/kg had no effect. With tobramycin 150 mg/kg and streptomycin 400 mg/kg a decrease in suppression was usually associated with a reduction of the ensemble background activity measured without acoustic stimulation, which may be a fist sign of alteration to cochlear function. There was no correlation between specificity and degree of aminoglycoside ototoxi-city and their action on the medial efferent system.

Possible mechanisms and preventive strategies have also been investigated in pigmented guinea-pigs (37–39). Animals that received alpha-lipoic acid (100 mg/kg/day), a powerful free radical scavenger, in combination with ami-kacin (450 mg/kg/day intramuscularly) had a less severe rise in compound action potential threshold than animals that received amikacin alone. In a similar study in pigmen-ted guinea-pigs, the iron chelator deferoxamine (150 mg/kg bd for 14 days) produced a significant protective effect against ototoxicity induced by neomycin (100 mg/kg/day for 14 days). The spin trap alpha-phenyl-tert-butyl-nitrone also protected against acute ototopical aminoglycoside oto-toxicity in guinea-pigs. These studies have provided further evidence for the hypothesis that aminoglycoside ototoxicity is mediated by the formation of an aminoglycoside-iron complex and reactive oxygen species.

Aminoglycoside-induced ototoxicity may be in part a process that involves the excitatory activation of cochlear NMDA receptors (40). In addition, the uncompetitive NMDA receptor antagonist dizocilpine attenuated the vestibular toxicity of streptomycin in a rat model, further stressing that excitotoxic mechanisms mediated by NMDA receptors also contribute to aminoglycoside-induced vestibular toxicity (41). In two studies in guinea-pigs, nitric oxide and free radicals, demonstrated by the beneficial effect of the antioxidant/free radical scavenger alpha-lipoic acid, have been suggested to be involved in aminoglycoside-induced ototoxicity (38,42). In contrast, insulin, transforming growth factor alpha, or retinoic acid may offer a protective potential against ototoxicity caused by aminoglycosides. However, they do not seem to promote cochlear hair cell repair (43). In guinea-pigs, brain-derived neurotrophic factor, neurotrophin-3, and the iron chelator and antioxidant 2-hydroxybenzoate (salicylate), at concentrations corresponding to anti-inflammatory concentrations in humans, attenuated aminoglycoside-induced ototoxicity (44,45). In rats,

concanavalin A attenuated aminoglycoside-induced oto-toxicity, and kanamycin increased the expression of the glutamate-aspartate transporter gene in the cochlea, which might play a role in the prevention of secondary deaths of spiral ganglion neurons (46,47). Finally, 4-methylcatechol, an inducer of nerve growth factor synthesis, enhanced spiral ganglion neuron survival after aminoglycoside treatment in mice (48).

In hatched chicks repeatedly injected with kanamycin, afferent innervation of the regenerated hair cells was related more to the recovery of hearing than efferent innervation (49).

Human studies
There is evidence that the site of ototoxic action is the mitochondrial ribosome (50,51). In some countries, such as China, aminoglycoside toxicity is a major cause of deafness. Susceptibility to ototoxicity in these populations appears to be transmitted by women, suggesting mito-chondrial inheritance. In Chinese, Japanese, and Arab-Israeli pedigrees a common mutation was found. A point mutation in a highly conserved region of the mitochon-drial 12S ribosomal RNA gene was common in all pedi-grees with maternally inherited ototoxic deafness (50). A mutation at nucleotide 1555 has been reported to confer susceptibility to aminoglycoside antibiotics, and to cause non-syndromic sensorineural hearing loss. Outside these susceptible families, sporadic cases also have this mutation in increased frequency. In patients bearing this mitochondrial mutation hearing loss was observed after short-term exposure to isepamicin sulfate (52). These findings might create a molecular baseline for preventive screening of patients when aminoglycosides are to be used (SEDA-18, 1) (50).

Differences between sera from patients with resistance or susceptibility to aminoglycoside ototoxicity have been described in vitro (53). Sera from sensitive but not from resistant individuals metabolized aminoglycosides to cytotoxins, whereas no sera were cytotoxic when tested without the addition of aminoglycosides. This effect per-sisted for up to 1 year after aminoglycoside treatment.

Susceptibility factors
Several factors predispose to ototoxic effects (Table 2). Drug-related toxicity is influenced by the quality of pre-scribing. Overdosage in patients with impaired renal func-tion, unnecessary prolongation of treatment, and the concomitant administration of other potentially ototoxic agents should be avoided. The exact mechanism of

Table 2 Factors that increase susceptibility to the adverse effects of aminoglycosides

Patient factors	Drug-related factors
Prior renal insufficiency	High temperature
Prior abnormal audiogram	Dose (blood concentration exceeding the usual target range)
Age (mainly older patients)	Total cumulative dose
Septicemia	Prolonged duration of therapy (2–3 weeks)
Dehydration	Prior aminoglycoside exposure

increased toxicity in patients with septicemia and a high temperature is not clear; the possible relevance of additive damage by bacterial endotoxins has been discussed (54). Dehydration with hypovolemia is probably the main reason for the increased toxicity experienced when aminoglycosides are given with loop diuretics, but furosemide itself does not seem to be an independent risk factor (55,56). Attempts have been made in animals to protect against ototoxicity by antioxidant therapy (for example glutathione and vitamin C), as well as iron chelators and neurotrophins (57).

Hereditary deafness is a heterogeneous group of disorders, with different patterns of inheritance and due to a multitude of different genes (58,59). The first molecular defect described was the A1555G sequence change in the mitochondrial 12S ribosomal RNA gene. A description of two families from Italy and 19 families from Spain has now suggested that this mutation is not as rare as was initially thought (60,61). The A1555G mutation is important to diagnose, since hearing maternal relatives who are exposed to aminoglycosides may lose their hearing. This predisposition is stressed by the fact that 40 relatives in 12 Spanish families and one relative in an Italian family lost their hearing after aminoglycoside exposure. Since the mutation can easily be screened, any patient with idiopathic sensorineural hearing loss may be screened for this and possible other mutations.

In an Italian family of whom five family members became deaf after aminoglycoside exposure, the nucleotide 961 thymidine deletion associated with a varying number of inserted cytosines in the mitochondrial 12S ribosomal RNA gene was identified as a second pathogenic mutation that could predispose to aminoglycoside ototoxicity (62). Molecular analysis excluded the A1555G mutation in this family.

The A1555G mutation in the human mitochondrial 12S RNA, which has been associated with hearing loss after aminoglycoside administration (63) and has been implicated in maternally inherited hearing loss in the absence of aminoglycoside exposure in some families, can be identified by a simple and rapid method for large-scale screening that uses one-step multiplex allele-specific PCR (64).

Using lymphoblastoid cell lines derived from five deaf and five hearing individuals from an Arab-Israeli family carrying the A1555G mutation, the first direct evidence has been provided that the mitochondrial 12S rRNA carrying the A1555G mutation is the main target of the aminoglycosides (65). This suggests that they exert their detrimental effect through altering mitochondrial protein synthesis, which exacerbates the inherent defect caused by the mutation and reduces the overall translation rate below the minimal level required for normal cellular function.

A second pathogenic mutation that could predispose to aminoglycoside ototoxicity has been identified in an Italian family, of whom five members became deaf after aminoglycoside exposure (62). In the mitochondrial 12S ribosomal RNA gene, the deletion of nucleotide 961 thymidine was associated with a varying number of inserted cytosines. Transient evoked otoacoustic emission has been suggested as a sensitive measure for the early effects of aminoglycosides on the peripheral auditory system and may be useful as a tool for the prevention of permanent ototoxicity (66).

In a case-control study in 15 children under 33 weeks gestation with significant sensorineural hearing loss and 30 matched controls, the children with sensorineural hearing loss had longer periods of intubation, ventilation, oxygen treatment, and acidosis, and more frequent treatment with dopamine or furosemide (67). However, neither peak nor trough aminoglycoside concentrations, nor duration of jaundice or bilirubin concentration varied between the groups. At 12 months of age, seven of the children with sensorineural hearing loss had evidence of cerebral palsy compared with two of the 30 controls. Therefore, preterm children with sensorineural hearing loss required more intensive care in the perinatal period and developed more neurological complications than controls, and the co-existence of susceptibility factors for hearing loss may be more important than the individual factors themselves.

Diagnosis
To recognize auditory damage at an early stage and avoid severe irreversible toxicity, repeated tests of cochlear and vestibular function should be carried out in all patients needing prolonged aminoglycoside treatment. Pure-tone audiometry at 250–8000 Hz and electronystagmography with caloric testing are the standard methods. The first detectable audiometric changes usually occur in the high-tone range (over 4000 Hz) and then progress to lower frequencies. Hearing loss of more than 15 db is usually considered as evidence of toxicity. Brainstem auditory-evoked potentials have been recommended as a means of monitoring ototoxicity in uncooperative, comatose patients (68,69). This technique is time-consuming and requires some expertise, but may become a useful tool for detecting damage at an early stage. It also provides information on pre-existing changes, which is otherwise rarely available in intensive care patients (69).

Prevention
In rats, ototoxicity caused by gentamicin or tobramycin was ameliorated by melatonin, which did not interfere with the antibiotic action of the aminoglycosides (70). The free radical scavenging agent alpha-lipoic acid has previously been shown to protect against the cochlear adverse effects of systemically administered aminoglycoside antibiotics, and in a recent animal study it also prevented cochlear toxicity after the administration of neomycin 5% directly to the round window membrane over 7 days (71).

Loss of spiral ganglion neurons can be prevented by neurotrophin 3, whereas hair cell damage can be prevented by N-methyl-D-aspartate (NMDA) receptor antagonists. In an animal study, an NMDA receptor antagonist (MK801) protected against noise-induced excitotoxicity in the cochlea; in addition, combined treatment with neurotrophin 3 and MK801 had a potent effect in preserving both auditory physiology and morphology against aminoglycoside toxicity induced by amikacin (72).

Metabolism

Aminoglycosides can stimulate the formation of reactive oxygen species (free radicals) both in biological and cell-free systems (73,74).

Electrolyte balance

Aminoglycoside-induced proximal tubular dysfunction, which causes some manifestations of Fanconi's syndrome, including electrolyte abnormalities, is rare.

- A 72-year-old man was treated with ceftriaxone (2 g bd) and gentamicin (80 mg tds) for a severe urinary tract infection (75). On day 5 his serum potassium concentration was 3 mmol/l with a normal serum creatinine and urine examination. Despite treatment with oral potassium chloride plus a high potassium diet, his serum potassium fell to 2.3 mmol/l 4 days later, accompanied by inappropriate kaliuresis, hypouricemia with inappropriate uricosuria, and hypophosphatemia with inappropriate phosphaturia. There was no bicarbonate wasting, but there was proteinuria 1.2 g/day, with a predominance of low molecular weight proteins; in contrast, serum creatinine was normal and creatinine clearance was 78 ml/minute. The aminoglycoside was withdrawn with subsequent progressive improvement in renal proximal tubular function, which normalized 9 days later.

Mineral balance

Hypomagnesemia is a well-recognized adverse effect of treatment with various drugs, including aminoglycosides (SEDA-16, 279). Gentamicin-induced magnesium depletion is most likely to occur in older patients when large doses are used over long periods of time (76). Under these circumstances, serum concentrations and urinary electrolyte losses should be monitored.

Metal metabolism

Aminoglycosides can cause renal magnesium wasting and hypomagnesemia, usually associated with acute renal insufficiency. However, animal studies have shown frequent renal magnesium wasting, even in the absence of renal insufficiency and abnormalities of renal tubular morphology. In 24 patients with cystic fibrosis, treatment with amikacin plus ceftazidime for exacerbation of pulmonary symptoms by *Pseudomonas aeruginosa* resulted in mild hypomagnesemia due to renal magnesium wasting, even in the absence of a significant rise in circulating creatinine and urea concentrations (77).

In five healthy volunteers gentamicin 5 mg/kg caused immediate but transient renal calcium and magnesium wasting (78).

Reversible hypokalemic metabolic alkalosis and hypomagnesemia can occur with gentamicin, and routine monitoring has been recommended (79).

The results of an in vitro study on immortalized mouse distal convoluted tubule cells have suggested that aminoglycosides act through an extracellular polyvalent cation-sensing receptor and that they inhibit hormone-stimulated magnesium absorption in the distal convoluted tubule (80).

In children with cystic fibrosis, aminoglycosides can cause hypomagnesemia due to excessive renal loss (81).

Hematologic

In an in vitro study both gentamicin sulfate and netilmicin sulfate showed competitive inhibition of glucose-6-phosphate dehydrogenase from human erythrocytes, whereas streptomycin sulfate showed non-competitive inhibition (82).

Liver

Certain aminoglycosides affect liver function tests. Increases in alkaline phosphatase after gentamicin and tobramycin have been described.

Urinary tract

Impairment of kidney function is a major adverse effect of the aminoglycoside antibiotics. In a survey of the use of antibiotics in a surgical service, aminoglycosides were given to 26 patients, of whom four developed nephrotoxicity (83).

In patients undergoing peritoneal dialysis, intraperitoneal or intravenous aminoglycosides can increase the rapidity of the fall in residual renal function. In an observational, non-randomized study, 72 patients on peritoneal dialysis were followed for 4 years (84). Patients who had been treated for peritonitis with intraperitoneal or intravenous aminoglycosides for more than 3 days had a more rapid fall in renal creatinine clearance and a more rapid fall in daily urine volume than patients without peritonitis or patients treated for peritonitis with antibiotics other than aminoglycosides. However, the use of other nephrotoxins or agents that may improve renal function was not quantified.

Incidence

Impairment of kidney function in different studies is highly variable. It depends on the study population and the definition of toxicity, and can range from a few percent to more than 30% in severely ill patients (85,86).

In a retrospective study, the rate of nephrotoxicity at the end of treatment with aminoglycosides was 7.5% (kanamycin 4.5%) (24). Patients who developed nephrotoxicity had a longer duration of treatment and received larger total doses.

Susceptibility factors

As in the case of ototoxicity, certain susceptibility factors have been identified for nephrotoxicity (87,88). Total dose, age, abnormal initial creatinine clearance, the 1-hour post-dose and trough aminoglycoside serum concentrations, duration of treatment, and co-existent liver disease were predictors of subsequent kidney damage. However, the clinical significance and utility of predictive nomograms based on such risk factors have been challenged (89). Other factors, such as dehydration, hypovolemia, potassium and magnesium depletion, and sepsis are also important. Gentamicin nephrotoxicity is increased in biliary obstruction (SEDA-20, 235). Nephrotoxicity is potentiated by ACE inhibitors, cephalosporins, ciclosporin, cisplatin, loop diuretics (secondary to volume depletion), methoxyflurane, non-steroidal anti-inflammatory drugs, and any basic amino acid such as lysine. Additional factors, such as previous aminoglycoside exposure, metabolic acidosis, female sex, and diabetes mellitus, are less clearly associated with renal damage (90,91).

In a prospective, non-interventional surveillance study of 249 patients receiving a once-daily aminoglycoside

(17% amikacin and 83% gentamicin), serum creatinine increased by more than 50% in 12%; none developed oliguric renal insufficiency (92). Renal damage correlated significantly with: a high aminoglycoside trough concentration (over 1.1 µg/ml); a hemoglobin concentration below 10 g/dl; hospital admission for more than 7 days before aminoglycoside treatment; and aminoglycoside treatment for more than 11 days.

Mechanism

The mechanism of nephrotoxicity has been studied in vitro, in animals, and in man. The data suggest that accumulation of aminoglycosides in the renal cortex is an important reason for functional damage. In addition, aminoglycoside-induced alterations of glomerular ultrastructure have been described (93). Tissue uptake is predominantly mediated by proximal tubular reabsorption of the filtered drug. The degree of renal injury caused by an aminoglycoside correlates with the amount of drug that accumulates in the renal cortex. However, intrinsic toxicity differs among the aminoglycosides. Endotoxins can increase intracortical accumulation (94). After the drug binds to an amino acid receptor site, there is pinocytotic entry into the tubular cells. Once the drug is within the cell, it persists there for a long time and is liberated only slowly, with a half-life of several days (95,96). Direct toxicity to tubular cells is mainly explained by inhibition of lysosomal activity, with accumulation of lamellar myeloid bodies consisting of phospholipids. Inhibition of lysosomal phospholipids can also be shown in purified liposomes in vitro (97). In renal biopsy specimens, vacuolization of the proximal tubular epithelium, clumped nuclear chromatin, and swollen mitochondria are seen. Patchy tubular cell necrosis, desquamation, and luminal obstruction are found at later stages.

The uptake of aminoglycosides into proximal renal tubular epithelial cells is limited to the luminal cell border and is saturable. Less frequent administration of doses larger than needed for saturation of this uptake may therefore reduce drug accumulation in the renal cortex (98). In vitro and in vivo data have provided evidence that partially reduced oxygen metabolites (superoxide anion, hydrogen peroxide, and hydroxyl radical), which are generated by renal cortical mitochondria, are important mediators of aminoglycoside-induced acute renal insufficiency (99).

A lipopeptide, daptomycin, which has bactericidal activity against Gram-positive bacteria by inhibition of the synthesis of lipoteichonic acid, prevents tobramycin-induced nephrotoxicity in rats. Fourier transformed infrared spectroscopy has been used to monitor the hydrolysis of phosphatidylcholine phospholipase A_2 in the presence of different aminoglycosides and/or daptomycin (100). Among the various aminoglycosides investigated there were major differences, directly related to chemical structure. The number of charges, the size, and the hydrophobicity of the substituents of an aminoglycoside determined the influence on the lag phase, on the maximal rate, and on the final extent of hydrolysis. Daptomycin alone eliminated the initial latency period, and reduced the maximal extent of hydrolysis. When daptomycin was combined with any of the aminoglycosides, the latency period also disappeared, but the phospholipase activity was higher than with the lipopeptide alone. The strongest activation of phospholipase A_2 activation was observed when daptomycin was combined with gentamicin.

Stress proteins seem to be actively involved in aminoglycoside-induced renal damage. In a study in Wistar rats, subcutaneous gentamicin caused tubular necrosis, followed by tubular regenerative changes and interstitial fibrosis (101). Both the regenerated and phenotypically altered tubulointerstitial cells were found to express heat-shock protein 47 in and around the fibrosis. Increased shedding of tubular membrane components, followed by rapid inductive repair processes with overshoot protein synthesis, can be detected by analysis of tubular marker protein in the urine of rats after administration of aminoglycosides (102).

Prevention

In a prospective, randomized, double-blind study of once-daily versus twice-daily aminoglycoside therapy in 123 patients (of whom 83 received treatment for over 72 hours), once-daily administration of aminoglycosides had a predictably lower probability of causing nephrotoxicity than twice-daily administration. In a Kaplan–Meier analysis, once-daily dosing provided a longer time of administration until the threshold for nephrotoxicity was met. The risk of nephrotoxicity was modulated by the daily AUC for aminoglycoside exposure, and the concurrent use of vancomycin significantly increased the probability of nephrotoxicity and shortened the time to its occurrence (98). In another study, once-daily aminoglycoside in 200 patients was prospectively compared with a retrospectively evaluated group of 100 patients treated with individualized traditional dosing. Patients with a baseline creatinine clearance below 40 ml/minute, meningitis, burns, spinal cord injury, endocarditis, or enterococcal infection were excluded. Clinical and microbial outcome was similar in the two groups. Nephrotoxicity occurred in 7.5% of the patients treated with once-daily aminoglycosides compared with 14% of the others. The cumulative AUC was significantly larger in patients on traditional dosing. Minimum serum concentrations, length of aminoglycoside therapy, and AUC over 24 hours were related to nephrotoxicity. Whereas vancomycin and concurrent nephrotoxic agents were independently related to toxicity, sex and age were not (103).

Careful tailoring of the dose can prevent nephrotoxicity. In 89 critically ill patients with a creatinine clearance over 30 ml/minute who were treated with gentamicin or tobramycin 7 mg/kg/day independent of renal function, with subsequent doses chosen on the basis of the pharmacokinetics of the first dose, signs of renal impairment occurred in 14%; in all survivors renal function recovered completely and hemofiltration was not needed (104).

Presentation and diagnosis

Nephrotoxicity can present as acute tubular necrosis or, more commonly, as gradually evolving non-oliguric renal failure. The time-course of toxicity is variable, but it usually develops only after several days of treatment. Early diagnosis is difficult, since there can be a reduction in glomerular filtration before a significant rise in serum creatinine concentration occurs (105). An increased number of casts in the urinary sediment can also precede the increase in serum creatinine (106). Measurement of phospholipids and urinary enzymes, such as beta$_2$-microglobulin or alanine aminopeptidase, has been proposed as a means of detecting early toxicity (107–109). However, data on these enzymes are not very useful, since they can be increased for various other reasons and raised concentrations do not reliably predict pending renal toxicity. Fortunately, recovery of renal function nearly always follows the withdrawal of aminoglycosides, although serum creatinine concentrations can continue to rise for several days after the last dose.

There is an increase in the urinary output of tubular marker proteins after aminoglycoside administration (102). Determination of *N*-acetyl-beta-D-glucosaminidase activity in the urine may be used as a screening test to facilitate early detection of the nephrotoxic effect of aminoglycosides (110). Urine chemiluminescence may aid in the detection of neonatal aminoglycoside-induced nephropathy (111).

Relative potency of different aminoglycosides

The nephrotoxicity of the various aminoglycosides has been compared in many animal experiments. The order of relative nephrotoxicity is as follows: neomycin > gentamicin > tobramycin > amikacin > netilmicin (112,113). However, in man conclusive data on the relative toxicity of the various aminoglycosides is still lacking. An analysis of 24 controlled trials showed the following average rates for nephrotoxicity: gentamicin 11%; tobramycin 11.5%; amikacin 8.5%; and netilmicin 2.8% (28). In contrast to this survey, direct comparison in similar patient groups showed no significant differences between the various agents in most trials (14,15,114–118). In fact, the relative advantage of lower nephrotoxicity rates observed with netilmicin in some studies may be limited to administration of low doses. In a prospective study there was significantly lower nephrotoxicity with amikacin 15 mg/kg/day (4% toxicity) compared with netilmicin 7 mg/kg/day (12%) (119). One prospective trial showed a significant advantage of tobramycin over gentamicin (120). However, these findings were not subsequently confirmed (121). Nephrotoxicity is a serious risk with all the currently available aminoglycoside antibiotics, and no drug in this series can be regarded as safe.

Skin

It is generally accepted that antibiotics that are important for systemic use should not be administered topically. This rule applies particularly to the aminoglycoside antibiotics. Even though neomycin and streptomycin are no longer often used systemically, the frequency of sensitization after topical administration of these drugs is particularly high.

Contact dermatitis due to arbekacin has been reported (122). The risk of sensitization by topically administered gentamicin seems to be smaller. Nevertheless, and in order to avoid resistance, topical use should be restricted to life-endangering thermal burns and to severe skin infections in which strains of *Pseudomonas* resistant to other antibiotics are involved.

Immunologic

In a prospective study of the results of skin patch testing in 149 patients who were scheduled for ear surgery, 14% of the patients had a positive skin reaction to one of the aminoglycosides (13% for gentamicin, 13% for neomycin) (123). In 16% of the patients with chronic otitis media and 6.7% of the patients with otosclerosis there was allergy to one of the aminoglycosides commonly found in antibiotic ear-drops. Patients who had previously received more than five courses of antibiotic ear-drops had a greater tendency to develop allergy to the aminoglycosides (35%).

Cross-reactivity between aminoglycoside antibiotics has long been known. Aminoglycoside antibiotics can be categorized in two groups, depending on the aminocycolitol nucleus: streptidine (streptomycin) and deoxystreptamine (neomycin, kanamycin, gentamicin, paromomycin, spectinomycin, and tobramycin). Another antigenic determinant is neosamine, a diamino sugar present in neomycin and, with minor changes, also in paromomycin, kanamycin, tobramycin, amikacin, and isepamicin. Streptomycin shares no common antigenic structures with the other aminoglycoside antibiotics, and cross-sensitivity with streptomycin has not been reported. Acute contact dermatitis was described in a 30-year-old man after rechallenge with gentamicin 80 mg; a patch test was positive for gentamicin, neomycin, and amikacin (124).

Occasional cases of anaphylactic shock have been reported, most of which have been due to streptomycin; other aminoglycosides have rarely been implicated, such as gentamicin (125,126) and neomycin (127).

Long-Term Effects

Drug resistance

During treatment of infections with either Gram-negative or Gram-positive bacteria, resistant subpopulations emerge, unless the peak to MIC ratio is high enough to reduce the bacterial inoculum drastically within a few hours (128). Similarly, rapid emergence of resistant subpopulations has been reported during aminoglycoside treatment in neutropenic animals. The virulence and clinical relevance of the relatively slow-growing resistant subpopulations (small colony variants) have been documented in both animal and clinical studies (129,130). Resistant subpopulations can be detected only by direct plating of specimens on aminoglycoside-containing agar plates, since resistance may be lost within one subculture. Combination therapy of an aminoglycoside plus a beta-lactam antibiotic has been successfully used to prevent selection of resistant subpopulations (131).

In a prospective surveillance study in France, the development of resistance to aminoglycosides and fluoroquinolones among Gram negative bacilli was assessed in 51 patients with a second infection due to Gram negative organisms at least 8 days after a first Gram negative infection (132). Treatment of the first infection with a beta-lactam antibiotic plus an aminoglycoside significantly reduced the susceptibility to amikacin (the most prescribed antibiotic). When the first infection was treated with a beta-lactam plus a fluoroquinolone, susceptibility to ciprofloxacin, pefloxacin, netilmicin, and tobramycin, but not gentamicin and amikacin, fell significantly.

A multidrug efflux system that appears to be a major contributor to intrinsic high-level resistance to aminoglycosides and macrolides has been identified in *Burkholderia pseudomallei* (133).

Out of 1102 consecutive clinical Gram negative blood isolates from Belgium and Luxembourg, 157 were "not susceptible" to aminoglycosides (134). The resistance levels were 5.9% for gentamicin, 7.7% for tobramycin, 7.5% for netilmicin, 2.8% for amikacin, and 1.2% for isepamicin. In a large European multinational study on 7057 Gram negative bacterial isolates, resistance levels were 0.4–3% for amikacin, 2–13% for gentamicin, and 2.5–15% for tobramycin among Enterobacteriaceae; 75% of *Staphylococcus aureus* isolates, but only 21% of enterococcal strains were susceptible to gentamicin (135). In a study from Spain, 9% of 1014 clinical *P. aeruginosa* isolates were resistant to amikacin or tobramycin (136). In the same country, resistance to amikacin rose from 21% to 84% and to tobramycin from 33% to 72% between 1991 and 1996 (137).

In a leading cancer center in Houston, 24% of 758 Gram negative clinical isolates were resistant to tobramycin and 12% were resistant to amikacin (138). In 3144 bacterial isolates causing urinary tract infections in Chile, 74% were identified as *Escherichia coli*; 4.2% of these strains were resistant to gentamicin, and 1.3% were resistant to amikacin (139). In contrast, the resistance levels were 30% and 17% respectively, in the other enterobacterial strains. In Brazil, all isolates of methicillin-resistant *S. aureus* were also resistant to gentamicin, amikacin, kanamycin, neomycin, and tobramycin (140), and 97% of such strains from Spain were resistant to tobramycin (141).

In mice, the bacterial neomycin phosphotransferase gene, which confers resistance to aminoglycoside antibiotics, prevented the loss of hair cells after neomycin treatment (142).

In in vitro susceptibility studies on 99 clinical isolates of *S. aureus*, 68 of 73 strains of methicillin-resistant *S. aureus* (MRSA) and two of 26 strains of methicillin-susceptible *S. aureus* were gentamicin-resistant (143). However, the combination of arbekacin plus vancomycin produced synergistic killing against 12 of 13 gentamicin-resistant MRSA isolates. Combinations of meropenem and aminoglycosides may be effective against strains of *P. aeruginosa* that are resistant to meropenem at clinically relevant concentrations; synergistic effects were observed in combinations that included arbekacin or amikacin (144).

Second-Generation Effects

Teratogenicity

During pregnancy the aminoglycosides cross the placenta and might theoretically be expected to cause otological and perhaps nephrological damage in the fetus. However, no proven cases of intrauterine damage by gentamicin and tobramycin have been recorded. In 135 mother/child pairs exposed to streptomycin during the first 4 months of pregnancy, there was no increase in the risk of any malformation (145). However, streptomycin and dihydrostreptomycin have caused severe otological damage (146).

Using the population-based dataset of the Hungarian Case-Control Surveillance of Congenital Abnormalities (1980–96), which includes 38 151 pregnant women who had newborn infants without any defects and 22 865 pregnant women who had fetuses or newborns with congenital abnormalities, no teratogenic risk of parenteral gentamicin, streptomycin, tobramycin, or oral neomycin was discovered when restricted to structural developmental disturbances (147).

Susceptibility Factors

Age

In a prospective study on the prevalence of hearing impairment in a neonatal intensive care unit population (a total of 942 neonates were screened), aminoglycoside administration did not seem to be an important risk factor for communication-related hearing impairment (148). In almost all cases, another factor was the more probable cause of the hearing loss (dysmorphism, prenatal rubella or cytomegaly, a positive family history of hearing loss, and severe perinatal and postnatal complications).

Other features of the patient

The main susceptibility factors are summarized in Table 2. The most important factors are renal insufficiency, high serum drug concentrations, and a long duration of treatment (54).

Drug Administration

Drug dosage regimens

Twice-daily or thrice-daily administration was for a long time standard in aminoglycoside therapy of systemic bacterial infections in patients with normal renal function. However, in vitro, in vivo, and clinical studies have suggested that once-daily dosing of the same total daily dose might be more beneficial with respect to both efficacy and toxicity (SEDA-21, 265) (149–152).

Less frequent administration of higher doses results in higher peak concentrations. Owing to the pronounced concentration dependence of bacterial killing, higher peaks potentiate the efficacy of the aminoglycosides. The importance of a high ratio of peak concentration to the minimal inhibitory concentration (MIC) has been shown in vitro for both bactericidal activity and prevention of the emergence of resistance (153). Clinically the predictive value of the peak to MIC ratio has been documented for aminoglycoside therapy of Gram-negative bacteremia (154). Although once-daily dosing can result in prolonged periods of subinhibitory concentrations, bacterial regrowth does not occur immediately after the aminoglycoside concentration drops below the MIC. The term "post-antibiotic effect" has been suggested to describe this hit-and-run effect, in which there is persistent suppression of bacterial regrowth after cessation of exposure of bacteria to an active antibiotic. This phenomenon has been observed both in vitro and in vivo (155).

Various in vivo models have been used to study the effect of the dosage regimen on aminoglycoside nephrotoxicity and ototoxicity. Renal uptake of aminoglycosides is not proportional to serum concentration, because of saturation at the high concentrations achieved with once-daily regimens. The degree of renal injury increases the more often the aminoglycoside is given in humans, dogs, rabbits, guinea-pigs, and rats, as long as the total daily dose is kept constant (156,157). Early auditory alterations also occur more often, or to a greater extent, the more often the aminoglycoside is given.

Once-daily regimens have been compared with multiple-daily regimens in at least 27 randomized clinical trials and eight meta-analyses and in a mega-analysis of meta-analyses (158). In all the studies, extended-interval dosing was at least as efficacious as multiple-daily dosing, and may have been slightly better; it was no more toxic, and may have been less nephrotoxic. Extended dosing is also less expensive than multiple-daily dosing and markedly reduces costs. An analysis of 24 randomized clinical trials of amikacin, gentamicin, and netilmicin, including 3181 patients, showed superior results with once-daily regimens with respect to clinical efficacy (90 versus 85%) and bacteriological efficacy (89 versus 83%) (151). There were no statistically significant differences for toxicity. Nevertheless, both nephrotoxicity and ototoxicity occurred less often during once-daily dosing (4.5 versus 5.5% and 4.2 versus 5.8% respectively). Finally, once-daily dosing is more economical, since less nursing time and infusion material are required and drug monitoring can be reduced. In conclusion, amikacin, gentamicin, and netilmicin can be given once a day.

In a randomized trial in 249 patients with suspected or proven serious infections, the safety and efficacy of gentamicin once-daily compared with three-times-a-day was assessed in 175 patients who were treated with ticarcillin–clavulanate combined with gentamicin once-daily or three times daily or with ticarcillin–clavulanate alone (159). The achievement of protocol-defined peak serum gentamicin concentrations was required for evaluability. There were no significant differences between treatment regimens with respect to clinical or microbiological efficacy; the incidence of nephrotoxicity was similar in the three groups. In a post-hoc analysis, renal function was better preserved in those treated with gentamicin once a day plus ticarcillin + clavulanate than ticarcillin + clavulanate only.

Once-daily amikacin was as effective and safe as twice-daily dosing in a prospective randomized study in 142 adults with systemic infections (160).

In 43 patients, once-daily tobramycin (4 mg/kg/day) was at least as effective and was no more and possibly even less toxic than a twice-daily regimen (161).

The pharmacokinetics of once-daily intravenous tobramycin have been investigated in seven children with cystic fibrosis (162). All responded well. There was one case of transient ototoxicity but no nephrotoxicity.

In a prospective study, only increasing duration of once-daily aminoglycoside therapy was recognized as risk factor for toxicity in 88 patients aged 70 years and over (163).

In controlled trials of once-daily aminoglycoside regimens patients with endocarditis have often been excluded, and therefore few clinical data are available on this topic. Based on pharmacokinetic data in experimental endocarditis and integrative computer modeling, it has been hypothesized that drug penetration into vegetations would be enhanced by once-daily aminoglycoside administration, resulting in a long residence time in the vegetations and a beneficial effect in providing synergistic bactericidal action in combination with another antibiotic (164). With the exception of two early studies using enterococci, results from animal studies have been promising in once-daily aminoglycoside treatment of endocarditis. Only two human studies of once-daily aminoglycoside therapy in streptococcal endocarditis were identified. The regimen was efficacious and safe. The authors concluded that there appeared to be sufficient promising evidence to justify large trials to further investigate once-daily aminoglycoside in the treatment of endocarditis due to viridans streptococci, whereas more preliminary investigations were needed for enterococcal endocarditis.

Once-daily dosing regimens of aminoglycosides are routinely used in critically ill patients with trauma, although there is a marked variability in pharmacokinetics in these patients, eventually leading to prolonged drug-free intervals, and individualized dosing on the basis of at least two serum aminoglycoside concentrations can be recommended when once-daily dosing regimens are chosen (165).

Not all populations of patients have been included or extensively studied in published trials. Therefore, conventional multiple-daily aminoglycoside dosing with individualized monitoring should be used in neonates and children, in patients with moderate to severe renal insufficiency (creatinine clearance below 40 ml/minute), serious burns (over 20% of body surface area), ascites, severe sepsis, endocarditis, and mycobacterial disease, in pregnancy, in patients on dialysis, in invasive *P. aeruginosa* infection in neutropenic patients, and with concomitant administration of other nephrotoxic agents (for example amphotericin, cisplatin, radiocontrast agents, and NSAIDs). Extended-interval aminoglycoside dosing may be safe and efficacious in patients with mild to moderate renal insufficiency (over 40 ml/minute) and febrile neutropenia, especially where the prevalence of *P. aeruginosa* is low. In other serious Gram-negative infections warranting aminoglycoside treatment, extended-interval dosing is strongly suggested (166).

Drug administration route

Intraocular

Aminoglycosides are often used in ophthalmology to treat or to prevent bacterial infections, and they can be toxic to retinal structures if high concentrations are reached in the vitreous. Retinal ultrastructure was examined at various intervals after a single intravitreal injection of 100–4000 µg of gentamicin into rabbit eyes. Three days after injection of 100–500 µg, numerous abnormal lamellar lysosomal inclusions were observed in the retinal pigment epithelium and in macrophages in the subretinal space. These changes were typical of drug-induced lipid storage and were comparable to inclusions reported in kidney and other tissues as manifestations of gentamicin toxicity. One week after similar injections, focal areas of retinal pigment epithelium necrosis and hyperplasia with disruption of outer segments appeared, but the inner segments and the inner retina were intact. Doses of 800–4000 µg produced a combined picture of lipidosis of the retinal pigment epithelium and macrophages within the first 3 days, with increasing superimposed inner retinal necrosis (167).

Intratympanic

Intratympanic gentamicin therapy has gained some popularity in the treatment of vertigo associated with Menière's disease, as it offers some advantages over traditional surgical treatment. However, although the vestibulotoxic effect of gentamicin is well documented, there is no general agreement about the dose needed to control attacks of vertigo without affecting hearing. In 27 patients treated with small doses of gentamicin delivered via a microcatheter in the round window niche and administered by an electronic micropump, vertigo was effectively controlled; however, the negative effect on hearing was unacceptable (168,169).

Intraperitoneal

Bolus intraperitoneal gentamicin or tobramycin (5 mg/kg ideal body weight) is safe, achieves therapeutic blood concentrations for extended intervals, causes no clinical ototoxicity or vestibular toxicity, is cost-effective, and is convenient for patients and nurses (170).

Drug overdose

Although aminoglycoside antibiotics are dialysable, peritoneal dialysis may not remove aminoglycosides from the blood after overdosage (171). However, hemodialysis is effective (172). In one study in eight patients hemodiafiltration removed more netilmicin than conventional hemodialysis (173).

Drug–Drug Interactions

Cephalosporins

There are many reports of acute renal insufficiency from combined treatment with gentamicin (or another aminoglycoside) and one of the cephalosporins (174–176). The potential nephrotoxic effect of the combinations seems to be related mainly to the nephrotoxic effect of the aminoglycosides. In contrast, there is some evidence, both experimental (177) and clinical (178), that ticarcillin may attenuate the renal toxicity of the aminoglycosides.

Cisplatin/carboplatin

The nephrotoxic and ototoxic effects of cisplatin and carboplatin can be potentiated by concurrent administration of aminoglycosides, as shown in animals (179).

Loop diuretics

Among the agents that promote the nephrotoxic effects of the aminoglycosides, the loop diuretics furosemide and etacrynic acid are often mentioned. However, this interaction is by no means clearly established (26). These agents are not nephrotoxic in themselves. This supposed interaction may only be a consequence of sodium and volume depletion. Other types of diuretics, such as mannitol, hydrochlorothiazide, and acetazolamide, do not produce this interaction (26).

- A 60-year-old white woman developed ototoxicity after only 5 days of gentamicin therapy (500 mg, 6.8 mg/kg/day) and one dose of furosemide 20 mg (180).

Loop diuretics greatly potentiate the cochleotoxic effects of aminoglycosides (181). In pigmented guinea-pigs the effects of high-dose topical (10 µl of a 100 mg/ml solution directly on to the round window) or single-dose systemic (100 mg/kg) gentamicin and intracardiac administration of the loop diuretic etacrynic acid (40 mg/kg) on cochlear function have been studied (182). Compound action potentials were elicited at 8 kHz. All animals that received etacrynic acid had an immediate and profound rise in hearing threshold, irrespective of the method of gentamicin administration. The maximum threshold shift occurred within 30 minutes. Animals that received topical gentamicin recovered after etacrynic acid treatment; by day 20 the mean threshold shift was 7 dB. This group did not differ statistically from animals that received etacrynic acid alone. In contrast, animals that received systemic gentamicin initially recovered within 2 hours after etacrynic acid, but subsequently deteriorated over the next 24 hours. The mean threshold shift was 70 dB at day 20. Animals that received topical gentamicin had a temporary shift that resolved within 24–48 hours; by day 20, the mean threshold shift was 7 dB. Animals treated with systemic gentamicin alone did not have hearing loss. This study suggests that the potentiating effect of etacrynic acid on aminoglycoside ototoxicity is only after systematic and not topical aminoglycoside administration. This may be due to an etacrynic acid-induced increase in leakiness of the stria vascularis, thereby facilitating diffusion of aminoglycosides from the systemic circulation into the endolymphatic fluid.

Neuromuscular blocking drugs

The aminoglycosides have a curare-like action, which can be antagonized by calcium ions and acetylcholinesterase inhibitors (8). In patients who require general anesthesia, the effect of muscle relaxants, such as D-tubocurarine, pancuronium, and suxamethonium, can be potentiated by aminoglycosides (183).

Penicillins

There is an in vitro interaction between aminoglycoside antibiotics and carbenicillin or ticarcillin, leading to a significant loss of aminoglycoside antibacterial activity if these antibiotics are mixed in the same infusion bottle (184). The extent of inactivation depends on the penicillin concentration, the contact time, and the temperature. Azlocillin and mezlocillin inactivate aminoglycosides in a similar manner to that described for carbenicillin (185,186). Aminoglycosides should not be mixed with penicillins or cephalosporins in the same infusion bottle.

However, the clinical significance of the presence of both types of antibiotics in the patient is debatable. In patients who received a combination of gentamicin and carbenicillin the measured serum gentamicin concentrations were lower than the pharmacokinetically predicted values (187). This interaction may be especially important in patients with severe renal impairment, in whom long in vivo incubation of these drug combinations takes place before supplemental doses of the aminoglycoside drugs are given.

Vancomycin

Combined use of vancomycin and an aminoglycoside can increase the risk of toxicity (188–190).

Monitoring Therapy

Serum concentrations have often been monitored during multiple-daily dosing of aminoglycosides, particularly when high doses are used and also during prolonged therapy. The main goals of individual dosing and monitoring are to reach high bactericidal drug concentrations and to avoid drug accumulation in the serum, to minimize the risk of toxicity. Since both goals are much more likely to be met with once-daily dosing it may be feasible to reduce monitoring efforts during such dosing regimens. However, more clinical experience needs to be accumulated to establish solid guidelines for monitoring once-daily dosing regimens. Although more clinicians are nowadays switching to once-daily dosing of aminoglycosides, some continue to use multiple-daily regimens. Therefore, two separate concepts of aminoglycoside monitoring have to be considered, depending on the dosing schedule.

In a retrospective case-control study, 2405 patients received aminoglycosides in doses that were decided either by individualized pharmacokinetic monitoring or by the physician (191). Those who received individualized pharmacokinetic monitoring were significantly less likely to develop aminoglycoside-associated nephrotoxicity. Women were also less likely to develop nephrotoxicity. Age 50 years and above, high initial aminoglycoside trough concentration, long duration of therapy, and concurrent therapy with piperacillin, clindamycin, or vancomycin increased the risk.

Monitoring multiple-daily dosing regimens

Peak serum concentrations of gentamicin and tobramycin over 5–7 μg/ml and of amikacin over 20–28 μg/ml are associated with improved survival in patients with septicemia and pneumonia caused by Gram-negative bacteria (192,193). On the other hand, excessive peak concentrations (over 10–12 μg/ml) and trough concentrations (over 2 μg/ml) of gentamicin and tobramycin increase the risk of ototoxicity and nephrotoxicity (194). Dosage requirements to obtain aminoglycoside concentrations in the target range can differ considerably, even in patients with normal renal function (195). Owing to the great individual variability in pharmacokinetics, dosage adjustments with the commonly used nomograms often result in suboptimal or potentially toxic aminoglycoside concentrations (196). An individualized treatment based on serum concentration monitoring is therefore necessary to achieve maximum bactericidal efficacy without a

concomitant high risk of adverse reactions. Measurements of peak and trough serum concentrations should be carried out during the first 24–48 hours in all patients and repeated after 3–5 days to detect any tendency to abnormal drug accumulation. However, one must realize that close monitoring alone cannot completely eliminate the danger of ototoxicity and nephrotoxicity, since aminoglycoside drug concentrations progressively increase in renal tissue and in the inner ear with repeated administration, even if optimum serum concentrations are maintained.

The relation between serum concentration of aminoglycosides and the two clinically important adverse effects, ototoxicity and nephrotoxicity, has been debated for many years. Whereas some authors have found a definite relation between the frequency of adverse effects and serum concentrations, others have not (194). This controversy can be partly explained by the pharmacokinetic behavior common to all aminoglycosides, which leads to drug accumulation in deep compartments, particularly in the renal cortex. Assuming that the extent of accumulation is a factor that relates to the frequency of adverse effects, it is not surprising to find a correlation between serum concentrations and toxicity in one group of patients but not in another. The amount accumulated depends not only on the dosing schedule and the serum concentration achieved during treatment, but also on the duration of drug administration. The same concentration in the same patient can be associated with a significantly different amount of drug in the body, depending on whether it was sampled during the second or the tenth day after the beginning of treatment.

In a survey of aminoglycoside treatment in 2022 patients in Saudi Arabia, 8.8%, 18%, and 12% had trough concentrations considered toxic for amikacin, gentamicin, and tobramycin respectively, whereas there were peak serum drug concentrations in the subtherapeutic range in 53%, 50%, and 57% respectively (197). Toxic concentrations were noticed mainly in patients aged over 60 years and in patients in the intensive care unit, coronary care unit, and burn unit.

Monitoring once-daily dosing regimens

In general, both peak and trough concentrations are determined during monitoring of multiple-daily dosing regimens, and doses are subsequently adjusted to achieve the target concentrations. However, peak and trough concentrations do not necessarily offer the most valuable information for dosage adjustments during once-daily dosing. The indication and frequency of monitoring and the timing of serum concentrations within the interval, along with their target ranges, have yet to be established. Different targets have been proposed and used clinically (198–200), including mid-dosage interval plasma concentration monitoring as an estimate of the AUC (201).

In one prospective study 8-hour concentrations have been considered for monitoring as an alternative to the measurement of peaks and troughs (202). In 51 adult patients given an average dose of 400 mg once a day, doses were adjusted during therapy if 8-hour concentrations were not within the target range of 1.5–6.0 μg/ml. Concentrations above or below this target range correlated significantly with nephrotoxicity, 24-hour trough concentrations, and AUCs. Determination of 8-hour concentrations was therefore useful for identifying patients with either low AUCs or an increased risk of nephrotoxicity. In other studies, aminoglycoside serum concentrations were determined in the second half of the dosing interval (198,200,203–205). However, trough concentrations do not allow for extrapolations of concentrations achieved in the period after infusion. Thus, patients with very low peak concentrations due to unusually high volumes of distribution cannot be identified. Similarly, very rapid elimination, as frequently happens in patients with burns or children, may not be noticed.

Depending on the goals of drug monitoring, peak 8-, 12- or 24-hour concentrations might be more important (151). Correlations of efficacy with high peak concentrations, high ratios of peak to MIC, and high AUCs suggest that drug concentrations should be determined during the first part of the dosing interval. In order to minimize toxicity, drug accumulation should be avoided. Therefore early detection of increased trough concentrations is of importance. It has been strongly suggested that the threshold values for troughs during once-daily dosing should be lowered, compared with multiple-daily dosing (203,206). To reduce the cost of aminoglycoside therapy, the indications for and frequency of monitoring serum concentrations should be minimal. Instead, serum creatinine concentrations might be used to monitor renal function. The strategy selected for monitoring aminoglycoside therapy must take a number of factors into account, including the type and severity of infection, the duration of therapy, or the presence of factors associated with increased risk of toxicity. In addition, local factors should be considered for the timing of blood samples, including the sensitivity of the drug assay available (207) and the time required for processing the specimens, in order to modify the subsequent dose, if necessary.

Major considerations in determining the appropriate dose of an aminoglycoside are its volume of distribution and rate of clearance. Concern has been raised regarding the use of the Cockcroft–Gault equation with either actual or ideal body weight, resulting in systematic errors, especially in malnourished patients (208). However, even extended-interval dosing should not obviate the need for monitoring drug concentrations. Even in patients with normal renal function in whom treatment is necessary for over 3 days, mid-interval or trough drug concentrations should be obtained once or twice a week to optimize the dosing regimen (166,209).

Economics of serum concentration monitoring

The economic impact of aminoglycoside toxicity and its prevention through therapeutic drug monitoring have been investigated in a cost-effectiveness study. It was estimated that to offset the cost of providing high-level drug monitoring, that is serum drug concentration monitoring with assessment and consultation by trained personnel using computerized resources to determine individualized pharmacokinetic parameters, for the purpose of achieving an optimum dosage regimen, by cost saving due to reducing nephropathy, the service should reduce the risk of nephrotoxicity by 6.6%. Therefore,

high-level therapeutic drug monitoring is only cost-justified in populations in which high rates of nephrotoxicity would be expected. Risk factors for a high rate of nephrotoxicity include age, duration of therapy, high drug concentrations, the presence of ascites or liver disease, and the concomitant use of nephrotoxic drugs (210). The economic significance of aminoglycoside peak concentrations has been assessed in 61 febrile neutropenic patients with hematological malignancies. Since the clinical outcome and average infection-related costs depended significantly on peak aminoglycoside concentration, it was concluded that successful pharmacokinetic intervention may save money (211).

A pharmacy-based active therapeutic drug monitoring service has been examined in a prospective study (63). In the patients that were not monitored, the gentamicin dosage regimen was determined by the physician; in the patients that were monitored, the regimen was calculated using a population model and measured serum gentamicin concentrations. This resulted in significantly different mean dosage intervals: 19 hours in the monitored patients and 14 hours in the others. Active monitoring resulted in higher peak concentrations of aminoglycosides, lower trough concentrations, a reduction in the length of hospitalization, a reduced duration of aminoglycoside therapy, reduced nephrotoxicity, and a trend toward reduced mortality that was significant for patients with an infection on admission. Costs were lower with active monitoring. Although all patients treated with an aminoglycoside profited from active monitoring, it was most beneficial in patients who were admitted to the hospital with a suspected or proven Gram negative infection.

References

1. Brewer NS. Antimicrobial agents—Part II. The aminoglycosides: streptomycin, kanamycin, gentamicin, tobramycin, amikacin, neomycin Mayo Clin Proc 1977;52(11):675–9.
2. Boselli E, Allaouchiche B. Diffusion osseuse des antibiotiques. [Diffusion in bone tissue of antibiotics.] Presse Méd 1999;28(40):2265–76.
3. John JF Jr. What price success? The continuing saga of the toxic:therapeutic ratio in the use of aminoglycoside antibiotics. J Infect Dis 1988;158(1):1–6.
4. Speich R, Imhof E, Vogt M, Grossenbacher M, Zimmerli W. Efficacy, safety, and tolerance of piperacillin/tazobactam compared to co-amoxiclav plus an aminoglycoside in the treatment of severe pneumonia. Eur J Clin Microbiol Infect Dis 1998;17(5):313–17.
5. Beringer PM, Wong-Beringer A, Rho JP. Economic aspects of antibacterial adverse effects. Pharmacoeconomics 1998;13(1 Pt 1):35–49.
6. Martin PD. ECG change associated with streptomycin. Chest 1974;65(4):478.
7. Emery ER. Neuromuscular blocking properties of antibiotics as a cause of post-operative apnoea. Anesthesia 1963;18:57.
8. Adams HR, Mathew BP, Teske RH, Mercer HD. Neuromuscular blocking effects of aminoglycoside antibiotics on fast- and slow-contracting muscles of the cat. Anesth Analg 1976;55(4):500–7.
9. Fiekers JF. Sites and mechanisms of antibiotic-induced neuromuscular block: a pharmacological analysis using quantal content, voltage clamped end-plate currents and

single channel analysis. Acta Physiol Pharmacol Ther Latinoam 1999;49(4):242–50.

10. Holtzman JL. Gentamicin and neuromuscular blockade. Ann Intern Med 1976;84(1):55.

11. Dzoljic M, Atanackovic D. Effect of neomycin on smooth muscle. Arch Int Pharmacodyn Ther 1966;162(2):493–6.

12. Caraffini S, Assalve D, Stingeni L, Lisi P. Allergic contact conjunctivitis and blepharitis from tobramycin. Contact Dermatitis 1995;32(3):186–7.

13. Tange RA. Ototoxicity. Adverse Drug React Toxicol Rev 1998;17(2–3):75–89.

14. Feld R, Valdivieso M, Bodey GP, Rodriguez V. Comparison of amikacin and tobramycin in the treatment of infection in patients with cancer. J Infect Dis 1977;135(1):61–6.

15. Barza M, Lauermann MW, Tally FP, Gorbach SL. Prospective, randomized trial of netilmicin and amikacin, with emphasis on eighth-nerve toxicity. Antimicrob Agents Chemother 1980;17(4):707–14.

16. Matz GJ, Lerner SA. Prospective studies of aminoglycoside ototoxicity in adults. In: Lerner SA, Matz GJ, Hawkins JE, editors. Aminoglycoside Ototoxicity. Boston: Little, Brown and Co, 1981:327.

17. Orts Alborch M, Morant Ventura A, Garcia Callejo J, Ferrer Baixauli F, Martinez Beneito MP, Marco Algarra J. Monitorizacion de la ototoxicidad por farmacos con productos de distorsion. [Monitoring drug ototoxicity with distortion products.] Acta Otorrinolaringol Esp 2000;51(5):387–95.

18. Walsh RM, Bath AP, Bance ML. Reversible tobramycin-induced bilateral high-frequency vestibular toxicity. ORL J Otorhinolaryngol Relat Spec 2000;62(3):156–9.

19. Tsuji K, Velazquez-Villasenor L, Rauch SD, Glynn RJ, Wall C 3rd, Merchant SN. Temporal bone studies of the human peripheral vestibular system. Aminoglycoside ototoxicity. Ann Otol Rhinol Laryngol Suppl 2000;181:20–5.

20. Brummett RE, Fox KE. Aminoglycoside-induced hearing loss in humans. Antimicrob Agents Chemother 1989;33(6):797–800.

21. Fee WE Jr. Aminoglycoside ototoxicity in the human. Laryngoscope 1980;90(10 Pt 2 Suppl 24):1–19.

22. Tablan OC, Reyes MP, Rintelmann WF, Lerner AM. Renal and auditory toxicity of high-dose, prolonged therapy with gentamicin and tobramycin in *Pseudomonas* endocarditis. J Infect Dis 1984;149(2):257–63.

23. Federspil P, Schatzle W, Tiesler E. Pharmakokinetische, histologische und histochemische Untersuchungen zur Ototoxizitat des Gentamicins, Tobramycins und Amikacins. [Pharmacokinetical, histological, and histochemical investigation on the ototoxicity of gentamicin, tobramycin, and amikacin.] Arch Otorhinolaryngol 1977;217(2):147–66.

24. de Jager P, van Altena R. Hearing loss and nephrotoxicity in long-term aminoglycoside treatment in patients with tuberculosis. Int J Tuberc Lung Dis 2002;6(7):622–7.

25. Mulheran M, Degg C, Burr S, Morgan DW, Stableforth DE. Occurrence and risk of cochleotoxicity in cystic fibrosis patients receiving repeated high-dose aminoglycoside therapy. Antimicrob Agents Chemother 2001;45(9):2502–9.

26. Brummett RE, Fox KE. Studies of aminoglycoside ototoxicity in animal models. In: Whelton A, Neu HC, editors. The Aminoglycosides. New York, Basel: Marcel Dekker, 1982:419.

27. Brummett RE, Fox KE, Brown RT, Himes DL. Comparative ototoxic liability of netilmicin and gentamicin. Arch Otolaryngol 1978;104(10):579–84.

28. Cone LA. A survey of prospective, controlled clinical trials of gentamicin, tobramycin, amikacin, and netilmicin. Clin Ther 1982;5(2):155–62.

29. Lerner AM, Reyes MP, Cone LA, Blair DC, Jansen W, Wright GE, Lorber RR. Randomised, controlled trial of the comparative efficacy, auditory toxicity, and nephrotoxicity of tobramycin and netilmicin. Lancet 1983;1(8334):1123–6.

30. Gatell JM, SanMiguel JG, Araujo V, Zamora L, Mana J, Ferrer M, Bonet M, Bohe M, Jimenez de Anta MT. Prospective randomized double-blind comparison of nephrotoxicity and auditory toxicity of tobramycin and netilmicin. Antimicrob Agents Chemother 1984;26(5):766–9.

31. Lange G, Keller R. Beidseitiger Funktionsverlust der peripheren Gleichgewichtsorgane. Beobachtungen zu 20 Fallen von Dandy-Syndrom. [Bilateral malfunction of peripheral vestibular organs. Observations of 20 cases of Dandy syndrome.] Laryngorhinootologie 2000;79(2):77–80.

32. Federspil P. Zur Ototoxizität der Aminoglykosid-Antibiotika. [Ototoxicity of the aminoglycoside antibiotics.] Infection 1976;4(4):239–48.

33. Henley CM 3rd, Schacht J. Pharmacokinetics of aminoglycoside antibiotics in blood, inner-ear fluids and tissues and their relationship to ototoxicity. Audiology 1988;27(3):137–46.

34. Rybak LP. Ototoxicity. Curr Opin Otolaryngol Head Neck Surg 1996;4:302–7.

35. Lima da Costa D, Erre JP, Pehourq F, Aran JM. Aminoglycoside ototoxicity and the medial efferent system: II. Comparison of acute effects of different antibiotics. Audiology 1998;37(3):162–73.

36. Lima da Costa D, Erre JP, Aran JM. Aminoglycoside ototoxicity and the medial efferent system: I. Comparison of acute and chronic gentamicin treatments. Audiology 1998;37(3):151–61.

37. Conlon BJ, Perry BP, Smith DW. Attenuation of neomycin ototoxicity by iron chelation. Laryngoscope 1998;108(2):284–7.

38. Conlon BJ, Aran JM, Erre JP, Smith DW. Attenuation of aminoglycoside-induced cochlear damage with the metabolic antioxidant alpha-lipoic acid. Hear Res 1999;128 (1–2):40–4.

39. Hester TO, Jones RO, Clerici WJ. Protection against aminoglycoside otic drop-induced ototoxicity by a spin trap: I. Acute effects. Otolaryngol Head Neck Surg 1998;119(6):581–7.

40. Segal JA, Harris BD, Kustova Y, Basile A, Skolnick P. Aminoglycoside neurotoxicity involves NMDA receptor activation. Brain Res 1999;815(2):270–7.

41. Basile AS, Brichta AM, Harris BD, Morse D, Coling D, Skolnick P. Dizocilpine attenuates streptomycin-induced vestibulotoxicity in rats. Neurosci Lett 1999;265(2):71–4.

42. Nakagawa T, Yamane H, Takayama M, Sunami K, Nakai Y. Involvement of nitric oxide in aminoglycoside vestibulotoxicity in guinea pigs. Neurosci Lett 1999;267(1):57–60.

43. Romand R, Chardin S. Effects of growth factors on the hair cells after ototoxic treatment of the neonatal mammalian cochlea in vitro. Brain Res 1999;825(1–2):46–58.

44. Ruan RS, Leong SK, Mark I, Yeoh KH. Effects of BDNF and NT-3 on hair cell survival in guinea pig cochlea damaged by kanamycin treatment. Neuroreport 1999;10(10):2067–71.

45. Vila J, Ruiz J, Navia M, Becerril B, Garcia I, Perea S, Lopez-Hernandez I, Alamo I, Ballester F, Planes AM, Martinez-Beltran J, de Anta TJ. Spread of amikacin resistance in *Acinetobacter baumannii* strains isolated in Spain due to an epidemic strain. J Clin Microbiol 1999;37(3): 758–61.

46. Matsuda K, Ueda Y, Doi T, Tono T, Haruta A, Toyama K, Komune S. Increase in glutamate-aspartate transporter (GLAST) mRNA during kanamycin-induced cochlear insult in rats. Hear Res 1999;133(1–2):10–16.

47. Zheng JL, Gao WQ. Concanavalin A protects hair cells against gentamicin ototoxicity in rat cochlear explant cultures. J Neurobiol 1999;39(1):29–40.

48. Kimura N, Nishizaki K, Orita Y, Masuda Y. 4-methylcatechol, a potent inducer of nerve growth factor synthesis, protects spiral ganglion neurons from aminoglycoside ototoxicity—preliminary report. Acta Otolaryngol Suppl 1999;540:12–15.

49. Xiang ML, Mu MY, Pao X, Chi FL. The reinnervation of regenerated hair cells in the basilar papilla of chicks after kanamycin ototoxicity. Acta Otolaryngol 2000;120(8):912–21.

50. Fischel-Ghodsian N, Prezant TR, Bu X, Oztas S. Mitochondrial ribosomal RNA gene mutation in a patient with sporadic aminoglycoside ototoxicity. Am J Otolaryngol 1993;14(6):399–403.

51. Jacobs HT. Mitochondrial deafness. Ann Med 1997;29(6):483–91.

52. Usami S, Abe S, Tono T, Komune S, Kimberling WJ, Shinkawa H. Isepamicin sulfate-induced sensorineural hearing loss in patients with the 1555 A→G mitochondrial mutation. ORL J Otorhinolaryngol Relat Spec 1998;60(3):164–9.

53. Wang S, Bian Q, Liu Z, Feng Y, Lian N, Chen H, Hu C, Dong Y, Cai Z. Capability of serum to convert streptomycin to cytotoxin in patients with aminoglycoside-induced hearing loss. Hear Res 1999;137(1–2):1–7.

54. Moore RD, Smith CR, Lietman PS. Risk factors for the development of auditory toxicity in patients receiving aminoglycosides. J Infect Dis 1984;149(1):23–30.

55. Smith CR, Lietman PS. Effect of furosemide on aminoglycoside-induced nephrotoxicity and auditory toxicity in humans. Antimicrob Agents Chemother 1983;23(1):133–7.

56. Schonenberger U, Streit C, Hoigne R. Nephro- und Ototoxizitat von Aminoglykosid-Antibiotica unter besonderer Berücksichtigung von Gentamicin. [Nephro- and ototoxicity of aminoglycoside-antibiotics, with special reference to gentamicin.] Schweiz Rundsch Med Prax 1981;70(5):169–73.

57. Schacht J. Aminoglycoside ototoxicity: prevention in sight? Otolaryngol Head Neck Surg 1998;118(5):674–7.

58. Hardisty RE, Fleming J, Steel KP. The molecular genetics of inherited deafness—current knowledge and recent advances. J Laryngol Otol 1998;112(5):432–7.

59. Steel KP. Progress in progressive hearing loss. Science 1998;279(5358):1870–1.

60. Casano RA, Bykhovskaya Y, Johnson DF, Hamon M, Torricelli F, Bigozzi M, Fischel-Ghodsian N. Hearing loss due to the mitochondrial A1555G mutation in Italian families. Am J Med Genet 1998;79(5):388–91.

61. Estivill X, Govea N, Barcelo E, Perello E, Badenas C, Romero E, Moral L, Scozzri R, D'Urbano L, Zeviani M, Torroni A. Familial progressive sensorineural deafness is mainly due to the mtDNA A1555G mutation and is enhanced by treatment of aminoglycosides. Am J Hum Genet 1998;62(1):27–35.

62. Casano RA, Johnson DF, Bykhovskaya Y, Torricelli F, Bigozzi M, Fischel-Ghodsian N. Inherited susceptibility to aminoglycoside ototoxicity: genetic heterogeneity and clinical implications. Am J Otolaryngol 1999;20(3):151–6.

63. Hutchin T. Sensorineural hearing loss and the 1555G mitochondrial DNA mutation. Acta Otolaryngol 1999; 119(1):48–52.

64. Scrimshaw BJ, Faed JM, Tate WP, Yun K. Rapid identification of an A1555G mutation in human mitochondrial DNA implicated in aminoglycoside-induced ototoxicity. J Hum Genet 1999;44(6):388–90.

65. Guan MX, Fischel-Ghodsian N, Attardi G. A biochemical basis for the inherited susceptibility to aminoglycoside ototoxicity. Hum Mol Genet 2000;9(12):1787–93.

66. Stavroulaki P, Apostolopoulos N, Dinopoulou D, Vossinakis I, Tsakanikos M, Douniadakis D. Otoacoustic emissions—an approach for monitoring aminoglycoside induced ototoxicity in children. Int J Pediatr Otorhinolaryngol 1999;50(3):177–84.

67. Marlow ES, Hunt LP, Marlow N. Sensorineural hearing loss and prematurity. Arch Dis Child Fetal Neonatal Ed 2000;82(2):F141–4.

68. Guerit JM, Mahieu P, Houben-Giurgea S, Herbay S. The influence of ototoxic drugs on brainstem auditory evoked potentials in man. Arch Otorhinolaryngol 1981; 233(2): 189–99.

69. Hotz MA, Allum JH, Kaufmann G, Follath F, Pfaltz CR. Shifts in auditory brainstem response latencies following plasma-level-controlled aminoglycoside therapy. Eur Arch Otorhinolaryngol 1990;247(4):202–5.

70. Lopez-Gonzalez MA, Guerrero JM, Torronteras R, Osuna C, Delgado F. Ototoxicity caused by aminoglycosides is ameliorated by melatonin without interfering with the antibiotic capacity of the drugs. J Pineal Res 2000;28(1):26–33.

71. Conlon BJ, Smith DW. Topical aminoglycoside ototoxicity: attempting to protect the cochlea. Acta Otolaryngol 2000;120(5):596–9.

72. Duan M, Agerman K, Ernfors P, Canlon B. Complementary roles of neurotrophin 3 and a N-methyl-D-aspartate antagonist in the protection of noise and aminoglycoside-induced ototoxicity. Proc Natl Acad Sci USA 2000;97(13):7597–602.

73. Lopez-Gonzalez MA, Delgado F, Lucas M. Aminoglycosides activate oxygen metabolites production in the cochlea of mature and developing rats. Hear Res 1999;136(1–2):165–8.

74. Sha SH, Schacht J. Stimulation of free radical formation by aminoglycoside antibiotics. Hear Res 1999;128(1–2):112–18.

75. Liamis G, Alexandridis G, Bairaktari ET, Elisaf MS. Aminoglycoside-induced metabolic abnormalities. Ann Clin Biochem 2000;37(Pt 4):543–4.

76. Kes P, Reiner Z. Symptomatic hypomagnesemia associated with gentamicin therapy. Magnes Trace Elem 1990;9(1):54–60.

77. von Vigier RO, Truttmann AC, Zindler-Schmocker K, Bettinelli A, Aebischer CC, Wermuth B, Bianchetti MG. Aminoglycosides and renal magnesium homeostasis in humans. Nephrol Dial Transplant 2000;15(6):822–6.

78. Elliott C, Newman N, Madan A. Gentamicin effects on urinary electrolyte excretion in healthy subjects. Clin Pharmacol Ther 2000;67(1):16–21.

79. Shetty AK, Rogers NL, Mannick EE, Aviles DH. Syndrome of hypokalemic metabolic alkalosis and hypomagnesemia associated with gentamicin therapy: case reports. Clin Pediatr (Phila) 2000;39(9):529–33.

80. Kang HS, Kerstan D, Dai L, Ritchie G, Quamme GA. Aminoglycosides inhibit hormone-stimulated Mg^{2+} uptake in mouse distal convoluted tubule cells. Can J Physiol Pharmacol 2000;78(8):595–602.

81. Akbar A, Rees JH, Nyamugunduru G, English MW, Spencer DA, Weller PH. Aminoglycoside-associated hypomagnesaemia in children with cystic fibrosis. Acta Paediatr 1999;88(7):783–5.

82. Ciftci M, Kufrevioglu OI, Gundogdu M, Ozmen I I. Effects of some antibiotics on enzyme activity of glucose-6-phosphate dehydrogenase from human erythrocytes. Pharmacol Res 2000;41(1):107–111.

83. English WP, Williams MD. Should aminoglycoside antibiotics be abandoned? Am J Surg 2000;180(6):512–16.

84. Shemin D, Maaz D, St Pierre D, Kahn SI, Chazan JA. Effect of aminoglycoside use on residual renal function in peritoneal dialysis patients. Am J Kidney Dis 1999;34(1):14–20.

85. Plaut ME, Schentag JJ, Jusko WJ. Aminoglycoside nephrotoxicity: comparative assessment in critically ill patients. J Med 1979;10(4):257–66.

86. Schentag JJ, Plaut ME, Cerra FB. Comparative nephrotoxicity of gentamicin and tobramycin: pharmacokinetic and clinical studies in 201 patients. Antimicrob Agents Chemother 1981;19(5):859–66.

87. Moore RD, Smith CR, Lipsky JJ, Mellits ED, Lietman PS. Risk factors for nephrotoxicity in patients treated with aminoglycosides. Ann Intern Med 1984;100(3):352–7.

88. Sawyers CL, Moore RD, Lerner SA, Smith CR. A model for predicting nephrotoxicity in patients treated with aminoglycosides. J Infect Dis 1986;153(6):1062–8.

89. Lam YW, Arana CJ, Shikuma LR, Rotschafer JC. The clinical utility of a published nomogram to predict aminoglycoside nephrotoxicity. JAMA 1986;255(5):639–42.

90. Thatte L, Vaamonde CA. Drug-induced nephrotoxicity: the crucial role of risk factors. Postgrad Med 1996;100(6):83–4, 87–8, 91 passim.

91. Samaniego-Picota MD, Whelton A. Aminoglycoside-induced nephrotoxicity in cystic fibrosis: a case presentation and review of the literature. Am J Ther 1996;3(3):248–57.

92. Raveh D, Kopyt M, Hite Y, Rudensky B, Sonnenblick M, Yinnon AM. Risk factors for nephrotoxicity in elderly patients receiving once-daily aminoglycosides. QJM 2002;95(5):291–7.

93. Luft FC, Evan AP. Comparative effects of tobramycin and gentamicin on glomerular ultrastructure. J Infect Dis 1980;142(6):910–14.

94. Tardif D, Beauchamp D, Bergeron MG. Influence of endotoxin on the intracortical accumulation kinetics of gentamicin in rats. Antimicrob Agents Chemother 1990;34(4):576–80.

95. Appel GB. Aminoglycoside nephrotoxicity: physiologic studies of the sites of nephron damage. In: Whelton A, Neu HC, editors. The Aminoglycosides. New York, Basel: Marcel Dekker, 1982:269.

96. Whelton A. Renal tubular transport and intrarenal aminoglycoside distribution. In: Whelton A, Neu HC, editors. The Aminoglycosides. New York, Basel: Marcel Dekker, 1982:191.

97. Carlier MB, Laurent G, Claes PJ, Vanderhaeghe HJ, Tulkens PM. Inhibition of lysosomal phospholipases by aminoglycoside antibiotics: in vitro comparative studies. Antimicrob Agents Chemother 1983;23(3):440–9.

98. Rybak MJ, Abate BJ, Kang SL, Ruffing MJ, Lerner SA, Drusano GL. Prospective evaluation of the effect of an aminoglycoside dosing regimen on rates of observed nephrotoxicity and ototoxicity. Antimicrob Agents Chemother 1999;43(7):1549–55.

99. Walker PD, Barri Y, Shah SV. Oxidant mechanisms in gentamicin nephrotoxicity. Ren Fail 1999;21(3–4):433–42.

100. Carrier D, Bou Khalil M, Kealey A. Modulation of phospholipase A2 activity by aminoglycosides and daptomycin: a Fourier transform infrared spectroscopic study. Biochemistry 1998;37(20):7589–97.

101. Cheng M, Razzaque MS, Nazneen A, Taguchi T. Expression of the heat shock protein 47 in gentamicin-treated rat kidneys. Int J Exp Pathol 1998;79(3):125–32.

102. Scherberich JE, Mondorf WA. Nephrotoxic potential of antiinfective drugs as assessed by tissue-specific proteinuria of renal antigens. Int J Clin Pharmacol Ther 1998;36(3):152–8.

103. Murry KR, McKinnon PS, Mitrzyk B, Rybak MJ. Pharmacodynamic characterization of nephrotoxicity associated with once-daily aminoglycoside. Pharmacotherapy 1999;19(11):1252–60.

104. Buijk SE, Mouton JW, Gyssens IC, Verbrugh HA, Bruining HA. Experience with a once-daily dosing program of aminoglycosides in critically ill patients. Intensive Care Med 2002;28(7):936–42.

105. Keys TF, Kurtz SB, Jones JD, Muller SM. Renal toxicity during therapy with gentamicin or tobramycin. Mayo Clin Proc 1981;56(9):556–9.

106. Schentag JJ, Gengo FM, Plaut ME, Danner D, Mangione A, Jusko WJ. Urinary casts as an indicator of renal tubular damage in patients receiving aminoglycosides. Antimicrob Agents Chemother 1979;16(4):468–74.

107. Schentag JJ, Sutfin TA, Plaut ME, Jusko WJ. Early detection of aminoglycoside nephrotoxicity with urinary beta-2-microglobulin. J Med 1978;9(3):201–10.

108. Tulkens PM. Pharmacokinetic and toxicological evaluation of a once-daily regimen versus conventional schedules of netilmicin and amikacin. J Antimicrob Chemother 1991;27(Suppl C):49–61.

109. Mondorf AW. Urinary enzymatic markers of renal damage. In: Whelton A, Neu HC, editors. The Aminoglycosides. New York, Basel: Marcel Dekker, 1982:283.

110. Marchewka Z, Dlugosz A. Enzymes in urine as markers of nephrotoxicity of cytostatic agents and aminoglycoside antibiotics. Int Urol Nephrol 1998;30(3):339–48.

111. Panova LD, Farkhutdinov RR, Akhmadeeva EN. [Urine chemiluminescence in preclinical diagnosis of neonatal drug-induced nephropathy.] Urol Nefrol (Mosk) 1998;(4):25–9.

112. Luft FC, Yum MN, Kleit SA. Comparative nephrotoxicities of netilmicin and gentamicin in rats. Antimicrob Agents Chemother 1976;10(5):845–9.

113. Hottendorf GH, Gordon LL. Comparative low-dose nephrotoxicities of gentamicin, tobramycin, and amikacin. Antimicrob Agents Chemother 1980;18(1):176–81.

114. Smith CR, Baughman KL, Edwards CQ, Rogers JF, Lietman PS. Controlled comparison of amikacin and gentamicin. N Engl J Med 1977;296(7):349–53.

115. Love LJ, Schimpff SC, Hahn DM, Young VM, Standiford HC, Bender JF, Fortner CL, Wiernik PH. Randomized trial of empiric antibiotic therapy with ticarcillin in combination with gentamicin, amikacin or netilmicin in febrile patients with granulocytopenia and cancer. Am J Med 1979;66(4):603–10.

116. Lau WK, Young LS, Black RE, Winston DJ, Linne SR, Weinstein RJ, Hewitt WL. Comparative efficacy and toxicity of amikacin/carbenicillin versus gentamicin/carbenicillin in leukopenic patients: a randomized prospective trial. Am J Med 1977;62(6):959–66.

117. Fong IW, Fenton RS, Bird R. Comparative toxicity of gentamicin versus tobramycin: a randomized prospective study. J Antimicrob Chemother 1981;7(1):81–8.

118. Bock BV, Edelstein PH, Meyer RD. Prospective comparative study of efficacy and toxicity of netilmicin and amikacin. Antimicrob Agents Chemother 1980;17(2):217–25.

119. Noone M, Pomeroy L, Sage R, Noone P. Prospective study of amikacin versus netilmicin in the treatment of severe infection in hospitalized patients. Am J Med 1989;86(6 Pt 2):809–13.

120. Smith CR, Lipsky JJ, Laskin OL, Hellmann DB, Mellits ED, Longstreth J, Lietman PS. Double-blind comparison of the nephrotoxicity and auditory toxicity of gentamicin and tobramycin. N Engl J Med 1980;302(20):1106–9.

121. Matzke GR, Lucarotti RL, Shapiro HS. Controlled comparison of gentamicin and tobramycin nephrotoxicity. Am J Nephrol 1983;3(1):11–17.

122. Akaki T, Dekio S. Contact dermatitis from arbekacin sulfate: report of a case. J Dermatol 2002;29(10):674–5.

123. Yung MW, Rajendra T. Delayed hypersensitivity reaction to topical aminoglycosides in patients undergoing middle ear surgery. Clin Otolaryngol Allied Sci 2002;27(5):365–8.

124. Paniagua MJ, Garcia-Ortega P, Tella R, Gaig P, Richart C. Systemic contact dermatitis to gentamicin. Allergy 2002;57(11):1086–7.

125. Schulze S, Wollina U. Gentamicin-induced anaphylaxis. Allergy 2003;58(1):88–9.

126. Hall FJ. Anaphylaxis after gentamycin. Lancet 1977;2(8035):455.

127. Goh CL. Anaphylaxis from topical neomycin and bacitracin. Australas J Dermatol 1986;27(3):125–6.

128. Blaser J, Stone BB, Zinner SH. Efficacy of intermittent versus continuous administration of netilmicin in a two-compartment in vitro model. Antimicrob Agents Chemother 1985;27(3):343–9.

129. Gerber AU, Craig WA. Aminoglycoside-selected subpopulations of *Pseudomonas aeruginosa*: characterization and virulence in normal and leukopenic mice. J Lab Clin Med 1982;100(5):671–81.

130. Olson B, Weinstein RA, Nathan C, Chamberlin W, Kabins SA. Occult aminoglycoside resistance in *Pseudomonas aeruginosa*: epidemiology and implications for therapy and control. J Infect Dis 1985;152(4):769–74.

131. Hilf M, Yu VL, Sharp J, Zuravleff JJ, Korvick JA, Muder RR. Antibiotic therapy for *Pseudomonas aeruginosa* bacteremia: outcome correlations in a prospective study of 200 patients. Am J Med 1989;87(5):540–6.

132. Mathon L, Decaillot F, Allaouchiche B. Impact de l'antibiothérapie initiale sur l'evolution des résistances aux fluoroquinolones et aux aminosides des bacilles a gram négatif isolés chez des patients de réanimation. [Impact of initial antibiotic therapy on the course of resistance to fluoroquinolones and aminoglycosides in Gram-negative bacilli isolated from intensive care patients.] Ann Fr Anesth Reanim 1999;18(10):1054–60.

133. Moore RA, DeShazer D, Reckseidler S, Weissman A, Woods DE. Efflux-mediated aminoglycoside and macrolide resistance in *Burkholderia pseudomallei*. Antimicrob Agents Chemother 1999;43(3):465–70.

134. Vanhoof R, Nyssen HJ, Van Bossuyt E, Hannecart-Pokorni E. Aminoglycoside resistance in Gram-negative blood isolates from various hospitals in Belgium and the Grand Duchy of Luxembourg. Aminoglycoside Resistance Study Group. J Antimicrob Chemother 1999;44(4):483–8.

135. Schmitz FJ, Verhoef J, Fluit AC. Prevalence of aminoglycoside resistance in 20 European university hospitals participating in the European SENTRY Antimicrobial Surveillance Programme. Eur J Clin Microbiol Infect Dis 1999;18(6):414–21.

136. Bouza E, Garcia-Garrote F, Cercenado E, Marin M, Diaz MS. *Pseudomonas aeruginosa*: a survey of resistance in 136 hospitals in Spain. The Spanish *Pseudomonas aeruginosa* Study Group. Antimicrob Agents Chemother 1999;43(4):981–2.

137. Ruiz J, Nunez ML, Perez J, Simarro E, Martinez-Campos L, Gomez J. Evolution of resistance among clinical isolates of *Acinetobacter* over a 6-year period. Eur J Clin Microbiol Infect Dis 1999;18(4):292–5.

138. Jacobson K, Rolston K, Elting L, LeBlanc B, Whimbey E, Ho DH. Susceptibility surveillance among Gram-negative bacilli at a cancer center. Chemotherapy 1999;45(5):325–34.

139. Valdivieso F, Trucco O, Prado V, Diaz MC, Ojeda A. Resistencia a los antimicrobianos en agentes causantes de infeccion del tracto urinario en 11 hospitales chilenos. [Antimicrobial resistance of agents causing urinary tract infections in 11 Chilean hospitals. PRONARES project.] Rev Med Chil 1999;127(9):1033–40.

140. Freitas FI, Guedes-Stehling E, Siqueira-Junior JP. Resistance to gentamicin and related aminoglycosides in *Staphylococcus aureus* isolated in Brazil. Lett Appl Microbiol 1999;29(3):197–201.

141. del Valle O, Trincado P, Martin MT, Gomez E, Cano A, Vindel A. Prevalencia de *Staphylococcus aureus* resistentes a meticilina fagotipo 95 en los Hospitales Vall d'Hebron de Barcelona. [The prevalence of methicillin-resistant *Staphylococcus aureus* phagotype 95 in the Hospitales Vall d'Hebron of Barcelona.] Enferm Infecc Microbiol Clin 1999;17(10):498–505.

142. Dulon D, Ryan AF. The bacterial Neo gene confers neomycin resistance to mammalian cochlear hair cells. Neuroreport 1999;10(6):1189–93.

143. You I, Kariyama R, Zervos MJ, Kumon H, Chow JW. In-vitro activity of arbekacin alone and in combination with vancomycin against gentamicin- and methicillin-resistant *Staphylococcus aureus*. Diagn Microbiol Infect Dis 2000;36(1):37–41.

144. Nakamura A, Hosoda M, Kato T, Yamada Y, Itoh M, Kanazawa K, Nouda H. Combined effects of meropenem and aminoglycosides on *Pseudomonas aeruginosa* in vitro. J Antimicrob Chemother 2000;46(6):901–4.

145. Heinonen OP, Slone D, Shapiro S. Birth defects and drugs in pregnancy. In: Kaufmann DW, editor. Antimicrobial and Parasite Agents. Littleton, MA: John Wright, 1982:296, 435.

146. Conway N, Birt BD. Streptomycin in pregnancy: effect on the foetal ear. BMJ 1965;5456:260–3.

147. Czeizel AE, Rockenbauer M, Olsen J, Sorensen HT. A teratological study of aminoglycoside antibiotic treatment during pregnancy. Scand J Infect Dis 2000;32(3):309–13.

148. Hess M, Finckh-Kramer U, Bartsch M, Kewitz G, Versmold H, Gross M. Hearing screening in at-risk neonate cohort. Int J Pediatr Otorhinolaryngol 1998;46 (1–2):81–9.

149. Mattie H, Craig WA, Pechere JC. Determinants of efficacy and toxicity of aminoglycosides. J Antimicrob Chemother 1989;24(3):281–93.

150. Gilbert DN. Once-daily aminoglycoside therapy. Antimicrob Agents Chemother 1991;35(3):399–405.

151. Blaser J, Konig C. Once-daily dosing of aminoglycosides. Eur J Clin Microbiol Infect Dis 1995;14(12):1029–38.

152. Lacy MK, Nicolau DP, Nightingale CH, Quintiliani R. The pharmacodynamics of aminoglycosides. Clin Infect Dis 1998;27(1):23–7.

153. Blaser J, Stone BB, Groner MC, Zinner SH. Comparative study with enoxacin and netilmicin in a pharmacodynamic model to determine importance of ratio of antibiotic peak concentration to MIC for bactericidal activity and emergence of resistance. Antimicrob Agents Chemother 1987;31(7):1054–60.

154. Moore RD, Lietman PS, Smith CR. Clinical response to aminoglycoside therapy: importance of the ratio of peak concentration to minimal inhibitory concentration. J Infect Dis 1987;155(1):93–9.

155. Vogelman B, Gudmundsson S, Turnidge J, Leggett J, Craig WA. In vivo postantibiotic effect in a thigh infection in neutropenic mice. J Infect Dis 1988;157(2):287–98.

156. Powell SH, Thompson WL, Luthe MA, Stern RC, Grossniklaus DA, Bloxham DD, Groden DL, Jacobs MR, DiScenna AO, Cash HA, Klinger JD. Once-daily vs. continuous aminoglycoside dosing: efficacy and toxicity in animal and clinical studies of gentamicin, netilmicin, and tobramycin. J Infect Dis 1983;147(5):918–32.

157. De Broe ME, Verbist L, Verpooten GA. Influence of dosage schedule on renal cortical accumulation of amikacin and tobramycin in man. J Antimicrob Chemother 1991;27(Suppl C):41–7.

158. Freeman CD, Strayer AH. Mega-analysis of meta-analysis: an examination of meta-analysis with an emphasis on once-daily aminoglycoside comparative trials. Pharmacotherapy 1996;16(6):1093–102.

159. Gilbert DN, Lee BL, Dworkin RJ, Leggett JL, Chambers HF, Modin G, Tauber MG, Sande MA. A randomized comparison of the safety and efficacy of once-daily gentamicin or thrice-daily gentamicin in combination with ticarcillin–clavulanate. Am J Med 1998;105(3):182–91.

160. Karachalios GN, Houpas P, Tziviskou E, Papalimneou V, Georgiou A, Karachaliou I, Halkiadaki D. Prospective randomized study of once-daily versus twice-daily amikacin regimens in patients with systemic infections. Int J Clin Pharmacol Ther 1998;36(10):561–4.

161. Sanchez-Alcaraz A, Vargas A, Quintana MB, Rocher A, Querol JM, Poveda JL, Hermenegildo M. Therapeutic drug monitoring of tobramycin: once-daily versus twice-daily dosage schedules. J Clin Pharm Ther 1998;23(5):367–73.

162. Bragonier R, Brown NM. The pharmacokinetics and toxicity of once-daily tobramycin therapy in children with cystic fibrosis. J Antimicrob Chemother 1998;42(1):103–6.

163. Paterson DL, Robson JM, Wagener MM. Risk factors for toxicity in elderly patients given aminoglycosides once daily. J Gen Intern Med 1998;13(11):735–9.

164. Tam VH, Preston SL, Briceland LL. Once-daily aminoglycosides in the treatment of Gram-positive endocarditis. Ann Pharmacother 1999;33(5):600–6.

165. Barletta JF, Johnson SB, Nix DE, Nix LC, Erstad BL. Population pharmacokinetics of aminoglycosides in critically ill trauma patients on once-daily regimens. J Trauma 2000;49(5):869–72.

166. Gerberding JL. Aminoglycoside dosing: timing is of the essence. Am J Med 1998;105(3):256–8.

167. Havener WH. Ocular Pharmacology. 4th ed. St Louis: CV Mosby, 1978.

168. Thomsen J, Charabi S, Tos M. Preliminary results of a new delivery system for gentamicin to the inner ear in patients with Menière's disease. Eur Arch Otorhinolaryngol 2000;257(7):362–5.

169. Quaranta A, Piazza F. Menière's disease: diagnosis and new treatment perspectives. [Mèniere's disease: diagnosis and new treatment perspectives.] Recenti Prog Med 2000;91(1):33–7.

170. Mars RL, Moles K, Pope K, Hargrove P. Use of bolus intraperitoneal aminoglycosides for treating peritonitis in end-stage renal disease patients receiving continuous ambulatory peritoneal dialysis and continuous cycling peritoneal dialysis. Adv Perit Dial 2000;16:280–4.

171. Green FJ, Lavelle KJ, Aronoff GR, Vander Zanden J, Brier GL. Management of amikacin overdose. Am J Kidney Dis 1981;1(2):110–12.

172. Lu CM, James SH, Lien YH. Acute massive gentamicin intoxication in a patient with end-stage renal disease. Am J Kidney Dis 1996;28(5):767–71.

173. Basile C, Di Maggio A, Curino E, Scatizzi A. Pharmacokinetics of netilmicin in hypertonic hemodiafiltration and standard hemodialysis. Clin Nephrol 1985;24(6):305–9.

174. Bailey RR. Renal failure in combined gentamicin and cephalothin therapy. BMJ 1973;2(5869):776–7.

175. Cabanillas F, Burgos RC, Rodriguez C, Baldizon C. Nephrotoxicity of combined cephalothin–gentamicin regimen. Arch Intern Med 1975;135(6):850–2.

176. Tobias JS, Whitehouse JM, Wrigley PF. Severe renal dysfunction after tobramycin/cephalothin therapy. Lancet 1976;1(7956):425.

177. English J, Gilbert DN, Kohlhepp S, Kohnen PW, Mayor G, Houghton DC, Bennett WM. Attenuation of experimental tobramycin nephrotoxicity by ticarcillin. Antimicrob Agents Chemother 1985;27(6):897–902.

178. Wade JC, Schimpff SC, Wiernik PH. Antibiotic combination-associated nephrotoxicity in granulocytopenic patients with cancer. Arch Intern Med 1981;141(13): 1789–93.

179. Caston J, Doinel L. Comparative vestibular toxicity of dibekacin, habekacin and cisplatin. Acta Otolaryngol 1987;104(3–4):315–21.

180. Bates DE, Beaumont SJ, Baylis BW. Ototoxicity induced by gentamicin and furosemide. Ann Pharmacother 2002;36(3):446–51.

181. Santucci RA, Krieger JN. Gentamicin for the practicing urologist: review of efficacy, single daily dosing and "switch" therapy. J Urol 2000;163(4):1076–84.

182. Conlon BJ, McSwain SD, Smith DW. Topical gentamicin and ethacrynic acid: effects on cochlear function. Laryngoscope 1998;108(7):1087–9.

183. Burkett L, Bikhazi GB, Thomas KC Jr, Rosenthal DA, Wirta MG, Foldes FF. Mutual potentiation of the neuromuscular effects of antibiotics and relaxants. Anesth Analg 1979;58(2):107–15.

184. Holt HA, Broughall JM, McCarthy M, Reeves DS. Interactions between aminoglycoside antibiotics and carbenicillin or ticarillin. Infection 1976;4(2):107–9.

185. Adam D, Haneder J. Studies on the inactivation of aminoglycoside antibiotics by acylureidopenicillins and piperacillin. Infection 1981;9:182.

186. Henderson JL, Polk RE, Kline BJ. In vitro inactivation of gentamicin, tobramycin, and netilmicin by carbenicillin, azlocillin, or mezlocillin. Am J Hosp Pharm 1981;38(8):1167–70.

187. Thompson MI, Russo ME, Saxon BJ, Atkin-Thor E, Matsen JM. Gentamicin inactivation by piperacillin or carbenicillin in patients with end-stage renal disease. Antimicrob Agents Chemother 1982;21(2):268–73.

188. Rybak MJ, Albrecht LM, Boike SC, Chandrasekar PH. Nephrotoxicity of vancomycin, alone and with an aminoglycoside. J Antimicrob Chemother 1990;25(4):679–87.

189. de Lemos E, Pariat C, Piriou A, Fauconneau B, Courtois P. Variations circadiennes de la nephrotoxicité de l'association vancomycine–gentamicine chez le rat. [Circadian variations in the nephrotoxicity of the vancomycin–gentamicin combination in rats.] Pathol Biol (Paris) 1991;39(1):12–15.

190. Pauly DJ, Musa DM, Lestico MR, Lindstrom MJ, Hetsko CM. Risk of nephrotoxicity with combination vancomycin–aminoglycoside antibiotic therapy. Pharmacotherapy 1990;10(6):378–82.

191. Streetman DS, Nafziger AN, Destache CJ, Bertino AS Jr. Individualized pharmacokinetic monitoring results in less aminoglycoside-associated nephrotoxicity and fewer associated costs. Pharmacotherapy 2001;21(4):443–51.

192. Moore RD, Smith CR, Lietman PS. The association of aminoglycoside plasma levels with mortality in patients with Gram-negative bacteremia. J Infect Dis 1984;149(3):443–8.

193. Moore RD, Smith CR, Lietman PS. Association of aminoglycoside plasma levels with therapeutic outcome in Gram-negative pneumonia. Am J Med 1984;77(4):657–62.

194. Wenk M, Vozeh S, Follath F. Serum level monitoring of antibacterial drugs. A review. Clin Pharmacokinet 1984;9(6):475–92.

195. Zaske DE, Cipolle RJ, Rotschafer JC, Solem LD, Mosier NR, Strate RG. Gentamicin pharmacokinetics in 1,640 patients: method for control of serum concentrations. Antimicrob Agents Chemother 1982;21(3):407–11.

196. Lesar TS, Rotschafer JC, Strand LM, Solem LD, Zaske DE. Gentamicin dosing errors with four commonly used nomograms. JAMA 1982;248(10):1190–3.

197. Adjepon-Yamoah KK, Al-Homrany M, Bahar Y, Ahmed ME. Aminoglycoside usage and monitoring in a Saudi Arabian teaching hospital: a ten-year laboratory audit. J Clin Pharm Ther 2000;25(4):303–7.

198. Konrad F, Wagner R, Neumeister B, Rommel H, Georgieff M. Studies on drug monitoring in thrice and once daily treatment with aminoglycosides. Intensive Care Med 1993;19(4):215–20.

199. Janknegt R. Aminoglycoside monitoring in the once- or twice-daily era. The Dutch situation considered. Pharm World Sci 1993;15(4):151–5.

200. Parker SE, Davey PG. Practicalities of once-daily aminoglycoside dosing. J Antimicrob Chemother 1993;31(1):4–8.

201. Barclay ML, Kirkpatrick CM, Begg EJ. Once daily aminoglycoside therapy. Is it less toxic than multiple daily doses and how should it be monitored? Clin Pharmacokinet 1999;36(2):89–98.

202. Blaser J, Konig C, Simmen HP, Thurnheer U. Monitoring serum concentrations for once-daily netilmicin dosing regimens. J Antimicrob Chemother 1994;33(2):341–8.

203. MacGowan AP, Reeves DS. Serum monitoring and practicalities of once-daily aminoglycoside dosing. J Antimicrob Chemother 1994;33(2):349–50.

204. Giamarellou H, Yiallouros K, Petrikkos G, Moschovakis E, Vavouraki E, Voutsinas D, Sfikakis P. Comparative kinetics and efficacy of amikacin administered once or twice daily in the treatment of systemic Gram-negative infections. J Antimicrob Chemother 1991;27(Suppl C):73–9.

205. Maller R, Ahrne H, Holmen C, Lausen I, Nilsson LE, Smedjegard J. Once- versus twice-daily amikacin regimen: efficacy and safety in systemic Gram-negative infections. Scandinavian Amikacin Once Daily Study Group. J Antimicrob Chemother 1993;31(6):939–48.

206. Reeves DS, MacGowan AP. Once-daily aminoglycoside dosing. Lancet 1993;341(8849):895–6.

207. Blaser J, Konig C, Fatio R, Follath F, Cometta A, Glauser M. Multicenter quality control study of amikacin assay for monitoring once-daily dosing regimens. International Antimicrobial Therapy Cooperative Group of the European Organization for Research and Treatment of Cancer. Ther Drug Monit 1995;17(2):133–6.

208. Kotler DP, Sordillo EM. Nutritional status and aminoglycoside dosing. Clin Infect Dis 1998;26(1):249–52.

209. Bailey TC, Reichley RM. Nutritional status and aminoglycoside dosing. Clin Infect Dis 1998;26:251–2.

210. Slaughter RL, Cappelletty DM. Economic impact of aminoglycoside toxicity and its prevention through therapeutic drug monitoring. Pharmacoeconomics 1998;14(4):385–94.

211. Binder L, Schiel X, Binder C, Menke CF, Schuttrumpf S, Armstrong VW, Unterhalt M, Erichsen N, Hiddemann W, Oellerich M. Clinical outcome and economic impact of aminoglycoside peak concentrations in febrile immunocompromised patients with hematologic malignancies. Clin Chem 1998;44(2):408–14.

Aminophenazone

General Information

Aminophenazone (amidopyrine) is the most toxic and most dangerous anti-inflammatory analgesic. Blood dyscrasias have been documented beyond any doubt, perhaps due to a hypersensitivity mechanism. The Committee on the Safety of Drugs of the Japanese Pharmaceutical Affairs Bureau has ordered its withdrawal because of its serious adverse effects (SEDA-12, 82) and it has been withdrawn in most developed countries. However, aminophenazone is still used in some developing countries (1).

Organs and Systems

Hematologic

Aminophenazone causes severe bone marrow depression, usually with a fulminant course and a high mortality (SED-9, 146) (2,3). Specific antibodies and leukoagglutinins are sometimes found (4). Agranulocytosis is caused by arrest of maturation at the metamyelocyte stage (5).

Fatal thrombocytopenia has been reported in a breastfeeding infant after the administration of aminophenazone suppositories (6).

Gastrointestinal

Gastrotoxicity with aminophenazone is less common than with other analgesic/anti-inflammatory drugs, probably because of its weaker anti-inflammatory effect.

Liver

Aminophenazone is not hepatotoxic, but liver damage can occur in the course of a general hypersensitivity reaction (7).

Urinary tract

Albuminuria, hematuria, and acute renal insufficiency have been observed, and aminophenazone causes direct renal damage even at therapeutic doses. It can also contribute to analgesic nephropathy (SED-8, 211) (8,9).

Skin

Toxic epidermal necrolysis, exfoliative dermatitis, and Stevens–Johnson syndrome have been described (SED-8, 210) (10–13).

Immunologic

A range of allergic skin reactions, acute anaphylactic shock, acute bronchospasm (in predisposed patients), and cross-sensitivity to aspirin have been reported (14).

Long-Term Effects

Tumorigenicity

Aminophenazone and its derivatives may be metabolized to carcinogenic nitrosamines. The clinical importance of this is not clear (SEDA-2, 389) (15).

Drug Administration

Drug overdose

In overdose, aminophenazone mainly affects the central nervous system, causing coma and convulsions, and the liver (16). Fatal intoxication has occurred in infants (17).

References

1. Epstein P, Yudkin JS. Agranulocytosis in Mozambique due to amidopyrine, a drug withdrawn in the west. Lancet 1980;2(8188):254–5.

2. Pisciotta AV. Drug-induced leukopenia and aplastic anemia. Clin Pharmacol Ther 1971;12(1):13–43.

3. Pisciotta V. Drug-induced agranulocytosis. Drugs 1978;15(2):132–43.
4. Barrett AJ, Weller E, Rozengurt N, Longhurst P, Humble JG. Amidopyrine agranulocytosis:drug inhibition of granulocyte colonies in the presence of patient's serum. BMJ 1976;2(6040):850–1.
5. Goudemand J, Plouvier J, Bauters F, Goudemand M. Les agranulocytoses aigues induites parle pyramidon ou les phenothiazines. A propos de 31 observations. [Acute agranulocytosis induced by pyramidon or phenothiazines. Apropos of 31 cases.] Sem Hop 1976;52(25–28):1513–20.
6. Ionescu D, Lunganoiu N. Sindrom hemoragipar trombocitopenic letal dupa aminofenazona la sugar. [A fatal thrombocytopenic hemorrhagiparous syndrome following aminophenazone in an infant.] Pediatrie (Bucur) 1991;40(1–2):169–72.
7. Scholz H, Meyer W. Akute Agranulozytose und intrahepatische Cholestase nach Aminophenazon bei einem 12 jahrigen Madchen. [Aminophenazone induced agranulocytosis and intrahepatic cholestasis in a 12-year-old girl.] Dtsch Gesundheitsw 1972;27(5):205–9.
8. Eknoyan G, Matson JL. Acute renal failure caused by aminopyrine. JAMA 1964;90:34–5.
9. Baumgartner H, Scheitlin W, von Rechenberg HK. [Bilateral renal cortical necrosis following pyrazolone treatment.] Dtsch Med Wochenschr 1967;2(23):1075–7.
10. Zombai E, Grof PA. Lyellbetegseg allergias jellegerol. Borgyogy Venerol Sz 1971;7:119.
11. Huriez C, Bergoend H, Bertez M. Vingt-trois cas de toxidermies bulleuses graves avec epidermolyse: part predominante d'anti-infectieux retard et de plurimedications. [23 cases of severe bullous toxicoderma with epidermolysis: predominant role of delayed-action anti-infectious agents and of plurimedications.] Bull Acad Natl Med 1972;156(1):12–18.
12. Kauppinen K. Lyellin syndrooma. [Lyell's syndrome.] Duodecim 1971;7(5):355–61.
13. Schmidt JG, Lischka G. Zur ophthalmologischen Symptomatologie, Therapie und Prognose des Fuchs- und Lyell-syndroms. [Ophthalmological symptomatology, therapy and prognosis of Fuch's and Lyell's syndromes.] Klin Monatsbl Augenheilkd 1970;157(3):342–57.
14. Bartoli E, Faedda in Masala R, Chiandussi L. Letter: Drug-induced asthma. Lancet 1976;1(7973):1357.
15. World Health Organisation. Aminophenazone a possible cancer hazard? WHO Drug Info 1977;Jul-Sep: 9.
16. Cervini C. Ipirazolonici: gli effetti indesiderati. [Pyrazolones: undesired effects.] Clin Ter 1972;60(4):305–18.
17. Tronzano L. Avvelenamento acuto mortale da iperdosaggio di piramidone in un lattante. [Fatal acute poisoning caused by an overdose of pyramidon in an infant.] Minerva Medicoleg 1968;88(1):71–6.

Aminorex

See also Anorectic drugs

General Information

Aminorex is an amfetamine analogue that was used as an anorectic agent, but was withdrawn from the market over 20 years ago because of its association with pulmonary hypertension, which sometimes proved fatal. Its adverse effects have been attributed predominantly to the release of noradrenaline and other catecholamines.

Organs and Systems

Respiratory

Aminorex can cause primary pulmonary hypertension, which can be fatal (1,2). The fulminant character and rapid development of the disease (characterized by dyspnea, dysrhythmias, peripheral edema, dizziness, cyanosis, chest pain, and syncope, in the absence of usual causes of pulmonary vascular disease) suggested the possibility of its being drug-induced. Long-term follow-up of aminorex-induced primary pulmonary hypertension showed that the syndrome has a chronic course, with long-term survival possible (3). Two cases of supposedly delayed reactions to aminorex have been described (4). Both concerned pulmonary hypertension, one in a subject who had taken aminorex 6 years before. In the other there was a reaction of limited duration 8 years after aminorex treatment.

In 16 patients polymorphic hydroxylation of debrisoquine was not related to the risk of aminorex-induced pulmonary hypertension (5).

Despite the withdrawal of aminorex, work to identify the mechanism of the pathogenic effect has continued, in view of the risk that other agents might behave similarly. In smooth muscle cells taken from the small resistance pulmonary arteries of the rat lung aminorex inhibited potassium current and in isolated, perfused rat lung, it caused a dose-related increase in perfusion pressure (6). However, long-term administration of aminorex fumarate to rats failed to cause hypertensive pulmonary vascular disease (7), although in dogs there was an increase in pulmonary pressure (8).

References

1. Hager W, Thiede D, Wink K. Primar vaskulare pulmonale Hypertonie und Appetitzugler. [Primary vascular pulmonary hypertension and appetite depressants.] Med Klin 1971;66(11):386–90.
2. Follath F, Burkart F, Schweizer W. Drug-induced pulmonary hypertension? BMJ 1971;1(5743):265–6.
3. Mlczoch J, Probst P, Szeless S, Kaindl F. Primary pulmonary hypertension: Follow-up of patients with and without anorectic drug intake. Cor Vasa 1980;22(4):251–7.
4. Simon H, Felix R. Reversibele pulmonalarterielle Hypertonie nach Einnahme von Menocil. [Reversible pulmonary arterial hypertension after aminorexfumarate.] Med Klin 1977;72(41):1685–8.
5. Saner H, Gurtner HP, Preisig R, Kupfer A. Polymorphic debrisoquine and mephenytoin hydroxylation in patients with pulmonary hypertension of vascular origin after aminorex fumarate. Eur J Clin Pharmacol 1986;31(4):437–42.
6. Weir EK, Reeve HL, Huang JM, Michelakis E, Nelson DP, Hampl V, Archer SL. Anorexic agents aminorex, fenfluramine, and dexfenfluramine inhibit potassium current in rat pulmonary vascular smooth muscle and cause pulmonary vasoconstriction. Circulation 1996;94(9):2216–20.
7. Engelhardt R, Kalbfleisch H. [Effect of chronic application of aminorex-fumarate on the pulmonary circulation of the rat]. Arzneimittelforschung 1973;23(8):1057–61.
8. Naeije R, Maggiorini M, Delcroix M, Leeman M, Melot C. Effects of chronic dexfenfluramine treatment on pulmonary hemodynamics in dogs. Am J Respir Crit Care Med 1996;154(54):1347–50.

Aminosalicylates

General Information

The aminosalicylates that are currently available are:

- mesalazine (rINN; 5-aminosalicylic acid mesalamine);
- sulfasalazine (rINN), a compound of mesalazine and sulfapyridine, the two compounds being linked by a diazo bond that is hydrolysed by intestinal bacteria; mesalazine is therapeutically effective in inflammatory bowel disease and sulfapyridine causes adverse effects;
- olsalazine (rINN), a compound of two molecules of mesalazine, linked by a diazo bond that is hydrolysed by intestinal bacteria;
- balsalazide (rINN), a prodrug of mesalazine linked to 4-amino-benzolylanine by an azo bond that is hydrolysed by intestinal bacteria.

Mesalazine can be administered using carriers that deliver it to the large bowel or on its own in the form of a modified-release formulation (1).

The pharmacological properties of aminosalicylates and their potential value in the treatment of inflammatory bowel disease have been reviewed (2). Aminosalicylates are the drugs of first choice in the acute treatment of ulcerative colitis and in maintaining remission. Their value in Crohn's disease is more modest. The variability in clinical results is at least partly caused by the different formulations and dosages of the drug used, as well as the high variation in drug disposition and topical availability of the active drug. The popularity of aminosalicylates is most likely due to the low incidence of adverse effects and good overall safety record.

Observational studies

Mesalazine caused apoptosis and reduced cell proliferation in the colorectal mucosa in 17 patients with sporadic polyps of the large bowel (3). This may be clinically relevant in lowering the rate of polyp recurrence after polypectomy, thereby contributing to chemoprevention of sporadic colonic carcinoma.

Comparative studies

In a randomized, double-blind study, balsalazide 3 g/day and mesalazine 1.2 g/day effectively maintained remission in 99 patients with ulcerative colitis (4). Adverse events were equally common in the two groups, the most common being headache, abdominal pain and diarrhea, respiratory infections, body pains, and flu-like symptoms.

In a 12-week trial in 168 patients with mild to moderate ulcerative colitis, olsalazine 3 g/day was as effective as mesalazine 3 g/day in inducing a remission (5). There were more adverse effects in patients taking olsalazine (41 of 88) than mesalazine (29 of 80). Most of the adverse effects related to bowel disturbances: diarrhea, vomiting, abdominal discomfort, heartburn, flatulence, and nausea. Diarrhea was more common in patients taking olsalazine. One patient taking mesalazine developed a lupus-like syndrome.

The effects of mesalazine and olsalazine in delivering active mesalazine to the colon and in producing a systemic load as a basis for potential long-term toxicity have been compared in a single-blind, randomized, crossover study in 15 patients with ulcerative colitis (6). The patients took either olsalazine 500 mg bd or mesalazine 500 mg tds, with a crossover after 7 days. Plasma and urine concentrations of mesalazine and acetylmesalazine were assayed. Olsalazine caused loose stools in one patient and diarrhea in two, whereas mesalazine caused diarrhea in one. The systemic load of active mesalazine was significantly higher after mesalazine than olsalazine, based on both therapeutically recommended doses and when calculated on an equimolar basis. Some patients treated with mesalazine had very high plasma and urinary concentrations of mesalazine and acetylmesalazine, which may have long-term safety implications.

The relapse-preventing effects and safety profiles of balsalazide 1.5 g bd, balsalazide 3 g bd, and mesalazine 0.5 g tds have been studied in a multicenter, randomized, double-blind trial in 133 patients with ulcerative colitis in remission (7). High-dose balsalazide was significantly more effective in maintaining remission compared with the other two treatments. All three treatments were well tolerated.

In a double-blind, multicenter study in 182 patients with active Crohn's disease affecting the ileum and/or ascending colon, a modified-release formulation of budesonide 9 mg/day was more effective in inducing remission than mesalazine 2 g bd (8). Adverse events were similar in the two groups. Mild abnormalities of adrenal function tests were slightly more common with budesonide, but the clinical significance of these was unclear.

In a randomized, multicenter study in 94 patients, mesalazine 4 g/day for 12 weeks in a microgranular formulation was as effective as a standard dose of a glucocorticoid (6-methylprednisolone 40 mg/day) in mild to moderate Crohn's ileitis (Crohn's Disease Activity Index 180-350) (9). The group treated with methylprednisolone had a higher number of adverse events than those given mesalazine. The only adverse effect related to mesalazine was acute pancreatitis, which resolved on withdrawal.

Short-chain fatty acids, especially butyrate, are a preferred source of energy for the colonic epithelium. There is evidence to suggest that butyrate enemas are effective in the treatment of ulcerative colitis. The seeds of *Plantago ovata* (a source of fermentable dietary fiber) increase fecal concentrations of butyrate and acetate. In a randomized, open, parallel-group, multicenter study in 105 patients with ulcerative colitis, *P. ovata* seeds 10 mg bd were as effective as mesalazine 500 mg tds in maintaining remission over 12 months (10). Adverse effects were similar in the two groups, and included constipation, flatulence, nausea, and diarrhea.

Placebo-controlled studies

In an 18-month, double-blind, randomized, placebo-controlled trial in 318 patients, mesalazine 4 g/day did not significantly affect the postoperative course of Crohn's disease compared with placebo (11). There was some relapse-preventing effect in patients with isolated small bowel disease. The overall incidence of adverse effects was similar with mesalazine and placebo. Of the serious adverse effects reported, only one case of alopecia was considered to be possibly or probably related to mesalazine.

In a double-blind, placebo-controlled, multicenter trial in 65 patients with ulcerative proctitis in clinical and endoscopic remission, mesalazine in suppositories 500 mg/day as sole treatment was effective, well tolerated, and safe for maintenance of remission over 24 months (12). The incidence of adverse effects was similar with mesalazine and placebo. The most frequent adverse effects with mesalazine were rectal disorders, abdominal pain, and headache.

Daily mesalazine 4 g orally plus placebo enema and mesalazine 2 g orally plus mesalazine 2 g rectally as a liquid enema have been compared in the treatment of mild to moderate ulcerative colitis in a multicenter, randomized, double-blind trial in 130 patients (7). The two treatments were equally effective in inducing disease remission. Both were well tolerated, and the frequencies of adverse effects were similar in the two groups.

In a randomized, double-blind, placebo-controlled trial in 328 patients with quiescent Crohn's disease, olsalazine 2 g/day given for 52 weeks was not superior to placebo in maintaining remission (13). Gastrointestinal adverse effects were significantly more frequent in the olsalazine group; diarrhea was the most commonly reported adverse effect.

General adverse effects

Adverse reactions with sulfasalazine are frequent, and the withdrawal rate for this reason can be as high as 30% (SEDA-16, 426). Common adverse effects related to sulfapyridine include headache, nausea, anorexia, and malaise. Other allergic or toxic adverse effects include fever, rash, hemolytic anemia, hepatitis, pancreatitis, paradoxical worsening of colitis, and reversible sperm abnormalities (14). Sulfasalazine appears to cause frequent severe adverse effects in adult-onset Still's disease and systemic-onset juvenile rheumatoid arthritis, as suggested by a long-term, follow-up study of 41 patients with adult-onset Still's disease and 109 consecutive patients with rheumatoid arthritis (15). Adverse effects included abdominal pain, nausea and vomiting, urticaria, facial flushing, high fever, hypotension, severe myelosuppression, and fulminant hepatitis, which resulted in death in one patient.

Skin reactions are common with sulfasalazine, and general sensitization can occur, as with other sulfa derivatives. The clinical features, besides skin rash, include granulomatous liver disease, positive lupus phenomenon, hypocomplementemia, and fever (16). More serious skin conditions can also occur. In the case of mild reactions, patients can often be desensitized by giving small (and then progressively increasing) doses. Various complex autoimmune syndromes can occur (SEDA-17, 423); in long-term studies of the use of sulfasalazine in rheumatoid arthritis, 12–20% of evaluable patients developed antinuclear antibodies during treatment (SEDA-16, 426) (SEDA-18, 375). Tumor-inducing effects have not been described.

The role of mesalazine in the acute and long-term treatment of ulcerative colitis has been reviewed (17). Mesalazine is equivalent to or better than sulfasalazine and better than placebo in inducing remission of acute disease, and comparable to sulfasalazine and better than placebo for long-term maintenance of remission. Adverse effects are uncommon, but include idiosyncratic worsening of colitis and renal toxicity. Mesalazine is safe during pregnancy and breastfeeding. In maintenance therapy, it may reduce the risk of developing colorectal carcinoma.

Crossover studies have shown that mesalazine has about a 10-fold lower potential than sulfasalazine for inducing allergic reactions or causing intolerance. Adverse effects with all aminosalicylates include (generally more frequent with sulfasalazine) headache, nausea, abdominal pain, dyspepsia, fatigue, rash, fever, rarely exacerbation of the disease, pancreatitis, pericarditis, pneumonitis, liver disease, nephritis, and bone marrow depression. Watery diarrhea is an adverse effect unique to olsalazine, while anorexia, folate malabsorption, hemolysis, neutropenia, agranulocytosis, male infertility, and neuropathy are unique to sulfasalazine.

The adverse effects of sulfasalazine 2–3 g/day and mesalazine 1.2–2.4 g/day in 685 patients have been reviewed for a median follow-up period of 7 and 5 years respectively (18). Adverse effects were observed overall in 20% of patients taking sulfasalazine and 6.5% of those taking mesalazine. The commonest adverse effects due to sulfasalazine (reported by more than 10% of patients) were dyspepsia, rash, and headache, while the commonest due to mesalazine were rash, diarrhea, headache, fever, abdominal pain, impaired renal function, dyspepsia, and edema. Fertility was affected in all 42 male patients taking sulfasalazine who were assessed, but improved when they changed to mesalazine.

A pharmacovigilance report from France reported 128 adverse events during 15.6 million days of therapy with Pentasa in 1993 and 1994. Adverse events with a high likelihood of causality included diarrhea, pancreatitis, liver abnormalities, blood dyscrasias, renal insufficiency, and cardiac disorders, including myocarditis. Most of these rare adverse events did not appear to be dose-related in the therapeutic range (SEDA-21, 364) A meta-analysis of studies of the effectiveness of mesalazine in maintaining remission in Crohn's disease showed an adverse effect frequency of 14% in patients taking mesalazine and 15% in patients taking placebo. The most frequent adverse effect attributable to mesalazine was diarrhea (SEDA-22, 394).

The dose response relation of oral mesalazine in inflammatory bowel disease has been briefly reviewed (19). Higher doses (3 g/day) are more effective in inducing and maintaining remission than lower doses (1.5 g/day). None of the known adverse effects of mesalazine is clearly dose-related in the therapeutic range of doses.

An analysis of suspected serious adverse reactions reported to the Committee on Safety of Medicines in the UK in 1991–98 has failed to show a safety advantage for mesalazine over sulfasalazine in the treatment of inflammatory bowel disease (20). Pancreatitis and interstitial nephritis were significantly more common with mesalazine.

The adverse effects of olsalazine would be expected to be those of mesalazine, and this is largely the case. However, diarrhea has been sufficiently common to suggest that it may be a particular problem with olsalazine, with an incidence of some 13%; it is probably a small-intestinal secretory diarrhea (SEDA-17, 425) (21). Similarly, cholestatic hepatitis, confirmed on rechallenge, did not recur with mesalazine in similar doses (SEDA-16, 428). In one case there was a marked hypersensitivity reaction in a man previously intolerant of sulfasalazine, but the circumstances suggested a reaction to mesalazine rather than to the double molecule (SEDA-18, 376).

Organs and Systems

Cardiovascular

A single Scandinavian case report has reliably attributed a fatal myocarditis to mesalazine (22).

The time between the start of treatment and the onset of mesalazine-associated pericarditis usually ranges from a few days to 7 months. However, the delay can be longer.

- A 53-year-old man with Crohn's disease, who had taken mesalazine 500 mg/day for the past 8 years, developed pericarditis with an effusion (23). The pericarditis resolved rapidly on drug withdrawal. Investigations excluded other common causes of pericarditis.
- Pericarditis in a 16-year-old boy with inflammatory bowel disease taking mesalazine resolved on withdrawal, but recurred after starting sulfasalazine 500 mg tds (24).
- Acute pericarditis has been reported in a 17-year-old man with severe ulcerative colitis who had taken mesalazine 1.5 g/day for 2 weeks (25). The pericarditis resolved on withdrawal and recurred on rechallenge with a low dose (62.5 mg) of mesalazine 3 weeks later.
- Constrictive pericarditis has been reported in a 37-year-old woman with chronic ulcerative colitis who had taken mesalazine 2 g/day for 2 weeks (26). She recovered after radical pericardiectomy.

Bradycardia has been attributed to mesalazine.

- Severe symptomatic bradycardia has been reported in a 29-year-old woman with ulcerative colitis who was taking mesalazine (27). The bradycardia resolved on withdrawal. Six weeks later mesalazine was restarted for a relapse of her colitis, and symptomatic bradycardia recurred. Again this resolved on withdrawal.

Chest pain has been attributed to mesalazine (28).

- A 37-year-old man with ulcerative colitis developed severe retrosternal chest pain with non-specific ST–T wave changes in the inferolateral leads of the electrocardiogram after taking mesalazine 800 mg qds for 1 week. Cardiac enzymes, coronary angiography, left ventricular function, and pulmonary angiography were normal. Mesalazine was omitted and glucocorticoids were tapered. He recovered completely and his electrocardiogram normalized. Two weeks later he was given mesalazine 800 mg qds and again developed retrosternal chest pain with T wave inversion in the lateral leads. Mesalazine was withdrawn and his symptoms resolved within 24 hours. His chest pain did not recur over an 18 month follow-up period while not taking mesalazine.

Raynaud's phenomenon has been attributed to sulfasalazine (29,30).

Respiratory

"Sulfasalazine lung," fibrosing alveolitis, and eosinophilic pleurisy are variants on a well-recognized although unusual lung complication. Most commonly it presents with cough, fever, eosinophilia, dyspnea, and pulmonary infiltrates (SEDA-15, 309) (31). Sputum production, a history of allergy, rash, chest pain, and weight loss are inconsistent findings. The disease usually develops 1–9 months after the start of treatment and the fibrosing alveolitis can be fatal (32). The lung pathology is variable, the commonest change being an eosinophilic pneumonia with peripheral eosinophilia and interstitial inflammation with or without fibrosis. In case reports, the majority of patients with suspected sulfasalazine-induced lung disease improved within weeks of drug withdrawal (33). Whether the salicylate or the sulfa moiety is responsible is unclear; both can cause pulmonary eosinophilia. Differentiation from lung disease simply associated with ulcerative colitis can be difficult, particularly because the drug-induced form sometimes causes an interstitial pneumonitis without evidence of an allergic reaction (34) and rechallenge can be dangerous (SEDA-16, 427).

Peripheral lung infiltrates with blood eosinophilia are rare effects of sulfasalazine. Sulfasalazine-induced hypersensitivity lung disease with simultaneous *Legionella pneumophila* infection has been reported for the first time (35).

- A 32-year-old woman with ulcerative colitis developed bilateral pulmonary infiltrates with peripheral eosinophilia 2 weeks after starting to take sulfasalazine and mesalazine enemas, and both drugs were withdrawn. Based on a high antibody titer, legionnaires' disease was diagnosed and empirical therapy with a macrolide antibiotic was started; she improved within a few days. Three months later sulfasalazine was restarted, followed 3 days later by acute pulmonary symptoms (bilateral confluent opacities) and blood eosinophilia. The abnormalities resolved completely after drug withdrawal and prophylactic antibiotic therapy.

Various adverse respiratory effects of mesalazine have been reported.

- A patient who took mesalazine for 2 years had a symptomatic bilateral lung reaction, with interstitial infiltrates and impaired function; the condition developed insidiously but recovered within 8 months after drug withdrawal (36). The condition was not necessarily identical to the lung reaction seen with sulfasalazine.
- Pleural effusion with pulmonary infiltration has been reported in a 72-year-old woman with ulcerative colitis taking mesalazine 800 mg tds (37). The lung pathology resolved after drug withdrawal.
- An eosinophilic pleural effusion has been reported in a 35-year-old male non-smoker who had taken mesalazine 2.4 g/day orally for 2 weeks for a diarrheal illness (38). He recovered after mesalazine was withdrawn.
- A 35-year-old woman with ulcerative colitis who had taken mesalazine 1.5 g/day for about 40 days developed a low-grade fever with bilateral eosinophilic pulmonary infiltrates (confirmed by transbronchial lung biopsy) (39). Spontaneous clinical and radiological resolution

occurred on withdrawal. A drug lymphocyte stimulation test was positive for mesalazine.

- A 29-year-old woman with ulcerative colitis taking mesalazine 1 g tds developed respiratory distress (40). Her respiratory symptoms (chest pain and respiratory distress, especially exertional dyspnea) occurred 48 hours after she started to take mesalazine and disappeared immediately on withdrawal. Similar symptoms recurred on rechallenge 3 weeks later in a lower dose of 500 mg bd. Chest X-ray and white cell count a day later were normal.
- Bronchiolitis obliterans has been reported in an 18-year-old female non-smoker with ulcerative colitis, 3 months after reintroduction of mesalazine 1.6 g/day orally (41). She recovered after mesalazine withdrawal and treatment with glucocorticoids.
- Interstitial pulmonary disease (lymphocytic alveolitis and mild interstitial pulmonary fibrosis) has been reported in a 70-year-old woman with ulcerative colitis who had taken mesalazine 2.4 g/day for 3 months (42). Halving the dose of mesalazine to 1.2 g/day led to resolution of her lung disorder without relapse of ulcerative colitis.

A limited form of Wegener's granulomatosis with a bronchiolitis obliterans organizing pneumonia-like variant has been reported in a 19-year-old man, a non-smoker, with ulcerative colitis, 6 months after the introduction of mesalazine 2.25 g tds orally (43). He recovered after mesalazine withdrawal and treatment with glucocorticoids.

Nervous system

An unusual but not unique case of transverse myelitis was reported in 1991, and other published case reports suggest links with chorea and ataxia (SEDA-16, 427).

Individual cases of other adverse effects on the nervous system have appeared.

- Vivid dreams and daytime hallucinations occurred in a woman taking sulfasalazine (44).
- Aseptic meningitis occurred in a patient with pre-existing Sjögren's syndrome; and the drug link was confirmed by positive rechallenge (45).
- In a slow acetylator, an axonal sensorimotor neuropathy could have been due to sulfasalazine (SEDA-17, 424).

Seizures with acute encephalopathy have been reported in a woman taking sulfasalazine for polyarthritis (46).

Hematologic

In a randomized, double-blind, placebo-controlled trial, 70 patients with established ankylosing spondylitis and a mean disease duration of 17 years were investigated in two centers for 26 weeks, comparing sulfasalazine 3 g/day with placebo. In the treatment group there were significantly more cases of anemia, leukopenia, eosinophilia, and thrombocytopenia (47).

Sulfasalazine causes Heinz body anemia in patients with abnormal hemoglobin and hemolysis in patients with glucose-6-phosphate dehydrogenase deficiency (48).

- A 79-year-old woman who had been taking sulfasalazine for ulcerative colitis for 5 years developed a positive Coombs' test and a hemoglobin of 8.2 g/dl.

Agglutination occurred when a mixture of sulfasalazine and the patient's serum was added to normal erythrocytes treated with the endopeptidase ficin, but there was no reactivity when control serum was used or when sulfasalazine was omitted. Preincubation of sulfasalazine with normal erythrocytes gave negative results on addition of the patient's serum, excluding the possibility of a penicillin-like reaction. The patient had normal glucose-6-phosphate dehydrogenase activity and there were no Heinz bodies in a blood smear.

However, about 1.7% of patients with ulcerative colitis develop immune hemolytic anemia, even in the absence of sulfasalazine, so cause and effect is not always possible to determine.

Agranulocytosis is very unusual but well described with sulfasalazine, and can occur suddenly and very early in treatment (49). The risk in sulfasalazine users with arthritic disorders (6/1000 users) was about 10 times higher than that in users with inflammatory bowel disease (0.6/1000 users) (SEDA-20, 320). Agranulocytosis is supposedly more common in slow acetylators (50). However, in one study the risk of agranulocytosis was not increased in slow acetylators (50). Leukopenia occurred in a patient taking mesalazine after a similar reaction to sulfasalazine (SEDA-17, 425).

Sulfasalazine reduces folic acid absorption, but rarely to a clinically significant extent, although megaloblastic anemia has rarely been documented (51,52).

Methemoglobinemia can occur in slow acetylators of sulfapyridine (53).

Thrombocytopenia has occasionally been attributed to mesalazine (54–56) and olsalazine (57).

- A possible association between mesalazine and pancytopenia has been reported in a 23-year-old man with Crohn's disease (58). The pancytopenia resolved after withdrawal.

Gastrointestinal

Nausea and vomiting, taste disturbances (SEDA-17, 424), anorexia, stomatitis, flatulence (59), and abdominal discomfort can occur in patients taking sulfasalazine and mesalazine. They are particularly common in slow acetylators, but symptoms remit with dosage reduction. Diarrhea is more common with olsalazine than with sulfasalazine.

Five cases of severe persistent diarrhea following the use of mesalazine in doses of 2.4–4.8 g/day have been reported (60). The diarrhea was made worse by increasing doses of the drug. Symptoms resolved on withdrawal or dosage reduction.

- Severe diarrhea that mimicked the effects expected with the use of non-steroidal anti-inflammatory drugs, associated with changes in fecal eicosanoid content, has been reported in a 57-year-old man with non-granulomatous enterocolitis who took mesalazine 4 g/day (61). The diarrhea resolved dramatically on withdrawal.

Exacerbation of existing colitis is rare but well recognized with sulfasalazine and it can also cause colitis de novo; pseudomembranous colitis with *Clostridium difficile* was reported in 1991, as was fatal neutropenic colitis with no evidence of *C. difficile* infection (SEDA-17, 424). Reports of exacerbation of colitic symptoms caused by intolerance of mesalazine are infrequent. Diarrhea, rectal bleeding, and weight loss have been described in three patients (aged 13, 14, and 17 years) with ulcerative colitis who were taking mesalazine 2–4 g/day (62). Their symptoms resolved dramatically after mesalazine withdrawal.

The finding of *Escherichia coli* on rectal swabs, with a range of resistance extending beyond the sulfa drugs, is difficult to evaluate. The clinical relevance is doubtful.

Liver

Exceptionally, fulminant hepatic failure with massive necrosis has been seen in patients taking sulfasalazine (63). Two fatal cases were reported in 1992 (SEDA-17, 424).

Cases of hepatitis have been observed in patients taking mesalazine; one such case was observed in a series of 103 patients taking mesalazine, and two further cases in another series of 44 patients (SEDA-20, 320).

- Severe hepatic injury with biopsy-proven cholestasis was reported in a man who had taken mesalazine in a dose of 4 g/day for 4 months (SEDA-22, 394) (64).

Mesalazine-induced chronic hepatitis and liver fibrosis, with raised serum IgG concentrations and autoantibodies, has been reported (65).

- A 57-year-old man with an unspecified abdominal complaint (later confirmed not to be inflammatory bowel disease), who was also taking simvastatin, developed abnormal liver function tests and antinuclear and anti-smooth muscle antibodies 13 months after starting to take mesalazine. Simvastatin hepatotoxicity was suspected and that drug was withdrawn, but there was no improvement in liver function. Mesalazine was withdrawn 21 months after the start of therapy, with rapid normalization of liver enzymes and serum IgG concentrations and disappearance of the autoantibodies.

Pancreas

Pancreatitis has several times been ascribed to sulfasalazine and may well be the expression of an allergic reaction; cases with positive rechallenge are on record.

Pancreatitis has been noted with mesalazine often enough to be taken seriously (66); it usually occurs within a short time of starting treatment, has occurred in children as well as adults, and has sometimes been confirmed by rechallenge (SEDA-18, 375).

- A 29-year-old man with Crohn's disease who had taken mesalazine 2 g/day for 3 days developed acute pancreatitis (67). Clinical and biochemical improvement occurred on drug withdrawal. Acute pancreatitis recurred on rechallenge.
- A 23-year-old man with ulcerative colitis developed acute pancreatitis after taking mesalazine 1.5 g/day for 4 days (68). Resolution occurred on withdrawal but rechallenge was not performed.
- A 10-year-old boy with ulcerative colitis developed acute pancreatitis 1 day after the dose of mesalazine was increased from 400 mg bd (which he has taken for 5 months without any adverse effect) to 800 mg bd for a

mild relapse (69). He became asymptomatic 3 days after drug withdrawal.
- A 34-year-old woman with colitis developed pancreatitis 1 week after starting mesalazine 1 g tds; she recovered after drug withdrawal (70). She was admitted 15 months later with a relapse of colitis and was given oral prednisolone 50 mg/day and mesalazine enemas (2 g bd). Although the colitis regressed, 10 days later she again developed acute pancreatitis. She recovered 3 days after prednisolone and mesalazine enemas were withdrawn. Symptoms of pancreatitis did not recur when prednisolone was restarted.
- A patient developed pancreatitis after taking mesalazine 2 g bd; the symptoms resolved when the drug was withdrawn, but recurred when azathioprine was given (71).

Two unusual cases of delayed-onset pancreatitis occurring 3 months and 2 years after starting mesalazine have been described (SEDA-22, 394) (72).

Urinary tract

Two patients with long-standing ulcerative colitis developed what seemed to be a drug-induced chronic interstitial nephritis after taking sulfasalazine for several years, with no other detectable cause (73); the same problem has arisen with mesalazine. However, in a long-term study (mean treatment time 10 years) in 36 patients taking sulfasalazine for ulcerative colitis, there was no nephrotoxicity (74).

Proximal renal tubular proteinuria is a possible complication in patients treated with high doses of mesalazine, and it is clearly important to monitor renal function in these patients (SEDA-22, 394) (75). Two studies in 21 (76) and 95 (77) patients with ulcerative colitis and Crohn's disease have shown that proteinuria of tubular marker proteins is common and is related to disease activity rather than to treatment with mesalazine. Thus, tubular proteins are not useful predictors of an adverse renal response to the drug. Nephrotic syndrome with minimal change nephropathy has been described with sulfasalazine and mesalazine (SEDA-16, 427).

Interstitial nephritis has been well documented in patients taking mesalazine (SEDA-17, 425) (8,78–81).

- Interstitial nephritis occurred in a 29-year-woman with ulcerative colitis and a 48-year-old woman with Crohn's disease who were taking mesalazine (82).

There have been three other reports of interstitial nephritis associated with mesalazine in patients with inflammatory bowel disease, two with ulcerative colitis and one with Crohn's disease (83–85). One patient continued to be dialysis-dependent and in two patients withdrawal of the drug and treatment with glucocorticoids resulted in partial improvement in renal function.

- Acute tubular necrosis has been reported in a 49-year-old man with Crohn's disease who had taken mesalazine 4 g/day for 1 month (86). Renal function normalized rapidly after withdrawal of mesalazine.

In addition, there has been a report of a possible association between mesalazine and nephrotic syndrome due to minimal change nephropathy, which resolved after withdrawal (87).

Serious renal impairment occurs in under 1 in 500 recipients of enteric-coated mesalazine (88), and early recognition and withdrawal (after up to 10 months of administration) has been reported to have resulted in complete recovery of renal function in five out of six patients. Monitoring renal function in patients taking mesalazine formulations is recommended. Oral enteric-coated mesalazine should not be used in patients with renal sensitivity to sulfasalazine, a history of hypersensitivity to salicylates, severe renal impairment, and children under 2 years old.

- A 23-year-old student with ulcerative colitis who took mesalazine 1.5 g/day for 15 days developed asymptomatic renal insufficiency (89). Renal function rapidly normalized after drug withdrawal.

Two other cases of interstitial nephritis have been reported in children with Crohn's disease who were taking mesalazine (90).

Nephrotoxicity has been described during treatment with olsalazine (SEDA-21, 364). To assess the effects of 9 months of treatment with oral mesalazine 1.2 g/day and olsalazine 1 g/day on renal function, a randomized trial has been performed in 40 patients with ulcerative colitis in complete remission (91). Neither drug had a significant effect on glomerular filtration rate. Adverse effects (all mild to moderate) were more common in the mesalazine group; they included abdominal pain and distension, dyspepsia, nausea, and diarrhea.

Skin

Simple rashes are not uncommon in patients taking sulfasalazine, including maculopapular rash, pruritus, urticaria, angioedema, eczematous dermatitis, photosensitivity, skin discoloration, and oral ulceration. Raynaud's phenomenon and toxic epidermal necrolysis associated with erythroid hypoplasia and agranulocytosis have occurred; in one case of toxic epidermal necrolysis there was marked immunosuppression (SEDA-18, 375).

- Acute generalized exanthematous pustulosis occurred in a 28-year-old man with ulcerative colitis taking sulfasalazine (92). A patch test was negative, but the lymphocyte stimulation assay for sulfasalazine showed a stimulation index of 541% (controls were not mentioned).

A rare case of skin hyperpigmentation (apparently a phototoxic reaction) has been associated with sulfasalazine lung (93).

Rashes have not generally proved an important problem with mesalazine, but two cases of oral and cutaneous lichen planus which had developed during sulfasalazine treatment recurred when the patients later took mesalazine (SEDA-17, 425).

Hair

Hair loss is rare in patients taking sulfasalazine (SEDA-16, 427).

Sexual function

Erectile impotence has often been described in patients taking sulfasalazine, sometimes with positive rechallenge (94).

Immunologic

The causes of ANCA-positive vasculitis with high titers of antimyeloperoxidase antibodies in 30 new patients have been reviewed (95). The findings illustrate that this type of vasculitis is predominantly drug-induced. Only 12 of the 30 cases were not related to a drug. The most frequently implicated drug was hydralazine ($n = 10$); the others were propylthiouracil ($n = 3$), penicillamine ($n = 2$), allopurinol ($n = 2$), and sulfasalazine ($n = 1$).

Treatment with sulfasalazine was associated with lupus-like symptoms and systemic lupus erythematosus-related autoantibody production in 10% of patients with early rheumatoid arthritis; risk factors included a systemic lupus erythematosus-related HLA haplotype, increased serum interleukin-10 concentrations, and a speckled pattern of antinuclear antibodies (96).

Sulfasalazine-induced angioimmunoblastic lymphadenopathy has been reported in a patient with juvenile chronic arthritis (97).

A Kawasaki-like syndrome has been reported in a patient taking sulfasalazine, who later reacted in the same way to mesalazine (SEDA-16, 427).

The possibility of allergic reactions to mesalazine has been suggested, but they may be rather less of a problem than with sulfasalazine.

- Angioedema has been reported in a 23-year-old man with inflammatory bowel disease 48 hours after he was given mesalazine 4 g/day (98).

A lupus-like syndrome has been described on several occasions (SEDA-15, 400) (99).

Second-Generation Effects

Fertility

Oligospermia, with reduced motility and a high frequency of abnormal forms, and male infertility are well documented in patients taking sulfasalazine. Oral and rectal treatments have the same effects, which reverse on withdrawal. Male infertility caused by sulfasalazine can be reversed by switching to mesalazine.

Pregnancy

Pregnant colitic patients generally fare better if they continued to take aminosalicylates. Though sulfasalazine crosses the placenta, competes for albumin-binding sites with bilirubin, and can be detected in breast milk, no adverse effects on offspring have been detected.

Lactation

Even in women taking large doses, only very small amounts of mesalazine enter the breast milk; toxic effects are unlikely but allergic effects can occur (SEDA-18, 376).

Susceptibility Factors

Genetic factors

Because sulfonamides are subject to polymorphic metabolism by *N*-acetyltransferase (NAT2), some of the adverse effects of sulfasalazine are more common in slow acetylators. Gastrointestinal adverse reactions occur more commonly in slow acetylators, and they should use lower doses.

Glucose-6-phosphate dehydrogenase deficiency can be associated with a tendency to hemolysis in patients taking sulfasalazine.

When chronic inflammatory bowel disease co-exists with acute intermittent porphyria, the bowel condition itself brings with it an increased risk of acute attacks of porphyria; sulfasalazine can trigger such an attack in this condition (SEDA-17, 425).

Drug Administration

Drug formulations

Oral enteric-coated mesalazine consists of ethylcellulose-coated microgranules from which mesalazine is released in the small and large intestines in a diffusion-dependent manner.

The use of oral enteric-coated mesalazine, which releases mesalazine in the terminal ileum and colon, has been reviewed (88,100). Dose-related improvements in clinical and endoscopic parameters have been reported with prolonged-release mesalazine 2–4 g/day in trials in patients with mild to moderately active ulcerative colitis. About 74% of patients with mild to moderate ulcerative colitis improve with enteric-coated mesalazine 2.4–4.8 g/day. There is a trend toward a better response with higher doses. Oral enteric-coated mesalazine 0.8–4.4 g/day appears to be as effective as sulfasalazine 2–4 g/day, modified-release mesalazine 1.5 g/day, and balsalazide 3 g/day in maintaining remission in ulcerative colitis.

Prolonged-release mesalazine also reduced disease activity in patients with mild to moderately active Crohn's disease. In Crohn's disease, mesalazine was more effective in preventing relapse in patients with isolated small bowel disease than in those with colonic involvement. Prolonged-release mesalazine appears to be as well tolerated as placebo, and the incidence of adverse effects does not appear to be dose related. Nausea/vomiting, diarrhea, abdominal pain, and dyspepsia are the most commonly reported. Reports of nephrotoxicity with this formulation are rare.

In a randomized, open trial in 227 patients with mild to moderate ulcerative colitis, mesalazine 4 g/day given as prolonged-release granules bd and qds was as effective as prolonged-release tablets given qds (101). All the treatments were well tolerated and the frequencies of adverse effects were similar in the treatment groups. The patients preferred twice-daily dosing.

In a 4-week, randomized trial in 103 patients with mild to moderate left-sided ulcerative colitis or proctosigmoiditis, mesalazine gel enema 2 g/day was as effective as mesalazine foam enema 2 g/day in inducing remission (102). Patients in the foam group had significantly more difficulty in retention and more abdominal bloating and discomfort during administration of the drug.

In an open, randomized trial in 266 patients with active distal ulcerative colitis, mesalazine foam enema 2 g/day was as effective as mesalazine standard liquid enema 4 g/day (103). The number of adverse effects attributable to medication was higher in the foam group than in the liquid enema group (14 versus 4). The most commonly reported adverse effect was flatulence.

Oral enteric-coated mesalazine is well tolerated in children aged 4–19 years and in adults who are intolerant of sulfasalazine. The most common adverse effects are headache, gas, nausea, diarrhea, and dyspepsia. The adverse effects can be severe enough to require withdrawal of the drug in up to 11% of patients.

Drug–Drug Interactions

Azathioprine and mercaptopurine

In a prospective, parallel-group study in 34 patients with Crohn's disease taking azathioprine or mercaptopurine, co-administration of mesalazine 4 g/day, sulfasalazine 4 g/day, or balsalazide 6.75 g/day for 8 weeks resulted in an increase in whole blood 6-thioguanine nucleotide concentrations and a high frequency of leukopenia (104). In 16 patients with quiescent Crohn's disease taking a stable dose of azathioprine plus sulfasalazine or mesalazine, mean 6-thioguanine nucleotide concentrations fell significantly after aminosalicylate withdrawal without significant changes in thiopurine methyltransferase activity (105).

Thiopurines are metabolized by thiopurine methyltransferase, whose activity is controlled by a common genetic polymorphism in the short arm of chromosome 6. Patients with low or intermediate activity who take azathioprine or 6-mercaptopurine are at risk of myelosuppression caused by excess accumulation of the active thiopurine metabolite 6-thioguanine nucleotide. Benzoic acid derivatives, such as mesalazine and its precursors, and prodrugs (sulfasalazine, olsalazine, and balsalazide) inhibit thiopurine methyltransferase activity in vitro. This action could explain the increase in whole blood concentrations of 6-thioguanine nucleotide, leading to leukopenia.

Digoxin

Sulfasalazine reduces the systemic availability of digoxin (106).

Ferrous sulfate

Ferrous sulfate interferes with the absorption of sulfasalazine, possibly by chelation (107). The significance of this phenomenon is doubtful, given that the beneficial effect of sulfasalazine depends on the release of mesalazine in the large intestine.

Warfarin

An interaction of mesalazine with warfarin has been reported (108).

- A 55-year-old woman taking warfarin 5 mg/day for deep venous thrombosis was also given mesalazine

800 mg tds for a solitary cecal ulcer. Four weeks later she developed worsening of her venous thrombosis. Her serum warfarin concentrations were undetectable and the INR was 0.9. Mesalazine was withdrawn; her INR rose to 1.8 on the following day and was 2.1 five days later.

The mechanism of this interaction is not known.

Interference with Diagnostic Tests

Iron

Sulfasalazine interferes with coulometry of serum iron (109).

References

1. Anonymous. Asacol: mesalazine for ulcerative colitis. Drug Ther Bull 1986;24(10):38–40.
2. Klotz U. The role of aminosalicylates at the beginning of the new millennium in the treatment of chronic inflammatory bowel disease. Eur J Clin Pharmacol 2000;56(5): 353–362.
3. Reinacher-Schick A, Seidensticker F, Petrasch S, Reiser M, Philippou S, Theegarten D, Freitag G, Schmiegel W. Mesalazine changes apoptosis and proliferation in normal mucosa of patients with sporadic polyps of the large bowel. Endoscopy 2000;32(3):245–54.
4. Green JR, Gibson JA, Kerr GD, Swarbrick ET, Lobo AJ, Holdsworth CD, Crowe JP, Schofield KJ, Taylor MD. Maintenance of remission of ulcerative colitis: a comparison between balsalazide 3 g daily and mesalazine 1.2 g daily over 12 months. ABACUS Investigator group. Aliment Pharmacol Ther 1998;12(12):1207–16.
5. Kruis W, Brandes JW, Schreiber S, Theuer D, Krakamp B, Schutz E, Otto P, Lorenz-Mayer H, Ewe K, Judmaier G. Olsalazine versus mesalazine in the treatment of mild to moderate ulcerative colitis. Aliment Pharmacol Ther 1998;12(8):707–15.
6. Stoa-Birketvedt G, Florholmen J. The systemic load and efficient delivery of active 5-aminosalicylic acid in patients with ulcerative colitis on treatment with olsalazine or mesalazine. Aliment Pharmacol Ther 1999;13(3):357–61.
7. Vecchi M, Meucci G, Gionchetti P, Beltrami M, Di Maurizio P, Beretta L, Ganio E, Usai P, Campieri M, Fornaciari G, de Franchis R. Oral versus combination mesalazine therapy in active ulcerative colitis: a double-blind, double-dummy, randomized multicentre study. Aliment Pharmacol Ther 2001;15(2):251–6.
8. Thomsen OO, Cortot A, Jewell D, Wright JP, Winter T, Veloso FT, Vatn M, Persson T, Pettersson E. A comparison of budesonide and mesalamine for active Crohn's disease. International Budesonide–Mesalamine Study Group. N Engl J Med 1998;339(6):370–4.
9. Prantera C, Cottone M, Pallone F, Annese V, Franze A, Cerutti R, Bianchi Porro G. Mesalamine in the treatment of mild to moderate active Crohn's ileitis: results of a randomized, multicenter trial. Gastroenterology 1999;116(3):521–6.
10. Fernandez-Banares F, Hinojosa J, Sanchez-Lombrana JL, Navarro E, Martinez-Salmeron JF, Garcia-Puges A, Gonzalez-Huix F, Riera J, Gonzalez-Lara V, Dominguez-Abascal F, Gine JJ, Moles J, Gomollon F, Gassull MA. Randomized clinical trial of Plantago ovata seeds (dietary fiber) as compared with mesalamine in maintaining remission in ulcerative colitis. Spanish Group for the Study of
11. Lochs H, Mayer M, Fleig WE, Mortensen PB, Bauer P, Genser D, Petritsch W, Raithel M, Hoffmann R, Gross V, Plauth M, Staun M, Nesje LB, Hinterleitner T, Holtz J, Plein K, Otto P, Thilo A, Raedler A, Jenss H, Kaskas B, Koop I, Frank M, Loeschke K, Dotzel W, Scheurien C, Gross V, Caesar I, Reissmann A. Prophylaxis of postoperative relapse in Crohn's disease with mesalamine: European Cooperative Crohn's Disease Study VI. Gastroenterology 2000;118(2):264–73.
12. Hanauer S, Good LI, Goodman MW, Pizinger RJ, Strum WB, Lyss C, Haber G, Williams CN, Robinson M. Long-term use of mesalamine (Rowasa) suppositories in remission maintenance of ulcerative proctitis. Am J Gastroenterol 2000;95(7):1749–54.
13. Mahmud N, Kamm MA, Dupas JL, Jewell DP, O'Morain CA, Weir DG, Kelleher D. Olsalazine is not superior to placebo in maintaining remission of inactive Crohn's colitis and ileocolitis: a double blind, parallel, randomised, multicentre study. Gut 2001;49(4):552–6.
14. Stein RB, Hanauer SB. Comparative tolerability of treatments for inflammatory bowel disease. Drug Saf 2000;23(5):429–48.
15. Jung JH, Jun JB, Yoo DH, Kim TH, Jung SS, Lee IH, Bae SC, Kim SY. High toxicity of sulfasalazine in adult-onset Still's disease. Clin Exp Rheumatol 2000;18 (2):245–8.
16. Pettersson T, Gripenberg M, Molander G, Friman C. Severe immunological reaction induced by sulphasalazine. Br J Rheumatol 1990;29(3):239–40.
17. Schroeder KW. Role of mesalazine in acute and long-term treatment of ulcerative colitis and its complications. Scand J Gastroenterol Suppl 2002;(236):42–7.
18. Di Paolo MC, Paoluzi OA, Pica R, Iacopini F, Crispino P, Rivera M, Spera G, Paoluzi P. Sulphasalazine and 5-aminosalicylic acid in long-term treatment of ulcerative colitis: report on tolerance and side-effects. Dig Liver Dis 2001;33(7):563–9.
19. Mulder CJ, van den Hazel SJ. Drug therapy: dose-response relationship of oral mesalazine in inflammatory bowel disease. Mediators Inflamm 1998;7(3):135–6.
20. Ransford RA, Langman MJ. Sulphasalazine and mesalazine: serious adverse reactions re-evaluated on the basis of suspected adverse reaction reports to the Committee on Safety of Medicines. Gut 2002;51(4):536–9.
21. Meyers S, Sachar DB, Present DH, Janowitz HD. Olsalazine sodium in the treatment of ulcerative colitis among patients intolerant of sulfasalazine. A prospective, randomized, placebo-controlled, double-blind, dose-ranging clinical trial. Gastroenterology 1987;93(6):1255–62.
22. Kristensen KS, Hoegholm A, Bohr L, Friis S. Fatal myocarditis associated with mesalazine. Lancet 1990;335 (8689):605.
23. Vayre F, Vayre-Oundjian L, Monsuez JJ. Pericarditis associated with longstanding mesalazine administration in a patient. Int J Cardiol 1999;68(2):243–5.
24. Sentongo TA, Piccoli DA. Recurrent pericarditis due to mesalamine hypersensitivity: a pediatric case report and review of the literature. J Pediatr Gastroenterol Nutr 1998;27(3):344–7.
25. Ishikawa N, Imamura T, Nakajima K, Yamaga J, Yuchi H, Ootsuka M, Inatsu H, Aoki T, Eto T. Acute pericarditis associated with 5-aminosalicylic acid (5-ASA) treatment for severe active ulcerative colitis. Intern Med 2001;40(9):901–4.
26. Oxentenko AS, Loftus EV, Oh JK, Danielson GK, Mangan TF. Constrictive pericarditis in chronic ulcerative colitis. J Clin Gastroenterol 2002;34(3):247–51.

27. Asirvatham S, Sebastian C, Thadani U. Severe symptomatic sinus bradycardia associated with mesalamine use. Am J Gastroenterol 1998;93(3):470–1.

28. Amin HE, Della Siega AJ, Whittaker JS, Munt B. Mesalamine-induced chest pain: a case report. Can J Cardiol 2000;16(5):667–9.

29. Reid J, Holt S, Housley E, Sneddon DJ. Raynaud's phenomenon induced by sulphasalazine. Postgrad Med J 1980;56(652):106–7.

30. Ahmad J, Siddiqui MA, Khan AS, Afzall S. Raynaud's phenomenon induced by sulphasalazine in a case of chronic ulcerative colitis. J Assoc Physicians India 1984;32(4):370.

31. Armentia L, Mar A, Ramos Dias F. Toxicidad pulmonar inducida por salazosulfapiridina. Farm Clin 1989;6:275.

32. Leino R, Liippo K, Ekfors T. Sulphasalazine-induced reversible hypersensitivity pneumonitis and fatal fibrosing alveolitis: report of two cases. J Intern Med 1991;229(6):553–6.

33. Parry SD, Barbatzas C, Peel ET, Barton JR. Sulphasalazine and lung toxicity. Eur Respir J 2002;19(4):756–64.

34. Hamadeh MA, Atkinson J, Smith LJ. Sulfasalazine-induced pulmonary disease. Chest 1992;101(4):1033–7.

35. Bielecki JW, Avar S, Joss R. Salazopyrin-induzierte Lungeninfiltrate und Legionellenpneumonie. [Sulfasalazine-induced pulmonary infiltrates and *Legionella* pneumonia.] Schweiz Med Wochenschr 2000;130(29-30):1078–83.

36. Reinoso MA, Schroeder KW, Pisani RJ. Lung disease associated with orally administered mesalamine for ulcerative colitis. Chest 1992;101(5):1469–71.

37. Sesin GP, Mucciardi N, Almeida S. Mesalamine-associated pleural effusion with pulmonary infiltration. Am J Health Syst Pharm 1998;55(21):2304–5.

38. Trisolini R, Dore R, Biagi F, Luinetti O, Pochetti P, Carrabino N, Luisetti M. Eosinophilic pleural effusion due to mesalamine. Report of a rare occurrence. Sarcoidosis Vasc Diffuse Lung Dis 2000;17(3):288–91.

39. Tanigawa K, Sugiyama K, Matsuyama H, Nakao H, Kohno K, Komuro Y, Iwanaga Y, Eguchi K, Kitaichi M, Takagi H. Mesalazine-induced eosinophilic pneumonia. Respiration 1999;66(1):69–72.

40. Guslandi M. Respiratory distress during mesalamine therapy. Dig Dis Sci 1999;44(1):48–9.

41. Haralambou G, Teirstein AS, Gil J, Present DH. Bronchiolitis obliterans in a patient with ulcerative colitis receiving mesalamine. Mt Sinai J Med 2001;68(6):384–8.

42. Sossai P, Cappellato MG, Stefani S. Can a drug-induced pulmonary hypersensitivity reaction be dose-dependent? A case with mesalamine. Mt Sinai J Med 2001;68(6):389–95.

43. Yano S, Kobayashi K, Kato K, Nishimura K. A limited form of Wegener's granulomatosis with bronchiolitis obliterans organizing pneumonitis-like variant in an ulcerative colitis patient. Intern Med 2002;41(11):1013–15.

44. Skeith KJ, Russell AS. Adverse reaction to sulfasalazine. J Rheumatol 1988;15(3):529–30.

45. Merrin P, Williams IA. Meningitis associated with sulphasalazine in a patient with Sjögren's syndrome and polyarthritis. Ann Rheum Dis 1991;50(9):645–6.

46. Chadenat ML, Morelon S, Dupont C, Dechy H, Raffin-Sanson ML, Dorra M, Rouveix E. Neurotoxicité à la sulfasalazine. [Sulfasalazine neurotoxicity.] Ann Med Interne (Paris) 2001;152(4):283–4.

47. Schmidt WA, Wierth S, Milleck D, Droste U, Gromnica-Ihle E. Sulfasalazin bei Spondylitis ankylosans: eine prospektive, randomisierte, doppelblinde, placebo-kontrollierte Studie und Vergleich mit und eren kontrollierten Studien. [Sulfasalazine in ankylosing spondylitis: a prospective, randomized, double-blind placebo-controlled study and comparison with other controlled studies.] Z Rheumatol 2002;61(2):159–67.

48. Teplitsky V, Virag I, Halabe A. Immune complex haemolytic anaemia associated with sulfasalazine. BMJ 2000;320(7242):1113.

49. Guillemin F, Aussedat R, Guerci A, Lederlin P, Trechot P, Pourel J. Fatal agranulocytosis in sulfasalazine treated rheumatoid arthritis. J Rheumatol 1989;16(8):1166–7.

50. Wadelius M, Stjernberg E, Wiholm BE, Rane A. Polymorphisms of NAT2 in relation to sulphasalazine-induced agranulocytosis. Pharmacogenetics 2000;10(1):35–41.

51. Kane SP, Boots MA. Megaloblastic anaemia associated with sulphasalazine treatment. BMJ 1977;2(6097):1287–8.

52. Hoshino J, Sugawara K, Ishikawa S, Hayami Y, Sakurazawa T, Tanaka T, Yamamoto N, Hashimoto M, Yamamoto T, Hoshihara Y. [A case of ulcerative colitis with folate deficient megaloblastic anemia induced by sulfasalazine.] Nippon Shokakibyo Gakkai Zasshi 1999;96(7): 840–5.

53. Pirmohamed M, Coleman MD, Hussain F, Breckenridge AM, Park BK. Direct and metabolism-dependent toxicity of sulphasalazine and its principal metabolites towards human erythrocytes and leucocytes. Br J Clin Pharmacol 1991;32(3):303–10.

54. Farrell RJ, Peppercorn MA, Fine SN, Michetti P. Mesalamine-associated thrombocytopenia. Am J Gastroenterol 1999;94(8):2304–6.

55. Daneshmend TK. Mesalazine-associated thrombocytopenia. Lancet 1991;337(8752):1297–8.

56. Seror P. Thrombopénie lors d'un traitement par mesalazine. [Thrombopenia in treatment with mesalazine.] Presse Méd 2000;29(27):1510–11.

57. Benoit R, Grobost O, Bichoffe A, Dol L. Thrombopénie au cours d'un traitement par 5-ASA (mesalazine puis olsalazine). [Thrombopenia during 5-ASA treatment (mesalazine and olsalazine).] Gastroenterol Clin Biol 1999;23 (3):410–11.

58. Kotanagi H, Ito M, Koyama K, Chiba M. Pancytopenia associated with 5-aminosalicylic acid use in a patient with Crohn's disease. J Gastroenterol 1998;33(4):571–4.

59. Jiang L, Zhao N, Ni L. Retrospective study of adverse events in patients with rheumatoid arthritis treated with second-line drugs. Zhonghua Liu Xing Bing Xue Za Zhi 2002;23(3):213–17.

60. Goldstein F, DiMarino AJ Jr. Diarrhea as a side effect of mesalamine treatment for inflammatory bowel disease. J Clin Gastroenterol 2000;31(1):60–2.

61. Fine KD, Sarles HE Jr, Cryer B. Diarrhea associated with mesalamine in a patient with chronic nongranulomatous enterocolitis. N Engl J Med 1998;338(13):923–5.

62. Iofel E, Chawla A, Daum F, Markowitz J. Mesalamine intolerance mimics symptoms of active inflammatory bowel disease. J Pediatr Gastroenterol Nutr 2002;34(1):73–6.

63. Schiemann U, Kellner H. Gastrointestinale Nebenwirkungen der Therapie rheumatischer Erkrankungen. [Gastrointestinal side effects in the therapy of rheumatologic diseases.] Z Gastroenterol 2002;40(11):937–43.

64. Stoschus B, Meybehm M, Spengler U, Scheurlen C, Sauerbruch T. Cholestasis associated with mesalazine therapy in a patient with Crohn's disease. J Hepatol 1997;26(2):425–8.

65. Deltenre P, Berson A, Marcellin P, Degott C, Biour M, Pessayre D. Mesalazine (5-aminosalicylic acid) induced chronic hepatitis. Gut 1999;44(6):886–8.

66. Sachedina B, Saibil F, Cohen LB, Whittey J. Acute pancreatitis due to 5-aminosalicylate. Ann Intern Med 1989;110(6):490–2.

67. Decocq G, Gras-Champel V, Vrolant-Mille C, Delcenserie R, Sauve L, Masson H, Andrejak M. Pancreatites aiguës induites par les medicaments derivés de l'acide 5-aminosalicylique: un cas et revue de la

litterature. [Acute pancreatitis induced by drugs derived from 5-aminosalicylic acid: case report and review of the literature.] Therapie 1999;54(1):41–8.

68. Mari B, Brullet E, Campo R, Bustamante E, Bombardo J. Pancreatitis aguda por acido 5-aminosalicilico. [5-Aminosalicylic acid-induced acute pancreatitis.] Gastroenterol Hepatol 1999;22(1):28–9.

69. Paul AC, Oommen SP, Angami S, Moses PD. Acute pancreatitis in a child with idiopathic ulcerative colitis on long-term 5-aminosalicylic acid therapy. Indian J Gastroenterol 2000;19(4):195–6.

70. Schworer H, Ramadori G. Akute Pankreatitis-unerwunschte Wirkung von Aminosalicylsäure (Mesalazin) in verschiedenen galenischen Applikationsformen. [Acute pancreatitis—adverse effect of 5-aminosalicylic acid (mesalazine) in various galenic dosage forms.] Dtsch Med Wochenschr 2000;125(44): 1328–30.

71. Glintborg B. Pancreatitis hos en patient med morbus Crohn behandlet med mesalazin og azathioprin. [Pancreatitis in a patient with Crohn disease treated with mesalazine and azathioprine.] Ugeskr Laeger 2000;162(34):4553–4.

72. Fernandez J, Sala M, Panes J, Feu F, Navarro S, Teres J. Acute pancreatitis after long-term 5-aminosalicylic acid therapy. Am J Gastroenterol 1997;92(12):2302–3.

73. Dwarakanath AD, Michael J, Allan RN. Sulphasalazine induced renal failure. Gut 1992;33(7):1006–7.

74. Birketvedt GS, Berg KJ, Fausa O, Florholmen J. Glomerular and tubular renal functions after long-term medication of sulphasalazine, olsalazine, and mesalazine in patients with ulcerative colitis. Inflamm Bowel Dis 2000;6(4):275–9.

75. Schreiber S, Hamling J, Zehnter E, Howaldt S, Daerr W, Raedler A, Kruis W. Renal tubular dysfunction in patients with inflammatory bowel disease treated with amino-salicylate. Gut 1997;40(6):761–6.

76. Fraser JS, Muller AF, Smith DJ, Newman DJ, Lamb EJ. Renal tubular injury is present in acute inflammatory bowel disease prior to the introduction of drug therapy. Aliment Pharmacol Ther 2001;15(8):1131–7.

77. Herrlinger KR, Noftz MK, Fellermann K, Schmidt K, Steinhoff J, Stange EF. Minimal renal dysfunction in inflammatory bowel disease is related to disease activity but not to 5-ASA use. Aliment Pharmacol Ther 2001;15(3):363–9.

78. UK Committee on Safety of Medicines. Nephrotoxicity associated with mesalazine (Asacol). Curr Probl 1990:30.

79. Calvino J, Romero R, Pintos E, Losada E, Novoa D, Guimil D, Mardaras J, Sanchez-Guisande D. Mesalazine-associated tubulo-interstitial nephritis in inflammatory bowel disease. Clin Nephrol 1998;49(4):265–7.

80. Popoola J, Muller AF, Pollock L, O'Donnell P, Carmichael P, Stevens P. Late onset interstitial nephritis associated with mesalazine treatment. BMJ 1998;317 (7161):795–7.

81. Howard G, Lynn KL. Renal dysfunction and the treatment of inflammatory bowel disease (IBD): a case for monitoring. Aust NZ J Med 1998;28(3):346.

82. Margetts PJ, Churchill DN, Alexopoulou I. Interstitial nephritis in patients with inflammatory bowel disease treated with mesalamine. J Clin Gastroenterol 2001;32 (2):176–8.

83. Frandsen NE, Saugmann S, Marcussen N. Acute interstitial nephritis associated with the use of mesalazine in inflammatory bowel disease. Nephron 2002;92(1):200–2.

84. Ohya M, Otani H, Kimura K, Kodama N, Minami Y, Liang XM, Maeshima E, Yamada Y, Mune M, Yukawa S. [Interstitial nephritis induced by mesalazine.] Nippon Jinzo Gakkai Shi 2002;44(4):414–19.

85. Laboudi A, Makdassi R, Cordonnier C, Fournier A, Choukroun G. Nephrite interstitielle chronique au 5-ASA: mise au point a partir d'un nouveau cas. [Chronic interstitial nephritis induced by 5-aminosalicylic acid: a new case report.] Nephrologie 2002;23(7):343–7.

86. Beaulieu S, Rocher P, Hillion D, Nochy D, Tennenbaum R, Vitte RL, Eugene C. Insuffisance rénale aiguë par necrose tubulaire aiguë au cours du premier mois de traitement par l'acide 5-amino-salicylique (Pentasa®). [Acute tubular necrosis with acute renal failure during the first month of treatment with 5-amino-salicylate (Pentasa®).] Gastroenterol Clin Biol 2002;26(4):412–14.

87. Skhiri H, Knebelmann B, Martin-Lefevre L, Grunfeld JP. Nephrotic syndrome associated with inflammatory bowel disease treated by mesalazine. Nephron 1998;79(2):236.

88. Prakash A, Markham A. Oral delayed-release mesalazine: a review of its use in ulcerative colitis and Crohn's disease. Drugs 1999;57(3):383–408.

89. Musil D. Casne renalni selhani vyvolane mesalazinem. [Early renal failure caused by mesalazine.] Vnitr Lek 2000;46(10):728–31.

90. Benador N, Grimm P, Lemire J, Griswold W, Billman G, Reznik V. Interstitial nephritis in children with Crohn's disease. Clin Pediatr (Phila) 2000;39(4):253–4.

91. Mahmud N, O'Toole D, O'Hare N, Freyne PJ, Weir DG, Kelleher D. Evaluation of renal function following treatment with 5-aminosalicylic acid derivatives in patients with ulcerative colitis. Aliment Pharmacol Ther 2002;16 (2):207–15.

92. Kawaguchi M, Mitsuhashi Y, Kondo S. Acute generalized exanthematous pustulosis induced by salazosulfapyridine in a patient with ulcerative colitis. J Dermatol 1999;26(6):359–62.

93. Gabazza EC, Taguchi O, Yamakami T, Machishi M, Ibata H, Suzuki S, Matsumoto K, Kitagawa T, Yamamoto J. Pulmonary infiltrates and skin pigmentation associated with sulfasalazine. Am J Gastroenterol 1992;87 (11):1654–7.

94. Ireland A, Jewell DP. Sulfasalazine-induced impotence: a beneficial resolution with olsalazine? J Clin Gastroenterol 1989;11(6):711.

95. Choi HK, Merkel PA, Walker AM, Niles JL. Drug-associated antineutrophil cytoplasmic antibody-positive vasculitis: prevalence among patients with high titers of antimyeloperoxidase antibodies. Arthritis Rheum 2000;43 (2):405–13.

96. Gunnarsson I, Nordmark B, Hassan Bakri A, Grondal G, Larsson P, Forslid J, Klareskog L, Ringertz B. Development of lupus-related side-effects in patients with early RA during sulphasalazine treatment-the role of IL-10 and HLA. Rheumatology (Oxford) 2000;39(8):886–93.

97. Pay S, Dinc A, Simsek I, Can C, Erdem H. Sulfasalazine-induced angioimmunoblastic lymphadenopathy developing in a patient with juvenile chronic arthritis. Rheumatol Int 2000;20(1):25–7.

98. Nguyen-Khac E, Le Baron F, Thevenot T, Tiry-Lescut C, Tiry F. Oedème de Quincke possiblement imputable à la mesalazine au cours de la maladie de Crohn. [Angioedema in Crohn's disease possibly due to mesalazine.] Gastroenterol Clin Biol 2002;26(5):535–6.

99. Pent MT, Ganapathy S, Holdsworth CD, Channer KC. Mesalazine induced lupus-like syndrome. BMJ 1992;305 (6846):159.

100. Clemett D, Markham A. Prolonged-release mesalazine: a review of its therapeutic potential in ulcerative colitis and Crohn's disease. Drugs 2000;59(4):929–56.

101. Farup PG, Hinterleitner TA, Lukas M, Hebuterne X, Rachmilewitz D, Campieri M, Meier R, Keller R, Rathbone B, Oddsson E. Mesalazine 4 g daily given as prolonged-release granules twice daily and five times daily is at least as effective as prolonged-release tablets four times daily in patients with ulcerative colitis. Inflamm Bowel Dis 2001;7(3):237–42.

102. Gionchetti P, Ardizzone S, Benvenuti ME, Bianchi Porro G, Biasco G, Cesari P, D'albasio G, De Franchis R, Monteleone G, Pallone F, Ranzi T, Trallori G, Valpiani D, Vecchi M, Campieri M. A new

mesalazine gel enema in the treatment of left-sided ulcerative colitis: a randomized controlled multicentre trial. Aliment Pharmacol Ther 1999;13(3):381–8.

103. Malchow H, Gertz B, CLAFOAM Study group. A new mesalazine foam enema (Claversal Foam) compared with a standard liquid enema in patients with active distal ulcerative colitis. Aliment Pharmacol Ther 2002;16(3):415–23.

104. Lowry PW, Franklin CL, Weaver AL, Szumlanski CL, Mays DC, Loftus EV, Tremaine WJ, Lipsky JJ, Weinshilboum RM, Sandborn WJ. Leucopenia resulting from a drug interaction between azathioprine or 6-mercaptopurine and mesalamine, sulphasalazine, or balsalazide. Gut 2001;49(5):656–64.

105. Dewit O, Vanheuverzwyn R, Desager JP, Horsmans Y. Interaction between azathioprine and aminosalicylates: an in vivo study in patients with Crohn's disease. Aliment Pharmacol Ther 2002;16(1):79–85.

106. Juhl RP, Summers RW, Guillory JK, Blaug SM, Cheng FH, Brown DD. Effect of sulfasalazine on digoxin bioavailability. Clin Pharmacol Ther 1976;20(4):387–94.

107. Das KM, Eastwood MA. Effect of iron and calcium on salicylazosulphapyridine metabolism. Scott Med J 1973;18(2):45–50.

108. Marinella MA. Mesalamine and warfarin therapy resulting in decreased warfarin effect. Ann Pharmacother 1998;32(7-8):841–2.

109. Jaynes P, Kapke GF. Sulfasalazine interferes with coulometry of serum iron. Clin Chem 1981;27(1):202–3.

Amiodarone

See also Antidysrhythmic drugs

General Information

Amiodarone is highly effective in treating both ventricular and supraventricular dysrhythmias (1). Its pharmacology, therapeutic uses, and adverse effects and interactions have been extensively reviewed (2–14).

General adverse effects

Amiodarone prolongs the QT interval and can therefore cause dysrhythmias; there have also been reports of conduction disturbances. Abnormalities of thyroid function tests can occur without thyroid dysfunction, typically increases in serum T4 and reverse T3 and a reduction in serum T3. However, in up to 6% of patients frank thyroid dysfunction can occur (either hypothyroidism or hyperthyroidism). Several of the adverse effects of amiodarone are attributable to deposition of phospholipids in the tissues. These include its effects on the eyes, nerves, liver, skin, and lungs. Almost all patients develop reversible corneal microdeposits, which can occasionally interfere with vision. There are reports of peripheral neuropathy and other neurological effects. Changes in serum activities of aspartate transaminase and lactate dehydrogenase can occur without other evidence of liver disease, but liver damage can occur in the absence of biochemical evidence. Skin sensitivity to light occurs commonly, possibly due to phototoxicity. There may also be a bluish pigmentation of the skin. Interstitial pneumonitis and alveolitis have been reported and may be fatal. Lung damage due to amiodarone may be partly due to hypersensitivity. Tumor-inducing effects have not been reported.

Studies in the prevention of dysrhythmias

In a study of the use of implantable defibrillators or antidysrhythmic drugs (amiodarone or metoprolol) in 288 patients resuscitated from cardiac arrest, the defibrillator was associated with a slightly lower rate of all-cause mortality than the antidysrhythmic drugs (15). However, the small difference was not statistically significant. There was hyperthyroidism in three of those given amiodarone. Drug withdrawal was required in nine of those given amiodarone and 10 of those given metoprolol. There were deaths in five patients fitted with a defibrillator and two patients given amiodarone. There was crossover to the other therapy in 6% in each group, usually because of recurrence of the dysrhythmia. When sudden cardiac death was analysed, the reduction in mortality with defibrillation was much larger (61%). There were no differences in all-cause mortality and sudden death rates between those given amiodarone and those given metoprolol.

Amiodarone and carvedilol have been used in combination in 109 patients with severe heart failure and left ventricular ejection fractions of 0.25 (16). They were given amiodarone 1000 mg/week plus carvedilol titrated to a target dose of 50 mg/day. A dual-chamber pacemaker was inserted and programmed in back-up mode at a basal rate of 40. Significantly more patients were in sinus rhythm after 1 year, and in 47 patients who were studied for at least 1 year the resting heart rate fell from 90 to 59. Ventricular extra beats were suppressed from 1 to 0.1/day and the number of bouts of tachycardia over 167 per minute was reduced from 1.2 to 0.3 episodes per patient per 3 months. The left ventricular ejection fraction increased from 0.26 to 0.39 and New York Heart Association Classification improved from 3.2 to 1.8. The probability of sudden death was significantly reduced by amiodarone plus carvedilol compared with 154 patients treated with amiodarone alone and even more so compared with 283 patients who received no treatment at all. However, the study was not randomized, and this vitiates the results. The main adverse effect was symptomatic bradycardia, which occurred in seven patients; two of those developed atrioventricular block and four had sinoatrial block and/or sinus bradycardia; one patient developed slow atrial fibrillation.

A meta-analysis of 13 randomized trials has shown that both total mortality and sudden death or dysrhythmic death was less common over 24 months after randomization to amiodarone than in control subjects (17).

Studies in atrial fibrillation

Cardiac glycosides such as digoxin are commonly used to treat uncomplicated atrial fibrillation. In those in whom digitalis is not completely effective or in whom symptoms (for example bouts of palpitation) persist despite adequate digitalization, a calcium antagonist, such as verapamil or diltiazem, can be added, or amiodarone used as an alternative.

The use of oral amiodarone in preventing recurrence of atrial fibrillation, for preventing recurrence after cardioversion or for pharmacological cardioversion of atrial fibrillation, has been reviewed (18). There is insufficient evidence to support its use as a first-line drug for preventing recurrence of atrial fibrillation or in preventing paroxysmal atrial fibrillation.

In 186 patients randomized equally to amiodarone 200 mg/day, sotalol 160–480 mg/day, or placebo, the incidence of atrial fibrillation after 6 months was higher in those taking placebo compared with amiodarone and sotalol and higher in those taking sotalol compared with amiodarone (19). Of the 65 patients who took amiodarone, 15 had significant adverse effects after an average of 16 months. There were eight cases of hypothyroidism, four of hyperthyroidism, two of symptomatic bradycardia, and one of ataxia. There were minor adverse effects in 9% of the patients, including gastrointestinal discomfort, nausea, photosensitivity, and eye problems. These patients had recurrent symptomatic atrial fibrillation. In contrast, only two patients using sotalol developed symptomatic bradycardia and one had severe dizziness.

In 208 patients with atrial fibrillation of various duration, including 50 with chronic atrial fibrillation, randomized to amiodarone or placebo, 80% converted to sinus rhythm after amiodarone compared with 40% of those given placebo (20). Amiodarone was given as an intravenous loading dose of 300 mg for 1 hour and 20 mg/kg for 24 hours, followed by 600 mg/day orally for 1 week and 400 mg/day for 3 weeks. Those who converted to sinus rhythm had had atrial fibrillation for a shorter duration and had smaller atria than those who did not convert. The shorter the duration of fibrillation and the smaller the atria the sooner conversion occurred. There was significant hypotension in 12 of the 118 patients who received amiodarone during the first hour of intravenous administration, but in all cases this responded to intravenous fluids alone. There was phlebitis at the site of infusion in 17 patients, and the peripheral catheter was replaced by a central catheter. There were no dysrhythmic effects.

In 40 patients with atrial fibrillation, some with severe heart disease (including cardiogenic shock in eight and pulmonary edema in 12), amiodarone 450 mg was given through a peripheral vein within 1 minute, followed by 10 ml of saline; 21 patients converted to sinus rhythm, 13 within 30 minutes and another 8 within 24 hours (21). There were two cases of hypotension, but in those that converted to sinus rhythm there was a slight increase in systolic blood pressure. There were no cases of thrombophlebitis. Efficacy is hard to judge from this study, because it was not placebo-controlled.

In 72 patients with paroxysmal atrial fibrillation randomized to either amiodarone 30 mg/kg or placebo, those who received amiodarone converted to sinus rhythm more often than those given placebo (22). The respective conversion rates were about 50 and 20% at 8 hours, and 87 and 35% after 24 hours. The time to conversion in patients who converted did not differ. One patient developed slow atrial fibrillation (35/minute) with a blood pressure of 75/55 mmHg. Three other patients who received amiodarone had diarrhea and one had nausea. In the control group two patients had headache, one had diarrhea, one had nausea, and two had episodes of sinus arrest associated with syncope during conversion to sinus rhythm; the last of these was thought to have sick sinus syndrome.

In a single-blind study 150 patients with acute atrial fibrillation were randomized to intravenous flecainide, propafenone, or amiodarone (23). At 12 hours there was conversion to sinus rhythm in 45 of 50 patients given flecainide, 36 of the 50 given propafenone, and 32 of the 50 given amiodarone. Thus, flecainide and propafenone were both more effective than amiodarone. There were no differences between the groups in the incidences of adverse effects; there was one withdrawal in each group, due to cerebral embolism in a patient given amiodarone, heart failure in a patient given propafenone, and atrial flutter in a patient given flecainide. There were no ventricular dysrhythmias during the study.

Amiodarone and magnesium have been compared in a placebo-controlled study to reduce the occurrence of atrial fibrillation in 147 patients after coronary artery bypass graft surgery (24). Amiodarone was given as a infusion of 900 mg/day for 3 days and magnesium by infusion of 4 g/day for 3 days. The cumulative occurrences of atrial fibrillation with placebo, amiodarone, and magnesium were 27, 14, and 23% respectively. These differences were not significant. Amiodarone delayed the onset of the first episode of dysrhythmia significantly, but the slight benefit was associated with a longer period of invasive monitoring and was not considered worthwhile. Patients who were more likely to develop atrial fibrillation were older and had a plasma magnesium concentration at 24 hours of under 0.95 mmol/l. Patients who were given amiodarone had a slightly higher rate of adverse events, including hypotension, atrioventricular block, and bradycardia; adverse events led to withdrawal in four cases.

Amiodarone, sotalol, and propafenone have been compared for the prevention of atrial fibrillation in 403 patients who had had at least one episode of atrial fibrillation within the previous 6 months; the study was not placebo-controlled (25). The rate of recurrence of atrial fibrillation was significantly higher in those given sotalol or propafenone than in those given amiodarone. During the study nine patients given amiodarone died, compared with eight given sotalol or propafenone. Four deaths were thought to be dysrhythmic, three in patients given amiodarone. There were major non-fatal adverse events in 36 of the 201 patients given amiodarone and in 35 of the 202 patients given propafenone or sotalol. These included one case of torsade de pointes in a patient who received propafenone, and congestive heart failure in 11 patients given amiodarone and nine given sotalol or propafenone. There were strokes and intracranial hemorrhages in one patient given amiodarone and nine patients given sotalol or propafenone, of whom most were taking warfarin at the time. In all, 68 of the patients who were given amiodarone and 93 of those given sotalol or propafenone withdrew from the study; 17 of those taking amiodarone withdrew because of lack of efficacy compared with 56 of those taking sotalol or propafenone; 36 of those who took amiodarone withdrew because of adverse events compared with 23 of those who took sotalol or propafenone, and this was almost statistically significant.

Amiodarone, propafenone, and sotalol have also been compared in the prevention of atrial fibrillation in 214 patients with recurrent symptomatic atrial fibrillation. They were randomized to amiodarone 200 mg/day, propafenone 450 mg/day, or sotalol 320 mg/day. There was recurrence of atrial fibrillation in 25 of the 75 patients who took amiodarone compared with the 51 of 75 who took sotalol and 24 of the 64 who took propafenone. There were adverse effects requiring withdrawal of treatment in 14 patients who took amiodarone, five who took sotalol and one who took propafenone while they were in sinus rhythm. These effects included symptomatic bradycardia in three patients, hyperthyroidism in six, hypothyroidism in four, and ataxia in one patient who took amiodarone. In those taking sotalol the adverse effects were bradycardia in three and severe dizziness in two. In the one patient in whom propafenone was withheld the reason was symptomatic bradycardia. Thus, amiodarone and propafenone were both more effective than sotalol, but amiodarone also caused more adverse effects requiring withdrawal (26).

In a meta-analysis of five randomized, placebo-controlled trials of amiodarone 200–1200 mg/day for 2–7 days in the treatment of postoperative atrial fibrillation and flutter in 764 patients, the incidence of adverse events with amiodarone was no greater than with placebo (27).

In a meta-analysis of five randomized, placebo-controlled trials of intravenous amiodarone about 500–2200 mg over 24 hours in the treatment of recent-onset atrial fibrillation in 410 patients, the incidence of adverse events was 27% with amiodarone and 11% with placebo (28). Intravenous amiodarone was significantly more effective than placebo in producing cardioversion. The most common adverse effects of intravenous amiodarone were phlebitis, bradycardia, and hypotension; most of these effects were not considered to be dose-limiting.

Of 85 patients with persistent atrial fibrillation after balloon mitral valvotomy given amiodarone (600 mg/day for 2 weeks and 200 mg/day thereafter), 33 converted to sinus rhythm (29). Of the other 52 patients, who underwent DC cardioversion at 6 weeks, 41 converted to sinus rhythm. Six patients had adverse effects attributable to amiodarone. Five had mild gastrointestinal symptoms, such as abdominal discomfort and nausea. One developed hypothyroidism after 3 months, which resolved when the dosage of amiodarone was reduced to 100 mg/day.

In 83 patients (27 women, 56 men; mean age 61 years) disopyramide, propafenone, or sotalol were used to prevent recurrence after elective electrical cardioversion for persistent atrial fibrillation (30). If there was recurrence cardioversion was repeated and the patient was given one of the other antidysrhythmic drugs. If there was further recurrence, amiodarone was used, a third cardioversion was performed, and, if sinus rhythm was restored, amiodarone 100–200 mg/day was continued. Patients in whom the initial cardioversion was not successful were given amiodarone and underwent repeated cardioversion. The follow-up duration was 12 months. The first electrical cardioversion was effective in 44 (53%) patients, and after 1 year 23 (52%) of them were still in sinus rhythm. None of the patients who underwent a second cardioversion and received a second antidysrhythmic drug stayed in sinus rhythm. Amiodarone as a third antidysrhythmic agent was effective in 10 (48%) patients. After 12 months of antidysrhythmic drug therapy sinus rhythm was maintained in 75% of patients in whom the first cardioversion had been effective, accounting for 40% of all the patients selected for cardioversion. In the 83 patients, sequential antidysrhythmic treatment effectively maintained sinus rhythm in 54 (65%), of whom 31 (57%) took amiodarone. The authors concluded that repeated electrical cardioversion and antidysrhythmic drug therapy enabled

maintenance of sinus rhythm in 68% of patients for 1 year, that there was limited efficacy of the first antidysrhythmic drug given after a first effective electrical cardioversion, regardless of the drug used, excluding amiodarone, and that when atrial fibrillation recurred, a second antidysrhythmic drug, other than amiodarone, was completely ineffective. There were very few adverse events in this study. One patient taking amiodarone developed hyperthyroidism and two had symptomatic bradycardia.

Amiodarone 30 mg/kg orally for the first 24 hours plus, if necessary, 15 mg/kg over 24 hours has been compared with propafenone 600 mg in the first 24 hours plus, if necessary, 300 mg in the next 24 hours in 86 patients with recent onset atrial fibrillation (31). Conversion to sinus rhythm occurred faster with propafenone (2.4 hours) than amiodarone (6.9 hours). However, by 24 hours and 48 hours the same proportions of patients were in sinus rhythm; one patient given amiodarone had a supraventricular tachycardia and one a non-sustained ventricular tachycardia.

Studies in atrial flutter

Antidysrhythmic drugs have been compared with radiofrequency ablation in 61 patients with atrial flutter (32). Drug treatment was with at least two drugs, one of which was amiodarone. Of the 30 patients who took drug therapy, 19 needed to come into hospital one or more times, whereas after radiofrequency ablation that happened in only seven of 31 cases. In those who took the antidysrhythmic drugs the mean number of drugs was 3.4 and the range of drugs used was very wide. Quality-of-life and symptoms scores improved significantly in those in whom radiofrequency ablation was used, but not in those who took the antidysrhythmic drugs, apart from the symptom of palpitation, which improved in both groups, but to a greater extent in the non-drug group. Adverse effects were not discussed in this study, but it is clear that it suggests that radiofrequency ablation is to be preferred in these patients.

Studies in ventricular dysrhythmias

The effects of amiodarone in 55 patients with sustained ventricular tachycardia after myocardial infarction have been assessed in a long-term follow-up study (33). The patients underwent programmed ventricular stimulation after having been loaded with amiodarone. They were divided into those in whom ventricular tachydysrhythmias could be induced or not, and all were then given amiodarone 200 mg/day. In 11 cases a cardioverter defibrillator was implanted, because the first episode of ventricular tachycardia had been poorly tolerated or had caused hemodynamic instability. A defibrillator was also implanted in five other cases during follow-up, because of recurrence of dysrhythmias. There was a non-significant trend to a difference between the cumulative rates of dysrhythmias during long-term follow-up, with more events in those in whom a dysrhythmia had been inducible after loading. However, mortality rates in the two groups did not differ, and was around 25% at a mean follow-up of 42 months. Survival was significantly higher in patients with a left ventricular ejection fraction over 0.4, and the lower the left ventricular ejection fractions the higher the mortality. Amiodarone was withdrawn in six patients after a mean of 34 months because of neuropathy ($n = 1$), hypothyroidism ($n = 1$), prodysrhythmia with incessant ventricular tachycardia ($n = 2$), and non-specific adverse effects ($n = 2$). There was no pulmonary toxicity and no cases of torsade de pointes. In two patients there was evidence of hypothyroidism, mild neuropathy, and skin discoloration, but these events did not lead to withdrawal. In two patients the doses of amiodarone was reduced to 100 mg/day because of sinus bradycardia.

In a comparison of amiodarone ($n = 23$) with sotalol ($n = 22$) in patients with spontaneous sustained ventricular tachydysrhythmias secondary to myocardial infarction, sotalol was much more effective, 75% of those taking it remaining free of dysrhythmias compared with 38% of those taking amiodarone (34). Adverse effects requiring withdrawal occurred in 17% of those taking amiodarone at a median time of 3.5 months. The adverse effects included malaise, rash, headaches, flushing, and dyspnea due to pulmonary fibrosis.

Studies in myocardial infarction and heart failure

There have been reviews of the results of major trials of amiodarone after myocardial infarction (35) and in chronic heart failure (36).

- In the Basel Antiarrhythmic Study of Infarct Survival (BASIS) amiodarone significantly reduced all-cause mortality from 13 to 5%, compared with no antidysrhythmic drug therapy (37).
- In the Polish Arrhythmia Trial (PAT) amiodarone reduced all-cause mortality from 10.7 to 6.9% compared with placebo and cardiac mortality from 10.7 to 6.2% (38).
- In the Spanish Study of Sudden Death (SSD) amiodarone reduced all-cause mortality from 15.4 to 3.5% compared with metoprolol; however, the mortality in those receiving no antidysrhythmic drugs at all was only 7.7%, and in those the effect of amiodarone was not significant (39).
- In the European Myocardial Infarction Arrhythmia Trial (EMIAT) amiodarone reduced the risk of dysrhythmic deaths from 8.5 to 4.1% compared with placebo (40).
- In the Canadian Amiodarone Myocardial Infarction Arrhythmia Trial (CAMIAT) amiodarone reduced dysrhythmic deaths from 6.0 to 3.3% compared with placebo; non-dysrhythmic deaths were not affected (41).

In a meta-analysis of 10 studies of the use of amiodarone in patients with heart failure, the overall odds ratio for mortality with amiodarone compared with placebo was 0.79 (95% CI = 0.68, 0.92). The corresponding odds ratio for adverse effects was 2.29 (1.97, 2.66) (36). The benefit to risk ratio of the use of amiodarone in these patients is not yet clear. The dosage of amiodarone in these studies varied from 50 to 400 mg/day, with an average of around 250 mg/day.

Organs and Systems

Cardiovascular

The incidence of cardiac dysrhythmias with amiodarone is under 3% (42), lower than with many other antidysrhythmic drugs, and several randomized controlled trials have failed to show any prodysrhythmic effect (43).

Other cardiac effects that have been reported include sinus bradycardia, atrioventricular block, infra-His block, asystole, and refractoriness to DC cardioversion (SEDA-10, 147).

There is a risk of hypotension and atrioventricular block when amiodarone is given intravenously.

Cardiogenic shock has been reported in 73-year-old woman with a dilated cardiomyopathy who had digitalis and amiodarone toxicity (44).

Ventricular dysrhythmias

Amiodarone can prolong the QT interval, and this can be associated with torsade de pointes, although this is uncommon. This effect is potentiated by hypokalemia (45).

Ventricular dysrhythmias due to drugs can be either monomorphic or polymorphic. The class Ia drugs are particularly likely to cause polymorphic dysrhythmias, as is amiodarone (although to a lesser extent). In contrast, the class Ic drugs are more likely to cause monomorphic dysrhythmias (46).

- A 40-year-old woman developed torsade de pointes within the first 24 hours of intravenous administration of amiodarone 150 mg followed by 35 mg/hour (47). The association with amiodarone was confirmed by subsequent rechallenge.
- Three boys with congenital cardiac defects developed polymorphous ventricular tachycardia after having been given intravenous amiodarone; two died (48).
- An 8-day-old boy was given intravenous amiodarone 5 mg/kg over 60 minutes followed by 10 mg/kg/day for a postoperative junctional ectopic tachycardia after a cardiac operation. He developed ventricular fibrillation 12 hours later, but recovered with defibrillation and internal cardiac massage. His serum amiodarone concentration was 1–2.5 mg/l, within the usual target range.
- A 3-month-old boy underwent a cardiac operation and 6 hours later developed a junctional ectopic tachycardia. He was given amiodarone as a continuous intravenous infusion of 10 mg/kg/day for 3 hours and developed ventricular fibrillation, from which he was not resuscitated. The serum amiodarone concentration was 0.3 mg/l.
- A 3-month-old boy developed a postoperative junctional ectopic tachycardia 48 hours after operation and was given a continuous intravenous infusion of amiodarone 10 mg/kg/day. After 2 hours he developed ventricular fibrillation and was not resuscitated. His serum amiodarone concentration was in the target range.

It is not clear that the dysrhythmias in these cases were due to amiodarone, particularly since the doses had been very low and the serum concentrations no higher than the usual target range; QT intervals were not reported.

- A 79-year-old woman took amiodarone 4800 mg over 6 days and developed a polymorphous ventricular tachycardia; the associated precipitating factors were a prolonged QT interval and hypokalemia (49).
- A 71-year-old Japanese man with bouts of sustained monomorphic ventricular tachycardia, in whom non-sustained polymorphic ventricular tachycardia was induced by rapid pacing during electrophysiological studies, was given amiodarone and developed three different types of sustained monomorphic ventricular

tachycardia, with slightly different cycle lengths, induced and terminated by rapid pacing (50).

The authors proposed that amiodarone had modulated the threshold of induction and/or termination of ventricular tachycardia.

Of 189 patients, five had torsade de pointes and all five had prolonged QT intervals (51). Two of the five, all women, also had raised blood glucose concentrations, and the authors suggested that hyperglycemia is a risk factor for torsade de pointes. However, the number of cases reported in this series was too small to justify such a conclusion.

It has been suggested that women are more likely to develop torsade de pointes than men in response to antidysrhythmic drugs (52), and this has been confirmed in the case of amiodarone in a study of 189 patients given intravenous amiodarone (51). This is also reminiscent of the finding that prolongation of the QT interval due to quinidine is greater in women than in men at equivalent serum concentrations (53).

T wave alternans is an occasional presentation, in association with ventricular dysrhythmias (SEDA-18, 201).

- A 65-year-old man with atrial fibrillation was given intravenous amiodarone 450 mg over 30 minutes followed by 900 mg over 24 hours (54). He reverted to sinus rhythm, but the electrocardiogram showed giant T wave alternans with a variable QT interval (0.52–0.84 seconds). He had a short bout of torsade de pointes and was given magnesium. Two days later the electrocardiogram was normal.
- In a 62-year-old man with dilated cardiomyopathy and an implantable cardioverter defibrillator for ventricular tachycardia, microvolt T wave alternans differed when amiodarone was added (55). The onset heart rate with T wave alternans was lower and the alternans voltage higher with amiodarone than without it.

The effects of amiodarone appeared to be related to exacerbations of ventricular tachycardia and an increased defibrillation threshold.

Atrial dysrhythmias

Amiodarone has been reported to cause atrial flutter in 10 patients who had been given it for paroxysmal atrial fibrillation (56). In nine of those the atrial flutter was successfully treated by catheter ablation. However, during a mean follow-up period of 8 months after ablation, atrial fibrillation occurred in two patients who had continued to take amiodarone; this was a lower rate of recurrence than in patients in whom atrial flutter was not associated with amiodarone. The authors therefore suggested that in patients with atrial flutter secondary to amiodarone given for atrial fibrillation, catheter ablation allows continuation of amiodarone therapy.

Amiodarone can sometimes cause atrial flutter, even though it is also used to treat it (SEDA-25, 180). There has been a report of seven cases (six men and one woman, aged 34–75 years) of 1:1 atrial flutter with oral amiodarone (57). Four of them had underlying cardiac disease; none had hyperthyroidism. The initial dysrhythmia was 2:1 atrial flutter ($n = 4$), 1:1 atrial flutter ($n = 2$), or atrial fibrillation ($n = 1$). One patient was taking amiodarone 200 mg/day and one was taking 400 mg/day plus

carvedilol. The other five all received loading doses of 9200 (sd 2400) mg over 10 (sd 4) days. There was an adrenergic trigger factor (exertion, fever, esophageal stimulation, or a beta-adrenoceptor agonist aerosol) in five patients. One required emergency cardioversion.

Of 136 patients with atrial fibrillation treated with either amiodarone ($n = 96$) or propafenone ($n = 40$), 15 developed subsequent persistent atrial flutter, nine of those taking amiodarone and six of those taking propafenone (58). In all cases radiofrequency ablation was effective. It is not clear to what extent these cases of atrial flutter were due to the drugs, although the frequency of atrial flutter in previous studies with propafenone has been similar. Atrial enlargement was significantly related to the occurrence of persistent atrial flutter in these patients.

Bradycardia

Bradycardia has been reported to occur in about 5% of patients taking amiodarone (SEDA-20, 176).

Of 2559 patients admitted to an intensive cardiac care unit over 3 years, 64 with major cardiac iatrogenic problems were reviewed (59). Of those, 58 had dysrhythmias, mainly bradydysrhythmias, secondary to amiodarone, beta-blockers, calcium channel blockers, electrolyte imbalance, or a combination of those. Amiodarone was implicated in 19 cases, compared with 44 cases attributed to beta-blockers and 28 to calcium channel blockers. Of the 56 patients with sinus bradycardia, 10 were taking a combination of amiodarone and a beta-blocker, six were taking amiodarone alone, and three were taking amiodarone plus a calcium channel blocker.

Heart block

- In a 66-year-old woman taking amiodarone 1200 mg/week there was marked prolongation of the QT interval, to 680 ms; the succeeding P waves fell within the refractory period of the preceding beat and were unable to institute conduction (60). This resulted in 2:1 atrioventricular block. Amiodarone was withdrawn and the QT interval normalized with a time-course consistent with the long half-life of amiodarone. A subsequent rechallenge with intravenous amiodarone caused further prolongation of the QT interval.

The authors hypothesized that this patient had a silent mutation in one of the genes coding for the two major potassium channel proteins (IK_r or IK_s) that are involved in the mode of action of amiodarone. However, they did not present any genetic studies to support this hypothesis.

Respiratory

There have been reviews of the lung complications of amiodarone toxicity (61,62) and of its mechanisms (63).

Frequency

The risk of lung toxicity is about 5–6% (64) and is greatest during the first 12 months of treatment and among patients over 40 years of age. The mortality rate in those who develop respiratory involvement is about 9% (about 0.5% of the total).

Mechanism

Amiodarone causes lung damage either by direct deposition of phospholipids in the lung tissue or by some immunologically mediated reaction. Other mechanisms have also been proposed, including oxidant-mediated damage, a direct detergent effect, and a direct toxic effect of iodide (SEDA-15, 168).

It has been suggested that the serum activity of lactate dehydrogenase (LDH) may be related to the occurrence of amiodarone-induced pneumonitis, as occurred in a 72-year-old woman in whom the serum LDH activity rose from a baseline of around 750 U/l to around 1500 U/l during acute pneumonitis and resolved with resolution of a clinical condition after withdrawal of amiodarone (65). The LDH activity in bronchoalveolar lavage fluid was also increased. The proposed mechanism was leakage of lactate dehydrogenase from the pulmonary interstitial cells into the blood. Of course, a rise in the serum LDH activity is highly non-specific, and it is not clear whether it might also rise in bronchoalveolar lavage fluid in other conditions.

Presentation

The commonest form of lung damage is an interstitial alveolitis, although pneumonitis and bronchiolitis obliterans have also been reported, as have solitary localized fibrotic lesions, non-cardiac pulmonary edema, pleural effusions, acute respiratory failure, acute pleuritic chest pain, and adult respiratory distress syndrome (SEDA-17, 220) (SEDA-18, 201) (66–68). Amiodarone has also been reported to cause impairment of lung function, even in patients who do not develop pneumonitis (69), and pre-existing impairment of lung function may constitute a contraindication to amiodarone.

Lung damage due to amiodarone usually develops slowly, but it can occasionally have a rapid onset, particularly in patients who are given high concentrations of inspired oxygen, and there is experimental evidence that amiodarone enhances the toxic effects of oxygen on the lungs (70).

- Adult respiratory distress syndrome occurred very rapidly in a 66-year-old man who took amiodarone 200 mg/day for a few weeks only (71).
- Pulmonary infiltrates occurred in a 72-year-old man after treatment with amiodarone (total dose 6800 mg) for only 7 days (72).
- Two patients with dilated cardiomyopathy developed pneumonitis after 6 weeks and 8 months while taking amiodarone 400 and 200 mg/day respectively (73).

Some cases of amiodarone-induced lung toxicity, some in patients who took very large doses, illustrate the wide variety of possible presentations.

- A 77-year-old man without a history of lung disease was given amiodarone 7 days after bypass surgery because of supraventricular dysrhythmias and non-sustained ventricular tachycardia (74). He had taken 1600 mg/day for a week followed by a maintenance dosage of 400 mg/day, and 15 days later became pale, sweaty, febrile, and tachypneic. His blood pressure was 100/60 and his heart rate 100/minute. There were reduced breath sounds and crackles throughout the lung fields.

A chest X-ray showed diffuse interstitial and alveolar infiltrates and small bilateral pleural effusions. A high-resolution CT scan of the chest showed diffuse ground-glass attenuation and patchy peripheral opacities, consistent with an acute hypersensitivity pneumonitis, and other diagnoses were ruled out. He responded to gluco-corticoids.

- A 72-year-old man developed hypoxemic respiratory failure while taking amiodarone 300 mg/day (74). He had no history of lung disease. His CT scan was similar to that of the first patient. He responded to treatment with corticosteroids.
- In a 79-year-old man with emphysema taking amiodarone 200 mg/day, the diagnosis of amiodarone-induced lung toxicity was complicated by the fact that emphysema has the opposite effect on lung volumes and spirometry from interstitial lung disease (75). His FEV_1, which had been reduced, became normal and then increased. However, the combination of emphysema with amiodarone-induced lung disease led to worsening dyspnea, and a chest X-ray showed patchy mixed interstitial and airspace disease, most marked in the mid to upper lung zones bilaterally, and ground-glass opacification in the left lower lobe, suggesting an acute alveolitis. He responded to prednisone after withdrawal of amiodarone. His carbon monoxide diffusing capacity, which had fallen, returned to normal. A CT scan showed marked bullous emphysema and ground-glass interstitial changes. The FEV_1 almost doubled, from being severely reduced to within the reference range.
- A 77-year-old man who had taken amiodarone 400 mg/day for 11 months developed crackles at the lung bases and scattered respiratory wheeze (76). His leukocyte count was raised at $13.5 \times 109/l$ and he had progressive reduction in carbon monoxide diffusing capacity, serially measured. A chest X-ray showed bilateral opacities in the upper zones, peripheral in distribution, and a CT scan showed dense bilateral lung parenchymal opacities. The symptoms of dyspnea on exertion, cough with minimal sputum, pleuritic chest pain, and low-grade fever abated after withdrawal, and the upper lobe densities resolved.
- A 62-year-old man took amiodarone 400 mg bd and developed several adverse effects, including bilateral apical opacities with left hilar lymphadenopathy (77). Amiodarone was withdrawn and he was given glucocorticoids, with good effect; there was dramatic radiographic resolution within 3 weeks and he was no longer breathless with 1 week. The lung biopsy showed typical foamy macrophages. He had fibrosis of the bronchioles and interstitium, foci of obliterative bronchiolitis, and thickening of the alveolar walls. He had an accompanying peripheral neuropathy, which improved after withdrawal, and impaired visual acuity, about which no further information was given. Biopsy of the right vastus lateralis muscle showed type II atrophy with vacuolization, which the authors suggested supported the suspicion of amiodarone toxicity.

Amiodarone can occasionally cause isolated lung masses (SEDA-15, 168). One case was associated with a vasculitis; the lesions resolved completely 4 months after amiodarone withdrawal (78). In another case an isolated mass was associated with multiple small nodules in both lungs; the lesions resolved completely 6 months after amiodarone withdrawal (79).

Diagnosis

Diagnosis of amiodarone-induced lung damage can be difficult. The clinical symptoms and signs, the changes on chest radiography, and abnormalities of lung function tests are all non-specific. The presence of lymphocytes and foamy macrophages in bronchial lavage fluids and of phospholipidosis in lung biopsies are all suggestive. Measurement of the diffusing capacity of carbon monoxide has been used, but is unreliable.

The sialylated carbohydrate antigen KL-6 has been reported to be a serum marker of the activity of interstitial pneumonitis in seven patients with amiodarone-induced pulmonary toxicity (80,81). The dosages of amiodarone were 200–800 mg as an oral loading dose followed by 75–200 mg/day. Pulmonary complications occurred at 17 days to 48 months of treatment. In two patients with severe dyspnea and interstitial shadows on chest X-ray the KL-6 concentrations were very high (2100 and 3000 U/ml). In one of these the concentration increased from 695 to 2100 U/ml at a time when the interstitial changes on the CT scan worsened. In contrast, in two patients in whom pneumonia resolved with antibiotic treatment and without withdrawal of amiodarone, the serum KL-6 concentrations were lower (120 and 330 U/ml). In a patient in whom congestion of the lungs due to congestive cardiac failure had been confused with interstitial shadows the KL-6 concentration was only 190 U/ml. In two patients with lung cancers the concentrations were 260 and 360 U/ml. The authors proposed that a KL-6 concentration above the reference range (more than 520 U/ml) might be useful in differentiating patients with amiodarone-induced pneumonitis from patients with similar features not associated with amiodarone.

In 25 patients, three had proven interstitial pneumonitis and KL-6 serum concentrations of 414, 848, and 1217 U/ml; in contrast, all of the other 22 patients had normal CT scans and normal KL-6 concentrations (under 500 U/ml) (82). In the same study the limitations of carbon monoxide diffusing capacity in the diagnosis of amiodarone-induced lung disease (SEDA-15, 168) were again demonstrated.

Several scanning techniques have been used in the diagnosis of amiodarone-induced lung damage.

Computed tomography

Computed tomography may show a typical pattern of basal peripheral high-density pleuroparenchymal linear opacities, although these may be absent (83). It has also been suggested that high-resolution CT scanning may be able to detect iodine deposition from the drug (84). Of 16 patients taking long-term amiodarone, eight had severe respiratory and other symptoms and eight either had no symptoms or had only mild or chronic respiratory symptoms. All eight controls had negative high-resolution CT scans with no areas of high attenuation, while all eight cases had a least one high-attenuation lesion.

[67]Gallium scintigraphy

[67]Gallium scintigraphy has been used to diagnose amiodarone-induced lung damage (SEDA-15, 168).

- A 75-year-old man, who had taken amiodarone 200 mg/day for 4 years, developed acute dyspnea, chest pain, fever, and sweats (85). The chest X-ray showed diffuse alveolar and interstitial infiltrates, particularly at the lung bases. No pathogenic organisms were isolated and antibiotics had no effect. There was no evidence of sarcoidosis. Pulmonary [67]gallium scintigraphy showed extensive uptake of tracer throughout both lungs, consistent with amiodarone pneumonitis on a background of asbestosis with interstitial fibrosis. Treatment with corticosteroids after withdrawal of amiodarone resulted in marked clinical improvement.

The authors said that the extensive changes on gallium scanning, not present on the chest X-ray, had helped them to make the diagnosis, although a high-resolution CT scan had also shown widespread changes.

[99m]Technetium-diethylene triamine penta-acetic acid (DPTA) aerosol scintigraphy

Another scanning technique, ^{99m}Tc-diethylene triamine penta-acetic acid (DPTA) aerosol scintigraphy, has been compared with ^{67}Ga scanning in 26 patients, seven with amiodarone-induced lung damage, eight taking amiodarone without lung damage, and 11 healthy controls (86). [67]Ga scintigraphy was positive in four of the seven patients with lung damage but normal in the others. There was a positive correlation between ^{99m}Tc-DTPA clearance and the cumulative dose of amiodarone. The mean clearance values were 2%/minute in those with amiodarone-induced lung damage, 1.3%/minute in those without lung damage, and 0.9%/minute in the controls. The authors concluded that ^{67}Ga lung scintigraphy is useful for detecting amiodarone-induced lung damage but that ^{99m}Tc-DTPA aerosol scintigraphy is better.

Management

Although early reports suggested that glucocorticoids might be beneficial in management, this has not been subsequently confirmed (87).

Nervous system

The most common forms of neurological damage attributed to amiodarone are tremor, peripheral neuropathy, and ataxia (88). Other effects that have been reported include delirium (89), Parkinsonian tremor (90), and pseudotumor cerebri (91). Acute myolysis has recently been described at high dose (92). The peripheral neuropathy is probably due to intracellular lipidosis (93).

- Periodic ataxia has been attributed to amiodarone in a 67-year-old man taking amiodarone 200 mg/day (94). The ataxia responded to acetazolamide and eventually to withdrawal of amiodarone. It recurred with rechallenge.

Amiodarone-induced neuromyopathy has been studied in three patients by a review of their records, electromyography, and histopathology of muscle and nerve (95). Two patients had a slightly asymmetric, mixed, but primarily demyelinating sensorimotor polyneuropathy and the third had an acute neuropathy resembling Guillain–Barré syndrome. Creatine kinase activity did not correlate with clinical or electromyographic evidence of myopathy. In the peripheral nerves there was demyelination, some axon loss, and a variable number of characteristic lysosomal inclusions. Muscle specimens from two patients showed evidence of a vacuolar myopathy. After withdrawal of amiodarone, two patients improved and one died with a cardiac dysrhythmia.

Benign orgasmic headache has been associated with amiodarone (96).

- A 52-year-old man, who had taken amiodarone 800 mg/day for 7 months, developed acute, severe, throbbing headaches precipitated by coitus and occasionally other forms of exertion. An MRI scan of the brain was normal. When the dose of amiodarone was reduced to 200 mg/day the headaches diminished in frequency and severity. When the dose was increased again to 400 mg/day they increased in frequency and severity. The amiodarone was withdrawn and the headaches resolved.

Amiodarone was originally developed as a vasodilator, and that may have been the cause of headaches in this case.

Sensory systems

The adverse effects of amiodarone on the eyes have been reviewed (97). The most common effect is corneal microdeposits. In some cases chronic blepharitis and conjunctivitis have been reported (98), but the relation of these to amiodarone is not clear.

Keratopathy

In almost all patients (99,100) corneal microdeposits of lipofuscin occur secondary to the deposition of amiodarone. These are generally of no clinical significance, but occasionally patients complain of haloes around lights, particularly at night, photophobia, blurring of vision, dryness of the eyes, or lid irritation. Occasionally amiodarone can cause anterior subcapsular deposits, which are usually asymptomatic. In 22 patients taking long-term amiodarone there were corneal drug deposits in all of the eyes, slight anterior subcapsular lens opacities in 22%, and dry eyes in 9% (101).

Verticillate epithelial keratopathy due to amiodarone, in which there is whorl-shaped pigmentation of the cornea, has been proposed to be worsened by soft contact lenses (SEDA-15, 171). Two patients with hard contact lenses and amiodarone-associated keratopathy both complained of increased sensitivity to sunlight and were fitted with ultraviolet light-blocking lenses instead, as a precaution against further corneal damage; however, the authors did not think that the contact lenses had contributed to the damage (102).

The eyes of 11 patients (eight men and three women) taking amiodarone have been compared with those of 10 healthy sex- and age-matched controls by confocal microscopy (103). All those taking amiodarone had bright, highly reflective intracellular inclusions in the epithelial layers, particularly in the basal cell layers. In eyes with advanced keratopathy there were bright microdots in the anterior and posterior stroma and on the endothelial cell layer. Keratocyte density in the anterior stroma was lower in the treated subjects than in the controls, and there was marked irregularity of the stromal nerve fibers. The authors concluded that in some patients taking long-term amiodarone corneal damage may penetrate deeper than has previously been suspected.

Color vision disturbances

Amiodarone can cause impaired color vision associated with keratopathy (SEDA-12, 153) (104). Of 22 patients taking long-term amiodarone, two who had otherwise healthy eyes had abnormal blue color vision (101). Otherwise, color vision, contrast sensitivity, and visual fields were normal or could be explained by eye diseases such as cataract.

Optic neuropathy

A more serious effect of amiodarone on the eye is an optic neuropathy (105) (SEDA-15, 171). Although this resolves on withdrawal there can be residual field defects (106,107). Blindness has been attributed to bilateral optic neuropathy in a patient taking amiodarone (108). The incidence of optic neuropathy with amiodarone (SEDA-23, 199) has been estimated at 1.8% (SEDA-13, 141). There has been a recent review of 73 cases of optic neuropathy associated with the use of amiodarone, including 16 published case reports and 57 other reports from the National Registry of Drug-Induced Ocular Side Effects, the US FDA, and the WHO (109). Amiodarone-induced optic neuropathy is of insidious onset, with slow progression, bilateral visual loss, and protracted disc swelling, which tends to stabilize within several months of withdrawal. These features all distinguish it from non-arteritic ischemic optic neuropathy. The pathology of amiodarone-induced optic neuropathy is associated with lipid deposition, as with other forms of adverse effects of amiodarone.

- A 51-year-old man developed blurred vision after having taken amiodarone 600 mg/day for 3 months and 400 mg/day for 5 months (110). There was mild optic disc palor and edema on the right side, with a nearby flame-shaped hemorrhage; the optic disc on the left side was normal. There were accompanying corneal opacities in both eyes. Amiodarone was withdrawn and the optic neuropathy and corneal opacities improved.
- A 48-year-old man developed bilateral blurred vision and visual field changes after having taken amiodarone 400 mg/day for 2 months; 3 weeks after withdrawal of amiodarone his symptoms improved (111). There was no optic disc edema.

Other effects

The absence of optic disc edema in the last case is unusual; most cases are accompanied by some form of swelling of the optic disc.

Rare effects include raised intracranial pressure with papilledema (SEDA-12, 153) (112), retinal maculopathy (113), and retinopathy (97).

Multiple chalazia have been reported on the eyelids, due to lipogranulomata that contained a lot of amiodarone (114).

Sicca syndrome has occasionally been reported (9,115–117).

Brown discoloration of implanted lenses has been attributed to amiodarone (118).

- A 66-year-old woman, who had had two silicone intra-ocular lenses inserted because of cataract, developed progressive brown discoloration of the lens while taking amiodarone (dosage not stated). The discoloration progressed markedly after vitrectomy, suggesting that it was due to leakage of the drug into the eye. She also had an amiodarone-induced keratopathy.

Psychological, psychiatric

Delirium has rarely been reported with amiodarone (SEDA-13, 140).

- A 54-year-old man with no previous psychiatric history took amiodarone 400 mg bd (119). After a few days he became depressed and paranoid, suffered from insomnia, and had rambling speech. The dosage of amiodarone was reduced to 200 mg bd and he improved. However, 3 days later he became confused, with tangential thinking, labile effect, and a macular rash on the limbs. His serum sodium was reduced at 127 mmol/l and his blood urea nitrogen was raised. A CT scan of the head was normal. Amiodarone was withdrawn and 4 days later he was alert and oriented. About a week later he started taking amiodarone again and within 4 days became increasingly agitated, confused, and paranoid. He once more recovered after withdrawal of amiodarone.
- Depression has been attributed to amiodarone in a 65-year-old woman who was taking amiodarone (dosage not stated) (120). Because the mode of presentation was atypical in onset, course, duration, and its response to antidepressant drugs, amiodarone was withdrawn, and she improved rapidly. There was no evidence of thyroid disease.

Endocrine

Testes
Amiodarone can cause endocrine testicular dysfunction, as judged by increases in serum concentrations of FSH and LH and hyper-responsiveness to GnRH (121).

Syndrome of inappropriate ADH secretion
Amiodarone-induced hyponatremia, due to the syndrome of inappropriate secretion of antidiuretic hormone, is rare (SEDA-21, 199) (122). The mechanism is unknown. Unlike other adverse effects of amiodarone, it seems to occur rapidly and to resolve rapidly after withdrawal.

- A 63-year-old man reduced his dietary sodium intake to combat fluid retention and was taking furosemide 40 mg/day, spironolactone 50 mg/day, and enalapril 2.5 mg/day (123). He then took amiodarone 800 mg/day for 7 days and his serum sodium concentration fell to 119 mmol/l; his plasma vasopressin concentration was raised at 2.6 pmol/l. The dose of amiodarone was reduced to 100 mg/day, with fluid restriction; his

sodium rose to 130 mmol/l and his vasopressin fell to 1.4 pmol/l.

- An 87-year-old man reduced his dietary sodium intake to combat fluid retention and was taking furosemide 40 mg/day and spironolactone 25 mg/day (123). He then took amiodarone 200 mg/day for 7 days and 100 mg/day for 8 days and his serum sodium concentration fell to 121 mmol/l; his plasma vasopressin concentration was raised at 11 pmol/l. Amiodarone was continued, with fluid restriction; his sodium rose to 133 mmol/l and his vasopressin fell to 2.4 pmol/l.
- A 67-year-old man, who had taken amiodarone 200 mg/day for 3 months, developed hyponatremia (serum sodium concentration 117 mmol/l) (124). He was also taking furosemide 20 mg/day, spironolactone 25 mg/day, and lisinopril 40 mg/day. His urine osmolality was 740 mosmol/kg with a normal serum osmolality. Fluid restriction was ineffective, but when amiodarone was withdrawn the sodium rose to 136 mmol/l.
- A 62-year-old woman with paroxysmal atrial fibrillation who had taken amiodarone 300 mg/day had a serum sodium concentration of 120 mmol/l with a normal serum potassium and a reduced serum osmolality (240 mmol/kg); the urinary sodium concentration was 141 mmol/l and the urine osmolality 422 mmol/kg (122). There was no evident cause of inappropriate secretion of ADH and within 5 days of withdrawal of amiodarone the serum sodium concentration had risen to 133 mmol/l and rose further to 143 mmol/l 14 days later. There was no rechallenge and no recurrence of hyponatremia during the next 6 months.

In some of these cases other factors may have contributed to the hyponatremia that amiodarone seems to have caused.

Thyroid gland
The effects of amiodarone on thyroid function tests and in causing thyroid disease, both hyperthyroidism and hypothyroidism, have been reviewed in the context of the use of perchlorate, which acts by inhibiting iodine uptake by the thyroid gland (125), and there have been several other reviews (126–130).

Effects on thyroid function tests
Amiodarone causes altered thyroid function tests, with rises in serum concentrations of T4 and reverse T3 and a fall in serum T3 concentration. This is due to inhibition of the peripheral conversion of T4 to T3, causing preferential conversion to reverse T3. These changes can occur in the absence of symptomatic abnormalities of thyroid function.

Hyperthyroidism
DoTS classification
Dose-relation: collateral effect
Time-course: delayed
Susceptibility factors: genetic (unoperated or palliated cyanotic congenital heart disease; beta-thalassemia major); sex (conflicting results); altered physiology (iodine intake, conflicting results)

Frequency

Apart from its effects on thyroid function tests, amiodarone is also associated with both functional hyperthyroidism and hypothyroidism, in up to 6% of patients. The frequency of thyroid disease in patients taking amiodarone has been retrospectively studied in 90 patients taking amiodarone 200 mg/day for a mean duration of 33 months (131). Hypothyroidism occurred in five patients and hyperthyroidism in 11. Hyperthyroidism became more frequent with time and was associated with recurrent supraventricular dysrhythmias in four of the 11 patients.

In a nested case-control analysis of 5522 patients with a first prescription for an antidysrhythmic drug and no previous use of thyroid drugs, cases were defined as all patients who had started a thyroid-mimetic or antithyroid drug no sooner than 3 months after the start of an antidysrhythmic drug and controls were patients with a comparable follow-up period who had not taken any thyroid drugs during the observation period (132). There were 123 patients who had started antithyroid drugs and 96 who had started a thyroid-mimetic drug. In users of amiodarone there was an adjusted odds ratios of 6.3 (95% CI = 3.9, 10) for hyperthyroidism compared with users of other antidysrhythmic drugs. Patients who were exposed to a cumulative dose of amiodarone over 144 g had an adjusted odds ratio of 13 (6, 27) for hyperthyroidism.

Mechanisms

Amiodarone causes two different varieties of hyperthyroidism (SEDA-23, 199), one by the effects of excess iodine in those with latent disease (so-called type 1 hyperthyroidism), the other through a destructive thyroiditis in a previously normal gland (so-called type 2 hyperthyroidism). The two varieties can be distinguished by differences in radio-iodine uptake by the gland: in type 1 hyperthyroidism radio-iodine uptake is normal or increased, whereas in type 2 it is reduced. In type 1 hyperthyroidism, thyroid ultrasound shows a nodular, hypoechoic gland of increased volume, whereas in type 2 the gland is normal.

Iodine intake may be important in determining the type of amiodarone-induced thyroid disease. In 229 patients taking long-term amiodarone hyperthyroidism was more common (9.6 versus 2%) in West Tuscany, where dietary iodine intake is low, and hypothyroidism more common (22 versus 5%) in Massachusetts, where iodine intake is adequate (SEDA-10, 148) (133). However, other factors may play a part. In a retrospective inter-regional study in France there was a greater incidence of amiodarone-induced hyperthyroidism in the maritime areas Aquitaine and Languedoc–Roussillon, and a greater incidence of amiodarone-induced hypothyroidism in Midi–Pyrenees, a non-maritime area, in which iodine intake is lower than in Languedoc–Roussillon (134).

There have also been reports of painful thyroiditis associated with amiodarone (SEDA-15, 170).

Susceptibility factors

There has been a retrospective study of the frequency of amiodarone-associated thyroid dysfunction in adults with congenital heart disease (135). Of 92 patients who had taken amiodarone for at least 6 months (mean age 35, range 18–60 years), 36% developed thyroid dysfunction—19 became hyperthyroid and 14 hypothyroid. The mean dosage was 194 (100–300) mg/day, and the median duration of therapy was 3 (0.5–15) years. Female sex (OR = 3) and unoperated or palliated cyanotic congenital heart disease (OR = 7) were significant susceptibility factors for thyroid dysfunction. The risk was also dose-related. Although the authors conceded that they may have over-estimated the risk of thyroid dysfunction, because of the selected nature of the population they studied, the risks were markedly higher than in previous studies of older patients with acquired heart disease, despite a lower maintenance dosage of amiodarone.

In contrast, it has been suggested that men are more susceptible to hyperthyroidism due to amiodarone (136). Of 122 600 patients in 12 practices in the West Midlands in the UK, 142 men and 74 women were taking amiodarone and 27 (12.5%) had thyroid disease. Of those, 11 men (7.7%) and 4 women (5.4%) had hypothyroidism, a nonsignificant difference; however, 12 men (8.5%) had hyperthyroidism compared with no women. This difference is particularly striking because hyperthyroidism is usually more common in women.

Patients with beta-thalassemia major have an increased risk of primary hypothyroidism. In 23 patients with beta-thalassemia amiodarone was associated with a high risk of overt hypothyroidism (33 versus 3% in controls) (137). This occurred at up to 3 months after starting amiodarone. The risk of subclinical hypothyroidism was similar in the two groups. In one case overt hypothyroidism resolved spontaneously after withdrawal, but the other patients were given thyroxine. After 21–47 months of treatment three patients developed thyrotoxicosis, with remission after withdrawal. There were no cases of hyperthyroidism in the controls. The authors proposed that patients with beta-thalassemia may be more susceptible to iodine-induced hypothyroidism, related to an underlying defect in iodine in the thyroid, perhaps associated with an effect of iron overload.

Presentation

Many examples of hyperthyroidism due to amiodarone have been published.

- A 72-year-old woman with dilated cardiomyopathy was given amiodarone for fast atrial flutter and 6 months later developed abnormal thyroid function tests, with a suppressed TSH and a raised serum thyroxine. The autoantibody profile was negative and a thyroid uptake scan showed reduced uptake (138).

Despite the fact that she was clinically euthyroid, the authors suggested that this patient had amiodarone-induced hyperthyroidism. However, amiodarone inhibits the peripheral conversion of thyroxine to triiodothyronine; it can therefore increase the serum thyroxine and suppress the serum TSH, as in this case. On the other hand, the reduced uptake by the thyroid gland is consistent with type 2 amiodarone-induced hyperthyroidism. The authors did not report the serum concentrations of free thyroxine and triiodothyronine.

- A 67-year-old man took amiodarone 200 mg/day for 20 months, after which it was withdrawn; 8 months later his serum TSH was suppressed and the free thyroxine and free triiodothyronine were both raised; there were no thyroid antibodies and an ultrasound scan showed a diffuse goiter with a nodule in the right lobe and reduced iodine uptake (139). Histological examination of the nodule showed a papillary cancer.

The authors attributed these changes to an effect of amiodarone, but it is not clear that amiodarone-induced changes would have taken so long to become manifest after withdrawal. However, the diagnosis of type 2 amiodarone-induced hyperthyroidism was supported by a poor response to prednisone, potassium perchlorate, and methimazole. Lithium produced temporary benefit, but thyroidectomy was required.

- In five patients who presented in Tasmania during 1 year, all of whom were taking amiodarone 200 mg/day, serum TSH was undetectable and the free thyroxine and triiodothyronine concentrations were raised (140). In one case there was a low titer of TSH receptor antibodies and in another a high titer of antithyroid peroxidase antibodies. In all cases the hyperthyroidism was severe and occurred after at least 2 years of treatment with amiodarone. In one of two patients in whom it was measured the serum concentration of interleukin-6 was raised, as has been previously shown (SEDA-19, 193). In two cases the hyperthyroidism was refractory to treatment with propylthiouracil, lithium, and dexamethasone; in these cases thyroidectomy was required. Two patients responded to propylthiouracil, lithium, and dexamethasone, and one responded to carbimazole.

Amiodarone-induced hyperthyroidism can occasionally be fatal (141).

- A 62-year-old man took amiodarone for 2 years and developed hyperthyroidism; carbimazole 40 mg/day, prednisolone, lithium, and colestyramine were ineffective and he died with hepatic encephalopathy and multiorgan failure.
- A 55-year-old man took amiodarone for 4 years and developed hyperthyroidism; carbimazole 60 mg/day, prednisolone, and lithium were ineffective and he died with septicemia and multiorgan failure.

In three other cases reported in the same paper, severe hyperthyroidism responded severally to treatment with carbimazole, carbimazole plus lithium, or propylthiouracil. In one case amiodarone therapy was restarted after prophylactic subtotal thyroidectomy.

Diagnosis
The diagnosis of amiodarone-induced thyroid disorders can be difficult, because amiodarone often alters thyroid function tests without disturbing clinical thyroid function. Although radio-iodine uptake by the thyroid gland is not helpful in making a diagnosis, the discharge of iodine from the thyroid gland in response to perchlorate is reduced in patients with hypothyroidism (142). The test is not abnormal in patients with hyperthyroidism and it is not clear how helpful it is in hypothyroidism.

Since the measurement of serum T3 and T4 concentrations may not be helpful, an alternative would be to measure metabolic status. Measurement of the serum concentration of co-enzyme Q10 may distinguish patients with clinical thyroid dysfunction from those who simply

have abnormalities of thyroid function tests (143), but the value of this test remains to be established.

Color-flow Doppler sonography of the thyroid and measurement of serum interleukin-6 (IL-6) have been studied as diagnostic tools in a retrospective case-note study of patients with amiodarone-associated hyperthyroidism (144). There were 37 patients with amiodarone-associated hyperthyroidism (mean age 65, range 20–86 years), and 25 underwent color-flow Doppler sonography. Of those, 10 were classified as type 1 (based on increased vascularity) and 10 as type 2 (based on patchy or reduced vascularity); 5 were indeterminate. In those with type 1 hyperthyroidism, free serum thyroxine tended to be lower (52 versus 75 pmol/l), free serum triiodothyronine was lower (8.8 versus 16 pmol/l), the cumulative amiodarone dose was lower (66 versus 186 g), and less prednisolone was used (because the diagnosis of type 1 disease encouraged steroid withdrawal); however, carbimazole doses were not different and the time to euthyroidism was the same in the two groups (81 versus 88 days). IL-6 was raised in two patients with type 1 and in one patient with type 2 hyperthyroidism. The authors proposed that color-flow Doppler sonography could be used to distinguish the two subtypes, confirming an earlier report (145), but that IL-6 measurement was unhelpful.

Management
The treatment of amiodarone-induced hyperthyroidism is difficult. It often does not respond to conventional therapy with carbimazole, methimazole, or radio-iodine. However, corticosteroids and the combination of methimazole with potassium perchlorate have been reported to be effective (146), even if amiodarone is continued (147). Other regimens that have been used include combinations of corticosteroids with carbimazole (148), corticosteroids and benzylthiouracil (149), or propylthiouracil (SEDA-15, 170). Potassium perchlorate has also been used (SEDA-21, 199). Other forms of treatment that have been successful have been plasma exchange and in very severe cases subtotal thyroidectomy (150) or total thyroidectomy (SEDA-15, 170) (SEDA-17, 220) (151).

It has been suggested that potassium perchlorate should be used in the treatment of type 1 hyperthyroidism and glucocorticoids in the treatment of type 2 (SEDA-21, 199). Since hypothyroidism due to amiodarone tends to occur in areas in which there is sufficient iodine in the diet, it has been hypothesized that an iodinated organic inhibitor of hormone synthesis is formed and that the formation of this inhibitor is inhibited by perchlorate to a greater extent than thyroid hormone iodination is inhibited, since the iodinated lipids that are thought to be inhibitors require about 10 times more iodide than the hormone. However, there is a high risk of recurrence after treatment with potassium perchlorate, and it can cause serious adverse effects (SED-13, 1281).

When five patients with type 2 amiodarone-induced hyperthyroidism were treated with a combination of an oral cholecystographic agent (sodium ipodate or sodium iopanoate, which are rich in iodine and potent inhibitors of 5′-deiodinase) plus a thionamide (propylthiouracil or methimazole) after amiodarone withdrawal, all improved substantially within a few days and became euthyroid or hypothyroid in 15–31 weeks (152). Four of the five became hypothyroid and required long-term treatment with levothyroxine.

In another study, three patients with type 1 disease, two of whom had not responded to methimazole plus perchlorate, were successfully treated with a short course of iopanoic acid 1 g/day, resulting in a marked reduction in the peripheral conversion of T4 to T3 (153). Euthyroidism was restored in 7–12 days, allowing uneventful thyroidectomy. The patients were then treated with levothyroxine for hypothyroidism and amiodarone was safely restarted. The authors suggested that iopanoic acid is the drug of choice for rapid restoration of normal thyroid function before thyroidectomy in patients with drug-resistant type 1 amiodarone-induced hyperthyroidism.

However, others have suggested that the differentiation of amiodarone-induced hyperthyroidism into two types is not helpful in determining suitable therapy (154). Of 28 consecutive patients there was spontaneous resolution of hyperthyroidism in 5 and 23 received carbimazole alone as first-line therapy. Long-term euthyroidism was achieved in 11, 5 became hypothyroid and required long-term thyroxine, and 5 relapsed after withdrawal of carbimazole and became euthyroid with either long-term carbimazole ($n = 3$) or radioiodine ($n = 2$). Four were intolerant of carbimazole and received propylthiouracil, with good effect in three. One was resistant to thionamides and responded to corticosteroids. There was no difference in presentation or outcome between those in whom amiodarone was continued or stopped or between possible type 1 or type 2 disease (defined clinically and by serum IL-6 measurement). The authors concluded that continuing amiodarone has no adverse effect on the response to treatment of hyperthyroidism and that first-line therapy with a thionamide alone, whatever the type of disease, is appropriate in iodine-replete areas, thus avoiding potential complications of other drugs. However, it is not clear how good their differentiation of types 1 and 2 disease was. A previous prospective study in 24 patients showed that differentiation predicted response to treatment (155).

It is generally recommended that amiodarone should be withdrawn. However, in some cases (156,157) worsening of thyrotoxic symptoms and heart function has been reported after withdrawal of amiodarone. When withdrawal of amiodarone is not an option, near-total thyroidectomy may be preferred. If surgery is not possible plasmapheresis can be helpful.

The use of local anesthesia for total thyroidectomy in patients with amiodarone-induced hyperthyroidism and cardiac impairment has been reviewed in the context of six patients (158).

Hypothyroidism
Amiodarone-induced hypothyroidism has been reviewed in the light of a case of 74-year-old woman (148).

In a nested case-control analysis of 5522 patients with a first prescription for an antidysrhythmic drug and no previous use of thyroid drugs, cases were defined as all patients who had started a thyroid-mimetic or antithyroid drug no sooner than 3 months after the start of an anti-dysrhythmic drug and controls were patients with a

comparable follow-up period who had not taken any thyroid drugs during the observation period (132). There were 123 patients who had started antithyroid drugs and 96 who had started a thyroid-mimetic drug. In users of amiodarone there was an adjusted odds ratios of 6.6 (3.9, 11) for hypothyroidism compared with users of other anti-dysrhythmic drugs.

The risk of amiodarone-induced hypothyroidism may be greater in patients who have pre-existing thyroid autoimmune disease (159). There is some evidence that the risk of hypothyroidism due to amiodarone is increased in elderly patients (160), but the data are not conclusive.

In amiodarone-induced hypothyroidism the simplest method of treatment is to continue with amiodarone and to add thyroxine as required.

Metabolism

Amiodarone can cause altered serum lipid concentrations (161). Serum cholesterol rises, as can blood glucose and serum triglyceride concentrations. The mechanisms of these effects are not known; nor is it known to what extent they are due to changes in thyroid function.

Hematologic

Although phospholipid inclusion bodies commonly occur in the neutrophils of patients taking amiodarone (162), adverse hematological effects have rarely been attributed to amiodarone. However, there have been reports of thrombocytopenia (163) and of impaired platelet aggregation, associated with gingival bleeding and ecchymoses of the legs (164). Coombs'-positive hemolytic anemia has also been reported (165).

Bone marrow granulomata have rarely been reported in patients taking amiodarone (166).

- A 53-year-old woman developed leukoerythroblastosis with giant thrombocytes in the peripheral blood and was subsequently given amiodarone. The bone marrow became hypocellular with atypical megakaryocytes and several granulomata.
- A 78-year-old woman with a raised erythrocyte sedimentation rate, a mild anemia, and a polyclonal gammopathy on serum immunoelectrophoresis. The bone marrow became hypocellular with atypical megakaryocytes and several granulomata.

In the first case amiodarone was given after the onset of the peripheral blood film abnormalities and the only change in the bone marrow was the occurrence of the granulomata. The authors proposed that the granulomata had occurred because of phospholipid accumulation.

- Bone marrow biopsy in a patient taking amiodarone 100 mg/day showed multiple non-caseating epithelioid granulomata, which resolved 3 months after the withdrawal of amiodarone in a 67-year-old man (167). Similar granulomas were found in a 77-year-old woman who had taken amiodarone 100 mg/day for many years and had thrombocytopenia; the bone marrow contained an increased number of megakaryocytes. Her platelet count normalized 1 month after amiodarone had been withdrawn, and after 3 months there were fewer granulomata in the bone marrow.

- A 76-year-old man, who had taken amiodarone for an unspecified time, developed a monoclonal gammopathy with bone marrow granulomata (168). After another 2 years he developed hepatic granulomata and the amiodarone was withdrawn. The bone marrow granulomata resolved within a few months. Infections were excluded and there was no evidence of sarcoidosis.

The mechanism of this effect is unknown.

Liver

Amiodarone often causes rises in the serum activities of aspartate transaminase and lactate dehydrogenase to about twice normal, without changes in alkaline phosphatase or bilirubin, and without clinical evidence of liver dysfunction (169). Changes of this kind were originally reported to be transient and dose-related, returning to normal when the dose was reduced (170).

However, amiodarone can also cause liver damage, which usually takes the form of a hepatitis associated with phospholipid deposition, and there can be changes similar to those of alcoholic hepatitis (171–173). In some cases there is progression of cirrhosis (174). The risk of hepatic impairment in patients taking amiodarone is not known, but relatively severe liver damage can occur even in the absence of symptoms and with only minor associated changes in liver function tests.

- A 40-year-old man who had taken amiodarone 400 mg/day for 6 weeks developed an acute hepatitis accompanied by clusters of light brown granular cells, which were identified as macrophages (175). There were phospholipid inclusions in the macrophages and hepatocytes.

The authors proposed that the granular macrophages represented an early marker of amiodarone-induced hepatotoxicity. Their unusual color was attributed to the deposition of a combination of phospholipid, lipofuscin, and bile breakdown products.

Other forms of liver damage that have been reported include a syndrome resembling Reye's syndrome (176). Severe hepatitis at low dosage and thought to be immunologically based has been described (177).

Chronic liver damage with amiodarone is much more common than acute hepatitis, but cholestatic jaundice is one of the relatively rare presentations (SEDA-19, 193) (178,179).

- An 84-year-old woman, who had taken amiodarone 400 mg/day for 4–5 years, developed weakness, fatigue, anorexia, and abnormal liver function tests, with an aspartate transaminase activity of 234 U/l, alanine transaminase 154 U/l, and alkaline phosphatase 316 U/l (180). She had a normal serum bilirubin and the serum concentrations of amiodarone and desethylamiodarone were both within the usual target ranges. Apart from gallstones, endoscopic retrograde cholangiography and abdominal ultrasound showed a normal biliary tree. After withdrawal of amiodarone her liver function tests improved, but 4 months later she developed a rapidly rising serum bilirubin concentration (142 mmol/l), her serum albumin

concentration fell to 30 g/l, and her serum cholesterol concentration was high (11 mmol/l). She had bilirubin and urobilinogen in the urine and there was no evidence of viral or immunological hepatitis. Abdominal ultrasonography was normal, as was a liver scan, but a CT scan of the abdomen showed a diffusely hyperdense liver consistent with the effects of amiodarone. Liver biopsy also showed findings consistent with amiodarone-induced cholestatic liver damage, with distorted architecture, portal fibrosis, pericellular sinusoidal fibrosis, and focally irregular lobular sinusoidal fibrosis, but without bridging fibrosis or cirrhosis. There was ductal proliferation and a mild lymphocytic infiltrate but no cholangitis. Electron microscopy showed lamella inclusions compatible with phospholipidosis.

If amiodarone was responsible in this case, it is hard to reconcile the improvement after amiodarone withdrawal with the cholestasis that occurred 4 months later. The patient was also taking felodipine, furosemide, potassium chloride, aspirin (500 mg/day), and cisapride, but the authors argued that the changes were not consistent with liver damage due to any of those drugs. In particular they thought that the felodipine was unlikely to have caused cholestasis, although that has been previously reported, because of the presence of Mallory bodies in the liver biopsy; however, Mallory bodies have previously been reported with felodipine, and although cholestatic liver injury caused by felodipine has not been reported before, that seems as likely a candidate in this case as amiodarone.

Acute hepatitis with liver failure can occur after intravenous administration and may be due to the solvent, polysorbate (SEDA-14, 149) (SEDA-16, 178) (SEDA-18, 202) (SEDA-22, 206) (181).

- A 69-year-old man was given amiodarone intravenously 1500 mg for multiple coupled ventricular extra beats and 24 hours later developed acute hepatitis, with a 50-fold increase in serum transaminase activities and simultaneous increases in lactate dehydrogenase, gamma-glutamyl transferase, bilirubin, and prothrombin time; there was a moderate leukocytosis and mild renal insufficiency (182). No further amiodarone was given and there was full recovery within 2 weeks. Other causes of acute hepatitis were excluded.

The mechanism of this effect is not known, but the histology includes Mallory bodies, steatosis, intralobular inflammatory infiltrates, and fibrosis; electron microscopy suggests phospholipidosis.

It has been suggested that liver injury due to amiodarone is either due to a direct biochemical action or perhaps metabolic idiosyncrasy. Because there have been cases in which oral administration has not led to a recurrence, it has also been suggested that the vehicle in which amiodarone is usually dissolved, polysorbate (Tween) 80, is responsible rather than the amiodarone itself (SEDA-18, 202).

Pancreas

There have been two reported cases of pancreatitis and in one the patient died of progressive liver failure (183,184). Whether this was a direct effect of amiodarone is unclear.

Urinary tract

Increases in serum creatinine concentrations, correlated with serum amiodarone concentrations, have been reported (185).

Skin

Amiodarone commonly causes phototoxicity reactions (186,187). The risk of phototoxicity increases with the duration of the exposure. Window glass and sun screens do not give protection, although zinc or titanium oxide formulations and narrow band UVB photo therapy can help (188–190). For most patients this adverse effect will be no more than a nuisance, and the benefit of therapy may be worthwhile. However, in a few cases treatment may have to be withdrawn. Histological examination of skin biopsies shows intracytoplasmic inclusions of phospholipids (191). There has been a single report of a severe case of photosensitivity in conjunction with a syndrome resembling porphyria cutanea tarda, resulting in bullous lesions (192).

Amiodarone can cause a cosmetically annoying bluish pigmentation of the skin (SEDA-15, 171) (SEDA-22, 207) (SEDA-23, 199) (193).

- A 54-year-old man who took the drug for 1 year developed bluish-gray discoloration of the face (194). The discoloration almost completely resolved within 9 months of withdrawal.
- A 55-year-old woman who had taken amiodarone 250 mg/day for about 10 years developed bluish-gray discoloration of the face (195). The pigmentation responded to treatment with a Q-switched ruby laser at an energy of 8 J/cm² and a wave length of 694 mm.

The authors suggested that the ruby laser had damaged pigment-containing cells. However, the amiodarone was continued, so presumably the laser also destroyed lipofuscin in situ.

- A 69-year-old white man who had taken amiodarone 400 mg/day for 3 years developed blue–gray discoloration of the face and other exposed areas (196). Areas that had been protected from the sun (the forehead by a broad-brimmed hat and the skin under his wrist watch) were not affected.
- A 70-year-old man developed grey–blue pigmentation on sun-exposed areas of his skin after taking amiodarone for 10 years and minocycline for 4 years (197).

Minocycline can also cause skin pigmentation and it is not clear in this last case what the interaction of amiodarone with minocycline was.

Grey–blue discoloration of the skin during amiodarone therapy has been presumed to be due to lipofucsin deposition. However, it has also been suggested that amiodarone may block the maturation of melanosomes, in view of a case of discoloration associated with a reduced number of mature melanosomes and an increased number of pre-melanosomes in sun-exposed areas of the skin, but normal numbers in non-exposed areas (198).

It has been suggested that the skin and mucosal toxicity of amiodarone may be enhanced by radiotherapy (SEDA-16, 178) (SEDA-17, 221). However, in a retrospective review of 10 patients who took amiodarone when having external beam radiation therapy there were no unexpected acute sequelae (199).

Other skin reactions that have been reported include iododerma (200), erythema nodosum, psoriasis (201), and exfoliative dermatitis (202).

Amiodarone can increase the risk of mucosal and skin toxicity due to radiotherapy and rarely causes hair loss (SEDA-17, 221) and vasculitis (203).

The severe form of erythema multiforme known as toxic epidermal necrolysis has rarely been attributed to amiodarone (204).

- A 71-year-old woman, who had taken amiodarone 200 mg/day for 3 months and diltiazem for 8 months, developed extensive erythema, blistering, and erosions affecting 50% of the body surface area, with a maculopapular rash on the limbs (205). She developed bilateral pneumonia and septicemia and died after 7 days.

Musculoskeletal

A proximal myopathy has occasionally been reported in patients taking amiodarone (69) and there has been a report of an acute necrotizing myopathy (206).

Sexual function

Epididymitis has been reported in patients taking high dosages of amiodarone, resolving with dosage reduction or withdrawal (SEDA-18, 203).

Reproductive system

Non-infective epididymitis has occasionally been reported in patients taking amiodarone (SEDA-10, 148) (SEDA-18, 203).

- A 25-year-old man who had taken amiodarone 200 mg bd for 1 year developed epididymitis, which resolved within 3 months of withdrawal of amiodarone and recurred within 2 months of its reintroduction (207).

This case was unusual in that it involved both testes. The mechanism of this effect is not known, but it has been reported to be dose-dependent, although anti-amiodarone antibodies have also been reported (208). The incidence is not known, but has been reported to be as high as 11%. The author of one very brief report (209) claimed to have seen 20 cases of epididymitis, some of which were bilateral, since the late 1980s. He claimed that withdrawal produced dramatic resolution of symptoms within 10–20 days, and that amiodarone in a dose of 200 mg/day did not usually cause symptoms, even in patients who had had epididymitis at higher dosages.

Immunologic

Lupus-like syndrome has rarely been attributed to amiodarone.

- A 71-year-old woman, who had been taking amiodarone 200 mg bd for 2 years, developed malaise, intermittent fever, arthralgia, and weight loss (210). She had a malar rash and hypoventilation at both lung bases. Her erythrocyte sedimentation rate was markedly raised (90 mm/hour), there was a mild normochromic normocytic anemia (10 g/dl), a slight lymphopenia, and otherwise normal routine tests. Her rheumatoid factor was raised in a titer of 1:320, and circulating complexes of IgG-C1q were positive. Antinuclear antibody was positive (1:640), but all other antibodies were negative. There was progressive improvement on withdrawal of amiodarone and all the biochemical tests returned to normal.

- A 59-year-old man, who had taken amiodarone 200 mg/day for 2 years, developed fever, pleuritic chest pain, dyspnea at rest, a non-productive cough, malaise, and joint pains (211). He had a verrucous endocarditis and a pleuropericardial effusion. He had raised titers of antinuclear antibodies (1:320) with anti-Ro specificity. Serum complement was normal and there were no circulating immune complexes, no cryoglobulins, and no anti-dsDNA, anti-La, anti-U1 ribonucleoprotein, anti-Sm, anti-Sc1, 70, anti-Jo 1, anti-histone, antiphospholipid, anticentromere, anticardiolipin, or anticytoplasmic antibodies. Within 7 days of withdrawal of amiodarone the signs and symptoms started to resolve, and he recovered fully with the addition of prednisolone.

Angioedema has been reported in a 70-year-old woman who had taken amiodarone 200 mg/day for 8 years (212). The amiodarone was withdrawn and the symptoms disappeared. Rechallenge produced facial flush and facial angioedema within 20 minutes of a 200 mg dose.

Death

The effect of intravenous and oral amiodarone on morbidity and mortality has been studied in 1073 patients during the first hours after the onset of acute myocardial infarction (213). The patients were randomized to receive amiodarone or placebo for 6 months. The interim analysis showed an increased mortality, albeit not significant, with high-dose amiodarone (16 versus 10%) and the dose was therefore reduced from 400 to 200 mg/day. Low-dose amiodarone was associated with a reduced death rate (6.6 versus 9.9%). There were non-fatal adverse events in 108 patients taking amiodarone and 73 taking placebo. The only non-fatal adverse effect that occurred significantly more often with amiodarone was hypotension during the initial intravenous loading phase, a well-known effect. In the context of this study, it should be remembered that in several previous studies amiodarone has been shown to reduce mortality after myocardial infarction (SEDA-23, 198) (SEDA-24, 206) (214).

Second-Generation Effects

Teratogenicity

There are no major teratogenic effects of amiodarone (215).

Fetotoxicity

Exposure to amiodarone in utero has only occasionally been described.

Cardiovascular

There have been reports of sinus bradycardia (SEDA-8, 179) (SEDA-20, 176) (216,217) and prolongation of the QT interval (215).

Nervous system

Congenital nystagmus has been described (SEDA-20, 176).

Psychological

In one child there was evidence of mental delay, hypotonia, hypertelorism, and micrognathia (SEDA-20, 176), although the authors thought that the link between amiodarone and neurotoxicity was speculative. However, there has also been a retrospective study of 10 children who were exposed to amiodarone during pregnancy, compared with matched controls (218). There was no change in IQ score, but the children who had been exposed to amiodarone had impaired expressive language skills and one child had global developmental delay. However, most of the mothers were not concerned about their children's development, and so any effect of amiodarone on neurological development was probably small. One child had transient neonatal hypothyroidism, which responded to a short course of thyroxine; another had mild transient neonatal hyperthyroidism; in neither case was there any difference in development from the other children who had been exposed to amiodarone. One child was born with a congenital jerk nystagmus and had relatively poor reading and comprehension skills for both words and passages, low scores on several of the verbal subtests of the WISC-R test for information, arithmetic, and vocabulary, and below average spelling.

Endocrine

The major adverse effect on the fetus is altered thyroid function (SEDA-13, 141) (SEDA-14, 149) (SEDA-19, 194) (SEDA-20, 176). There have been individual reports of neonatal hyperthyroxinemia (219), goiter (216), and hypothyroidism (220). In the patient with goiter there was associated hypotonia, bradycardia, large fontanelles, and macroglossia (216).

Two neonates who had been given intravenous amiodarone as fetuses at 26 and 29 weeks and whose mothers had also taken it orally developed hypothyroidism (221). The authors suggested that low dietary iodine intake by the mothers may have contributed, by enhancing the Wolff–Chaikoff effect.

Susceptibility Factors

Age

The safety and efficacy of amiodarone for supraventricular tachycardia have been studied in 50 infants (mean age 1.0 month, 35 boys) (222). They had congenital heart disease (24%), congestive heart failure (36%), or ventricular dysfunction (44%). Six, who were critically ill, received a loading dose of intravenous amiodarone 5 mg/kg over 1 hour, and all took 20 mg/kg/day orally for 7–10 days, followed by 100 mg/day; if this failed to control the dysrhythmia, oral propranolol (2 mg/kg/day) was added. Follow-up was for an average of 16 months. Rhythm control was achieved in all patients. Growth and development were normal. The higher dose of amiodarone was associated with an increase in the QT_c interval to over 0.44 seconds, but there were no dysrhythmias. Two infants had hypotension during intravenous loading, as has previously been reported in infants (SEDA-19, 194). Aspartate transaminase and alanine transaminase activities and thyrotropin (TSH) concentrations all increased, but remained within their reference ranges. There were no adverse effects that necessitated drug withdrawal.

Young patients are more likely to develop adverse effects in the skin (223).

In children under 10 years of age the risk of adverse effects is less than in adults (224,225). It is not clear whether older children are at greater or lesser risks of adverse effects than are adults.

The safety of antidysrhythmic drugs in children has not been thoroughly studied. However, the risk of prolongation of the QT interval seems to be considerably less than that in adults (226), although it has been reported with quinidine, disopyramide, amiodarone, sotalol, and diphemanil.

Other features of the patient

Amiodarone-induced liver damage is more common in those with reduced left ventricular function (223).

Anesthesia and surgery

It has been reported that there is an increased risk of adverse reactions to amiodarone in patients undergoing anesthesia (SEDA-15, 171). However, in a retrospective survey of 12 patients who underwent anesthesia for urgent thyroidectomy due to amiodarone there were no anesthetic complications or deaths (227).

There is an increased risk of some of the adverse effects of amiodarone (including dysfunction of the liver and lungs) in patients who have had or who are having surgery (228). In addition the perioperative mortality in these patients is higher than in controls (229). The factors that increase the risks of amiodarone-associated adverse cardiovascular effects during surgery (230) include pre-existing ventricular dysfunction, too rapid a rate of intravenous infusion, hypocalcemia, and an interaction between amiodarone and both the general anesthetics used and other drugs with negative inotropic or chronotropic effects. It has therefore been recommended (230) that serum concentrations of calcium, amiodarone, and digoxin should be within the reference or target ranges before operation, and that other drugs with negative inotropic or chronotropic effects should be withdrawn before surgery.

The use of amiodarone in the prevention of atrial fibrillation after cardiac surgery has been reviewed (231). When an intravenous loading dose of amiodarone was used, bradycardia was a common adverse effect but was rarely severe enough to warrant withdrawal. When only oral amiodarone was used there were no serious adverse reactions.

Drug Administration

Drug formulations

The steady-state plasma concentrations of amiodarone and desethylamiodarone in 77 patients taking two different formulations, a new generic formulation and Cordarone, were comparable (232).

Drug administration route

In contrast to its effects during oral administration, the therapeutic and short-term unwanted effects of amiodarone during intravenous administration arise within minutes or hours (2). The reason for this is not clear; plasma concentrations after single oral and intravenous doses of 400 mg are very similar (2), but that does not rule out a pharmacokinetic explanation for the paradox. The possible role of the solvent used in the intravenous formulation, polysorbate (Tween) 80, has not been fully elucidated. Amiodarone certainly has different electrophysiological effects when it is given intravenously. For example, intravenous amiodarone prolongs the AH interval, while oral amiodarone prolongs atrial and ventricular refractory periods and the HV interval (233). Furthermore, the blocking effects of amiodarone on sodium and calcium channels and its beta-adrenoceptor blocking action occur earlier than its Class III action (234). An anecdotal report of torsade de pointes after both intravenous and oral administration of amiodarone on different occasions has underlined this difference.

- A 70-year-old woman with dilated cardiomyopathy, ventricular tachydysrhythmia, and a QT_c interval of 0.49 seconds was given intravenous amiodarone 240 mg over 15 minutes, and 30 minutes later developed a junctional escape rhythm (48/minute) with QT_c prolongation to 0.68 seconds; 8 hours later she developed torsade de pointes (235). A few years later she was given oral amiodarone 100 mg/day and 7 weeks later presented with congestive heart failure. Her QT_c interval was prolonged (0.50 seconds) and increased further to 0.64 seconds after the addition of dopamine 3 micrograms/kg/minute; torsade de pointes again developed. Amiodarone was withdrawn and the QT_c interval shortened, but she continued to have recurrent episodes of sustained ventricular tachycardia.

The authors suggested that torsade de pointes induced by intravenous amiodarone depended on heart rate during a bout of bradycardia, while that after oral amiodarone depended on increased sympathetic nervous system activity, and that therefore different electrophysiological mechanisms had been at play. However, it is by no means clear from their description of this case that that was so. They did not report plasma concentrations of amiodarone or desethylamiodarone, its active metabolite.

After rapid intravenous administration hypotension, shock, and atrioventricular block can occur and can be fatal (2). The rate of infusion should not exceed 5 mg/minute. Other adverse effects reported during intravenous infusion include sinus bradycardia (236), facial flushing, and thrombophlebitis (236–239). The risk of this last complication can be reduced by infusing the drug into as large a vein as possible and preferably via a central venous catheter, or perhaps by using a very dilute solution of the drug (240).

The use of intravenous amiodarone for atrial fibrillation has been reviewed (241). The most commonly reported adverse effects in all studies have been hypotension and bradycardia. Other effects include worsening of heart failure, thrombophlebitis at the site of infusion, non-sustained ventricular tachycardia, facial rash, and nightmares.

A few studies have also reported the effects and adverse effects of intravenous amiodarone in patients with atrial fibrillation. Of 67 patients with atrial fibrillation, of whom 33 received amiodarone and 34 received placebo, conversion to sinus rhythm occurred in 16 of the patients who received amiodarone and in none of those who received placebo (242). In five patients the systolic blood pressure fell significantly during the first trial of intravenous drug administration. There were no cardiac dysrhythmias. Thrombophlebitis occurred in 12 patients who received amiodarone.

In a randomized, placebo-controlled trial of 100 patients with paroxysmal atrial fibrillation, intravenous amiodarone 125 mg/hour was compared with placebo (243). There were no serious adverse effects; five patients given amiodarone developed significant sinus bradycardia, in all cases after conversion to sinus rhythm. In this series there were no significant episodes of hypotension. Thrombophlebitis occurred in eight patients who received amiodarone.

Drug overdose

The features of amiodarone overdose and its management have been reviewed (244).

- There has been a report of acute self-poisoning with 8 g of amiodarone orally (245). Initially the only abnormal physical sign was profuse sweating; the electrocardiogram showed sinus rhythm with a normal QT_c interval and the blood pressure was normal. No active measures were taken. The QT_c interval subsequently lengthened on the third and fourth days after overdosage, and there was sinus bradycardia between the second and fifth days. Over 3 months of follow-up there were no effects on thyroid or liver function and no evidence of lung, skin, or corneal involvement.

Drug–Drug Interactions

Anesthetics

The risks of cardiovascular adverse effects in patients undergoing surgery may be partly related to an interaction of amiodarone with anesthetics, either directly or via some interaction with the catecholamines that are released during anesthesia (246). The risk of hypotension during cardiopulmonary bypass in patients taking amiodarone can be increased by the concurrent administration of an ACE inhibitor. There is a high incidence of lung complications when patients treated with amiodarone are ventilated with 100% oxygen, including acute adult respiratory distress syndrome.

Beta-blockers

The combination of amiodarone with beta-adrenoceptor antagonists can be beneficial in the treatment of refractory ventricular tachycardia, especially when low doses of the beta-blockers are used. However, there have also been reports of adverse interactions in these circumstances, and various correspondents have commented on the possibility that beta-blockers may enhance the effects of amiodarone in reducing mortality in patients who have

had a myocardial infarction or are in heart failure (190,247,248).

In a systematic review, the beneficial interaction has been confirmed (249). Four groups of patients who had been studied in EMIAT and CAMIAT (SEDA-21, 198) were defined: patients who had taken amiodarone plus beta-blockers, patients who had taken beta-blockers or amiodarone alone, and patients who had taken neither. The relative risks for all-cause mortality and all forms of cardiac death or resuscitated cardiac arrest were lower in the patients who had taken amiodarone plus beta-blockers than in the other three groups. The results of this post hoc analysis should be regarded with caution, but in view of previous similar reports they are suggestive of a beneficial interaction of amiodarone with beta-blockers in patients who have had a previous myocardial infarction. The interaction was statistically significant for cardiac deaths and for dysrhythmic deaths or resuscitated cardiac arrest. In all other cases the relative risk was reduced, although not significantly. The risk was not affected by heart rate. This interaction has been reviewed (250).

Budesonide

The corticosteroid budesonide undergoes a high degree of first-pass elimination in the liver after oral administration, and therefore causes few systemic adverse effects. It was therefore surprising that Cushing's syndrome occurred in an 81-year-old man taking oral budesonide 9 mg/day and amiodarone 100 mg/day (251). When amiodarone was withdrawn the clinical effects of Cushing's syndrome disappeared. The authors suggested that amiodarone had inhibited the metabolism of budesonide by hepatic CYP3A.

Ciclosporin

Amiodarone can increase the blood concentrations of ciclosporin and thus impair renal function.

- A 66-year-old developed a ventricular tachycardia after kidney transplantation and was given amiodarone. Maintenance immunosuppression included prednisone, azathioprine, and ciclosporin. Ciclosporin concentrations before amiodarone initiation were stable (range 100–150 ng/ml). During amiodarone therapy, the ciclosporin concentration increased more than two-fold.

The authors proposed that changes in protein binding or metabolism might have explained this interaction.

Class I antidysrhythmic drugs

Amiodarone can potentiate the dysrhythmogenic actions of some Class I antidysrhythmic drugs (SEDA-18, 203), particularly because of the risk of QT interval prolongation (SEDA-19, 194). In 26 patients taking mexiletine plus amiodarone for 1 month and 155 taking mexiletine alone, there was no significant difference in the apparent oral clearance of mexiletine (252). However, the lack of a pharmacokinetic interaction does not reduce the risk that dangerous QT interval prolongation may occur with a combination such as this.

Cyclophosphamide

Both amiodarone and cyclophosphamide can cause lung damage.

- Interstitial pneumonitis has been reported in a 59-year-old man, who had taken amiodarone for 18 months, 18 days after a single dose of cyclophosphamide; 1 year before he had also received six cycles of chemotherapy containing cyclophosphamide, vincristine, and prednisone, followed by four cycles of cisplatin, cytarabine, and dexamethasone (253).

The authors suggested that the lung damage had been due to the cyclophosphamide, enhanced by the presence of amiodarone, but in view of the fact that previous similar exposure on six occasions had not resulted in the same effect, it is perhaps more likely that this was a long-term adverse effect of amiodarone alone. The presence of foamy histiocytes in the lung biopsy was consistent with this interpretation (SEDA-15, 168). It is true, however, that lung damage due to amiodarone is usually of a more insidious onset than was reported in this case, although a more rapid onset can occur in patients who are given high concentrations of inspired oxygen. On the other hand, lung damage has occasionally been reported to occur rapidly (71).

Digoxin

Amiodarone reduces both the renal and non-renal clearances of digoxin and prolongs its half-life, without changing its apparent volume of distribution. It has also been suggested that amiodarone increases the extent of absorption of digoxin (SEDA-10, 144) (SEDA-12, 150). Digoxin dosages should be halved as soon as amiodarone is introduced. This interaction may also occur with acetyldigitoxin (254).

Diltiazem

Sinus arrest with hypotension has been reported in a patient with a congestive cardiomyopathy when diltiazem was added to amiodarone (255).

Indinavir

Indinavir inhibits CYP3A4, which is responsible for the de-ethylation of amiodarone to desethylamiodarone.

- A 38-year-old man, who had taken amiodarone 200 mg/day for more than 6 months, was given postexposure prophylaxis for HIV infection after a needle injury; this included zidovudine, lamivudine, and indinavir (256). During the 4 weeks of therapy his serum amiodarone concentration rose from 0.9 to 1.3 mg/l, with only a small rise in the serum concentration of desethylamiodarone from 0.4 to 0.5 mg/l. After withdrawal of the prophylactic therapy the plasma amiodarone concentration gradually fell to the pretreatment value, and there was no further change in the concentration of desethylamiodarone.

No adverse effects of this interaction were reported.

Meglumine antimoniate

A pharmacodynamic interaction has been described between amiodarone and meglumine antimoniate, both of which prolong the QT interval; the interaction resulted in torsade de pointes (257).

- A 73-year-old man with visceral leishmaniasis was given meglumine antimoniate intramuscularly 75 mg/kg/day. At that time his QT_c interval was normal at 0.42 seconds. Three weeks later his QT_c interval was prolonged to 0.64 seconds and he was given methyldigoxin 0.4 mg and amiodarone 450 mg intravenously over 8.25 hours; 12 hours later he had a cardiac arrest with torsade de pointes, which was cardioverted by two direct shocks of 300 J and lidocaine 100 mg in two bolus injections. Because he had frequent episodes of paroxysmal atrial fibrillation, he was given amiodarone 100 mg over the next 40 hours, and developed recurrent self-limiting episodes of torsade de pointes associated with QT_c interval prolongation, which responded to intravenous magnesium 1500 mg. After withdrawal of amiodarone there was no recurrence and a week later the QT_c interval was 0.48 seconds. The plasma potassium concentration was not abnormal in this case.

In view of this report it is probably wise to avoid co-administration of these two drugs.

Phenazone (antipyrine)

The clearance of phenazone (antipyrine) is reduced by amiodarone (258).

Phenytoin

Amiodarone increases the plasma concentrations of phenytoin, probably by inhibiting its metabolism (259,260), while phenytoin increases the metabolism of amiodarone and perhaps also of its metabolite desethylamiodarone (261).

Rifampicin

- In a 33-year-old woman taking amiodarone 400 mg/day the addition of rifampicin 600 mg/day resulted in paroxysms of atrial fibrillation and atrial flutter, with a very low serum amiodarone concentration and an undetectable concentration of desethylamiodarone (262). This was attributed to induction of the metabolism of amiodarone and desethylamiodarone, and after withdrawal of rifampicin the concentrations of the two compounds rose to within the target ranges.

This interaction has been demonstrated in human liver microsomes (263).

Warfarin

That amiodarone can potentiate the action of warfarin by inhibiting its metabolism is well known (SEDA-11, 156). However, potentiation of the action of warfarin has been attributed to amiodarone-induced thyrotoxicosis (264). A metabolic interaction in this case was unlikely, because the patient had taken both drugs together for 2 years before the increase in response to warfarin, coincident with the emergence of thyrotoxicosis.

In a study of this interaction in 43 patients who took both amiodarone and warfarin for at least 1 year, the interaction peaked at 7 weeks and the mean dosage of warfarin fell by 44% from 5.2 to 2.9 mg/day (265). The dosage of warfarin correlated inversely with the maintenance dose of amiodarone. There were minor bleeding episodes in five patients. The authors recommended reducing the daily warfarin dose by about 25, 30, 35, and 40% in patients taking amiodarone 100, 200, 300, and 400 mg/day respectively.

Interference with Diagnostic Tests

Serum creatinine

Amiodarone has been reported to cause a small and reversible increase in serum creatinine concentration (266). It is not clear whether this effect is due to true renal impairment, or to some effect on either the kinetics of creatinine or its measurement in the blood.

Thyroid function tests

Amiodarone causes altered thyroid function tests, with rises in serum concentrations of T4 and reverse T3 and a fall in serum T3 concentration (267). This is due to inhibition of the peripheral conversion of T4 to T3, causing preferential conversion to reverse T3. These changes can occur in the absence of symptomatic abnormalities of thyroid function.

Blood urea nitrogen

Amiodarone has also been reported to cause a small and reversible increase in blood urea nitrogen concentration (266). It is not clear whether this effect is due to true renal impairment, or to some effect on either the kinetics of urea or its measurement in the blood.

Diagnosis of Adverse Drug Reactions

The differences in the rates of onset of effects of amiodarone after oral and intravenous administration in the face of similar plasma concentrations suggest that there can be no simple relation between the plasma concentrations of amiodarone and its therapeutic effects. Matters are further complicated by metabolism of amiodarone to desethylamiodarone, which has pharmacological activity. However, evidence (2,268) suggests that a plasma amiodarone concentration of around 1.0–2.5 mg/ml is associated with a high likelihood of therapeutic efficacy in patients with dysrhythmias. However, adverse effects can still occur when the plasma concentration is within this range, and there is no clear limit to the concentration above which toxicity starts to become important. Similarly, the therapeutic range of concentrations for desethylamiodarone is unclear, although it has been suggested to be around 0.5–1.0 mg/ml (SEDA-10, 146).

In one careful study EC_{50} values for certain effects of amiodarone were calculated (269). The respective concentrations of amiodarone and desethylamiodarone that were associated with effects were as follows: reduction in heart rate 1.2 and 0.5 mg/ml; QT_c prolongation 2.6 and 1.4 mg/ml; corneal microdeposits 2.2 and 1.1 mg/ml.

Because amiodarone prolongs the QT_c interval, it has been suggested that this might be a useful measure of its efficacy. The percentage prolongation of the QT_c interval correlates well with both daily dose and the plasma and myocardial concentrations of amiodarone (270), although this is not a universal finding during long-term

administration (237,271), and the QT_c interval is not prolonged after short-term intravenous use (2).

Since amiodarone inhibits the peripheral conversion of thyroxine (T4) to tri-iodothyronine (T3), there is an increase in serum concentrations of reverse tri-iodothyronine (rT3). However, there have been conflicting results in studies of the relation between serum concentrations of rT3 and the therapeutic and adverse effects of amiodarone (SEDA-15, 172).

References

1. Rosenbaum MB, Chiale PA, Halpern MS, Nau GJ, Przybylski J, Levi RJ, Lazzari JO, Elizari MV. Clinical efficacy of amiodarone as an antiarrhythmic agent. Am J Cardiol 1976;38(7):934–44.
2. McGovern B, Garan H, Ruskin JN. Serious adverse effects of amiodarone. Clin Cardiol 1984;7(3):131–7.
3. Latini R, Tognoni G, Kates RE. Clinical pharmacokinetics of amiodarone. Clin Pharmacokinet 1984;9(2):136–56.
4. Heger JJ, Prystowsky EN, Miles WM, Zipes DP. Clinical use and pharmacology of amiodarone. Med Clin North Am 1984;68(5):1339–66.
5. Cetnarowski AB, Rihn TL. A review of adverse reactions to amiodarone. Cardiovasc Rev Rep 1985;6:1206–22.
6. Kadish A, Morady F. The use of intravenous amiodarone in the acute therapy of life-threatening tachyarrhythmias. Prog Cardiovasc Dis 1989;31(4):281–94.
7. Kopelman HA, Horowitz LN. Efficacy and toxicity of amiodarone for the treatment of supraventricular tachyarrhythmias. Prog Cardiovasc Dis 1989;31(5):355–66.
8. Heger JJ. Monitoring and treating side effects of amiodarone therapy. Cardiovasc Rev Rep 1988;9:47.
9. Kerin NZ, Aragon E, Faitel K, Frumin H, Rubenfire M. Long-term efficacy and toxicity of high- and low-dose amiodarone regimens. J Clin Pharmacol 1989;29(5):418–23.
10. Somani P. Basic and clinical pharmacology of amiodarone: relationship of antiarrhythmic effects, dose and drug concentrations to intracellular inclusion bodies. J Clin Pharmacol 1989;29(5):405–12.
11. Vorperian VR, Havighurst TC, Miller S, January CT. Adverse effects of low dose amiodarone: a meta-analysis. J Am Coll Cardiol 1997;30(3):791–8.
12. Marcus FI. Drug combinations and interactions with class III agents. J Cardiovasc Pharmacol 1992;20(Suppl 2):S70–4.
13. Tsikouris JP, Cox CD. A review of class III antiarrhythmic agents for atrial fibrillation: maintenance of normal sinus rhythm. Pharmacotherapy 2001;21(12):1514–29.
14. Trappe HJ. Amiodarone. Intensivmed Notf Med 2001;38:169–78.
15. Kuck KH, Cappato R, Siebels J, Ruppel R. Randomized comparison of antiarrhythmic drug therapy with implantable defibrillators in patients resuscitated from cardiac arrest: the Cardiac Arrest Study Hamburg (CASH). Circulation 2000;102(7):748–54.
16. Nagele H, Bohlmann M, Eck U, Petersen B, Rodiger W. Combination therapy with carvedilol and amiodarone in patients with severe heart failure. Eur J Heart Fail 2000;2(1):71–9.
17. Connolly SJ. Meta-analysis of antiarrhythmic drug trials. Am J Cardiol 1999;84(9A):R90–3.
18. Levy S. Amiodarone in atrial fibrillation. Int J Clin Pract 1998;52(6):429–31.
19. Kochiadakis GE, Igoumenidis NE, Marketou ME, Kaleboubas MD, Simantirakis EN, Vardas PE. Low dose amiodarone and sotalol in the treatment of recurrent, symptomatic atrial fibrillation: a comparative, placebo controlled study. Heart 2000;84(3):251–7.

20. Vardas PE, Kochiadakis GE, Igoumenidis NE, Tsatsakis AM, Simantirakis EN, Chlouverakis GI. Amiodarone as a first-choice drug for restoring sinus rhythm in patients with atrial fibrillation: a randomized, controlled study. Chest 2000;117(6):1538–45.

21. Hofmann R, Wimmer G, Leisch F. Intravenous amiodarone bolus immediately controls heart rate in patients with atrial fibrillation accompanied by severe congestive heart failure. Heart 2000;84(6):635.

22. Peuhkurinen K, Niemela M, Ylitalo A, Linnaluoto M, Lilja M, Juvonen J. Effectiveness of amiodarone as a single oral dose for recent-onset atrial fibrillation. Am J Cardiol 2000;85(4):462–5.

23. Martinez-Marcos FJ, Garcia-Garmendia JL, Ortega-Carpio A, Fernandez-Gomez JM, Santos JM, Camacho C. Comparison of intravenous flecainide, propafenone, and amiodarone for conversion of acute atrial fibrillation to sinus rhythm. Am J Cardiol 2000;86(9):950–3.

24. Treggiari-Venzi MM, Waeber JL, Perneger TV, Suter PM, Adamec R, Romand JA. Intravenous amiodarone or magnesium sulphate is not cost-beneficial prophylaxis for atrial fibrillation after coronary artery bypass surgery. Br J Anaesth 2000;85(5):690–5.

25. Roy D, Talajic M, Dorian P, Connolly S, Eisenberg MJ, Green M, Kus T, Lambert J, Dubuc M, Gagne P, Nattel S, Thibault B. Amiodarone to prevent recurrence of atrial fibrillation. Canadian Trial of Atrial Fibrillation Investigators. N Engl J Med 2000;342(13):913–20.

26. Kochiadakis GE, Marketou ME, Igoumenidis NE, Chrysostomakis SI, Mavrakis HE, Kaleboubas MD, Vardas PE. Amiodarone, sotalol, or propafenone in atrial fibrillation: which is preferred to maintain normal sinus rhythm? Pacing Clin Electrophysiol 2000;23(11 Pt 2):1883–7.

27. Wurdeman RL, Mooss AN, Mohiuddin SM, Lenz TL. Amiodarone vs. sotalol as prophylaxis against atrial fibrillation/flutter after heart surgery: a meta-analysis. Chest 2002;121(4):1203–10.

28. Hilleman DE, Spinler SA. Conversion of recent-onset atrial fibrillation with intravenous amiodarone: a meta-analysis of randomized controlled trials. Pharmacotherapy 2002;22(1):66–74.

29. Kapoor A, Kumar S, Singh RK, Pandey CM, Sinha N. Management of persistent atrial fibrillation following balloon mitral valvotomy: safety and efficacy of low-dose amiodarone. J Heart Valve Dis 2002;11(6):802–9.

30. Kosior D, Karpinski G, Wretowski D, Stolarz P, Stawicki S, Rabczenko D, Torbicki A, Opolski G. Sequential prophylactic antiarrhythmic therapy for maintenance of sinus rhythm after cardioversion of persistent atrial fibrillation—one year follow-up. Kardiol Pol 2002;56:361–7.

31. Blanc JJ, Voinov C, Maarek M. Comparison of oral loading dose of propafenone and amiodarone for converting recent-onset atrial fibrillation. PARSIFAL Study Group. Am J Cardiol 1999;84(9):1029–32.

32. Natale A, Newby KH, Pisano E, Leonelli F, Fanelli R, Potenza D, Beheiry S, Tomassoni G. Prospective randomized comparison of antiarrhythmic therapy versus first-line radiofrequency ablation in patients with atrial flutter. J Am Coll Cardiol 2000;35(7):1898–904.

33. Maury P, Zimmermann M, Metzger J, Reynard C, Dorsaz P, Adamec R. Amiodarone therapy for sustained ventricular tachycardia after myocardial infarction: long-term follow-up, risk assessment and predictive value of programmed ventricular stimulation. Int J Cardiol 2000;76(2–3):199–210.

34. Kovoor P, Eipper V, Byth K, Cooper MJ, Uther JB, Ross DL. Comparison of sotalol with amiodarone for long-term treatment of spontaneous sustained ventricular tachyarrhythmia based on coronary artery disease. Eur Heart J 1999;20(5):364–74.

35. Cairns JA. Antiarrhythmic therapy in the post-infarction setting: update from major amiodarone studies. Int J Clin Pract 1998;52(6):422–4.

36. Piepoli M, Villani GQ, Ponikowski P, Wright A, Flather MD, Coats AJ. Overview and meta-analysis of randomised trials of amiodarone in chronic heart failure. Int J Cardiol 1998;66(1):1–10.

37. Pfisterer ME, Kiowski W, Brunner H, Burckhardt D, Burkart F. Long-term benefit of 1-year amiodarone treatment for persistent complex ventricular arrhythmias after myocardial infarction. Circulation 1993;87(2):309–11.

38. Ceremuzynski L, Kleczar E, Krzeminska-Pakula M, Kuch J, Nartowicz E, Smielak-Korombel J, Dyduszynski A, Maciejewicz J, Zaleska T, Lazarczyk-Kedzia E, et al. Effect of amiodarone on mortality after myocardial infarction: a double-blind, placebo-controlled, pilot study. J Am Coll Cardiol 1992;20(5):1056–62.

39. Navarro-Lopez F, Cosin J, Marrugat J, Guindo J, Bayes de Luna A. Comparison of the effects of amiodarone versus metoprolol on the frequency of ventricular arrhythmias and on mortality after acute myocardial infarction. SSSD Investigators. Spanish Study on Sudden Death. Am J Cardiol 1993;72(17):1243–8.

40. Julian DG, Camm AJ, Frangin G, Janse MJ, Munoz A, Schwartz PJ, Simon P. Randomised trial of effect of amiodarone on mortality in patients with left-ventricular dysfunction after recent myocardial infarction: EMIAT. European Myocardial Infarct Amiodarone Trial Investigators. Lancet 1997;349(9053):667–74.

41. Cairns JA, Connolly SJ, Roberts R, Gent M. Randomised trial of outcome after myocardial infarction in patients with frequent or repetitive ventricular premature depolarisations: CAMIAT. Canadian Amiodarone Myocardial Infarction Arrhythmia Trial Investigators. Lancet 1997;349(9053):675–82.

42. Kerin NZ, Blevins RD, Kerner N, Faitel K, Frumin H, Maciejko JJ, Rubenfire M. A low incidence of proarrhythmia using low-dose amiodarone. J Electrophysiol 1988;2:289–95.

43. Hohnloser SH. Proarrhythmia with class III antiarrhythmic drugs: types, risks, and management. Am J Cardiol 1997;80(8A):G82–9.

44. Crocco F, Severino M, Scrivano P, Calcaterra R, Cristiano G. Cardiogenic shock in a case of amiodarone intoxication. Gazz Med Ital Arch Sci Med 1999;158:159–63.

45. Krikler DM, McKenna WJ, Chamberlain DA, editors. Amiodarone and Arrhythmias. Oxford: Pergamon Press, 1983.

46. Hilleman DE, Larsen KE. Proarrhythmic effects of antiarrhythmic drugs. PT 1991;June:520–4.

47. Tomcsanyi J, Merkely B, Tenczer J, Papp L, Karlocai K. Early proarrhythmia during intravenous amiodarone treatment. Pacing Clin Electrophysiol 1999;22(6 Pt 1):968–70.

48. Yap SC, Hoomtje T, Sreeram N. Polymorphic ventricular tachycardia after use of intravenous amiodarone for postoperative junctional ectopic tachycardia. Int J Cardiol 2000;76(2–3):245–7.

49. Nkomo VT, Shen WK. Amiodarone-induced long QT and polymorphic ventricular tachycardia. Am J Emerg Med 2001;19(3):246–8.

50. Shimoshige S, Uno K, Miyamoto K, Nakahara N, Wakabayashi T, Tsuchihashi K, Shimamoto K, Murakami H. Amiodarone modulates thresholds of induction and/or termination of ventricular tachycardia and ventricular fibrillation—a case of VT with previous myocardial infarction. Ther Res 2001;22:861–6.

51. Psirropoulos D, Lefkos N, Boudonas G, Efthimiadis A, Eklissiarhos D, Tsapas G. Incidence of and predicting factors for torsades de pointes during intravenous administration of amiodarone. Heart Drug 2001;1:186–91.

52. Makkar RR, Fromm BS, Steinman RT, Meissner MD, Lehmann MH. Female gender as a risk factor for torsades de pointes associated with cardiovascular drugs. JAMA 1993;270(21):2590–7.

53. Benton RE, Sale M, Flockhart DA, Woosley RL. Greater quinidine-induced QTc interval prolongation in women. Clin Pharmacol Ther 2000;67(4):413–18.

54. Tomcsanyi J, Somloi M, Horvath L. Amiodarone-induced giant T wave alternans hastens proarrhythmic response. J Cardiovasc Electrophysiol 2002;13(6):629.

55. Matsuyama T, Tanno K, Kobayashi Y, Obara C, Ryu S, Adachi T, Ezumi H, Asano T, Miyata A, Koba S, Baba T, Katagiri T. T wave alternans for predicting adverse effects of amiodarone in a patient with dilated cardiomyopathy. Jpn Circ J 2001;65(5):468–70.

56. Reithmann C, Hoffmann E, Spitzlberger G, Dorwarth U, Gerth A, Remp T, Steinbeck G. Catheter ablation of atrial flutter due to amiodarone therapy for paroxysmal atrial fibrillation. Eur Heart J 2000;21(7):565–72.

57. Aouate P, Elbaz N, Klug D, Lacotte J, Raguin D, Frank R, Lelouche D, Dubois-Rande JL, Tonet J, Fontaine G. Flutter atrial à conduction nodo-ventricular 1/1 sous amiodarone. De la physiopathologie au dépistage. [Atrial flutter with 1/1 nodo-ventricular conduction with amiodarone. From physiopathology to diagnosis.] Arch Mal Coeur Vaiss 2002;95(12):1181–7.

58. Tai CT, Chiang CE, Lee SH, Chen YJ, Yu WC, Feng AN, Ding YA, Chang MS, Chen SA. Persistent atrial flutter in patients treated for atrial fibrillation with amiodarone and propafenone: electrophysiologic characteristics, radiofrequency catheter ablation, and risk prediction. J Cardiovasc Electrophysiol 1999; 10(9):1180–7.

59. Hammerman H, Kapeliovich M. Drug-related cardiac iatrogenic illness as the cause for admission to the intensive cardiac care unit. Isr Med Assoc J 2000;2(8):577–9.

60. Ravina T, Gutierrez J. Amiodarone-induced AV block and ventricular standstill. A forme fruste of an idiopathic long QT syndrome. Int J Cardiol 2000;75(1):105–8.

61. Dunn M, Glassroth J. Pulmonary complications of amiodarone toxicity. Prog Cardiovasc Dis 1989;31(6):447–53.

62. Kennedy JI Jr. Clinical aspects of amiodarone pulmonary toxicity. Clin Chest Med 1990;11(1):119–29.

63. Martin WJ 2nd. Mechanisms of amiodarone pulmonary toxicity. Clin Chest Med 1990;11(1):131–8.

64. Dusman RE, Stanton MS, Miles WM, Klein LS, Zipes DP, Fineberg NS, Heger JJ. Clinical features of amiodarone-induced pulmonary toxicity. Circulation 1990;82(1):51–9.

65. Drent M, Cobben NA, Van Dieijen-Visser MP, Braat SH, Wouters EF. Serum lactate dehydrogenase activity: indicator of the development of pneumonitis induced by amiodarone. Eur Heart J 1998;19(6):969–70.

66. Gonzalez-Rothi RJ, Hannan SE, Hood CI, Franzini DA. Amiodarone pulmonary toxicity presenting as bilateral exudative pleural effusions. Chest 1987;92(1):179–82.

67. Carmichael LC, Newman JH. Lymphocytic pleural exudate in a patient receiving amiodarone. Br J Clin Pract 1996;50(4):228–30.

68. Valle JM, Alvarez D, Antunez J, Valdes L. Bronchiolitis obliterans organizing pneumonia secondary to amiodarone: a rare aetiology. Eur Respir J 1995;8(3):470–1.

69. Kudenchuk PJ, Pierson DJ, Greene HL, Graham EL, Sears GK, Trobaugh GB. Prospective evaluation of amiodarone pulmonary toxicity. Chest 1984;86(4):541–8.

70. Donica SK, Paulsen AW, Simpson BR, Ramsay MA, Saunders CT, Swygert TH, Tappe J. Danger of amiodarone therapy and elevated inspired oxygen concentrations in mice. Am J Cardiol 1996;77(1):109–10.

71. Liverani E, Armuzzi A, Mormile F, Anti M, Gasbarrini G, Gentiloni N. Amiodarone-induced adult respiratory distress syndrome after nonthoracotomy subcutaneous defibrillator implantation. J Intern Med 2001;249(6):565–6.

72. Kaushik S, Hussain A, Clarke P, Lazar HL. Acute pulmonary toxicity after low-dose amiodarone therapy. Ann Thorac Surg 2001;72(5):1760–1.

73. Alter P, Grimm W, Maisch B. Amiodaron-induzierte Pneumonitis bei dilatativer Kardiomyopathie. [Amiodarone induced pulmonary toxicity.] Pneumologie 2002;56(1):31–5.

74. Kanji Z, Sunderji R, Gin K. Amiodarone-induced pulmonary toxicity. Pharmacotherapy 1999;19(12):1463–6.

75. Cockcroft DW, Fisher KL. Near normalization of spirometry in a subject with severe emphysema complicated by amiodarone lung. Respir Med 1999;93(8):597–600.

76. Kagawa FT, Kirsch CM, Jensen WA, Wehner JH. A 77-year-old man with bilateral pulmonary infiltrates and shortness of breath. Semin Respir Infect 2000;15(1):90–2.

77. Burns KE, Piliotis E, Garcia BM, Ferguson KA. Amiodarone pulmonary, neuromuscular and ophthalmological toxicity. Can Respir J 2000;7(2):193–7.

78. Scharf C, Oechslin EN, Salomon F, Kiowski W. Clinical picture: Amiodarone-induced pulmonary mass and cutaneous vasculitis. Lancet 2001;358(9298):2045.

79. Rodriguez-Garcia JL, Garcia-Nieto JC, Ballesta F, Prieto E, Villanueva MA, Gallardo J. Pulmonary mass and multiple lung nodules mimicking a lung neoplasm as amiodarone-induced pulmonary toxicity. Eur J Intern Med 2001;12(4):372–6.

80. Endoh Y, Hanai R, Uto K, Uno M, Nagashima H, Takizawa T, Narimatsu A, Ohnishi S, Kasanuki H. [Diagnostic usefulness of KL-6 measurements in patients with pulmonary complications after administration of amiodarone.] J Cardiol 2000;35(2):121–7.

81. Endoh Y, Hanai R, Uto K, Uno M, Nagashima H, Narimatsu A, Takizawa T, Onishi S, Kasanuki H. KL-6 as a potential new marker for amiodarone-induced pulmonary toxicity. Am J Cardiol 2000;86(2):229–31.

82. Esato M, Sakurada H, Okazaki H, Kimura T, Nomizo A, Endou M, Tamura T, Hiyoshi Y, Mishizaki M, Teshima T, Yanase O, Hiraoka M. Evaluation of pulmonary toxicity by CT, pulmonary function tests, and KL-6 measurements in amiodarone-treated patients. Ther Res 2001;22:867–73.

83. Nicholson AA, Hayward C. The value of computed tomography in the diagnosis of amiodarone-induced pulmonary toxicity. Clin Radiol 1989;40(6):564–7.

84. Siniakowicz RM, Narula D, Suster B, Steinberg JS. Diagnosis of amiodarone pulmonary toxicity with high-resolution computerized tomographic scan. J Cardiovasc Electrophysiol 2001;12(4):431–6.

85. Lim KK, Radford DJ. Amiodarone pneumonitis diagnosed by gallium-67 scintigraphy. Heart Lung Circ 2002;11:59–62.

86. Dirlik A, Erinc R, Ozcan Z, Atasever A, Bacakoglu F, Nalbantgil S, Ozhan M, Burak Z. Technetium-99m-DTPA aerosol scintigraphy in amiodarone induced pulmonary toxicity in comparison with Ga-67 scintigraphy. Ann Nucl Med 2002;16(7):477–81.

87. Biour M, Hugues FC, Hamel JD, Cheymol G. Les effets indésirables pulmonaires de l'amiodarone: analyse de 162 observations. [Adverse pulmonary effects of amiodarone. Analysis of 162 cases.] Therapie 1985;40(5):343–8.

88. Palakurthy PR, Iyer V, Meckler RJ. Unusual neurotoxicity associated with amiodarone therapy. Arch Intern Med 1987;147(5):881–4.

89. Trohman RG, Castellanos D, Castellanos A, Kessler KM. Amiodarone-induced delirium. Ann Intern Med 1988;108(1):68–9.

90. Werner EG, Olanow CW. Parkinsonism and amiodarone therapy. Ann Neurol 1989;25(6):630–2.

91. Borruat FX, Regli F. Pseudotumor cerebri as a complication of amiodarone therapy. Am J Ophthalmol 1993;116(6):776–7.

92. Itoh K, Kato R, Hotta N. A case report of myolysis during high-dose amiodarone therapy for uncontrolled ventricular tachycardia. Jpn Circ J 1998;62(4):305–8.

93. Jacobs JM, Costa-Jussa FR. The pathology of amiodarone neurotoxicity. II. Peripheral neuropathy in man. Brain 1985;108(Pt 3):753–69.

94. Onofrj M, Thomas A. Acetazolamide-responsive periodic ataxia induced by amiodarone. Mov Disord 1999;14(2):379–81.

95. Pulipaka U, Lacomis D, Omalu B. Amiodarone-induced neuromyopathy: three cases and a review of the literature. J Clin Neuromuscular Dis 2002;3:97–105.

96. Biran I, Steiner I. Coital headaches induced by amiodarone. Neurology 2002;58(3):501–2.

97. Mantyjarvi M, Tuppurainen K, Ikaheimo K. Ocular side effects of amiodarone. Surv Ophthalmol 1998;42(4):360–6.

98. Duff GR, Fraser AG. Impairment of colour vision associated with amiodarone keratopathy. Acta Ophthalmol (Copenh) 1987;65(1):48–52.

99. Ingram DV, Jaggarao NS, Chamberlain DA. Ocular changes resulting from therapy with amiodarone. Br J Ophthalmol 1982;66(10):676–9.

100. Ingram DV. Ocular effects in long-term amiodarone therapy. Am Heart J 1983;106(4 Pt 2):902–5.

101. Ikaheimo K, Kettunen R, Mantyjarvi M. Visual functions and adverse ocular effects in patients with amiodarone medication. Acta Ophthalmol Scand 2002;80(1):59–63.

102. Astin CLK. Amiodarone keratopathy and rigid contact lens wear. Contact Lens Anterior Eye 2001;24:80–2.

103. Ciancaglini M, Carpineto P, Zuppardi E, Nubile M, Doronzo E, Mastropasqua L. In vivo confocal microscopy of patients with amiodarone-induced keratopathy. Cornea 2001;20(4):368–73.

104. Feiner LA, Younge BR, Kazmier FJ, Stricker BH, Fraunfelder FT. Optic neuropathy and amiodarone therapy. Mayo Clin Proc 1987;62(8):702–17.

105. Mansour AM, Puklin JE, O'Grady R. Optic nerve ultrastructure following amiodarone therapy. J Clin Neuroophthalmol 1988;8(4):231–7.

106. Dewachter A, Lievens H. Amiodarone and optic neuropathy. Bull Soc Belge Ophtalmol 1988;227:47–50.

107. Garret SN, Kearney JJ, Schiffman JS. Amiodarone optic neuropathy. J Clin Neuro-ophthalmol 1988;8:105.

108. Mindel JM. Amiodarone and optic neuropathy—a medicolegal issue. Surv Ophthalmol 1998;42(4):358–9.

109. Macaluso DC, Shults WT, Fraunfelder FT. Features of amiodarone-induced optic neuropathy. Am J Ophthalmol 1999;127(5):610–12.

110. Eryilmaz T, Atilla H, Batioglu F, Gunalp I. Amiodarone-related optic neuropathy. Jpn J Ophthalmol 2000;44(5):565–8.

111. Speicher MA, Goldman MH, Chrousos GA. Amiodarone optic neuropathy without disc edema. J Neuroophthalmol 2000;20(3):171–2.

112. Fikkers BG, Bogousslavsky J, Regli F, Glasson S. Pseudotumor cerebri with amiodarone. J Neurol Neurosurg Psychiatry 1986;49(5):606.

113. Thystrup JD, Fledelius HC. Retinal maculopathy possibly associated with amiodarone medication. Acta Ophthalmol (Copenh) 1994;72(5):639–41.

114. Reifler DM, Verdier DD, Davy CL, Mostow ND, Wendt VE. Multiple chalazia and rosacea in a patient treated with amiodarone. Am J Ophthalmol 1987;103(4):594–5.

115. Dickinson EJ, Wolman RL. Sicca syndrome associated with amiodarone therapy. BMJ (Clin Res Ed) 1986;293:510.

116. Vrobel TR, Miller PE, Mostow ND, Rakita L. A general overview of amiodarone toxicity: its prevention, detection, and management. Prog Cardiovasc Dis 1989;31(6):393–426.

117. Greene HL, Graham EL, Werner JA, Sears GK, Gross BW, Gorham JP, Kudenchuk PJ, Trobaugh GB. Toxic and therapeutic effects of amiodarone in the treatment of cardiac arrhythmias. J Am Coll Cardiol 1983;2(6):1114–28.

118. Katai N, Yokoyama R, Yoshimura N. Progressive brown discoloration of silicone intraocular lenses after vitrectomy in a patient on amiodarone. J Cataract Refract Surg 1999;25(3):451–2.

119. Barry JJ, Franklin K. Amiodarone-induced delirium. Am J Psychiatry 1999;156(7):1119.

120. Ambrose A, Salib E. Amiodarone-induced depression. Br J Psychiatry 1999;174:366–7.

121. Dobs AS, Sarma PS, Guarnieri T, Griffith L. Testicular dysfunction with amiodarone use. J Am Coll Cardiol 1991;18(5):1328–32.

122. Odeh M, Schiff E, Oliven A. Hyponatremia during therapy with amiodarone. Arch Intern Med 1999;159(21):2599–600.

123. Ikegami H, Shiga T, Tsushima T, Nirei T, Kasanuki H. Syndrome of inappropriate antidiuretic hormone secretion (SIADH) induced by amiodarone: a report on two cases. J Cardiovasc Pharmacol Ther 2002;7(1):25–8.

124. Patel GP, Kasiar JB. Syndrome of inappropriate antidiuretic hormone-induced hyponatremia associated with amiodarone. Pharmacotherapy 2002;22(5):649–51.

125. Wolff J. Perchlorate and the thyroid gland. Pharmacol Rev 1998;50(1):89–105.

126. Wiersinga WM, Trip MD. Amiodarone and thyroid hormone metabolism. Postgrad Med J 1986;62(732):909–14.

127. Mason JW. Amiodarone. N Engl J Med 1987;316(8):455–66.

128. Tajiri J, Higashi K, Morita M, Umeda T, Sato T. Studies of hypothyroidism in patients with high iodine intake. J Clin Endocrinol Metab 1986;63(2):412–17.

129. Nademanee K, Piwonka RW, Singh BN, Hershman JM. Amiodarone and thyroid function. Prog Cardiovasc Dis 1989;31(6):427–37.

130. Newman CM, Price A, Davies DW, Gray TA, Weetman AP. Amiodarone and the thyroid: a practical guide to the management of thyroid dysfunction induced by amiodarone therapy. Heart 1998;79(2):121–7.

131. Rouleau F, Baudusseau O, Dupuis JM, Victor J, Geslin P. Incidence et delai d'apparition des dysthyroïdies sours traitement chronique par amiodarone. [Incidence and timing of thyroid dysfunction with long-term amiodarone therapy.] Arch Mal Coeur Vaiss 2001;94(1):39–43.

132. Bouvy ML, Heerdink ER, Hoes AW, Leufkens HG. Amiodarone-induced thyroid dysfunction associated with cumulative dose. Pharmacoepidemiol Drug Saf 2002;11(7):601–6.

133. Martino E, Safran M, Aghini-Lombardi F, Rajatanavin R, Lenziardi M, Fay M, Pacchiarotti A, Aronin N, Macchia E, Haffajee C, et al. Environmental iodine intake and thyroid dysfunction during chronic amiodarone therapy. Ann Intern Med 1984;101(1):28–34.

134. Bagheri H, Lapeyre-Mestre M, Levy C, Haramburu F, Hillaire-Buys D, Blayac JP, Montastruc JL. Dysthyroidism due to amiodarone: comparison of spontaneous reporting in Aquitaine, Midi–Pyrenees and Languedoc–Roussillon. [Inter-regional differences in dysthyroidism due to amiodarone: comparison of spontaneous notifications in Aquitaine, Midi–Pyrenees and Languedoc–Roussillon.] Therapie 2001;56(3):301–6.

135. Thorne SA, Barnes I, Cullinan P, Somerville J. Amiodarone-associated thyroid dysfunction: risk factors in adults with congenital heart disease. Circulation 1999;100(2):149–54.

136. Sidhu J, Jenkins D. Men are at increased risk of amiodarone-associated thyrotoxicosis in the UK. QJM 2003;96(12):949–50.

137. Mariotti S, Loviselli A, Murenu S, Sau F, Valentino L, Mandas A, Vacquer S, Martino E, Balestrieri A, Lai ME. High prevalence of thyroid dysfunction in adult patients with beta-thalassemia major submitted to amiodarone treatment. J Endocrinol Invest 1999;22(1):55–63.

138. Findlay PF, Seymour DG. Hyperthyroidism in an elderly patient. Postgrad Med J 2000;76(893):173–5.

139. Cattaneo F. Type II amiodarone-induced thyrotoxicosis and concomitant papillary cancer of the thyroid. Eur J Endocrinol 2000;143(6):823–4.

140. Claxton S, Sinha SN, Donovan S, Greenaway TM, Hoffman L, Loughhead M, Burgess JR. Refractory amiodarone-associated thyrotoxicosis: an indication for thyroidectomy. Aust NZ J Surg 2000;70(3):174–8.

141. Leung PM, Quinn ND, Belchetz PE. Amiodarone-induced thyrotoxicosis: not a benign condition. Int J Clin Pract 2002;56(1):44–6.

142. Martino E, Bartalena L, Mariotti S, Aghini-Lombardi F, Ceccarelli C, Lippi F, Piga M, Loviselli A, Braverman L, Safran M, et al. Radioactive iodine thyroid uptake in patients with amiodarone-iodine-induced thyroid dysfunction. Acta Endocrinol (Copenh) 1988;119(2):167–73.

143. Mancini A, De Marinis L, Calabro F, Sciuto R, Oradei A, Lippa S, Sandric S, Littarru GP, Barbarino A. Evaluation of metabolic status in amiodarone-induced thyroid disorders: plasma coenzyme Q10 determination. J Endocrinol Invest 1989;12(8):511–16.

144. Eaton SE, Euinton HA, Newman CM, Weetman AP, Bennet WM. Clinical experience of amiodarone-induced thyrotoxicosis over a 3-year period: role of colour-flow Doppler sonography. Clin Endocrinol (Oxf) 2002; 56(1):33–8.

145. Bogazzi F, Bartalena L, Brogioni S, Mazzeo S, Vitti P, Burelli A, Bartolozzi C, Martino E. Color flow Doppler sonography rapidly differentiates type I and type II amiodarone-induced thyrotoxicosis. Thyroid 1997;7(4):541–5.

146. Martino E, Aghini-Lombardi F, Mariotti S, Lenziardi M, Baschieri L, Braverman LE, Pinchera A. Treatment of amiodarone associated thyrotoxicosis by simultaneous administration of potassium perchlorate and methimazole. J Endocrinol Invest 1986;9(3):201–7.

147. Reichert LJ, de Rooy HA. Treatment of amiodarone induced hyperthyroidism with potassium perchlorate and methimazole during amiodarone treatment. BMJ 1989;298(6687):1547–8.

148. Stephens JW, Baynes C, Hurel SJ. Amiodarone and thyroid dysfunction. A case-illustrated guide to management. Br J Cardiol 2001;8:499–506.

149. Broussolle C, Ducottet X, Martin C, Barbier Y, Bornet H, Noel G, Orgiazzi J. Rapid effectiveness of prednisone and thionamides combined therapy in severe amiodarone iodine-induced thyrotoxicosis. Comparison of two groups of patients with apparently normal thyroid glands. J Endocrinol Invest 1989;12(1):37–42.

150. Marketou ME, Simantirakis EN, Manios EG, Vardas PE. Electrical storm due to amiodarone induced thyrotoxicosis in a young adult with dilated cardiomyopathy: thyroidectomy as the treatment of choice. Pacing Clin Electrophysiol 2001;24(12):1827–8.

151. Daniels GH. Amiodarone-induced thyrotoxicosis. J Clin Endocrinol Metab 2001;86(1):3–8.

152. Chopra IJ, Baber K. Use of oral cholecystographic agents in the treatment of amiodarone-induced hyperthyroidism. J Clin Endocrinol Metab 2001;86(10):4707–10.

153. Bogazzi F, Aghini-Lombardi F, Cosci C, Lupi I, Santini F, Tanda ML, Miccoli P, Basolo F, Pinchera A, Bartalena L, Braverman LE, Martino E. Lopanoic acid rapidly controls type I amiodarone-induced thyrotoxicosis prior to thyroidectomy. J Endocrinol Invest 2002;25(2):176–80.

154. Osman F, Franklyn JA, Sheppard MC, Gammage MD. Successful treatment of amiodarone-induced thyrotoxicosis. Circulation 2002;105(11):1275–7.

155. Bartalena L, Brogioni S, Grasso L, Bogazzi F, Burelli A, Martino E. Treatment of amiodarone-induced thyrotoxicosis, a difficult challenge: results of a prospective study. J Clin Endocrinol Metab 1996;81(8):2930–3.

156. Leger AF, Massin JP, Laurent MF, Vincens M, Auriol M, Helal OB, Chomette G, Savoie JC. Iodine-induced thyrotoxicosis: analysis of eighty-five consecutive cases. Eur J Clin Invest 1984;14(6):449–55.

157. Brennan MD, van Heerden JA, Carney JA. Amiodarone-associated thyrotoxicosis (AAT): experience with surgical management. Surgery 1987;102(6):1062–7.

158. Williams M, Lo Gerfo P. Thyroidectomy using local anesthesia in critically ill patients with amiodarone-induced thyrotoxicosis: a review and description of the technique. Thyroid 2002;12(6):523–5.

159. Martino E, Aghini-Lombardi F, Bartalena L, Grasso L, Loviselli A, Velluzzi F, Pinchera A, Braverman LE. Enhanced susceptibility to amiodarone-induced hypothyroidism in patients with thyroid autoimmune disease. Arch Intern Med 1994;154(23):2722–6.

160. Hyatt RH, Sinha B, Vallon A, Bailey RJ, Martin A. Noncardiac side-effects of long-term oral amiodarone in the elderly. Age Ageing 1988;17(2):116–22.

161. Pollak PT, Sharma AD, Carruthers SG. Elevation of serum total cholesterol and triglyceride levels during amiodarone therapy. Am J Cardiol 1988;62(9):562–5.

162. Adams PC, Sloan P, Morley AR, Holt DW. Peripheral neutrophil inclusions in amiodarone treated patients. Br J Clin Pharmacol 1986;22(6):736–8.

163. Weinberger I, Rotenberg Z, Fuchs J, Ben-Sasson E, Agmon J. Amiodarone-induced thrombocytopenia. Arch Intern Med 1987;147(4):735–6.

164. Berrebi A, Shtalrid M, Vorst EJ. Amiodarone-induced thrombocytopathy. Acta Haematol 1983;70(1):68–9.

165. Arpin MP, Alt M, Kheiralla JC, Chabrier G, Welsch M, Imbs JL, Imler M. Hyperthyroïdie et anémie hémolytique immune après traitement par amiodarone. [Hyperthyroidism and immune hemolytic anemia following amiodarone therapy.] Rev Med Interne 1991;12(4):309–11.

166. Rosenbaum H, Ben-Arie Y, Azzam ZS, Krivoy N. Amiodarone-associated granuloma in bone marrow. Ann Pharmacother 1998;32(1):60–2.

167. Boutros NY, Dilly S, Bevan DH. Amiodarone-induced bone marrow granulomas. Clin Lab Haematol 2000;22(3):167–70.

168. Moran SK, Manoharan A. Amiodarone-induced bone marrow granulomas. Pathology 2002;34(3):267–9.

169. Heger JJ, Prystowsky EN, Jackman WM, Naccarelli GV, Warfel KA, Rinkenberger RL, Zipes DP. Amiodarone. N Engl J Med 1982;305:539–45.

170. Bexton RS, Camm AJ. Drugs with a class III antiarrhythmic action. Pharmacol Ther 1982;17(3):315–55.

171. Freneaux E, Larrey D, Pessayre D. Phospholipidose et lesions pseudoalcooliques hepatiques medicamenteuses. Rev Fr Gastroenterol 1988;24:879–84.

172. Adams PC, Bennett MK, Holt DW. Hepatic effects of amiodarone. Br J Clin Pract Suppl 1986;44:81–95.

173. Geneve J, Zafrani ES, Dhumeaux D. Amiodarone-induced liver disease. J Hepatol 1989;9(1):130–3.

174. Harrison RF, Elias E. Amiodarone-associated cirrhosis with hepatic and lymph node granulomas. Histopathology 1993;22(1):80–2.

175. Jain D, Bowlus CL, Anderson JM, Robert ME. Granular cells as a marker of early amiodarone hepatotoxicity. J Clin Gastroenterol 2000;31(3):241–3.

176. Jones DB, Mullick FG, Hoofnagle JH, Baranski B. Reye's syndrome-like illness in a patient receiving amiodarone. Am J Gastroenterol 1988;83(9):967–9.

177. Breuer HW, Bossek W, Haferland C, Schmidt M, Neumann H, Gruszka J. Amiodarone-induced severe hepatitis mediated by immunological mechanisms. Int J Clin Pharmacol Ther 1998;36(6):350–2.

178. Tilz GP, Liebig E, Pristautz H. Cholestase bei Amiodaron-eine seltene Komplikation der antiarrhythmischen Therapie. Med Welt 1989;40:985.

179. Salti Z, Cloche P, Weber P, Houssemand G, Vollmer F. A propos d'un cas d'hepatite choléstatique à l'amiodarone. [A case of cholestatic hepatitis caused by amiodarone.] Ann Cardiol Angeiol (Paris) 1989;38(1):13–16.

180. Chang CC, Petrelli M, Tomashefski JF Jr, McCullough AJ. Severe intrahepatic cholestasis caused by amiodarone toxicity after withdrawal of the drug: a case report and review of the literature. Arch Pathol Lab Med 1999;123(3):251–6.

181. Rhodes A, Eastwood JB, Smith SA. Early acute hepatitis with parenteral amiodarone: a toxic effect of the vehicle? Gut 1993;34(4):565–6.

182. Iliopoulou A, Giannakopoulos G, Mayrikakis M, Zafiris E, Stamatelopoulos S. Reversible fulminant hepatitis following intravenous amiodarone loading. Amiodarone hepatotoxicity. Int J Clin Pharmacol Ther 1999;37(6):312–3.

183. Sastri SV, Diaz-Arias AA, Marshall JB. Can pancreatitis be associated with amiodarone hepatotoxicity? J Clin Gastroenterol 1990;12(1):70–3.

184. Bosch X, Bernadich O. Acute pancreatitis during treatment with amiodarone. Lancet 1997;350(9087):1300.

185. Pollak PT, Sharma AD, Carruthers SG. Creatinine elevation in patients receiving amiodarone correlates with serum amiodarone concentration. Br J Clin Pharmacol 1993;36(2):125–7.

186. Anonymous. Amiodarone—a new type of antiarrhythmic drug. Drug Ther Bull 1981;19(22):86–8.

187. Chalmers RJ, Muston HL, Srinivas V, Bennett DH. High incidence of amiodarone-induced photosensitivity in Northwest England. BMJ (Clin Res Ed) 1982;285(6338):341.

188. Ferguson J, de Vane PJ, Wirth M. Prevention of amiodarone-induced photosensitivity. Lancet 1984;2(8399):414.

189. Ferguson J, Addo HA, Jones S, Johnson BE, Frain-Bell W. A study of cutaneous photosensitivity induced by amiodarone. Br J Dermatol 1985;113(5):537–49.

190. Collins P, Ferguson J. Narrow-band UVB (TL-01) phototherapy: an effective preventative treatment for the photodermatoses. Br J Dermatol 1995;132(6):956–63.

191. Waitzer S, Butany J, From L, Hanna W, Ramsay C, Downar E. Cutaneous ultrastructural changes and photosensitivity associated with amiodarone therapy. J Am Acad Dermatol 1987;16(4):779–87.

192. Parodi A, Guarrera M, Rebora A. Amiodarone-induced pseudoporphyria. Photodermatol 1988;5(3):146–7.

193. Beukema WP, Graboys TB. Spontaneous disappearance of blue-gray facial pigmentation during amiodarone therapy (out of the blue). Am J Cardiol 1988;62(16):1146–7.

194. Sra J, Bremner S. Images in cardiovascular medicine: amiodarone skin toxicity. Circulation 1998;97(11):1105.

195. Karrer S, Hohenleutner U, Szeimies RM, Landthaler M, Hruza GJ. Amiodarone-induced pigmentation resolves after treatment with the Q-switched ruby laser. Arch Dermatol 1999;135(3):251–3.

196. Rogers KC, Wolfe DA. Amiodarone-induced blue-gray syndrome. Ann Pharmacother 2000;34(9):1075.

197. Erdmann SM, Poblete P. Hyperpigmentation in a patient under treatment with amiodarone and minocycline. H G Z Hautkr 2001;76:746–8.

198. Haas N, Schadendorf D, Hermes B, Henz BM. Hypomelanosis due to block of melanosomal maturation in amiodarone-induced hyperpigmentation. Arch Dermatol 2001;137(4):513–14.

199. Wilkinson CM, Weidner GJ, Paulino AC. Amiodarone and radiation therapy sequelae. Am J Clin Oncol 2001;24(4):379–81.

200. Zantkuyl CF, Weemers M. Iododerma caused by amiodarone (Cordarone). Dermatologia (Basel) 1975;151:311.

201. Muir AD, Wilson M. Amiodarone and psoriasis. NZ Med J 1982;95(717):711.

202. Moots RJ, Banerjee A. Exfoliative dermatitis after amiodarone treatment. BMJ (Clin Res Ed) 1988;296(6632):1332–3.

203. Dootson G, Byatt C. Amiodarone-induced vasculitis and a review of the cutaneous side-effects of amiodarone. Clin Exp Dermatol 1994;19(5):422–4.

204. Bencini PL, Crosti C, Sala F, Bertani E, Nobili M. Toxic epidermal necrolysis and amiodarone treatment. Arch Dermatol 1985;121(7):838.

205. Yung A, Agnew K, Snow J, Oliver F. Two unusual cases of toxic epidermal necrolysis. Australas J Dermatol 2002;43(1):35–8.

206. Clouston PD, Donnelly PE. Acute necrotising myopathy associated with amiodarone therapy. Aust NZ J Med 1989;19(5):483–5.

207. Gabal-Shehab LL, Monga M. Recurrent bilateral amiodarone induced epididymitis. J Urol 1999;161(3):921.

208. Sadek I, Biron P, Kus T. Amiodarone-induced epididymitis: report of a new case and literature review of 12 cases. Can J Cardiol 1993;9(9):833–6.

209. Kirkali Z. Re: Recurrent bilateral amiodarone induced epididymitis. J Urol 1999;162(3 Pt 1):808–9.

210. Susano R, Caminal L, Ramos D, Diaz B. Amiodarone induced lupus. Ann Rheum Dis 1999;58(10):655–6.

211. Sheikhzadeh A, Schafer U, Schnabel A. Drug-induced lupus erythematosus by amiodarone. Arch Intern Med 2002;162(7):834–6.

212. Burches E, Garcia-Verdegay F, Ferrer M, Pelaez A. Amiodarone-induced angioedema. Allergy 2000;55(12):1199–200.

213. Elizari MV, Martinez JM, Belziti C, Ciruzzi M, Perez de la Hoz R, Sinisi A, Carbajales J, Scapin O, Garguichevich J, Girotti L, Cagide A. Morbidity and mortality following early administration of amiodarone in acute myocardial infarction. GEMICA study investigators, GEMA Group, Buenos Aires, Argentina. Grupo de Estudios Multicentricos en Argentina. Eur Heart J 2000;21(3): 198–205.

214. Scheinman MM. Amiodarone after acute myocardial infarction. Eur Heart J 2000;21(3):177–8.

215. Foster CJ, Love HG. Amiodarone in pregnancy. Case report and review of the literature. Int J Cardiol 1988;20(3):307–16.

216. De Wolf D, De Schepper J, Verhaaren H, Deneyer M, Smitz J, Sacre-Smits L. Congenital hypothyroid goiter and amiodarone. Acta Paediatr Scand 1988; 77(4):616–18.

217. Hofmann R, Leisch E. Symptomatische Bradykardien unter Amiodaron bei Patienten mit praexistenter Reizleitungs storung. [Symptomatic bradycardia with amiodarone in patients with pre-existing conduction disorders.] Wien Klin Wochenschr 1995;107(21):640–4.

218. Magee LA, Nulman I, Rovet JF, Koren G. Neurodevelopment after in utero amiodarone exposure. Neurotoxicol Teratol 1999;21(3):261–5.

219. Tubman R, Jenkins J, Lim J. Neonatal hyperthyroxinaemia associated with maternal amiodarone therapy: case report. Ir J Med Sci 1988;157(7):243.

220. De Catte L, De Wolf D, Smitz J, Bougatef A, De Schepper J, Foulon W. Fetal hypothyroidism as a complication of amiodarone treatment for persistent fetal supraventricular tachycardia. Prenat Diagn 1994;14(8):762–5.

221. Vanbesien J, Casteels A, Bougatef A, De Catte L, Foulon W, De Bock S, Smitz J, De Schepper J. Transient fetal hypothyroidism due to direct fetal administration of amiodarone for drug resistant fetal tachycardia. Am J Perinatol 2001;18(2):113–16.

222. Etheridge SP, Craig JE, Compton SJ. Amiodarone is safe and highly effective therapy for supraventricular tachycardia in infants. Am Heart J 2001;141(1):105–10.

223. Tisdale JE, Follin SL, Ordelova A, Webb CR. Risk factors for the development of specific noncardiovascular adverse

effects associated with amiodarone. J Clin Pharmacol 1995;35(4):351–6.

224. Garson A Jr, Gillette PC, McVey P, Hesslein PS, Porter CJ, Angell LK, Kaldis LC, Hittner HM. Amiodarone treatment of critical arrhythmias in children and young adults. J Am Coll Cardiol 1984;4(4):749–55.

225. Guccione P, Paul T, Garson A Jr. Long-term follow-up of amiodarone therapy in the young: continued efficacy, unimpaired growth, moderate side effects. J Am Coll Cardiol 1990;15(5):1118–24.

226. Villain E. Les syndromes de QT long chez l'enfant. [Long QT syndromes in children.] Arch Fr Pediatr 1993;50(3):241–7.

227. Sutherland J, Robinson B, Delbridge L. Anaesthesia for amiodarone-induced thyrotoxicosis: a case review. Anaesth Intensive Care 2001;29(1):24–9.

228. Kupferschmid JP, Rosengart TK, McIntosh CL, Leon MB, Clark RE. Amiodarone-induced complications after cardiac operation for obstructive hypertrophic cardiomyopathy. Ann Thorac Surg 1989;48(3):359–64.

229. Andersen HR, Bjorn-Hansen LS, Kimose HH, et al. Amiodaronebehandling og arytmikirurgi. Ugeskr Laeger 1989;151:2264.

230. Perkins MW, Dasta JF, Reilley TE, Halpern P. Intraoperative complications in patients receiving amiodarone: characteristics and risk factors. DICP 1989;23(10):757–63.

231. Morady F. Prevention of atrial fibrillation in the postoperative cardiac patient: significance of oral class III antiarrhythmic agents. Am J Cardiol 1999;84(9A):R156–60.

232. Sauro SC, DeCarolis DD, Pierpont GL, Gornick CC. Comparison of plasma concentrations for two amiodarone products. Ann Pharmacother 2002;36(11):1682–5.

233. Wellens HJ, Brugada P, Abdollah H, Dassen WR. A comparison of the electrophysiologic effects of intravenous and oral amiodarone in the same patient. Circulation 1984;69(1):120–4.

234. Mitchell LB, Wyse DG, Gillis AM, Duff HJ. Electropharmacology of amiodarone therapy initiation. Time courses of onset of electrophysiologic and antiarrhythmic effects. Circulation 1989;80(1):34–42.

235. Yamada S, Kuga K, Yamaguchi I. Torsade de pointes induced by intravenous and long-term oral amiodarone therapy in a patient with dilated cardiomyopathy. Jpn Circ J 2001;65(3):236–8.

236. Morady F, Scheinman MM, Shen E, Shapiro W, Sung RJ, DiCarlo L. Intravenous amiodarone in the acute treatment of recurrent symptomatic ventricular tachycardia. Am J Cardiol 1983;51(1):156–9.

237. Holt P, Curry PVL, Way B, Storey G, Holt DW. Intravenous amiodarone in the management of tachyarrhythmias. In: Breithardt H, Loogen F, editors. New Aspects in the Medical Treatment of Tachyarrhythms. Munich; Urban and Schwartzenberg, 1983:136–41.

238. Faniel R, Schoenfeld P. Efficacy of i.v. amiodarone in converting rapid atrial fibrillation and flutter to sinus rhythm in intensive care patients. Eur Heart J 1983;4(3):180–5.

239. Antonelli D, Barzilay J. Acute thrombophlebitis following IV amiodarone administration. Chest 1983;84(1):120.

240. Kerin NZ, Blevins R, Rubenfire M, Faital K, Householder S. Acute thrombophlebitis following IV amiodarone administration. Chest 1983;84(1):120.

241. Reiffel JA. Intravenous amiodarone in the management of atrial fibrillation. J Cardiovasc Pharmacol Ther 1999;4(4):199–204.

242. Kochiadakis GE, Igoumenidis NE, Solomou MC, Kaleboubas MD, Chlouverakis GI, Vardas PE. Efficacy of amiodarone for the termination of persistent atrial fibrillation. Am J Cardiol 1999;83(1):58–61.

243. Cotter G, Blatt A, Kaluski E, Metzkor-Cotter E, Koren M, Litinski I, Simantov R, Moshkovitz Y, Zaidenstein R, Peleg E, Vered Z, Golik A. Conversion of recent onset paroxysmal atrial fibrillation to normal sinus rhythm: the effect of no treatment and high-dose amiodarone. A randomized, placebo-controlled study. Eur Heart J 1999;20(24):1833–42.

244. Leatham EW, Holt DW, McKenna WJ. Class III antiarrhythmics in overdose. Presenting features and management principles. Drug Saf 1993;9(6):450–62.

245. Bonati M, D'Aranno V, Galletti F, Fortunati MT, Tognoni G. Acute overdosage of amiodarone in a suicide attempt. J Toxicol Clin Toxicol 1983;20(2):181–6.

246. Liberman BA, Teasdale SJ. Anaesthesia and amiodarone. Can Anaesth Soc J 1985;32(6):629–38.

247. Landray MJ, Kendall MJ. Effect of amiodarone on mortality. Lancet 1998;351(9101):523.

248. McCullough PA, Redle JD, Zaman AG, Archbold A, Alamgir F, Ulahannan TJ, Daoud EG, Morady F. Amiodarone prophylaxis for atrial fibrillation after cardiac surgery. N Engl J Med 1998;338(19):1383–4.

249. Boutitie F, Boissel JP, Connolly SJ, Camm AJ, Cairns JA, Julian DG, Gent M, Janse MJ, Dorian P, Frangin G. Amiodarone interaction with beta-blockers: analysis of the merged EMIAT (European Myocardial Infarct Amiodarone Trial) and CAMIAT (Canadian Amiodarone Myocardial Infarction Trial) databases. The EMIAT and CAMIAT Investigators. Circulation 1999;99(17):2268–75.

250. Ogunyankin KO, Singh BN. Mortality reduction by antiadrenergic modulation of arrhythmogenic substrate: significance of combining beta blockers and amiodarone. Am J Cardiol 1999;84(9A):R76–82.

251. Ahle GB, Blum AL, Martinek J, Oneta CM, Dorta G. Cushing's syndrome in an 81-year-old patient treated with budesonide and amiodarone. Eur J Gastroenterol Hepatol 2000;12(9):1041–2.

252. Yonezawa E, Matsumoto K, Ueno K, Tachibana M, Hashimoto H, Komamura K, Kamakura S, Miyatake K, Tanaka K. Lack of interaction between amiodarone and mexiletine in cardiac arrhythmia patients. J Clin Pharmacol 2002;42(3):342–6.

253. Bhagat R, Sporn TA, Long GD, Folz RJ. Amiodarone and cyclophosphamide: potential for enhanced lung toxicity. Bone Marrow Transplant 2001;27(10):1109–11.

254. Lelarge P, Bauer P, Royer-Morrot MJ, Meregnani JL, Larcan A, Lambert H. Intoxication digitalique après administration conjointe d'acétyl digitoxine et d'amiodarone. Ann Med Nancy Est 1993;32:307.

255. Lee TH, Friedman PL, Goldman L, Stone PH, Antman EM. Sinus arrest and hypotension with combined amiodarone–diltiazem therapy. Am Heart J 1985;109(1):163–4.

256. Lohman JJ, Reichert LJ, Degen LP. Antiretroviral therapy increases serum concentrations of amiodarone. Ann Pharmacother 1999;33(5):645–6.

257. Segura I, Garcia-Bolao I. Meglumine antimoniate, amiodarone and torsades de pointes: a case report. Resuscitation 1999;42(1):65–8.

258. Staiger C, Jauernig R, de Vries J, Weber E. Influence of amiodarone on antipyrine pharmacokinetics in three patients with ventricular tachycardia. Br J Clin Pharmacol 1984;18(2):263–4.

259. McGovern B, Geer VR, LaRaia PJ, Garan H, Ruskin JN. Possible interaction between amiodarone and phenytoin. Ann Intern Med 1984;101(5):650–1.

260. Lesko LJ. Pharmacokinetic drug interactions with amiodarone. Clin Pharmacokinet 1989;17(2):130–40.

261. Nolan PE Jr, Marcus FI, Karol MD, Hoyer GL, Gear K. Effect of phenytoin on the clinical pharmacokinetics of amiodarone. J Clin Pharmacol 1990;30(12):1112–19.

262. Zarembski DG, Fischer SA, Santucci PA, Porter MT, Costanzo MR, Trohman RG. Impact of rifampin on serum

amiodarone concentrations in a patient with congenital heart disease. Pharmacotherapy 1999;19(2):249–51.

263. Fabre G, Julian B, Saint-Aubert B, Joyeux H, Berger Y. Evidence for CYP3A-mediated N-deethylation of amiodarone in human liver microsomal fractions. Drug Metab Dispos 1993;21(6):978–85.

264. Woeber KA, Warner I. Potentiation of warfarin sodium by amiodarone-induced thyrotoxicosis. West J Med 1999;170(1):49–51.

265. Sanoski CA, Bauman JL. Clinical observations with the amiodarone/warfarin interaction: dosing relationships with long-term therapy. Chest 2002;121(1):19–23.

266. Jacobs MB. Serum creatinine increase associated with amiodarone therapy. NY State J Med 1987;87(6):358–9.

267. Davies PH, Franklyn JA. The effects of drugs on tests of thyroid function. Eur J Clin Pharmacol 1991;40(5):439–51.

268. Rotmensch HH, Belhassen B, Swanson BN, Shoshani D, Spielman SR, Greenspon AJ, Greenspan AM, Vlasses PH, Horowitz LN. Steady-state serum amiodarone concentrations: relationships with antiarrhythmic efficacy and toxicity. Ann Intern Med 1984;101(4):462–9.

269. Pollak PT, Sharma AD, Carruthers SG. Correlation of amiodarone dosage, heart rate, QT interval and corneal microdeposits with serum amiodarone and desethylamiodarone concentrations. Am J Cardiol 1989;64(18):1138–43.

270. Debbas NM, du Cailar C, Bexton RS, Demaille JG, Camm AJ, Puech P. The QT interval: a predictor of the plasma and myocardial concentrations of amiodarone. Br Heart J 1984;51(3):316–20.

271. Willems J, De Geest H. Digitalis intoxicatie. Ned Tijdschr Geneeskd 1968;24:617.

Amiphenazole

General Information

Amiphenazole is a respiratory stimulant. It increases ventilation by accelerating the frequency at increased CO_2 partial pressures above 6 kPa (45 mmHg) (1).

Its adverse effects include restlessness, prolonged and forced expiration, nausea and vomiting, sweating, and skin reactions; the last include rashes (2), occasionally oral lichenoid eruptions (3), and ulceration (4). Muscle twitching and mental disorientation can also occur in the elderly. With large doses, convulsions can occur (5).

In a double-blind randomized study in 30 women in the recovery room a single intravenous bolus injection of amiphenazole 150 mg was compared with placebo; amiphenazole did not improve ventilation (6). However, in a double-blind study amiphenazole reversed respiratory depression and analgesia due to morphine (7).

References

1. Wiessmann KJ, Steinijans VW, Brossmann D. The efficacy of four respiratory analeptics on healthy young men in a CO_2 rebreathing experiment. Arzneimittelforschung 1979;29(2):329–33.

2. Moon W, Shaw FH, Bruce DW. Rashes with amiphenazole. Br Med J 1964;5384:698.

3. Simpson JD. Amiphenazole and lichen planus. BMJ 1963;5373:1655.

4. Dinsdale RC, Walker AE. Amiphenazole sensitivity with oral ulceration. Br Dent J 1966;121(10):460–2.

5. Today's drugs. Drugs for respiratory insufficiency. BMJ 1963;1:731.

6. Lehmann KA, Asoklis S, Grond S, Schroeder B. Kontinuierliches monitoring der Spontanatmung in der postoperativen Phase. Teil 3. Einfluss von amiphenazol auf kutane Sauerstoff- und Kohlendioxidpartialdrucke nach gynakologischen Eingriffen unter Halothannarkosen. [Continuous monitoring of spontaneous postoperative respiration. 3. The effect of amiphenazole on cutaneous oxygen and carbon dioxide partial pressure following gynecologic surgery under halothane anesthesia.] Anaesthesist 1993;42(4):227–31.

7. Gairola RL, Gupta PK, Pandley K. Antagonists of morphine-induced respiratory depression. A study in postoperative patients. Anaesthesia 1980;35(1):17–21.

Amisulpride

See also Neuroleptic drugs

General Information

Amisulpride is an atypical antipsychotic drug, a benzamide derivative, which may have a low propensity to cause extrapyramidal symptoms (SEDA-22, 55).

Amisulpride 600–1200 mg/day for 3 months was effective and well tolerated in 445 patients with schizophrenia aged 18–45 years (1). During this time, 124 patients (28%) dropped out of the study; 21% reported adverse events, neurological (35%), psychiatric (15%), or endocrine (9.1%). Seven adverse events were assessed as serious: two suicides, two suicide attempts, one neuroleptic malignant syndrome, one somnolence, and one worsening of arteritis.

A lower dose of amisulpride (50 mg) has been tested in 20 healthy elderly volunteers (aged 65–79 years) (2). There were no serious adverse events, but one subject reported a moderate headache for 18 hours, a second subject vomited 9 hours after dosing, and a further subject complained of mild somnolence for 12 hours starting 4 hours after dosing; however, there were no extrapyramidal symptoms, clinically significant hemodynamic variations, or electrocardiographic abnormalities.

Comparisons with placebo and other antipsychotic drugs

In a randomized double-blind study, there were no differences in the numbers of patients with at least one adverse effect with amisulpride 100 mg (24%; $n = 18$), amisulpride 50 mg (25%; $n = 21$), or placebo (33%; $n = 27$) (3). Few patients had endocrine symptoms (2 out of 160 in the amisulpride groups).

Two narrative reviews of amisulpride have been published (4,5). The authors emphasized that amisulpride in low dosages (below 300 mg/day) causes a similar incidence of adverse effects to placebo; nevertheless, at higher dosages (400–1200 mg/day), the overall incidence of adverse events in those taking amisulpride was similar to that in patients taking haloperidol, flupenthixol, or risperidone. The most commonly reported adverse events associated with higher dosages of amisulpride were extrapyramidal symptoms, insomnia, hyperkinesia, anxiety, increased body weight, and agitation. The incidence of extrapyramidal symptoms was dose-related. In elderly people, amisulpride can cause hypotension and sedation. There are no systematic published data on efficacy in children aged under 15 years.

In an extensive review of 19 randomized studies for the Cochrane Library ($n = 2443$), most of the trials were small and of short duration (6). The data from four trials with 514 participants with predominantly negative symptoms suggested that low-dose amisulpride (up to 300 mg/day) was more acceptable than placebo ($n = 514$; RR = 0.6; 95% CI = 0.5, 0.8).

A meta-analysis of 10 randomized controlled clinical trials of amisulpride in "acutely ill patients" ($n = 1654$) has been published, supported in part by a grant from Sanofi-Synthélabo, the marketing authorization holder (7). Amisulpride was significantly better than conventional antipsychotic drugs by about 11 percentage points on the Brief Psychiatric Rating Scale. In four studies in patients with "persistent negative symptoms," amisulpride was significantly better than placebo ($n = 514$), but there was no significant difference between amisulpride and conventional drugs (only three trials; $n = 130$). Low doses of amisulpride (50–300 mg/day) were not associated with significantly more use of antiparkinsonian drugs than placebo ($n = 507$), and usual doses caused fewer extrapyramidal adverse effects than conventional antipsychotic drugs ($n = 1599$). In studies in acutely ill patients, significantly fewer patients taking amisulpride dropped out compared with patients taking conventional drugs, mainly owing to fewer adverse events; there were no significant differences in dropout rates between amisulpride and conventional antipsychotic drugs (three small studies).

Comparisons with antidepressants

Amisulpride has been compared with amitriptyline ($n = 250$; 6 months) (8) and with amineptine ($n = 323$; 3 months) in randomized double-blind trials in the treatment of dysthymia (9). In both trials, amisulpride was more efficacious than placebo but equal to amineptine and amitriptyline. Endocrine symptoms (such as galactorrhea and menstrual disorders) and weight gain were more frequent with amisulpride. There was galactorrhea in 8.4% and 11% respectively. In one of the studies (8), serious adverse events occurred in 13 of 165 patients taking amisulpride (15 events). Sudden death, probably secondary to myocardial infarction, occurred in a patient taking amisulpride 7 days after withdrawal. In the other cases, admission to hospital was required for fracture (two cases) and gastric pain, neuralgia, hyperglycemia, eczema, an injury, and an erythematous rash (one case each).

In a randomized, double-blind, multicenter trial for 8 weeks in 278 patients with depression, there were no differences in efficacy or tolerability between amisulpride 50 mg and SSRIs (10).

Organs and Systems

Cardiovascular

QT interval prolongation has been attributed to amisulpride.

- Sinus bradycardia and QT interval prolongation occurred in a 25-year-old man taking amisulpride 800 mg/day (11). The dosage of amisulpride was reduced to 600 mg/day and the electrocardiogram normalized within a few days.

Psychological, psychiatric

In a randomized, double-blind, crossover study in 21 healthy volunteers who took amisulpride 50 mg/day, amisulpride 400 mg/day, haloperidol 4 mg/day, or placebo, amisulpride 400 mg had several adverse effects on psychomotor performance and cognitive performance, similar to those of haloperidol, at the end of the 5-day course of treatment; however, there were no signs of mental disturbances on clinical rating scales or during a structured psychiatric interview (12).

References

1. Wetzel H, Grunder G, Hillert A, Philipp M, Gattaz WF, Sauer H, Adler G, Schroder J, Rein W, Benkert O. Amisulpride versus flupentixol in schizophrenia with predominantly positive symptomatology—a double-blind controlled study comparing a selective D2-like antagonist to a mixed D1-/D2-like antagonist. The Amisulpride Study Group. Psychopharmacology (Berl) 1998;137(3):223–32.
2. Hamon-Vilcot B, Chaufour S, Deschamps C, Canal M, Zieleniuk I, Ahtoy P, Chretien P, Rosenzweig P, Nasr A, Piette F. Safety and pharmacokinetics of a single oral dose of amisulpride in healthy elderly volunteers. Eur J Clin Pharmacol 1998;54(5):405–9.
3. Danion JM, Rein W, Fleurot O. Improvement of schizophrenic patients with primary negative symptoms treated with amisulpride. Amisulpride Study Group. Am J Psychiatry 1999;156(4):610–16.
4. Curran MP, Perry CM. Spotlight on amisulpride in schizophrenia. CNS Drugs 2002;16(3):207–11.
5. Green B. Focus on amisulpride. Curr Med Res Opin 2002;18(3):113–17.
6. Mota NE, Lima MS, Soares BG. Amisulpride for schizophrenia. Cochrane Database Syst Rev 2002;(2):CD001357.
7. Leucht S, Pitschel-Walz G, Engel RR, Kissling W. Amisulpride, an unusual "atypical" antipsychotic: a meta-analysis of randomized controlled trials. Am J Psychiatry 2002;159(2):180–90.
8. Ravizza L. Amisulpride in medium-term treatment of dysthymia: a six-month, double-blind safety study versus amitriptyline. AMILONG investigators. J Psychopharmacol 1999;13(3):248–54.
9. Boyer P, Lecrubier Y, Stalla-Bourdillon A, Fleurot O. Amisulpride versus amineptine and placebo for the treatment of dysthymia. Neuropsychobiology 1999;39(1):25–32.
10. Cassano GB, Jori MC. AMIMAJOR Group. Efficacy and safety of amisulpride 50 mg versus paroxetine 20 mg in major depression: a randomized, double-blind, parallel group study Int Clin Psychopharmacol 2002;17(1):27–32.
11. Pedrosa Gil F, Grohmann R, Ruther E. Asymptomatic bradycardia associated with amisulpride. Pharmacopsychiatry 2001;34(6):259–61.
12. Ramaekers JG, Louwerens JW, Muntjewerff ND, Milius H, de Bie A, Rosenzweig P, Patat A, O'Hanlon JF. Psychomotor, cognitive, extrapyramidal, and affective functions of healthy volunteers during treatment with an atypical (amisulpride) and a classic (haloperidol) antipsychotic. J Clin Psychopharmacol 1999;19(3):209–21.

Amitriptylinoxide

See also Tricyclic antidepressants

General Information

Amitriptylinoxide, a metabolite of amitriptyline, has been compared with the parent drug (1). The antidepressant effects were comparable, but the metabolite was thought to have fewer adverse effects, especially cardiotoxic ones. This conclusion was based on the absence of cardiographic abnormalities in 15 patients, but this is a very small series on which to base such a conclusion.

Reference

1. Godt HH, Fredslund-Andersen K, Edlund AH. Amitriptyline N-oxid, et nyt antidepressivum: sammenlignende klinisk vurdering i forhold til amitriptylin. [Amitriptyline N-oxide. A new antidepressant. A clinical double-blind comparison with amitriptyline.] Nord Psykiatr Tidsskr 1971;25(3):237–46.

Amlodipine

See also Calcium channel blockers

General Information

Amlodipine is a long-acting dihydropyridine calcium channel blocker. It has an adverse effects profile similar to those of other dihydropyridines, but at a lower frequency (1). Along with felodipine (2), but unlike other calcium channel blockers, it may also be safer in severe chronic heart failure when there is concurrent angina or hypertension (3).

The effects of amlodipine and isosorbide-5-mononitrate for 3 weeks on exercise-induced myocardial stunning have been compared in a randomized, double-blind, crossover study in 24 patients with chronic stable angina and normal left ventricular function (4). Amlodipine attenuated stunning, evaluated by echocardiography, significantly more than isosorbide, without difference in anti-ischemic action or hemodynamics. Amlodipine was better tolerated than isosorbide, mainly because of a lower incidence of headache (4).

Vasodilatory calcium channel blockers have been reported to improve exercise tolerance in some preliminary studies. A multicenter, randomized, placebo-controlled trial was therefore performed in 437 patients with mild to moderate heart failure to assess the effects of amlodipine 10 mg/day in addition to standard therapy (5). Over 12 weeks amlodipine did not improve exercise time and did not increase the incidence of adverse events.

Mental stress is a risk factor for cardiovascular disease. In 24 patients with mild to moderate hypertension, amlodipine reduced the blood pressure rise during mental stress compared with placebo, but increased plasma noradrenaline concentrations (6).

Hypertension leading to cardiac dysfunction is very frequent in patients with the inherited syndrome called Ribbing's disease, which is characterized by multiple epiphyseal dystrophy. In a randomized, double-blind comparison of amlodipine (10 mg/day) and enalapril (20 mg/day) in 50 patients for 6 months, both drugs significantly reduced blood pressure, but amlodipine increased heart rate and plasma concentrations of noradrenaline and angiotensin II (7). These undesired effects make ACE inhibitors a better choice for prevention of cardiac dysfunction.

Organs and Systems

Nervous system

- A 35-year-old woman with benign intracranial hypertension and high blood pressure was given amlodipine, with good control of her blood pressure (8). However, her headache worsened and she developed papilledema. The CSF pressure was 30 cm. Her symptoms disappeared shortly after amlodipine withdrawal.

Liver

Hepatitis has been attributed to amlodipine.

- A 77-year-old man took amlodipine for 1 month and developed jaundice and raised aspartate transaminase, alanine transaminase, and bilirubin (9). A liver biopsy suggested a drug-induced hepatitis and the amlodipine was withdrawn. His symptoms and laboratory values normalized. Other drugs (metformin, fluindione, and omeprazole) were not withdrawn.
- A 69-year-old hypertensive man who had taken amlodipine for 10 months abruptly developed jaundice, choluria, raised serum bilirubin, and increased transaminases (10). After amlodipine withdrawal he progressively recovered in a few weeks without sequelae or relapses. However, after several months he presented again with jaundice and an enlarged liver, having started to take diltiazem 5 months before. He recovered completely in a few weeks after drug withdrawal.

In the second case the authors hypothesized an idiosyncratic mechanism.

Skin

Recognized skin eruptions associated with amlodipine include erythematous and maculopapular rashes, skin discoloration, urticaria, dryness, alopecia, dermatitis, erythema multiforme, and lichen planus. A granuloma annulare-like eruption has been reported (11).

- A 64-year-old Caucasian woman, with a history of ankylosing spondylitis, hypertension, and osteoporosis, took amlodipine for 13 days and developed a rash on her lower legs. Amlodipine was withdrawn, but the rash progressed to involve both of her hands. The eruption consisted of multiple erythematous pruritic papules. Histology showed focal collagen degeneration and a significant interstitial histiocytic dermal infiltrate, suggestive of granuloma annulare. Within 3 months of withdrawal of amlodipine the reaction cleared and did not recur during follow-up for 3 years.

Amlodipine can cause generalized pruritus, which usually happens within 24 hours and resolves within 24 hours of withdrawal (12).

Photosensitivity presenting with telangiectasia can be caused by calcium channel blockers.

- A 57-year-old hypertensive man developed telangiectasia, initially on the forehead and rapidly extending to the upper back, shoulders, and chest, particularly during the summer (13). The eruption began 1 month after starting amlodipine and diminished considerably 3 months after withdrawal.
- A 3-year-old girl developed telangiectases on the cheeks and gingival hyperplasia while taking furosemide, captopril, and amlodipine for hypertension due to hemolytic–uremic syndrome (14). Both lesions disappeared on withdrawal of amlodipine.

Calcium channel blockers can cause lichen planus.

- A 56-year-old Nigerian woman, with a previous history of sickle cell trait, osteoarthritis, and non-insulin-dependent diabetes mellitus, took amlodipine 5 mg/day for hypertension for 2 weeks and developed a lichenoid eruption (15). Histological examination confirmed the diagnosis of lichen planus. Amlodipine was withdrawn and there was rapid symptomatic and clinical improvement after treatment with glucocorticoids and antihistamines.

Musculoskeletal

A patient presented with severe, generalized muscle stiffness, joint pain, and fatigue while taking amlodipine for hypertension and zafirlukast for asthma. Stopping zafirlukast did not change her symptoms; the dose of amlodipine was increased at different times up to 15 mg to control blood pressure better. The neurological symptoms worsened, in the absence of any evidence of immunological or neurological disorders, and so amlodipine was withdrawn: the symptoms disappeared within 4 days (16).

Second-Generation Effects

Pregnancy

Subcutaneous fat necrosis in a neonate has been attributed to maternal use of amlodipine during pregnancy (17).

- A boy weighing 4 kg was born by spontaneous normal delivery at 39 weeks to a 38-year-old Afro-Caribbean woman, whose pregnancy was complicated by essential hypertension treated with amlodipine. On day 1 the child developed firm, red, pea-sized nodular lesions on the face, buttocks, back, shoulders, and arms.

Subcutaneous fat necrosis of the newborn is relatively uncommon. It is said to be benign and painless and to resolve within a few weeks. However, in this case it was extremely painful and was relieved only by opiates. The skin changes persisted beyond the age of 6 months and remained extremely symptomatic until the age of 9 months, when the skin had become normal. Calcium abnormalities have often been reported in association with subcutaneous fat necrosis, and exposure to amlodipine during pregnancy may have resulted in impairment of enzyme systems dependent on calcium fluxes for their action; it may also have affected calcium homeostasis in the neonate. Since previous reports of teratogenicity in animals have been published, few women take calcium channel blockers during

pregnancy and there are no reports to date of an association between these drugs and subcutaneous fat necrosis (17).

Drug Administration

Drug overdose

Amlodipine overdose has been reported (18).

- A 23-year-old woman took 60 tablets of amlodipine intentionally and developed tachycardia and severe hypotension. She did not improve with intensive therapy and developed left ventricular failure and oliguria and underwent hemodiafiltration. Her condition slowly improved over 4 days.

Drug–Drug Interactions

Chloroquine

A possible interaction of amlodipine with chloroquine has been reported (19).

- A 48-year-old hypertensive physician, who had optimal blood pressure control after taking oral amlodipine 5 mg/day for 3 months, developed a slight frontal headache and fever, thought that he had malaria, and took four tablets of chloroquine sulfate (total 600 mg base). Two hours later he became nauseated and dizzy and collapsed; his systolic blood pressure was 80 mmHg and his diastolic pressure was unrecordable, suggesting vasovagal syncope, which was corrected by dextrose–saline infusion.

There was no malaria parasitemia in this case, and hence the syncope may have resulted from the acute synergistic hypotensive, venodilator, and cardiac effects of chloroquine plus amlodipine, possibly acting via augmented nitric oxide production and calcium channel blockade. Since malaria fever is itself associated with orthostatic hypotension, this possible interaction may be unrecognized and unreported in these patients.

Ciclosporin

Ciclosporin increases the survival of allografts in man. However, it causes renal vasoconstriction and increases proximal tubular reabsorption, leading in some cases to hypertension (20). The concomitant use of calcium channel blockers can prevent most of these adverse effects of ciclosporin. However, some calcium channel blockers (verapamil, diltiazem, nicardipine) can increase plasma concentrations of ciclosporin up to three-fold through inhibition of cytochrome P450. Eight different studies have been performed on the combination of amlodipine and ciclosporin given for 1–6 months to kidney transplant recipients, and the results have been reviewed (21). In three studies, in a total of 41 patients, amlodipine increased ciclosporin concentrations, while in the others, a total of 85 patients, there was no evidence of an interaction.

In normotensive renal transplant recipients treated for 2 months with amlodipine there was a small but significant nephroprotective effect (22). Thus, amlodipine, in contrast to other calcium channel blockers, does not affect ciclosporin blood concentrations and can be safely added in transplant recipients.

Sildenafil

The effect of sildenafil on arterial pressure has been tested in 16 hypertensive men taking amlodipine 5–10 mg/day (23). Sildenafil did not affect amlodipine pharmacokinetics, but caused a further additive fall in blood pressure. Adverse events with the combination of sildenafil and amlodipine, headache, dyspepsia, and nausea, did not require drug withdrawal.

References

1. Osterloh I. The safety of amlodipine. Am Heart J 1989;118(5 Pt 2):1114–19.
2. Cohn JN, Ziesche S, Smith R, Anand I, Dunkman WB, Loeb H, Cintron G, Boden W, Baruch L, Rochin P, Loss L. Effect of the calcium antagonist felodipine as supplementary vasodilator therapy in patients with chronic heart failure treated with enalapril: V-HeFT III. Vasodilator-Heart Failure Trial (V-HeFT) Study Group. Circulation 1997;96(3):856–63.
3. Packer M, O'Connor CM, Ghali JK, Pressler ML, Carson PE, Belkin RN, Miller AB, Neuberg GW, Frid D, Wertheimer JH, Cropp AB, DeMets DL. Effect of amlodipine on morbidity and mortality in severe chronic heart failure. Prospective Randomized Amlodipine Survival Evaluation Study Group. N Engl J Med 1996;335 (15):1107–14.
4. Rinaldi CA, Linka AZ, Masani ND, Avery PG, Jones E, Saunders H, Hall RJ. Randomized, double-blind crossover study to investigate the effects of amlodipine and isosorbide mononitrate on the time course and severity of exercise-induced myocardial stunning. Circulation 1998; 98(8):749–56.
5. Udelson JE, DeAbate CA, Berk M, Neuberg G, Packer M, Vijay NK, Gorwitt J, Smith WB, Kukin ML, LeJemtel T, Levine TB, Konstam MA. Effects of amlodipine on exercise tolerance, quality of life, and left ventricular function in patients with heart failure from left ventricular systolic dysfunction. Am Heart J 2000;139(3):503–10.
6. Spence JD, Munoz C, Huff MW, Tokmakjian S. Effect of amlodipine on hemodynamic and endocrine responses to mental stress. Am J Hypertens 2000;13(5 Pt 1):518–22.
7. Cocco G, Ettlin T, Baumeler HR. The effect of amlodipine and enalapril on blood pressure and neurohumoral activation in hypertensive patients with Ribbing's disease (multiple epiphysal dystrophy). Clin Cardiol 2000;23(2):109–14.
8. Gurm HS, Farooq M. Calcium channel blockers and benign hypertension. Arch Intern Med 1999;159(9):1011.
9. Khemissa-Akouz F, Ouguergouz F, Sulem P, Tkoub el M, Vaucher E. Hepatite aiguë a l'amlodipine. [Amlodipine-induced acute hepatitis.] Gastroenterol Clin Biol 2002;26(6–7):637–8.
10. Lafuente NG, Egea AM. Calcium channel blockers and hepatotoxicity. Am J Gastroenterol 2000;95(8):2145.
11. Lim AC, Hart K, Murrell D. A granuloma annulare-like eruption associated with the use of amlodipine. Australas J Dermatol 2002;43(1):24–7.
12. Orme S, da Costa D. Generalised pruritus associated with amlodipine. BMJ 1997;315(7106):463.
13. Grabczynska SA, Cowley N. Amlodipine induced-photosensitivity presenting as telangiectasia. Br J Dermatol 2000;142(6):1255–6.
14. van der Vleuten CJ, Trijbels-Smeulders MA, van de Kerkhof PC. Telangiectasia and gingival hyperplasia as side-effects of amlodipine (Norvasc) in a 3-year-old girl. Acta Dermatol Venereol 1999;79(4):323–4.
15. Swale VJ, McGregor JM. Amlodipine-associated lichen planus. Br J Dermatol 2001;144(4):920–1.
16. Phillips BB, Muller BA. Severe neuromuscular complications possibly associated with amlodipine. Ann Pharmacother 1998;32(11):1165–7.
17. Rosbotham JL, Johnson A, Haque KN, Holden CA. Painful subcutaneous fat necrosis of the newborn associated with intra-partum use of a calcium channel blocker. Clin Exp Dermatol 1998;23(1):19–21.
18. Feldman R, Glinska-Serwin M. Gleboka hipotensja z przemijajaca oliguria oraz ciezka niewydolnosc serca W przebiegu ostrego zamierzonego zatrucia amlodypina. [Deep hypotension with transient oliguria and severe heart failure in course of acute intentional poisoning with amlodipine.] Pol Arch Med Wewn 2001;105(6):495–9.
19. Ajayi AA, Adigun AQ. Syncope following oral chloroquine administration in a hypertensive patient controlled on amlodipine. Br J Clin Pharmacol 2002;53(4):404–5.
20. Curtis JJ. Hypertension following kidney transplantation. Am J Kidney Dis 1994;23(3):471–5.
21. Schrama YC, Koomans HA. Interactions of cyclosporin A and amlodipine: blood cyclosporin A levels, hypertension and kidney function. J Hypertens Suppl 1998;16(4):S33–8.
22. Venkat Raman G, Feehally J, Coates RA, Elliott HL, Griffin PJ, Olubodun JO, Wilkinson R. Renal effects of amlodipine in normotensive renal transplant recipients. Nephrol Dial Transplant 1999;14(2):384–8.
23. Knowles S, Gupta AK, Shear NH. The spectrum of cutaneous reactions associated with diltiazem: three cases and a review of the literature. J Am Acad Dermatol 1998;38(2 Pt 1): 201–6.

Ammonium chloride

General Information

Ammonium chloride, which is used as an expectorant in productive cough, can cause gastric irritation, acidosis, and hypokalemia in large doses (1).

Reference

1. Bushinsky DA, Coe FL. Hyperkalemia during acute ammonium chloride acidosis in man. Nephron 1985;40(1):38–40.

Ammonium tetrathiomolybdate

General Information

Ammonium tetrathiomolybdate can be used as a chelator of copper in Wilson's disease.

Organs and Systems

Hematologic

Several reports suggest that ammonium tetrathiomolybdate can cause reversible hypoplastic anemia (1,2).

References

1. Brewer GJ, Johnson V, Dick RD, Kluin KJ, Fink JK, Brunberg JA. Treatment of Wilson disease with ammonium tetrathiomolybdate. II. Initial therapy in 33 neurologically affected patients and follow-up with zinc therapy. Arch Neurol 1996;53(10):1017–25.
2. Walshe JM, Yealland M. Chelation treatment of neurological Wilson's disease. Q J Med 1993;86(3):197–204.

Amocarzine

General Information

Amocarzine is an antifilarial antihelminthic drug, derived from amoscanate, that is active against the adult worms of *Onchocerca volvulus*.

Although ivermectin is very effective in the treatment of onchocerciasis, a fully effective and safe macrofilaricidal drug is still lacking. In animal studies of filarial infections, amocarzine showed promise as a macrofilaricidal drug and was afterward extensively tried in humans. Promising results were obtained in the early 1990s in Ecuador with amocarzine 3 mg/kg bd for 3 days and with acceptable adverse effects, including dizziness, itching, and rash. There were reversible neurological symptoms, such as impaired coordination and a positive Romberg's sign, in 4–12% of patients (1). Amocarzine was later tried in Africa in higher doses, with less good results. In a study from Ghana (2), the combination of ivermectin and amocarzine was not more effective than ivermectin alone. Adverse effects were more severe with amocarzine alone compared with ivermectin alone or with amocarzine preceded by ivermectin. Mazzotti-type reactions, such as itching, rash, peripheral sensory phenomena, and swellings, were all more severe or frequent after amocarzine than after ivermectin. Pretreatment with ivermectin markedly reduced these adverse reactions but did not affect other symptoms, such as dizziness and gaze-evoked nystagmus, suggesting that these adverse effects were probably directly drug-related and not a reaction to dying worms.

References

1. Guderian RH, Anselmi M, Proano R, Naranjo A, Poltera AA, Moran M, Lecaillon JB, Zak F, Cascante S. Onchocercacidal effect of three drug regimens of amocarzine in 148 patients of two races and both sexes from Esmeraldas, Ecuador. Trop Med Parasitol 1991;42(3):263–85.
2. Awadzi K, Opoku NO, Attah SK, Addy ET, Duke BO, Nyame PK, Kshirsagar NA. The safety and efficacy of amocarzine in African onchocerciasis and the influence of ivermectin on the clinical and parasitological response to treatment. Ann Trop Med Parasitol 1997;91(3):281–96.

Amodiaquine

General Information

Amodiaquine is a Mannich base derivative related to chloroquine. While it is generally considered equivalent to chloroquine, more recent studies have shown that amodiaquine is superior to chloroquine in tackling resistant strains of *Plasmodium falciparum*, although there may be cross-resistance to chloroquine (SEDA-20, 260).

Compared with chloroquine, amodiaquine was more effective and better tolerated in outpatients with uncomplicated malaria tropica in Kenya (SEDA-20, 260).

Because of its adverse effects, amodiaquine is no longer in use in the countries of the European Union or the USA, and was dropped from malaria control programs by the WHO in 1990 (SEDA-20, 260). However, it remains in use in other areas, including Africa and Oceania (SEDA-18, 287).

Organs and Systems

Cardiovascular

Prolongation of the QT interval is a recognized effect of 4-aminoquinolines. In 20 adult Cameroonian patients with non-severe falciparum malaria treated with amodiaquine (total dose 30 mg/kg or 35 mg/kg over 3 days) there was asymptomatic sinus bradycardia ($n = 16$) and prolongation of the PQ, QRS, and QT intervals at the time of maximum cumulative concentration of drug (day 2 of treatment) (1).

Sensory systems

Corneal and conjunctival changes, which included intralysosomal membranous and amorphous inclusions in the epithelial cells, as well as abnormal retinal test responses, were reported in a man who took amodiaquine for 1 year. Follow-up over the years after withdrawal showed a reduction in the abnormalities. There are no data on possible retinal changes similar to those seen with chloroquine.

In 69 children given 35 mg/kg over 3 days (SEDA-16, 306), parasitemia was cleared in all but one case. Tolerance was good, except that there was a fairly high incidence of conjunctival hyperemia.

Hematologic

The principal reason against recommending amodiaquine for malaria prophylaxis is the reporting of agranulocytosis, occasionally associated with hepatitis (SEDA-12, 241) (SED-12, 692). Since specific IgG antibodies, which lead to leukopenia, can be detected, all this suggests that the agranulocytosis is immune-mediated.

It takes substantial doses for a couple of weeks to cause the adverse hematological effects (SEDA-16, 692) (SEDA-17, 327). If this is correct, amodiaquine could still be of use for short intensive courses of treatment in areas of chloroquine resistance.

Gastrointestinal

Gastrointestinal complaints (nausea, vomiting, diarrhea, or constipation) are not uncommon with amodiaquine (SEDA-11, 587).

Skin

Abnormal pigmentation of the palate, nail beds, and the skin of the face and neck has been reported. The duration of such pigmentation after withdrawal is unknown. The effects on the nails resemble those seen with chloroquine (SEDA-12, 692) (SEDA-12, 241).

Nails

Abnormal pigmentation of nail beds has been reported. The duration of such pigmentation after withdrawal is unknown. The effects on the nails resemble those seen with chloroquine (SEDA-12, 692) (SEDA-12, 241).

Reference

1. Ngouesse B, Basco LK, Ringwald P, Keundjian A, Blackett KN. Cardiac effects of amodiaquine and sulfadoxine-pyrimethamine in malaria-infected African patients. Am J Trop Med Hyg 2001;65(6):711–16.

Amopyroquine

General Information

Amopyroquine is a 4-aminoquinoline, structurally related to amodiaquine. It is not a new compound, but it is of renewed interest as a result of the extensive occurrence of resistance to chloroquine and the adverse effects of prophylactic amodiaquine. In a study in 152 patients with malaria, the efficacy of a 12 mg/kg, given as two intramuscular injections of 6 mg/kg 24 hours apart, was described as good (1). All the patients became apyrexial and there was clearance of parasites on day 7 in 143 cases; the nine who retained a low level of parasitemia were all children. In 50% of the cases, the parasite had been chloroquine-resistant. The drug was well tolerated, and there were no major adverse effects.

Reference

1. Gaudebout C, Pussard E, Clavier F, Gueret D, Le Bras J, Brandicourt O, Verdier F. Efficacy of intramuscular amopyroquin for treatment of *Plasmodium falciparum* malaria in the Gabon Republic. Antimicrob Agents Chemother 1993;37(5): 970–4.

Amoxapine

See also Tricyclic antidepressants

General Information

In a major review of amoxapine and its pharmacology it was concluded that it is similar in efficacy and potency to standard tricyclic compounds, with a sedative action intermediate between amitriptyline and imipramine (1).

As previously noted (SEDA-4, 21) (SEDA-5, 17), amoxapine has a tricyclic nucleus with a modified piperazine side chain and is closely related to the neuroleptic drug loxapine. In animals, amoxapine has no antiserotonergic properties and less anticholinergic activity than prototype drugs. Peak plasma concentrations are achieved in less than 2 hours, and the half-lives of the parent drug and its two active metabolites are 8, 6, and 30 hours respectively.

Overall, amoxapine appears to have some advantage over other tricyclic antidepressants: possible earlier onset of action and relative freedom from serious cardiotoxic effects. Its major drawbacks are the potential for neuroleptic adverse effects, a high incidence of seizures, deaths in overdose (2), and the possibility of long-term neurological damage.

Amoxapine is less potent than other tricyclic antidepressants, with a therapeutic dosage range of 75–600 mg/day (usually 200–400 mg/day). Clinical effects have not been consistently correlated with plasma concentrations, but amoxapine has similar efficacy to other tricyclic antidepressants in heterogeneous populations of depressed patients. Controlled comparisons have shown that its clinical profile is very similar to that of imipramine (3) and that it is somewhat less sedative than amitriptyline (4–6). In two of these studies (4,6) the results confirmed the suggestion of a somewhat earlier onset of action.

Amoxapine appears to have the same common adverse effects as other tricyclic compounds, including those attributable to anticholinergic activity. Its structural similarity to the classic neuroleptic drugs appears to confer an additional hazard of adverse effects usually found in that category of drugs, such as galactorrhea and extrapyramidal disorders (SEDA-9, 20). In a study of its potential neuroleptic properties (7), using a radioreceptor assay in vivo and using plasma drawn from patients taking neuroleptic drugs or antidepressants, amoxapine and its metabolite, 7-hydroxyamoxapine, had potent neuroleptic activity. In patients taking amoxapine, there was neuroleptic activity comparable to that in patients taking loxapine, while none of the other tricyclic antidepressants (amitriptyline, nortriptyline, imipramine, and desipramine) had this property. Further reports of adverse effects attributable to its neuroleptic profile continue to appear, including tardive dyskinesia (8,9), acute torticollis (10), and malignant neuroleptic syndrome (SEDA-16, 9) (SEDA-17, 18) (11).

Organs and Systems

Metabolism

A further reminder of the structural resemblance of amoxapine to the neuroleptic drugs has been provided by an adverse effect reported with both amoxapine and its close congener, loxapine (12).

- A 49-year-old woman with no history of diabetes was admitted in unexplained hyperglycemic coma (blood glucose 26 mmol/l) while taking lithium 1500 mg/day and loxapine 150 mg/day. She responded to insulin, but insulin responses on testing were not delayed and suggested an iatrogenic rather than a diabetic cause. The fasting glucose fell to 4.2 mmol/l after withdrawal of loxapine but continuing lithium. Two weeks later amoxapine 150 mg/day was started and she became acutely confused, with a serum glucose of 5.7 mmol/l. Two weeks after stopping amoxapine the serum glucose returned to normal.

The authors speculated that a common metabolite of both drugs, 7-hydroxyamoxapine, was responsible for the hyperglycemia, owing to its antidopaminergic properties.

Drug Administration

Drug overdose

A bleak picture has rapidly evolved for amoxapine with regard to its toxicity in overdosage. Over 18 months, 33 cases were reported from Washington, DC, and New Mexico Poison Centers (2). These cases included 5 patients who died and 12 who developed seizures. Thus, the mortality rate of 15% greatly exceeds that of 0.7% for other antidepressants in the same centers, and the seizure rate is 36% compared to 4.3%. The authors noted that "the striking CNS toxicity of amoxapine overdose with frequent, persistent, and poorly controlled seizure activity is disconcerting." In a retrospective comparison of deaths from antidepressant overdosage in Scotland, England, and Wales between 1987 and 1992, the number of deaths per million prescriptions of amoxapine was significantly higher than expected (13).

Renal damage has occurred in cases of amoxapine overdose.

- Acute renal insufficiency and rhabdomyolysis were reported in a 27-year-old man who took 1–2 g of amoxapine (14). The authors recommended aggressive volume expansion and diuresis with loop diuretics, because of the futility of hemodialysis.
- A 24-year-old man took 4 g of amoxapine and developed gross hematuria and a high serum uric acid concentration on the second day of hospitalization (15). As in previously reported cases, serum creatine phosphokinase was grossly raised. The patient remained obtunded and stuporose for 7 days but eventually recovered.

References

1. Jue SG, Dawson GW, Brogden RN. Amoxapine: a review of its pharmacology and efficacy in depressed states. Drugs 1982;24(1):1–23.
2. Litovitz TL, Troutman WG. Amoxapine overdose. Seizures and fatalities. JAMA 1983;250(8):1069–71.
3. Bagodia VN, Shah LP, Pradan PV, Gada MT. A double-blind controlled study of amoxapine and imipramine in cases of depression. Curr Ther Res Clin Exp 1979; 26:417.
4. Sethi BB, Sharma I, Singh H, Metha VK. Amoxapine and amitriptyline: a double-blind study in depressed patients. Curr Ther Res Clin Exp 1979;25:726.
5. Fruensgaard K, Hansen CE, Korsgaard S, Nymgaard K, Vaag UH. Amoxapine versus amitriptyline in endogenous depression. A double-blind study. Acta Psychiatr Scand 1979;59(5):502–8.
6. Kaumeier HS, Haase HJ. A double-blind comparison between amoxapine and amitriptyline in depressed in-patients. Int J Clin Pharmacol Ther Toxicol 1980;18(4):177–84.
7. Cohen BM, Harris PQ, Altesman RI, Cole JO. Amoxapine: neuroleptic as well as antidepressant? Am J Psychiatry 1982;139(9):1165–7.
8. Huang CC. Persistent tardive dyskinesia associated with amoxapine therapy. Am J Psychiatry 1986;143(8):1069–70.
9. Price WA, Giannini AJ. Withdrawal dyskinesia following amoxapine therapy. J Clin Psychiatry 1986;47(6):329–30.
10. Matot JP, Ziegler M, Olie JP, Rondot P. Amoxapine. Un antidepresseur responsable d'effets secondaires extrapyramidaux? [Amoxapine. An antidepressant responsible for extrapyramidal side effects?] Therapie 1985;40(3):187–90.
11. Burch EA Jr., Downs J. Development of neuroleptic malignant syndrome during simultaneous amoxapine treatment and alprazolam discontinuation. J Clin Psychopharmacol 1987;7(1):55–6.
12. Tollefson G, Lesar T. Nonketotic hyperglycemia associated with loxapine and amoxapine: case report. J Clin Psychiatry 1983;44(9):347–8.
13. Henry JA, Alexander CA, Sener EK. Relative mortality from overdose of antidepressants. BMJ 1995;310(6974): 221–4.
14. Jennings AE, Levey AS, Harrington JT. Amoxapine-associated acute renal failure. Arch Intern Med 1983;143(8):1525–7.
15. Thompson M, Dempsey W. Hyperuricemia, renal failure, and elevated creatine phosphokinase after amoxapine overdose. Clin Pharm 1983;2(6):579–81.

Amphetamines

See also Individual agents

General Information

Note on spelling

In International Non-proprietary Names the digraph -ph- is usually replaced by -f-, although usage is not consistent, and -ph- is used at the beginnings of some drug names (for example, compare fenfluramine and phentermine) or when a name that beings with a ph- is modified by a prefix (for example, chlorphentermine). For the amphetamines we have used the following spellings: amfetamine, benzfetamine, dexamfetamine, metamfetamine (methylamphetamine), and methylenedioxymetamfetamine (ecstasy).

Pharmacology and general adverse effects

Amfetamine is a sympathomimetic compound derived from phenylethylamine. However, the word amphetamines has become generic for the entire group of related substances, including benzfetamine, dexamfetamine, metamfetamine, and methylenedioxymetamfetamine (MDMA, ecstasy). Metamfetamine, a popular drug of abuse, is also known as "speed," "meth," "chalk," "crank," "ice," "crystal," or "glass." Other amfetamine-like drugs include fenfluramine (used as an appetite suppressant) and methylphenidate (used in narcolepsy and attention deficit hyperactivity disorder (ADHD)). When it was first introduced, one of the most frequent uses of amfetamine was as an anorexigenic agent in the treatment of obesity. A number of anorectic agents, many of them related to amfetamine, have since been manufactured. Most are stimulants of the central nervous system; in descending order of approximate stimulatory potency, they are dexamfetamine, phentermine, chlorphentermine, mazindol, amfepramone (diethylpropion), and fenfluramine.

The amfetamine epidemic of the 1960s and early 1970s has now been superseded by cocaine abuse in the USA and many other Western countries. Realization of the risk of abuse and of dependence has led to the present attitude that there may be only a restricted place for amphetamines in medicine. Perhaps low-dose, short-term use in combating fatigue and altering depressed mood could be justified, but only for specific indications and under continuous medical supervision. However, in the USA there has been a resurgence of metamfetamine abuse on the West coast and in the Southwest and Midwest. This geographical distribution is thought to reflect the traffic from Mexico of ephedrine, a precursor for the synthesis of metamfetamine in the quick-bake method. Because primitive labs can be established in trailers, the spread to adjacent locals has been very rapid, resulting in escalation of migrating epidemics.

Adverse effects of "catecholaminergic stimulants," such as amfetamine and cocaine, fall into several categories, based on dose, time after dose, chronicity of use, and pattern of use/abuse (for example 4–5 day bingeing episodes). Adverse effects include not only responses during the period of use but also intermediate and long-term residual effects after withdrawal. For example, in some abusers once an amfetamine psychosis has developed with chronic abuse, only one or two moderate doses are required to induce the full-blown psychosis in its original form, even long after withdrawal (1). This is also evidenced by the precipitous slide to severe re-addiction in former abusers who are re-introduced to stimulants.

Even with therapeutic use of stimulants, usually in moderate doses, careful monitoring for emergent psychosis, agitation, and abuse is important. Periodic checks for monodelusional syndromes are important with doses in the mid-to-high range (2).

The use of amfetamine-type stimulants for depression, fatigue, and psychasthenia has fallen into disfavor since the early 1970s, because of the potential for abuse and the low rates of success, especially after tolerance is established. However, there have been reports and reviews of successes in carefully selected groups of patients (3–5). The underlying symptoms of patients who respond to stimulants are mild anhedonia, lack of mental and physical energy, easy fatiguability, and low self-esteem, but in the absence of the marked depressed mood disturbance, guilt, and hopelessness that are associated with major depression. Examples include patients with dysthymic disorders, medically ill patients (especially after a stroke), depressed patients, hospitalized cancer patients, and patients with significant cardiovascular disorders, all of whom can have anergia and easy fatiguability. HIV-related neuropsychiatric symptoms, including depression, respond to psychostimulants (4–6). Withdrawn apathetic geriatric patients without major dementia have positive responses (7). General adverse effects, such as tachycardia and agitation, are relatively mild and all reverse on withdrawal (SEDA-17, 1). The combination of stimulants with monoamine oxidase inhibitors in treatment-resistant depressed patients has been reported (8). However, this use should be restricted to patients in whom there is careful monitoring by specialists, because of the potential for hypertensive crisis.

The relative reinforcing effects or abuse potential of these drugs is thought to be related to their potency in releasing dopamine from nerve terminals, compared with serotonin release. Amfetamine, metamfetamine, and phenmetrazine are potent dopamine releasers with high euphoriant and stimulant properties, whereas the compounds with halide substitution in the phenol ring, for example chlorphentermine, are more potent releasers of serotonin and have greater sedative action in anorectic doses. Thus, in summary, those drugs with relatively strong serotonergic to dopaminergic releasing properties seem to provide anorectic effects without euphoria, except at high doses, and might be considered first in any patient who has potential for abuse (2,9,10).

In a study of extended treatment (15 months) of ADHD, amfetamine was clearly superior to placebo in reducing inattention, hyperactivity, and other disruptive behavioral problems. The treatment failure rate was considerably lower and the time to treatment failure was longer in the treated group; adverse effects were few and relatively mild (11).

There is an association between the illicit use of metamfetamine and traumatic accidents. A retrospective review of trauma patients in California showed that metamfetamine rates doubled between 1989 and 1994, while cocaine showed a minimal increase and alcohol a fall. Metamfetamine-positive patients were most likely to be Caucasian or Hispanic and were most commonly injured in motor vehicle collisions. The authors recommended intervention strategies, similar to those used for preventing alcohol consumption and driving, in order to minimize morbidity and mortality (12).

Traumatic shock can be complicated by metamfetamine intoxication (13). Identifying the cause of shock is a key step in the management of patients with severe injuries. This is a challenge, because shock is occasionally caused by more than one mechanism; among the many causes, metabolic derangement attributable to drug abuse should be considered, and masked metabolic acidosis may be a clue to metamfetamine intoxication (14). With the increased emergence of metamfetamine abuse, clinicians should consider it in the differential diagnosis of any patient exhibiting violence, psychosis, seizures, or cardiovascular abnormalities.

Organs and Systems

Cardiovascular

Tachycardia, dysrhythmias, and a rise in blood pressure have been described after the administration of centrally acting sympathomimetic amines. Amfetamine acutely administered to men with a history of amfetamine abuse enhanced the pressor effects of tyramine and noradrenaline, while continuous amfetamine led to tolerance of the pressor response to tyramine. As with intravenous amphetamines, cardiomyopathy, cardiomegaly, and pulmonary edema have been reported with smoking of crystal metamfetamine (15–17).

The cardiovascular response to an oral dose of d-amfetamine 0.5 mg/kg has been determined in 81 subjects with schizophrenia, 8 healthy controls who took amfetamine, and 7 subjects with schizophrenia who took a placebo (18). Blood pressure increased in both amphetamine groups, whereas placebo had no effect. However, pulse rate did not change in the schizophrenic group and only increased after 3 hours in the controls. Intramuscular haloperidol 5 mg produced a more rapid fall in systolic blood pressure in six subjects, compared with 12 subjects who did not receive haloperidol. The authors concluded that increased blood pressure due to amfetamine may have a dopaminergic component. They also suggested that haloperidol may be beneficial in the treatment of hypertensive crises caused by high doses of amfetamine or metamfetamine.

Two cases of myocardial infarction after the use of amfetamine have been reported (19,20).

- A 34-year-old man who smoked a pack of cigarettes a day took amfetamine for mild obesity. He developed an acute myocardial infarction 1 week later. Echocardiography showed inferior left ventricular hypokinesia and a left ventricular ejection fraction of 50%. Coronary cineangiography showed normal coronary arteries but confirmed the inferior left ventricular hypokinesia. Blood and urine toxicology were positive only for amfetamine.
- A 31-year-old man developed generalized discomfort after injecting four doses of amfetamine and metamfetamine over 48 hours, but no chest pain or tightness or shortness of breath. Electrocardiography showed inverted T-waves and left bundle branch block. Echocardiography showed reduced anterior wall motion.

The authors reviewed other reported cases of myocardial infarction associated with amphetamines. The patients were in their mid-thirties and most were men. The interval from the use of amphetamines to the onset of symptoms varied from a few minutes to years. No specific myocardial site was implicated. Coronary angiography in most cases showed non-occlusion. The cause of myocardial ischemia in these cases was uncertain, even though coronary artery spasm followed by thrombus formation was considered the most likely underlying mechanism. Some have suggested that electrocardiographic and biochemical cardiac marker testing should be considered in every patient, with or without symptoms suggesting acute coronary syndrome, after the use of amphetamines. Others have suggested that calcium channel blockers may play an important role in the treatment of myocardial infarction due to amfetamine use or abuse. In one patient, administration of beta-blockers caused anginal pain, suggesting that they should be avoided. All the patients except one had a good outcome.

Vertebral artery dissection has been described in a previously healthy man with a 3-year history of daily oral amfetamine abuse (21).

- A healthy 40-year-old right-handed man presented with a 3-day history of an occipital headache and imbalance. He had a 3-year history of daily oral amfetamine abuse with escalating quantities, the last occasion being 12 hours before the onset of the symptoms. He had a history of "speed" abuse and a 20-pack-year history of tobacco use. He had mild right arm dysmetria without ataxia. His brain CT scan without contrast was

normal. He then developed nausea, vomiting, visual loss, and progressive obtundation. He had hypertension (160/90 mmHg), bilateral complete visual loss, right lower facial weakness, mild dysarthria without tongue deviation, divergent gaze attenuated by arousal, bilateral truncal and appendicular dysmetria with inability to stand and walk, and generalized symmetrical hyperreflexia with extensor plantar reflexes. His urine screen was positive for metamfetamine. A brain MRI scan showed infarction of both medial temporal lobes, the left posteromedial thalamus, and the right superior and left inferior cerebellum. Magnetic resonance angiography and fat saturation MRI showed reduced flow in the left vertebral artery and a ring of increased signal within its lumen, consistent with hematoma and dissection. He was treated with anticoagulants and made a partial recovery.

Since this patient had no known risk factors for vertebral artery dissection and had abused amfetamine daily for 3 years with escalating amounts, an association between metamfetamine and vertebral artery dissection cannot be excluded. The local and systemic vascular impacts of amfetamine could have contributed to initial changes (along with smoking), resulting in dissection.

Of the other central stimulants, aminorex, doxapram, fenfluramine, and fenfluramine plus phentermine can cause chronic pulmonary hypertension, as can chlorphentermine, phentermine, phenmetrazine, and D-norpseudoephedrine (SED-9, 8). A genetic predisposition may be involved (SED-9, 8). Pulmonary hypertension may develop or be diagnosed a long time after the drug has been withdrawn.

Nervous system

Metamfetamine toxicity in infants can mimic scorpion (*Centruroides sculpturatus*) envenomation (22,23). However, the neurotoxic effect of envenomation can be distinguished from amfetamine-induced toxicity by the presence of cholinergic stimulation in scorpion envenomation, producing hypersalivation, bronchospasm, fasciculation of the tongue, purposeless motor agitation, involuntary and conjugate slow and roving eye movements, and often extraocular muscle dysfunction (24). Failure of the antivenin would bring scorpion neurotoxicity into great question (25).

Concentrations of metamfetamine and its metabolite amfetamine were measured in autopsied brain regions of 14 human metamfetamine abusers (26). There was no evidence of variation in the regional distribution of amphetamines in the brain. Post-mortem redistribution of metamfetamine in the heart and lung has been reported before, although peripheral blood concentrations appear to remain constant (27,28).

Stereotyped behavior

A type of automatic behavior, which can continue for hours, has been observed in addicts who inject large doses of central nervous system stimulants. Dyskinesias can occur, with strange facial and tongue movements or jerky motions of the arms and legs and a never-ending repetition of certain actions. Such stereotyped activity is induced in laboratory animals with high doses of amfetamine.

Amphetamines and brain damage

The question of whether amphetamines in large doses can cause permanent brain damage has repeatedly been raised by animal studies (29,30), but definitive studies in man have not been performed. Vasculitis of large elastic vessels, found in chronic animal studies, has been reported to involve the internal carotid artery in man (31); intravenous administration is secondarily implicated. In man and animals, behavioral changes continue for several months after withdrawal of amphetamines; chronic residual changes have been reported mainly in monoaminergic neurons or terminals, either as structural changes or as residual depletion of monoamines and synthesizing enzymes (32). In post-mortem studies (33,34) chronic metamfetamine abusers had significantly lower concentrations of dopamine, tyrosine hydroxylase, and dopamine transporters in the caudate and putamen. It has been suggested that the reduced dopamine concentrations (up to 50% of control), even if not indicative of neurotoxicity, are consistent with amotivational changes reported by metamfetamine abusers after withdrawal (33).

Metamfetamine-induced neurotoxicity in animals, especially involving effects on the mitochondrial membrane potential and electron transport chain and subsequent apoptotic cascade, has been comprehensively reviewed (35). Metamfetamine increases the activity of dopamine, mainly by inhibiting the dopamine transporter. However, this does not explain why psychosis persists even when the metamfetamine is no longer present in the body (36). Chronic metamfetamine use has been reported to reduce dopamine transporter density in the caudate/putamen and nucleus accumbens. However, previous studies have been criticized for not controlling for other drug use.

Dopamine transporter density in the brain has been investigated during a period of abstinence in 11 metamfetamine monodrug users and nine healthy subjects, all men (37). The dopamine transporter density of metamfetamine users was significantly lower in the caudate/putamen, nucleus accumbens, and prefrontal cortex than in the controls. The severity of psychiatric symptoms correlated with the duration of metamfetamine use. The reduction in dopamine transporter density in the caudate/putamen and nucleus accumbens was significantly associated with the duration of metamfetamine use and closely related to the severity of persistent psychiatric symptoms. The reduction in dopamine transporters may be long lasting, even if metamfetamine is withdrawn.

Only some metamfetamine users develop psychosis, not all (36). In laboratory animals, metamfetamine is toxic to dopamine terminals. In 15 subjects (six men and nine women, mean age 32 years), who met the criteria for metamfetamine abuse, and 18 healthy volunteers (12 men and six women), there was a significant reduction in the number of dopamine transporters in detoxified metamfetamine abusers compared with controls (mean values of 28% in the caudate and 21% in the putamen) (38). This was associated with poor motor and memory performance. The reductions in dopamine transporters in the metamfetamine abusers were smaller than those found in patients with Parkinson's disease and occurred in subjects who had been abstinent for 11 months. Since significant reductions in dopamine transporters occur with both age

and metamfetamine use, it is possible that metamfetamine will be associated with a higher risk of parkinsonian symptoms in abusers later in life.

Glucose metabolism in the brain has been studied using positron emission tomography after administration of ^{18}F-fluorodeoxyglucose, to look for evidence of functional changes in regions other than those innervated by dopamine neurons in 15 detoxified metamfetamine abusers and 21 controls (39). Whole-brain metabolism in the metamfetamine abusers was 14% higher than in the controls. The difference was largest in the parietal cortex (20%), but there was significantly lower metabolism in the thalamus (17%) and striatum (12% caudate and 6% putamen). The authors suggested that metamfetamine, in doses abused by humans, causes long-lasting metabolic changes in brain regions connected with dopamine pathways, but also in areas that are not innervated by dopamine.

The effects of protracted abstinence on loss of dopamine transporters in the striatum in five metamfetamine abusers have been evaluated during short-term abstinence and then retested during protracted abstinence (12–17 months) (40). The dopamine transporters increased in number, providing hope for effective treatment; however, this regeneration was not sufficient to provide complete functional recovery, as measured by neuropsychological tests.

Chronic amfetamine abusers, chronic opiate abusers, and patients with focal lesions of the orbital prefrontal cortex or dorsal lateral/medial prefrontal cortex were subjected to a computerized decision-making task, in order to compare their capacity for making decisions (41). Chronic amfetamine abusers made suboptimal decisions (correlated with years of abuse) and deliberated significantly longer before making their choices. The opiate abusers had only the second of these behavioral changes. Both the suboptimal choices and the increased deliberation times were also evident in patients with damage to the orbital frontal prefrontal cortex but not other areas. These data are consistent with the hypothesis that chronic amfetamine abusers have similar decision-making deficits to those seen after focal damage to the orbital frontal prefrontal cortex.

The use of proton magnetic resonance scanning (^{1}H MRS) in detecting long-term cerebral metabolite abnormalities in abstinent metamfetamine users has been studied in 26 subjects (13 men) with a history of metamfetamine dependence (mean age 33 years) and 24 healthy subjects with no history of drug dependence (42). The neuronal marker N-acetylaspartate was reduced by 6% in the frontal white matter and by 5% in the basal ganglia of the abstinent metamfetamine users. N-acetylaspartate is a marker for mature neurons, and reduced N-acetylaspartate is thought to indicate reduced neuronal density or neuronal content. According to the authors, these findings suggest neuronal loss or persistent neuronal damage in the absence of significant brain atrophy in metamfetamine users. They speculated that these abnormalities may underlie the persistent abnormal forms of behavior, such as violence, psychosis, and personality changes, seen in some individuals months or even years after their last drug use. Metamfetamine users in the study also had increased concentrations of choline-containing compounds and myoinositol in the frontal gray matter. Myoinositol is a glial cell marker, while the increase in choline-containing compounds reflects increased cell membrane turnover. Thus, these increases in the frontal cortex in drug users may have reflected glial proliferation (astrocytosis). The authors suggested that the finding of reduced N-acetylaspartate accompanied by increased myoinositol, which has been observed in many active brain disorders, indicated glial proliferation in response to neuronal injury. However, they noted that neurotoxicity may not be present in subjects who use amounts of the drugs that are much lower than the amounts used by the chronic abusers they studied. They suggested that future studies should observe whether treatments or long periods of abstinence could reverse these abnormalities.

These findings have given further support to an earlier observation of long-term neurotoxicity associated with MDMA (ecstasy) in animals (SEDA-14, 3). However, it is uncertain whether the reported abnormalities suggestive of neuronal damage are reversible despite continued treatment or beyond 21 months of abstinence.

Dyskinesias

Although controversial, there is a growing consensus that stimulants can provoke, cause, or exacerbate Gilles de la Tourette's syndrome (SEDA-7, 10), based on the observation that stimulants such as the amphetamines, methylphenidate, and pemoline facilitate dopamine retention in the synaptic cleft. There is much evidence that in children with ADHD vulnerable to Tourette's syndrome, stimulants exacerbate motor and phonic tics (43). These studies suggest that Tourette's syndrome and a family history of dyskinesias should be contraindications to stimulant use. However, there is virtually no evidence that stimulants in clinically appropriate doses provoke Tourette's syndrome, and it has been suggested that dyskinesias are a function of high doses (44). Nevertheless, patients taking stimulants should be carefully examined periodically for dyskinesias. It is not known whether structural changes in the central nervous system accompany stimulant-induced dyskinesias.

Stroke

Intracerebral hemorrhage associated with amfetamine has been reported for more than five decades. Eight cases were associated with amfetamine over a period of 3.5 years (45). All had undergone head CT scans and cerebral digital subtraction angiography. Seven had a parenchymal hematoma, three in the frontal lobe and one each in the parietal lobe, frontoparietal region, temporal lobe, and brain stem. One patient had a subarachnoid hemorrhage. The time from exposure to onset of symptoms ranged from less than 10 minutes to about 2 months (median 1 day). The authors reviewed the literature and found 37 other cases. They observed that young people, mean age 28 years, were at high risk. While most were repeat abusers, one-third claimed to be first time or infrequent users. Intracerebral hemorrhage was seen with all routes of drug use, 57% from oral use, 34% from intravenous use, and 5% after inhalation. Of those who had a CT scan, 84% had a proven intracerebral

hemorrhage, three had a subarachnoid hemorrhage, and one had a brainstem hemorrhage. In one patient, with a negative CT scan, the diagnosis of subarachnoid hemorrhage was confirmed by lumbar puncture. In 35 patients who had angiography, 20 were normal or showed only mass effect from a hematoma, 16 had vasculitic beading, and 1 had an arteriovenous malformation. Seven patients died and only 14 had a good recovery.

- A previously healthy 16-year-old schoolboy had mesencephalic ischemia, most probably caused by vasospasm, after combined abuse of amfetamine and cocaine (46). There was a close temporal relation between intake of the drug and the onset of symptoms. Thus, combining these drugs, even in small amounts, may be harmful.

Psychological, psychiatric

Amphetamines release monoamines from the brain and thereby stimulate noradrenergic, serotonergic, and particularly dopaminergic receptors. Under certain circumstances this leads to psychosis and compulsive behavior, as well as auditory hallucinations similar to those experienced in paranoid schizophrenia. In addition, amphetamines cause an acute toxic psychosis with visual hallucinations, usually after one or two extremely large doses (47).

When an amfetamine is taken, even in a therapeutic dose, most people experience a sensation of enhanced energy or vitality, which, with repetitive administration, follows different patterns. Most often euphoria will develop, usually with a sense of heightened function or perception, and occasionally compulsive behavior as well as hallucinogenic delusions. Dysphoria occurs in some (especially older) individuals. The euphoric effect may enhance craving for amfetamine, and repeated reinforcement can lead to conditioned drug responses, which may facilitate dependence. Progression to severe dependence depends highly on individual vulnerability, the circumstances, the setting, the pattern of use, and especially escalation to high-dose patterns of use. Although most people probably use amphetamines for the original reason they were prescribed, and do not escalate the dosage, a significant proportion do, highlighting the abuse potential. The amphetamines are sometimes used recreationally for years in moderate doses. However, once inhalation and intravenous administration or higher doses are used, a "high-dose transition" into abuse usually occurs, and the capacity for low-dose occasional use is lost, presumably, forever (see the sections on Drug abuse and Drug dependence in this monograph).

Personality degeneration

In a double-blind, placebo-controlled, short-term study there was significant deterioration of personality in five of 26 children treated with dexamfetamine (48).

Phobias

Social phobia has been attributed to amfetamine (49).

- A 26-year-old woman reported flushing, sweating, palpitation, and shortness of breath, in a range of social situations. She was described as a confident and extroverted woman, with no history of psychiatric problems.

She reported daily oral consumption of street amfetamine 1.6 g. At the time of assessment, she had given up her work. Initially, she felt good while taking the drug, but more recently she had been using it to "get going"; there were no symptoms of psychosis or affective disorder.

The authors speculated that dopaminergic dysfunction, reported by some to underlie social phobia, could have resulted in this case from chronic amfetamine-related striatal dopamine depletion.

Psychoses

Psychotic reactions in people taking amphetamines were first reported many years ago and the question was posed whether it was due to the amphetamines or to co-existing and exacerbated paranoid schizophrenia. In one study, most of the psychotic symptoms remitted before the excretion of amines had fallen to its normal basal value (SED-9, 8). The psychotic syndrome was indistinguishable from paranoid schizophrenia, with short periods of disorientation, and could occur after a single dose (many had taken the equivalent of some 500 mg of amfetamine or metamfetamine orally) with or without simultaneous alcohol, and was most pronounced in addicts (SED-9, 9). Amfetamine psychosis was also seen in 14 people in Australia (1); the predominant hallucinations were visual, which is unusual for schizophrenia (SED-8, 11). Similarly, in contrast to schizophrenia, vision was the primary sensory mode in thinking disorders and body schema distortions in 25 amfetamine addicts (50).

In other studies, volunteers previously dependent on amphetamines were dosed to a level at which amfetamine psychosis was produced, in order to examine the mechanism of action and pharmacokinetics of amfetamine and its possible relation to schizophrenia (51,52). Psychosis was induced by moderately high doses of amfetamine and the psychotic symptoms were often a replication of the chronic amfetamine psychosis, raising the question of whether the establishment of chronic stimulant psychosis leaves residual vulnerability to psychosis precipitated by stimulants. The mechanism might be similar to that which operates in the reverse tolerance that has been seen in experimental animals (53). In some cases an underlying psychosis can be precipitated; an increase in schizophrenic symptoms (SED-8, 12) was observed in 17 actively ill schizophrenic patients after a single injection of amfetamine.

Amfetamine psychosis is relatively rare in children, even in hyperactive children taking large doses of amfetamine; amfetamine psychosis has been reported in an 8-year-old child with a hyperkinetic syndrome (SED-8, 12). Large doses of amfetamine can cause disruption of thinking, but amfetamine psychosis is not usually accompanied by the degree of disorganization normally seen in schizophrenia (SED-9, 8).

Increased sensitivity to stress may be related to spontaneous recurrence of metamfetamine psychosis, triggering flashbacks. Stressful experiences, together with metamfetamine use, induce sensitization to stress associated with noradrenergic hyperactivity, involving increased dopamine release (54,55). This hypothesis has been investigated by determining plasma noradrenaline metabolite concentrations in 26 flashbackers (patients with spontaneous recurrence of metamfetamine psychosis) (11 taking neuroleptic drugs before and during the study and 15 during the course of the study), 18 non-flashbackers with a history of metamfetamine psychosis, 8 with persistent metamfetamine psychosis, and 34 controls (23 metamfetamine users and 11 non-users). The 26 flashbackers had had stressful events and/or metamfetamine-induced, fear-related, psychotic symptoms during previous metamfetamine use. Mild psychosocial stressors then triggered flashbacks. During flashbacks, plasma noradrenaline concentrations increased markedly. Flashbackers with a history of stressful events, whether or not they had had fear-related symptoms, had a further increase in 3-methoxytyramine concentrations. Thus, robust noradrenergic hyperactivity, involving increased dopamine release in response to mild stress, may predispose to further episodes of flashbacks. The authors pointed out the limitations of their study: (a) plasma noradrenaline concentrations do not accurately reflect central monoamine neurotransmitter function; (b) raised noradrenaline concentrations may reflect heightened autonomic arousal secondary to stress or anxiety; (c) the neuroleptic drugs used may have altered the concentrations of noradrenaline and 3-methoxytyramine; and (d) the study was retrospective and carried out in women in prison.

A paranoid hallucinatory state similar to schizophrenia has been reported in women with a history of metamfetamine abuse in a study of flashbacks in 81 female inmates in Japan (56). Details of symptoms of initial metamfetamine psychosis, stressful experiences, and patterns of abuse were obtained. Plasma monoamine concentrations were also measured during flashback states and in control abusers who had never experienced them. The researchers reported that concreteness of abstract thought and impaired goal-directed thought characteristic of schizophrenia was not usually seen in metamfetamine-induced psychosis. Moreover, it was the use of metamfetamine and not a severe stressor that caused the initial psychotic state, but the flashbacks appeared to be due to mild environmental stressors. The authors described this pattern as "spontaneous psychosis due to previous metamfetamine psychosis." They also observed that plasma concentrations of noradrenaline were significantly higher in women with flashbacks both during flashbacks and during remissions. This suggests a possible role of noradrenergic hyperactivity in sensitivity to mild stress and susceptibility to flashbacks. Furthermore, these noradrenergic findings could be used to predict relapse to a paranoid hallucinatory state in schizophrenia.

Chlorpromazine has been used to treat amfetamine psychosis due to acute poisoning in children who did not respond to barbiturates (57).

Management

Reports have suggested that atypical antipsychotic drugs, such as risperidone (58–60) and olanzapine (61), can be effective in the treatment of acute and residual metamfetamine-induced psychosis. Moreover, adherence to olanzapine for about 8 weeks also effectively controlled cravings for metamfetamine. Rigorous controlled studies are needed to establish the therapeutic efficacy of atypical antipsychotic drugs in the treatment of the psychosis and cravings of metamfetamine addiction.

- A 76-year-old woman, who had taken dexamfetamine since the age of 28 years for narcolepsy, developed an acute schizophreniform psychosis with paranoid delusions and auditory hallucinations. She was initially treated with sulpiride while continuing to take dexamfetamine. Five months later, sulpiride was withdrawn, and her psychotic symptoms recurred. She was given risperidone 3 mg/day and continued to take dexamfetamine 15 mg/day.
- A 24-year-old man, with a history of intravenous metamfetamine abuse since the age of 19 years, developed psychotic symptoms characterized by auditory hallucinations and persecutory delusions. He had no insight and was given haloperidol and levomepromazine. His symptoms disappeared after 4 months of treatment and he then stopped using metamfetamine. A year and a half later, "odd ideas" recurred, and he became anxious but had insight. He was treated with bromperidol 9 mg/day for 6 months, but the odd ideas persisted. On referral, he was found to fulfil the criteria for obsessive-compulsive disorder according to DSM-IV. No abused substances, including metamfetamine, were identified in his urine. Risperidone 2 mg/day was started and then increased to 5 mg/day. After 3 weeks, the intrusive thoughts and symptoms of "anxious-restless state" gradually subsided and eventually disappeared. His symptoms recurred within a week of stopping risperidone and resolved on reintroduction.

Metabolism

Amphetamines can cause retardation of growth (height and weight) in hyperactive children (SED-9, 9).

Hematologic

Acute myeloblastic leukemia occurred in a 24-year-old man who had taken massive doses of amfetamine for more than 2 years (SED-8, 13).

Mouth and teeth

Dental wear has been evaluated prospectively in metamfetamine users at an urban university hospital (62). Information was collected from 43 patients (26 men, 40 tobacco smokers), mean age 39 years, who admitted to having used metamfetamine for more than 1 year. Patients who regularly snorted metamfetamine had higher "tooth-wear" scores for anterior maxillary teeth than patients who injected, smoked, or ingested metamfetamine. The authors suggested that the anatomy of the blood supply to this area possibly explained the association of the regional differences in tooth wear with snorted metamfetamine. The anterior maxillary teeth and the nasal mucosa have a common blood supply. Thus, snorting may cause vasoconstriction, impairing the blood supply both to the nasal mucosa as well as the teeth.

Skin

The severe form of erythema multiforme known as toxic epidermal necrolysis has been attributed to a mixture of dexamfetamine and ephedrine (63).

- A 27-year-old woman developed peripheral target plaques, papules, blisters, and lip erosions, consistent with erythema multiforme, 9 days after using "speed" (dexamfetamine and ephedrine), and 3 days later developed widespread lesions with large areas of blistering affecting 40% of her body surface area. She was given intravenous ciclosporin and improved within 24 hours.

Musculoskeletal

There may be an association between metamfetamine abuse and rhabdomyolysis. In a retrospective review of 367 patients with rhabdomyolysis, 166 were positive for metamfetamine (64). They had higher mean initial and lower mean peak activities of creatine phosphokinase. There was no significant difference in the incidence of acute renal insufficiency. The authors suggested screening all patients with rhabdomyolysis of unclear cause for metamfetamine and measuring creatine phosphokinase activity.

Sexual function

Reports of the effects of amfetamine on sexual behavior refer variously to unchanged, reduced, mixed, and heightened sexual performance, but long-term abusers often have sexual dysfunction (SED-9, 9).

Immunologic

An anaphylactic reaction after the injection of crushed tablets equivalent to 45 mg of amfetamine occurred in a young woman; in others injected with the same solution and at the same time there were no adverse effects (SED-9, 8). The reaction may have involved amfetamine or excipients. Scleroderma is a potential consequence of various stimulants used for appetite control (65).

Infection risk

- A 34-year-old woman who had taken intranasal metamfetamine weekly for 15 years developed osteomyelitis of the frontal bone and a subperiosteal abscess. The authors proposed that this was due to chronic abuse of metamfetamine (66).

A rare case of Pott's puffy tumor, anterior extension of a frontal sinus infection that results in frontal bone osteomyelitis and subperiosteal abscess, has been associated with metamfetamine use (67).

- A 34-year-old woman presented with a 9-day history of fever, chills, photophobia, and neck pain. Nine months earlier, she had developed a swelling on her forehead, which enlarged and spontaneously drained pus. Over the next weeks, a fistula developed at the site of the swelling, accompanied by an intermittent bloody purulent drainage that lasted for about 9 months. She had either inhaled metamfetamine or had used it intranasally weekly for 15 years and reported continued use immediately before the development of the forehead lesion. She had a sinocutaneous fistula in the midline of the forehead, with seropurulent discharge but no local erythema or tenderness. A CT scan of the head showed complete opacification of all sinuses, with a 1 cm connection between the anterior frontal sinus and the skin. Cultures grew *Streptococcus milleri* and *Candida albicans*. She responded to extensive medical and surgical treatment.

The authors proposed that intranasal metamfetamine had contributed to chronic sinus inflammation and subsequent complications. Furthermore, the vasoconstriction induced by metamfetamine in the mucosal vessels may have resulted in ischemic injury to the sinus mucosa, providing an environment conducive to bacterial growth.

Death

There has been a retrospective investigation of metamfetamine-related fatalities during a 5-year period (1994–1998) in Southern Osaka city in Japan (68). Among 646 autopsy cases, methamphetamine was detected in 15, most of whom were men in their late thirties. The cause and manner of death were methamphetamine poisoning ($n = 4$), homicide ($n = 4$), accidental falls and aspiration from drug abuse ($n = 4$), death in an accidental fire, myocardial infarction, and cerebral hemorrhage (one each). Blood metamfetamine concentrations were 23–170 µmol/l in fatal poisoning, 4.4–38 µmol/l in deaths from other extrinsic causes, and 14–22 µmol/l in cardiovascular and cerebrovascular accidents. The common complications were cardiomyopathy, cerebral perivasculitis, and liver cirrhosis/interstitial hepatitis. The general profile of patients reported in this series compares with that of a previous study from Taiwan (SEDA-24, 2).

Long-Term Effects

Drug abuse

The most important problem encountered with amphetamines is abuse and the development of dependence. The most rapid amfetamine epidemic occurred in Japan after World War II, where there had been little or no previous abuse (69). Although a high proportion of amfetamine users probably already have emotional and social difficulties, sustained abuse can result in serious psychiatric complications, ranging from severe personality disorders to chronic psychoses (70,71). Whereas signs of intense physical dependence are not thought to occur (SED-9, 9), withdrawal may be associated with intense depression (SED-9, 9) (72), and relapses in psychiatric disorders have often been noted. Some countries in which the problem became widespread banned amphetamines, and Australia restricted their use to narcolepsy and behavioral disorders in children. Amfetamine dependence developed into a serious problem in the USA (and to a lesser extent in the UK), where it followed the typical pattern of drug dependence (SED-9, 7, 10).

Continuing critical re-assessment of the usefulness versus the harmfulness of amphetamines has led to further restrictions in their use (SED-9, 10). They have been subjected to rigid legislative control in many countries, accompanied by recommendations that they should not be prescribed. The World Health Organization and the United Nations have also stressed the need for strict control of amphetamines (SED-9, 10) (73).

There is a high prevalence of the use of amfetamine-like drugs in Brazil, particularly among women, owing to the "culture of slimness as a symbol of beauty" (74). Of 2370 subjects in São Paulo and Brasilia, 72% had already undergone from one to more than 10 previous courses of treatment, usually with amfetamine-like anorectic drugs. Over half of them had taken amfetamine-like drugs in compound formulations containing four or more substances, such as benzodiazepines and/or laxatives, diuretics, and thyroid hormones. There were adverse reactions to the amfetamine-like drugs in 86% and 37% sought medical advice; 3.9% required hospitalization. The authors argued the need for more rigorous legislation and enforcement strategies to stop such misuse of drugs.

Further evidence concerning increased metamfetamine abuse has come from Taiwan (75). Between 1991 and 1996, of 3958 deaths with autopsies, 244 were related to metamfetamine (mean age 31 years, 73% men). The manner of death was natural (13%), accidental (59%), suicidal (11%), homicidal (14%), or uncertain (3%). Owing to the endemic problem and public hazard created by illicit metamfetamine abuse, the authors urged stronger antidrug programs.

Drug dependence

The role of dopamine in the addictive process has been explored (76). The authors raised the possibility that the orbitoprefrontal cortex is linked to compulsive drug abuse. They recruited 15 metamfetamine users and 20 non-drug user controls. The metamfetamine abusers had significantly fewer dopamine D_2 receptors than the controls. There was an association between lower numbers of dopamine D_2 receptors and metabolism in the orbitofrontal cortex in the metamfetamine users. These findings are similar to those observed in cocaine, alcohol, and heroin users. The authors suggested that D_2 receptor-mediated dysregulation of the orbitofrontal cortex could be a common mechanism underlying loss of control and compulsive abuse of drugs.

Second-Generation Effects

Pregnancy

In pregnant women who reported for prenatal care between 1959 and 1966 there was an excess of oral clefts in the offspring of mothers who had taken amphetamines in the first 56 days from their last menstrual period, but this was considered to be either a chance finding or one element in a multifactorial situation (SED-9, 9).

Teratogenicity

The possible neurotoxic effect of prenatal metamfetamine exposure on the developing brain has been studied using ^1H magnetic resonance spectroscopy in 12 metamfetamine-exposed children and 14 age-matched unexposed controls (77). There was an increased creatinine concentration in the striatum, with relatively normal concentrations of *N*-acetyl-containing compounds in children exposed to metamfetamine. These findings suggest that exposure to metamfetamine in utero causes abnormal energy metabolism in the brain of children. However, there were no differences in reported behavioral problems among metamfetamine-exposed children compared with controls.

Susceptibility Factors

Genetic factors

A study in 93 unrelated metamfetamine-dependent subjects and 131 controls did not prove any association between metamfetamine dependence in Caucasians of Czech origin and TaqI A polymorphism of the DRD2 gene, I/D polymorphism of the ACE gene, or M235T polymorphism of the AGT gene (78).

Age

Special care should be taken when using amphetamines in elderly patients, in view of the likelihood of stimulation of adrenoceptors and in particular of cardiovascular and respiratory function. Periodic users especially need to be wary of acute use under circumstances of exercise and environmental heat, owing to the risk of heat stroke.

Other features of the patient

The existence of a previous neurological disorder may be a risk factor for treatment-resistant psychosis in metamfetamine abusers (79). It is of particular interest that most of these patients sustained their disorder during childhood. It is not uncommon for metamfetamine patients to continue with psychotic symptoms despite extended periods of abstinence (80). These patients often are labeled as being schizophrenic. This study has shown the importance of considering a history of neurological disorders, especially during childhood, in such patients.

Drug Administration

Drug administration route

Injection as a method of delivery of illicit drugs carries its own special risks. Metamfetamine-dependent subjects ($n = 427$) participated in a study to detect differences between injecting metamfetamine users (13%) and non-injecting users (87%) (81). The patients entered treatment at a center in California between 1988 and 1995. Injectors reported significantly more years of heavy use. Psychological problems were more common in the injectors, more of whom reported depression, suicidal ideation, hallucinations, and episodes of feeling that their body parts "disconnect and leave." Moreover, injectors reported more problems concerning sexual functioning and more episodes of loss of consciousness. The injectors were more commonly HIV-positive and they had more felony convictions and were on parole more often than other users. Although individuals who inject metamfetamine use it more often than non-injectors, the number of grams used per week did not differ between the groups. Thus, injectors use a smaller amount of drug per dose than non-injectors. Eighty percent of the injectors were unemployed, possibly reflecting the extent of impairment related to addiction in

this group. The injectors, who had more psychiatric and medical morbidity, warrant special attention and carefully designed treatment plans.

Drug overdose

Overdosage of amphetamines can cause restlessness, dizziness, tremor, increased reflexes, talkativeness, tenseness, irritability, and insomnia; less common effects include euphoria, confusion, anxiety, delirium, hallucinations, panic states, suicidal and homicidal tendencies, excessive sweating, dry mouth, metallic taste, anorexia, nausea, vomiting, diarrhea, and abdominal cramps. Fatal poisoning is usually associated with hyperpyrexia, convulsions, coma, or cerebral hemorrhage. In addition, peripheral excitation of smooth muscle or blood vessels supplying skeletal muscle has been described. Excitatory actions can cause increased heart rate, palpitation, dysrhythmias, and metabolic effects, such as glycogenolysis in liver and adipose tissue.

The problem of fatal overdose is central to the problem of frequently repeated intravenous high-dose abuse of stimulants of unknown quality and quantity. Fatal overdose is less frequent among experienced chronic users than in naive or episodic high-dose users (82–84), in part because of the establishment of tolerance to hyperpyrexia and hypertension. Fatal hypertension can be potentiated by high ambient temperatures and vigorous exercise, as in the use of these drugs by athletes. Rare individuals have used up to 1–3 g/day of oral amfetamine for many years without problems of overdosing, yet acute toxic overdoses have been reported at 100–200 mg (53). Hyperpyrexia, seizures, hypertensive cerebrovascular hemorrhage, ventricular fibrillation, left ventricular failure, and complications of intravenous drug abuse have all been reported as causes of death (83–86). An autopsy study of amfetamine abusers in San Francisco showed that 54% died of drug toxicity, 10% of accidental trauma, 12% by suicide, and 10% by homicide (87).

Two deaths from metamfetamine overdose in drug dealers have been reported from Thailand, which has experienced an increase in metamfetamine abuse (88).

- A 43-year-old male drug dealer swallowed a number of metamfetamine tablets at the time of his arrest. When seen in the emergency room, he was comatose with reactive pupils. He died 6 hours after consuming the tablets. The autopsy findings were non-specific.
- Another 33-year-old female drug dealer, while at the police station, swallowed a number of metamfetamine pills that had been hidden in her undergarments. At the hospital, a gastric lavage was done but she died 10 hours after ingestion.

As described in these cases, there may be an increased risk of death in drug dealers who, in attempting to prevent arrest, may consume toxic amounts without anticipating the consequences.

Drug–Drug Interactions

Adrenergic neuron blocking drugs

Amphetamines and other stimulatory anorectic agents, apart from fenfluramine, would be expected to impair the hypotensive effects of adrenergic neuron blocking drugs such as guanethidine. Not only do they release noradrenaline from stores in adrenergic neurons and block the reuptake of released noradrenaline into the neuron, but they also impair re-entry of the antihypertensive drugs (89).

Alcohol

Alcohol increases blood concentrations of amphetamines (SED-9, 9).

Barbiturates

Barbiturates can enhance amfetamine hyperactivity (SED-8, 9).

Benzodiazepines

Benzodiazepines can enhance amfetamine hyperactivity (SED-8, 9).

Estradiol

Preclinical studies (as well as anecdotal clinical reports) have shown that estrogens, through effects on the central nervous system, can influence behavioral responses to psychoactive drugs. In an unusual crossover study, the subjective and physiological effects of oral D-amfetamine 10 mg were assessed after pretreatment with estradiol (90). One group of healthy young women used estradiol patches (Estraderm TTS, total dose 0.8 mg), which raised plasma estradiol concentrations to about 750 pg/ml, and a control group used placebo patches. Most of the subjective and physiological effects of amfetamine were not affected by acute estradiol treatment, but the estrogen did increase the magnitude of the effect of amfetamine on subjective ratings of "pleasant stimulation" and reduced ratings of "want more." Estradiol also produced some subjective effects when used alone, raising ratings of "feel drug," "energy and intellectual efficiency," and "pleasant stimulation." Some limitations of the study were:

(a) plasma amfetamine concentrations were not measured, so an effect of estradiol on the pharmacokinetics of amfetamine cannot be ruled out;
(b) only single doses of amfetamine and estradiol were tested;
(c) the dose of amfetamine was relatively low and that of estradiol relatively high, maximizing the chances of detecting estradiol-dependent increases in two subjective effects of amfetamine.

Monoamine oxidase inhibitors

The amphetamines should not be used together with or within 14 days of any monoamine oxidase inhibitors; severe hypertensive reactions and on occasion confusional states (for example with fenfluramine) can occur (SED-9, 9).

Ritonavir

A fatal interaction between ritonavir and metamfetamine has been described (91).

- A 49-year-old HIV-positive Caucasian man had taken ritonavir (400 mg bd), saquinavir (400 mg bd), and stavudine (40 mg bd) for 4 months. His CD4 cell count was 617×10^6 cells/l and HIV-1 RNA less than 400 copies/ml. He had previously taken zidovudine for 7 months. He self-injected twice with metamfetamine and sniffed amyl nitrite and was found dead a few hours later. At autopsy, there was no obvious cause of death. Metamfetamine was detected in the bile (0.5 mg/l) and cannabinoids and traces of benzodiazepines were detected in the blood.

Nitric oxide formed from amyl nitrite inhibits cytochrome P450 (92) and ritonavir inhibits CYP2D6 (93), which has a major role in metamfetamine detoxification (94). This interaction could have led to fatal plasma concentrations of metamfetamine. It is therefore suggested that patients who take protease inhibitors are made aware of the potential risk of using any form of recreational drugs metabolized by CYP2D6, particularly metamfetamine.

SSRIs

A man taking long-term dexamfetamine had two episodes of serotonin syndrome while taking first venlafaxine and later citalopram (95).

- A 32-year-old man, who was taking dexamfetamine 5 mg tds for adult ADHD, developed marked agitation, anxiety, shivering, and tremor after taking venlafaxine for 2 weeks (75 mg/day increased after a week to 150 mg/day). His heart rate was 140/minute, blood pressure 142/93 mmHg, and temperature 37.3°C. His pupils were dilated but reactive. There was generalized hypertonia, hyper-reflexia, and frequent myoclonic jerking. Dexamfetamine and venlafaxine were withdrawn and cyproheptadine (in doses of 8 mg up to a total of 32 mg over 3 hours) was given. His symptoms completely resolved within a few hours.

Dexamfetamine was restarted 3 days later and citalopram was started a few days later. Two weeks later he reported similar symptoms and stopped taking citalopram. He was successfully treated again with cyproheptadine.

Tricyclic antidepressants

Tricyclic antidepressants increase blood concentrations of amfetamine (96,97).

References

1. Bell DS. The experimental reproduction of amphetamine psychosis. Arch Gen Psychiatry 1973;29(1):35–40.
2. Ellinwood EH, Jr. Emergency treatment of acute adverse reactions to CNS stimulants. In: Bourne P, editor. Acute Drug Abuse Emergencies: A Treatment Manual. New York: Academic Press, 1976:115.
3. Fawcett JF, Busch KA. Stimulants in psychiatry. In: Schatzberg AF, Nemeroff CB, editors. The American Psychiatric Press Textbook of Psychopharmacology. Washington, DC: American Psychiatric Press, 1995:417.
4. Angrist B, d'Hollosy M, Sanfilipo M, Satriano J, Diamond G, Simberkoff M, Weinreb H. Central nervous system stimulants as symptomatic treatments for

AIDS-related neuropsychiatric impairment. J Clin Psychopharmacol 1992;12(4):268–72.

5. Satel SL, Nelson JC. Stimulants in the treatment of depression: a critical overview. J Clin Psychiatry 1989;50(7):241–9.

6. Holmes VF, Fernandez F, Levy JK. Psychostimulant response in AIDS-related complex patients. J Clin Psychiatry 1989;50(1):5–8.

7. Chiarello RJ, Cole JO. The use of psychostimulants in general psychiatry. A reconsideration. Arch Gen Psychiatry 1987;44(3):286–95.

8. Fawcett J, Kravitz HM, Zajecka JM, Schaff MR. CNS stimulant potentiation of monoamine oxidase inhibitors in treatment-refractory depression. J Clin Psychopharmacol 1991;11(2):127–32.

9. Jonsson S, O'Meara M, Young JB. Acute cocaine poisoning. Importance of treating seizures and acidosis. Am J Med 1983;75(6):1061–4.

10. Barinerd H, Krupp M, Chatton J, et al. Current Medical Diagnosis and Treatment. Los Altos CA: Lange Medical Publishers, 1970.

11. Gillberg C, Melander H, von Knorring AL, Janols LO, Thernlund G, Hagglof B, Eidevall-Wallin L, Gustafsson P, Kopp S. Long-term stimulant treatment of children with attention-deficit hyperactivity disorder symptoms. A randomized, double-blind, placebo-controlled trial. Arch Gen Psychiatry 1997;54(9):857–64.

12. Pacifici R, Zuccaro P, Farre M, Pichini S, Di Carlo S, Roset PN, Ortuno J, Segura J, de la Torre R. Immunomodulating properties of MDMA alone and in combination with alcohol: a pilot study. Life Sci 1999;65(26):PL309–16.

13. Schneider HJ, Jha S, Burnand KG. Progressive arteritis associated with cannabis use. Eur J Vasc Endovasc Surg 1999;18(4):366–7.

14. Stracciari A, Guarino M, Crespi C, Pazzaglia P. Transient amnesia triggered by acute marijuana intoxication. Eur J Neurol 1999;6(4):521–3.

15. Karch SB, Billingham ME. The pathology and etiology of cocaine-induced heart disease. Arch Pathol Lab Med 1988;112(3):225–30.

16. Ellenhorn DJ, Barceloux DG. Amphetamines. In: Medical Toxicology: Diagnosis and Treatment of Human Poisoning. New York: Elsevier Science Publishers, 1988:625.

17. Call TD, Hartneck J, Dickinson WA, Hartman CW, Bartel AG. Acute cardiomyopathy secondary to intravenous amphetamine abuse. Ann Intern Med 1982;97(4):559–60.

18. Angrist B, Sanfilipo M, Wolkin A. Cardiovascular effects of 0.5 milligrams per kilogram oral d-amphetamine and possible attenuation by haloperidol. Clin Neuropharmacol 2001;24(3):139–44.

19. Waksman J, Taylor RN Jr., Bodor GS, Daly FF, Jolliff HA, Dart RC. Acute myocardial infarction associated with amphetamine use. Mayo Clin Proc 2001;76(3):323–6.

20. Costa GM, Pizzi C, Bresciani B, Tumscitz C, Gentile M, Bugiardini R. Acute myocardial infarction caused by amphetamines: a case report and review of the literature. Ital Heart J 2001;2(6):478–80.

21. Zaidat OO, Frank J. Vertebral artery dissection with amphetamine abuse. J Stroke Cerebrovasc Dis 2001; 10:27–9.

22. Sewell RA, Cozzi NV. More about parkinsonism after taking ecstasy. N Engl J Med 1999;341(18):1400.

23. Baggott M, Mendelson J, Jones R. More about parkinsonism after taking ecstasy. N Engl J Med 1999;341(18):1400–1.

24. Mintzer S, Hickenbottom S, Gilman S. More about parkinsonism after taking ecstasy. N Engl J Med 1999;341:1401.

25. Borg GJ. More about parkinsonism after taking ecstasy. N Engl J Med 1999;341(18):1400.

26. Kalasinsky KS, Bosy TZ, Schmunk GA, Reiber G, Anthony RM, Furukawa Y, Guttman M, Kish SJ. Regional distribution of methamphetamine in autopsied brain of chronic human methamphetamine users. Forensic Sci Int 2001;116(2–3):163–9.

27. Barnhart FE, Fogacci JR, Reed DW. Methamphetamine—a study of postmortem redistribution. J Anal Toxicol 1999;23(1):69–70.

28. Moriya F, Hashimoto Y. Redistribution of methamphetamine in the early postmortem period. J Anal Toxicol 2000;24(2):153–5.

29. Escalante OD, Ellinwood EH Jr. Central nervous system cytopathological changes in cats with chronic methedrine intoxication. Brain Res 1970;21(1):151–5.

30. Wagner GC, Ricaurte GA, Seiden LS, Wagner GC, Ricaurte GA, Seiden LS, Schuster CR, Miller RJ, Westley J. Long-lasting depletions of striatal dopamine and loss of dopamine uptake sites following repeated administration of methamphetamine. Brain Res 1980;181(1):151–60.

31. Bostwick DG. Amphetamine-induced cerebral vasculitis. Hum Pathol 1981;12(11):1031–3.

32. Napiorkowski B, Lester BM, Freier MC, Brunner S, Dietz L, Nadra A, Oh W. Effects of in utero substance exposure on infant neurobehavior. Pediatrics 1996;98(1):71–5.

33. Wilson JM, Kalasinsky KS, Levey AI, Bergeron C, Reiber G, Anthony RM, Schmunk GA, Shannak K, Haycock JW, Kish SJ. Striatal dopamine nerve terminal markers in human, chronic methamphetamine users. Nat Med 1996;2(6):699–703.

34. McCann UD, Wong DF, Yokoi F, Villemagne V, Dannals RF, Ricaurte GA. Reduced striatal dopamine transporter density in abstinent methamphetamine and methcathinone users: evidence from positron emission tomography studies with (^{11}C)WIN-35,428. J Neurosci 1998;18(20):8417–22.

35. Davidson C, Gow AJ, Lee TH, Ellinwood EH. Methamphetamine neurotoxicity: necrotic and apoptotic mechanisms and relevance to human abuse and treatment. Brain Res Brain Res Rev 2001;36(1):1–22.

36. Volkow ND. Drug abuse and mental illness: progress in understanding comorbidity. Am J Psychiatry 2001; 158(8):1181–3.

37. Sekine Y, Iyo M, Ouchi Y, Matsunaga T, Tsukada H, Okada H, Yoshikawa E, Futatsubashi M, Takei N, Mori N. Methamphetamine-related psychiatric symptoms and reduced brain dopamine transporters studied with PET. Am J Psychiatry 2001;158(8):1206–14.

38. Volkow ND, Chang L, Wang GJ, Fowler JS, Leonido-Yee M, Franceschi D, Sedler MJ, Gatley SJ, Hitzemann R, Ding YS, Logan J, Wong C, Miller EN. Association of dopamine transporter reduction with psychomotor impairment in methamphetamine abusers. Am J Psychiatry 2001; 158(3):377–82.

39. Volkow ND, Chang L, Wang GJ, Fowler JS, Franceschi D, Sedler MJ, Gatley SJ, Hitzemann R, Ding YS, Wong C, Logan J. Higher cortical and lower subcortical metabolism in detoxified methamphetamine abusers. Am J Psychiatry 2001;158(3):383–9.

40. Volkow ND, Chang L, Wang GJ, Fowler JS, Franceschi D, Sedler M, Gatley SJ, Miller E, Hitzemann R, Ding YS, Logan J. Loss of dopamine transporters in methamphetamine abusers recovers with protracted abstinence. J Neurosci 2001;21(23):9414–18.

41. Rogers RD, Everitt BJ, Baldacchino A, Blackshaw AJ, Swainson R, Wynne K, Baker NB, Hunter J, Carthy T, Booker E, London M, Deakin JF, Sahakian BJ, Robbins TW. Dissociable deficits in the decision-making cognition of chronic amphetamine abusers, opiate abusers,

patients with focal damage to prefrontal cortex, and tryptophan-depleted normal volunteers: evidence for monoaminergic mechanisms. Neuropsychopharmacology 1999;20(4):322–39.

42. Ernst T, Chang L, Leonido-Yee M, Speck O. Evidence for long-term neurotoxicity associated with methamphetamine abuse: a ^{1}H MRS study. Neurology 2000;54(6):1344–9.

43. Lowe TL, Cohen DJ, Detlor J, Kremenitzer MW, Shaywitz BA. Stimulant medications precipitate Tourette's syndrome. JAMA 1982;247(12):1729–31.

44. Shapiro AK, Shapiro E. Do stimulants provoke, cause, or exacerbate tics and Tourette syndrome? Compr Psychiatry 1981;22(3):265–73.

45. Buxton N, McConachie NS. Amphetamine abuse and intracranial haemorrhage. J R Soc Med 2000;93(9):472–7.

46. Strupp M, Hamann GF, Brandt T. Combined amphetamine and cocaine abuse caused mesencephalic ischemia in a 16-year-old boy—due to vasospasm? Eur Neurol 2000;43(3):181–2.

47. Kramer JC, Fischman VS, Littlefield DC. Amphetamine abuse. Pattern and effects of high doses taken intravenously. JAMA 1967;201(5):305–9.

48. Greenberg LM, McMahon SA, Deem MA. Side effects of dextroamphetamine therapy of hyperactive children. West J Med 1974;120:105.

49. Williams K, Argyropoulos S, Nutt DJ. Amphetamine misuse and social phobia. Am J Psychiatry 2000;157(5):834–5.

50. Ellinwood EH Jr. Amphetamine psychosis. 1. Description of the individuals and process. J Nerv Ment Dis 1967;144:273.

51. Griffith JD, Cavanaugh JH, Held J, et al. Experimental psychosis induced by the administration of d-amphetamine. In: Costa E, Garattini S, editors. Amphetamines and Related Compounds. New York: Raven Press, 1970:897.

52. Griffith JD, Cavanaugh J, Held J, Oates JA. Dextroamphetamine. Evaluation of psychomimetic properties in man. Arch Gen Psychiatry 1972;26(2):97–100.

53. Ellinwood EH, Jr. Kilbey MM. Fundamental mechanisms underlying altered behavior following chronic administration of psychomotor stimulants. Biol Psychiatry 1980;15(5):749–57.

54. Yui K, Goto K, Ikemoto S, Ishiguro T. Stress induced spontaneous recurrence of methamphetamine psychosis: the relation between stressful experiences and sensitivity to stress. Drug Alcohol Depend 2000;58(1–2):67–75.

55. Yui K, Ishiguro T, Goto K, Ikemoto S. Susceptibility to subsequent episodes in spontaneous recurrence of methamphetamine psychosis. Ann NY Acad Sci 2000; 914:292–302.

56. Yui K, Ikemoto S, Goto K, Nishijima K, Yoshino T, Ishiguro T. Spontaneous recurrence of methamphetamine-induced paranoid-hallucinatory states in female subjects: susceptibility to psychotic states and implications for relapse of schizophrenia. Pharmacopsychiatry 2002; 35(2):62–71.

57. Espelin DE, Done AK. Amphetamine poisoning. Effectiveness chlorpromazine N Engl J Med 1968; 278(25):1361–5.

58. Bertram M, Egelhoff T, Schwarz S, Schwab S. Toxic leukencephalopathy following "ecstasy" ingestion. J Neurol 1999;246(7):617–8.

59. Semple DM, Ebmeier KP, Glabus MF, O'Carroll RE, Johnstone EC. Reduced in vivo binding to the serotonin transporter in the cerebral cortex of MDMA ("ecstasy") users. Br J Psychiatry 1999;175:63–9.

60. Misra L, Kofoed L, Oesterheld JR, Richards GA. Risperidone treatment of methamphetamine psychosis. Am J Psychiatry 1997;154(8):1170.

61. Misra LK, Kofoed L, Oesterheld JR, Richards GA. Olanzapine treatment of methamphetamine psychosis. J Clin Psychopharmacol 2000;20(3):393–4.

62. Richards JR, Brofeldt BT. Patterns of tooth wear associated with methamphetamine use. J Periodontol 2000;71(8):1371–4.

63. Yung A, Agnew K, Snow J, Oliver F. Two unusual cases of toxic epidermal necrolysis. Australas J Dermatol 2002;43(1):35–8.

64. O'Connor A, Cluroe A, Couch R, Galler L, Lawrence J, Synek B. Death from hyponatraemia-induced cerebral oedema associated with MDMA ("ecstasy") use. NZ Med J 1999;112(1091):255–6.

65. Aeschlimann A, de Truchis P, Kahn MF. Scleroderma after therapy with appetite suppressants. Report on four cases. Scand J Rheumatol 1990;19(1):87–90.

66. Hall W, Lynskey M, Degenhardt L. Trends in opiate-related deaths in the United Kingdom and Australia, 1985–1995. Drug Alcohol Depend 2000;57(3):247–54.

67. Banooni P, Rickman LS, Ward DM. Pott puffy tumor associated with intranasal methamphetamine. JAMA 2000;283(10):1293.

68. Heinemann A, Iwersen-Bergmann S, Stein S, Schmoldt A, Puschel K. Methadone-related fatalities in Hamburg 1990–1999: implications for quality standards in maintenance treatment? Forensic Sci Int 2000;113(1–3): 449–55.

69. Masaki T. The amphetamine problem in Japan: annex to Sixth Report of Expert Committee on Drugs Liable to Produce Addiction. World Health Organ Tech Rep Series 1956;102:14.

70. Unwin JR. Illicit drug use among Canadian youth. I. Can Med Assoc J 1968;98(8):402–7.

71. Kosman ME, Unna DR. Effects of chronic administration of the amphetamines and other stimulants on behavior. Clin Pharmacol Ther 1968;9(2):240–54.

72. Ellinwood EH Jr, Petrie WM. Drug induced psychoses. In: Pickens RW, Heston LL, editors. Psychiatric Factors in Drug Abuse. New York: Grune and Stratton, 1979:301.

73. Ellinwood EH, Jr. Assault and homicide associated with amphetamine abuse. Am J Psychiatry 1979;3:25.

74. Niki Y, Watanabe S, Yoshida K, Miyashita N, Nakajima M, Matsushima T. Effect of pazufloxacin mesilate on the serum concentration of theophylline. J Infect Chemother 2002;8(1):33–6.

75. Ashton CH. Adverse effects of cannabis and cannabinoids. Br J Anaesth 1999;83(4):637–49.

76. Volkow ND, Chang L, Wang GJ, Fowler JS, Ding YS, Sedler M, Logan J, Franceschi D, Gatley J, Hitzemann R, Gifford A, Wong C, Pappas N. Low level of brain dopamine D_2 receptors in methamphetamine abusers: association with metabolism in the orbitofrontal cortex. Am J Psychiatry 2001;158(12):2015–21.

77. Smith LM, Chang L, Yonekura ML, Grob C, Osborn D, Ernst T. Brain proton magnetic resonance spectroscopy in children exposed to methamphetamine in utero. Neurology 2001;57(2):255–60.

78. Sery O, Vojtova V, Zvolsky P. The association study of DRD2, ACE and AGT gene polymorphisms and metamphetamine dependence. Physiol Res 2001;50(1):43–50.

79. Fujii D. Risk factors for treatment-resistive methamphetamine psychosis. J Neuropsychiatry Clin Neurosci 2002;14(2):239–40.

80. Iwanami A, Sugiyama A, Kuroki N, Toda S, Kato N, Nakatani Y, Horita N, Kaneko T. Patients with methamphetamine psychosis admitted to a psychiatric hospital in Japan. A preliminary report. Acta Psychiatr Scand 1994;89(6):428–32.

81. Domier CP, Simon SL, Rawson RA, Huber A, Ling W. A comparison of injecting and noninjecting methamphetamine users. J Psychoactive Drugs 2000;32(2):229–32.

82. Ellinwood EH Jr. Emergency treatment of acute reactions to CNS stimulants. J Psychedelic Drugs 1972;5:147.

83. Nausieda PA. Central stimulant toxicity. In: Vinken PJ, Bruyn GW, editors. Handbook of Clinical Neurology. Intoxications of the Nervous System. Part 11. Amsterdam: Elsevier/North-Holland Biomedical Press, 1979:223.

84. Kalant H, Kalant OJ. Death in amphetamine users: causes and rates. Can Med Assoc J 1975;112(3):299–304.

85. Delaney P, Estes M. Intracranial hemorrhage with amphetamine abuse. Neurology 1980;30(10):1125–8.

86. Olsen ER. Intracranial hemorrhage and amphetamine usage. Review of the effects of amphetamines on the central nervous system. Angiology 1977;28(7):464–71.

87. Karch SB, Stephens BG, Ho CH. Methamphetamine-related deaths in San Francisco: demographic, pathologic, and toxicologic profiles. J Forensic Sci 1999;44(2):359–68.

88. Sribanditmongkol P, Chokjamsai M, Thampitak S. Methamphetamine overdose and fatality: 2 case reports. J Med Assoc Thai 2000;83(9):1120–3.

89. Simpson FO. Antihypertensive drug therapy. Drugs 1973;6(5):333–63.

90. Justice AJ, de Wit H. Acute effects of estradiol pretreatment on the response to d-amphetamine in women. Neuroendocrinology 2000;71(1):51–9.

91. Cullen W, Bury G, Langton D. Experience of heroin overdose among drug users attending general practice. Br J Gen Pract 2000;50(456):546–9.

92. Christie B. Gangrene bug killed 35 heroin users. West J Med 2000;173(2):82–3.

93. Dettmeyer R, Schmidt P, Musshoff F, Dreisvogt C, Madea B. Pulmonary edema in fatal heroin overdose: immunohistological investigations with IgE, collagen IV and laminin—no increase of defects of alveolar-capillary membranes. Forensic Sci Int 2000;110(2):87–96.

94. McCreary M, Emerman C, Hanna J, Simon J. Acute myelopathy following intranasal insufflation of heroin: a case report. Neurology 2000;55(2):316–17.

95. Prior FH, Isbister GK, Dawson AH, Whyte IM. Serotonin toxicity with therapeutic doses of dexamphetamine and venlafaxine. Med J Aust 2002;176(5):240–1.

96. Wharton RN, Perel JM, Dayton PG, Malitz S. A potential clinical use for methylphenidate with tricyclic antidepressants. Am J Psychiatry 1971;127(12):1619–25.

97. Cooper TB, Simpson GM. Concomitant imipramine and methylphenidate administration: a case report. Am J Psychiatry 1973;130(6):721.

Amphotericin

General Information

Having a broad-spectrum fungicidal activity, amphotericin remains the mainstay of treatment of most invasive fungal infections. Compared with conventional amphotericin B deoxycholate, other lipid formulations of amphotericin (amphotericin B colloidal dispersion, amphotericin B lipid complex, and liposomal amphotericin B) facilitate treatment in patients with suspected and proven invasive mycoses, who are intolerant of or refractory to conventional amphotericin.

Mechanism of action

The principal mechanism of action of amphotericin is based on its binding to lipids of the cell membrane of target cells, particularly to ergosterol, the predominant lipid in fungal cells, and cholesterol, the predominant lipid of the vertebrate cell membrane. The principle of selectivity is based on a higher affinity of amphotericin to ergosterol than cholesterol, but peroxidation of the membrane appears to be of equal importance (1–3).

Different formulations of amphotericin

Because of nephrotoxicity from amphotericin, which is common when amphotericin is given as the deoxycholate, lipid formulations have been developed. The formulations that are currently available are:

- amphotericin B deoxycholate (DAMB);
- amphotericin B colloidal dispersion (ABCD);
- amphotericin B lipid complex (ABLC);
- liposomal amphotericin B (L-Amb, AmBisome).

Pharmacokinetics

The pharmacokinetics of amphotericin are highly variable and depend on the formulation used and the infusion rate (4,5). Amphotericin, when administered as the deoxycholate complex, is highly bound to lipoproteins, mainly LDL and VLDL, and to a lesser extent to HDL (6,7) as well as to cell membranes of circulating blood cells. Binding is so avid that after spiking human plasma, no unbound amphotericin is detectable (7). Concentrations in peritoneal, pleural, and synovial fluids are usually less than half of those in serum, while cerebrospinal fluid concentrations range from undetectable to some 4% of the serum concentration, but over 40% in neonates (8). For DAMB the half-life is 1–2 days. Concentrations in bile are detectable for up to 12 days and in urine for 27–35 days. Clearance is faster and the volume of distribution smaller in neonates and infants (9) There is marked tissue storage of amphotericin, again depending on the formulation and the rate of infusion. Liver, spleen, kidneys, and lungs accumulate large amounts. Tissue storage plays a major role in the pharmacokinetics of amphotericin, which can be detected in tissues much more than a year after the completion of therapy (10–12). Up to 40% of amphotericin is ultimately excreted unchanged in urine. Elimination via the bile plays a lesser role, and metabolism appears to be unimportant. Elimination is so slow that dosages need not be altered in patients with renal insufficiency.

Lipid formulations of amphotericin have individually variable pharmacokinetics. The use of DAMB in 20% Intralipid results in marked changes, with lower antifungally active blood concentrations (13). Infusion of ABLC, ABCD, or L-Amb, AmBisome results in plasma amphotericin concentrations specific to the individual formulation. The half-life of amphotericin after lipid formulations is prolonged compared with the deoxycholate formulation (14): 4–10 days for ABCD (15) and about 5 days for ABLC (16). The importance of these differences is unknown, because they do not reflect the biologically active concentration of amphotericin, which also varies with formulation. On a weight for weight basis amphotericin in lipid formulations is less active than in the deoxycholate formulation, because of lower systemic availability (5). One factor that complicates the interpretation of blood concentrations is the sparse data discriminating between amphotericin bound to the original lipid formula and to plasma lipoproteins, and the minute amount of unbound amphotericin not detectable by available analytical methods (7).

The interaction of amphotericin with serum lipoproteins (6) suggests that manipulations of blood lipids and blood lipoproteins might affect the pharmacokinetics of amphotericin, and therefore also alter its activity, including toxic effects, as suggested in animal studies (17).

Observational studies

Amphotericin is highly effective in the treatment of visceral leishmaniasis (18). In a prospective study of 938 patients from Bihar, India, who received the drug in a dosage of 1 mg/kg/day infused over 2 hours for 20 days, serum creatinine values over 177 µmol/l were noted in 6.3%, and acute renal insufficiency developed in three patients. Two patients died, possibly related to amphotericin, one with renal insufficiency and one with hypokalemia and cardiac arrest. Infusion-related chills occurred in 92% and fever in 40% of patients. The parasitological cure rate (no relapse within 6 months) exceeded 99%.

Amphotericin deoxycholate

The adverse effects of amphotericin deoxycholate have been reviewed in a retrospective analysis of 102 adult patients (median age 61 years) with a variety of underlying conditions who were admitted to a small community hospital in Honolulu and who received the drug for treatment of presumed or proven fungal infections that were mostly due to *Candida* species (19). The average total dose of amphotericin deoxycholate was comparatively low at 162 (range 10–840) mg. The initial dose averaged 16 (range 1–50) mg and the total duration of therapy was 8.3 (range 1–46) days. Chills, fever, and/or nausea were noted in 25% of the patients. Hypokalemia (a serum potassium concentration below 3.5 mmol/l) occurred in 19%, and nephrotoxicity (defined as a serum creatinine concentration of at least 141 µmol/l (1.6 mg/dl) with an increase of at least 44 µmol/l (0.5 mg/dl) during amphotericin deoxycholate therapy) in 15% of the patients. Nephrotoxicity increased with increasing total dose of amphotericin, while infusion-associated toxicity decreased with advancing age. The overall response rate to therapy with amphotericin deoxycholate was 83%.

Amphotericin colloidal dispersion

The safety and efficacy of amphotericin colloidal dispersion have been evaluated in 148 immunocompromised patients with candidemia (20). ABCD was given intravenously in a median daily dose of 3.9 (range 0.1–9.1) mg/kg for a median of 12 (range 1–72) days. In the safety analysis ($n = 148$ patients), nephrotoxicity occurred in 16% of the patients, with either doubling of the baseline serum creatinine concentration or an increase of 88 µmol/l (1.0 mg/dl) or a 50% fall in calculated creatinine clearance. Severe adverse events were believed to be probably or possibly related to ABCD in 36 patients (24%), including chills and fever (9.5%), hypotension and abnormal kidney function (4%), tachycardia, asthma, hypotension (3%), and dyspnea (2%). ABCD was withdrawn in 12%

because of toxicity. The overall response rate in 89 evaluable patients was 66% with candidemia alone and 14% with disseminated candidiasis.

The safety and efficacy of ABCD have been studied in 133 patients with invasive fungal infections and renal impairment due to either amphotericin deoxycholate or pre-existing renal disease (21). The mean daily dose of ABCD was 3.4 (range 0.1–5.5) mg/kg, and the mean duration of therapy was 21 (range 1–207) days. Although individual patients had increases in serum creatinine concentrations, ABCD did not have an adverse effect on renal function: the mean serum creatinine concentration tended to fall slightly with days on therapy, and increases were not dose-related. Six patients discontinued ABCD therapy because of nephrotoxicity. Infusion-related adverse events occurred at least once in 74 patients (56%); however, while 43% of patients had infusion-related toxic effects on day 1, only 18% reported these events by day 7. There were complete or partial responses in 50% of the intention-to-treat population and in 67% of the 58 evaluable patients.

The safety of ABCD has been reviewed using data from 572 immunocompromised patients refractory to or intolerant of standard therapies enrolled in five phase I/II clinical trials (22). The mean daily dose of ABCD was 3.85 (median 3.8, range 0.1–9.1) mg/kg and the mean duration of treatment was 25 (median 16, range 1–409) days. Overall, the principal adverse events associated with ABCD therapy were chills (52%), fever (39%), and hypotension (19%). These infusion-related reactions were dose-related and were the dose-limiting adverse events, defining the maximum tolerated dosage at 7.5 mg/kg. ABCD did not adversely affect renal function, as measured by overall changes in serum creatinine from baseline to the end of therapy, even in patients with pre-existing renal impairment; only 3.3% of patients discontinued therapy because of nephrotoxicity. Complete or partial responses to treatment were reported in 149 of 260 evaluable patients (57%).

The safety and efficacy of ABCD have been studied in 220 bone marrow transplant recipients enrolled in the same five phase I or phase II studies (23). The median dose in this population was 4 (range 0.4–8.0) mg/kg, and the median duration of treatment was 16 (range 1–409) days. Overall, 37 (19%) of the patients had nephrotoxicity, defined as a doubling of serum creatinine from baseline, an increase of 88 µmol/l from baseline, or at least a 50% fall in calculated creatinine clearance. There were no significant changes in hepatic transaminases, alkaline phosphatase, or total bilirubin. Fever and chills were reported by 12 and 11% of patients respectively. Other acute, severe, infusion-related adverse events were hypoxia (4.1%), hypertension (2.7%), and hypotension (2.7%).

Mucormycosis has an exceedingly high mortality rate in immunocompromised patients. In five phase I and phase II studies of ABCD, 21 patients were given ABCD (mean dose 4.8 mg/kg per infusion for a mean duration of 37 days) on the basis of pre-existing renal insufficiency, nephrotoxicity during amphotericin B therapy, or refractory infections (24). Of 20 evaluable patients, 12 responded to ABCD, and there was no renal or hepatic toxicity. However, a previous randomized, comparative trial showed an at least similar if not increased frequency and severity of infusion-related reactions compared with conventional amphotericin B (25).

Amphotericin lipid complex

The safety and efficacy of ABLC have been evaluated in 556 cases of proven or presumptive invasive fungal infection treated in an open, single-patient, US emergency-use study of patients who were refractory to or intolerant of conventional antifungal therapy (26). The daily dosage was either 5 mg/kg (87%) or 3 mg/kg. The investigators had the option of reducing the daily dosage as clinically warranted. Treatment was for 7 days in 540 patients (97%). During the course of ABLC therapy, serum creatinine concentrations in all patients fell significantly from baseline. In 162 patients with serum creatinine concentrations of at least 221 µmol/l (2.5 mg/dl) at baseline, the mean serum creatinine concentration fell significantly from the first week to the sixth week. The serum creatinine concentration increased from baseline to the end of therapy in 132 patients (24%). Hypokalemia (serum potassium concentration of less than 3 mmol/l) developed in 4.6%, and hypomagnesemia (serum magnesium concentration of less than 0.75 mmol/l) in 18%. There was a rise in serum bilirubin in 142/284 patients (33%); the overall increase was from 79 to 112 µmol/l (4.66–6.59 mg/dl) at the end of therapy. The mean alkaline phosphatase activity rose from 273 to 320 IU/l. There was no significant change overall in alanine transaminase activity, but the activity increased by the end of treatment in 16% of patients with initially normal values. There were complete or partial responses to therapy with ABLC in 167 of 291 mycologically confirmed cases evaluable for therapeutic response (57%).

The safety and efficacy of ABLC 5 mg/kg/day in patients with neutropenia and intolerance or refractoriness to amphotericin deoxycholate have been reported in two smaller series of 25 treatment courses from the UK. In one, the mean serum creatinine at the start of therapy was 139 µmol/l and at the end of therapy 132 µmol/l; there were no infusion-related adverse events (27). There was an increase in alanine transaminase activity in 12 of the 22 analysed treatment courses. In the other, there was an increase in serum creatinine in 5 of 18 courses (28%), and hypokalemia (less than 2.5 mmol/l) in two courses (11%); premedication for infusion-associated reactions was required in three courses (17%) (28). There were modest increases in serum alanine transaminase activities in five patients (30%).

In contrast to these reports, there was a high prevalence of adverse events with ABLC in the treatment of suspected or documented invasive fungal infections in 19 Scandinavian patients with mostly hematological malignancies (29). The mean starting dose of ABLC was 4.1 mg/kg/day, given for a median of 3 (range 1–19) days. ABLC was withdrawn because of adverse events in 14/19 patients (74%). These included rising creatinine concentrations ($n = 12$), increased serum bilirubin ($n = 7$), erythema ($n = 6$), increased alanine transaminase ($n = 6$), fever and chills ($n = 5$), hypoxemia ($n = 3$), hemolysis ($n = 2$), and back pain and increased serum alkaline phosphatase activity ($n = 1$

each). In patients with renal adverse effects, there were significantly increased serum creatinine concentration (from 85 to 199 mmol/l) and increased bilirubin concentration (from 17 to 77 µmol/l) in seven patients. The authors stated that while all the patients were very ill at the time of the start of ABLC therapy, in all cases the adverse effects had a direct and obvious correlation with the administration of ABLC. However, the reason for this unusual high rate of adverse events remains unclear.

Safety data have been published in a retrospective analysis of 551 patients with invasive fungal infections intolerant of or refractory to conventional antifungal therapy, 73 of whom received ABLC initially at 3 mg/kg/day instead of 5 mg/kg/day, as recommended in the protocol (30). There were no notable differences in adverse events (increased serum creatinine, infusion-related chills) between the two groups. Serum creatinine values were improved or stable at the end of therapy in 78 and 70% of patients respectively.

Two smaller series have addressed the safety of ABLC in immunocompromised patients (31,32). Each included about 30 patients who were treated with median dosages of 4.8 and 5.0 mg/kg for a median of 8 and 14 days. In contrast to a previous retrospective analysis that showed a 74% withdrawal rate, mostly due to infusion-related reactions (29), ABLC was well tolerated, with withdrawal rates of 6 and 0% and an overall trend for stable or improved serum creatinine values at the end of therapy. Similarly, 13 infusion-related reactions have been reported among 308 infusions in four of ten patients with hematological malignancies receiving ABLC 3 mg/kg/day (33). These reactions (fever, rigors, myalgias), occurred during the first infusions, were judged to be mild, and resolved during later infusions. ABLC was well tolerated by 30 persistently febrile neutropenic patients with hematological malignancies who received it in a low dosage of 1 mg/kg/day for a median of 7.5 (range 2–19) days (34). Seven patients (23%) had mild to moderate infusion-related reactions, and no patient had nephrotoxicity. In one patient, ABLC was discontinued owing to intolerable infusion-related fever and chills.

The safety and efficacy of low dose ABLC (1 mg/kg/day) for empirical treatment of fever and neutropenia have been studied in 69 episodes in 61 patients with hematological malignancies (35). The median duration of therapy was 8 (range 2–19) days and 13 patients had mild to moderate infusion-related adverse events. Creatinine concentrations remained stable in 42 cases, improved in 9, and deteriorated in 18. There were no other toxic effects. The response rate (resolution of fever during neutropenia and absence of invasive fungal infection) was 67%.

Fungal infection remains an important cause of morbidity and mortality in lung transplant patients. In a prospective non-comparative evaluation in lung or heart-lung transplant recipients, ventilated patients received undiluted aerosolized ABLC 100 mg, and extubated patients received 50 mg; in all, 381 treatments were given (98 in ventilated patients and 283 in extubated patients) (36). The treatment was administered by face mask jet nebulizer with compressed oxygen at a flow rate of 7–8 l/minute and inhaled over 15–30 minutes. Treatments were delivered once every day for four consecutive days, then once a week for 2 months. In all, 381 treatments were given to 51 patients, and ABLC was subjectively well tolerated in 98%. Pulmonary function worsened by 20% or more in under 5% of all treatments. There were no significant adverse events.

Liposomal amphotericin

The safety, tolerance, and pharmacokinetics of liposomal amphotericin have been evaluated in an open, sequential dose escalation, multiple-dose phase I/II study in 36 patients with neutropenia and persistent fever requiring empirical antifungal therapy (37). The patients received doses of 1, 2.5, 5.0, or 7.5 mg/kg/day of liposomal amphotericin for a mean of 9.2 days. Liposomal amphotericin was well tolerated: infusion-related adverse effects (fever, chills, rigor) occurred in 15 (5%) of all 331 infusions, and only two patients (5%) required premedication (dyspnea and generalized flushing; facial urticaria). Hypotension (one infusion) and hypertension (three infusions) were infrequent. One patient each had sharp flank pain and dyspnea during one infusion; these symptoms did not recur during subsequent infusions. Serum creatinine, potassium, and magnesium concentrations were not significantly changed from baseline, and there were no net increases in serum transaminases. There was, however, a significant increase in serum alkaline phosphatase activity and increase in bilirubin concentration in the overall population as well as in individual dosage groups. One patient who received concomitant L-asparaginase had increases in serum lipase and amylase activities in association with symptoms of pancreatitis while receiving liposomal amphotericin; however, as he continued to receive the drug, the serum lipase and amylase returned to baseline. Liposomal amphotericin had non-linear pharmacokinetics consistent with reticuloendothelial uptake and redistribution. There were no breakthrough fungal infections during therapy.

The efficacy of two dosages of liposomal amphotericin in the treatment of proven or probable invasive aspergillosis in neutropenic patients with cancer or those undergoing bone marrow transplantation has been studied in a prospective, randomized, open, multicenter trial in 120 patients randomized to receive either 1 mg/kg/day or 4 mg/kg/day of liposomal amphotericin; 87 patients were available for evaluation (38). There was at least one toxic event during treatment in 15 of 41 patients given 1 mg/kg/day and 25 of 46 given 4 mg/kg/day, but the numbers of events per patient were similar. These events included headache, nausea, diarrhea, rash, liver toxicity, myalgia, dyspnea, fever, chills, and back pain. Renal toxicity definitely related to liposomal amphotericin occurred in 1/41 patients treated with 1 mg/kg/day and 5/46 patients treated with 4 mg/kg/day. Only in one case was treatment permanently discontinued because of toxicity related to liposomal amphotericin (4 mg/kg/day). No patient died from liposomal amphotericin toxicity. Overall, liposomal amphotericin was effective in 50–60% of patients; however, the number of cases with proven invasive aspergillosis was too small to allow a meaningful comparison of the two dosages regarding efficacy in this life-threatening disease.

The safety and efficacy of liposomal amphotericin have been compared with that of ABLC in a retrospective analysis of 59 adult patients with hematological malignancies who received 68 courses of either liposomal amphotericin ($n = 32$) or ABLC ($n = 36$) for a variety of presumed or confirmed invasive fungal infections (39). The median daily dosages were 1.9 (range 0.7–4.0) mg/kg for liposomal amphotericin and 4.8 (range 1.9–5.8) mg/kg for ABLC. There was no statistically significant difference in the overall outcome; febrile reactions were significantly more common with ABLC (36 versus 6%), but there were no significant differences in the median creatinine concentrations at baseline and at the end of therapy or in the number of patients with urinary loss of potassium or magnesium.

In an open, sequential phase II clinical study of three different regimens of liposomal amphotericin for visceral leishmaniasis (2 mg/kg on days 1–6 and on day 10; 2 mg/kg on days 1–4 and on day 10; 2 mg/kg on days 1, 5, and 10) in Indian and Kenyan patients in three developing countries, there were few infusion-associated adverse effects (40). Of 32 Brazilian patients (15 of whom received 2 mg/kg on days 1–10 because of poor responses to the first regimen, 37% had a fever with one or more infusions, 9% had chills, and 6% had back pain; in addition, three patients had respiratory distress and/or cardiac dysrhythmias. There were different response rates to the three regimens in the different countries, leading to the recommendation of 2 mg/kg on days 1–4 and day 10 in India and Kenya, and 2 mg/kg on days 1–10 in Brazil.

In order to determine the maximum tolerated dosage of liposomal amphotericin B, a phase I/II study was conducted in 44 adult patients with proven ($n = 21$) or probable ($n = 23$) infections due to *Aspergillus* species and other filamentous fungi (41). The dosages were 7.5, 10, 12.5, and 15 mg/kg/day. The number of infusions was 1–83 with a median duration of 11 days. The maximum tolerated dosage was at least 15 mg/kg. Infusion-related reactions included fever in 8 and chills and rigors in 5 of 43 patients. Three patients developed a syndrome of substernal chest tightness, dyspnea, and flank pain, which was relieved by diphenhydramine. Serum creatinine increased two times above baseline in 32% of patients, but this increase was not dose-related. Hepatotoxicity developed in one patient. Altogether, the most common adverse events included fever (48%), increased creatinine concentration (46%), hypokalemia (39%), chills (32%), and abdominal pain (25%), with no obvious dose-dependency. Nine patients (20%) stopped taking the drug because of an adverse event. The reasons included raised serum creatinine, renal insufficiency, pancreatitis, hyperbilirubinemia, hypotension associated with the infusion, cardiorespiratory failure, multiorgan failure, and relapse of the primary malignancy. The last three events were attributed to the underlying disease process. Discontinuation was unrelated to dosage. Pharmacokinetic analysis showed dose-related non-linear kinetics at dosages of 7.5 mg/kg/day and over.

Aerosolized amphotericin

In a prospective, randomized, multicenter trial, inhalation of aerosolized amphotericin (10 mg bd) has been investigated as prophylaxis against invasive aspergillosis in 382 cancer patients with an anticipated duration of neutropenia of at least 10 days (42). While there was no difference in the incidence of invasive aspergillosis, infection-related mortality, and overall mortality, 31% of the patients discontinued amphotericin prophylaxis prematurely owing to adverse effects (55%; most commonly cough, bad taste, nausea), inability to cooperate further (30%), violation of the study protocol (11%), and non-adherence (4%).

Comparative studies

Comparisons of different formulations of amphotericin

Amphotericin deoxycholate in glucose versus amphotericin deoxycholate in Intralipid

The safety of two formulations of intravenous amphotericin deoxycholate has been investigated in a randomized, open comparison in neutropenic patients with refractory fever of unknown origin or pulmonary infiltrates (43). Amphotericin deoxycholate was given in a dose of 0.75 mg/kg/day either in 250 ml of a 5% glucose solution or mixed with 250 ml of a 20% lipid emulsion (Intralipid 20%) on eight consecutive days and then on alternate days as a 1–4 hour infusion. The mean number of days of treatment was 11.3 versus 9.9 days. There were no statistically significant differences between the two cohorts with respect to the incidence of infusion-related adverse events, such as fever and chills, renal impairment, or treatment failure. However, grade 3–4 acute dyspnea occurred slightly more often with the lipid emulsion formulation, and there were significantly more other severe respiratory events in patients receiving lipid emulsion, raising the possibility of a causal relation via fat overload or incompatibility between amphotericin deoxycholate and the lipid emulsion.

The efficacy and tolerability of amphotericin prepared in Intralipid 20% have been evaluated in 16 patients with HIV infection and esophageal candidiasis or cryptococcosis and compared with standard amphotericin in a matched group of 24 patients (44). While both formulations had apparently similar clinical and microbiological efficacy, fewer patients receiving the lipid emulsion formulation required premedication or symptomatic therapy for infusion-associated adverse events, and fewer patients were withdrawn because of adverse effects. Renal adverse effects (a rise in serum creatinine and/or electrolyte loss) were more common in patients who received the conventional formulation.

The efficacy and safety of amphotericin in Intralipid 20% or 5% glucose has been evaluated in a retrospective case analysis in 30 patients with AIDS and cryptococcal meningitis who received either formulation 1 mg/kg/day for 20 days with or without flucytosine (*n* = 20) or fluconazole (*n* = 4), followed by maintenance therapy with fluconazole 400 mg/day (45). Twenty patients received amphotericin deoxycholate in 500 ml 5% glucose over 5 hours, and 10 received amphotericin deoxycholate in 100 ml of 20% Intralipid given over 2 hours. Complete clinical resolution was obtained in 55 and 60% of the patients respectively. There were no differences regarding infusion-related adverse effects, nephrotoxicity, or anemia.

Amphotericin deoxycholate versus amphotericin B colloidal dispersion

Amphotericin colloidal dispersion has been compared with amphotericin deoxycholate in a prospective, randomized, double-blind study in the empirical treatment of fever and neutropenia in 213 patients (25). Patients were stratified by age and concomitant use of ciclosporin or tacrolimus and then randomized to receive ABCD (4 mg/kg/day) or amphotericin deoxycholate (0.8 mg/kg/day) for 14 days. Renal dysfunction was less likely to develop and occurred later with ABCD than with amphotericin deoxycholate. Likewise, the absolute and percentage fall in the serum potassium concentration from baseline to the end of therapy was greater with amphotericin deoxycholate than ABCD. However, probable or possible infusion-related hypoxia and chills were more common with ABCD than amphotericin deoxycholate. There was a therapeutic response in 50% of the patients who received ABCD and 43% of those who received amphotericin deoxycholate. Thus, ABCD was of comparable efficacy and less nephrotoxic than amphotericin deoxycholate, but infusion-related events were more common with ABCD.

Amphotericin deoxycholate versus liposomal amphotericin

Liposomal amphotericin 5 mg/kg/day and amphotericin deoxycholate 1 mg/kg/day have been compared in the treatment of proven or suspected invasive fungal infections in neutropenic patients in a randomized, multicenter study (46). Significantly more patients given amphotericin deoxycholate had a greater than 100% increase in baseline serum creatinine. Treatment was temporarily discontinued or the dosage reduced because of an increase in serum creatinine in 18/54 (33%) patients treated with amphotericin deoxycholate versus 2/51 (4%) treated with liposomal amphotericin. There was no statistically significant difference in the number of patients with infusion-related toxicity (fever/chills), hypokalemia, or increases in serum transaminases, alkaline phosphatase, or serum bilirubin. In 66 patients eligible for analysis of efficacy, there was a trend to an improved overall response rate and a significant difference in the rate of complete responses in favor of liposomal amphotericin; death rates were also lower in patients treated with liposomal amphotericin.

The results of a randomized, double-blind, multicenter comparison of liposomal amphotericin (3.0 mg/kg/day) with conventional amphotericin deoxycholate (0.6 mg/kg/day) for empirical antifungal therapy in patients with persistent fever and neutropenia have been reported (47). The mean duration of therapy was 10.8 days for liposomal amphotericin (343 patients) and 10.3 days for amphotericin deoxycholate (344 patients). While the composite rates of successful treatment were similar (50% for liposomal amphotericin and 49% for amphotericin deoxycholate), significantly fewer of the patients who received the liposomal preparation had infusion-related fever (17 versus 44%), chills or rigors (18 versus 54%), or other reactions, including hypotension, hypertension, and hypoxia. Nephrotoxicity (defined by a serum creatinine concentration twice the upper limit of normal) was significantly less frequent among patients treated with liposomal amphotericin (19%) than among those treated with conventional amphotericin deoxycholate (34%).

Amphotericin lipid complex versus liposomal amphotericin

Liposomal amphotericin and ABLC have been compared in an open randomized study in 75 adults with leukemia and 82 episodes of suspected or documented mycosis (48). The median durations of treatment and dosages were 15 days at 4 mg/kg/day for liposomal amphotericin and 10 days at 3 mg/kg/day for ABLC. Acute but not dose-limiting infusion-related adverse events occurred in 36 versus 70%. Bilirubin increased to over 1.5 times baseline in 59 versus 38%. There was no difference in the effects of either agent on renal function and drug-related withdrawals. The overall response rate to therapy in documented fungal infections (29 and 30% respectively) was not different between the two drugs.

Amphotericin deoxycholate in glucose versus amphotericin in nutritional fat emulsion

The safety of DAMB prepared in nutritional fat emulsion (a non-approved mode of amphotericin administration) has been reviewed (SEDA-21, 282) (SEDA-22, 285). It is not clear whether it has a better therapeutic index than other formulations, and methods of preparing it have not been standardized. The adverse effects of amphotericin prepared in nutritional fat emulsion have been compared with those of amphotericin prepared in 5% dextrose in two studies. While one of the studies showed a significantly lower frequency of infusion-related reactions and hypokalemia in patients receiving the fat emulsion (49), there were no differences in safety and tolerance between the two formulations in the other study (50). The safety of amphotericin prepared in nutritional fat emulsions has been reviewed (SEDA-21, 282) (SEDA-22, 285). Because of stability concerns and lack of systematic safety data, this form of amphotericin cannot be recommended.

Comparisons of amphotericin with other antifungal drugs

Antifungal azoles

Fluconazole

There has been an open, randomized comparison of amphotericin deoxycholate 0.5 mg/kg/day intravenously versus fluconazole 400 mg/day orally for empirical antifungal therapy in neutropenic patients with cancer and fever refractory to broad-spectrum antibiotics (51). Patients with abnormal hepatic or renal function were excluded, as were those with proven or suspected invasive fungal infection. The mean duration of therapy was 8.3 days with amphotericin deoxycholate and 7.9 days

with fluconazole. Altogether, 32/48 patients randomized to amphotericin deoxycholate and 19/52 randomized to fluconazole had adverse affects (67 versus 36%). Two patients developed immediate hypersensitivity reactions (flushing, hypotension, bronchospasm) to amphotericin deoxycholate and had to be withdrawn. Hypokalemia was noted in 25 patients (52%), and nephrotoxicity, defined as a rise in serum creatinine of 44 μmol/l (0.5 mg/dl) or more compared with the baseline value, in nine patients (19%). The corresponding frequencies with fluconazole were 23 and 6% respectively. Treatment success rates and mortality were similar (46 versus 56% and 33 versus 27% respectively).

Fluconazole and amphotericin as empirical antifungal drugs in febrile neutropenic patients have been investigated in a prospective, randomized, multicenter study in 317 patients randomized to either fluconazole (400 mg qds) or amphotericin deoxycholate (0.5 mg/kg qds) (52). Adverse events (fever, chills, renal insufficiency, electrolyte disturbances, and respiratory distress) occurred significantly more often in patients who were given amphotericin (128/151 patients, 81%) than in those given fluconazole (20/158 patients, 13%). Eleven patients treated with amphotericin, but only one treated with fluconazole, were withdrawn because of an adverse event. Overall mortality and mortality from fungal infections were similar in both groups. There was a satisfactory response in 68% of the patients treated with fluconazole and 67% of those treated with amphotericin. Thus, fluconazole may be a safe and effective alternative to amphotericin for empirical therapy of febrile neutropenic patients; however, since fluconazole is ineffective against opportunistic molds, the possibility of an invasive infection by a filamentous fungus should be excluded before starting empirical therapy. Similarly, patients who take azoles for prophylaxis are not candidates for empirical therapy with fluconazole.

Conventional amphotericin deoxycholate (0.2 mg/kg qds) and fluconazole (400 mg qds) have been compared in a prospective randomized study in 355 patients with allogeneic and autologous bone marrow transplantation (53). The drugs were given prophylactically from day 1 until engraftment. There was no difference in the occurrence of invasive fungal infections, but amphotericin was significantly more toxic than fluconazole, especially in related allogeneic transplantation, after which 19% of patients developed toxicity compared with none of those who received fluconazole.

Itraconazole

Amphotericin and itraconazole have been compared in a multicenter, open, randomized study in 277 adults with cancer and neutropenia (54). Itraconazole oral solution (100 mg bd, $n = 144$) was compared with a combination of amphotericin capsules and nystatin oral suspension ($n = 133$). Adverse events were reported in about 45% of patients in each group. The most frequent were vomiting (14 versus 12 patients), diarrhea (12 versus 9 patients), nausea (5 versus 12 patients), and rash (2 versus 13 patients). There were no differences in liver function test abnormalities. Treatment had to be withdrawn because of adverse events (including death) in 34 patients who took itraconazole and 33 of those who took amphotericin plus nystatin; there were 17 deaths in each group and death was recorded as adverse event in 13 and nine patients respectively.

Intravenous amphotericin deoxycholate (0.7–1.0 mg/kg) and itraconazole (400 mg intravenously for 2 days, 200 mg intravenously for up to 12 days, then 400 mg/day orally) have been compared in 384 granulocytopenic patients with persistent fever in a randomized, multicenter trial (55). The median duration of therapy was 8.5 days. The incidence of drug-related adverse events (54 versus 5%) and the rate of withdrawal due to toxicity (38 versus 19%) were significantly higher with amphotericin. The most frequent reasons for withdrawal in patients taking itraconazole were nausea and vomiting (5%), rash (3%), and abnormal liver function tests (3%). Significantly more of the patients who received amphotericin had nephrotoxicity (24 versus 5%); however, fewer had hyperbilirubinemia (5 versus 10%). There was no difference in gastrointestinal adverse events between the two groups.

Amphotericin in capsules 500 mg qds has been compared with itraconazole elixir 2.5 mg/kg bd for the prophylaxis of systemic and superficial fungal infections in a double-blind, randomized, placebo-controlled, multicenter trial for 1–59 days (56). While itraconazole significantly reduced the frequency of superficial fungal infections, it was not superior in reducing invasive fungal infections or in improving mortality. Adverse events were reported in 222 patients taking itraconazole (79%) and in 205 patients taking amphotericin (74%). The commonest adverse events were gastrointestinal, followed by rash and hypokalemia, with no differences between the two regimens. In both groups, 5% of the adverse events were considered to be definitely drug-related. Comparable numbers of patients in the two groups permanently stopped treatment because of adverse events (including death), 78 (28%) in the amphotericin group and 75 (27%) in the itraconazole group. Nausea (11 and 9%) and vomiting (7 and 8%) were the most frequently reported adverse events that led to withdrawal. Biochemical changes were comparable in the two groups.

Echinocandins

In a randomized, double-blind comparison of amphotericin (0.5 mg/kg intravenously) and caspofungin acetate (35, 50, or 70 mg) once daily for 7–14 days in 140 patients with oropharyngeal and/or esophageal candidiasis, 63% had esophageal involvement and 98% were infected with HIV (57). Response rates were 63% with amphotericin and 74–91% with caspofungin. More patients receiving amphotericin had drug-related adverse effects (fever, chills, nausea, vomiting) than those receiving any dose of caspofungin. Two patients who took caspofungin 35 mg and one who was given amphotericin withdrew because of adverse effects. Drug-related laboratory abnormalities were also more common in patients who received amphotericin. The most common drug-related laboratory abnormalities in

patients who received caspofungin were raised alanine transaminase, aspartate transaminase, and alkaline phosphatase, which were typically less than five times the upper limit of normal and resolved despite continued treatment. None of the patients receiving caspofungin and nine of those who received amphotericin developed drug-related increases in serum creatinine concentrations. No patient withdrew because of drug-related laboratory adverse effects.

Amphotericin has been compared with caspofungin in a multicenter, double-blind, randomized trial in 128 adults with endoscopically documented symptomatic *Candida* esophagitis (58). There was endoscopically verified clinical success in 63% of patients given amphotericin deoxycholate 0.5 mg/kg/day and in 74 and 89% of the patients who received caspofungin 50 and 70 mg/day respectively. Therapy was withdrawn because of drug-related adverse events in 24% of the patients who were given amphotericin and in 4 and 7% of those who were given caspofungin 50 and 70 mg/day respectively. More patients who received amphotericin had drug-related fever, chills, or nausea than those who received caspofungin. More patients who received amphotericin (91%) than caspofungin (61 and 32%) developed drug-related laboratory abnormalities. There were drug-related increases in blood urea–nitrogen concentrations in 15% of the patients who received amphotericin but none of those who received caspofungin. Likewise, serum creatinine concentrations increased in 16 patients who received amphotericin but in only one who received caspofungin. In summary, caspofungin was as effective as amphotericin but better tolerated in the treatment of esophageal candidiasis.

In a double-blind, randomized trial, amphotericin deoxycholate was compared with caspofungin for the primary treatment of invasive candidiasis (59). Patients who had clinical evidence of infection and a positive culture for *Candida* species from blood or another site were enrolled. They were stratified according to the severity of disease, as indicated by the presence or absence of neutropenia and the Acute Physiology and Chronic Health Evaluation (APACHE II) score, and were randomly assigned to receive either amphotericin (0.6–0.7 mg/kg/day or 0.7–1.0 mg/kg/day for patients with neutropenia) or caspofungin (50 mg/day with a loading dose of 70 mg on day 1). Of the 239 patients enrolled, 224 were included in the modified intention-to-treat analysis. Baseline characteristics, including the percentage of patients with neutropenia and the mean APACHE II score, were similar in the two treatment groups. The efficacy of amphotericin was similar to that of caspofungin, with successful outcomes in 62% of the patients treated with amphotericin and in 73% of those treated with caspofungin. There were significantly more drug-related adverse events (fever, chills, and infusion-related events) associated with amphotericin. Amphotericin caused more nephrotoxicity, as defined by an increase in serum creatinine of at least twice the baseline value or an increase of at least 88 µmol/l) (8.4 versus 25%). Only 2.6% of those who were given caspofungin were withdrawn because of adverse events, compared with 23% of those who were given amphotericin. Thus, caspofungin was at least as effective as amphotericin for the treatment of mostly non-neutropenic patients with invasive candidiasis but significantly better tolerated.

Comparisons with antimonials

Amphotericin might be useful in the treatment of leishmaniasis, as suggested by a comparative study (amphotericin in 14 doses of 0.5 mg/kg infused in 5% glucose on alternate days) against sodium stibogluconate (20 mg/kg in two divided doses daily for 40 days). All 40 patients taking amphotericin were cured, whereas in the stibogluconate group 28 of the 40 showed an initial cure but only 25 a definite cure (60).

Placebo-controlled studies

In a small randomized, double-blind, placebo-controlled study, liposomal amphotericin (2 mg/kg three times weekly) was investigated as prophylaxis against fungal infections in 161 patients undergoing chemotherapy or bone marrow transplantation for hematological malignancies (61). There were no statistically significant differences between the two study arms in the incidences of the most frequently reported adverse events or in changes in renal and hepatic laboratory parameters. Despite a sizable rate of suspected or documented fungal infections in the placebo arm, prophylactic therapy with liposomal amphotericin did not lead to a significant reduction in fungal infections or the requirement for systemic antifungal therapy.

General adverse effects

Fever, rigors, nausea, vomiting, headaches, muscle pains, and joint pains are common. The incidence and severity of these reactions are highest with rapidly increasing blood concentrations, and are frequent during the start of therapy (62). Hypersensitivity reactions have been described in case reports. Reports of rashes have been rare. The UK Committee on Safety of Medicines received 20 reports of the occurrence of rash over a 17-year period (SEDA-16, 289). However, with increased use of lipid formulations this could change (63–65). Tumor-inducing effects have not been demonstrated in animals or humans.

Organs and Systems

Cardiovascular

Electrolyte disturbances (hyperkalemia, hypomagnesemia, renal tubular acidosis) due to renal toxicity can be additional factors that precipitate cardiac reactions.

Effects on blood pressure

Changes in blood pressure (hypotension as well as hypertension) have been reported (66,67).

- A 67-year-old man with multiple intraperitoneal and urinary fungal pathogens and a history of well-controlled chronic hypertension developed severe hypertension associated with an infusion of ABLC (68). He received a 5 mg test dose, which was tolerated without incident. About 60 minutes into the infusion (5 mg/kg), his blood pressure rapidly increased to 262/110 mmHg from a baseline of 150/80 mmHg. His temperature increased to 39.8°C, and tachycardia developed (up to 121/minute). The infusion was stopped, and he was given morphine, propranolol, and paracetamol. His blood pressure returned to baseline over the next 2 hours. Rechallenge with ABLC on the next day resulted in an identical reaction despite premedication with pethidine, diphenhydramine, and morphine. ABLC was permanently withdrawn, and the infection was managed with high dosages of fluconazole.

The etiology of amphotericin-associated hypertension has not been elucidated, but it may be related to vasoconstriction. Of note, the traditional test dose appears not to identify individuals predisposed to hypertensive reactions; four of six cases of amphotericin-associated hypertension received test doses without incident.

Cardiac dysrhythmias

In 6 of 90 children given intravenous amphotericin there was a significant fall in heart rate, and monitoring of heart rate was recommended in children with underlying heart disease (69). These immediate reactions follow intravenous administration and occur particularly with excessively rapid infusion of DAMB.

Ventricular dysrhythmias have been reported after rapid infusion of large doses of DAMB (70) in patients with hyperkalemia and renal insufficiency, but not in patients with normal serum creatinine and potassium concentrations, even if they have received the drug over a period of 1 hour. Slower infusion rates and infusion during hemodialysis have been advocated in patients with terminal kidney insufficiency, in order to avoid hyperkalemia.

Chest pain

Three cases of chest discomfort associated with infusion of L-AmB at a dosage of 3 mg/kg/hour for 1 hour have been reported (71).

- The first patient had chest tightness and difficulty in breathing and the second had dyspnea and acute hypoxia (PaO$_2$ 55 mmHg; 7.3 kPa), both within 10 minutes of the start of the infusion. The third complained of chest pain 5 minutes after the start of two infusions. In all cases the symptoms resolved on terminating therapy. Two patients were later rechallenged with slower infusions and tolerated the drug well.

A review of the literature showed that similar reactions had been reported anecdotally in several clinical trials of L-AmB, with all other formulations, and with liposomal daunorubicin and doxorubicin. While the pathophysiology of such reactions is yet unclear, the authors recommended infusing L-AmB over at least 2 hours with careful monitoring of adverse events.

Myocardial ischemia

Rare instances of cardiac arrest have been reported (72).

Vascular effects

Phlebitis occurs in over 5% of patients receiving amphotericin deoxycholate through peripheral veins, which limits the concentration advisable for this route of administration.

Raynaud's syndrome has been attributed to DAMB phenomenon (73).

Extravasation can cause severe local reactions, including tissue necrosis. Safe venous access, preferably via a central line is advisable. The recommendation to use sodium heparin or buffered dextrose is not supported by clinical data.

Respiratory

Inhaled DAMB, and to a lesser extent inhaled liposomal amphotericin, can provoke pulmonary reactions, including bronchospasm, cough, and dyspnea (74–77).

Original suggestions that DAMB in combination with granulocyte transfusions (78) result in pulmonary toxicity have subsequently not been confirmed in prospective observations (62,79). Pulmonary reactions, including dyspnea, hemoptysis, and new infiltrates, have also been suspected to be caused by the combined use of blood platelet transfusions and DAMB (SEDA-12, 227). It therefore appears advisable to space transfusions of blood products and amphotericin if possible (80).

Intravenous administration of DAMB has been associated with pulmonary reactions, including dyspnea, bronchospasm, fever, and chills; in contrast to rare reports of dyspnea after liposomal amphotericin (5), dyspnea was not associated with general toxic reactions. The possibility that liposome overload is the explanation of this reaction should be considered.

A life-threatening event has been reported after the use of ABLC in a patient previously treated with amphotericin deoxycholate (81).

- Tachycardia, tachypnea, dyspnea, and severe hypoxemia occurred 90 minutes after the start of the first dose of ABLC, with radiological evidence of bilateral interstitial infiltrates, and required transient mechanical ventilation. After the event, treatment was continued with amphotericin deoxycholate without undesirable effects.

Nervous system

Headache is common during the immediate infusion reaction. Neuropathy, convulsions, tremor, and paresis have also been attributed to amphotericin. It is difficult to assess these reports, because in systemic fungal infections, with the possibility of central nervous system involvement, the symptoms may be due to the underlying disease.

Reversible parkinsonism has been attributed to ABLC (82).

- A 10-year-old bone marrow recipient was given ABLC 7 mg/kg/day for prolonged periods of time. Ablation therapy before transplantation included cytosine arabinoside, cyclophosphamide, and total body irradiation. He developed progressive parkinsonian features; an MRI scan showed non-specific frontal cortex white matter abnormalities, and brain MR spectroscopy was consistent with significant neuronal loss in the left insular cortex, left basal ganglia, and left frontal white matter. He was given co-careldopa (carbidopa + levodopa) and made a slow recovery within 4 months. A follow-up MRI scan again showed frontal white matter changes, but repeat MR spectroscopy showed marked improvement in the areas previously examined.

This case shows that, regardless of the formulation of amphotericin, severe neurological adverse effects can occur, in particular in patients who receive large dosages of amphotericin after cranial irradiation. A clinical syndrome of akinetic mutism, incontinence, and parkinsonism has been described in patients who received large doses of amphotericin deoxycholate in association with central nervous system irradiation or infection (67).

Electrolyte balance

Selective distal tubular epithelial toxicity by amphotericin can cause hypokalemia, and hypokalemia can cause further tubular damage. There is some evidence that hypokalemia due to amphotericin is mitigated by both spironolactone (83) and amiloride (84).

Infusion of amphotericin deoxycholate can cause hyperkalemia, in particular in the setting of renal insufficiency (67). The primary mechanism is not known.

- Fatal cardiopulmonary arrest occurred in a 4-year-old boy with acute leukemia and disseminated invasive candidiasis after the third infusion of ABLC 5 mg/kg/day, infused over 1 hour (85). During resuscitation he had a serum potassium concentration of 16 mmol/l; there was no evidence of hemolysis or rhabdomyolysis and serum creatinine and potassium concentrations had been within the reference ranges earlier in the day. Autopsy showed numerous fungal abscesses, including several in the myocardium.
- Serum potassium concentrations were determined at the end of a 2-hour infusion of amphotericin deoxycholate (1 mg/kg/day) in a 2-year-old girl with systemic candidiasis receiving long-term hemodialysis for renal dysplasia (85). The potassium concentration was 6.7 mmol/l, despite dialysis against a 1.5 mmol/l potassium bath just before the infusion. The next dose was given during dialysis, and the serum potassium concentration was 2.6 mmol/l after the infusion.

When giving amphotericin to dialysed patients, it may be necessary to give it during dialysis in order to avoid hyperkalemia.

Hematologic

A normochromic, normocytic, usually mild anemia develops regularly during therapy with DAMB. The erythropoietin response to anemia appears to be blunted during DAMB therapy, and survival of erythrocytes may be reduced by toxic effects of amphotericin on the cell membrane (86).

Frank hemolysis has also been reported in rare instances, including, rarely, immune-mediated hemolysis (87,88).

Leukopenia has been reported (SED-12, 673).

Thrombocytopenia has been reported in several instances and also occurs with lipid formulations (89,90).

During amphotericin therapy, the response of platelet counts to thrombocyte transfusions was reduced, as was platelet survival (91,92).

Gastrointestinal

Anorexia, nausea, and vomiting are common effects of parenteral administration of amphotericin. Gastrointestinal complaints are markedly less common with liposomal amphotericin than with ABCD(5).

Liver

Cholestasis has been reported in infants treated with amphotericin for systemic *Candida* infections (SEDA-14, 230). Most of the above reports were incidental, and amphotericin cannot be regarded as a known cause of liver damage. This does not necessarily also apply to liposomal amphotericin and other lipid formulations. Therapy with L-Amb, AmBisome was associated with a rise in alkaline phosphatase in over a third of children treated with AmBisome (93) and with hepatic dysfunction in a little under 20% of adolescents and adults. In a small retrospective study, ABLC was withdrawn in 27% of patients because of rises in serum bilirubin and alkaline phosphatase, a finding confirmed in a larger prospective study. Cholestasis has also been observed with ABCD, in contrast to reports that L-AmB does not increase transaminases (5).

Acute hepatic damage has rarely been reported with DAMB. Asymptomatic increases in hepatic serum enzyme activities were seen in one case (94).

- A 26-year-old previously healthy man with life-threatening pulmonary blastomycosis developed increased hepatic transaminases to a maximum of ten times (aspartate transaminase) and 20 times (alanine transaminase), the upper limit of the reference ranges, 10 days after the addition of amphotericin (0.5 mg/kg) to his initial itraconazole therapy (200 mg bd) (95). The serum transaminase activities returned to normal within 4 days after withdrawal of amphotericin, and the blastomycosis was successfully treated with itraconazole alone. A liver biopsy showed mild focal fatty changes but no evidence of blastomycosis.

The authors speculated that amphotericin may have facilitated the uptake of itraconazole into mammalian cells by its membrane-damaging action, leading to increased interaction of itraconazole with CYP450 enzymes and hepatocellular damage.

Pancreas

In a retrospective analysis, 5 of 31 children with cancers, who had received liposomal amphotericin in dosages of 1–3 mg/kg/day, had an isolated transient rise in the serum lipase activity during or shortly after therapy with liposomal amphotericin (96). Three of these patients had signs of pancreatitis. While the exact pathogenesis is unclear, the authors proposed fat overload or toxic damage to the pancreas by the liposomes or amphotericin itself as potential mechanisms.

Urinary tract

Amphotericin can cause both glomerular and tubular damage. Lipid-based formulations (colloidal dispersion, lipid complex, and liposomal amphotericin) are less nephrotoxic than conventional amphotericin deoxycholate (97). However, several caveats have to be kept in mind in making such comparisons. For example, there are no defined equivalent doses for amphotericin deoxycholate and its lipid-based counterparts.

Presentation
The clinical and laboratory findings include reductions in glomerular filtration rate and renal plasma flow, proteinuria, cylindruria, and hematuria; the last three are frequent but usually discrete. The reductions in renal plasma flow and filtration fraction occur early. Changes in tubular function can cause increased excretion of uric acid (an effect that can be used to monitor the tubular damage). Excessive loss of potassium, magnesium, and bicarbonate result in hypokalemia, hypomagnesemia, and renal tubular acidosis (98,99). Severe hypokalemia is common, and requires parenteral potassium replacement. Acidosis can also be severe, requiring bicarbonate. Hypomagnesemia, which may be symptomatic, can cause secondary hypocalcemia, resulting in tetany (100–102).

Amphotericin can cause an inability to form a concentrated urine (hyposthenuria) although this rarely becomes clinically important (67).

Nephrogenic diabetes insipidus, resistant to vasopressin, following damage to the distal renal tubule, may be more common than reported (103,104). Careful monitoring of electrolytes is therefore recommended in all instances of amphotericin therapy.

- A 43-year-old HIV-infected patient presented with nephrogenic diabetes insipidus associated with amphotericin deoxycholate therapy for ocular candidiasis; rechallenge was positive (105).

Mechanism
The exact mechanisms involved in amphotericin-induced uremia are not yet fully understood. Changes in tubular ion permeability have been demonstrated both in vitro and in vivo (12,100,106). The uremia can be caused by tubuloglomerular feedback, a mechanism whereby increased delivery and re-absorption of chloride ions in the distal tubule initiates a reduction in the glomerular filtration rate. Tubuloglomerular feedback is amplified by sodium deprivation and suppressed by sodium loading. Other possible mechanisms are renal arteriolar spasm, calcium deposition during periods of ischemia, and direct cellular toxicity (12). Yet other lines of research have looked at the roles of prostaglandins and TNFα, with evidence that indometacin may abate prostaglandin-mediated toxicity (107), an approach that is not practical in most patients requiring antifungal drugs.

- Renal damage due to amphotericin has also been reportedly caused by a tumor lysis-like syndrome in a 41-year-old woman with visceral leishmaniasis, with hyperkalemia, hyperphosphatemia, hyperuricemia, and acute renal insufficiency (108).

Differences among formulations
The nephrotoxicity of lipid formulations of amphotericin varies from formulation to formulation.

Amphotericin B deoxycholate
The epidemiology of the nephrotoxicity of conventional amphotericin B has been investigated in a retrospective study in 494 adult inpatients who received two or more doses (109). Nephrotoxicity was defined as a 50–100% increase in the baseline creatinine concentration. The median cumulative dose was 240 mg and most of the patients received it for empirical therapy. Overall, 139 patients (28%) had renal toxicity, including 58 (12%) with moderate to severe nephrotoxicity. For each 10 mg increase in the mean daily dose, the adjusted rate of renal toxicity increased by a factor of 1.13. Five risk factors were defined: a mean daily dose of 35 mg or more, male sex, weight 90 kg or more, chronic renal disease, and concurrent use of amikacin or ciclosporin. The incidence of moderate to severe nephrotoxicity was 4% in patients with none of these risk factors, 8% in those with one, 18% in those with two, and 29% in those with three or more. Nephrotoxicity rarely led to hemodialysis ($n = 3$). However, at the time of discharge or death, 70% of the patients with moderate to severe nephrotoxicity had a serum creatinine concentration that was at least 44 µmol/l above baseline. This study shows dose-dependency of nephrotoxicity related to DAMB, accentuated by other nephrotoxic drugs and patient risk factors. The authors suggested that in patients with more than two risk factors alternative antifungal drugs should be considered.

The nephrotoxicity of amphotericin deoxycholate has been investigated in a retrospective multicenter study in 239 immunosuppressed patients with suspected or proven aspergillosis for a median duration of 15 days (110). The serum creatinine concentration doubled in 53% of the patients and exceeded 221 µmol/l in 29%; 15% underwent dialysis, and 60% died. Multivariate Cox proportional hazards analysis showed that patients whose creatinine concentration exceeded 221 µmol/l, and patients with allogeneic and autologous bone marrow transplants were at greatest risk of requiring hemodialysis. The use of hemodialysis, the duration of amphotericin therapy, and the use of nephrotoxic agents were associated with a greater risk of death, whereas patients who underwent solid organ transplantation were at lowest risk. The findings of this study suggest that raised creatinine concentrations during therapy with amphotericin are associated with a substantial risk of hemodialysis and a higher mortality rate, but these risks vary in different patients.

Amphotericin-associated nephrotoxicity has been studied in a retrospective analysis of 69 recipients of blood stem-cell transplants with multiple myeloma who received at least two doses of amphotericin deoxycholate during 1992–95 (111). Nephrotoxicity occurred in 30 patients (43%) and developed rapidly. Patients who developed nephrotoxicity were similar to those who did not in many aspects associated with their treatment. However, baseline-estimated creatinine clearance, ciclosporin therapy, nephrotoxic drug therapy within 30 days of starting amphotericin, and the number of concomitant nephrotoxic drugs were significant predictors of amphotericin-associated nephrotoxicity. The authors concluded that recipients of bone marrow or peripheral blood stem-cell transplants who have multiple myeloma and are receiving ciclosporin or multiple nephrotoxic drugs at the start of amphotericin therapy should be considered at high risk of amphotericin-associated nephrotoxicity.

In a retrospective study, renal function was investigated in patients receiving ciclosporin alone or in combination with amphotericin (24-hour infusion) after allogeneic stem-cell transplantation (112). Of 84 patients, 22 were treated with amphotericin. There was a statistically significant reduction in renal function compared with the 62 patients who received ciclosporin alone. However, renal insufficiency in all patients remained in a clinically acceptable range and was reversible in patients who survived to 1 year after transplantation.

Continuous infusion of amphotericin has been assessed in an open study in six lung transplant recipients with invasive or semi-invasive bronchopulmonary azole-resistant candidal infections who were treated for 40 (17–73) days by 24-hour continuous infusions of amphotericin 1 mg/kg (113). They received at least 1000 ml/day of 0.9% saline intravenously. Apart from ciclosporin, five patients received aminoglycosides for at least 2 weeks, and four received ganciclovir. Calculated creatinine clearance fell from 57 (43–73) ml/minute to a nadir of 35 (28–39) and recovered to 52 (33–60) after the end of therapy. One patient needed temporary hemofiltration for 7 days. Besides three episodes of mild hypokalemia there were no adverse effects attributable to amphotericin. Asymptomatic colonization with *Candida* persisted for 10 months in one case, but the other five patients were cured.

Amphotericin B colloidal dispersion
During ABCD therapy 8.5% of patients developed nephrotoxicity compared with 21% in those given amphotericin deoxycholate (5).

In a randomized, double-blind, multicenter trial, ABCD (Amphotec; 6 mg/kg/day) was compared with liposomal amphotericin (1.0–1.5 mg/kg/day) for the first-line treatment of invasive aspergillosis in 174 patients (114). The median duration of therapy was 13 (1–357) days in those given ABCD, and 15 (1–87) days in those given liposomal amphotericin. For evaluable patients ($n = 103$) given ABCD or liposomal amphotericin, the respective rates of therapeutic response (52 versus 51%), mortality (36 versus 45%), and death due to fungal infection (32 versus 26%) were similar. Renal toxicity was significantly lower (25 versus 49%) and the median time to onset of nephrotoxicity longer (301 versus 22 days;) in the patients who received ABCD. Rates of drug-related toxicity in the patients who received ABCD and liposomal amphotericin were respectively 53 versus 30% (chills), 27 versus 16% (fever), 1 versus 4% (hypoxia), and 22 versus 24% (toxicity requiring study drug withdrawal). Based on the results of this trial, ABCD appears to have equivalent efficacy to liposomal amphotericin, and superior renal safety in the treatment of invasive aspergillosis.

However, infusion-related chills and fever occurred more often with ABCD.

Amphotericin B lipid complex (ABLC)
A comparison of ABLC with amphotericin deoxycholate showed significant differences, with a doubling of baseline creatinine in 28% during ABLC compared with 47% during conventional therapy (5).

There has been a retrospective comparison of the renal effects of ABLC with amphotericin deoxycholate in the treatment of invasive candidiasis and cryptococcosis in dosages of 0.6–5 mg/kg/day; most patients received 5 mg/kg/day (115). Changes in serum creatinine were evaluated in three ways: doubling of the baseline value, an increase from below 132 μmol/l (1.5 mg/dl) at baseline to over 132 μmol/l, and an increase from below 132 μmol/l at baseline to at least 177 μmol/l (2.0 mg/dl). These endpoints were achieved significantly more often with amphotericin deoxycholate than with ABLC, and the time needed to reach each of the endpoints was significantly shorter with amphotericin deoxycholate. An increased serum creatinine concentration was reported as an adverse event more often in patients receiving amphotericin deoxycholate than in patients receiving ABLC (24 versus 43%).

The rates of ABLC-associated nephrotoxicity in various clinical settings at a university hospital have been estimated retrospectively and compared with previously reported rates of nephrotoxicity (116). Data from 33 adult patients (20 men, 13 women; mean age 49 years) with and without neutropenia receiving ABLC were collected, and the degree of nephrotoxicity was determined using two definitions: (1) doubling of baseline serum creatinine concentration using the peak value within the first 7 days and (2) end-of-therapy doubling of baseline serum concentration using the end-of-therapy value. Using the selected definitions of ABLC-associated nephrotoxicity, there were only two cases. This rate was significantly below the 42% rate reported in the only large published study (95% CI = 1.7, 19.6). The median change in serum creatinine concentration was 8.9 (–97 to 380) μmol/l. The concomitant use of nephrotoxic agents was not associated with significant changes in serum creatinine concentration. The authors concluded that ABLC infrequently causes clinically significant nephrotoxicity, and that earlier data derived from a single study in febrile patients with neutropenia should be interpreted cautiously.

Liposomal amphotericin B (L-Amb, AmBisome)
In a prospective double-blind study of more than 600 patients, 0.6 mg/kg of DAMB was compared with 3.0 mg/kg of L-Amb, a dose relation at the lower limit of equivalent doses determined in an animal model (117). At these dosages, in a large prospective double-blind study, there was a doubling of serum creatinine concentration in 19% of neutropenic patients receiving empirical therapy with L-AmB and 34% receiving conventional amphotericin (47).

Liposomal amphotericin has been given to an immunosuppressed renal transplant patient with cerebral aspergillosis for almost 10 months at a cumulative dose of 42 g with no apparent changes in the function of the renal allograft, as measured by serum creatinine, creatinine clearance, and potassium concentrations (118). Therapy was ultimately successful and was discontinued after surgical resection of a residual sclerotic lesion.

Liposomal amphotericin (3 mg/kg/day) has been compared with conventional amphotericin (0.7 mg/kg/day) for induction therapy of moderate to severe disseminated histoplasmosis in a randomized, double-blind, multicenter trial in 81 patients with AIDS (119). The duration of induction was 2 weeks, to be followed by 10 weeks of itraconazole in the case of a response. Clinical success was achieved in 14 of 22 patients treated with conventional amphotericin compared with 45 of 51 patients who received liposomal amphotericin (difference, 24%; 95% CI = 1%, 52%). Culture conversion rates were similar. Three patients treated with conventional amphotericin and one treated with liposomal amphotericin died during induction. Infusion-related adverse effects were more common with conventional amphotericin (63%) than with liposomal amphotericin (25%). Nephrotoxicity occurred in 37% of patients treated with conventional amphotericin and 9% of patients treated with liposomal amphotericin. The results of this study suggest that liposomal amphotericin is less toxic than conventional amphotericin and is associated with improved survival.

Prevention
Avoidance of salt depletion and a salt load (500–1000 ml of 0.9% saline) reduce the renal toxicity of DAMB (120–126). Also the maintenance of adequate serum potassium concentrations by replacement therapy may be important and may contribute to "kidney sparing" (127). Other preventive measures, including dopamine infusion, are of no value (128).

It has been suggested that amphotericin-induced nephrotoxicity may be mitigated by increasing renal blood flow and glomerular filtration rate with low-dose dopamine (1–3 μg/kg/minute). The efficacy of low-dose dopamine in preventing nephrotoxicity associated with amphotericin deoxycholate has been evaluated in a prospective randomized study in 71 patients after antineoplastic chemotherapy for autologous bone marrow transplantation or acute leukemia (128). The patients were randomly assigned to receive low-dose dopamine by continuous infusion (3 μg/kg/minute) or no dopamine. Amphotericin deoxycholate 0.5 or 1.0 mg/kg/day was given for respectively 8 and 13 days on average. Nephrotoxicity, defined as a 1.5-fold or greater increase in baseline serum creatinine concentration, was slightly less common, but not significantly so, in those given dopamine (67 versus 80%). The grade of nephrotoxicity was the same. Ten patients developed grade IV nephrotoxicity and were withdrawn from the study. The authors concluded that dopamine offers little benefit in preventing amphotericin deoxycholate-associated nephrotoxicity.

In a randomized, controlled, single-center study, continuous infusion of amphotericin reduced nephrotoxicity and infusion-associated reactions compared with the standard infusion over 2–4 hours in patients with neutropenia, refractory fever, and suspected or proven invasive fungal infections (129). However, the concentration-dependent pharmacodynamics of antifungal polyenes raise concerns about the antifungal effectiveness of this mode of administration in particular, as its therapeutic efficacy has not been adequately studied in animals or in patients with documented infections.

Skin

An allergic skin reaction to amphotericin has been reported (130).

- A 3-year-old child had a severe allergic reaction during treatment with liposomal amphotericin for persistent neutropenic fever following unrelated allogeneic cord blood stem-cell transplantation. The patient developed an extensive maculopapular rash and severe itching that was unresponsive to antihistamine and glucocorticoid medication and resolved only after drug withdrawal. Continuation of therapy with conventional amphotericin for 20 days was well tolerated, suggesting that the lipid carrier was responsible for the adverse event.

Immunologic

A literature review found no support for the routine use of a test dose of amphotericin before the first therapeutic dose of amphotericin deoxycholate, as is still recommended by the manufacturers (131). The mechanism of common infusion-related adverse effects does not appear to be allergic in nature, and true allergic reactions are rare. Moreover, the absence of a reaction to a test dose does not necessarily indicate that patients will not have a severe infusion-related reaction later in the course of therapy, and the procedure of administering a test dose can lead to a detrimental delay in adequate antifungal therapy. The authors recommended starting therapy with amphotericin deoxycholate at the full therapeutic target dose, with careful bedside monitoring for infusion-related adverse events throughout therapy.

Anaphylaxis is rare with amphotericin (67). It is important to note that a patient may tolerate one formulation and respond with anaphylaxis to another.

- Anaphylaxis after ABCD occurred in a patient who had previously been treated with both amphotericin deoxycholate and ABLC without infusion-related adverse effects (65). During the first infusion of ABCD he developed spontaneously reversible severe back pain and then swelling of his lips, respiratory distress, and left-sided hemiparesis, which resolved after 24 hours. An MRI scan suggested an ischemic event in the right putamen, lending support to the hypothesis that he had had an anaphylactic reaction to ABCD, hypoperfusion, and a subsequent stroke.
- In another patient, serious adverse events (fever, severe rigors, a fall in blood pressure, worsening mental status, increasing creatinine concentration, and leukocytosis) occurred after unrecognized substitution of one amphotericin formulation (ABLC) by another (ABCD) (132). After discovery of the switch, ABLC therapy was reinstituted and tolerated without incident.

These cases underscore the need to monitor patients closely when infusing the first dose of a different formulation of amphotericin.

Second-Generation Effects

Pregnancy

Experience with amphotericin in pregnancy is limited. Amphotericin crosses the placenta and can increase creatinine concentrations in the neonate. High tissue concentrations of amphotericin persist weeks after treatment has been stopped (133).

Susceptibility Factors

Age

Neonates

The safety and efficacy of liposomal amphotericin in 40 preterm and 4 full-term neonates with invasive yeast infections have been studied retrospectively (134). The initial dosage was 1 mg/kg/day, and was increased stepwise by 1 mg/kg to a maximum of 5 mg/kg, depending on the clinical condition. There were no infusion-associated reactions. Blood pressure, hepatic, renal, and hematological indices were not altered. Hypokalemia was noted in 16 infants but was always transient and responsive to potassium supplementation. Treatment with liposomal amphotericin was successful in 72% of the children. However, 12 of the 40 preterm infants succumbed to the fungal infection; all had a birth weight of less than 1.5 kg.

Changes in serum creatinine and serum potassium have been measured in 21 neonates of very low birth weight who received amphotericin for presumed or documented yeast infections (135). The median dosage was 2.6 (range 1–5) mg/kg/day, and the median duration of therapy was 2 (11–79) days. Hypokalemia (below 3 mmol/l) was observed in 30% before treatment and in 15% during treatment. However, 21 days after the end of therapy, hypokalemia was not present in any patient. The maximum creatinine concentration fell from 121 (71–221) μmol/l to 68 (31–171) μmol/l during treatment and 46 (26–62) μmol/l at 21 days after the end of therapy. However, creatinine concentrations were available for only 10, 18, and 15 of the 21 patients respectively, and no information was provided on the number of patients who had an increase in serum creatinine during therapy. All patients responded to therapy with liposomal amphotericin, although the number of proven invasive fungal infections was small (7/21).

Infants

The safety and efficacy of ABLC in 11 neonates with systemic *Candida* infections have been reported (136). The infants were aged 3–14 (median 7) weeks and weighed 0.7–5 (median 1.4) kg. The median duration of ABLC treatment was 23 (range 4–41) days at an average dose of 4.9 (range 3.2–6.5) mg/kg/day. Nine of the eleven patients improved clinically, and eight of nine evaluable patients had a mycological cure. No infant discontinued treatment because of adverse drug reactions, and none had appreciable hepatic or hematological toxicity. Renal function improved or did not change in 8 of the 11. The median pretreatment serum creatinine concentration was 80 (range 35–522) μmol/l and the median creatinine concentration at the end of treatment was 44 (range 18–628) µmol/l.

Children

The disposition of liposomal amphotericin in children and adolescents is similar to that in adults. Liposomal amphotericin and conventional amphotericin have been compared in a randomized, multicenter study in 204 children with cancers, pyrexia, and neutropenia (137). There was a 2.6 times lower incidence of adverse effects with the liposomal formulation. There were severe adverse effects in 1% of those who received liposomal amphotericin and 12% of those who received the conventional formulation.

Data on the safety of amphotericin deoxycholate have been reported for 50 therapeutic courses in 44 children and adolescents with cancer and a median age of 6.8 years (range 9 months to 18 years) (50). Amphotericin deoxycholate was given in a dose of 1 mg/kg over 2 hours for a mean duration of 7.8 days. Most of the patients received the drug as empirical antifungal therapy in the setting of persistent fever and neutropenia. Nephrotoxicity, defined as a 100% increase in the serum creatinine from baseline, was observed in only one patient. Infusion-related reactions (fevers and/or rigors) occurred in 24% of treatment courses. Thus, amphotericin deoxycholate was relatively well tolerated in this population, although the mean duration of therapy was comparatively short.

The safety and efficacy of ABLC have been studied in an open, emergency-use, multicenter study in 111 treatment episodes in children with invasive mycoses refractory to or intolerant of conventional antifungal drugs (138). The mean daily dosage was 4.85 (range 1.1–9.5) mg/kg, and the mean duration of therapy was 33 (range 1–191) days. While the proportion of patients with deteriorating renal function was not mentioned, the mean serum creatinine concentration in the entire study population did not change significantly between baseline (109 µmol/l) and withdrawal of ABLC (117 µmol/l) over 6 weeks. Similarly, there were no significant differences between initial and end-of-therapy concentrations of serum potassium, magnesium, transaminases, alkaline phosphatase, and hemoglobin. However, there was a significant increase in mean total bilirubin (from 63 to 91 µmol/l) at the end of therapy. ABLC was withdrawn because of toxicity in 7 of the 111 children; adverse events leading to withdrawal included intolerable infusion-related reactions and allergic reactions. Among the 54 evaluable patients, a complete or partial therapeutic response was obtained in 38.

Drug Administration

Drug dosage regimens

By lowering the infusion rate and using continuous infusion, fewer toxic reactions have been observed. In contrast, varying the infusion time of daily doses between 1 and 6 hours made no important change in regard to toxicity (139–144). Alternatively, smaller starting doses have been suggested to reduce toxicity, a strategy that is often not advisable in acute severe

mycoses. The use of lipid formulations reduces the incidence and severity of general toxic reactions and of nephrotoxicity (22,47,49). It is currently unclear, however, whether lipid formulations of amphotericin have a broader therapeutic index than conventional DAMB. It has to be borne in mind that lipid formulations, while affecting the pharmacokinetics of amphotericin, have no targeting properties that discriminate between the cell membrane of the pathogen and that of host cells. It therefore appears possible that some, if not all, of their advantages are in the avoidance of high concentrations of reactive amphotericin, an effect that could also be obtained by continuous infusion of the conventional formula (62). Monitoring of blood concentrations of amphotericin B is not practical, and there are no validated recommendations for its use, neither for avoidance of toxicity nor for monitoring of efficacy.

Drug administration route

Amphotericin given intravenously does not lead to adequate CSF concentrations, and it can rarely be given intrathecally in cases of cerebral infection. Nevertheless, amphotericin is effective even in cryptococcal meningitis, in the absence of marked meningeal inflammation. Continuous infusion may be associated with less toxicity, but experience is limited.

Delirium (145) and parkinsonism (146) have been described after intrathecal or intraventricular therapy.

Drug–Drug Interactions

Aminoglycoside antibiotics

Amphotericin prolongs the half-life of aminoglycoside antibiotics (147).

Antifungal azoles

In evaluating possible antagonism between amphotericin and antifungal azoles, details of the experimental set-up are crucial. When filamentous fungi were exposed to subfungicidal concentrations of azoles, before exposure to an amphotericin + azole combination, antagonism could always be shown both in vitro and in vivo (148–150).

In vitro studies and experiments in animals have given conflicting results relating to potential antagonism between the effects of fluconazole and amphotericin on *Candida* species (149). However, large, randomized, double-blind comparisons of fluconazole with and without amphotericin for 5 days in non-neutropenic patients with candidemia showed no evidence of antagonism, but faster clearance of the organism from the blood and a trend toward an improved outcome in those who received the combination (151).

The combination of amphotericin with ketoconazole appears to lead to antagonism (148). A study of the effects of combinations of amphotericin with fluconazole, itraconazole, or ketoconazole against strains of *Aspergillus fumigatus* in vitro showed antagonistic effects in some strains, but different effects in other strains (152). In one group of mice infected with *Candida*, combinations of amphotericin with fluconazole were more effective than fluconazole alone; in another group the combination showed no interaction, but was not better than either drug given alone (153).

Although there are no clinical data, it can be expected that similar antagonism occurs between amphotericin and squalene oxidase inhibitors, which also eliminate the primary target ergosterol from the fungal cell membrane.

Ciclosporin

Because ciclosporin causes a reduction in renal function, there is increased nephrotoxicity if amphotericin is also given (112,147).

Cisplatin

Amphotericin-induced hypomagnesemia may be more profound in patients who develop a divalent cation-losing nephropathy associated with cisplatin (12).

Cytotoxic drugs

Amphotericin can enhance the risk of adverse effects from cytotoxic drugs (154).

Digitalis

Hypokalemia due to amphotericin can enhance the toxicity of digitalis (12,127).

Diuretics

The concurrent use of diuretics is associated with a higher risk of nephrotoxicity from amphotericin (155).

Flucytosine

Amphotericin in combination with flucytosine results in an increased risk of hematological complications, because amphotericin often impairs renal function, causing retention of flucytosine (10).

Neuromuscular blocking drugs

Hypokalemia due to amphotericin can enhance the curariform effect of neuromuscular blocking agents (12,127,154).

Tacrolimus

Tacrolimus (FK 506), a macrolide immunosuppressant, has adverse effects similar to those of ciclosporin, including nephrotoxicity. Increased nephrotoxicity can be expected when it is given with amphotericin (156).

References

1. Bolard J. How do the polyene macrolide antibiotics affect the cellular membrane properties? Biochim Biophys Acta 1986;864(3–4):257–304.
2. Vertut-Croquin A, Bolard J, Chabbert M, Gary-Bobo C. Differences in the interaction of the polyene antibiotic amphotericin B with cholesterol- or ergosterol-containing phospholipid vesicles. A circular dichroism and permeability study. Biochemistry 1983;22(12):2939–44.
3. Sokol-Anderson ML, Brajtburg J, Medoff G. Amphotericin B-induced oxidative damage and killing of *Candida albicans*. J Infect Dis 1986;154(1):76–83.
4. Edmonds LC, Davidson L, Bertino JS. Effect of variation in infusion time and macrophage blockade on organ uptake of amphotericin B-deoxycholate. J Antimicrob Chemother 1991;28(6):919–24.
5. Wong-Beringer A, Jacobs RA, Guglielmo BJ. Lipid formulations of amphotericin B: clinical efficacy and toxicities. Clin Infect Dis 1998;27(3):603–18.
6. Brajtburg J, Elberg S, Bolard J, Kobayashi GS, Levy RA, Ostlund RE Jr, Schlessinger D, Medoff G. Interaction of plasma proteins and lipoproteins with amphotericin B. J Infect Dis 1984;149(6):986–97.
7. Ridente Y, Aubard J, Bolard J. Absence in amphotericin B-spiked human plasma of the free monomeric drug, as detected by SERS. FEBS Lett 1999;446(2–3):283–6.
8. Baley JE, Meyers C, Kliegman RM, Jacobs MR, Blumer JL. Pharmacokinetics, outcome of treatment, and toxic effects of amphotericin B and 5-fluorocytosine in neonates. J Pediatr 1990;116(5):791–7.
9. Starke JR, Mason EO Jr, Kramer WG, Kaplan SL. Pharmacokinetics of amphotericin B in infants and children. J Infect Dis 1987;155(4):766–74.
10. Polak A. Pharmacokinetics of amphotericin B and flucytosine. Postgrad Med J 1979;55(647):667–70.
11. Atkinson AJ Jr, Bennett JE. Amphotericin B pharmacokinetics in humans. Antimicrob Agents Chemother 1978;13(2):271–6.
12. Lyman CA, Walsh TJ. Systemically administered antifungal agents. A review of their clinical pharmacology and therapeutic applications. Drugs 1992;44(1):9–35.
13. Chavanet PY, Garry I, Charlier N, Caillot D, Kisterman JP, D'Athis M, Portier H. Trial of glucose versus fat emulsion in preparation of amphotericin for use in HIV infected patients with candidiasis. BMJ 1992;305(6859):921–5.
14. Janknegt R, de Marie S, Bakker-Woudenberg IA, Crommelin DJ. Liposomal and lipid formulations of amphotericin B. Clinical pharmacokinetics. Clin Pharmacokinet 1992;23(4):279–91.
15. Sanders SW, Buchi KN, Goddard MS, Lang JK, Tolman KG. Single-dose pharmacokinetics and tolerance of a cholesteryl sulfate complex of amphotericin B administered to healthy volunteers. Antimicrob Agents Chemother 1991;35(6):1029–34.
16. Adedoyin A, Bernardo JF, Swenson CE, Bolsack LE, Horwith G, DeWit S, Kelly E, Klasterksy J, Sculier JP, DeValeriola D, Anaissie E, Lopez-Berestein G, Llanos-Cuentas A, Boyle A, Branch RA. Pharmacokinetic profile of ABELCET (amphotericin B lipid complex injection): combined experience from phase I and phase II studies. Antimicrob Agents Chemother 1997;41(10):2201–8.
17. Vita E, Schroeder DJ. Intralipid in prophylaxis of amphotericin B nephrotoxicity. Ann Pharmacother 1994;28(10):1182–3.
18. Thakur CP, Singh RK, Hassan SM, Kumar R, Narain S, Kumar A. Amphotericin B deoxycholate treatment of visceral leishmaniasis with newer modes of administration and precautions: a study of 938 cases. Trans R Soc Trop Med Hyg 1999;93(3):319–23.
19. Pathak A, Pien FD, Carvalho L. Amphotericin B use in a community hospital, with special emphasis on side effects. Clin Infect Dis 1998;26(2):334–8.
20. Noskin GA, Pietrelli L, Coffey G, Gurwith M, Liang LJ. Amphotericin B colloidal dispersion for treatment of candidemia in immunocompromised patients. Clin Infect Dis 1998;26(2):461–7.
21. Anaissie EJ, Mattiuzzi GN, Miller CB, Noskin GA, Gurwith MJ, Mamelok RD, Pietrelli LA. Treatment of invasive fungal infections in renally impaired patients with amphotericin B colloidal dispersion. Antimicrob Agents Chemother 1998;42(3):606–11.

22. Herbrecht R, Letscher V, Andres E, Cavalier A. Safety and efficacy of amphotericin B colloidal dispersion. An overview. Chemotherapy 1999;45(Suppl 1):67–76.

23. Noskin G, Pietrelli L, Gurwith M, Bowden R. Treatment of invasive fungal infections with amphotericin B colloidal dispersion in bone marrow transplant recipients. Bone Marrow Transplant 1999;23(7):697–703.

24. Herbrecht R, Letscher-Bru V, Bowden RA, Kusne S, Anaissie EJ, Graybill JR, Noskin GA, Oppenheim BA, Andrès E, Pietrelli LA. Treatment of 21 cases of invasive mucormycosis with amphotericin B colloidal dispersion. Eur J Clin Microbiol Infect Dis 2001;20(7):460–6.

25. White MH, Bowden RA, Sandler ES, Graham ML, Noskin GA, Wingard JR, Goldman M, van Burik JA, McCabe A, Lin JS, Gurwith M, Miller CB. Randomized, double-blind clinical trial of amphotericin B colloidal dispersion vs. amphotericin B in the empirical treatment of fever and neutropenia. Clin Infect Dis 1998;27(2):296–302.

26. Walsh TJ, Hiemenz JW, Seibel NL, Perfect JR, Horwith G, Lee L, Silber JL, DiNubile MJ, Reboli A, Bow E, Lister J, Anaissie EJ. Amphotericin B lipid complex for invasive fungal infections: analysis of safety efficacy in 556 cases. Clin Infect Dis 1998;26(6):1383–96.

27. Allsup D, Chu P. The use of amphotericin B lipid complex in 15 patients with presumed or proven fungal infection. Br J Haematol 1998;102(4):1109–10.

28. Myint H, Kyi AA, Winn RM. An open, non-comparative evaluation of the efficacy and safety of amphotericin B lipid complex as treatment of neutropenic patients with presumed or confirmed pulmonary fungal infections. J Antimicrob Chemother 1998;41(3):424–6.

29. Ringden O, Jonsson V, Hansen M, Tollemar J, Jacobsen N. Severe and common side-effects of amphotericin B lipid complex (Abelcet). Bone Marrow Transplant 1998;22(7):733–4.

30. Linden P, Lee L, Walsh TJ. Retrospective analysis of the dosage of amphotericin B lipid complex for the treatment of invasive fungal infections. Pharmacotherapy 1999;19(11):1261–8.

31. Singhal S, Hastings JG, Mutimer DJ. Safety of high-dose amphotericin B lipid complex. Bone Marrow Transplant 1999;24(1):116–17.

32. Cook G, Franklin IM. Adverse drug reactions associated with the administration of amphotericin B lipid complex (Abelcet). Bone Marrow Transplant 1999:23(12):1325–6.

33. Martino R, Subira M, Sureda A, Sierra J. Amphotericin B lipid complex at 3 mg/kg/day for treatment of invasive fungal infections in adults with haematological malignancies. J Antimicrob Chemother 1999;44(4):569–72.

34. Martino R, Subira M, Domingo-Albos A, Sureda A, Brunet S, Sierra J. Low-dose amphotericin B lipid complex for the treatment of persistent fever of unknown origin in patients with hematologic malignancies and prolonged neutropenia. Chemotherapy 1999;45(3):205–12.

35. Subira M, Martino R, Sureda A, Altes A, Briones J, Brunet S, Sierra J. Safety and efficacy of low-dose amphotericin B lipid complex for empirical antifungal therapy of neutropenic fever in patients with hematologic malignancies. Methods Find Exp Clin Pharmacol 2001;23(9):505–10.

36. Palmer SM, Drew RH, Whitehouse JD, Tapson VF, Davis RD, McConnell RR, Kanj SS, Perfect JR. Safety of aerosolized amphotericin B lipid complex in lung transplant recipients. Transplantation 2001;72(3):545–8.

37. Walsh TJ, Yeldandi V, McEvoy M, Gonzalez C, Chanock S, Freifeld A, Seibel NI, Whitcomb PO, Jarosinski P, Boswell G, Bekersky I, Alak A, Buell D, Barret J, Wilson W. Safety, tolerance, and pharmacokinetics of a small unilamellar liposomal formulation of amphotericin B (AmBisome) in neutropenic patients. Antimicrob Agents Chemother 1998;42(9):2391–8.

38. Ellis M, Spence D, de Pauw B, Meunier F, Marinus A, Collette L, Sylvester R, Meis J, Boogaerts M, Selleslag D, Krcmery V, von Sinner W, MacDonald P, Doyen C, Vandercam B. An EORTC international multicenter randomized trial (EORTC number 19923) comparing two dosages of liposomal amphotericin B for treatment of invasive aspergillosis. Clin Infect Dis 1998;27(6):1406–12.

39. Clark AD, McKendrick S, Tansey PJ, Franklin IM, Chopra R. A comparative analysis of lipid-complexed and liposomal amphotericin B preparations in haematological oncology. Br J Haematol 1998;103(1):198–204.

40. Berman JD, Badaro R, Thakur CP, Wasunna KM, Behbehani K, Davidson R, Kuzoe F, Pang L, Weerasuriya K, Bryceson AD. Efficacy and safety of liposomal amphotericin B (AmBisome) for visceral leishmaniasis in endemic developing countries. Bull World Health Organ 1998;76(1):25–32.

41. Walsh TJ, Goodman JL, Pappas P, Bekersky I, Buell DN, Roden M, Barrett J, Anaissie EJ. Safety, tolerance, and pharmacokinetics of high-dose liposomal amphotericin B (AmBisome) in patients infected with *Aspergillus* species and other filamentous fungi: maximum tolerated dose study. Antimicrob Agents Chemother 2001;45(12):3487–96.

42. Schwartz S, Behre G, Heinemann V, Wandt H, Schilling E, Arning M, Trittin A, Kern WV, Boenisch O, Bosse D, Lenz K, Ludwig WD, Hiddemann W, Siegert W, Beyer J. Aerosolized amphotericin B inhalations as prophylaxis of invasive *Aspergillus* infections during prolonged neutropenia: results of a prospective randomized multicenter trial. Blood 1999;93(11):3654–61.

43. Schoffski P, Freund M, Wunder R, Petersen D, Kohne CH, Hecker H, Schubert U, Ganser A. Safety and toxicity of amphotericin B in glucose 5% or Intralipid 20% in neutropenic patients with pneumonia or fever of unknown origin: randomised study. BMJ 1998;317(7155):379–84.

44. Manfredi R, Chiodo F. Case-control study of amphotericin B in a triglyceride fat emulsion versus conventional amphotericin B in patients with AIDS. Pharmacotherapy 1998;18(5):1087–92.

45. Torre D, Banfi G, Tambini R, Speranza F, Zeroli C, Martegani R, Airoldi M, Fiori G. A retrospective study on the efficacy and safety of amphotericin B in a lipid emulsion for the treatment of cryptococcal meningitis in AIDS patients. J Infect 1998;37(1):36–8.

46. Leenders AC, Daenen S, Jansen RL, Hop WC, Lowenberg B, Wijermans PW, Cornelissen J, Herbrecht R, van der Lelie H, Hoogsteden HC, Verbrugh HA, de Marie S. Liposomal amphotericin B compared with amphotericin B deoxycholate in the treatment of documented and suspected neutropenia-associated invasive fungal infections. Br J Haematol 1998;103(1):205–12.

47. Walsh TJ, Finberg RW, Arndt C, Hiemenz J, Schwartz C, Bodensteiner D, Pappas P, Seibel N, Greenberg RN, Dummer S, Schuster M, Holcenberg JS. Liposomal amphotericin B for empirical therapy in patients with persistent fever and neutropenia. National Institute of Allergy and Infectious Diseases Mycoses Study Group. N Engl J Med 1999;340(10):764–71.

48. Fleming RV, Kantarjian HM, Husni R, Rolston K, Lim J, Raad I, Pierce S, Cortes J, Estey E. Comparison of amphotericin B lipid complex (ABLC) vs. ambisome in the treatment of suspected or documented fungal infections in patients with leukemia. Leuk Lymphoma 2001;40(5–6):511–20.

49. Nucci M, Loureiro M, Silveira F, Casali AR, Bouzas LF, Velasco E, Spector N, Pulcheri W. Comparison of the toxicity of amphotericin B in 5% dextrose with that of amphotericin B in fat emulsion in a randomized trial with cancer patients. Antimicrob Agents Chemother 1999;43(6):1445–8.

50. Nath CE, Shaw PJ, Gunning R, McLachlan AJ, Earl JW. Amphotericin B in children with malignant disease: a comparison of the toxicities and pharmacokinetics of amphotericin B administered in dextrose versus lipid emulsion. Antimicrob Agents Chemother 1999;43(6):1417–23.

51. Malik IA, Moid I, Aziz Z, Khan S, Suleman M. A randomized comparison of fluconazole with amphotericin B as empiric anti-fungal agents in cancer patients with prolonged fever and neutropenia. Am J Med 1998;105(6):478–83.

52. Winston DJ, Hathorn JW, Schuster MG, Schiller GJ, Territo MC. A multicenter, randomized trial of fluconazole versus amphotericin B for empiric antifungal therapy of febrile neutropenic patients with cancer. Am J Med 2000;108(4):282–9.

53. Wolff SN, Fay J, Stevens D, Herzig RH, Pohlman B, Bolwell B, Lynch J, Ericson S, Freytes CO, LeMaistre F, Collins R, Pineiro L, Greer J, Stein R, Goodman SA, Dummer S. Fluconazole vs low-dose amphotericin B for the prevention of fungal infections in patients undergoing bone marrow transplantation: a study of the North American Marrow Transplant Group. Bone Marrow Transplant 2000;25(8):853–9.

54. Boogaerts M, Maertens J, van Hoof A, de Bock R, Fillet G, Peetermans M, Selleslag D, Vandercam B, Vandewoude K, Zachee P, De Beule K. Itraconazole versus amphotericin B plus nystatin in the prophylaxis of fungal infections in neutropenic cancer patients. J Antimicrob Chemother 2001;48(1):97–103.

55. Boogaerts M, Winston DJ, Bow EJ, Garber G, Reboli AC, Schwarer AP, Novitzky N, Boehme A, Chwetzoff E, De Beule K; Itraconazole Neutropenia Study Group. Intravenous and oral itraconazole versus intravenous amphotericin B deoxycholate as empirical antifungal therapy for persistent fever in neutropenic patients with cancer who are receiving broad-spectrum antibacterial therapy. A randomized, controlled trial. Ann Intern Med 2001;135(6):412–22.

56. Harousseau JL, Dekker AW, Stamatoullas-Bastard A, Fassas A, Linkesch W, Gouveia J, De Bock R, Rovira M, Seifert WF, Joosen H, Peeters M, De Beule K. Itraconazole oral solution for primary prophylaxis of fungal infections in patients with hematological malignancy and profound neutropenia: a randomized, double-blind, double-placebo, multicenter trial comparing itraconazole and amphotericin B. Antimicrob Agents Chemother 2000;44(7):1887–93.

57. Arathoon EG, Gotuzzo E, Noriega LM, Berman RS, DiNubile MJ, Sable CA. Randomized, double-blind, multicenter study of caspofungin versus amphotericin B for treatment of oropharyngeal and esophageal candidiases. Antimicrob Agents Chemother 2002;46(2):451–7.

58. Villanueva A, Arathoon EG, Gotuzzo E, Berman RS, DiNubile MJ, Sable CA. A randomized double-blind study of caspofungin versus amphotericin for the treatment of candidal esophagitis. Clin Infect Dis 2001;33(9):1529–35.

59. Mora-Duarte J, Betts R, Rotstein C, Colombo AL, Thompson-Moya L, Smietana J, Lupinacci R, Sable C, Kartsonis N, Perfect J. Caspofungin Invasive Candidiasis Study Group. Comparison of caspofungin and amphotericin B for invasive candidiasis. N Engl J Med 2002;347(25):2020–9.

60. Mishra M, Biswas UK, Jha AM, Khan AB. Amphotericin versus sodium stibogluconate in first-line treatment of Indian kala-azar. Lancet 1994;344(8937):1599–600.

61. Kelsey SM, Goldman JM, McCann S, Newland AC, Scarffe JH, Oppenheim BA, Mufti GJ. Liposomal amphotericin (AmBisome) in the prophylaxis of fungal infections in neutropenic patients: a randomised, double-blind, placebo-controlled study. Bone Marrow Transplant 1999;23(2):163–8.

62. Chabot GG, Pazdur R, Valeriote FA, Baker LH. Pharmacokinetics and toxicity of continuous infusion amphotericin B in cancer patients. J Pharm Sci 1989;78(4):307–10.

63. Ringden O, Andstrom E, Remberger M, Svahn BM, Tollemar J. Allergic reactions and other rare side-effects of liposomal amphotericin. Lancet 1994;344(8930):1156–7.

64. Laing RB, Milne LJ, Leen CL, Malcolm GP, Steers AJ. Anaphylactic reactions to liposomal amphotericin. Lancet 1994;344(8923):682.

65. Kauffman CA, Wiseman SW. Anaphylaxis upon switching lipid-containing amphotericin B formulations. Clin Infect Dis 1998;26(5):1237–8.

66. Le Y, Rana KZ, Dudley MN. Amphotericin B-associated hypertension. Ann Pharmacother 1996;30(7–8):765–7.

67. Groll AH, Piscitelli SC, Walsh TJ. Clinical pharmacology of systemic antifungal agents: a comprehensive review of agents in clinical use, current investigational compounds, and putative targets for antifungal drug development. Adv Pharmacol 1998;44:343–500.

68. Rowles DM, Fraser SL. Amphotericin B lipid complex (ABLC)-associated hypertension: case report and review. Clin Infect Dis 1999;29(6):1564–5.

69. Levy M, Domaratzki J, Koren G. Amphotericin-induced heart-rate decrease in children. Clin Pediatr (Phila) 1995;34(7):358–64.

70. el-Dawlatly AA, Gomaa S, Takrouri MS, Seraj MA. Amphotericin B and cardiac toxicity—a case report. Middle East J Anesthesiol 1999;15(1):107–12.

71. Johnson MD, Drew RH, Perfect JR. Chest discomfort associated with liposomal amphotericin B: report of three cases and review of the literature. Pharmacotherapy 1998;18(5):1053–61.

72. DeMonaco HJ, McGovern B. Transient asystole associated with amphotericin B infusion. Drug Intell Clin Pharm 1983;17(7–8):547–8.

73. Zernikow B, Fleischhack G, Hasan C, Bode U. Cyanotic Raynaud's phenomenon with conventional but not with liposomal amphotericin B: three case reports. Mycoses 1997;40(9–10):359–61.

74. Griese M, Schams A, Lohmeier KP. Amphotericin B and pulmonary surfactant. Eur J Med Res 1998;3(8):383–6.

75. Gryn J, Goldberg J, Johnson E, Siegel J, Inzerillo J. The toxicity of daily inhaled amphotericin. B. Am J Clin Oncol 1993;16(1):43–6.

76. Erjavec Z, Woolthuis GM, de Vries-Hospers HG, Sluiter WJ, Daenen SM, de Pauw B, Halie MR. Tolerance and efficacy of amphotericin B inhalations for prevention of invasive pulmonary aspergillosis in haematological patients. Eur J Clin Microbiol Infect Dis 1997;16(5):364–8.

77. Dubois J, Bartter T, Gryn J, Pratter MR. The physiologic effects of inhaled amphotericin. B. Chest 1995;108(3):750–3.

78. Wright DG, Robichaud KJ, Pizzo PA, Deisseroth AB. Lethal pulmonary reactions associated with the combined use of amphotericin B and leukocyte transfusions. N Engl J Med 1981;304(20):1185–9.

79. Dutcher JP, Kendall J, Norris D, Schiffer C, Aisner J, Wiernik PH. Granulocyte transfusion therapy and

amphotericin B: adverse reactions? Am J Hematol 1989;31(2): 102–8.

80. Hussein MA, Fletcher R, Long TJ, Zuccaro K, Bolwell BJ, Hoeltge A. Transfusing platelets 2 h after the completion of amphotericin-B decreases its detrimental effect on transfused platelet recovery and survival. Transfus Med 1998;8(1):43–7.

81. Garnacho-Montero J, Ortiz-Leyba C, Garcia Garmendia JL, Jimenez Jimenez F. Life-threatening adverse event after amphotericin B lipid complex treatment in a patient treated previously with amphotericin B deoxycholate. Clin Infect Dis 1998;26(4):1016.

82. Manley TJ, Chusid MJ, Rand SD, Wells D, Margolis DA. Reversible parkinsonism in a child after bone marrow transplantation and lipid-based amphotericin B therapy. Pediatr Infect Dis J 1998;17(5):433–4.

83. Ural AU, Avcu F, Cetin T, Beyan C, Kaptan K, Nazaroglu NK, Yalcin A. Spironolactone: is it a novel drug for the prevention of amphotericin B-related hypokalemia in cancer patients? Eur J Clin Pharmacol 2002;57(11):771–3.

84. Bearden DT, Muncey LA. The effect of amiloride on amphotericin B-induced hypokalaemia. J Antimicrob Chemother 2001;48(1):109–11.

85. Barcia JP. Hyperkalemia associated with rapid infusion of conventional and lipid complex formulations of amphotericin B. Pharmacotherapy 1998;18(4):874–6.

86. Blum SF, Shohet SB, Nathan DG, Gardner FH. The effect of amphotericin B on erythrocyte membrane cation permeability: its relation to in vivo erythrocyte survival. J Lab Clin Med 1969;73(6):980–7.

87. Salama A, Burger M, Mueller-Eckhardt C. Acute immune hemolysis induced by a degradation product of amphotericin B. Blut 1989;58(2):59–61.

88. Juliano RL, Grant CW, Barber KR, Kalp MA. Mechanism of the selective toxicity of amphotericin B incorporated into liposomes. Mol Pharmacol 1987;31(1):1–11.

89. Charak BS, Iyer RS, Rajoor BG, Saikia TK, Gopal R, Advani SH. Amphotericin B-related thrombocytopenia. A report of two cases. J Assoc Physicians India 1990; 38(3):235–6.

90. Chan CS, Tuazon CU, Lessin LS. Amphotericin-B-induced thrombocytopenia. Ann Intern Med 1982;96(3):332–3.

91. Bock M, Muggenthaler KH, Schmidt U, Heim MU. Influence of antibiotics on posttransfusion platelet increment. Transfusion 1996;36(11–12):952–4.

92. Kulpa J, Zaroulis CG, Good RA, Kutti J. Altered platelet function and circulation induced by amphotericin B in leukemic patients after platelet transfusion. Transfusion 1981;21(1):74–6.

93. Ringden O, Andstrom EE, Remberger M, Dahllof G, Svahn BM, Tollemar J. Prophylaxis and therapy using liposomal amphotericin B (AmBisome) for invasive fungal infections in children undergoing organ or allogeneic bone-marrow transplantation. Pediatr Transplant 1997;1(2):124–9.

94. Miller MA. Reversible hepatotoxicity related to amphotericin B. Can Med Assoc J 1984;131(10):1245–7.

95. Gill J, Sprenger HR, Ralph ED, Sharpe MD. Hepatotoxicity possibly caused by amphotericin B. Ann Pharmacother 1999;33(6):683–5.

96. Stuecklin-Utsch A, Hasan C, Bode U, Fleischhack G. Pancreatic toxicity after liposomal amphotericin B. Mycoses 2002;45(5–6):170–3.

97. Groll AH, Gea-Banacloche JC, Glasmacher A, Just-Nuebling G, Maschmeyer G, Walsh TJ. Clinical pharmacology of antifungal compounds. Infect Dis Clin North Am 2003;17(1):159–91.

98. McCurdy DK. Distal tubule affected by amphotericin B. N Engl J Med 1969;280(4):220–1.

99. McCurdy DK, Frederic M, Elkinton JR. Renal tubular acidosis due to amphotericin B. N Engl J Med 1968;278(3):124–30.

100. Sabra R, Branch RA. Amphotericin B nephrotoxicity. Drug Saf 1990;5(2):94–108.

101. Barton CH, Pahl M, Vaziri ND, Cesario T. Renal magnesium wasting associated with amphotericin B therapy. Am J Med 1984;77(3):471–4.

102. Tsau YK, Tsai WY, Lu FL, Tsai WS, Chen CH. Symptomatic hypomagnesemia in children. Zhonghua Min Guo Xiao Er Ke Yi Xue Hui Za Zhi 1998; 39(6):393–7.

103. Spath-Schwalbe E, Koschuth A, Dietzmann A, Schanz J, Possinger K. Successful use of liposomal amphotericin B in a case of amphotericin B-induced nephrogenic diabetes insipidus. Clin Infect Dis 1999;28(3):680–1.

104. Barbour GL, Straub KD, O'Neal BL, Leatherman JW. Vasopressin-resistant nephrogenic diabetes insipidus. A result of amphotericin B therapy. Arch Intern Med 1979;139(1):86–8.

105. Araujo JJ, Dominguez A, Bueno C, Rodriguez J, Rios MJ, Muniain MA, Perez R. Diabetes insipida nefrogenica secundaria a la administracion de anfortericina B y anfotericina B liposomal. [Nephrogenous diabetes insipidus secondary to the administration of amphotericin B and liposomal amphotericin B.] Enferm Infecc Microbiol Clin 1998;16(4):204–5.

106. Burges JL, Birchall R. Nephrotoxicity of amphotericin B, with emphasis on changes in tubular function. Am J Med 1972;53(1):77–84.

107. Hohler T, Teuber G, Wanitschke R, Meyer zum Buschenfeld KH. Indomethacin treatment in amphotericin B induced nephrogenic diabetes insipidus. Clin Investig 1994;72(10):769–71.

108. Liberopoulos E, Alexandridis G, Elisaf M. A tumor lysis-like syndrome during therapy of visceral leishmaniasis. Ann Clin Lab Sci 2002;32(4):419–21.

109. Harbarth S, Pestotnik SL, Lloyd JF, Burke JP, Samore MH. The epidemiology of nephrotoxicity associated with conventional amphotericin B therapy. Am J Med 2001;111(7):528–34.

110. Wingard JR, Kubilis P, Lee L, Yee G, White M, Walshe L, Bowden R, Anaissie E, Hiemenz J, Lister J. Clinical significance of nephrotoxicity in patients treated with amphotericin B for suspected or proven aspergillosis. Clin Infect Dis 1999;29(6):1402–7.

111. Gubbins PO, Penzak SR, Polston S, McConnell SA, Anaissie E. Characterizing and predicting amphotericin B-associated nephrotoxicity in bone marrow or peripheral blood stem cell transplant recipients. Pharmacotherapy 2002;22(8):961–71.

112. Furrer K, Schaffner A, Vavricka SR, Halter J, Imhof A, Schanz U. Nephrotoxicity of cyclosporine A and amphotericin B-deoxycholate as continuous infusion in allogenic stem cell transplantation. Swiss Med Wkly 2002;132(23–24):316–20.

113. Speich R, Dutly A, Naef R, Russi EW, Weder W, Boehler A. Tolerability, safety and efficacy of conventional amphotericin B administered by 24-hour infusion to lung transplant recipients. Swiss Med Wkly 2002;132(31–32):455–8.

114. Bowden R, Chandrasekar P, White MH, Li X, Pietrelli L, Gurwith M, van Burik JA, Laverdiere M, Safrin S, Wingard JR. A double-blind, randomized, controlled trial of amphotericin B colloidal dispersion versus amphotericin B for treatment of invasive aspergillosis in immunocompromised patients. Clin Infect Dis 2002;35(4):359–66.

115. Luke RG, Boyle JA. Renal effects of amphotericin B lipid complex. Am J Kidney Dis 1998;31(5):780–5.

116. Slain D, Miller K, Khakoo R, Fisher M, Wierman T, Jozefczyk K. Infrequent occurrence of amphotericin B lipid complex-associated nephrotoxicity in various clinical settings at a university hospital: a retrospective study. Clin Ther 2002;24(10):1636–42.

117. Pahls S, Schaffner A. Comparison of the activity of free and liposomal amphotericin B in vitro and in a model of systemic and localized murine candidiasis. J Infect Dis 1994;169(5):1057–61.

118. Carlini A, Angelini D, Burrows L, De Quirieo G, Antonelli A. Cerebral aspergillosis: long term efficacy and safety of liposomal amphotericin B in kidney transplant. Nephrol Dial Transplant 1998;13(10):2659–61.

119. Johnson PC, Wheat LJ, Cloud GA, Goldman M, Lancaster D, Bamberger DM, Powderly WG, Hafner R, Kauffman CA, Dismukes WE. U.S. National Institute of Allergy and Infectious Diseases Mycoses Study Group. Safety and efficacy of liposomal amphotericin B compared with conventional amphotericin B for induction therapy of histoplasmosis in patients with AIDS. Ann Intern Med 2002;137(2):105–9.

120. Branch RA. Prevention of amphotericin B-induced renal impairment. A review on the use of sodium supplementation. Arch Intern Med 1988;148(11):2389–94.

121. Gardner ML, Godley PJ, Wasan SM. Sodium loading treatment for amphotericin B-induced nephrotoxicity. DICP 1990;24(10):940–6.

122. Llanos A, Cieza J, Bernardo J, Echevarria J, Biaggioni I, Sabra R, Branch RA. Effect of salt supplementation on amphotericin B nephrotoxicity. Kidney Int 1991;40(2):302–8.

123. Stein RS, Alexander JA. Sodium protects against nephrotoxicity in patients receiving amphotericin B. Am J Med Sci 1989;298(5):299–304.

124. Arning M, Scharf RE. Prevention of amphotericin-B-induced nephrotoxicity by loading with sodium chloride: a report of 1291 days of treatment with amphotericin B without renal failure. Klin Wochenschr 1989;67(20):1020–8.

125. Anderson CM. Sodium chloride treatment of amphotericin B nephrotoxicity. Standard of care? West J Med 1995;162(4):313–17.

126. Heidemann HT, Gerkens JF, Spickard WA, Jackson EK, Branch RA. Amphotericin B nephrotoxicity in humans decreased by salt repletion. Am J Med 1983;75(3):476–81.

127. Bernardo JF, Murakami S, Branch RA, Sabra R. Potassium depletion potentiates amphotericin-B-induced toxicity to renal tubules. Nephron 1995;70(2):235–41.

128. Camp MJ, Wingard JR, Gilmore CE, Lin LS, Dix SP, Davidson TG, Geller RB. Efficacy of low-dose dopamine in preventing amphotericin B nephrotoxicity in bone marrow transplant patients and leukemia patients. Antimicrob Agents Chemother 1998;42(12):3103–6.

129. Eriksson U, Seifert B, Schaffner A. Comparison of effects of amphotericin B deoxycholate infused over 4 or 24 hours: randomised controlled trial. BMJ 2001;322(7286):579–82.

130. Cesaro S, Calore E, Messina C, Zanesco L. Allergic reaction to the liposomal component of liposomal amphotericin B. Support Care Cancer 1999;7(4):284–6.

131. Griswold MW, Briceland LL, Stein DS. Is amphotericin B test dosing needed? Ann Pharmacother 1998;32(4):475–7.

132. Johnson JR, Kangas PJ, West M. Serious adverse event after unrecognized substitution of one amphotericin B lipid preparation for another. Clin Infect Dis 1998;27(5):1342–3.

133. Dean JL, Wolf JE, Ranzini AC, Laughlin MA. Use of amphotericin B during pregnancy: case report and review. Clin Infect Dis 1994;18(3):364–8.

134. Scarcella A, Pasquariello MB, Giugliano B, Vendemmia M, de Lucia A. Liposomal amphotericin B treatment for neonatal fungal infections. Pediatr Infect Dis J 1998;17(2):146–8.

135. Weitkamp JH, Poets CF, Sievers R, Musswessels E, Groneck P, Thomas P, Bartmann P. Candida infection in very low birth-weight infants: outcome and nephrotoxicity of treatment with liposomal amphotericin B (AmBisome). Infection 1998;26(1):11–15.

136. Adler-Shohet F, Waskin H, Lieberman JM. Amphotericin B lipid complex for neonatal invasive candidiasis. Arch Dis Child Fetal Neonatal Ed 2001;84(2):F131–3.

137. Prentice HG, Hann IM, Herbrecht R, Aoun M, Kvaloy S, Catovsky D, Pinkerton CR, Schey SA, Jacobs F, Oakhill A, Stevens RF, Darbyshire PJ, Gibson BE. A randomized comparison of liposomal versus conventional amphotericin B for the treatment of pyrexia of unknown origin in neutropenic patients. Br J Haematol 1997;98(3):711–18.

138. Walsh TJ, Seibel NL, Arndt C, Harris RE, Dinubile MJ, Reboli A, Hiemenz J, Chanock SJ. Amphotericin B lipid complex in pediatric patients with invasive fungal infections. Pediatr Infect Dis J 1999;18(8):702–8.

139. Cruz JM, Peacock JE Jr, Loomer L, Holder LW, Evans GW, Powell BL, Lyerly ES, Capizzi RL. Rapid intravenous infusion of amphotericin B: a pilot study. Am J Med 1992;93(2):123–30.

140. Arning M, Dresen B, Aul C, Schneider W. Influence of infusion time on the acute toxicity of amphotericin B: results of a randomized double-blind study. Recent Results Cancer Res 1991;121:347–52.

141. Ellis ME, al-Hokail AA, Clink HM, Padmos MA, Ernst P, Spence DG, Tharpe WN, Hillier VF. Double-blind randomized study of the effect of infusion rates on toxicity of amphotericin B. Antimicrob Agents Chemother 1992;36(1):172–9.

142. Nicholl TA, Nimmo CR, Shepherd JD, Phillips P, Jewesson PJ. Amphotericin B infusion-related toxicity: comparison of two- and four-hour infusions. Ann Pharmacother 1995;29(11):1081–7.

143. Spitzer TR, Creger RJ, Fox RM, Lazarus HM. Rapid infusion amphotericin B: effective and well-tolerated therapy for neutropenic fever. Pharmatherapeutica 1989;5(5):305–11.

144. Gales MA, Gales BJ. Rapid infusion of amphotericin B in dextrose. Ann Pharmacother 1995;29(5):523–9.

145. Winn RE, Bower JH, Richards JF. Acute toxic delirium. Neurotoxicity of intrathecal administration of amphotericin B. Arch Intern Med 1979;139(6):706–7.

146. Fisher JF, Dewald J. Parkinsonism associated with intraventricular amphotericin B. J Antimicrob Chemother 1983;12(1):97–9.

147. Goren MP, Viar MJ, Shenep JL, Wright RK, Baker DK, Kalwinsky DK. Monitoring serum aminoglycoside concentrations in children with amphotericin B nephrotoxicity. Pediatr Infect Dis J 1988;7(10):698–703.

148. Schaffner A, Frick PG. The effect of ketoconazole on amphotericin B in a model of disseminated aspergillosis. J Infect Dis 1985;151(5):902–10.

149. Pahls S, Schaffner A. Aspergillus fumigatus pneumonia in neutropenic patients receiving fluconazole for infection due to Candida species: is amphotericin B combined with

fluconazole the appropriate answer? Clin Infect Dis 1994;18(3):484–6.

150. Schaffner A, Bohler A. Amphotericin B refractory aspergillosis after itraconazole: evidence for significant antagonism. Mycoses 1993;36(11–12):421–4.
151. Rex JH, Pappas PG, Karchmer AW, Sobel J, Edwards JE, Hadley S, Brass C, Vazquez JA, Chapman SW, Horowitz HW, Zervos M, McKinsey D, Lee J, Babinchak T, Bradsher RW, Cleary JD, Cohen DM, Danziger L, Goldman M, Goodman J, Hilton E, Hyslop NE, Kett DH, Lutz J, Rubin RH, Scheld WM, Schuster M, Simmons B, Stein DK, Washburn RG, Mautner L, Chu TC, Panzer H, Rosenstein RB, Booth J; National Institute of Allergy and Infectious Diseases Mycoses Study Group. A randomized and blinded multicenter trial of high-dose fluconazole plus placebo versus fluconazole plus amphotericin B as therapy for candidemia and its consequences in nonneutropenic subjects. Clin Infect Dis 2003;36(10):1221–8.
152. Maesaki S, Kohno S, Kaku M, Koga H, Hara K. Effects of antifungal agent combinations administered simultaneously and sequentially against *Aspergillus fumigatus*. Antimicrob Agents Chemother 1994; 38(12):2843–5.
153. Sugar AM, Hitchcock CA, Troke PF, Picard M. Combination therapy of murine invasive candidiasis with fluconazole and amphotericin B. Antimicrob Agents Chemother 1995;39(3):598–601.
154. Bickers DR. Antifungal therapy: potential interactions with other classes of drugs. J Am Acad Dermatol 1994;31(3 Pt 2):S87–90.
155. Fisher MA, Talbot GH, Maislin G. McKeon BP, Tynan KP, Strom BL. Risk factors for amphotericin B-associated nephrotoxicity. Am J Med 1989;87(5):547–52.
156. Peters DH, Fitton A, Plosker GL, Faulds D. Tacrolimus. A review of its pharmacology, and therapeutic potential in hepatic and renal transplantation. Drugs 1993;46(4):746–94.

Ampiroxicam

See also Non-steroidal anti-inflammatory drugs

General Information

Ampiroxicam is a piroxicam prodrug, which is completely converted to piroxicam after oral administration. Its adverse effects profile is expected to be similar to that of piroxicam. A few cases of photosensitivity have been reported (1–5).

References

1. Carty TJ, Marfat A, Moore PF, Falkner FC, Twomey TM, Weissman A. Ampiroxicam, an anti-inflammatory agent which is a prodrug of piroxicam. Agents Actions 1993;39(3–4):157–65.
2. Falkner FC, Twomey TM, Borgers AP, Garg D, Weidler D, Gerber N, Browder IW. Disposition of ampiroxicam, a prodrug of piroxicam, in man. Xenobiotica 1990;20(6):645–52.
3. Chishiki M, Kawada A, Fujioka A, Hiruma M, Ishibashi A, Banba H. Photosensitivity due to ampiroxicam. Dermatology 1997;195(4):409–10.

4. Toyohara A, Chen KR, Miyakawa S, Inada M, Ishiko A. Ampiroxicam-induced photosensitivity. Contact Dermatitis 1996;35(2):101–2.
5. Kurumaji Y. Ampiroxicam-induced photosensitivity. Contact Dermatitis 1996;34(4):298–9.

Amprenavir

See also Protease inhibitors

General Information

Amprenavir is an HIV protease inhibitor with an enzyme inhibitory constant of 0.6 nmol/l, similar to the inhibitory constants of other protease inhibitors. Its in vitro IC_{50} against wild-type clinical HIV isolates is 115 ng/ml. It has a long half-life (7–10 hours). It can be given twice-daily without food restrictions and had high potency when given as monotherapy in dose-finding studies (1). The recommended doses are 1200 mg bd for adults and 20 mg/kg bd or 15 mg/kg tds for children under 13 years of age or adolescents under 50 kg. Capsules and solution do not have equal systemic availability, and the recommended dose for amprenavir oral solution is 1.5 ml/kg bd or 1.1 ml/kg tds. The systemic availability increases with increasing doses. Amprenavir is about 90% bound to alpha$_1$ acid glycoprotein and 40% to albumin. It does not penetrate the brain well, because it is exported by P glycoprotein. It is mainly metabolized by CYP3A4 and its clearance is reduced in liver disease. The clinical pharmacology of amprenavir has been reviewed (2).

The use of amprenavir has been limited to patients who are highly motivated, because of the high capsule burden (16/day).

Fosamprenavir is a prodrug of amprenavir with better systemic availability. In large clinical trials the most common adverse events in patients taking fosamprenavir, with or without ritonavir, plus abacavir and lamivudine were diarrhea, nausea, vomiting, abdominal pain, drug hypersensitivity, and skin rashes (3).

Observational studies

In a monotherapy trial ($n = 37$), adverse effects were frequent but generally mild, and included rash, diarrhea or loose stools, and headache. In general, these adverse effects tend to disappear or weaken in severity within the first 2–4 weeks of treatment.

General adverse effects

The adverse effects of amprenavir in patients treated with combination therapy included nausea, vomiting, diarrhea, epigastric pain, flatulence, paresthesia, headache, rash, and fatigue (4). The contribution of a single drug to the observed adverse effects is difficult to establish. Amprenavir inhibits CYP3A4 to a greater extent than saquinavir, and to a much lesser extent than ritonavir (5). Co-administration with rifampicin and rifabutin should be avoided. Those who take amprenavir have complained of diarrhea, nausea, headache, and fatigue (6). The frequency of diarrhea may be as high as 50%.

Organs and Systems

Nervous system

Neurotoxicity has been attributed to amprenavir (7).

- A 61-year-old man, who had taken various antiretroviral drugs, took amprenavir 750 mg bd and after the first dose had hallucinations, disorientation, tinnitus, and vertigo. The symptoms abated within 2 hours and recurred after the next dose.

Drug–Drug Interactions

Clarithromycin

A pharmacokinetic study has shown a minor interaction of amprenavir with clarithromycin in healthy men (8). The mean AUC, $C_{max.ss}$ and $C_{min.ss}$ of amprenavir increased by 18, 15, and 39% respectively. Amprenavir had no effect on the AUC of clarithromycin, but the median $t_{max.ss}$ increased by 2 hours, renal clearance increased by 34%, and the AUC for 14-(R)-hydroxy-clarithromycin fell by 35%. These effects were felt not to be clinically important and dosage adjustment was not recommended.

Efavirenz

Four HIV-infected children undergoing intense antiretroviral combination therapy were switched to regimens including amprenavir and efavirenz after the failure of other drugs (9). Pharmacokinetic studies suggested that combinations of these drugs can result in suboptimal concentrations of amprenavir. This was evident in two of the children taking amprenavir and efavirenz, in combination with two NRTIs, who had undetectable concentrations of amprenavir within 4 hours of administration. The addition of ritonavir to the combination restored the blood concentrations of amprenavir to those normally recorded (median 3500 ng/ml). The most probable reason for this effect is enhanced metabolism of amprenavir due to induction by efavirenz.

Indinavir

In an open, randomized study of amprenavir combined with indinavir, nelfinavir, and saquinavir (10) the amprenavir AUC increased by 35% when it was combined with indinavir, and indinavir concentrations also fell, suggesting that this protease inhibitor combination should be avoided. There was no significant interaction of amprenavir with nelfinavir.

Methadone

Amprenavir is extensively metabolized by and induces CYP3A4. Plasma methadone concentrations fell by 35% when amprenavir was used (11).

Rifamycins

Co-administration of amprenavir with rifampicin and rifabutin should be avoided (12).

Ritonavir

In attempts to lower the amprenavir capsule burden, low-dose ritonavir has been used as a pharmacokinetic booster. When ritonavir was added to amprenavir, the amprenavir AUC increased 3–4 times (13), which should allow the total daily capsule burden to be reduced. Adverse effects included diarrhea, nausea, paresthesia, rash, increased cholesterol, and increased triglycerides. The frequency of adverse events correlated with the dose of ritonavir.

Saquinavir

In an open, randomized study of amprenavir combined with indinavir, nelfinavir, and saquinavir (10), saquinavir lowered the amprenavir AUC by 32%; amprenavir did not alter the pharmacokinetics of saquinavir.

Food–Drug Interactions

Grapefruit juice

In 12 healthy volunteers, co-administration of a single dose of amprenavir 1200 mg with grapefruit juice slightly reduced the C_{max} compared with water (7.11 versus 9.10 µg/ml) and slightly increased the t_{max} (1.13 versus 0.75 hours), but did not affect the AUC (14). Thus, grapefruit juice has no clinically important effect on amprenavir pharmacokinetics.

References

1. Sadler BM, Hanson CD, Chittick GE, Symonds WT, Roskell NS. Safety and pharmacokinetics of amprenavir (141W94), a human immunodeficiency virus (HIV) type 1 protease inhibitor, following oral administration of single doses to HIV-infected adults. Antimicrob Agents Chemother 1999;43(7):1686–92.
2. Sadler BM, Stein DS. Clinical pharmacology and pharmacokinetics of amprenavir. Ann Pharmacother 2002;36(1):102–18.
3. Chapman TM, Plosker GL, Perry CM. Fosamprenavir: a review of its use in the management of antiretroviral therapy-naive patients with HIV infection. Drugs 2004;64(18):2101–24.
4. Adkins JC, Faulds D. Amprenavir. Drugs 1998;55(6):837–42.
5. Decker CJ, Laitinen LM, Bridson GW, Raybuck SA, Tung RD, Chaturvedi PR. Metabolism of amprenavir in liver microsomes: role of CYP3A4 inhibition for drug interactions. J Pharm Sci 1998;87(7):803–7.
6. Kost RG, Hurley A, Zhang L, Vesanen M, Talal A, Furlan S, Caldwell P, Johnson J, Smiley L, Ho D, Markowitz M. Open-label phase II trial of amprenavir, abacavir, and fixed-dose zidovudine/lamivudine in newly and chronically HIV-1-infected patients. J Acquir Immune Defic Syndr 2001;26(4):332–9.
7. James CW, McNelis KC, Matalia MD, Cohen DM, Szabo S. Central nervous system toxicity and amprenavir oral solution. Ann Pharmacother 2002;36(1):174.
8. Brophy DF, Israel DS, Pastor A, Gillotin C, Chittick GE, Symonds WT, Lou Y, Sadler BM, Polk RE. Pharmacokinetic interaction between amprenavir and

clarithromycin in healthy male volunteers. Antimicrob Agents Chemother 2000;44(4):978–84.

9. Wintergerst U, Engelhorn C, Kurowski M, Hoffmann F, Notheis G, Belohradsky BH. Pharmacokinetic interaction of amprenavir in combination with efavirenz or delavirdine in HIV-infected children. AIDS 2000;14(12):1866–8.

10. Sadler BM, Gillotin C, Lou Y, Eron JJ, Lang W, Haubrich R, Stein DS. Pharmacokinetic study of human immunodeficiency virus protease inhibitors used in combination with amprenavir. Antimicrob Agents Chemother 2001;45(12):3663–8.

11. Bart PA, Rizzardi PG, Gallant S, Golay KP, Baumann P, Pantaleo G, Eap CB. Methadone blood concentrations are decreased by the administration of abacavir plus amprenavir. Ther Drug Monit 2001;23(5):553–5.

12. Polk RE, Brophy DF, Israel DS, Patron R, Sadler BM, Chittick GE, Symonds WT, Lou Y, Kristoff D, Stein DS. Pharmacokinetic interaction between amprenavir and rifabutin or rifampin in healthy males. Antimicrob Agents Chemother 2001;45(2):502–8.

13. Sadler BM, Gillotin C, Lou Y, Stein DS. Pharmacokinetic and pharmacodynamic study of the human immunodeficiency virus protease inhibitor amprenavir after multiple oral dosing. Antimicrob Agents Chemother 2001;45(1):30–7.

14. Demarles D, Gillotin C, Bonaventure-Paci S, Vincent I, Fosse S, Taburet AM. Single-dose pharmacokinetics of amprenavir coadministered with grapefruit juice. Antimicrob Agents Chemother 2002;46(5):1589–90.

Amrinone

See also Phosphodiesterase type III, selective inhibitors of

General Information

Amrinone is an inhibitor of phosphodiesterase type III, and has a positive inotropic effect. Its adverse effects (1–5) include thrombocytopenia (10%), hypotension, tachydysrhythmias (sometimes resulting in syncope and death) (9%), worsening cardiac ischemia (7%), worsening heart failure (15%), gastrointestinal disturbances (39%), neurological complications (17%), liver damage (7%), fever (6%), nephrogenic diabetes insipidus, hyperuricemia, flaking of the skin, brown discoloration of the nails, and reduced tear secretions. The figures in parentheses are taken from a study of the use of amrinone in 173 patients with chronic ischemic heart disease or idiopathic cardiomyopathies (3).

Other reported adverse effects include acute pleuropericardial effusions, perforated duodenal ulcer, acute myositis and pulmonary infiltrates, vasculitis with pulmonary infiltrates and jaundice, influenza-like illnesses, chest pain, headache, dizziness, anxiety, maculopapular rash, and night sweats (6).

Organs and Systems

Cardiovascular

There has been one report of paroxysmal supraventricular tachycardia in one of 16 patients with cardiogenic shock given amrinone (7).

Hematologic

Thrombocytopenia due to amrinone has been briefly reviewed (8).

References

1. Wilsmhurst PT, Webb-Peploe MM. Side effects of amrinone therapy. Br Heart J 1983;49(5):447–51.

2. DiBianco R, Shabetai R, Silverman BD, Leier CV, Benotti JR. Oral amrinone for the treatment of chronic congestive heart failure: results of a multicenter randomized double-blind and placebo-controlled withdrawal study. J Am Coll Cardiol 1984;4(5):855–66.

3. Johnston DL, Humen DP, Kostuk WJ. Amrinone therapy in patients with heart failure. Lack of improvement in functional capacity and left ventricular function at rest and during exercise. Chest 1984;86(3):394–400.

4. Packer M, Medina N, Yushak M. Hemodynamic and clinical limitations of long-term inotropic therapy with amrinone in patients with severe chronic heart failure. Circulation 1984;70(6):1038–47.

5. Klepzig M, Kleinhans E, Bull U, Strauer BE. Amrinone in Akut- und Langzeittherapie. [Amrinone in acute and long-term therapy.] Z Kardiol 1985;74(2):85–90.

6. Leier CV, Dalpiaz K, Huss P, Hermiller JB, Magorien RD, Bashore TM, Unverferth DV. Amrinone therapy for congestive heart failure in outpatients with idiopathic dilated cardiomyopathy. Am J Cardiol 1983;52(3):304–8.

7. Bichel T, Steinbach G, Olry L, Lambert H. Utilisation de l'amrinone intraveineux dans le traitement du choc cardiogenique. [Use of intravenous amrinone in the treatment of cardiogenic shock.] Agressologie 1988;29(3):187–92.

8. Patnode NM, Gandhi PJ. Drug-induced thrombocytopenia in the coronary care unit. J Thromb Thrombolysis 2000;10(2):155–67.

Amtolmetin guacil

See also Non-steroidal anti-inflammatory drugs

General Information

Amtolmetin guacil (2-[2[1-methyl-5-(4-methylbenzoyl)-2-yl] acetamido] acetic acid 2-methoxyphenyl ester) is a non-acid prodrug of tolmetin. It has been introduced in various countries, and its launch was characterized by claims of better gastrointestinal tolerability than older compounds (1,2). Clinical and endoscopic comparative studies have been carried out in patients with various osteoarticular diseases (3–5). In most of these studies amtolmetin showed similar anti-inflammatory activity to other NSAIDs (diclofenac, flurbiprofen, ibuprofen, indometacin, naproxen) but less gastrotoxicity at endoscopic evaluation, with no difference in the incidence of gastrointestinal symptoms. Unfortunately, the clinical studies were small and of short duration, and the prognostic value of endoscopic studies with respect to severe gastrointestinal complications (bleeding, perforation, and obstruction) is debatable. It has been suggested that the mechanism of the gastric sparing effect of amtolmetin might be related to the local production of nitric oxide, which can counteract the damaging effects of prostaglandin inhibition (6,7).

A renal sparing effect has also been reported, but clinical experience with this compound is limited (8).

References

1. Marcolongo R, Frediani B, Biasi G, Minari C, Barreca C. Metanalisi sulla tollerabilità di amtolmetina guacil, un nuovo, efficace farmaco antinfiammatorio non steroideo, confrontato con FANS tradizionali. Clin Drug Invest 1999;17:89–96.
2. Caruso A, Cutuli VM, De Bernardis E, Attaguile G, Amico-Roxas M. Pharmacological properties and toxicology of MED-15, a prodrug of tolmetin. Drugs Exp Clin Res 1992;18(11–12):481–5.
3. Tavella A, Ursini G. Studio clinico sull'attivita antiinfiammatoria e sulla tollerabilita gastro-enterica di amtolmetineguacil, un nuovo FANS, in confronto a diclofenac su pazienti anziani con patologie osteoarticolari. [A clinical study on the anti-inflammatory activity and gastrointestinal tolerability of amtolmetin guacyl, a new NSAID, compared with diclofenac in aged patients with osteoarticular diseases.] Clin Ter 1997;148(11):543–8.
4. Montrone F, Santandrea S, Caruso I, Gerli R, Cesarotti ME, Frediani P, Bassani R. Amtolmetin guacyl versus piroxicam in patients with osteoarthritis. J Int Med Res 2000;28(2):91–100.
5. Bianchi Porro G, Montrone F, Lazzaroni M, Manzionna G, Caruso I. Clinical and gastroscopic evaluation of amtolmetin guacyl versus diclofenac in patients with rheumatoid arthritis. Ital J Gastroenterol Hepatol 1999;31(5):378–85.
6. Tubaro E, Belogi L, Mezzadri CM. The mechanism of action of amtolmetin guacyl, a new gastroprotective non-steroidal anti-inflammatory drug. Eur J Pharmacol 2000;387(2):233–44.
7. Pisano C, Grandi D, Morini G, Coppelli G, Vesci L, Lo Giudice P, Pace S, Pacifici L, Longo A, Coruzzi G, Carminati P. Gastrosparing effect of new antiinflammatory drug amtolmetin guacyl in the rat: involvement of nitric oxide. Dig Dis Sci 1999;44(4):713–24.
8. Niccoli L, Bellino S, Cantini F. Renal tolerability of three commonly employed non-steroidal anti-inflammatory drugs in elderly patients with osteoarthritis. Clin Exp Rheumatol 2002;20(2):201–7.

Amylin analogues

General Information

Amylin is a hormone produced in the beta-cells of the islets of Langerhans and is co-secreted with insulin. It has glucoregulatory effects that may complement the actions of insulin.

Pramlintide (rINN) is a non-aggregating analogue of amylin. It reduces postprandial glucose excursions, probably by reducing stomach emptying, not by stimulating the release of glucagon-like peptide (GLP-1) (1). It can only be given by injection.

The most common adverse effect of pramlintide is nausea. Hypoglycemia can occur if the dose of insulin is not reduced when pramlintide is added. In no studies was there evidence of cardiac, hepatic, or renal toxicity or hypersensitivity reactions.

Pramlintide has been studied in a double-blind, placebo-controlled, multicenter study in 480 patients with type 1 diabetes for 1 year, followed by an 1-year open extension (2). Glucose control improved with pramlintide. Hypoglycemia was less frequent with pramlintide, but nausea and anorexia doubled in frequency and constituted the most common reason for withdrawal.

In a comparable study, 656 patients with type 2 diabetes took preprandial pramlintide 60 micrograms tds, 90 micrograms bd, or 120 micrograms bd (3). Only 120 micrograms bd gave a sustained reduction in HbA_{1c}. In the first 4 weeks there was an increase in the risk of hypoglycemia, but not thereafter. Mild to moderate nausea and headache were the most frequent adverse effects; nausea abated during treatment.

Insulin + pramlintide

Pramlintide 30 micrograms was given to 16 patients using insulin pumps as an injection at meal times (4). Mealtime insulin was reduced by 17%. Serum fructosamine improved. Nausea was the most common adverse effect. There was no hypoglycemia.

References

1. Ahren B, Adner N, Svartberg J, Petrella E, Holst JJ, Gutniak MK. Anti-diabetogenic effect of the human amylin analogue, pramlintide, in Type 1 diabetes is not mediated by GLP-1. Diabet Med 2002;19(9):790–2.
2. Whitehouse F, Kruger DF, Fineman M, Shen L, Ruggles JA, Maggs DG, Weyer C, Kolterman OG. A randomized study and open-label extension evaluating the long-term efficacy of pramlintide as an adjunct to insulin therapy in type 1 diabetes. Diabetes Care 2002;25(4):724–30.
3. Hollander PA, Levy P, Fineman MS, Maggs DG, Shen LZ, Strobel SA, Weyer C, Kolterman OG. Pramlintide as an adjunct to insulin therapy improves long-term glycemic and weight control in patients with type 2 diabetes: a 1-year randomized controlled trial. Diabetes Care 2003;26(3):784–90.
4. Levetan C, Want LL, Weyer C, Strobel SA, Crean J, Wang Y, Maggs DG, Kolterman OG, Chandran M, Mudaliar SR, Henry RR. Impact of pramlintide on glucose fluctuations and postprandial glucose, glucagon, and triglyceride excursions among patients with type 1 diabetes intensively treated with insulin pumps. Diabetes Care 2003;26(1):1–8.

Anacardiaceae

See also Herbal medicines

General Information

The genera in the family of Anacardiaceae (Table 1) include pistachio, poison ivy, and sumac.

Rhus species

Rhus is used as a traditional remedy for gastrointestinal complaints in Korea.

Table 1 The genera of Anacardiaceae

Anacardium (anacardium)
Buchanania (buchanania)
Campnospera
Comocladia (maidenplum)
Cotinus (smoke tree)
Dracontomelon (dracontomelon)
Gluta (gluta)
Lithrea (lithrea)
Malosma (laurel sumac)
Mangifera (mango)
Melanorrhoea (melanorrhoea)
Metopium (Florida poison tree)
Pistacia (pistachio)
Rhus (sumac)
Schinus (pepper tree)
Schinopsis (schinopsis)
Sclerocarya (sclerocarya)
Semecarpus (semecarpus)
Spondias (mombin)
Toxicodendron (poison oak)

Adverse effects
Skin
Contact dermatitis has been attributed to *Rhus* species (1,2), including a case that followed exposure to a homeopathic remedy (3).

Oral or parenteral exposure to certain contact allergens can elicit an eczematous skin reaction in sensitized individuals. This phenomenon has been called systemic contact dermatitis (SCD) and is relatively rare compared with classical contact dermatitis.

In 42 patients with systemic contact dermatitis caused by ingestion of *Rhus* (24 men and 18 women, average age 44 years, range 24–72), 14 of whom had a history of allergy to lacquer, there were skin lesions such as generalized maculopapular eruptions (50%), erythroderma (29%), vesiculobullous lesions (14%), and erythema multiforme-like lesions (7%) (4). Many patients (57%) developed a leukocytosis with a neutrophilia (74%). In some patients (5%) there were abnormalities of liver function. The lymphocyte subsets of 12 patients studied were within the reference ranges with no differences between patients with or without a history of allergy to lacquer. The authors concluded that the skin eruptions were caused by toxic reactions to *Rhus* rather than by immunological mechanisms.

In 31 patients with *Rhus* allergy over a 10-year period the clinical manifestations included maculopapular eruptions (65%), erythema multiforme (32%), erythroderma (19%) pustules, purpura, wheals, and blisters (5). All the patients had generalized or localized pruritus, and other symptoms included gastrointestinal problems (32%), fever (26%), chills, and headache. Many developed a leukocytosis (70%) with neutrophilia (88%), and some had toxic effects on the liver or kidneys. All responded to glucocorticoids or antihistamines.

Erythema multiforme in a photodistribution has been attributed to *Rhus verniciflua*, the Japanese lacquer tree (6). The rash was reproduced by challenge with the drug and sunlight. On contact with *R. verniciflua* the patient had a flare of the eruption, which was limited to the areas previously exposed to sun. Immunohistochemical studies suggested that the keratinocytes in the skin that retain the photoactivated substances may facilitate epidermal invasion of lymphocytes by persistent expression of intercellular adhesion molecules.

References

1. Powell SM, Barrett DK. An outbreak of contact dermatitis from *Rhus verniciflua (Toxicodendron vernicifluum)*. Contact Dermatitis 1986;14(5):288–9.
2. Sasseville D, Nguyen KH. Allergic contact dermatitis from *Rhus toxicodendron* in a phytotherapeutic preparation. Contact Dermatitis 1995;32(3):182–3.
3. Cardinali C, Francalanci S, Giomi B, Caproni M, Sertoli A, Fabbri P. Contact dermatitis from *Rhus toxicodendron* in a homeopathic remedy. J Am Acad Dermatol 2004;50(1):150–1.
4. Oh SH, Haw CR, Lee MH. Clinical and immunologic features of systemic contact dermatitis from ingestion of *Rhus (Toxicodendron)*. Contact Dermatitis 2003;48(5):251–4.
5. Park SD, Lee SW, Chun JH, Cha SH. Clinical features of 31 patients with systemic contact dermatitis due to the ingestion of *Rhus* (lacquer). Br J Dermatol 2000;142(5):937–42.
6. Shiohara T, Chiba M, Tanaka Y, Nagashima M. Drug-induced, photosensitive, erythema multiforme-like eruption: possible role for cell adhesion molecules in a flare induced by *Rhus* dermatitis. J Am Acad Dermatol 1990;22(4):647–50.

Anakinra

General Information

Anakinra is an interleukin-1 receptor antagonist. It has been used to treat rheumatoid arthritis (1,2). It has been tried in graft-versus-host disease, but without success (3). According to published trial data, moderate injection site reactions were the primary adverse effect and required treatment withdrawal in under 5% of patients. An erythematous rash was seldom observed. Although a few patients have developed antibodies to anakinra, these have not so far been associated with lack of efficacy or allergic skin reactions.

Drug–Drug Interactions

Etanercept

Regulatory agencies have issued an important post-marketing warning of an increased risk of serious infections and neutropenia in patients who receive concomitant anakinra and etanercept (4). This warning was based on an analysis of a randomized clinical trial in 242 patients with rheumatoid arthritis, in which 7% of patients receiving concomitant treatment had serious infections, compared with none in those treated with etanercept alone. Concurrent administration of these two drugs was therefore not recommended.

References

1. Cohen SB. The use of anakinra, an interleukin-1 receptor antagonist, in the treatment of rheumatoid arthritis. Rheum Dis Clin North Am 2004;30(2):365–80.
2. Bresnihan B. The safety and efficacy of interleukin-1 receptor antagonist in the treatment of rheumatoid arthritis. Semin Arthritis Rheum 2001;30(5 Suppl 2):17–20.
3. Antin JH, Weisdorf D, Neuberg D, Nicklow R, Clouthier S, Lee SJ, Alyea E, McGarigle C, Blazar BR, Sonis S, Soiffer RJ, Ferrara JL. Interleukin-1 blockade does not prevent acute graft-versus-host disease: results of a randomized, double-blind, placebo-controlled trial of interleukin-1 receptor antagonist in allogeneic bone marrow transplantation. Blood 2002;100(10):3479–82.
4. EMEA/31631/02 Public Statement. Increased risk of serious infection and neutropenia in patients treated concurrently with Kineret (anakinra) and Enbrel (etanercept). http://www.emea.eu.int/pdfs/human/press/pus/3163102en.pdf.

Androgens and anabolic steroids

See also Hormonal contraceptives—male

General Information

The classic androgen is natural testosterone, which can be given orally in micronized form, but has much more often been used as the orally active 17-methyl derivative or an injectable ester. Androgens are used to some extent in male hypogonadism, when they can promote libido and potency and increase the frequency of erections and the volume of the ejaculate (1). The use of androgens by either sex as "sexual tonics" is a matter of dispute. Some centers have used androgens to treat postmenopausal women complaining of weak libido, poor energy, or a feeling of malaise (2); workers who use this contentious approach have suggested that they should be given in association with estrogens, because of the adverse effects of androgens on serum lipids.

While some anabolic steroids are still available in the legitimate trade, others are manufactured and distributed illegally, and the contents and potency of these are unknown; some adverse effects could be due to impurities or content variation.

From about 1955 onwards, a number of so-called anabolic steroids were developed for which it was claimed, on the basis of animal experiments, that the virilizing effects had been reduced compared with testosterone, whereas the effects on tissue build-up and nitrogen retention had been maintained. These compounds were therefore promoted for such purposes as the promotion of appetite and weight increase in children and the advancement of convalescence. In fact, it has never been at all clear that these compounds are anything other than weak and expensive androgens. Even in these "tonic" doses, they can cause virilization in women and precocious development of secondary characteristics in children. In the much higher doses later developed for use in such conditions as aplastic anemia, mammary carcinoma, terminal uremia, and even hereditary angioedema (3), their androgenic

effects are very pronounced indeed, and other serious complications can occur, for example in the liver (SED-12, 1038) (4–10). One formerly well-known "anabolic" steroid, metandienone (Dianabol), was withdrawn as early as 1982, and other withdrawals have followed.

When androgen therapy is used in postmenopausal women who complain of poor libido, poor energy, or a feeling of malaise (2), it should be given in association with estrogens, because of its adverse effects on serum lipids.

Hormonal contraception in men

The use of intramuscular testosterone + oral desogestrel for hormonal contraception in men is discussed in a separate monograph (Hormonal contraceptives—male).

General adverse reactions

Adverse effects of pharmacological doses of androgens include, as one would expect from male hormones, hirsutism with acne and other signs of virilization, along with adverse lipoprotein profiles, endometrial hyperplasia in women, and an increased risk of cardiovascular disease. Some compounds are particularly likely to cause liver disorders.

Male hormone replacement therapy has been reviewed (11). Hypogonadism can be accompanied by hot flushes, similar to those seen in postmenopausal women, and gynecomastia. The potential risks of testosterone replacement in adult men are precipitation or worsening of sleep apnea, hastened onset of clinical significant prostate disease, benign prostatic hyperplasia, prostatic carcinoma, gynecomastia, fluid retention, polycythemia, exacerbation of hypertension, edema, and an increased risk of cardiovascular disease.

The adverse effects of long-term testosterone therapy in HIV-positive men are irritability, weight gain, fatigue, hair loss, reduced volume of ejaculate, testicular atrophy, truncal acne, breast tenderness, and increased aggression (12).

Supraphysiological concentrations of androgen hormones can cause acne, hirsutism, and deepening of the voice.

Adverse effects of androgens in women

There are clear differences of opinion about the use of androgens in women. An Australian reviewer has argued that women may have symptoms secondary to androgen deficiency and that "prudent" androgen replacement can be effective in relieving both the physical and psychological symptoms of such insufficiency (13). The reviewer suggested that testosterone replacement for women is safe, with the caveat that doses should be restricted to the "therapeutic" window for androgen replacement in women, such that the beneficial effects on well-being and quality of life are achieved without incurring undesirable virilizing effects. The predominant symptom of women with androgen deficiency is claimed to be loss of sexual desire after a premature or natural menopause, while other indications for androgens include premenopausal iatrogenic androgen deficiency states, glucocorticoid-induced bone loss, management of wasting syndromes, and possibly premenopausal bone loss, premenopausal loss of libido, and the treatment of the premenstrual syndrome.

Some reservations about this approach arise when one considers the possible adverse effects and the doubts that have been raised as to whether there is in fact a safe therapeutic window when treating women with androgens. This comes clearly to the fore in a thoughtful paper by another Australian author, a speech therapist (14). For women treated with androgens or related compounds for any reason, virilization of the voice, which soon becomes permanent, is a distressing complication that has not received a great deal of specific study. This review provides some pointers for clinical practice. She reports on four women aged 27–58 years who sought otolaryngological examination because of significant alterations to their voices, the primary concerns being hoarseness, lowering of habitual pitch, difficulty in projecting their speaking voices, and loss of control over their singing voices. Otolaryngological examination with a mirror or flexible laryngoscope showed no apparent abnormality of vocal fold structure or function, and the women were referred for speech pathology with diagnoses of functional dysphonia. Objective acoustic measures using the Kay Visipitch showed significant lowering of the mean fundamental frequency in each woman, and perceptual analysis of the patients' voices during quiet speaking, projected voice use, and comprehensive singing activities showed a constellation of features typically noted in pubescent men. The original diagnosis of functional dysphonia was queried, prompting further exploration of each woman's medical history. In each case the vocal symptoms had started shortly after the beginning of treatment with medications containing virilizing agents, notably danazol, nandrolone decanoate, and testosterone. Although some of the vocal symptoms abated in severity with 6 months of voice therapy and after withdrawal of the drugs, a number of symptoms remained permanent, suggesting that each subject had suffered significant alterations in vocal physiology, including muscle tissue changes, muscle coordination dysfunction, and proprioceptive dysfunction. The study showed that both the projected speaking voice and the singing voice proved highly sensitive to virilizing effects.

It has been known for more than 30 years that some 50% of women have voice changes with anabolic steroids. While it has sometimes been thought that safe doses can be identified, studies of individual patients, including one of the cases documented here, throw doubt on this. The effects can be disastrous for any woman and incapacitating to a singer; clearly the use in women of any product having any androgenic potency must be undertaken with great reticence.

Organs and Systems

Cardiovascular

Particularly when androgens/anabolics are misused to promote extreme muscular development, there is a risk of cardiomegaly and ultimate cardiac failure. Androgen-induced hypertension may be due to a hypertensive shift in the pressure-natriuresis relation, either by an increase in proximal tubular reabsorption or by activation of the renin–angiotensin system (15). This effect is not related to higher doses or longer treatment and can develop after a few months but can also be delayed for many years.

Respiratory

There has been a single published report, which could have been coincidental, of obstructive sleep apnea during use of testosterone (16).

Nervous system

Use of androgenic steroids is likely to produce a sensation of energy and euphoria, but also with a tendency to sleeplessness and irritability (1). More extreme changes in mental state can result in extreme swings in mood, ranging from depression to aggressive elation. An unusual complication in one case was a toxic confusional state and choreiform movements caused by an anabolic steroid (SED-12, 1038) (17), but it may have been due to the non-specific results of endocrine stress in a susceptible individual.

- A 40-year-old Korean woman who had taken oxymetholone for aplastic anemia (doses not stated) developed cerebral venous thrombosis accompanied by a tentorial subdural hematoma (18).

Hiccups have been classified as a neurological reaction that can be triggered by many factors. There have been a few published reports of persistent hiccups associated with oral and intravenous glucocorticoids and one of progesterone-induced hiccups, which were thought to be secondary to the glucocorticoid-like effects of progesterone on the brainstem.

- Anabolic steroid-induced hiccups have been reported in a champion power lifter (19). The hiccups occurred within 12 hours of an increase in the dose of oral methandrostenolone from 50 to 75 mg/day, and persisted for 12 consecutive hours until medical attention was sought. The hiccups abated rapidly after the dose of methandrostenolone was reduced, but he was unwilling to abandon it completely.

Psychological, psychiatric

Apart from the physical effects of exogenous anabolics and androgens, they can also have behavioral effects, including promotion of sexual behavior (which may or may not be regarded as an unwanted effect) and perhaps enhanced aggressiveness. Men who use androgenic anabolic steroids to enhance their sporting achievements seem to be more likely to have cyclic depression (20), but young men who have stopped using anabolic steroids can also develop depression and fatigue as withdrawal effects (21).

Androgens can rarely cause psychotic mania.

- A 28-year-old man with AIDS and a history of bipolar disorder was given a testosterone patch to counter progressive weight loss and developed worsening mania with an elevated mood, racing thoughts, grandiose delusions, and auditory hallucinations (22). His condition improved in hospital after removal of the patch and the administration of antipsychotic drugs. No cause for the psychosis, other than the use of testosterone, was found.

Suicide—or attempted suicide—in eight users of anabolic steroids has been described in Germany; the cases were related variously to hypomanic states during use of anabolic steroids or depression after withdrawal (23). Some of the users had committed acts of violence while using the drugs. In all cases, there were risk factors for suicidality and the drugs may simply have triggered the suicidal decision.

Endocrine

While both androgens and anabolic steroids have male hormone effects, resulting in virilization, they suppress endogenous secretion of follicle-stimulating hormone (FSH) and luteinizing hormone (LH); the result is that on withdrawal the system is for a time deprived of sufficient amounts of male hormone (24); this can lead to hypogonadism until endogenous secretions recover. A transdermal product has a particularly marked effect on circulating concentrations of serum dehydrotestosterone, and this may prove to be the case with other forms of administration; the effects of dehydrotestosterone on the prostate and other systems do not appear to have been systematically studied.

Metabolism

Androgens alone have unfavorable effects on lipids and are atherogenic (2). However, the simultaneous administration of estrogens appears to have a protective effect on the lipid profile. Androgen implants combined with estrogens cause a fall in total cholesterol and LDL cholesterol, without significant effects on HDL cholesterol or triglycerides. There is a similar reduction in total cholesterol in postmenopausal women treated with estrogen plus methyltestosterone, with a reduction in HDL2 cholesterol and triglycerides but no change in LDL cholesterol. Testosterone replacement therapy should therefore be given to women only if they are concurrently using estrogen replacement therapy.

In sufficient doses, androgens can alter regional fat distribution, with a reduction in subcutaneous fat; despite their body-building effects they have therefore been used as part of slimming programs in men (25). In women, testosterone causes an increase in lean body mass with a reduction in total body fat (26).

One residual medical use for oxandrolone in some centers is as a growth-promoting treatment for girls with Turner's syndrome, in which it is regarded by certain workers as an acceptable supplement (in a dose of 0.06 mg/kg/day) to recombinant human growth hormone. A risk of this treatment is altered glucose metabolism, but this effect is usually transient. In a series of 18 patients, one girl developed non-ketotic hyperglycemia 50 months after the end of treatment; in the other 17 girls the effect of treatment on glucose metabolism was reversible (27). There was a moderate, but not significant, rise in fasting blood glucose throughout the course of the longitudinal study. Fasting insulin increased continuously during treatment but fell after the end of treatment; subsequent concentrations were slightly higher than before treatment, but this could have been an effect of age.

Fluid balance

Androgens, particularly oxymetholone, can lead to increased water retention (28), but it is not clear whether this occurs via a mineralocorticoid or an estrogenic effect.

Hematologic

Hemoglobin can increase with high doses of androgens (29). Severe aplastic anemia has been reported.

- A 26-year-old woman developed severe aplastic anemia, complicated by superior sagittal sinus thrombosis, while taking fluoxymesterone 30 mg/day (30).

Anabolic steroids have been reported to be thrombogenic (31–33). Stanozolol, fluomesterone, metandienone, methyltestosterone, oxymesterone, and oxymetholone all reduce the synthesis or increase the degradation of clotting factors; as a rule this effect is not clinically significant, but it can result in an interaction with anticoagulants.

Liver

Particularly because the bulk of oral treatment with androgens has been with a 17-substituted compound (methyltestosterone) there have been considerable problems with liver toxicity (5). Liver dysfunction, first indicated by a rise in alkaline phosphatase and then by increases in other enzymes, transaminases and lactate dehydrogenase, is the earliest and most common sign of dysfunction. Peliosis hepatis (characterized by blood-filled cysts in the liver), hepatomas, and hepatocellular carcinoma can follow with prolonged treatment. Large hepatocellular carcinomas have been described on various occasions (8). The anabolic steroids are as risky in this respect as more traditional androgens; a case of a liver cell adenoma in a child (9) and two cases of nodular hepatocellular carcinoma (10) have been reported in patients who took oxymetholone, metenolone acetate, or other anabolic steroids for 5–15 years. It must be stressed that the complication is not limited to the 17-substituted compounds; other anabolic steroids and androgens, if given in sufficient doses (which are likely to be in excess of physiological amounts), can also damage liver function. Early damage to liver function, for example by methyltestosterone, has been shown to be reversible (6), but longer-term effects are not. The reversibility however depends on the nature of the derangement. Patients with severe cholestasis occurring late with stanozolol recovered biochemically over 3–6 months after drug withdrawal (7).

- A Japanese girl aged 20 years, who had been legitimately treated with oxymetholone (30 mg/day) for 6 years for aplastic anemia, developed a hepatic adenoma (34). In this case, in contrast to some earlier reports, there was a predisposing factor in the form of familial adenomatous polyposis.
- Reversible hepatotoxicity, in the form of abnormal liver function tests, led to the withdrawal of stanozolol in a patient with lipodermatosclerosis (35). Since some dermatologists continue to have faith in anabolic steroids in this condition, the patient was then given oxandrolone, which is reputed to be less hepatotoxic. The

hepatic problems did not recur, although several months later the patient developed a cardiomyopathy, which may have been coincidental.

Skin

Acne is common in patients taking androgens (36). When the effect of testosterone and anabolic steroids on the size of sebaceous glands was studied in a series of male athletes, high doses of all the products tested were found to enlarge the glands (37).

It has been claimed that testosterone implants are much less likely to cause acne than are injections of testosterone enanthate in equivalent doses; it is not clear why this might be expected and the claim seems dubious.

Multiple halo nevi have been described in a patient who took oxymetholone (SED-12, 1038) (38).

Hair

Hirsutism is common in patients taking androgens, and is often irreversible (39,40). In contrast, in women, loss of scalp hair can occur (41). Of 81 female-to-male transsexual subjects, mean age 37 years (range 21–61), treated with testosterone esters ($n = 61$; 250 mg intramuscularly every 2 weeks) or testosterone undecanoate ($n = 20$; 160–240 mg/day orally), 31 developed male-pattern baldness; thinning of the hair was related to the duration of androgen administration and was present in about half of the transsexuals after 13 years (42).

Musculoskeletal

The ability of androgens to counter osteoporosis is the basis of their use as a supplement to estrogens in one version of hormone replacement therapy. Testosterone can increase markers of bone formation (43). However, the early closure of epiphyses, with an arrest of growth, is a risk if children are exposed to these substances; this latter effect may be produced by the estrogen to which testosterone is metabolized. In some patients with excessive growth (such as Klinefelter's syndrome or Marfan syndrome) the effect is exploited therapeutically (SEDA-21, 434). Follow-up in these subjects at the age of 21–30 years showed no abnormalities of testicular function as a consequence of treatment.

A potential adverse effect of oxandrolone is acceleration of puberty and skeletal maturation (44).

- A 9-year-old boy with early puberty took oxandrolone for 22 months because of constitutional delay of growth. His height velocity increased above the 97th percentile and his bone age developed twice as fast as his chronological age. The oxandrolone was withdrawn, but his growth velocity did not decrease and his bone age continued to accelerate.

The authors hypothesized that oxandrolone could have induced early puberty. They concluded that in young children oxandrolone should be used with caution for short periods only.

Sexual function

In men, the (often desired) effects can include an increase in libido. After some time, androgenic treatment in men will lead to a reduction in the volume of the testes and azoospermia or oligospermia because of suppression of gonadotropins. Severe priapism occasionally occurs.

- A 20-year-old man with idiopathic hypogonadotrophic hypogonadism receiving a testosterone ester in a dose of 250 mg intramuscularly every 2 weeks developed priapism (46).

Reproductive system

In women and children, the main effect will be one of virilization in its various forms, ranging from hirsutism and deepening of the voice to enlargement of the female clitoris and male pattern baldness; the effect on the voice rapidly becomes irreversible because of changes in the larynx; laryngeal polyps have also been observed (46). In women, menstrual abnormalities are likely. Short-term treatment can produce increases in estradiol, dihydrotestosterone, testosterone (total and unbound), and the ratio of dihydrotestosterone to testosterone.

When ill-advisedly used to promote growth in boys by administration for some years, oxandrolone caused gynecomastia in a high proportion of subjects treated; 23 of the 33 patients affected subsequently required mastectomy (47,48).

Long-Term Effects

Drug abuse

There is a persistent illegal market in androgenic anabolic steroids, to promote physical strength. A difficulty in determining the ultimate consequences of anabolic steroid abuse for body-building or to advance sporting achievement is that individuals who are susceptible to such abuse may well have taken several different types of substance at the same time or in succession. Indeed, an analysis of the hair of seven body-builders showed what the authors termed a "complete pharmacopeia" of drug residues, ranging from glucocorticoids, anabolic steroids, and androgens to beta-adrenoceptor agonists, antidepressants, diuretics, and human chorionic gonadotropin (49).

The claimed body-building effect of the so-called anabolic compounds reflects their ability to promote muscular development, even beyond physiological limits, and this can bring with it cardiovascular complications. Surreptitious misuse by athletes remains a recurrent problem in professional sport (50); apart from the cardiovascular risks, one observes numerous physiological changes, including effects on plasma levels of enzymes, minerals and vitamins and reduced concentrations of HDL cholesterol (51).

- Poststeroid balance disorder was diagnosed in a 20-year-old Polish athlete who had been given two courses of metandienone, oxymetholone, and nandrolone phenylpropionate (52). Vertigo occurred twice just after "doping" and persisted in spite of a 1.5-year break in taking anabolic steroids. There was positional nystagmus, the eye-tracking test was abnormal, and there were abnormal responses in caloric tests. In computed dynamic posturography, the incidence and degree of body sway were increased and consequently the field of the outspread area was enlarged. These findings pointed to a permanent poststeroid disorder of the central part of the equilibrium organ.

- A German report of a 22-year-old male body-builder who had taken both testosterone propionate and nandrolone decanoate in rising doses over a period of 4 months detailed the emergence of fulminant acne, a sternoclavicular bone lesion, and loss of libido (53). Severe acne after excessive androgen use has been reported before, and the apparently osteoarthritic complication in this case was probably secondary to the acne.
- A Texas group observed erythrocytosis in a young body-builder taking androgens and followed up this observation by examining hematological measures in nine male competitive body-builders who admitted to using these steroids illicitly (54). Although erythropoietin concentrations were normal (and even tended to be low), six subjects had a raised hematocrit with erythrocytosis.
- Cholestasis and renal insufficiency occurred together in a German body-builder who had been taking two anabolic steroids together over a period of 80 days (55).
- A large hepatic hematoma led to intra-abdominal hemorrhage in a 24-year-old man who for 2 years had taken two anabolic steroids as well as clomiphene and human chorionic gonadotropin (56). The authors obtained information from health clubs that users commonly took some 300 mg of nandrolone weekly, whereas the recommended dose was only 50 mg monthly.

An Australian study of 41 past and present users of anabolic steroids, together with controls from a similar population ("potential users") has vividly portrayed the risks that prolonged use of these products brings (57). Complications included alterations in libido (61%), changes in mood (48%), reduced testicular volume (46%), and acne (43%). The mean systolic and diastolic blood pressures were raised in 29% of current users, 37% of past users, and only 8% of controls, although these differences were not significant. Gynecomastia was found in 10 past users (37%), two current users (12%), and none of the controls, while mean testicular volume was significantly smaller in current users (18 ml). There were abnormal liver function tests in 20 past users (83%), eight present users (62%), and five potential users (71%).

- A partial empty sella syndrome occurred in an elite 39-year-old body-builder with a 17-year history of drug abuse involving growth hormone, anabolic steroids, testosterone, and thyroid hormone (58).

The pituitary is a hormone-responsive gland, but it has not previously been shown to suffer negative feedback in response to any of these substances. Any one of them could in principle have contributed to the effect, or it could have been an indirect consequence of drug abuse, by way of an increase in intracranial pressure, which is a known cause of empty sella syndrome.

Drug withdrawal

Withdrawal of high doses of androgens or anabolic steroids after the system has become accustomed to them can lead to menopause-like reactions, such as anxiety, chills, tachycardia, anorexia, piloerection, insomnia, sweats, hypertension, myalgia, nausea, vomiting, irritability, and hot flushes. Young men who have used these compounds can experience depression and fatigue for a time after withdrawal.

Tumorigenicity

Danazol is a weak androgen and also has a series of other hormonal and anti-hormonal properties. It inhibits pituitary gonadotropin and has been used in the treatment of endometriosis, fibrocystic disease of the breast, idiopathic thrombocytopenic purpura, and hereditary angioedema. Its hepatotoxic effects include reversible rises in serum transaminases and cholestatic hepatitis; a few cases of hepatocellular tumors have been reported.

- A 34-year-old woman who had taken danazol 400 mg/day for 13 years for hereditary angioedema developed a mass in the right hypochondrium. Her alcohol intake was under 20 g/day. She had a large heterogeneous hepatic tumor, a well-differentiated hepatocellullar carcinoma in a non-cirrhotic liver.

The hypothesis that hepatocellular carcinoma had been caused by danazol was accepted in the absence of other causes (59).

Susceptibility Factors

Age

In children, who may be exposed to androgens or anabolic steroids accidentally or in ill-advised therapy (for example to improve appetite), there will be a particular risk of virilization, premature sexual development, and early closure of the epiphyses. Virilization has even been reported after topical androgen administration (60).

Interest in the use of androgens in elderly men continues, with on the one hand the long-standing hope that potency and libido may be restored, and, on the other hand, the belief that cardiovascular prospects might be improved. The uncertainties that exist in this latter respect have been well reviewed in a paper that merits reading in full; it is best summarized in the author's own conclusion that "··· overall, the androgens are as likely to prevent arterial disease as they are to cause it ···" (61).

Other features of the patient

One possible use of anabolic agents is in the treatment of the physical wasting associated with HIV infection. Some experience has been gained, but it is still not clear whether such treatment is warranted, bearing in mind the limited benefits that can be expected and the well-documented risks of anabolic drug therapy (62). The effects and adverse effects of testosterone replacement with a non-genital transdermal system, Androderm, have been studied in 41 HIV-positive men with low testosterone concentrations (63). Nine men taking placebo and 11 taking testosterone reported adverse events. Five men taking testosterone had reactions at the site of administration; other adverse events in this group included problems related to resistance mechanisms ($n = 2$), gastrointestinal system ($n = 2$), and skin and appendages ($n = 1$); there was one severe adverse event (a suicidal amitriptyline overdose). There were skin reactions at the site of application of the placebo or testosterone patch in 19% of the participants. One man had blisters on one occasion, related to rupture of the patch. The mean erythrocyte count increased with testosterone and fell with placebo. Hemoglobin concentration increased with testosterone and fell with placebo.

Older data pointed to some reduction in insulin requirements when patients with diabetes mellitus received androgens, and it is wise to avoid these drugs altogether in patients with diabetes.

Drug Administration

Drug formulations

Testosterone is available as oral testosterone undecanoate, buccal testosterone, intramuscular testosterone esters, testosterone implants, and testosterone transdermal patches and gel.

After oral administration there is large variability in systemic availability, which makes this route generally unsuitable.

Buccal testosterone tablets provide sustained release of testosterone and also bypass first-pass metabolism in the liver. Common adverse effects include gum irritation, pain, and tenderness, and edema (64) and headache (65).

Intramuscular testosterone is given as a deep intramuscular injection of single testosterone esters or a mixture of testosterone propionate, testosterone phenylpropionate, testosterone isocaproate, and testosterone decanoate (Sustanon), every 2–3 weeks. In one series of 551 injections, 162 were associated with pain and bleeding; injection in the gluteal site caused fewer complaints and was less susceptible to bleeding, but was painful more often than injection in the deltoid muscle or thigh (66). There were no serious adverse effects and the only systemic adverse effect was episodes of sudden non-productive cough associated with faintness after eight injections which the authors thought might have been due to pulmonary oil microembolism. Systemic availability of testosterone after intramuscular administration is variable and there can be fluctuations in mood and sexual function (67). High testosterone concentrations can cause raised lipid concentrations (68).

Topical application of testosterone, as a gel or from transdermal patches, can lead to absorption and systemic effects (SEDA-16, 158). Transdermal absorption of testosterone (usually from treatment of vulvar lichen sclerosus et atrophicus) can lead to increased libido, clitoral hypertrophy, pubic hirsutism, thinning of the scalp hair, facial acne, voice change, hirsutism, and even virilization (69).

The use of transdermal patches for administering testosterone to hypogonadal men ("Andropatch") seems logical and convenient, but a British study in 50 treated patients showed that patient acceptance was surprisingly poor (70). There were adverse effects in 84%, mostly skin problems; 72% requested a return to depot injections, and 5% returned to oral therapy. The reservoir patches, 6 cm in diameter, were, to quote the report literally, judged to be too large,

uncomfortable, and visually obtrusive, while the noise they made on bodily movement distracted dogs, wives, and children; they fell off in showers and attracted ribald remarks from sports partners; they could only be removed with difficulty and left bald red marks on the body. The nature of the complaints suggests that they might be accommodated by further technical development of the product.

One unusual variant involves applying a transdermal preparation to the scrotum (71), a technique that has been claimed to mimic more closely the natural pattern of release of endogenous testosterone. It is not clear that applying it at this site has any special merit, although some work suggests that the scrotal skin is less likely than other skin areas to exhibit local reactions. Certainly topical preparations of testosterone can elicit such reactions, with pruritus and blistering being common, while induration, erythema, and allergic reactions can also occasionally occur.

Testosterone implants, like implants of other substances, can be subject to extrusion, probably in about a tenth of cases treated, and can also give rise to local irritation (72).

Drug–Drug Interactions

Anticoagulants

Many androgens and anabolic steroids reduce the dose of oral anticoagulant that a patient requires, sometimes by as much as 25% (73), and hemorrhage has sometimes resulted from their use. From the results of a study in which stanozolol reduced warfarin requirements, the investigators concluded that stanozolol increased fibrinolysis, reduced the production of vitamin K-dependent clotting factors, and increased the amount of the natural anticoagulant antithrombin III (74).

References

1. Birkhauser MH. Chemistry, physiology and pharmacology of sex steroids. J Cardiovasc Pharmacol 1996;28(Suppl 5):S1–13.
2. Vermeulen A. Plasma androgens in women. J Reprod Med 1998;43(Suppl 8):725–33.
3. Cicardi M, Castelli R, Zingale LC, Agostoni A. Side effects of long-term prophylaxis with attenuated androgens in hereditary angioedema: comparison of treated and untreated patients. J Allergy Clin Immunol 1997;99(2):194–6.
4. Pandita R, Quadri MI. Constitutional aplastic anemia. Indian Pediatr 1988;25(5):469–72.
5. Kaunitz AM. The role of androgens in menopausal hormonal replacement. Endocrinol Metab Clin North Am 1997;26(2):391–7.
6. Lowdell CP, Murray-Lyon IM. Reversal of liver damage due to long term methyltestosterone and safety of non-17 alpha-alkylated androgens. BMJ (Clin Res Ed) 1985;291(6496):637.
7. Evely RS, Triger DR, Milnes JP, Low-Beer TS, Williams R. Severe cholestasis associated with stanozolol. BMJ (Clin Res Ed) 1987;294(6572):612–13.
8. McCaughan GW, Bilous MJ, Gallagher ND. Long-term survival with tumor regression in androgen-induced liver tumors. Cancer 1985;56(11):2622–6.
9. Sanchez JMC, Becerra EP, Martin AA, et al. Adenoma hepatico después del tratamiento con oximetolona. Rev Esp Pediatr 1988;44:195.
10. Oda K, Oguma N, Kawano M, Kimura A, Kuramoto A, Tokumo K. Hepatocellular carcinoma associated with long-

term anabolic steroid therapy in two patients with aplastic anemia. Nippon Ketsueki Gakkai Zasshi 1987;50(1):29–36.

11. Tenover JL. Male hormone replacement therapy including "andropause". Endocrinol Metab Clin North Am 1998;27(4):969–87.

12. Maguen S, Wagner GJ, Rabkin JG. Long-term testosterone therapy in HIV-positive men: side-effects and maintenance of clinical benefit. AIDS 1998;12(3):327–8.

13. Davis SR. The therapeutic use of androgens in women. J Steroid Biochem Mol Biol 1999;69(1–6):177–84.

14. Baker J. A report on alterations to the speaking and singing voices of four women following hormonal therapy with virilizing agents. J Voice 1999;13(4):496–507.

15. Reckelhoff JF, Granger JP. Role of androgens in mediating hypertension and renal injury. Clin Exp Pharmacol Physiol 1999;26(2):127–31.

16. Sandblom RE, Matsumoto AM, Schoene RB, Lee KA, Giblin EC, Bremner WJ, Pierson DJ. Obstructive sleep apnea syndrome induced by testosterone administration. N Engl J Med 1983;308(9):508–10.

17. Tilzey A, Heptonstall J, Hamblin T. Toxic confusional state and choreiform movements after treatment with anabolic steroids. BMJ (Clin Res Ed) 1981;283(6287):349–50.

18. Chu K, Kang DW, Kim DE, Roh JK. Cerebral venous thrombosis associated with tentorial subdural hematoma during oxymetholone therapy. J Neurol Sci 2001;185(1):27–30.

19. Dickerman RD, Jaikumar S. The hiccup reflex arc and persistent hiccups with high-dose anabolic steroids: is the brainstem the steroid-responsive locus? Clin Neuropharmacol 2001;24(1):62–4.

20. Copeland J, Peters R, Dillon P. Anabolic–androgenic steroid use disorders among a sample of Australian competitive and recreational users. Drug Alcohol Depend 2000;60(1):91–6.

21. Christiansen K. Behavioural effects of androgen in men and women. J Endocrinol 2001;170(1):39–48.

22. Weiss EL, Bowers MB Jr, Mazure CM. Testosterone-patch-induced psychotic mania. Am J Psychiatry 1999;156(6):969.

23. Thiblin I, Runeson B, Rajs J. Anabolic androgenic steroids and suicide. Ann Clin Psychiatry 1999;11(4):223–31.

24. Anderson SJ, Bolduc SP, Coryllos E, Griesemer B, McLain L. Adolescents and anabolic steroids: a subject review. American Academy of Pediatrics. Committee on Sports Medicine and Fitness. Pediatrics 1997;99(6):904–8.

25. Lovejoy JC, Bray GA, Greeson CS, Klemperer M, Morris J, Partington C, Tulley R. Oral anabolic steroid treatment, but not parenteral androgen treatment, decreases abdominal fat in obese, older men. Int J Obes Relat Metab Disord 1995;19(9):614–24.

26. Davis SR, Burger HG. Androgens and the postmenopausal woman. J Clin Endocrinol Metab 1996;81(8):2759–63.

27. Joss EE, Zurbrugg RP, Tonz O, Mullis PE. Effect of growth hormone and oxandrolone treatment on glucose metabolism in Turner syndrome. A longitudinal study. Horm Res 2000;53(1):1–8.

28. International Programme on Chemical Safety. Poisons Information Monograph 915.

29. Bebb RA, Anawalt BD, Christensen RB, Paulsen CA, Bremner WJ, Matsumoto AM. Combined administration of levonorgestrel and testosterone induces more rapid and effective suppression of spermatogenesis than testosterone alone: a promising male contraceptive approach. J Clin Endocrinol Metab 1996;81(2):757–62.

30. Kaito K, Kobayashi M, Otsubo H, Ogasawara Y, Sekita T, Shimada T, Hosoya T. Superior sagittal sinus thrombosis in a patient with aplastic anemia treated with anabolic steroids. Int J Hematol 1998;68(2):227–9.

31. Ferenchick GS. Are androgenic steroids thrombogenic? N Engl J Med 1990;322(7):476.

32. Lowe GD, Thomson JE, Reavey MM, Forbes CD, Prentice CR. Mesterolone: thrombosis during treatment, and a study of its prothrombotic effects. Br J Clin Pharmacol 1979;7(1):107–9.

33. Toyama M, Watanabe S, Kobayashi T, Iida K, Koseki S, Yamaguchi I, Sugishita Y. Two cases of acute myocardial infarction associated with aplastic anemia during treatment with anabolic steroids. Jpn Heart J 1994;35(3):369–73.

34. Nakao A, Sakagami K, Nakata Y, Komazawa K, Amimoto T, Nakashima K, Isozaki H, Takakura N, Tanaka N. Multiple hepatic adenomas caused by long-term administration of androgenic steroids for aplastic anemia in association with familial adenomatous polyposis. J Gastroenterol 2000;35(7):557–62.

35. Segal S, Cooper J, Bolognia J. Treatment of lipodermatosclerosis with oxandrolone in a patient with stanozolol-induced hepatotoxicity. J Am Acad Dermatol 2000;43(3):558–9.

36. Zouboulis CC, Degitz K. Androgen action on human skin—from basic research to clinical significance. Exp Dermatol 2004;13(Suppl 4):5–10.

37. Kiraly CL, Collan Y, Alen M. Effect of testosterone and anabolic steroids on the size of sebaceous glands in power athletes. Am J Dermatopathol 1987;9(6):515–19.

38. Jhung JW, Edelstein LM, Church A. Multiple halo nevi developing after oxymetholone treatment of "aplastic anemia". Cutis 1973;12:56.

39. Muller SA. Hirsutism. Am J Med 1969;46(5):803–17.

40. Muller OA. Hirsutismus und Androgenexzess: Diagnostische Probleme, therapeutische Schwierigkeiten. [Hirsutism and androgen excess: diagnostic problems, therapeutic difficulties.] Med Monatsschr Pharm 1982;5(11):329–36.

41. Birch MP, Lalla SC, Messenger AG. Female pattern hair loss. Clin Exp Dermatol 2002;27(5):383–8.

42. Giltay EJ, Toorians AW, Sarabdjitsingh AR, de Vries NA, Gooren LJ. Established risk factors for coronary heart disease are unrelated to androgen-induced baldness in female-to-male transsexuals. J Endocrinol 2004;180(1):107–12.

43. Wang C, Eyre DR, Clark R, Kleinberg D, Newman C, Iranmanesh A, Veldhuis J, Dudley RE, Berman N, Davidson T, Barstow TJ, Sinow R, Alexander G, Swerdloff RS. Sublingual testosterone replacement improves muscle mass and strength, decreases bone resorption, and increases bone formation markers in hypogonadal men—a clinical research center study. J Clin Endocrinol Metab 1996;81(10):3654–62.

44. Doeker B, Muller-Michaels J, Andler W. Induction of early puberty in a boy after treatment with oxandrolone? Horm Res 1998;50(1):46–8.

45. Zelissen PM, Stricker BH. Severe priapism as a complication of testosterone substitution therapy. Am J Med 1988;85(2):273–4.

46. Keul J, Deus B, Kindermann W. Anabole Hormone: Schädigung, Leistungsfähigkeit und Stoffwechsel. [Anabolic steroids: damages, effect on performance, and on metabolism.] Med Klin 1976;71(12):497–503.

47. Joss EE, Schmidt HA, Zuppinger KA. Oxandrolone in constitutionally delayed growth, a longitudinal study up to final height. J Clin Endocrinol Metab 1989;69(6):1109–15.

48. Moore DC, Ruvalcaba RHA. Late onset gynecomastia associated with oxandrolone therapy in adolescents with short stature. J Pediatr Endocrinol 1991;4:249.

49. Dumestre-Toulet V, Kintz P, Cirimele V, Gromb S, Ludes BJ. Analyse des cheveux de 7 culturistes: toute une pharmacopée. J Med Leg Droit Med 2001;44:38–44.

50. Perlmutter G, Lowenthal DT. Use of anabolic steroids by athletes. Am Fam Physician 1985;32(4):208–10.

51. Costill DL, Pearson DR, Fink WJ. Anabolic steroids use among athletes: changes in HDL-C levels. Phys Sportsmed 1984;12:113.

52. Bochnia M, Medras M, Pospiech L, Jaworska M. Poststeroid balance disorder—a case report in a body builder. Int J Sports Med 1999;20(6):407–9.

53. Assmann T, Arens A, Becker-Wegerich PM, Schuppe HC, Lehmann P. Acne fulminans with sternoclavicular bone lesions and azoospermia after abuse of anabolic steroids. H G Z Hautkr 1999;74:570–2.

54. Dickerman RD, Pertusi R, Miller J, Zachariah NY. Androgen-induced erythrocytosis: is it erythropoietin? Am J Hematol 1999;61(2):154–5.

55. Habscheid W, Abele U, Dahm HH. Schwere Cholestase mit Nierenversagen durch Anabolika bei einem Bodybuilder. [Severe cholestasis with kidney failure from anabolic steroids in a body builder.] Dtsch Med Wochenschr 1999;124(36):1029–32.

56. Schumacher J, Muller G, Klotz KF. Large hepatic hematoma and intraabdominal hemorrhage associated with abuse of anabolic steroids. N Engl J Med 1999;340(14):1123–4.

57. O'Sullivan AJ, Kennedy MC, Casey JH, Day RO, Corrigan B, Wodak AD. Anabolic–androgenic steroids: medical assessment of present, past and potential users. Med J Aust 2000;173(6):323–7.

58. Dickerman RD, Jaikumar S. Secondary partial empty sella syndrome in an elite bodybuilder. Neurol Res 2001;23(4):336–8.

59. Crampon D, Barnoud R, Durand M, Ponard D, Jacquot C, Sotto JJ, Letoublon C, Zarski JP. Danazol therapy: an unusual aetiology of hepatocellular carcinoma. J Hepatol 1998;29(6):1035–6.

60. Kunz GJ, Klein KO, Clemons RD, Gottschalk ME, Jones KL. Virilization of young children after topical androgen use by their parents. Pediatrics 2004;114(1):282–4.

61. Crook D. Androgen therapy in the aging male: assessing the effect on heart disease. Aging Male 1999;2:151–6.

62. Taiwo BO. HIV-associated wasting: brief review and discussion of the impact of oxandrolone. AIDS Patient Care STDS 2000;14(8):421–5.

63. Bhasin S, Storer TW, Asbel-Sethi N, Kilbourne A, Hays R, Sinha-Hikim I, Shen R, Arver S, Beall G. Effects of testosterone replacement with a nongenital, transdermal system, Androderm, in human immunodeficiency virus-infected men with low testosterone levels. J Clin Endocrinol Metab 1998;83(9):3155–62.

64. Wang C, Swerdloff R, Kipnes M, Matsumoto AM, Dobs AS, Cunningham G, Katznelson L, Weber TJ, Friedman TC, Snyder P, Levine HL. New testosterone buccal system (Striant) delivers physiological testosterone levels: pharmacokinetics study in hypogonadal men. J Clin Endocrinol Metab 2004;89(8):3821–9.

65. Ross RJ, Jabbar A, Jones TH, Roberts B, Dunkley K, Hall J, Long A, Levine H, Cullen DR. Pharmacokinetics and tolerability of a bioadhesive buccal testosterone tablet in hypogonadal men. Eur J Endocrinol 2004;150(1):57–63.

66. Mackey MA, Conway AJ, Handelsman DJ. Tolerability of intramuscular injections of testosterone ester in oil vehicle. Hum Reprod 1995;10(4):862–5.

67. Jockenhovel F. Testosterone supplementation: what and how to give. Aging Male 2003;6(3):200–6.

68. Whitsel EA, Boyko EJ, Matsumoto AM, Anawalt BD, Siscovick DS. Intramuscular testosterone esters and plasma lipids in hypogonadal men: a meta-analysis. Am J Med 2001;111(4):261–9.

69. Parker LU, Bergfeld WF. Virilization secondary to topical testosterone. Cleve Clin J Med 1991;58(1):43–6.

70. Parker S, Armitage M. Experience with transdermal testosterone replacement therapy for hypogonadal men. Clin Endocrinol (Oxf) 1999;50(1):57–62.

71. Jordan WP Jr. Allergy and topical irritation associated with transdermal testosterone administration: a comparison of scrotal and nonscrotal transdermal systems. Am J Contact Dermat 1997;8(2):108–13.

72. Handelsman DJ, Mackey MA, Howe C, Turner L, Conway AJ. An analysis of testosterone implants for androgen replacement therapy. Clin Endocrinol (Oxf) 1997;47(3):311–16.

73. Weser JK, Sellers E. Drug interactions with coumarin anticoagulants. 2. N Engl J Med 1971;285(10):547–58.

74. Acomb D, Shaw PW. A significant interaction between warfarin and stanozolol. Pharm J 1985;234:73.

Anesthetic ether

See also General anesthetics

General Information

Diethyl ether (SED-9, 172) is obsolete as a general anesthetic (1). It is highly inflammable and therefore incompatible with modern surgical and anesthetic techniques. It has an unpleasant smell and irritates mucous membranes; this can cause coughing, straining, laryngeal spasm, and hypersalivation. Recovery is slow and accompanied by nausea and vomiting in up to 85% of patients. Liver damage is as frequent as with halothane. Ether raises intracranial pressure and can cause convulsions. It can cause impaired immune responsiveness and contact dermatitis has been reported, together with a systemic allergic reaction (SEDA-5, 120).

Reference

1. Whaten FX, Bacon DR, Smith HM. Inhaled anesthetics: an historical overview. Best Pract Res Clin Anaesthesiol 2005;19(3):323–30.

Angiotensin II receptor antagonists

See also Individual agents

General Information

Inhibition of the renin–angiotensin system by ACE inhibitors has proved efficacious in the treatment of hypertension, cardiac failure, myocardial infarction, in secondary prevention after myocardial infarction, and for kidney protection in diabetic and non-diabetic nephropathy. The development of specific antagonists to subtype 1 of the angiotensin II receptor (AT_1) has provided a new tool for inhibiting the renin–angiotensin system.

Experimental data and preliminary clinical experience have suggested that the efficacy of AT_1 receptor antagonists in the treatment of hypertension is similar to that of ACE inhibitors. However, the two drug categories also have potential differences, because of their different mechanisms of action. Since they have an action that is exclusively targeted at angiotensin II, the AT_1 receptor antagonists should lack the effects of ACE inhibitors that are mediated through the accumulation of bradykinin and other peptides. Furthermore, since a significant amount of angiotensin II can be generated by enzymes other than ACE, particularly the chymases, AT_1 receptor antagonists achieve more complete blockade of the effects of angiotensin than ACE inhibitors do. Nevertheless, whether these differences are clinically important is still being investigated.

The first attempt at blocking the AT_1 receptor with the peptide analogues of angiotensin II resulted in the discovery of saralasin, an antagonist that lacked oral activity and had partial agonist properties. Losartan was the first agent in the new class of orally active AT_1 receptor antagonists. Other agents with different receptor affinities and binding kinetics, such as candesartan, eprosartan, irbesartan, losartan, tasosartan, telmisartan, and valsartan, have since become available (1). Variations in chemical structure may lead to marginal but potentially clinically significant differences in the time-effect profile. Non-competitive antagonists may have longer durations of action than competitive antagonists, because they bind irreversibly to angiotensin II receptors. There have been several reviews of this class of agents (2,3). All have emphasized their remarkable tolerance profile. In double-blind, placebo-controlled trials, the type and frequency of reported adverse effects were consistently no different from placebo (4).

The angiotensin II receptor antagonists are being considered for the treatment of diseases other than hypertension (heart failure with or without left ventricular systolic dysfunction, during and after acute myocardial infarction, diabetic nephropathy, other forms of glomerulopathy, restenosis after coronary angioplasty, and atherosclerosis).

Comparative studies

The RESOLVD (Randomized Evaluation of Strategies for Left Ventricular Dysfunction) trial was a pilot study investigating the effects of candesartan, enalapril, and their combination on exercise tolerance, ventricular function, quality of life, neurohormone concentrations, and tolerability in congestive heart failure (5). Candesartan alone was as effective, safe, and well tolerated as enalapril. The combination of candesartan with enalapril was more beneficial in preventing left ventricular remodelling than either alone. Although the trial was not powered to assess effects on cardiovascular events, it was terminated prematurely because of a trend toward a greater number of events in the candesartan alone and combination groups compared with enalapril alone.

In the ELITE study losartan produced greater survival benefit in elderly patients with heart failure than captopril (6). ELITE II was performed in order to confirm this. It included 3152 patients aged 60 years and over with NYHA class II–IV heart failure and was powered to detect a clinically significant effect on all-cause mortality. Median follow up was 555 days. Losartan was not superior to captopril in improving survival; however, it was better tolerated. Significantly fewer patients taking losartan

withdrew because of adverse effects, including effects attributed to the study drug, or because of cough. Fewer patients discontinued treatment because of adverse effects (10 versus 15%), including effects attributed to the study drug (3 versus 8%) or because of cough (0.4 versus 2.8%) (6).

The results of SPICE (The Study of Patients Intolerant of Converting Enzyme Inhibitors) and of the previously published RESOLVD led to the design of the current CHARM trial, which is investigating the effect of candesartan in 6600 patients with heart failure in three different ways: versus an ACE inhibitor in patients with preserved left ventricular function; versus placebo in patients intolerant of ACE inhibitors; and in addition to ACE inhibitors in all other patients. While waiting for the results of this trial it is advisable to continue to use ACE inhibitors as the initial therapy for heart failure. In patients with documented intolerance of ACE inhibitors (which may represent 10–20% of patients with heart failure) angiotensin receptor antagonists may be useful as a substitute to block the renin–angiotensin–aldosterone system.

Placebo-controlled studies

The SPICE was a smaller trial (270 patients, 12 weeks follow-up) which evaluated the use of candesartan versus placebo in patients with heart failure and a history of intolerance of ACE inhibitors (most commonly because of cough, symptomatic hypotension, or renal insufficiency). Titration to the highest dose of candesartan 16 mg was possible in 69% of the patients (84% in the placebo group). Death and cardiovascular events tended to be lower with candesartan (7).

The results of another trial in heart failure with another angiotensin receptor antagonist (valsartan) are now available but are still to be published. In the VAL-HeFT (Valsartan in Heart Failure Trial) valsartan 160 mg bd was compared with placebo in 5010 patients with heart failure and left ventricular systolic dysfunction receiving optimal conventional therapy, including ACE inhibitors. The results showed a non-significant effect on mortality (19% on placebo, 20% on valsartan), but a highly significant effect on the primary endpoint of all-cause mortality and morbidity (32% on placebo, 29% on valsartan). A subgroup analysis suggested that the combination of valsartan, an ACE inhibitor, and a beta-blocker was not beneficial and might even be harmful, whereas the combination of valsartan and an ACE inhibitor caused a reduction of 45% (8).

General adverse effects

The safety profile of angiotensin II receptor antagonists is so far remarkably good. Except for hypotension, virtually no dose-related adverse effects have been reported. Headache, dizziness, weakness, and fatigue are the most common adverse effects. There have been reports of raised liver enzymes (9), cholestatic hepatitis (10), and pancreatitis (11) with losartan. Several cases of angioedema have been reported but no other obvious hypersensitivity reactions.

Organs and Systems

Cardiovascular

The action of angiotensin II receptor antagonists in interfering with the activity of the renin–angiotensin system is so similar to the action of the ACE inhibitor drugs that episodes of first-dose hypotension, renal impairment, and hyperkalemia would be anticipated. However, there have been only a few such reports to date, although this may reflect the careful screening of patients for clinical trials, from which, by inference, obviously high-risk patients may have been excluded.

Respiratory

Cough has been specifically studied, because the mechanism of action of losartan differs from the ACE inhibitors, in that there is no accumulation of kinins, which have been implicated in the non-productive cough associated with ACE inhibitors (12). In 135 patients known to have ACE inhibitor-induced cough, lisinopril, losartan, or hydrochlorothiazide were given. Of the patients rechallenged with lisinopril, 72% developed a cough compared with only 29 and 34% challenged with losartan and hydrochlorothiazide respectively (13). However, in a Prescription Event Monitoring (PEM) study in four cohorts of 9000 patients exposed to losartan, enalapril, lisinopril, or perindopril, the rate of cough was high even with losartan. The authors attributed this to a carry-over effect, since presumably patients taking losartan have previously had cough with an ACE inhibitor (14).

A compilation of three controlled trials in 1200 patients showed incidence rates of cough of 3.6% with valsartan versus 9.5% with ACE inhibitors and 0.4% with placebo (1).

In a PEM study in 9000 patients cough occurred in 3.1% of patients taking losartan, compared with 3.9, 14, and 16% in patients taking enalapril, lisinopril, and perindopril respectively (14). The unusual low rate of cough with enalapril was surprising and emphasizes the limitations of PEM studies. Worthy of remark is a possible confounding effect, discussed by the authors, related to the fact that a large number of patients were given losartan because they had had cough with an ACE inhibitor. Because of a carry-over effect, cough may still be reported, especially in the first week when patients change to losartan. This carry-over effect may have been the cause of cough reported with losartan in other cases (15).

In a multicenter controlled study in patients with hypertension and a history of ACE inhibitor-induced cough, eprosartan significantly reduced the risk of cough by 88% compared with enalapril (16).

Immunologic

Because ACE inhibitor-induced anaphylaxis is thought to be related to accumulation of bradykinin, it was assumed that angiotensin II receptor antagonists would not cause this reaction. However, angioedema has been described within 30 minutes of a first dose of losartan 50 mg in a 52-year-old man (17). The author also referred to a single case of losartan-induced angioedema mentioned in the manufacturers' package insert from among 4058 patients

treated with losartan. In an international safety update report based on 200 000 patients there were 13 cases of angioedema (18). Two had also taken an ACE inhibitor and three others had previously developed angioedema when taking ACE inhibitors.

References

1. Birkenhager WH, de Leeuw PW. Non-peptide angiotensin type 1 receptor antagonists in the treatment of hypertension. J Hypertens 1999;17(7):873–81.
2. Bakris GL, Giles TD, Weber MA. Clinical efficacy and safety profiles of AT1 receptor antagonists. Cardiovasc Rev Rep 1999;20:77–100.
3. Burnier M. Angiotensin II type 1 receptor blockers. Circulation 2001;103(6):904–12.
4. Hedner T, Oparil S, Rasmussen K, Rapelli A, Gatlin M, Kobi P, Sullivan J, Oddou-Stock P. A comparison of the angiotensin II antagonists valsartan and losartan in the treatment of essential hypertension. Am J Hypertens 1999;12(4 Pt 1):414–17.
5. McKelvie RS, Yusuf S, Pericak D, Avezum A, Burns RJ, Probstfield J, Tsuyuki RT, White M, Rouleau J, Latini R, Maggioni A, Young J, Pogue J. Comparison of candesartan, enalapril, and their combination in congestive heart failure: randomized evaluation of strategies for left ventricular dysfunction (RESOLVD) pilot study. The RESOLVD Pilot Study Investigators. Circulation 1999;100(10):1056–64.
6. Pitt B, Poole-Wilson PA, Segal R, Martinez FA, Dickstein K, Camm AJ, Konstam MA, Riegger G, Klinger GH, Neaton J, Sharma D, Thiyagarajan B. Effect of losartan compared with captopril on mortality in patients with symptomatic heart failure: randomised trial—the Losartan Heart Failure Survival Study ELITE II. Lancet 2000;355(9215):1582–7.
7. Granger CB, Ertl G, Kuch J, Maggioni AP, McMurray J, Rouleau JL, Stevenson LW, Swedberg K, Young J, Yusuf S, Califf RM, Bart BA, Held P, Michelson EL, Sellers MA, Ohlin G, Sparapani R, Pfeffer MA. Randomized trial of candesartan cilexetil in the treatment of patients with congestive heart failure and a history of intolerance to angiotensin-converting enzyme inhibitors. Am Heart J 2000;139(4):609–17.
8. Cohn JN, Tognoni G, Glazer RD, Spormann D, Hester A. Rationale and design of the Valsartan Heart Failure Trial: a large multinational trial to assess the effects of valsartan, an angiotensin-receptor blocker, on morbidity and mortality in chronic congestive heart failure. J Card Fail 1999;5(2):155–60.
9. Losartan potassium prescribing information. Merck & Co Inc., West Point, PA 19486, USA, April 1995.
10. Bosch X, Goldberg AL, Smith IS, Stephenson WP. Losartan-induced hepatotoxicity. JAMA 1997;278(19):1572.
11. Bosch X. Losartan-induced acute pancreatitis. Ann Intern Med 1997;127(11):1043–4.
12. Lacourciere Y, Brunner H, Irwin R, Karlberg BE, Ramsay LE, Snavely DB, Dobbins TW, Faison EP, Nelson EB. Effects of modulators of the renin–angiotensin–aldosterone system on cough. Losartan Cough Study Group. J Hypertens 1994;12(12):1387–93.
13. Lacourciere Y, Lefebvre J. Modulation of the renin–angiotensin–aldosterone system and cough. Can J Cardiol 1995;11(Suppl F):F33–9.
14. Mackay FJ, Pearce GL, Mann RD. Cough and angiotensin II receptor antagonists: cause or confounding? Br J Clin Pharmacol 1999;47(1):111–14.
15. Conigliaro RL, Gleason PP. Losartan-induced cough after lisinopril therapy. Am J Health Syst Pharm 1999;56(9):914–15.

16. Oparil S. Eprosartan versus enalapril in hypertensive patients with angiotensin-converting enzyme inhibitor-induced cough. Curr Ther Res Clin Exp 1999;60:1–4.
17. Acker CG, Greenberg A. Angioedema induced by the angiotensin II blocker losartan. N Engl J Med 1995;333(23):1572.
18. Hansson L. Medical and cost-economy aspects of modern antihypertensive therapy—with special reference to 2 years of clinical experience with losartan. Blood Press Suppl 1997;1:52–5.

Angiotensin-converting enzyme inhibitors

See also Individual agents

General Information

Angiotensin-converting enzyme (ACE) inhibitors inhibit the conversion of angiotensin I to angiotensin II. The ACE is also a kininase, and so ACE inhibitors inhibit the breakdown of kinins. Some of the adverse effects of these drugs are related to these pharmacological effects. For example, cough is thought to be due to the action of kinins on axon fibers in the lungs and hypotension is due to vasodilatation secondary to reduced concentrations of the vasoconstrictor angiotensin II.

Our knowledge of the use of ACE inhibitors has expanded dramatically during recent years, thanks to the publication of the results of a number of large clinical trials (1).

The Heart Outcomes Prevention Evaluation (HOPE) study showed that virtually all patients with a history of cardiovascular disease, not only those who have had an acute myocardial infarction or who have heart failure, benefit from ACE inhibitor therapy (2). The authors selected 9297 patients at increased risk of cardiovascular disease, defined as a history of a cardiovascular event or evidence of disease, such as angina. People with diabetes but no indication of heart disease were included, but they had to have an additional risk factor. They were allocated to receive the ACE inhibitor ramipril 10 mg/day or placebo. The trial was stopped early, according to the pre-defined rules, because of an overwhelming effect of ramipril on the primary end-point, a 22% reduction in a composite measure of myocardial infarction, stroke, and death from cardiovascular causes. Significance was also achieved on outcomes as diverse as myocardial infarction, revascularization, heart failure, cardiac arrest, and worsening angina. Patients with diabetes had a similar 25% reduction for the composite cardiovascular end-point. Moreover, patients taking ramipril had 16% less overt nephropathy (defined as urine albumin over 300 mg/24 hours, or urine total protein excretion over 500 mg/24 hours, or a urine albumin/creatinine ratio over 36 mg/mmol). They also needed 22% less laser therapy for retinopathy. Since all the patients in the HOPE study were not hypertensive, and since the cardiovascular benefit was greater than that attributable to the fall in blood pressure, the authors suggested that ACE inhibitors are cardioprotective, vasculoprotective, and renal protective, independently of their blood pressure lowering effect.

Relative to the dosage issue, the dosage–plasma concentration relation for enalaprilat (the active metabolite of enalapril) in patients with heart failure and its relation to drug-related adverse effects has been investigated (3). In patients taking enalapril for more than 3 months, in dosages of 5–20 mg bd, there were highly variable trough concentrations of enalaprilat. They were affected by serum creatinine, the severity of heart failure, and body weight. Adverse effects, such as cough and rises in serum creatinine and potassium, were more common at high enalaprilat trough concentrations. The authors concluded that these results provide a rationale for individually adjusting ACE inhibitor doses in case of adverse effects.

Use in hypertension

In hypertension, the Captopril Prevention Project (CAPPP) trial evaluated an ACE inhibitor as an alternative first-line agent in mild to moderate hypertension. It was a prospective randomized open study with blinded end point evaluation (PROBE design), comparing an antihypertensive strategy based on either captopril or conventional therapy with a beta-blocker or a diuretic in patients with mild to moderate hypertension. At the end of follow-up the incidence of cardiovascular events was equal with the two strategies. However, imbalances in the assignment of treatment resulted in a 2 mmHg higher average diastolic blood pressure at entry in the group assigned to captopril. This difference in blood pressure alone would be sufficient to confer an excess of cardiovascular risk within this group, could mask real differences between the regimens in their effects on coronary events, and could explain the greater risk of stroke among patients who took captopril. The authors claimed that the overall results support the position that from now on one should consider ACE inhibitors as first-line agents, equal to diuretics and beta-blockers (4). The CAPPP study also reported a reduced risk of diabetes with captopril, which may be explained by the fact that thiazides and beta-blockers cause changes in glucose metabolism and by favorable effects of ACE inhibition on insulin responsiveness.

The second Swedish Trial in Old Patients with hypertension, STOP-2, was designed to compare the effects of conventional antihypertensive drugs on cardiovascular mortality and morbidity with those of newer antihypertensive drugs, including ACE inhibitors, in elderly patients (5). The study was prospective, randomized, and open, but with a blinded end-point evaluation. It included 6614 patients aged 70–84 years with hypertension (blood pressure over 180 mmHg systolic, or over 105 mmHg diastolic, or both). The patients were randomly assigned to conventional drugs (atenolol 50 mg/day, metoprolol 100 mg/day, pindolol 5 mg/day, or hydrochlorothiazide 25 mg/day plus amiloride 2.5 mg/day) or to newer drugs (enalapril 10 mg/day or lisinopril 10 mg/day, or felodipine 2.5 mg/day or isradipine 2.5 mg/day). Blood pressure fell similarly in all treatment groups. There were equal incidences of the primary end-points (fatal stroke, fatal myocardial infarction, and other fatal cardiovascular disease combined) in all groups (20 events per 1000 patient years). Subgroup analyses showed that conventional therapy,

ACE inhibitors, and calcium antagonists had similar efficacy in preventing cardiovascular mortality and major morbidity. This finding argues against the hypothesis that some classes of antihypertensive drugs have efficacy advantages over others, at least in this population of elderly hypertensive patients. Therefore, the choice of antihypertensive treatment will be related to other factors, such as cost, co-existing disorders, and adverse effects. With respect to the reported adverse effects, since the study was open, causality cannot be established. Nevertheless, the size of the study and its naturalistic design allowed accurate assessment of the incidence of adverse effects in this population of elderly hypertensive patients. With ACE inhibitors the most frequently reported adverse effects were cough 30%, dizziness 28%, ankle edema 8.7%, headache 7.7%, shortness of breath 7.3%, and palpitation 5.5%. Actually, little detail was given in the section devoted to safety in the main publication of the results of the trial.

Use in heart failure

In heart failure much debate has been generated by the observation of general "under-use" of ACE inhibitors and the use of smaller doses than have been beneficial in clinical trials. This was partly related to concern about safety with the highest doses, especially in high-risk groups, such as the elderly and patients with renal insufficiency (6). Actually, outcome trials effectively excluded elderly patients (75–80 years and over) and usually patients with renal insufficiency. As elderly patients have poorer renal function, they are more likely to have vascular disease in their renal and carotid arteries, and may be more prone to symptomatic hypotension, it cannot be assumed that the benefit to harm balance observed in younger patients will be the same, at the same doses, in elderly people. The NETWORK trial, a comparison of small and large doses of enalapril in heart failure, was poorly designed and is not conclusive. However, it suggested that apart from a trend to more fatigue with higher doses (10 mg bd), the incidence of adverse effects, including symptomatic hypotension, was similar across the three dosages (2.5, 5, and 10 mg bd) (7).

In heart failure the issue of whether it is justified to use doses of ACE inhibitors substantially smaller than the target doses used in the large-scale studies that established the usefulness of these drugs has been examined in the ATLAS (Assessment of Treatment with Lisinopril and Survival) trial (8). This trial randomized 3164 patients with New York Heart Association (NYHA) class II–IV heart failure and ejection fractions less than 30% to double-blind treatment with either low doses (2.5–5.0 mg/day) or high doses (32.5–35 mg/day) of the ACE inhibitor lisinopril for 39–58 months, while background therapy for heart failure was continued. When compared with the low-dose group, patients in the high-dose group had a non-significant 8% lower risk of death but a significant 12% lower risk of death plus hospitalization for any reason and 24% fewer hospitalizations for heart failure. Dizziness and renal insufficiency were more frequent in the high-dose group, but the two groups were similar in the number of patients who required withdrawal of the study medication. These findings suggest that patients with heart failure should not generally be maintained on very low doses of an ACE inhibitor, unless higher doses cannot be tolerated. However, the ATLAS trial did not address this issue properly. The doses in the small-dose arm were actually very small, and much smaller than those used in routine practice, as reported in several other studies (9). The doses in the large-dose arm may have been unnecessarily high. The recommendation of using target doses proven to be effective in large-scale trials remains unchallenged.

In the studies of left ventricular dysfunction (SOLVD), adverse effects related to the long-term use of enalapril have been thoroughly investigated (10).

Use in myocardial infarction

In the acute infarction ramipril efficacy (AIRE) study, oral ramipril in 2006 patients with heart failure after acute myocardial infarction resulted in a substantial reduction in deaths within 30 days (11).

More trials during and after myocardial infarction have been published and subjected to meta-analysis (12). This very large database provides valuable information on the rate of the most common adverse effects. Of all trials of the effects of ACE inhibitors on mortality in acute myocardial infarction, only the CONSENSUS II trial did not show a positive effect. In this trial, enalaprilat was infused within 24 hours after the onset of symptoms, followed by oral enalapril. The reasons for the negative result of CONSENSUS II remain unresolved, but hypotension and a proischemic effect linked to a poorer prognosis have been suggested.

Use in nephropathy

The results of two trials in patients with chronic nephropathy have reinforced the benefit of ACE inhibitors in slowing the progression of chronic renal insufficiency due to renal diseases other than diabetic nephropathy (13–15) and have provided sufficient information on the safety profile of these agents in chronic renal insufficiency. This was found to be essentially the same as in patients with normal renal function. The current practice of avoiding ACE inhibitors in severe renal insufficiency, to prevent further renal impairment and hyperkalemia, is no longer justified, although careful monitoring should still be observed.

Ramipril has a renal protective effect in non-diabetic nephropathies with nephrotic and non-nephrotic proteinuria (14). It also improves cardiovascular morbidity and all-cause mortality in patients with some cardiovascular risk (2).

The Ramipril Efficacy in Nephropathy (REIN) trial was designed to test whether glomerular protein traffic, and its modification by an ACE inhibitor, influenced disease progression in non-diabetic chronic nephropathies (13). Patients were stratified before randomization by 24-hour proteinuria. Treatment with ramipril or placebo plus conventional antihypertensive therapy was targeted at the same bloodpressure control. At the second interim analysis, ramipril had slowed the fall in glomerular filtration rate (GFR) more than expected from the degree of blood pressure reduction. In the follow-up study GFR almost stabilized in patients who had been originally randomized to ramipril and had continued to take it for more than 36 months. The combined risk of doubling of the serum creatinine or end-stage renal insufficiency was half that found in those taking placebo plus conventional therapy. In patients with proteinuria of 1–3 g/day the fall in GFR per month was not significantly affected, but progression to end-stage renal insufficiency was significantly less common with ramipril (9/99 versus 18/87) for a relative risk of 2.72 (CI = 1.22, 6.08) (14); and so was progression to overt proteinuria (15/99 versus 27/87; RR = 2.40; CI = 1.27, 4.52).

The results of this trial show that ramipril was well tolerated and even protective in cases of advanced renal insufficiency. One major reason for the current practice of underprescription and of prescription of suboptimal doses of ACE inhibitors, especially in patients with heart failure, is the presence of renal insufficiency (16). In such patients, not only should ACE inhibitors no longer be avoided, they are indeed indicated for preservation of renal function.

General adverse effects

The commonest unwanted effects of ACE inhibitors are related to their pharmacological actions (that is inhibition of angiotensin-converting enzyme and kininase II): renal insufficiency, potassium retention, pronounced first-dose hypotension, cough, and the serious but less common angioedema. Skin rashes and taste disturbances are uncommon, but may be more likely with sulfhydryl-containing drugs, particularly captopril. Rare hypersensitivity reactions include rashes, bone-marrow suppression, hepatitis, and alveolitis. If administered in the second or third term of pregnancy, ACE inhibitors can cause a number of fetal anomalies, including growth retardation, renal impairment, oligohydramnios, hypocalvaria, fetal pulmonary hypoplasia, and fetal death. Neonatal anuria and neonatal death can also occur (17,18). Tumor-inducing effects have not been reported.

The frequencies and the profile of adverse effects of five major classes of antihypertensive agents have been assessed in an unselected group of 2586 chronically drug-treated hypertensive patients (19). This was accompanied by a questionnaire-based survey among patients visiting a general practitioner. The percentages of patients who reported adverse effects spontaneously, on general inquiry, and on specific questioning were 16, 24, and 62% respectively. With ACE inhibitors the figures were 15, 22, and 55%. The percentage of patients in whom discontinuation was due to adverse effects was 8.1% with ACE inhibitors (significantly higher than diuretics). Compared with beta-blockers, ACE inhibitors were associated with less fatigue (RR = 0.57; 95% CI = 0.38, 0.85), cold extremities (RR = 0.11; CI = 0.07, 0.18), sexual urge (RR = 0.52; CI = 0.33, 0.82), insomnia (RR = 0.10; CI = 0.04, 0.26), dyspnea (RR = 0.38; CI = 0.17, 0.85), and more coughing (RR = 13; CI = 5.6, 30). The authors did not find a significant effect of age on the pattern of adverse effects. Women reported more effects and effects that were less related to the pharmacological treatment.

Organs and Systems

Cardiovascular

Marked reductions in blood pressure, without any significant change in heart rate, can occur at the start of ACE inhibitor therapy. Such reductions, which are not orthostatic, are sometimes symptomatic but rarely fatal. The volume of evidence is greatest with the longer established agents, but continues to suggest that the problems of first-dose hypotension are most likely to occur in patients whose renin–angiotensin system is stimulated (renin-dependent states), such as in renovascular hypertension or other causes of renal hypoperfusion, dehydration, or previous treatment with other vasodilators (20). These conditions can co-exist, particularly in severe heart failure (21–23). Similar problems have occurred in the treatment of hypertensive neonates and infants (24), but again were particularly likely in the setting of high plasma renin activity associated with either renovascular disease or concurrent diuretic treatment.

The use of very low doses to avoid first-dose hypotension is common, although the rationale remains unclear (25). It is even less clear whether or not there are differences between different ACE inhibitors, that is whether first-dose hypotension is agent-specific or a class effect (26,27).

Respiratory

Cough
DoTS classification
   Dose-relation: collateral effect
   Time-course: time-independent
   Susceptibility factors: genetic (polymorphisms of the bradykinin B_2 receptor gene and the ACE gene); sex (men); exogenous factors (non-smokers).

A non-productive irritant cough is associated with ACE inhibitors (28,29). The dose-relatedness of this adverse effect is not clear.

Frequency
In different studies there has been large variability in the absolute incidence of cough (0.7–48%), the discontinuation rate (1–10%), and the relative incidences with different ACE inhibitors (30). However, the placebo-controlled, randomized, HOPE study has provided a remarkable database, with the largest cohort and the longest follow-up ever reported with such therapy (over 9000 patients followed for 5 years on average). Compared with placebo, ACE inhibitor therapy with ramipril caused cough leading to drug withdrawal in 7.3% of patients (compared with 1.8% for placebo) (13).

Mechanism
The mechanism of this effect has been explored (31–33). It may be more complicated than just an increase in concentrations of bradykinin and substance P, increased microvasculature leakage, and stimulation of vagal C fibers (34). Sulindac and indometacin may abolish or reduce the intensity and frequency of cough, supposedly because of inhibition of prostaglandin synthesis (35,36). Common variant genetics of ACE, chymase, and the bradykinin B_2 receptor do not explain the occurrence of ACE inhibitor-related cough (37). In general, bronchial hyper-reactivity has been causally implicated and may also be associated with exaggerated dermal responses to

histamine (31,33). However, in one report, airways hyper-responsiveness was not a consistent finding (38).

Susceptibility factors
Cough is more common in non-smokers (39) and in women (39,40). It has been speculated that the risk of cough is genetically predetermined. The possibility that polymorphisms of the human bradykinin B_2 receptor gene may be involved in ACE inhibitor-related cough has been investigated in a case-control study (41). The DNA of 60 subjects with and without cough who were treated with ACE inhibitors was compared with that of 100 patients with untreated essential hypertensive and 100 normotensive subjects. The frequencies of the TT genotype and T allele were significantly higher in the subjects with cough than in subjects without. These tendencies were more pronounced in women. Subjects with the CC genotype were less susceptible to cough. According to the authors, high transcriptional activity of the bradykinin B_2 receptor promoter may be related to the risk of ACE inhibitor-related cough. This is the first demonstration that a genetic variant is involved in ACE inhibitor-related cough. It may therefore be possible to predict the occurrence of cough related to ACE inhibitor use.

The genetic basis of ACE inhibitor-induced cough and its relation to bradykinin have been further explored in a study of the effect of cilazapril in two groups of healthy volunteers genotyped for ACE insertion/deletion (I/D) polymorphism (42). The cough threshold to inhaled capsaicin was significantly lower in the genotype II group than in the DD group. Skin responses to intradermal bradykinin were significantly enhanced in the genotype II group. There was no difference in responsiveness to intradermal substance P. The authors suggested that these findings provide further evidence of the link between ACE inhibitor-induced cough and I/D polymorphism of the ACE gene, and that this supports the hypothesis that ACE inhibitors cause cough by modulating tissue concentrations of bradykinin.

Chinese patients experience more cough from ACE inhibitors than Caucasians. A review of the pharmacokinetics and blood pressure-lowering efficacy of ACE inhibitors as well as of ACE and angiotensinogen gene polymorphism did not find significant differences between Chinese and Caucasians to account for the difference in cough incidence (43).

Management
ACE inhibitor-associated cough seems to be a class effect: switching to another ACE inhibitor rarely solves the problem, although there are occasional anecdotal reports (40,44). However, most patients who develop a cough related to an ACE inhibitor are able and willing to continue therapy. In a small randomized study inhaled sodium cromoglicate relieved the symptom (45). In those in whom the symptom is intolerable, a switch to an angiotensin receptor antagonist is justified.

Obstructive airways disease
It has been suggested that ACE inhibitors are also associated with an increased incidence of symptomatic obstructive airways disease, leading to bronchospasm and asthma (46). However, a prescription event monitoring study of more than 29 000 patients taking ACE inhibitors, compared with 278 000 patients taking other drugs, failed to confirm this association (47).

Endocrine

Gynecomastia has been reported in a patient taking captopril 75 mg/day; it resolved when captopril was withdrawn but recurred when the patient was given enalapril (48). This suggests that gynecomastia may not be simply attributable to the sulfhydryl group of captopril.

Metabolism

ACE inhibition has been associated with increased insulin sensitivity in diabetic patients, and it has therefore been hypothesized that ACE inhibitors can precipitate hypoglycemia in such patients. A Dutch case-control study suggested that among users of insulin or oral hypoglycemic drugs, the use of ACE inhibitors was significantly associated with an increased risk of hospital admission for hypoglycemia (49). However, a French case/non-case study from the pharmacovigilance database did not confirm this finding (50).

In a matched case-control study of 404 cases of hospitalization for hypoglycemia in diabetic patients and 1375 controls, the risk of hypoglycemia was greater in those who used insulin versus a sulfonylurea and was not influenced by the use of ACE inhibitors (51). However, the use of enalapril was associated with an increased risk of hypoglycemia (OR = 2.4; CI = 1.1, 5.3) in sulfonylurea users. Although the authors emphasized the fact that previous reports of ACE inhibitor-related hypoglycemia were more frequent with enalapril, it is unclear why only enalapril, and not ACE inhibitors as a class, was associated with a significantly increased risk of hypoglycemia, and why this occurred only in sulfonylurea users.

Conversely, it has been suggested that the protective effect of ACE inhibitors against severe hypoglycemia should be tested in high-risk patients with high ACE activity. About 10–20% of patients with type 1 diabetes mellitus have a risk of severe hypoglycemia. In 307 unselected consecutive diabetic outpatients, those with the ACE DD genotype had a relative risk of severe hypoglycemia of 3.2 (95% CI = 1.4, 7.4) compared with those with the genotype II (52). There was a significant relation between serum ACE activity and the risk of severe hypoglycemia.

Electrolyte balance

ACE inhibitors can cause hyperkalemia because they inhibit the release of aldosterone. The effect is usually not significant in patients with normal renal function. However, in patients with impaired kidney function and/or in patients taking potassium supplements (including salt substitutes) or potassium-sparing diuretics, and especially aldosterone antagonists, hyperkalemia can occur. In two cases, hypoaldosteronism with diabetes was implicated (53,54).

Hyponatremia, defined as a plasma sodium concentration of 133 mmol/l or under, has been investigated in a prospective study of elderly patients with hip fractures. ACE inhibitors were the most frequently used drugs (five of 14 cases) (55). Of course, this does not prove a cause and effect relation, since in elderly people ACE inhibitors are likely to be among the most frequently prescribed drugs. However, hypoaldosteronism would be a likely mechanism.

Hematologic

ACE inhibitors are used to treat erythrocytosis, for example after transplantation (56). Efficacy in treating erythrocytosis in chronic obstructive pulmonary disease has also been described with the angiotensin II receptor antagonist losartan (57). ACE inhibitors can also lower normal erythrocyte counts and cause anemia (58). This effect has been assessed in a retrospective study of 92 patients after transplantation with and without erythrocytosis, comparing patients taking the same anti-rejection therapy (steroids plus ciclosporin or steroids, ciclosporin, and azathioprine) taking ACE inhibitors with those not taking ACE inhibitors (59). There were significantly lower hemoglobin and erythropoietin concentrations in patients taking ACE inhibitors. When enalapril was given to those who had not previously taken an ACE inhibitor, the hemoglobin concentration fell by around 10% and erythropoietin by around 40%. These effects were not affected by the presence or absence of azathioprine. Although the hemoglobin-lowering effect of ACE inhibition is not a new finding, the lack of an influence of azathioprine adds some further understanding to the effect.

Liver

Hepatic injury is a rare adverse effect of the ACE inhibitors (60,61). Both acute and chronic hepatitis and cholestatic jaundice can occur (62,63), as can cross-reactivity, as identified in a report involving enalapril and captopril (64).

Pancreas

Acute pancreatitis has been reported with both enalapril and lisinopril (65,66).

Urinary tract

The ACE inhibitors can cause reversible impairment of renal function in the setting of reduced renal perfusion, whether due to bilateral renal artery stenosis, severe congestive heart failure, volume depletion, hyponatremia, high dosages of diuretics, combined treatment with NSAIDs, or diabetes mellitus (67). Beyond treatment of the cause, preventive measures include withholding diuretics for a few days, beginning therapy with very small doses of ACE inhibitors, and cautious dosage titration. Therapy involves increasing dietary sodium intake and reducing dosages of diuretics or temporarily withdrawing them. The ACE inhibitor may have to be given in reduced dosages or withdrawn for a time. Because they prolong survival in heart failure and after myocardial infarction, if withdrawal is deemed necessary ACE inhibitors should be reintroduced after a brief respite.

The agreed mechanism of renal function impairment with ACE inhibitors is as follows: when perfusion pressure or afferent arteriolar pressure is reduced in the glomerulus, glomerular filtration is maintained by efferent arteriolar vasoconstriction, an effect of angiotensin II. Blocking the formation of angiotensin II, and perhaps increasing the formation of bradykinin, causes selective efferent arteriolar vasodilatation and results in a reduction in glomerular filtration (68).

In a retrospective study of 64 patients, mean age 71 years, with acute renal insufficiency associated with an ACE inhibitor, over 85% presented with overt dehydration due to diuretics or gastrointestinal fluid loss (69). Bilateral renal artery stenosis or stenosis in a solitary kidney was documented in 20% of cases. In seven patients dialysis was required, but none became dialysis dependent. After resolution of acute renal insufficiency, the plasma creatinine concentration returned to baseline and renal function was not significantly worsened. Two-year mortality was the highest in a subgroup of patients with pre-existing chronic renal insufficiency.

Skin

There have been numerous reports of different rashes in association with ACE inhibitors. The most common skin reaction is a pruritic maculopapular eruption, which is reportedly more common with captopril (2–7%) than with enalapril (about 1.5%). This rash occurs in the usual dosage range and is more common in patients with renal insufficiency (70). Lichenoid reactions, bullous pemphigoid, exfoliative dermatitis, flushing and erythroderma, vasculitis/purpura, subcutaneous lupus erythematosus, and reversible alopecia have all been reported (70–72).

The ACE inhibitors can worsen psoriasis by a mechanism mediated by inhibition of the activity of leukotrienes, which are implicated in the pathogenesis of psoriasis (73).

The ACE inhibitor-related pemphigus has been reviewed in the light of two cases of pemphigus attributed to fosinopril and quinapril (74). Drug-related pemphigus can be classified into two major types, based on the clinical course: induced pemphigus and triggered pemphigus, in which endogenous factors are more important and the drug plays a secondary role. The first type is usually related to thiol drugs. It is impossible to distinguish drug-related pemphigus reliably from idiopathic pemphigus on the basis of clinical findings, histopathology, or immunofluorescence. Captopril tends to be associated with pemphigus foliaceus, whereas the non-thiol ACE inhibitors are more often associated with pemphigus vulgaris, although there are exceptions. A transition from pemphigus vulgaris to pemphigus foliaceus is more common than the reverse. Several mechanisms have been proposed to be involved in the induction of pemphigus: interaction of the thiol group with sulfur-containing groups on the keratinocyte membrane, leading to acantholysis by biochemical interference with adhesion mechanisms; antigen modification resulting in antibody formation; inhibition of suppressor T cells, resulting in pathogenic autoantibody formation by B cell clones; or enzyme activation or inhibition. The maximum latency to the development of pemphigus reported for ACE inhibitors is 2 years. It can take up to 17 months for lesions to resolve after drug withdrawal. A significant proportion of cases will not improve or resolve spontaneously on drug withdrawal alone. It is important to withdraw the offending drug, treat the bullous reaction appropriately, and advise avoidance of ACE inhibitors, although substitution of enalapril for captopril or vice versa has been successful in some cases.

Immunologic

Angioedema

Angioedema is a potentially fatal complication that has been associated with several different ACE inhibitors, with a reported incidence of 0.1–0.5%.

Presentation

Angioedema due to ACE inhibitors can manifest as recurrent episodes of facial swelling, which resolves on withdrawal, or as acute oropharyngeal edema and airways obstruction, which requires emergency treatment with an antihistamine and corticosteroids. It may be life-threatening (75) and may need tracheostomy (76). It is occasionally fatal (77). An unusual presentation with subglottic stenosis has also been reported (78). A variant form is angioedema of the intestine, which tends to occur within the first 24–48 hours of treatment (79,80).

- Two patients presented with isolated visceral angioedema with episodes of recurrent abdominal symptoms (81). Each had undergone surgical procedures for symptoms that persisted after surgery and were ultimately relieved by withdrawal of their ACE inhibitors.
- Another similar case was diagnosed as angioedema of the small bowel after an abdominal CT scan (82). Angioedema occurred in a 58-year-old woman 3 hours after biopsy of a hypopharyngeal mass under general anesthesia and was accompanied by transient electrocardiographic features of anterior myocardial infarction with severe hypokinesis of the anterior wall regions on echocardiography but no significant change in creatinine kinase activity (83). Only T wave inversion persisted on follow-up. Repeat echocardiography showed significant spontaneous improvement and coronary angiography showed normal coronary arteries. Hypotension and hypoxemia did not seem to occur, and the authors could not therefore speculate on the mechanism of the concomitant cardiac changes.
- Recurrent episodes of tongue swelling have been reported with cilazapril (84) and perindopril (85).
- A 74-year-old man with a permanent latex condom catheter developed penile swelling that was non-pitting and involved the subcutaneous tissue of a normal scrotum, after taking lisinopril 5 mg/day for 6 days (86). Removal of the catheter had no effect. After other possible causes were ruled out, ACE inhibitor-induced angioedema was suspected and lisinopril was withdrawn. Within a few days, the swelling, which had not spread, resolved.

Time-course

Angioedema can occur within the day after the start of treatment (87) and the risk is highest within the first month of ACE inhibitor use. However, it can occur many months after the start of therapy (88,89) or even years after (90).

Susceptibility factors

Black Americans are at increased risk of angioedema (91), with an overall rate of 1.6 per 1000 person years of ACE inhibitor use.

Anaphylactoid reactions, with hypotension, and flushing, occasionally associated with abdominal cramping, diarrhea, nausea, and sweating, have been reported in patients taking ACE inhibitors undergoing hemodialysis. Angioedema can also occur in these patients; it is occasionally life-threatening and is usually associated with the concurrent use of ACE inhibitors and dialysers in which the membrane is made of polyacrylonitrile (also known as AN69) (92,93). This combination should be avoided, since well-established alternatives are available.

For unclear reasons, ACE inhibitor-induced angioedema was more prevalent among immunosuppressed patients after cardiac or renal transplantation than among other patients (94). In 156 cardiac patients and 341 patients with renal transplants, this adverse effect was observed in 4.8 and 1% respectively, that is 24 times and 5 times higher than in the general population (0.1–0.2%).

Mechanism

The exact mechanism of angioedema associated with ACE inhibitors has not been determined. Although the reaction may be immune mediated, IgE antibodies or other specific antibodies have not been detected. Some authors have speculated that it may be related to a deficiency of carboxypeptidase N and complement components, because of its parallel role with that of ACE in enzymatic inactivation of bradykinin. The involvement of high concentrations of bradykinin in the pathogenesis of angioedema related to the use of ACE inhibitors is still hypothetical, since no definitive increase in bradykinin plasma concentration during attacks of angioedema has been shown. However, kinin concentrations are difficult to measure. In a well-documented study, a newly developed reliable assay for specific measurement of plasma bradykinin, excluding other immunoreactive kinins, detected a very high concentration of bradykinin (47 pmol/l) during an acute attack of angioedema in a patient taking captopril (95).

There have been reports of a lupus-like syndrome with captopril (96) and lisinopril (97).

Second-Generation Effects

Fetotoxicity

Enalapril, captopril, and lisinopril (and presumably other ACE inhibitors) cross the placenta in pharmacologically significant amounts (17). There is clear evidence of fetotoxicity when ACE inhibitors are used beyond the first trimester of pregnancy. Since continuation of treatment beyond the first trimester carries an excess risk of low fetal birth weight and other more severe complications, it is important to withdraw the ACE inhibitor at this time. Intrauterine growth retardation, oligohydramnios, and neonatal renal impairment, often with a serious outcome, are characteristic (98); failure of ossification of the skull or hypocalvaria also appear to be part of the pattern (17). There is also evidence that persistence of a patent ductus arteriosus is also more likely to occur.

Susceptibility Factors

Renal disease

Enalapril has been specifically studied in patients who are resistant to other drugs and intolerant of captopril (99) and in patients with collagen vascular disease and renal disease known to be at high risk of adverse effects (100). In the first study (99), the major reasons for discontinuing captopril were a low white blood cell count, proteinuria, taste disturbance, and rash. In the vast majority of the 281 patients, these adverse effects did not recur during enalapril treatment. The main adverse events that warranted withdrawal of enalapril were impairment of renal function (5%), hypotension (2%), and rashes (2%). The authors noted that patients with angioedema should not be given alternative ACE inhibitors.

In the second study (100) of 738 high-risk patients the main reasons for the withdrawal of enalapril were increases in serum creatinine (4%), hypotension (1%), and nausea (1%).

The long-term safety of enalapril in patients with severe renal insufficiency and hypertension has been evaluated in a pooled analysis of three similar, randomized, placebo-controlled clinical trials in 317 patients with renal insufficiency (101). Only patients without diabetes were included. Follow-up was for 2 and 3 years. One protocol used a fixed dose (5 mg/day) and the other two allowed titration up to 40 mg/day. Cough occurred in 18% of the patients taking enalapril and in 6.1% of those taking placebo. Hypotension (5.9 versus 1.2%) and paresthesia (7.8 versus 2.4%) were more frequent with enalapril. Angioedema (1.3 versus 0.6%) and first-dose hypotension (1.3 versus 0%) tended to occur more often with enalapril. Hyperkalemia, defined as any increase from baseline and left to the judgement of the investigators, was excessive in the enalapril-treated patients (28 versus 8.8%). Finally, the hematocrit fell more often with enalapril (7.1 versus 2.0%).

It is important to stress that although it is a risk factor, renal insufficiency is a good indication for ACE inhibitors, which slow the progression of chronic renal insufficiency (102). In trials in patients with chronic renal insufficiency (13–15,17), the safety profile was essentially the same as in patients with normal renal function. The current practice of avoiding ACE inhibitors in severe renal insufficiency, to prevent further renal impairment and hyperkalemia, seems no longer justified. However, patients with bilateral renal artery stenosis carry an excess risk of renal insufficiency when treated with ACE inhibitors. These agents are therefore contraindicated in such patients.

Drug–Drug Interactions

Aspirin

Antagonistic effects of cyclo-oxygenase inhibitors (indometacin or aspirin) have been repeatedly reported both in hypertension and in heart failure, strongly suggesting that there may be prostaglandin participation in the clinical response to ACE inhibitors (103,104). In animals, although not in all experimental models, aspirin can attenuate the beneficial effects of ACE inhibitors on ventricular remodelling after myocardial infarction.

However, there are conflicting reports on the clinical significance of this interaction (105).

Positive studies

From a post-hoc analysis of the SOLVD trial, it appears that in patients with left ventricular systolic dysfunction, the use of aspirin was associated with improved survival and reduced morbidity. In aspirin users, benefit from enalapril was retained but reduced (106).

The WASH pilot study (Warfarin/Aspirin Study in Heart Failure) compared the effects on cardiovascular events of warfarin and aspirin, and on antithrombotic therapy in patients with heart failure, most of whom were also taking an ACE inhibitor. Patients taking aspirin had more events and hospitalizations related to worsening heart failure than patients in the two other groups (unpublished data, reported at the 1999 annual meeting of the European Society of Cardiology, John Cleland, personal communication). The authors speculated that this may have been related to a negative interaction between ACE inhibitor therapy and aspirin, which would counteract the beneficial effects of ACE inhibitors. The Warfarin-Antiplatelet Trial in Chronic Heart Failure (WATCH) is indirectly addressing the issue. It is based on the hypothesis that warfarin or clopidogrel (an antiplatelet agent that acts by a pathway independent of cyclo-oxygenase) may be preferred to aspirin as antithrombotic therapy in patients with heart failure. It will randomize 4500 patients, most of whom will be taking ACE inhibitors. Meanwhile, it may be advisable to avoid aspirin in patients with heart failure and no clear indication for aspirin (no evidence of atherosclerosis), and to consider substituting warfarin or clopidogrel for aspirin in patients with refractory or rapidly progressive heart failure (107). In all other cases, because each drug is clearly associated with a substantial clinical benefit, it would be excessive to deny patients aspirin or ACE inhibitors.

In a series of studies of ACE inhibitor-induced improvement in pulmonary function, treatment with aspirin 325 mg/day for 8 weeks in patients with mild to moderate heart failure due to primitive dilated cardiomyopathy did not affect ventilation and peak oxygen consumption during exercise when the patients were not taking an ACE inhibitor but worsened pulmonary diffusion capacity and made the ventilatory response to exercise (tidal volume, ventilation to carbon dioxide production) less effective in those who were, regardless of the duration of ACE inhibition (108).

A systematic overview of major ACE inhibitor trials (CONSENSUS II, AIRE, TRACE, SMILE) found a trend toward less benefit from ACE inhibitors among aspirin users (109). Although the interaction was not statistically significant, the authors concluded that the data did not "refute the hypothesis of a major aspirin interaction with ACE inhibitors," especially because patients taking aspirin had only 60% of the benefit seen in patients not taking it.

GUSTO-1 and EPILOG, two different antithrombotic trials, GUSTO-1 and EPILOG, the first in acute myocardial infarction and the second during coronary stenting, compared the event rates in patients taking aspirin, an ACE inhibitor, or both (110). In each of these trials, events were more frequent in patients taking the combination than in those taking aspirin alone. The authors interpreted these findings as suggesting that ACE inhibitors may reduce the benefit of aspirin in these patients, whereas the results of the ACE inhibitor trials suggested that aspirin may interfere with the effect of ACE inhibitors.

Negative studies

A post-hoc analysis of the CATS trial database in patients with acute myocardial infarction suggested that aspirin does not attenuate the acute and long-term effects of captopril (111). Because of the demonstrated benefit on morbidity and mortality with each agent, textbooks and official guidelines do not recommend withholding either aspirin or ACE inhibitors in patients with heart failure or myocardial infarction. With no sufficient proof of lack of interaction, the use of small doses of aspirin (100 mg/day or less) is recommended.

In a study of the effects of aspirin 325 mg/day, both acute (4 hours after the dose) and chronic (6 weeks), in 62 patients with mild to moderate heart failure taking enalapril (more than 10 mg/day for at least 3 months), there were no significant changes in mean arterial pressure or in forearm blood flow and vascular resistance measured by venous plethysmography (112). In another arm of the study the same results were observed with ifetroban 250 mg/day, a thromboxane A_2 receptor antagonist.

Conclusions

Two post-hoc analyses of clinical trials (110) have added to the confusion engendered by these conflicting results. GUSTO-1 and EPILOG, two different antithrombotic trials, the first in acute myocardial infarction and the second during coronary stenting, compared the event rates in patients taking aspirin, an ACE inhibitor, or both (110). In each of these trials, events were more frequent in patients taking the combination than in those taking aspirin alone. The authors interpreted these findings as suggesting that ACE inhibitors may reduce the benefit of aspirin in these patients, whereas the results of the ACE inhibitor trials suggested that aspirin may interfere with the effect of ACE inhibitors.

These conflicting results may be partly explained by the various mechanisms of the vasodilatory action of ACE inhibitors, which may differ according to the regional peripheral circulation. In none of the studies was central hemodynamics or cardiac output assessed.

However, none of the trials post-hoc analysis, which suggested that there is an interaction between aspirin and ACE inhibitors, was specifically designed to examine this question. Post-hoc and subgroup analyses may be heavily biased, and multivariate adjustment may not have been able to account fully for confounding factors. Aspirin in itself may be harmful in certain patients, such as those with heart failure, because of its antiprostaglandin activity, rather than because it interferes with the actions of ACE inhibitors, a phenomenon that would also manifest as an aspirin–ACE inhibitor interaction.

The interaction between aspirin and ACE inhibitors in patients with heart failure is probably clinically important (105). Both drugs are often prescribed for a large number of patients with a variety of cardiovascular diseases. These agents have mechanisms of action that interact at the physiological level, and there are consequently many theoretical reasons to expect important clinical consequences. In animals, although not in all experimental models, aspirin can attenuate the beneficial effects of ACE inhibitors on ventricular remodelling after myocardial infarction. Some clinical studies have suggested that there is minimal, if any, adverse peripheral hemodynamic effect. In the most recent such study, the acute (4 hours after the dose) and chronic (6 weeks) effects of aspirin 325 mg/day were investigated in 62 patients with mild to moderate heart failure treated with enalapril (more than 10 mg/day for at least 3 months) (112). This did not produce significant changes in mean arterial pressure or in forearm blood flow and vascular resistance measured by venous plethysmography. In another arm of the study the same results were observed with ifetroban 250 mg/day, a thromboxane A_2 receptor antagonist. These conflicting results may be explained by the various mechanisms of the vasodilatory action of ACE inhibitors, which may differ according to the regional peripheral circulation. In none of the studies was central hemodynamics or cardiac output assessed. There is evidence that co-administration of aspirin and ACE inhibitors can be detrimental to renal function in patients with heart failure.

Beta-lactams

Intestinal absorption of beta-lactams occurs at least in part by an active mechanism involving a dipeptide carrier, and this pathway can be inhibited by dipeptides and tripeptides (113,114), which reduce the rate of absorption of the beta-lactams. ACE inhibitors, which have an oligopeptide structure, are absorbed by the same carrier (115) and interact with beta-lactams in isolated rat intestine (116).

A second potential site of interaction between ACE inhibitors and beta-lactams is the renal anionic transport system, and concomitant administration sometimes results in pronounced inhibition of the elimination of beta-lactams (117).

Diuretics

Because of dehydration, patients taking diuretics can be particularly sensitive to the hypotensive effect of ACE inhibitors (20).

Potassium supplements, potassium-sparing diuretics, or salt substitutes

Concurrent administration of potassium supplements, potassium-sparing diuretics, or salt substitutes can precipitate hyperkalemia in ACE inhibitor-treated patients, in whom aldosterone is suppressed (SED-14, 674). Regular monitoring of serum potassium is essential in these patients, because of the risk of hyperkalemia in patients given potassium (or potassium-sparing diuretics) and ACE inhibitors or angiotensin receptor antagonists.

In a retrospective study, five patients developed extreme hyperkalemia (9.4–11 mmol/l) within 8–18 days of starting combination therapy with co-amilozide and an ACE inhibitor (118).

In eight healthy subjects, treatment with spironolactone and losartan increased mean plasma potassium concentration by 0.8 mmol/l (up to 5.0 mmol/l) and reduced mean urinary potassium excretion from 108 to 87 mmol/l (119).

Until more data are available, it is prudent to consider angiotensin II receptor antagonists similar to ACE inhibitors as risk factors for hyperkalemia in patients taking potassium-sparing diuretics.

Selective cyclo-oxygenase-2 (COX-2) inhibitors

Non-selective non-steroidal inflammatory drugs can attenuate the antihypertensive effects of ACE inhibitors and increase the risk of renal insufficiency. In 2278 patients taking NSAIDs, 328 taking ACE inhibitors, and 162 taking both, no nephrotoxicity was found in patients taking monotherapy, but there were three cases of reversible renal insufficiency in patients taking the combination (120).

This effect is more prominent in patients with low renin concentrations. The interaction of COX-2 inhibitors with ACE inhibitors has been much less well investigated. In a review of Phase II/III studies of COX-2 inhibitors, it was reported that the co-administration of rofecoxib 25 mg/day and benazepril 10–40 mg/day for 4 weeks was associated with an average increase in mean arterial pressure of about 3 mmHg compared with ACE inhibitor monotherapy (121).

One report has described a case of increased blood pressure in a patient taking rofecoxib and lisinopril (122).

- The blood pressure of a 59-year-old man with hypertension and normal renal function rose when rofecoxib 25 mg/day was added to lisinopril 10 mg/day (from an average of 135/80–85 to 168/98 mmHg within 5 weeks). Four days after rofecoxib was withdrawn the blood pressure was 127/78 mmHg. Rechallenge with the same dose of rofecoxib produced the same effect and the blood pressure fell when the dosage of lisinopril was increased to 20 mg/day on continuous rofecoxib. The authors did not report on the course of renal function.

The increase in blood pressure with COX-2 inhibitors from interaction with ACE inhibitors may be greater in some patients than has previously been reported.

References

1. Brown NJ, Vaughan DE. Angiotensin-converting enzyme inhibitors. Circulation 1998;97(14):1411–20.
2. Yusuf S, Sleight P, Pogue J, Bosch J, Davies R, Dagenais G. Effects of an angiotensin-converting-enzyme inhibitor, ramipril, on cardiovascular events in high-risk patients. The Heart Outcomes Prevention Evaluation Study Investigators. N Engl J Med 2000;342(3):145–53.
3. Brunner-La Rocca HP, Weilenmann D, Kiowski W, Maly FE, Follath F. Plasma levels of enalaprilat in chronic therapy of heart failure: relationship to adverse events. J Pharmacol Exp Ther 1999;289(1):565–71.
4. Hansson L, Lindholm LH, Niskanen L, Lanke J, Hedner T, Niklason A, Luomanmaki K, Dahlof B, de Faire U, Morlin C, Karlberg BE, Wester PO, Bjorck JE. Effect of angiotensin-converting-enzyme inhibition compared with conventional therapy on cardiovascular morbidity and mortality in hypertension: the Captopril Prevention Project (CAPPP) randomised trial. Lancet 1999;353(9153):611–16.
5. Hansson L, Lindholm LH, Ekbom T, Dahlof B, Lanke J, Schersten B, Wester PO, Hedner T, de Faire U. Randomised trial of old and new antihypertensive drugs in elderly patients: cardiovascular mortality and morbidity the Swedish Trial in Old Patients with Hypertension-2 study. Lancet 1999;354(9192):1751–6.
6. Cleland JG. ACE inhibitors for the prevention and treatment of heart failure: why are they "under-used"? J Hum Hypertens 1995;9(6):435–42.
7. Poole-Wilson PA; on behalf of the NETWORK investigators. The NETWORK study. The effect of dose of an ACE inhibitor on outcome in patients with heart failure. J Am Coll Cardiol 1996;27(Suppl A):141A.
8. Packer M, Poole-Wilson PA, Armstrong PW, Cleland JG, Horowitz JD, Massie BM, Ryden L, Thygesen K, Uretsky BF. Comparative effects of low and high doses of the angiotensin-converting enzyme inhibitor, lisinopril, on morbidity and mortality in chronic heart failure. ATLAS Study Group. Circulation 1999;100(23):2312–18.
9. Gerstein HC, Yusuf S, Mann JFE. Effects of ramipril on cardiovascular and microvascular outcomes in people with diabetes mellitus: results of the HOPE study and MICRO-HOPE substudy. Heart Outcomes Prevention Evaluation Study Investigators. Lancet 2000;355(9200):253–9.
10. Kostis JB, Shelton B, Gosselin G, Goulet C, Hood WB Jr, Kohn RM, Kubo SH, Schron E, Weiss MB, Willis PW 3rd, Young JB, Probstfield J. Adverse effects of enalapril in the Studies of Left Ventricular Dysfunction (SOLVD). SOLVD Investigators. Am Heart J 1996;131(2):350–5.
11. The Acute Infarction Ramipril Efficacy (AIRE) Study Investigators. Effect of ramipril on mortality and morbidity of survivors of acute myocardial infarction with clinical evidence of heart failure. Lancet 1993;342(8875):821–8.
12. Latini R, Maggioni AP, Flather M, Sleight P, Tognoni G. ACE inhibitor use in patients with myocardial infarction. Summary of evidence from clinical trials. Circulation 1995;92(10):3132–7.
13. Ruggenenti P, Perna A, Gherardi G, Gaspari F, Benini R, Remuzzi G. Renal function and requirement for dialysis in chronic nephropathy patients on long-term ramipril: REIN follow-up trial. Gruppo Italiano di Studi Epidemiologici in Nefrologia (GISEN). Ramipril Efficacy in Nephropathy. Lancet 1998;352(9136):1252–6.
14. Ruggenenti P, Perna A, Gherardi G, Garini G, Zoccali C, Salvadori M, Scolari F, Schena FP, Remuzzi G. Renoprotective properties of ACE-inhibition in non-diabetic nephropathies with non-nephrotic proteinuria. Lancet 1999;354(9176):359–64.
15. Maschio G, Alberti D, Janin G, Locatelli F, Mann JF, Motolese M, Ponticelli C, Ritz E, Zucchelli P, Marai P, Marcelli D, Tentori F, Oldrizzi L, Rugiu C, Salvadeo A, Villa G, Picardi L, Borghi M, Moriggi M, et al. Effect of the angiotensin-converting-enzyme inhibitor benazepril on the progression of chronic renal insufficiency. The Angiotensin-Converting-Enzyme Inhibition in Progressive Renal Insufficiency Study Group. N Engl J Med 1996;334(15):939–45.
16. Echemann M, Zannad F, Briancon S, Juilliere Y, Mertes PM, Virion JM, Villemot JP. Determinants of angiotensin-converting enzyme inhibitor prescription in severe heart failure with left ventricular systolic dysfunction: the EPICAL study. Am Heart J 2000;139(4):624–31.
17. Barr M Jr. Teratogen update: angiotensin-converting enzyme inhibitors. Teratology 1994;50(6):399–409.

18. Sedman AB, Kershaw DB, Bunchman TE. Recognition and management of angiotensin converting enzyme inhibitor fetopathy. Pediatr Nephrol 1995;9(3):382–5.

19. Olsen H, Klemetsrud T, Stokke HP, Tretli S, Westheim A. Adverse drug reactions in current antihypertensive therapy: a general practice survey of 2586 patients in Norway. Blood Press 1999;8(2):94–101.

20. Scott RA, Barnett DB. Lower than conventional doses of captopril in the initiation of converting enzyme inhibition in patients with severe congestive heart failure. Clin Cardiol 1989;12(4):225–6.

21. Kjekshus J, Swedberg K. Enalapril for congestive heart failure. Am J Cardiol 1989;63(8):D26–32.

22. Francis GS, Rucinska EJ. Long-term effects of a once-a-day versus twice-a-day regimen of enalapril for congestive heart failure. Am J Cardiol 1989;63(8):D17–21.

23. Lewis GR. Comparison of lisinopril versus placebo for congestive heart failure. Am J Cardiol 1989;63(8):D12–16.

24. Perlman JM, Volpe JJ. Neurologic complications of captopril treatment of neonatal hypertension. Pediatrics 1989;83(1):47–52.

25. Reznik V, Griswold W, Mendoza S. Dangers of captopril therapy in newborns. Pediatrics 1989;83(6):1076.

26. MacFadyen RJ, Lees KR, Reid JL. Differences in first dose response to angiotensin converting enzyme inhibition in congestive heart failure: a placebo controlled study. Br Heart J 1991;66(3):206–11.

27. Mullen PJ. Unexpected first dose hypotensive reaction to enalapril. Postgrad Med J 1990;66(782):1087–8.

28. Strocchi E, Malini PL, Valtancoli G, Ricci C, Bassein L, Ambrosiani E. Cough during treatment with angiotensin converting enzyme inhibitors. Analysis of predisposing factors. Drug Invest 1992;4:69–72.

29. Simon SR, Black HR, Moser M, Berland WE. Cough and ACE inhibitors. Arch Intern Med 1992;152(8):1698–700.

30. Kaplan NM. The CARE Study: a postmarketing evaluation of ramipril in 11,100 patients. The Clinical Altace Real-World Efficacy (CARE) Investigators. Clin Ther 1996;18(4):658–70.

31. Lindgren BR, Andersson RG. Angiotensin-converting enzyme inhibitors and their influence on inflammation, bronchial reactivity and cough. A research review. Med Toxicol Adverse Drug Exp 1989;4(5):369–80.

32. Kaufman J, Casanova JE, Riendl P, Schlueter DP. Bronchial hyperreactivity and cough due to angiotensin-converting enzyme inhibitors. Chest 1989;95(3):544–8.

33. Lindgren BR, Rosenqvist U, Ekstrom T, Gronneberg R, Karlberg BE, Andersson RG. Increased bronchial reactivity and potentiated skin responses in hypertensive subjects suffering from coughs during ACE-inhibitor therapy. Chest 1989;95(6):1225–30.

34. Emanueli C, Grady EF, Madeddu P, Figini M, Bunnett NW, Parisi D, Regoli D, Geppetti P. Acute ACE inhibition causes plasma extravasation in mice that is mediated by bradykinin and substance P. Hypertension 1998;31(6):1299–304.

35. Ohya Y, Kumamoto K, Fujishima M. Effects of crossover application of sulindac and azelastine on enalapril-induced cough. J Hum Hypertens 1992;6(1):81–2.

36. Fogari R, Zoppi A, Tettamanti F, Malamani GD, Tinelli C, Salvetti A. Effects of nifedipine and indomethacin on cough induced by angiotensin-converting enzyme inhibitors: a double-blind, randomized, cross-over study. J Cardiovasc Pharmacol 1992;19(5):670–3.

37. Zee RY, Rao VS, Paster RZ, Sweet CS, Lindpaintner K. Three candidate genes and angiotensin-converting enzyme inhibitor-related cough: a pharmacogenetic analysis. Hypertension 1998;31(4):925–8.

38. Boulet LP, Milot J, Lampron N, Lacourciere Y. Pulmonary function and airway responsiveness during long-term therapy with captopril. JAMA 1989;261(3):413–16.

39. Os I, Bratland B, Dahlof B, Gisholt K, Syvertsen JO, Tretli S. Female sex as an important determinant of lisinopril-induced cough. Lancet 1992;339(8789):372.

40. Israili ZH, Hall WD. Cough and angioneurotic edema associated with angiotensin-converting enzyme inhibitor therapy. A review of the literature and pathophysiology. Ann Intern Med 1992;117(3):234–42.

41. Mukae S, Aoki S, Itoh S, Iwata T, Ueda H, Katagiri T. Bradykinin B(2) receptor gene polymorphism is associated with angiotensin-converting enzyme inhibitor-related cough. Hypertension 2000;36(1):127–31.

42. Takahashi T, Yamaguchi E, Furuya K, Kawakami Y. The ACE gene polymorphism and cough threshold for capsaicin after cilazapril usage. Respir Med 2001;95(2):130–5.

43. Ding PY, Hu OY, Pool PE, Liao W. Does Chinese ethnicity affect the pharmacokinetics and pharmacodynamics of angiotensin-converting enzyme inhibitors? J. Hum Hypertens 2000;14(3):163–70.

44. Sharif MN, Evans BL, Pylypchuk GB. Cough induced by quinapril with resolution after changing to fosinopril. Ann Pharmacother 1994;28(6):720–2.

45. Hargreaves MR, Benson MK. Inhaled sodium cromoglycate in angiotensin-converting enzyme inhibitor cough. Lancet 1995;345(8941):13–16.

46. Lunde H, Hedner T, Samuelsson O, Lotvall J, Andren L, Lindholm L, Wiholm BE. Dyspnoea, asthma, and bronchospasm in relation to treatment with angiotensin converting enzyme inhibitors. BMJ 1994;308(6920):18–21.

47. Inman WH, Pearce G, Wilton L, Mann RD. Angiotensin Converting Enzyme Inhibitors and Asthma. Southampton: Drug Safety Research Unit, 1994.

48. Nakamura Y, Yoshimoto K, Saima S. Gynaecomastia induced by angiotensin converting enzyme inhibitor. BMJ 1990;300(6723):541.

49. Herings RM, de Boer A, Stricker BH, Leufkens HG, Porsius A. Hypoglycaemia associated with use of inhibitors of angiotensin converting enzyme. Lancet 1995;345(8959):1195–8.

50. Moore N, Kreft-Jais C, Haramburu F, Noblet C, Andrejak M, Ollagnier M, Begaud B. Reports of hypoglycaemia associated with the use of ACE inhibitors and other drugs: a case/non-case study in the French pharmacovigilance system database. Br J Clin Pharmacol 1997;44(5):513–18.

51. Thamer M, Ray NF, Taylor T. Association between antihypertensive drug use and hypoglycemia: a case-control study of diabetic users of insulin or sulfonylureas. Clin Ther 1999;21(8):1387–400.

52. Pedersen-Bjergaard U, Agerholm-Larsen B, Pramming S, Hougaard P, Thorsteinsson B. Activity of angiotensin-converting enzyme and risk of severe hypoglycaemia in type 1 diabetes mellitus. Lancet 2001;357(9264):1248–53.

53. Uchida K, Azukizawa S, Nakano S, Kaneko M, Kigoshi T, Morimoto S, Matsui A. Reversible hyperkalemia during antihypertensive therapy in a hypertensive diabetic patient with latent hypoaldosteronism and mild renal failure. South Med J 1994;87(11):1153–5.

54. Bonnet F, Thivolet CH. Reversible hyperkalemia at the initiation of ACE inhibitors in a young diabetic patient with latent hyporeninemic hypoaldosteronism. Diabetes Care 1996;19(7):781.

55. Schwab M, Roder F, Morike K, Thon KP, Klotz U. Drug-induced hyponatraemia in elderly patients. Br J Clin Pharmacol 1999;48(1):105–6.

56. Mazzali M, Filho GA. Use of aminophylline and enalapril in posttransplant polycythemia. Transplantation 1998;65(11):1461–4.

57. Olger AF, Ozlem OK, Ozgur K, Peria A, Doganay A. Effects of losartan on the renin–angiotensin–aldosterone system and erythrocytosis in patients with chronic obstructive pulmonary diseases and systemic hypertension. Clin Drug Invest 2001;21:337–43.

58. Gossmann J, Kachel HG, Schoeppe W, Scheuermann EH. Anemia in renal transplant recipients caused by concomitant therapy with azathioprine and angiotensin-converting enzyme inhibitors. Transplantation 1993;56(3):585–9.

59. Montanaro D, Gropuzzo M, Tulissi P, Boscutti G, Risaliti A, Baccarani U, Mioni G. Angiotensin-converting enzyme inhibitors reduce hemoglobin concentrations, hematocrit, and serum erythropoietin levels in renal transplant recipients without posttransplant erythrocytosis. Transplant Proc 2001;33(1–2):2038–40.

60. Deira JL, Corbacho L, Bondia A, Lerma JL, Gascon A, Martin B, Garcia P, Tabernero JM. Captopril hepatotoxicity in a case of renal crisis due to systemic sclerosis. Nephrol Dial Transplant 1997;12(8):1717–18.

61. Nissan A, Spira RM, Seror D, Ackerman Z. Captopril-associated "pseudocholangitis." A case report and review of the literature. Arch Surg 1996;131(6):670–1.

62. Valle R, Carrascosa M, Cillero L, Perez-Castrillon JL. Enalapril-induced hepatotoxicity. Ann Pharmacother 1993;27(11):1405.

63. Droste HT, de Vries RA. Chronic hepatitis caused by lisinopril. Neth J Med 1995;46(2):95–8.

64. Hagley MT, Benak RL, Hulisz DT. Suspected cross-reactivity of enalapril- and captopril-induced hepatotoxicity. Ann Pharmacother 1992;26(6):780–1.

65. Maringhini A, Termini A, Patti R, Ciambra M, Biffarella P, Pagliaro L. Enalapril-associated acute pancreatitis: recurrence after rechallenge. Am J Gastroenterol 1997;92(1):166–7.

66. Standridge JB. Fulminant pancreatitis associated with lisinopril therapy. South Med J 1994;87(2):179–81.

67. Packer M. Identification of risk factors predisposing to the development of functional renal insufficiency during treatment with converting-enzyme inhibitors in chronic heart failure. Cardiology 1989;76(Suppl 2):50–5.

68. Kon V, Fogo A, Ichikawa I. Bradykinin causes selective efferent arteriolar dilation during angiotensin I converting enzyme inhibition. Kidney Int 1993;44(3):545–50.

69. Wynckel A, Ebikili B, Melin JP, Randoux C, Lavaud S, Chanard J. Long-term follow-up of acute renal failure caused by angiotensin converting enzyme inhibitors. Am J Hypertens 1998;11(9):1080–6.

70. Kuechle MK, Hutton KP, Muller SA. Angiotensin-converting enzyme inhibitor-induced pemphigus: three case reports and literature review. Mayo Clin Proc 1994;69(12):1166–71.

71. Gilleaudeau P, Vallat VP, Carter DM, Gottlieb AB. Angiotensin-converting enzyme inhibitors as possible exacerbating drugs in psoriasis. J Am Acad Dermatol 1993;28(3):490–2.

72. Butt A, Burge SM. Pemphigus vulgaris induced by captopril. Dermatology 1993;186:315.

73. Ikai K. Exacerbation and induction of psoriasis by angiotensin-converting enzyme inhibitors. J Am Acad Dermatol 1995;32(5 Pt 1):819.

74. Ong CS, Cook N, Lee S. Drug-related pemphigus and angiotensin converting enzyme inhibitors. Australas J Dermatol 2000;41(4):242–6.

75. Sadeghi N, Panje WR. Life-threatening perioperative angioedema related to angiotensin-converting enzyme inhibitor therapy. J Otolaryngol 1999;28(6):354–6.

76. Maestre ML, Litvan H, Galan F, Puzo C, Villar Landeira JM. Imposibilidad de intubacion por angioedema secundario a IECA. [Impossibility of intubation due to angioedema secondary to an angiotensin-converting enzyme inhibitor.] Rev Esp Anestesiol Reanim 1999;46(2):88–91.

77. Hedner T, Samuelsson O, Lunde H, Lindholm L, Andren L, Wiholm BE. Angio-oedema in relation to treatment with angiotensin converting enzyme inhibitors. BMJ 1992;304(6832):941–6.

78. Martin DJ, Grigg RG, Tomkinson A, Coman WB. Subglottic stenosis: an unusual presentation of ACE inhibitor-induced angioedema. Aust NZ J Surg 1999;69(4):320–1.

79. Jacobs RL, Hoberman LJ, Goldstein HM. Angioedema of the small bowel caused by an angiotensin-converting enzyme inhibitor. Am J Gastroenterol 1994;89(1):127–8.

80. Dupasquier E. Une forme clinique rare d'oedème angioneurotique sous énalapril: l'abdomen aigu. [A rare clinical form of angioneurotic edema caused by enalapril: acute abdomen.] Arch Mal Coeur Vaiss 1994;87(10):1371–4.

81. Byrne TJ, Douglas DD, Landis ME, Heppell JP. Isolated visceral angioedema: an underdiagnosed complication of ACE inhibitors? Mayo Clin Proc 2000;75(11):1201–4.

82. Chase MP, Fiarman GS, Scholz FJ, MacDermott RP. Angioedema of the small bowel due to an angiotensin-converting enzyme inhibitor. J Clin Gastroenterol 2000;31(3):254–7.

83. Blomberg PJ, Surks HK, Long A, Rebeiz E, Mochizuki Y, Pandian N. Transient myocardial dysfunction associated with angiotensin-converting enzyme inhibitor-induced angioedema: recognition by serial echocardiographic studies. J Am Soc Echocardiogr 1999;12(12):1107–9.

84. Kyrmizakis DE, Papadakis CE, Fountoulakis EJ, Liolios AD, Skoulas JG. Tongue angioedema after long-term use of ACE inhibitors. Am J Otolaryngol 1998;19(6):394–6.

85. Lapostolle F, Borron SW, Bekka R, Baud FJ. Lingual angioedema after perindopril use. Am J Cardiol 1998;81(4):523.

86. Henson EB, Bess DT, Abraham L, Bracikowski JP. Penile angioedema possibly related to lisinopril. Am J Health Syst Pharm 1999;56(17):1773–4.

87. Jae Joo Cho, Woo Seok Koh, Bang Soon Kim. A case of angioedema probably induced by captopril. Korean J Dermatol 1999;37:404–6.

88. Mchaourab A, Sarantopoulos C, Stowe DF. Airway obstruction due to late-onset angioneurotic edema from angiotensin-converting enzyme inhibition. Can J Anaesth 1999;46(10):975–8.

89. Maliekal J, Del Rio G. Acute angioedema associated with long-term benazepril therapy. J Pharm Technol 1999;15:208–11.

90. Brown NJ, Ray WA, Snowden M, Griffin MR. Black Americans have an increased rate of angiotensin converting enzyme inhibitor-associated angioedema. Clin Pharmacol Ther 1996;60(1):8–13.

91. Burkhart DG, Brown NJ, Griffin MR, Ray WA, Hammerstrom T, Weiss S. Angiotensin converting enzyme inhibitor-associated angioedema: higher risk in blacks than whites. Pharmacoepidemiol Drug Saf 1996;5(3):149–54.

92. Committee on Safety of Medicines. Anaphylactoid reactions to high-flux polyacrylonitrile membranes in combination with ACE inhibitors. Curr Probl 1992:33.

93. Kammerl MC, Schaefer RM, Schweda F, Schreiber M, Riegger GA, Kramer BK. Extracorporeal therapy with AN69 membranes in combination with ACE inhibition causing severe anaphylactoid reactions: still a current problem? Clin Nephrol 2000;53(6):486–8.

94. Abbosh J, Anderson JA, Levine AB, Kupin WL. Angiotensin converting enzyme inhibitor-induced angioedema more

prevalent in transplant patients. Ann Allergy Asthma Immunol 1999;82(5):473–6.

95. Nussberger J, Cugno M, Amstutz C, Cicardi M, Pellacani A, Agostoni A. Plasma bradykinin in angio-oedema. Lancet 1998;351(9117):1693–7.

96. Sieber C, Grimm E, Follath F. Captopril and systemic lupus erythematosus syndrome. BMJ 1990;301(6753):669.

97. Leak D. Absence of cross-reaction between lisinopril and enalapril in drug-induced lupus. Ann Pharmacother 1997;31(11):1406–7.

98. Pryde PG, Sedman AB, Nugent CE, Barr M Jr. Angiotensin-converting enzyme inhibitor fetopathy. J Am Soc Nephrol 1993;3(9):1575–82.

99. Rucinska EJ, Small R, Mulcahy WS, Snyder DL, Rodel PV, Rush JE, Smith RD, Walker JF, Irvin JD. Tolerability of long term therapy with enalapril maleate in patients resistant to other therapies and intolerant to captopril. Med Toxicol Adverse Drug Exp 1989;4(2):144–52.

100. Rucinska EJ, Small R, Irvin J. High-risk patients treated with enalapril maleate: safety considerations. Int J Cardiol 1989;22(2):249–59.

101. Keane WF, Polis A, Wolf D, Faison E, Shahinfar S. The long-term tolerability of enalapril in hypertensive patients with renal impairment. Nephrol Dial Transplant 1997;12(Suppl 2):75–81.

102. Zanchetti A. Contribution of fixed low-dose combinations to initial therapy in hypertension. Eur Heart J 1999;1(Suppl L):L5–9.

103. Guazzi MD, Campodonico J, Celeste F, Guazzi M, Santambrogio G, Rossi M, Trabattoni D, Alimento M. Antihypertensive efficacy of angiotensin converting enzyme inhibition and aspirin counteraction. Clin Pharmacol Ther 1998;63(1):79–86.

104. Spaulding C, Charbonnier B, Cohen-Solal A, Juilliere Y, Kromer EP, Benhamda K, Cador R, Weber S. Acute hemodynamic interaction of aspirin and ticlopidine with enalapril: results of a double-blind, randomized comparative trial. Circulation 1998;98(8):757–65.

105. Teerlink JR, Massie BM. The interaction of ACE inhibitors and aspirin in heart failure: torn between two lovers. Am Heart J 1999;138(2 Pt 1):193–7.

106. Al-Khadra AS, Salem DN, Rand WM, Udelson JE, Smith JJ, Konstam MA. Antiplatelet agents and survival: a cohort analysis from the Studies of Left Ventricular Dysfunction (SOLVD) trial. J Am Coll Cardiol 1998;31(2):419–25.

107. Massie BM, Teerlink JR. Interaction between aspirin and angiotensin-converting enzyme inhibitors: real or imagined. Am J Med 2000;109(5):431–3.

108. Guazzi M, Pontone G, Agostoni P. Aspirin worsens exercise performance and pulmonary gas exchange in patients with heart failure who are taking angiotensin-converting enzyme inhibitors. Am Heart J 1999;138(2 Pt 1):254–60.

109. Flather MD, Yusuf S, Kober L, Pfeffer M, Hall A, Murray G, Torp-Pedersen C, Ball S, Pogue J, Moye L, Braunwald E. Long-term ACE-inhibitor therapy in patients with heart failure or left-ventricular dysfunction: a systematic overview of data from individual patients. ACE-Inhibitor Myocardial Infarction Collaborative Group. Lancet 2000;355(9215):1575–81.

110. Peterson JG, Topol EJ, Sapp SK, Young JB, Lincoff AM, Lauer MS. Evaluation of the effects of aspirin combined with angiotensin-converting enzyme inhibitors in patients with coronary artery disease. Am J Med 2000;109(5):371–7.

111. Oosterga M, Anthonio RL, de Kam PJ, Kingma JH, Crijns HJ, van Gilst WH. Effects of aspirin on angiotensin-converting enzyme inhibition and left ventricular dilation one year after acute myocardial infarction. Am J Cardiol 1998;81(10):1178–81.

112. Katz SD, Radin M, Graves T, Hauck C, Block A, LeJemtel TH. Effect of aspirin and ifetroban on skeletal muscle blood flow in patients with congestive heart failure treated with Enalapril. Ifetroban Study Group. J Am Coll Cardiol 1999;34(1):170–6.

113. Sugawara M, Toda T, Iseki K, Miyazaki K, Shiroto H, Kondo Y, Uchino J. Transport characteristics of cephalosporin antibiotics across intestinal brush-border membrane in man, rat and rabbit J Pharm Pharmacol 1992;44(12):968–72.

114. Dantzig AH, Bergin L. Uptake of the cephalosporin, cephalexin, by a dipeptide transport carrier in the human intestinal cell line, Caco-2. Biochim Biophys Acta 1990;1027(3):211–17.

115. Friedman DI, Amidon GL. Intestinal absorption mechanism of dipeptide angiotensin converting enzyme inhibitors of the lysyl-proline type: lisinopril and SQ 29,852. J Pharm Sci 1989;78(12):995–8.

116. Hu M, Amidon GL. Passive and carrier-mediated intestinal absorption components of captopril. J Pharm Sci 1988;77(12):1007–11.

117. Padoin C, Tod M, Perret G, Petitjean O. Analysis of the pharmacokinetic interaction between cephalexin and quinapril by a nonlinear mixed-effect model. Antimicrob Agents Chemother 1998;42(6):1463–9.

118. Chiu TF, Bullard MJ, Chen JC, Liaw SJ, Ng CJ. Rapid life-threatening hyperkalemia after addition of amiloride HCl/hydrochlorothiazide to angiotensin-converting enzyme inhibitor therapy. Ann Emerg Med 1997;30(5):612–15.

119. Henger A, Tutt P, Hulter HM, Krapf R. Acid-base effects of inhibition of aldosterone and angiotensin II action in chronic metabolic acidosis in humans. J Am Soc Nephrol 1999;10:121A.

120. Seelig CB, Maloley PA, Campbell JR. Nephrotoxicity associated with concomitant ACE inhibitor and NSAID therapy. South Med J 1990;83(10):1144–8.

121. Kaplan-Machlis B, Klostermeyer BS. The cyclooxygenase-2 inhibitors: safety and effectiveness. Ann Pharmacother 1999;33(9):979–88.

122. Brown CH. Effect of rofecoxib on the antihypertensive activity of lisinopril. Ann Pharmacother 2000;34(12):1486.

Animal products

General Information

Drug substances of animal origin can produce anaphylactic or anaphylactoid reactions, particularly after parenteral administration (1). Animal products can also transmit an infectious disease because of the presence of a pathogenic microbe.

The following products are covered in this monograph:

- bear bile
- bee products (bee pollen, propolis, and royal jelly)
- carp bile
- fish oils
- gangliosides (from bovine brain)
- ghee
- glycosaminoglycans (Arumalon, chitosan, chondroitin, and glucosamine)
- green-lipped mussel
- Imedeen
- Kombucha "mushroom"

- oyster extract
- rattlesnake meat
- shark products (shark cartilage and squalene)
- Spanish fly
- toad venom

Bear bile

Bear bile contains bile acids, cholesterol, and phospholipids (phosphatidylcholine, phosphatidylethanolamine, and phosphatidylinositol). It has been used for centuries in traditional Chinese medicine to treat liver and eye complaints and convulsions, and, in combination with curcuma and capillaris, gallstones and cholecystitis. More recently it has been touted as a treatment for stroke on the basis of animal experiments. It has few or no adverse effects, but by the same token probably has little or no efficacy, although it does contain ursodeoxycholic acid, which in purified form is effective in managing gallstones.

Bee products

Bee pollen

Bee pollen products are used as general tonics. Their use has been associated with allergic reactions, including anaphylaxis (2).

Propolis

Propolis (SEDA-12, 410) (SEDA-13, 459) (SEDA-18, 4) or bee-glue is a resinous material used by bees to seal hive walls and to strengthen the borders of the combs and the hive entrance. It has antiseptic, antimycotic, and bacteriostatic properties and is found in cosmetics and "natural products" for self-treatment.

Oral mucositis with ulceration caused by propolis has been reported in an HIV-negative man (3). Infectious stomatitis is common in HIV-positive patients. Therefore, the first approach is usually the administration of antiviral therapy, antimycotic therapy, or both. However, other causes, such as contact allergy, should be suspected if the patient is exposed to a potentially allergenic substance.

Propolis can cause allergic contact dermatitis (4), and have been reported in HIV-infected patients (5–7). It has been associated with allergy after its use in cosmetics and in the self-treatment of various diseases. Although most cases involve allergic contact dermatitis arising from topical application, a few reports have described an allergic reaction after oral ingestion. Adulteration of propolis capsules with excessive amounts of lead has been reported from New Zealand (8).

Royal jelly

Royal jelly (SEDA-21, 494) is a viscous secretion produced by the pharyngeal glands of the worker bee, *Apis mellifera*. It is widely used in alternative medicine as a health tonic. Its internal use by atopic individuals can cause severe, sometimes even fatal, asthma and anaphylaxis (9–11). Topical application can lead to contact dermatitis (12).

Two patients who were sensitized to a member of the Asteraceae (Compositae) family, mugwort, had severe systemic reactions (anaphylaxis and generalized urticaria/angioedema) due to honey and royal jelly (13). Both had positive skin tests and RAST to mugwort, and in one case

the RAST inhibition assay showed strong cross-reactivity between the proteins of honey and mugwort. The authors suggested that there is a link between sensitization to Asteraceae and adverse reactions to honey and royal jelly.

Of 1472 hospital employees of a teaching hospital in Hong Kong, 461 had taken royal jelly in the past (14). Nine subjects reported 14 adverse reactions to royal jelly, including urticaria, eczema, rhinitis, and acute asthma. Of 176 subjects who responded to a questionnaire, 13 (7.4%) had positive skin tests to pure royal jelly, as did 23 of 300 consecutive asthma clinic attendees (7.3%). All but one of the 36 subjects with positive royal jelly skin tests was atopic to other common allergens. There were associations between positive royal jelly skin tests and atopy (OR = 33, 95% CI = 4.5, 252) and between adverse reactions to royal jelly and a history of clinical allergy (OR = 2.88, 95% CI = 0.72, 12), but not between royal jelly symptoms and previous royal jelly intake.

Carp bile

In Asia, the raw bile of the grass carp (*Ctenopharyngodom idellus*) is believed by some to be health promoting. However, eating it can result in hepatic dysfunction and nephrotoxicity (15). The former usually resolves within a few days, but the latter is more serious, culminating in acute renal insufficiency within 2–3 days after ingestion (16). Experiments in rats have shown that the bile of the grass carp loses its lethality when treated with colestyramine, which forms insoluble complexes with bile acids (17).

Fish oils

Fish oil supplements (SEDA-13, 460) (SEDA-18, 3), rich in long-chain polyunsaturated ω-3 fatty acids (eicosapentaenoic acid, docosahexaenoic acid), can reduce plasma concentrations of triglycerides and VLDL cholesterol, reduce platelet aggregation, prolong bleeding time, reduce blood pressure, increase the fluidity of the blood, and affect leukotriene production. Reported adverse effects include fullness and epigastric discomfort, diarrhea, and a fishy taste after belching. In addition to these mild symptoms, certain areas have been identified in which problems of a more serious nature could arise:

- a potential risk that the favorable changes in plasma lipids could be offset by a deleterious increase in LDL cholesterol or LDL apoprotein B;
- the possible adverse consequence of the capacity to increase bleeding time and to reduce platelet aggregation, especially in patients with pre-existing bleeding and platelet abnormalities and in those taking other antithrombotic agents;
- preliminary evidence that a detrimental effect on patients with aspirin-sensitive asthma is possible;
- an adverse effect on the metabolic control of patients with non-insulin-dependent diabetes mellitus, when these patients are not being treated with a sulfonylurea derivative (18);
- prothrombotic effects through changes on clotting factor concentration (19);
- possible contamination.

Gangliosides

Gangliosides extracted from bovine brain tissue (Cronassial, Sygen) have been widely used in Western Europe and South America for several neurological disorders.

Reported adverse effects of gangliosides, other than discomfort at the injection site, include a motor neuron disease-like illness, cutaneous erythema (with or without fever and nausea), and anaphylaxis. After evaluation of reported associations between the use of gangliosides and Guillain–Barré syndrome (20,21), the Committee for Proprietary Medicinal Products (CPMP) of the European Commission recommended in September 1994 that the marketing authorizations for Cronassial (a mixture of gangliosides for treating peripheral neuropathies) should be withdrawn. At the same time, the CPMP recommended that marketing authorizations for Sygen (a monosialoganglioside known as GM-1, used for the treatment of cerebral vascular insufficiency) should be suspended.

In 65 patients with ischemic stroke treated for 6 weeks with intramuscular Sygen (monosialoganglioside 40 mg/day) in a double-blind, placebo-controlled study, there were no significant differences between the groups (22). A subsequent double-blind, sequential, multicenter, randomized, placebo-controlled trial of two doses of Sygen did not provide convincing evidence of efficacy (23).

Ghee

Ghee is clarified butter from the milk of water buffaloes or cows. Although the butter is heated enough to eliminate non-sporulating organisms, the process is unlikely to kill the spores of *Clostridium tetani*. This may explain why a case-control study in rural areas of Pakistan identified its traditional use as an umbilical cord dressing as a risk factor for the development of neonatal tetanus (24).

Glycosaminoglycans

Glycosaminoglycans include chondroitin-4-sulfate, chondroitin-6-sulfate, and disaccharide polymers composed of equimolar quantities of D-glucuronic acid, N-acetylglucosamine, and sulfates.

Arumalon

Arumalon (Rumalon) (SEDA-14, 440) is a glycosaminoglycan-peptide complex, a "chondroprotective" agent containing a watery extract of cartilage and an extract of the red bone marrow of calves. Parenteral use has been associated with local reactions at the site of the injection and with allergic symptoms (such as fever, malaise, symptoms of pronounced inflammation, nephrotic syndrome). Polymyositis and fatal dermatomyositis are also alleged to be associated with it.

- After 18 intramuscular injections of Arumalon, a 62-year-old woman with degenerative hip-joint changes developed a severe illness, with fever up to 39°C, swellings of the finger, hand, and knee joints, a rash, leukopenia (1.9×10^9/l), thrombocytopenia (113×10^9/l), and increased transaminases and lactate dehydrogenase activity (25). There was a positive lymphocyte transformation test with Arumalon and its constituents, and Arumalon-specific antibodies in the cultured

lymphocyte fluid but not the serum. She became completely free of symptoms only after 1 year while taking a maintenance dose of prednisone 15 mg/day.

Chitosan

Chitosan is a polymer of glucosamine and N-acetylglucosamine, obtained from crustacean shells. It has been used to lower blood lipid concentrations, for body weight reduction (26), and as an excipient in pharmaceutical formulations.

Chondroitin

Chondroitin (Arteparon) (SEDA-14, 441) is a glycosaminoglycan, a "chondroprotective" agent prepared from bovine lung and tracheal cartilage. Mucopolysaccharide polysulfuric acid ester (also known as glycosaminoglycan polysulfate), said to be its major principle, resembles heparin in its molecular structure and can have the same effect on platelet aggregation. Chondroitin has been associated with life-threatening thromboembolic complications (myocardial infarction, pulmonary embolism, hemiplegic apoplexia, cerebral hemorrhage, death). Other reported adverse effects include local reactions at the site of the injection, serious allergic symptoms, arthropathy, subcutaneous fat necrosis, and reversible alopecia.

Glucosamine

Glucosamine is 2-amino-2-deoxy-D-chitin glucopyranose, which is present in joint cartilage. It has been used to treat osteoarthritis and has a small beneficial effect (27).

Asthma has reportedly been exacerbated by the use of a glucosamine-chondroitin supplement for osteoarthritis (28).

Interactions of glucosamine with warfarin (29,30) and acenocoumarol (31) have been described.

Green-lipped mussel

An extract of the New Zealand green-lipped mussel (*Perna canaliculus*) (SED-11, 1021) has been advocated for the treatment of arthritic symptoms. Reported adverse effects include flare-up of the disease, epigastric discomfort, flatulence, and nausea. Jaundice some weeks after starting treatment has been reported.

Imedeen

Imedeen is the trade name of an oral health food product containing freeze-dried proteins from the cartilage of deep-sea fish, which is advocated as an anti-wrinkling agent. Its use has been associated with generalized skin reactions and extensive Quincke's edema (32).

Kombucha "mushroom"

Kombucha "mushroom" (SEDA-20, 430) is a symbiotic yeast/bacteria aggregate surrounded by a permeable membrane. It has no proven efficacy for any indication and has serious adverse effects (33).

Liver damage has been reported after the ingestion of Kombucha tea (34). No other cause of the liver problem could be found. The patient recovered after withdrawal of Kombucha tea.

Anti-Jo1 antibody-positive myositis, associated with pleural effusions, pericardial effusion with tamponade, and "mechanic's hands," was attributed to the consumption of Kombucha "mushroom" (35).

Oyster extract

A food supplement consisting of oyster extract, ginseng, taurine, and zinc (Ostrin plus GTZ 611) has been associated with Quincke's facial edema. The reaction developed immediately after intake of the food supplement, and the oyster extract was considered to be its most likely cause (36).

Rattlesnake meat

Dried rattlesnake meat (SEDA-14, 442) (SEDA-18, 2) is a well-known folk remedy that can be purchased without prescription in Mexico, El Salvador, and the South-western part of the USA. It is available as such and in the form of powder, capsules, or pills, which may be labeled in Spanish as "víbora de cascabel," "pulvo de víbora," or "carne de víbora."

All of 16 different formulations of rattlesnake powder capsules, obtained in six different cities in Mexico, were significantly contaminated with Gram-negative coliform bacteria: *Escherichia coli*, *Klebsiella pneumoniae*, *Enterobacter agglomerans*, *Enterobacter cloacae*, *Salmonella arizona*, and *Salmonella* of groups B, E4, and G; 81% of the capsules were contaminated with *Salmonella* species, the most frequent being *S. arizona* (37). Contamination was probably derived from both the flesh of the snake and fecal contamination during domestic preparation of the powder to produce the capsules.

Rattlesnake products can therefore cause serious systemic infections, particularly with *S. arizona*. Typical victims are Hispanic patients with an immunocompromising illness, such as systemic lupus erythematosus (38,39), AIDS (40), or cancer (41).

Of 22 Latino patients with *S. arizona* infection in Los Angeles County in 1986 and 1987, 18 reported taking snake capsules compared with two of 24 matched Latino controls with non-subgroup three salmonellosis or shigellosis (OR = 18.0, CI = 4.2, 76) (42). An average of 18 cases per year of *S. arizona* infection were reported in the county between 1980 and 1987. In this investigation most of the patients with *S. arizona* infection after snake capsule ingestion had underlying illnesses, such as AIDS, diabetes, arthritis, or cancer. The capsules were obtained primarily from Tijuana, Mexico and from Los Angeles pharmacies in Latino neighborhoods.

Although most patients respond well to intravenous therapy with ampicillin or co-trimoxazole, deaths have occurred. *S. arizona* peritonitis has been reported.

Shark products

Shark cartilage

Shark cartilage powder, prepared from cartilage from the fins of hammerhead sharks (*Sphyrna lewini*) or spiny dogfish (*Squalus acanthias*), is promoted as a treatment for arthritis and cancer (43), based on antiangiogenic properties, but crude extracts are ineffective (44), presumably because the active constituents, such as sphyrnastatins are not absorbed.

- A 38-year-old white man worked in a factory that ground shark cartilage (45). After 10 months of exposure, he reported chest symptoms at work in association with exposure to shark cartilage dust, and a physician diagnosed

asthma. Six months later, he complained of shortness of breath at work and died from autopsy-confirmed asthma.

Symptomatic hypercalcemia has been reported in patients taking shark cartilage supplements (46).

There has been one report of hepatitis associated with the use of a shark cartilage product (47).

Occupational asthma has been attributed to shark cartilage dust (48).

Squalene

Squalene is a popular over-the-counter Asian folk remedy derived from shark liver oil. Oral capsules are readily available in Asian health food stores and the substance is also widely used in cosmetics.

Ingestion of squalene capsules has been associated with severe lipoid pneumonia due to aspiration; the patient also had abnormal liver function, which raised the possibility of hepatotoxicity (49). In nine patients with squalene-induced extrinsic lipoid pneumonia the most common pattern of parenchymal abnormalities on chest X-ray was areas of ground-glass opacity ($n = 9$, bilateral 6), followed by consolidation ($n = 7$, bilateral 3), and poorly defined small nodules ($n = 4$, bilateral 2) (50). The abnormalities were distributed in the right lower zone ($n = 9$), left lower zone ($n = 6$), and right middle zone ($n = 6$). Initial CT scans ($n = 8$) showed bilateral areas of ground-glass attenuation ($n = 8$), poorly defined centrilobular nodules ($n = 8$), crazy paving ($n = 6$), and consolidation ($n = 3$). The abnormalities were distributed in the right middle lobe ($n = 8$) and in both lower lobes ($n = 5$). Follow-up chest X-rays ($n = 9$) showed complete disappearance ($n = 2$) or reduction ($n = 7$) in the extent of the parenchymal abnormalities, and follow-up CT scans ($n = 3$) showed improvement ($n = 2$) or no change ($n = 1$).

Spanish fly

Spanish fly (SED-11, 1023), also known as cantharides, is the dried blistering beetle (*Cantharis vesicatoria* and related species), which contains cantharidin as a major active constituent. A related insect, which serves as an alternative source of cantharidin in the East, is the Chinese blistering beetle (*Mylabris* species). Spanish fly has gained a considerable reputation as an aphrodisiac, following observations that nearly toxic doses could cause priapism in men and pelvic congestion, occasionally with uterine bleeding, in women. These effects are due to an irritant effect on the genitourinary tract, which could be misinterpreted as increased sensuality. Cantharidin was formerly used medicinally as a counter-irritant and vesicant, but this use has been abandoned because of toxicity.

The effects of cantharidin poisoning include local vesicobullous formation, burning of the mouth, dysphagia, nausea, hematemesis, hepatotoxicity, gross hematuria, and dysuria. Mucosal erosion and hemorrhage occur in the upper gastrointestinal tract. Renal dysfunction is common and related to acute tubular necrosis and glomerular destruction. Priapism, seizures, and cardiac abnormalities are less common. Deaths have occurred (51). However, the lethal dose is not well established; one patient died after taking only 10 mg, while another survived even after taking 50 mg. Four patients with cantharidin poisoning had dysuria and dark urine, three had abdominal pain, one had flank pain, three had hematuria, two had occult rectal bleeding, and one woman had vaginal bleeding; there was low-grade disseminated intravascular coagulation in two patients (52).

A report from Hong Kong described a fatal case due to the ingestion of a decoction of more than 200 dried *Mylabris* beetles as an abortifacient (53).

Toad venom

The dried venom of the Chinese toad (*Bufo bufo gargarizans*) is one of the ingredients of the traditional Chinese medicine kyushin. It has been used as an aphrodisiac and contains the bufadienolides bufalin and cinobufaginal, which are structurally related to cardenolides, such as digoxin, and create the false impression of high plasma digoxin concentrations (54). Digoxin Fab fragments have therefore been used to treat toad venom poisoning (55).

Poisoning with toad venom presents like digitalis toxicity (56). A deliberate overdose of kyushin in an attempt to commit suicide resulted in nausea, vomiting, general malaise, and electrocardiographic changes (for example atrioventricular block) (57). Fatal poisoning with toad venom presented with gastrointestinal symptoms, severe bradycardia, hyperkalemia, acidosis, and cardiac dysrhythmias (58).

The Chinese medicine Ch'an su, which is derived from dried toad venom, also contains bufalin and cinobufaginal, and has repeatedly been linked with serious, even fatal, cardiotoxicity (59).

References

1. de Smet PA, Pegt GW, Meyboom RH. Acute circulatoire shock na toepassing van het niet-reguliere enzympreparaat Wobe-Mugos. [Acute circulatory shock following administration of the non-regular enzyme preparation Wobe-Mugos.] Ned Tijdschr Geneeskd 1991;135(49):2341–4.
2. Chivato T, Juan F, Montoro A, Laguna R. Anaphylaxis induced by ingestion of a pollen compound. J Investig Allergol Clin Immunol 1996;6(3):208–9.
3. Bernier PA, Zimmern PE, Saboorian MH, Chassagne S. Female outlet obstruction after repeated collagen injections. Urology 1997;50(4):618–21.
4. Bellegrandi S, D'Offizi G, Ansotegui IJ, Ferrara R, Scala E, Paganelli R. Propolis allergy in an HIV-positive patient. J Am Acad Dermatol 1996;35(4):644.
5. Rietmeijer CA, Cohn DL. Severe allergic contact dermatitis from dinitrochlorobenzene in a patient with human immunodeficiency virus infection. Arch Dermatol 1988;124(4):490–1.
6. Sadick NS, McNutt NS. Cutaneous hypersensitivity reactions in patients with AIDS. Int J Dermatol 1993;32(9):621–7.
7. Finesmith TH, Seaman S, Rietschel R. Paradoxical coexistence of contact dermatitis and anergy in a man with AIDS. J Am Acad Dermatol 1995;32(3):526–7.
8. Anonymous. Propolis-recalled because of lead contamination. WHO Pharm Newslett 1995;1:3.
9. Harwood M, Harding S, Beasley R, Frankish PD. Asthma following royal jelly. NZ Med J 1996;109(1028):325.
10. Bullock RJ, Rohan A, Straatmans JA. Fatal royal jelly-induced asthma. Med J Aust 1994;160(1):44.
11. Perharic L, Shaw D, Colbridge M, House I, Leon C, Murray V. Toxicological problems resulting from exposure to traditional remedies and food supplements. Drug Saf 1994;11(4):284–94.
12. Takahashi M, Matsuo I, Ohkido M. Contact dermatitis due to honeybee royal jelly. Contact Dermatitis 1983;9(6):452–5.
13. Lombardi C, Senna GE, Gatti B, Feligioni M, Riva G, Bonadonna P, Dama AR, Canonica GW, Passalacqua G.

14. Leung R, Ho A, Chan J, Choy D, Lai CK. Royal jelly consumption and hypersensitivity in the community. Clin Exp Allergy 1997;27(3):333–6.
15. Centers for Disease Control and Prevention (CDC). Acute hepatitis and renal failure following ingestion of raw carp gallbladders—Maryland and Pennsylvania, 1991 and 1994. MMWR Morb Mortal Wkly Rep 1995;44(30):565–6.
16. Chan DW, Yeung CK, Chan MK. Acute renal failure after eating raw fish gall bladder. BMJ (Clin Res Ed) 1985;290(6472):897.
17. Chen CF, Lin MC, Liu HM. Plasma electrolyte changes after ingestion of bile extract of the grass carp (*Ctenopharyngodon idellus*) in rats. Toxicol Lett 1990;50(2–3):221–8.
18. Sorisky A, Robbins DC. Fish oil and diabetes. The net effect. Diabetes Care 1989;12(4):302–4.
19. Haines AP, Sanders TA, Imeson JD, Mahler RF, Martin J, Mistry M, Vickers M, Wallace PG. Effects of a fish oil supplement on platelet function, haemostatic variables and albuminuria in insulin-dependent diabetics. Thromb Res 1986;43(6):643–55.
20. Anonymous. Ganglioside (Cronassial u.a.) und neurologische Erkrankungen. Arznei-Telegramm 1992;12:126.
21. Nobile-Orazio E, Carpo M, Scarlato G. Gangliosides. Their role in clinical neurology. Drugs 1994;47(4):576–85.
22. Wender M, Mularek J, Godlewski A, Losy J, Michalowska-Wender G, Sniatala-Kamasa M, Wojcicka M. Proby leczenia monosialogangliozydem (Sygenem) chorych z niedokrwiennym udarem mozgu. [Trials of monosialoganglioside (Sygen) treatment in ischemic stroke.] Neurol Neurochir Pol 1993;27(1):31–8.
23. Geisler FH, Coleman WP, Grieco G, Poonian D; Sygen Study Group. The Sygen multicenter acute spinal cord injury study. Spine 2001;26(Suppl 24):S87–98.
24. Traverso HP, Bennett JV, Kahn AJ, Agha SB, Rahim H, Kamil S, Lang MH. Ghee applications to the umbilical cord: a risk factor for neonatal tetanus. Lancet 1989;1(8636):486–8.
25. Berg PA, Kaboth U, Becker EW, Klein R. Analyse einer schweren Nebenwirkung auf ein Chondroprotektivum mit Hilfe immunologischer Untersuchungen. [The analysis of a severe side effect of a cartilage-protective agent by immunological studies.] Dtsch Med Wochenschr 1992;117(42):1589–93.
26. Ernst E, Pittler MH. Chitosan as a treatment for body weight reduction? A meta-analysis. Perfusion 1998;11:461–5.
27. McAlindon TE, LaValley MP, Gulin JP, Felson DT. Glucosamine and chondroitin for treatment of osteoarthritis: a systematic quality assessment and meta-analysis. JAMA 2000;283(11):1469–75.
28. Tallia AF, Cardone DA. Asthma exacerbation associated with glucosamine–chondroitin supplement. J Am Board Fam Pract 2002;15(6):481–4.
29. Scott GN. Interaction of warfarin with glucosamine–chondroitin. Am J Health Syst Pharm 2004;61(11):1186.
30. Rozenfeld V, Crain JL, Callahan AK. Possible augmentation of warfarin effect by glucosamine–chondroitin. Am J Health Syst Pharm 2004;61(3):306–7.
31. Garrote Garcia M, Iglesias Pineiro MJ, Martin Alvarez R, Perez Gonzalez J. Interaccion farmacologica del sulfato de glucosamina con acenocumarol. [Pharmacological interaction of glucosamine sulphate and acenocoumarol.] Aten Primaria 2004;33(3):162–3.
32. Anonymous. Imedeen, bron der eeuwige jeugd? Gebu Prikbord 1993;27:68.
33. Ernst E. Kombucha: a systematic review of the clinical evidence. Forsch Komplementarmed Klass Naturheilkd 2003;10(2):85–7.

34. Perron AD, Patterson JA, Yanofsky NN. Kombucha "mushroom" hepatotoxicity. Ann Emerg Med 1995;26(5):660–1.

35. Derk CT, Sandorfi N, Curtis MT. A case of anti-Jo1 myositis with pleural effusions and pericardial tamponade developing after exposure to a fermented Kombucha beverage. Clin Rheumatol 2004;23(4):355–7.

36. Anonymous. Quincke's oedeem bij gebruik van oesterextract in Ostrin plus GTZ 611. Gebu Prikbord 1994;28:67.

37. Marquez-Davila G, Martinez-Barreda C, Suarez-Ramirez I. Capsulas de vibora desecada: una fuente potencial de infeccion por bacterias Gram negativas. [Desiccated rattlesnake capsules: a potential source of Gram-negative bacterial infection.] Rev Invest Clin 1991;43(4):315–17.

38. Kraus A, Guerra-Bautista G, Alarcon-Segovia D. Salmonella arizona arthritis and septicemia associated with rattlesnake ingestion by patients with connective tissue diseases. A dangerous complication of folk medicine. J Rheumatol 1991;18(9):1328–31.

39. Bhatt BD, Zuckerman MJ, Foland JA, Polly SM, Marwah RK. Disseminated *Salmonella arizona* infection associated with rattlesnake meat ingestion Am J Gastroenterol 1989;84(4):433–5.

40. Noskin GA, Clarke JT. *Salmonella arizonae* bacteremia as the presenting manifestation of human immunodeficiency virus infection following rattlesnake meat ingestion Rev Infect Dis 1990;12(3):514–17.

41. Cortes E, Zuckerman MJ, Ho H. Recurrent *Salmonella arizona* infection after treatment for metastatic carcinoma J Clin Gastroenterol 1992;14(2):157–9.

42. Waterman SH, Juarez G, Carr SJ, Kilman L. *Salmonella arizona* infections in Latinos associated with rattlesnake folk medicine Am J Public Health 1990;80(3):286–9.

43. Markman M. Shark cartilage: the Laetrile of the 1990s. Cleve Clin J Med 1996;63(3):179–80.

44. Ostrander GK, Cheng KC, Wolf JC, Wolfe MJ. Shark cartilage, cancer and the growing threat of pseudoscience. Cancer Res 2004;64(23):8485–91.

45. Ortega HG, Kreiss K, Schill DP, Weissman DN. Fatal asthma from powdering shark cartilage and review of fatal occupational asthma literature. Am J Ind Med 2002;42(1):50–4.

46. Lagman R, Walsh D. Dangerous nutrition? Calcium, vitamin D, and shark cartilage nutritional supplements and cancer-related hypercalcemia. Support Care Cancer 2003;11(4):232–5.

47. Ashar B, Vargo E. Shark cartilage-induced hepatitis. Ann Intern Med 1996;125(9):780–1.

48. San-Juan S, Garces M, Caballero ML, Monzon S, Moneo I. Occupational asthma caused by shark cartilage dust. J Allergy Clin Immunol 2004;114(5):1227–8.

49. Asnis DS, Saltzman HP, Melchert A. Shark oil pneumonia. An overlooked entity. Chest 1993;103(3):976–7.

50. Lee JY, Lee KS, Kim TS, Yoon HK, Han BK, Han J, Chung MP, Kwon OJ. Squalene-induced extrinsic lipoid pneumonia: serial radiologic findings in nine patients. J Comput Assist Tomogr 1999;23(5):730–5.

51. Hundt HK, Steyn JM, Wagner L. Post-mortem serum concentration of cantharidin in a fatal case of cantharides poisoning. Hum Exp Toxicol 1990;9(1):35–40.

52. Karras DJ, Farrell SE, Harrigan RA, Henretig FM, Gealt L. Poisoning from "Spanish fly" (cantharidin). Am J Emerg Med 1996;14(5):478–83.

53. Cheng KC, Lee HM, Shum SF, Yip CP. A fatality due to the use of cantharides from *Mylabris phalerata* as an abortifacient Med Sci Law 1990;30(4):336–40.

54. Fushimi R, Tachi J, Amino N, Miyai K. Chinese medicine interfering with digoxin immunoassays. Lancet 1989;1(8633):339.

55. Brubacher JR, Ravikumar PR, Bania T, Heller MB, Hoffman RS. Treatment of toad venom poisoning with digoxin-specific Fab fragments. Chest 1996;110(5):1282–8.

56. Kwan T, Paiusco AD, Kohl L. Digitalis toxicity caused by toad venom. Chest 1992;102(3):949–50.

57. Lin CS, Lin MC, Chen KS, Ho CC, Tsai SR, Ho CS, Shieh WH. A digoxin-like immunoreactive substance and atrioventricular block induced by a Chinese medicine "kyushin." Jpn Circ J 1989;53(9):1077–80.

58. Gowda RM, Cohen RA, Khan IA. Toad venom poisoning: resemblance to digoxin toxicity and therapeutic implications. Heart 2003;89(4):e14.

59. Ko RJ, Greenwald MS, Loscutoff SM, Au AM, Appel BR, Kreutzer RA, Haddon WF, Jackson TY, Boo FO, Presicek G. Lethal ingestion of Chinese herbal tea containing ch'an su. West J Med 1996;164(1):71–5.

Anorectic drugs

See also Individual agents

General Information

Anorectic drugs, which are structurally related to the amphetamines, act mainly on the satiety centre in the hypothalamus and also increase general physical activity (1). All of them, except fenfluramine, stimulate the central nervous system and can cause restlessness, nervousness, irritability, and insomnia. Adverse effects also occur through sympathetic stimulation and gastrointestinal irritation. Drug interactions can occur with monoamine oxidase inhibitors. Dexamfetamine, phenmetrazine, and benzfetamine can cause dependence. Some of them have been associated with cardiac valvulopathy and primary pulmonary hypertension (2).

Anorectic drugs act mainly on the satiety centre in the hypothalamus (1). They also have metabolic effects involving fat and carbohydrate metabolism. Most of them are structurally related to amfetamine and increase physical activity. Their therapeutic effect tends to abate after some months, and part of this reduction in effect may be due to chemical alterations in the brain. Fenfluramine commonly produces drowsiness in normal doses, but has stimulant effects in overdosage. Dexamfetamine, phenmetrazine, and benzfetamine all tend to cause euphoria, with a risk of addiction. Euphoria occasionally occurs with amfepramone (diethylpropion), phentermine, and chlorphentermine, but to a much lesser extent. Some adverse effects are due to sympathetic stimulation and gastrointestinal irritation; these may necessitate withdrawal but are never serious. There are interactions with monoamine oxidase inhibitors and antihypertensive drugs.

References

1. Craddock D. Anorectic drugs: use in general practice. Drugs 1976;11(5):378–93.

2. Rothman RB, Ayestas MA, Dersch CM, Baumann MH. Aminorex, fenfluramine, and chlorphentermine are serotonin transporter substrates. Implications for primary pulmonary hypertension. Circulation 1999;100(8):869–75.

Antacids

General Information

Antacids are alkalis, such as aluminium hydroxide, magnesium salts (magnesium hydroxide and magnesium trisilicate), sodium bicarbonate, and calcium hydroxide. They are generally formulated in combinations (for example magnesium hydroxide + aluminium hydroxide, known as co-magaldrox), often with other components, such as simeticone (activated dimeticone, an anti-foaming agent), alginates (anti-reflux agents), and hydrotalcite (another type of antacid, the addition of which does not improve efficacy (1).

Comparative studies

Effervescent ranitidine 150 mg bd has been compared with as-needed calcium carbonate antacids 750 mg in a randomized study in 115 subjects who frequently self-treated heartburn (2). Effervescent ranitidine was significantly more effective than antacids in reducing heartburn, healing erosive esophagitis, alleviating pain, and improving quality of life. The overall incidences of adverse events were not significantly different in the two groups; 12% in the antacid group and 3% in the ranitidine group had adverse events related to the gastrointestinal system: nausea, vomiting, diarrhea, constipation, gas, fecal incontinence; and 1% in the antacid group and 4% in the ranitidine group had adverse events related to the central nervous system: headache, dizziness, insomnia, malaise, fatigue, weakness, nervousness.

Placebo-controlled studies

In a randomized, placebo-controlled, four-way, crossover study of the effects of low-dose ranitidine and an antacid on meal-induced heartburn and acidity in 26 subjects, ranitidine 75 mg significantly reduced gastric but not esophageal acidity, calcium carbonate 420 mg significantly reduced esophageal but not gastric acidity, and ranitidine plus calcium carbonate reduced both esophageal and gastric acidity (3). Both drugs given alone reduced heartburn severity compared with placebo.

General adverse effects

When they are given in conventional doses for symptomatic relief, antacids are safe, and adverse effects seldom limit the choice of formulation, except when troublesome diarrhea occurs (4). Change of bowel habit, usually in the form of mild diarrhea, is common, especially with magnesium salts. Other adverse effects usually occur as a direct consequence of ion absorption. They include alkalosis (particularly with large doses of soluble antacids), milk alkali syndrome when calcium is included, and the consequences of absorbing individual ions, particularly sodium but also bismuth and aluminium. Heart failure can be precipitated in susceptible patients by antacids with a high sodium content (see the Cardiovascular section). Antacids can interfere with the absorption of other drugs to a clinically important extent. Allergic reactions and tumor-inducing effects have not been described.

Alginates
The use, efficacy, and adverse effects of non-prescription alginate-containing formulations and H_2 receptor antagonists obtained from community pharmacies have been evaluated in 767 customers with dyspepsia (5). Most obtained some or complete symptom relief (75%) and were completely satisfied with the product (78%). H_2 receptor antagonists were more likely to produce complete relief of symptoms than alginate-containing formulations. Only 3% reported adverse effects: diarrhea, constipation, bloating, and flatulence from alginate formulations, and dry mouth, altered bowel habit, diarrhea, and constipation from H_2 receptor antagonists.

Simeticone
No specific adverse effects have been attributed to dimeticone and its activated form simeticone, which are commonly compounded with antacids. Its use has been associated with reduced hydrogen concentrations in the breath (6), but this has not been confirmed (7).

Organs and Systems

Cardiovascular

The sodium content of antacids varies greatly; a daily dose of some products may contain sodium equivalent to more than 1 g of salt. This may not be clear from the labeling or the name of the formulation. However, the amount can be sufficient to precipitate heart failure in predisposed individuals (8).

Nervous system

Absence seizures have been described during treatment with sodium bicarbonate (9).

Metabolism

Some antacids contain enough sugar to affect diabetic control (10). Since the sugar is not an active component, it will not be declared on the packaging in many countries.

Gastrointestinal

Formulations that contain alginates can cause gastric bezoars, as can tube-feed thickening when antacids are added (11).

With sodium bicarbonate, gastric rupture due to massive carbon dioxide release has been described, though it is very rare (12).

Second-Generation Effects

Lactation

Antacids are generally regarded as safe to use during pregnancy (13) and lactation (14), particularly those that are poorly absorbed from the gastrointestinal tract.

Table 1   The effects of aluminium-containing antacids on the absorption of some other drugs

Drug	Effect
Of probable or known clinical significance	
Diflunisal	Reduced absorption
Digoxin	Reduced absorption
Ferrous ions	Reduced absorption
Ketoconazole	Reduced absorption
Tetracycline	Reduced absorption
^{99m}TcPYP	Altered distribution[a]
Quinolone antibiotics	Reduced circulating concentrations (15)
Of dubious or unlikely clinical significance	
Aminophylline	Absorption retarded
Oral antidiabetic agents	Partly adsorbed by antacids
Cimetidine	Reduced peak concentration
Diazepam	Absorption retarded but complete
Indometacin	Reduced absorption
Isoniazid	Reduced peak concentration
Levodopa	Reduced absorption
Phenothiazines	Adsorbed in vitro
Phenytoin	Absorption retarded

[a] Accumulation of the radiopharmaceutical in the liver and reticuloendothelial system (16)

Drug–Drug Interactions

General

Concurrent antacid intake can alter the absorption of many other drugs. Antacids can reduce the peak concentration (C_{max}) by reducing the speed of absorption, and/or reduce the amount of absorption (that is the systemic availability). However, the effects are not always of clinical importance (Table 1). Interactions can be minimized by giving antacids and other medications 2–3 hours apart.

Oral anticoagulants

Since dimeticone is a surfactant, one might expect it to enhance the absorption of drugs, and there are some reports that this happens with ethyl biscoumacetate (17).

References

1. Vatier J, Ramdani A, Vitre MT, Mignon M. Antacid activity of calcium carbonate and hydrotalcite tablets. Comparison between in vitro evaluation using the "artificial stomach-duodenum" model and in vivo pH-metry in healthy volunteers. Arzneimittelforschung 1994;44(4): 514–18.
2. Earnest D, Robinson M, Rodriguez-Stanley S, Ciociola AA, Jaffe P, Silver MT, Kleoudis CS, Murdock RH. Managing heartburn at the "base" of the GERD "iceberg": effervescent ranitidine 150 mg b.d. provides faster and better heartburn relief than antacids. Aliment Pharmacol Ther 2000;14(7):911–18.
3. Robinson M, Rodriguez-Stanley S, Ciociola AA, Filinto J, Zubaidi S, Miner PB Jr, Gardner JD. Synergy between low-dose ranitidine and antacid in decreasing gastric and oesophageal acidity and relieving meal-induced heartburn. Aliment Pharmacol Ther 2001;15(9):1365–74.
4. Sewing KF. Tolerance of antacids. J Physiol Pharmacol 1993;44(3 Suppl 1):75–7.
5. Krska J, John DN, Hansford D, Kennedy EJ. Drug utilization evaluation of nonprescription H2-receptor antagonists and alginate-containing preparations for dyspepsia. Br J Clin Pharmacol 2000;49(4):363–8.
6. Lifschitz CH, Irving CS, Smith EO. Effect of a simethicone-containing tablet on colonic gas elimination in breath. Dig Dis Sci 1985;30(5):426–30.
7. Friis H, Bode SH, Rumessen JJ, Gudmand-Hoyer E. Dimetikon ved laktuloseinduceret dyspepsi. Effekt pa H2-produktion og symptomer. [Dimethicone in lactulose-induced dyspepsia. Effect on H2 production and symptoms.] Ugeskr Laeger 1993;155(42):3378–80.
8. Barry RE, Ford J. Sodium content and neutralising capacity of some commonly used antacids. BMJ 1978;1(6110):413.
9. Reif S, Holzman M, Barak S, Spirer Z. Absence seizures associated with bicarbonate therapy and normal serum pH. JAMA 1989;262(10):1328–9.
10. Stolinsky DC. Sugar and saccharin content of antacids. N Engl J Med 1981;305(3):166–7.
11. Schulthess HK, Valli C, Escher F, Asper R, Hacki WH. Ösophagusobstruktion wahrend Sondenernahrung: Folge von Eiweissfallung durch Antazida? [Esophageal obstruction in tube feeding: a result of protein precipitation caused by antacids?] Schweiz Med Wochenschr 1986;116(29):960–2.
12. Brismar B, Strandberg A, Wiklund B. Stomach rupture following ingestion of sodium bicarbonate. Acta Chir Scand Suppl 1986;530:97–9.
13. Hagemann TM. Gastrointestinal medications and breast-feeding. J Hum Lact 1998;14(3):259–62.
14. Broussard CN, Richter JE. Treating gastro-oesophageal reflux disease during pregnancy and lactation: what are the safest therapy options? Drug Saf 1998;19(4):325–37.
15. Moreno I, Rosell R, Abad-Esteve A, Barnadas A, Carles J, Ribelles N. Randomized trial for the control of acute vomiting in cisplatin-treated patients: high-dose metoclopramide with dexamethasone and lorazepam as adjuncts versus high-dose alizapride plus dexamethasone and lorazepam. Study of the incidence of delayed emesis. Oncology 1991;48 (5):397–402.
16. McGeown MG. Renal disease associated with drugs. In: D'Arcy PF, Griffin JP, editors. Iatrogenic Diseases. 3rd ed. Oxford-New York-Tokyo: Oxford University Press, 1986:790.
17. Copie X, Pinquier JL, Letrait M, Paltiat MH, Pello JY, Rey E, Chanteclair G, de Lauture D, Olive G, Strauch G. Effet du diméticone sur la pharmacocinétique et la pharmacodynamie du biscoumacétate d'éthyle. [Effect of dimethicone on pharmacokinetics and pharmacodynamics of ethyl biscoumacetate.] Therapie 1993;48(2): 119–23.

Antazoline

See also Antihistamines

General Information

Antazoline is a first-generation antihistamine.

Organs and Systems

Hematologic

Antazoline has sometimes produced thrombocytopenic purpura when used in normal doses (1). Antibodies to antazoline were present, obviously as a result of previous, yet uneventful, use.

- Antazoline-induced thrombocytopenic purpura occurred on three occasions in a 21-year-old woman (2). After withdrawal of the drug she recovered promptly. In vitro investigations showed the presence of an antibody in her serum, which in association with antazoline caused complement fixation when added to test platelets. Platelet agglutinins were also detected in her serum when antazoline was added.

The reactions in this case were drug specific and could still be demonstrated 9 months after the last exposure to the drug.

References

1. Slipko Z, Walewska I, Bragiel J, Jonas S. Purpura thrombopénique par sensibilisation à un médicament antihistaminique. Presse Méd 1966;74:1193.
2. Lanng Nielsen J, Dahl R, Kissmeyer-Nielsen F. Immune thrombocytopenia due to antazoline (Antistina). Allergy 1981;36(7):517–19.

Anthracyclines and related compounds

See also Cytostatic and immunosuppressant drugs

General Information

Anthracyclines form a broad group of antitumor drugs within the group of cytotoxic antibiotics. The lead compounds were doxorubicin and daunorubicin; analogues include epirubicin, idarubicin, and aclarubicin. Mitoxantrone and pixantrone are related compounds of the anthracenedione family. Amsacrine is a related compound of the aminoacridine family.

Liposomal forms of doxorubicin (Caelyx, Myocet) and daunorubicin (DaunoXome) are in use. These drugs are licensed for the treatment of a wide range of tumors (Table 1). Much information regarding the anthracyclines has been previously published in major reviews and textbooks (1,2). With this in mind, their major toxic effects are outlined here, but concentrating in more detail on new findings, such as the interaction with trastuzumab.

Organs and Systems

Cardiovascular

Cardiomyopathy

Anthracyclines can cause the late complication of a cardiomyopathy, which can be irreversible and can proceed to congestive cardiac failure, ventricular dysfunction, conduction disturbances, or dysrhythmias several months or years after the end of treatment (3,4). Doxorubicin can cause abnormalities of right ventricular wall motion (5). A significant number of patients receiving anthracyclines develop cardiac autonomic dysfunction (6).

Table 1 Licensed indications for anthracyclines

Drug	Where licensed	Licensed for the treatment of
Doxorubicin	USA and EU	Acute leukemia, lymphomas, soft tissue and osteogenic sarcomas, pediatric malignancies, and adult solid tumors (particularly lung and breast cancers)
Epirubicin	EU	Breast, ovarian, gastric, and lung cancers; malignant lymphomas, leukemias, and multiple myeloma; superficial and in-situ bladder carcinomas
Daunorubicin	USA and EU	Acute leukemias
Idarubicin	USA and EU	Relapsed or first-line treatment refractory advanced breast cancer, acute leukemias
Liposomal doxorubicin (Caelyx, Doxil)	USA and EU	Kaposi's sarcoma in AIDS
Liposomal pegylated daunorubicin (DaunoXome)	USA and EU	Kaposi's sarcoma in AIDS
Liposomal doxorubicin (Myocet)	EU	Breast cancer

Dose-relatedness

The development of anthracycline-induced cardiomyopathy is closely related to the cumulative lifetime dose of the anthracycline. The recommended maximum cumulative lifetime dose of doxorubicin is 450–550 mg/m^2 (7) and of daunorubicin 400–550 mg/m^2 intravenously in adults (1,2). About 5% of doxorubicin-treated patients develop congestive cardiac failure at this dose; however, the incidence approaches 50% at cumulative doses of 1000 mg/m^2 (7–9). These figures are derived from experience with doxorubicin administered as a bolus or by infusion of very short duration (under 30 minutes). The incidence of clinical cardiotoxicity falls dramatically with other schedules of administration (that is weekly doses or continuous infusion for more than 24 hours).

In a randomized study of adjuvant chemotherapy comparing bolus against continuous intravenous infusion of doxorubicin 60 mg/m^2, cardiotoxicity, defined as a 10% or greater reduction in left ventricular ejection fraction, occurred in 61% of patients on a bolus median dose equal to 420 mg/m^2 compared with 42% on the continuous infusion schedule with a median dose of 540 mg/m^2; the rate of cardiotoxicity as a function of the cumulative dose of doxorubicin was significantly higher in the bolus treatment arm (10).

In 11 patients with anthracycline cardiotoxicity studied by heart catheterization and endomyocardial biopsy, myocytic damage correlated linearly with cumulative dose (11). There was a non-linear relation between electron microscopic changes and the extent of hemodynamic impairment. There was pronounced fibrous thickening of the endocardium in most patients, especially in the left ventricle. Endocardial fibrosis may be the first morphological sign of cardiotoxicity.

Susceptibility factors
The risk of cardiotoxicity is greater in children and patients with pre-existing cardiac disease or concomitant or prior mediastinal or chest wall irradiation (12,13).

Of 682 patients, 144 who were over 65 years of age all had doses up to but not exceeding the usual cumulative dose for doxorubicin (14). The authors concluded that older patients without cardiovascular co-morbidity are at no greater risk of congestive heart failure.

The use of doxorubicin in childhood impairs myocardial growth, resulting in a progressive increase in left ventricular afterload, sometimes associated with impaired myocardial contractility (15). Of 201 children who received doxorubicin and/or daunorubicin $200–1275$ mg/m^2, 23% had abnormal cardiac function 4–20 years afterwards. Of those who were followed for more than 10 years, 38% had abnormal cardiac function compared with 18% in those who were followed for less than 10 years (16,17). In another study, more than half of the children studied by serial echocardiography after doxorubicin therapy for acute lymphoblastic leukemia developed increased left ventricular wall stress due to reduced wall thickness. This stress progressed with time (18).

Predisposing factors to mitoxantrone cardiotoxicity include increasing age, prior anthracycline therapy, previous cardiovascular disease, mediastinal radiotherapy, and a cumulative dose of the drug exceeding 120 mg/m^2. In 801 patients treated with mitoxantrone, prior treatment with doxorubicin and mitoxantrone was significantly associated with risk of cardiotoxicity; however, age, sex, and prior mediastinal radiotherapy were not useful predictors (19).

Anesthesia is difficult in patients with cumulative anthracycline-induced cardiotoxicity, and it has proved fatal on occasions (20).

Comparative studies of anthracyclines
All anthracyclines have cardiotoxic potential. However, because only a few cycles of treatment are administered in most regimens, few patients reach the cardiotoxic threshold of cumulative anthracycline dose. There is therefore limited information about the comparative cardiotoxic potential of these agents.

Epirubicin is considered to cause substantially less cardiotoxicity than doxorubicin on a molar basis (4,21). This has been attributed to its more rapid clearance rather than a different action (22). In a randomized, double-blind comparison of epirubicin and doxorubicin, there was a significant reduction in left ventricle ejection fraction with doxorubicin but not with epirubicin (23). However, data from large clinical series and from morphological examination of endomyocardial biopsies in smaller series of patients suggest that the incidence and severity of cumulative cardiac toxicity associated with epirubicin 900 mg/m^2 is similar to that associated with doxorubicin 450–550 mg/m^2 (24). In 29 patients treated with epirubicin in cumulative doses ranging from 147 to 888 mg/m^2 the ultrastructural myocardial lesions were similar to those produced by doxorubicin (partial and total myofibrillar loss in individual myocytes) (25). With both drugs, severe lesions were associated with replacement fibrosis. None of the patients who received epirubicin in the study developed congestive cardiac failure.

Both mitoxantrone and the oral formulation of idarubicin have been thought to be less cardiotoxic than doxorubicin (26,27). The South West Oncology Group reported on 801 patients treated with mitoxantrone; 1.5% developed congestive cardiac failure, an additional 1.5% had a reduced left ventricular ejection fraction (LVEF), and 0.25% developed acute myocardial infarction (19). Idarubicin has been reported to cause short-term cardiac toxicity when used in high doses in leukemia, and there is no doubt that it causes cumulative dose-related toxicity as well (28). Electrocardiographic changes occurred in 7% of adults with acute leukemia receiving aclarubicin (29).

Presentation
The main effects of anthracycline-induced cardiotoxicity are reduced left ventricular function and chronic congestive heart failure. Other cardiotoxic events occur only rarely. Occasionally, acute transient electrocardiographic changes (ST–T wave changes, prolongation of the QT interval) and dysrhythmias can occur. Acute conduction disturbances, acute myopericarditis, and acute cardiac failure are also rare. In a study of the effects of anthracyclines on myocardial function in 50 long-term survivors of childhood cancer, there was cardiac failure in one patient and electrocardiographic abnormalities (non-specific ST segment and T wave changes) in two (13). In one patient with a VVI pacemaker, who received the combination of vincristine, doxorubicin, and dexamethasone, the pacemaker had to be reset after each cycle of treatment, as the pacing threshold had increased, resulting in bradycardia (30).

Hypokinetic heart wall motion abnormalities and early signs of chronic cardiomyopathy have been identified as a significant toxic effect of mitoxantrone in patients who received cumulative doses of 32–174 mg (31). Electrocardiographic T wave inversion and cardiac complications have been described from intensive therapy with mitoxantrone 40 mg/m^2 over 5 days and cyclophosphamide 1550 mg/m^2 for 4 days, given before bone marrow transplantation for metastatic breast cancer. All the patients had had previous exposure to doxorubicin in cumulative doses that did not exceed 442 mg/m^2 (19).

The authors of a study of the use of MRI scans to assess the subclinical effects of the anthracyclines concluded that increased MRI enhancement equal to or greater than 5 on day 3 compared with the baseline predicted significant reduction in ejection fraction at day 28 (32). In 1000 patients given doxorubicin chemotherapy and irradiation there were six cases of congestive heart failure and three cases of myocardial infarction; there was a cumulative cardiac mortality of 0.4% in all anthracycline-exposed patients (33).

Diagnosis
The diagnosis of anthracycline cardiomyopathy is based on the clinical presentation and investigations such as

radionuclide cardiac angiography, which can show a reduced ejection fraction (34), and echocardiography, which can show reduced or abnormal ventricular function (35,36). Dysrhythmias can be detected by electrocardiography, and QT_c interval prolongation may offer an easy, non-invasive test to predict patients who are at special risk of late cardiac decompensation after anthracycline treatment for childhood cancer (37). Radioimmunoscintigraphy can be used to highlight damaged myocytes, and changes such as myocardial fibrosis are characteristic on endomyocardial biopsy (13,38,39).

The subtle chronic abnormalities in myocardial function that occur 10–20 years after anthracycline exposure in childhood are best detected by exercise echocardiography, since these patients may have normal resting cardiac function (40).

It has been suggested that monitoring B type natriuretic peptide concentrations after anthracycline administration can reflect cardiac tolerance, and through serial monitoring allow a picture of the degree of left ventricular dysfunction to be established (41).

Mechanisms
Several mechanisms contribute to anthracycline cardiotoxicity. The principal mechanism is thought to be oxidative stresses placed on cardiac myocytes by reactive oxygen species. Amelioration of this toxicity is possible using dexrazoxane, an intracellular metal-chelating agent of the dioxopiperazine class (3). Dexrazoxane acts by depleting intracellular iron, thus reducing the formation of cardiotoxic hydroxyl anions and radicals. In patients without heart failure, in-vivo measurements of myocardial oxidative metabolism and blood flow did not change in patients with cancer receiving doxorubicin (42).

Anthracyclines have the ability inherent in their quinone structure to form free-radical semiquinones which result in very reactive oxygen species, causing peroxidation of the lipid membranes of the heart. However, this reaction has not been demonstrated with mitoxantrone, and the mechanism of its cardiotoxicity is unknown.

Abnormalities of left ventricular ejection fraction have been described in 46% of patients ($n = 14$) treated with mitoxantrone (14 mg/m^2) and with vincristine and prednisolone (43). A history of cardiac disease or of previous anthracycline exposure was excluded. Only one patient developed clinically overt congestive cardiac failure. Other reports have described less cardiotoxicity compared with the parent compound, doxorubicin (4,44).

Management
Anthracycline cardiomyopathy, although reportedly difficult to treat, often responds to current methods used to manage congestive cardiac failure.

Severe anthracycline-induced cardiotoxicity is generally considered irreversible, and it is associated with a poor prognosis and high mortality. However, in four cases the advanced cardiac dysfunction associated with doxorubicin recovered completely after withdrawal (45). Of 19 patients with anthracycline-induced congestive cardiac failure, 12 recovered after withdrawal, although reversal was modest (46).

The prolongation of the QT interval that occurs in patients who have recently finished doxorubicin therapy is slowly reversible over at least 3 years and the degree of prolongation is related to the cumulative dose (47).

Heart transplantation has been successful in patients with late, progressive cardiomyopathy without recurrence of the underlying malignant disease (48).

Cardiac dysrhythmias
Cardiac dysrhythmias have been reported after amsacrine therapy in association with hypokalemia. Pre-existing supraventricular dysrhythmias or ventricular extra beats are not absolute contraindications to its use (49). Of 5430 patients treated with amsacrine, 65 developed cardiotoxicity, including prolongation of the QT interval, non-specific ST–T wave changes, ventricular tachycardia, and ventricular fibrillation (50). There were serious ventricular dysrhythmias resulting in cardiopulmonary arrest in 31 patients; 14 died as a result. The dysrhythmias occurred within minutes to several hours after drug administration. The cardiotoxicity was not related to total cumulative dose, and hypokalemia was possibly a risk factor for dysrhythmias.

Sensory systems

Doxorubicin can cause conjunctivitis, periorbital edema, lacrimation, blepharospasm, keratitis, and reduced visual acuity (51). There have been two reports of persistent photophobia and chronic inflammation of the eye following accidental topical exposure to doxorubicin (52).

Hematologic

Myelosuppression, principally neutropenia, occurs in 60–80% of patients who receive conventional doses of anthracyclines (single-agent standard doses: doxorubicin 60–75 mg/m^2, epirubicin 60–90 mg/m^2 given 3-weekly) (53). On an equimolar basis, in both the single-agent and combination regimens, epirubicin causes less hematological toxicity than doxorubicin (24). The incidence and severity of myelosuppression is related to dose; it has been suggested that severe neutropenia occurs in all patients who are given high-dose anthracyclines (doxorubicin 100 mg/m^2 or more and epirubicin 120 mg/m^2 or more) (54). Neutrophil nadirs occur at 7–10 days after treatment, and full neutrophil recovery usually occurs by day 21 (24). Platelets are less affected; about 35% of patients receiving epirubicin 120 mg/m^2 have grade-3 thrombocytopenia (55). Anemia occurs rarely (24).

Although the extent of leukopenia is not related to cumulative anthracycline dose, patients who have received extensive prior chemotherapy develop more severe leukopenia, possibly because of diminished bone marrow reserve (24). There was a strong correlation between dose and both leukocyte nadirs and platelet nadirs in 287 patients who received single-agent epirubicin 40, 60, 90, or 135 mg/m^2 every 3 weeks (56). Myelosuppression correlates with exposure to epirubicin, as reflected by the plasma AUC (57).

Myelosuppression is not prevented by prolonged doxorubicin infusion (53), although this can mitigate other adverse effects. Hematological toxicity associated with high-dose regimens can be partially ameliorated by giving hemopoietic growth factors, with or without autologous bone marrow or peripheral blood progenitor cell rescue (58–60). However, other adverse effects, mainly mucositis, then become dose-limiting. It has been suggested that mitoxantrone 14 mg/m^2 is more myelosuppressive than doxorubicin 70 mg/m^2, which in turn is more myelosuppressive than epirubicin 70 mg/m^2, each given at 3-week intervals (61).

Secondary acute myeloid leukemia, with or without a preleukemic phase, has been rarely reported in patients being concurrently treated with epirubicin or doxorubicin in association with DNA-damaging antineoplastic agents; such cases have a short latency period (1–3 years) (62,63). In one study, three of 77 patients who received epirubicin plus cisplatin and two who received other epirubicin-containing combinations developed acute myelogenous leukemia 15–33 months after the start of epirubicin treatment for advanced breast cancer (62). However, all had received prior treatment with alkylating agents and/or radiotherapy, which are recognized independent leukemogenic risk factors. Despite high mean lifetime epirubicin doses in this study (mean 800 mg/m^2), there was no relation between cumulative dose and the risk of acute myelogenous leukemia. In a second study, four of 351 patients with metastatic breast cancer who received fluorouracil + epirubicin + cyclophosphamide, but none of 359 who received cyclophosphamide + methotrexate + 5-fluorouracil, developed leukemia (three acute myelogenous leukemia, one acute lymphoblastic leukemia) (63). No secondary leukemias were documented in other large comparative studies of epirubicin-containing regimens (64,65). Nevertheless, a retrospective analysis of case reports, published in abstract form without references or methods, concluded that when epirubicin was combined with alkylating agents it was associated with an increased risk of secondary acute myelogenous leukemia in women with breast cancer (66).

Prolongation of the prothrombin time after the use of amsacrine 1200 mg/m^2 for acute myeloid leukemia was related to transient deficiency of factor X (67).

Mouth and teeth

Mucositis is a well-documented toxic effect of anthracyclines; it has been reported in 8% of combination chemotherapeutic courses including epirubicin in a dose of 180 mg/m^2 (68).

Gastrointestinal

The anthracyclines are classed as moderately to strongly emetogenic. Nausea and vomiting occurs in 21–55% of patients, but is substantially reduced by pretreatment with antiemetic drugs (53,55). In one randomized study, epirubicin 70 mg/m^2, doxorubicin 70 mg/m^2, and mitoxantrone 14 mg/m^2 were compared (61). The first cycles of epirubicin and mitoxantrone were given without antiemetic drugs, unless specifically requested, but thereafter antiemetic drugs were given as required; doxorubicin was given with antiemetic drugs from cycle one. Doxorubicin and epirubicin were significantly more emetogenic than mitoxantrone; there was grade 3 nausea and vomiting in 22% of those who received doxorubicin, 18% of those who

received epirubicin, and none of those who received mitoxantrone. Oral idarubicin may cause more emesis, which is quoted as occurring in 25–86% of patients; however, these effects are said to be usually mild to moderate (27).

With the advent of the 5-hydroxytryptamine (5-HT$_3$) receptor antagonists (ondansetron, granisetron, tropisetron), used in conjunction with dexamethasone, nausea and vomiting can be ameliorated in most patients.

Mucositis and stomatitis are potentially severe and dose-limiting adverse effects of the anthracyclines. Both the frequency and the severity are dose-dependent (56,69). Their onset and recovery generally parallel the hematological toxicity, but they can occur earlier (5–10 days after treatment starts). Areas of painful erosions, mainly along the side of the tongue and on the sublingual mucosa, are common. Mucositis occurs in about 9% of patients who receive oral idarubicin in standard doses (27).

Diarrhea has also been reported with the anthracyclines. In a typical study, in which epirubicin 100 mg/m^2 was given for 1–8 cycles, one of 39 patients had grade 1/2 diarrhea and two of 39 had grade 3/4 diarrhea (70). Of patients who take oral idarubicin 10–38% are said to develop diarrhea, again generally mild to moderate (27).

Urinary tract

All anthracyclines can cause discoloration of the urine and other body fluids (that is tears) (1,2).

Skin

Anthracyclines can cause local irritant reactions. These range from erythema and phlebitis at the injection site to potentially severe vesicant reactions requiring skin grafting (24). Care appropriate to the administration of a vesicant must be observed during infusion. Various treatments have been used immediately after extravasation in an attempt to lessen the injury, including ice, steroids, vitamin E, and bicarbonate. The current recommended treatment is by intermittent cooling of the affected area, together with intermittent use of topical dimethylsulfoxide 99% (71). There is also evidence of the efficacy of intravenous dexrazoxane, and the first dose should preferably be given within 6 hours (72). In three patients who had extravasation of epirubicin or doxorubicin, healing occurred without sequelae (73,74); all three received three doses of intravenous dexrazoxane over 3 days (1000 mg/m^2 on the first two days and 500 mg/m^2 on day 3), the first dose being administered at 2–5 hours after extravasation. A fourth patient received dexrazoxane 1500 mg 1 hour after extravasation of doxorubicin and repeated 5 hours later, and 750 mg on day 2; the wound healed slowly and required surgery after 3 months (75). A fifth patient received dexrazoxane more than 6 hours after extravasation of epirubicin; the wound healed slowly and with a crusted center (76).

Reactivation of skin damage can also occur at sites of prior radiation therapy ("radiation recall") (77).

- Widespread allergic contact dermatitis occurred in a 73-year-old man after intravesical administration of epirubicin; a patch test with an aqueous solution of the drug (0.1%) was positive (78).

A syndrome of palmar–plantar erythema (progressing in some patients to blistering and desquamation) has been reported in seven of eight patients with advanced breast or ovarian cancer who received high-dose doxorubicin (125–150 mg/m^2) (79). By contrast, in a similar dose intensification study in which patients received epirubicin 200 mg/m^2 with cyclophosphamide and growth factor support, the palmar–plantar syndrome did not occur (80).

In 60 patients receiving polyethylene glycol-coated liposomal doxorubicin (Doxil) 35–70 mg/m^2 by infusion over 1–2 hours there were four patterns of skin eruption: hand–foot syndrome (40%), a diffuse follicular rash (10%), an intertrigo-like eruption (8%), and new melanotic macules (0.5%) (81).

Hair

Complete or partial alopecia occurs in the majority (60–90%) of patients who receive anthracyclines, and although it is reversible it can be distressing (24). Scalp cooling during chemotherapy to minimize hair loss is now little used, because of limited efficacy, the discomfort of scalp cooling techniques, and concern about the potential creation of a "sanctuary" for circulating tumor cells. Alopecia is less frequent (about 35% of patients) in patients who take oral idarubicin 40–45 mg/m^2 every 3 weeks (27).

Nails

Painful onycholysis, blue discoloration of the nails (82), and reversible loss of fingernails (83) have been attributed to mitoxantrone.

Sweat glands

There has been a single report of hidradenitis associated with mitoxantrone (84).

Long-Term Effects

Mutagenicity

There was an increased number of chromosomally aberrant lymphocytes in nurses who handled cytostatic agents (doxorubicin, cyclophosphamide, vincristine, fluorouracil, and methotrexate) many years ago, before modern facilities for the preparation of chemotherapeutic drugs were in use (85). No long-term fertility problems were identified in 205 men who were treated with doxorubicin during childhood (86).

Tumorigenicity

In 604 women who were given six cycles of epirubicin after 4 years of tamoxifen, there were 12 non-breast second malignancies (87). Although the authors did not analyse these in respect to population expectation, they thought that the frequency was relatively high.

Second-Generation Effects

Teratogenicity

There is no conclusive evidence about whether anthracyclines adversely affect human fertility or are teratogenic.

In 26 of 28 pregnancies, three or more chemotherapeutic agents were used to treat acute leukemia ($n = 20$), non-Hodgkin's lymphoma ($n = 3$), Ewing's sarcoma ($n = 2$), breast cancer ($n = 2$), and myoblastoma ($n = 1$) (88). The anthracyclines were introduced at various gestational ages, ranging from time of conception to 38 weeks, but in most cases chemotherapy was started in the second trimester. The outcomes were 24 normal infants, including a set of twins. Four of the five cases of infant death occurred in those with hematological malignancies (acute leukemia and non-Hodgkin's lymphoma), one each due to maternal death and therapeutic abortion and two resulting from spontaneous abortion. Neonatal pathological examination showed no congenital anomalies or organ defects, one case of marrow hypoplasia, and one case of neonatal sepsis. These findings suggest that anthracyclines have no detectable effect on the offspring up to the age of 54 months. However, bias inherent in reporting pregnancies with a successful outcome is obvious, so extreme caution must be exercised in the use of anthracyclines in pregnancy, and they should be avoided if at all possible.

Fetotoxicity

Cardiac failure occurred in a 3-day-old neonate whose mother had been given idarubicin 9 mg/m^2 as part of induction therapy for acute lymphoblastic leukemia at 22 weeks; the baby was delivered at 28 weeks (89). In the absence of another known cause, the cardiotoxicity was attributed to idarubicin exposure 6 weeks before.

Susceptibility Factors

Hepatic disease

Since the main route of metabolism and elimination of anthracyclines is via the bile, dosage reduction is recommended if there is hepatic impairment. This was first suggested after a report of increased toxicity in patients with liver metastases who received full-dose anthracycline treatment, followed by a second report that suggested that the clearance of anthracyclines is reduced in patients with hepatic metastases (90,91). These reports led to the current recommendations for anthracycline doses, based on serum bilirubin concentration or sulfobromophthalein clearance. However, the question of whether liver dysfunction significantly affects anthracycline clearance is unclear, and the dosage modifications suggested (see Table 2) have never been validated. Indeed, there is evidence that anthracycline kinetics are altered in patients with raised serum transaminases alone,

Table 2 Effects of liver function on doses of doxorubicin and epirubicin

Drug	Serum bilirubin concentration	BSP retention	Recommended dose
Doxorubicin	20–50 µmol/l	9–15%	50% of normal
	>50 µmol/l	>15%	25% of normal
Epirubicin	20–50 µmol/l		50% of normal
	>50 µmol/l		25% of normal

which may be a better basis for dosage modification (92). In practice, many clinicians make empirical dosage modifications in patients with abnormal liver biochemistry tests (57).

Drug Administration

Drug formulations

The anthracyclines have been formulated in liposomal formulations in order to alter their pharmacokinetics and improve their therapeutic index. Examples include:

- pegylated liposomal doxorubicin (Caelyx/Doxil);
- liposomal doxorubicin (Myocet);
- liposomal daunorubicin (DaunoXome).

These formulations are dealt with in a separate monograph.

Drug administration route

The anthracyclines are most commonly given intravenously, either as bolus doses or, less often, as infusions over varying lengths of time. Alternative routes have been tried, such as the intraperitoneal, intrapleural, and intravesical routes (93,94).

Intraperitoneal

Intraperitoneal instillation of doxorubicin has been used in the early postoperative period in patients with retroperitoneal or visceral sarcoma, in an attempt to eradicate microscopic residual disease after complete macroscopic surgical excision (95). Three of 17 patients had pyrexia, one peritoneal sclerosis, one a pancreatic fistula, and two abdominal pain. There were no anastomotic disruptions or intra-abdominal hemorrhages.

Intrapleural

Adverse effects associated with the intrapleural instillation of doxorubicin in doses of 10–40 mg consist of fever (11–15%), anorexia (24–29%), nausea (20–29%), and chest pain (28–29%) (94,96). Cardiomyopathy and myelosuppression were not reported (96).

Intravesical

Intravesical epirubicin has been used to treat superficial bladder cancers. At a dose of 50 mg, the overall incidence of adverse events was 16–25% (93). The frequency of adverse events tended to increase with dose but not the number of instillations. Most adverse events were mild and transient; the commonest were localized to the bladder and included chemical cystitis (10–38%), urinary tract infection (2–13%), and hematuria (2–33%). Contracted bladder or hemorrhagic cystitis have been reported in 1–6% of patients (93).

Adverse events occurred in 31 of 194 patients who received epirubicin 80 mg intravesically compared with 12 of 205 who received placebo after transurethral resection (97). Systemic adverse events (usually cardiac or hematological adverse events or hypersensitivity) generally occurred in under 5% of patients. In two studies of intravesical epirubicin, there were reports of myocardial infarction (9%), stroke (3%), angina pectoris (3%), or

atrioventricular block (2%) (98,99). There were no reports of myelosuppression in clinical trials of intravesical epirubicin, apart from thrombocytopenia in one of 37 patients in one cancer trial (98) and hemoglobinemia in two of 40 patients in another (100).

Biochemical abnormalities have been reported in trials of intravesical epirubicin. In one trial, liver function tests were impaired in seven of 40 patients who received epirubicin and in 10 of 35 patients who received epirubicin and verapamil concomitantly (101). In another study, liver function tests were impaired in one of 69 patients who received combination prophylaxis with epirubicin 50 mg and BCG 150 mg after transurethral resection (102).

Hypersensitivity has been reported in 0–8% of patients in trials of intravesical epirubicin; the symptoms included generalized skin rash, vulval irritation, or urinary frequency and dysuria, or were not stated (100,103,104). One of 34 patients developed symptoms characterized as allergic (dizziness, nausea, hypotension) 1 hour after instillation of epirubicin (105). Two patients who received epirubicin developed severe allergic reactions and one died (106,107).

Non-specific systemic adverse events (flu-like symptoms, malaise, fever, nausea, vomiting, anorexia, rash) occurred in under 5% of patients who received intravesical epirubicin (98,103,108). Alopecia was reported in one of 37 patients (98).

Intravesical epirubicin and doxorubicin appear to have similar tolerability profiles (104,109–112).

Valrubicin (a novel *N*-trifluoroacetyl, 14-valerate derivative of doxorubicin) is currently licensed in the USA for intravesical use in prophylaxis in patients with BCG-refractory carcinoma in situ after transurethral resection. It has a similar toxicity profile to that of epirubicin and doxorubicin (113).

Drug overdose

Very high single doses of anthracyclines can cause acute myocardial degeneration within 24 hours and severe myelosuppression within 10–14 days. Treatment should aim to support the patient during this period and should include such measures as blood transfusion and reverse barrier nursing. Delayed cardiac failure can occur up to 6 months after overdosage.

Drug–Drug Interactions

Etoposide

The combination of idarubicin plus etoposide (total doses 180 mg and 5760 mg respectively) was associated with a case of acute promyelocytic leukemia (114).

Taxanes

The combination of doxorubicin plus paclitaxel is cardiotoxic.

Of 57 patients who had received at least three courses of chemotherapy with a combination of doxorubicin 50 mg/m^2 plus paclitaxel 175–225 mg/m^2, left ventricular ejection fraction did not fall overall but was significantly reduced in eight patients; it fell by more than 14% in three cases and by 33–48% in the other five; none of the patients developed clinical heart failure (115).

Two studies of the combination of epirubicin plus paclitaxel have shown less reduction in left ventricular ejection fraction and no clinical evidence of cardiac failure (116,117).

Clinically significant cardiac insufficiency has been reported in a patient who was given epirubicin (316 mg/m^2) followed by six cycles of docetaxel (100 mg/m^2/cycle) (118).

Trastuzumab

An interaction of doxorubicin with the anti-HER_2 receptor humanized monoclonal antibody, trastuzumab (Herceptin), has been reported. Most patients who received trastuzumab in early trials had been pretreated with anthracyclines. Despite this, preliminary information suggested that reduced systolic cardiac function was an adverse effect of trastuzumab (119). More recently, this problem has been further highlighted in a study of women with metastatic breast cancer (120). Patients who had not received prior anthracycline-containing adjuvant chemotherapy were at greater risk of cardiotoxicity when they received trastuzumab in combination with doxorubicin or cyclophosphamide (27 and 75% respectively), compared with only 11% of patients who received trastuzumab in combination with paclitaxel (120,121). The risk of cardiac events in patients treated with doxorubicin, cyclophosphamide, and trastuzumab increased markedly after a cumulative doxorubicin dose of 360 mg/m^2. This suggests synergistic cardiotoxicity with trastuzumab and doxorubicin. Trastuzumab is therefore currently licensed only for use in conjunction with paclitaxel or docetaxel and not with conventional doxorubicin.

The mechanism of trastuzumab-induced cardiotoxicity and its synergy with doxorubicin is as yet unknown. However, the cardiac failure responds to standard medical management (122).

Since trastuzumab is active as a single agent and in combination with chemotherapy in patients whose tumors overexpress HER_2, the interaction with doxorubicin is clearly of concern. Although it is possible to avoid this problem by not combining trastuzumab with doxorubicin, there are compelling reasons for further exploring its use with anthracyclines. For example, follow-up results from the CALGB 8541 study have shown that patients who received high and moderate (standard) doses of cyclophosphamide plus doxorubicin plus fluorouracil survived longer than those who received low doses (123). Moreover, examination of patients' HER_2 status in this trial showed that those whose tumors expressed large amounts of the HER_2 protein had a significantly worse survival if treated with moderate or low doses of cyclophosphamide plus doxorubicin plus fluorouracil, compared with high doses (124). These results suggest that patients whose tumors express large amounts of the HER_2 receptor protein may require high-dose anthracyclines, presenting the problem of how then to treat them with trastuzumab without causing cardiotoxicity.

In an attempt to avoid cardiotoxicity after the administration of trastuzumab with doxorubicin, alternative adjuvant regimens have been suggested. Trastuzumab could be combined with other anthracyclines (epirubicin or liposomal formulations), which are inherently less cardiotoxic, or given sequentially rather than concomitantly with the anthracycline. Alternatively, non-anthracycline combinations, such as cyclophosphamide plus doxorubicin plus fluorouracil or based around taxanes, cisplatin, and vinorelbine are being investigated (125).

Caution should of course be exercised when giving other cytotoxic drugs, especially myelotoxic agents or agents that cause significant mucositis/stomatitis, in combination with anthracyclines.

References

1. Chabner BA, Longo DL. Cancer Chemotherapy and Biotherapy: Principles and Practice. 2nd ed. Lippincott Williams and Wilkins, 2001.
2. Souhami RL, Tannock I, Hohenberger P, Horiot JC. Oxford Textbook of Oncology. 2nd ed. Oxford: Oxford University Press, 2002.
3. Wiseman LR, Spencer CM. Dexrazoxane. A review of its use as a cardioprotective agent in patients receiving anthracycline-based chemotherapy. Drugs 1998;56(3):385–403.
4. Okuma K, Ariyoshi Y, Ota K. [Clinical study of acute cardiotoxicity of anti-cancer agents—analysis using Holter ECG monitoring.] Gan To Kagaku Ryoho 1988;15(6):1893–900.
5. Barendswaard EC, Prpic H, Van der Wall EE, Camps JA, Keizer HJ, Pauwels EK. Right ventricle wall motion abnormalities in patients treated with chemotherapy. Clin Nucl Med 1991;16(7):513–16.
6. Viniegra M, Marchetti M, Losso M, Navigante A, Litovska S, Senderowicz A, Borghi L, Lebron J, Pujato D, Marrero H, et al. Cardiovascular autonomic function in anthracycline-treated breast cancer patients. Cancer Chemother Pharmacol 1990;26(3):227–31.
7. Launchbury AP, Habboubi N. Epirubicin and doxorubicin: a comparison of their characteristics, therapeutic activity and toxicity. Cancer Treat Rev 1993;19(3):197–228.
8. Shan K, Lincoff AM, Young JB. Anthracycline-induced cardiotoxicity. Ann Intern Med 1996;125(1):47–58.
9. Von Hoff DD, Layard MW, Basa P, Davis HL Jr, Von Hoff AL, Rozencweig M, Muggia FM. Risk factors for doxorubicin-induced congestive heart failure. Ann Intern Med 1979;91(5):710–17.
10. Casper ES, Gaynor JJ, Hajdu SI, Magill GB, Tan C, Friedrich C, Brennan MF. A prospective randomized trial of adjuvant chemotherapy with bolus versus continuous infusion of doxorubicin in patients with high-grade extremity soft tissue sarcoma and an analysis of prognostic factors. Cancer 1991;68(6):1221–9.
11. Mortensen SA, Olsen HS, Baandrup U. Chronic anthracycline cardiotoxicity: haemodynamic and histopathological manifestations suggesting a restrictive endomyocardial disease. Br Heart J 1986;55(3):274–82.
12. Pihkala J, Saarinen UM, Lundstrom U, Virtanen K, Virkola K, Siimes MA, Pesonen E. Myocardial function in children and adolescents after therapy with anthracyclines and chest irradiation. Eur J Cancer 1996;32A(1):97–103.
13. Hesseling PB, Kalis NN, Wessels G, van der Merwe PL. The effect of anthracyclines on myocardial function in 50 long-term survivors of childhood cancer. Cardiovasc J South Afr 1999;89(Suppl 1):C25–8.
14. Ibrahim NK, Hortobagyi GN, Ewer M, Ali MK, Asmar L, Theriault RL, Fraschini G, Frye DK, Buzdar AU. Doxorubicin-induced congestive heart failure in elderly patients with metastatic breast cancer, with long-term

follow-up: the M.D. Anderson experience. Cancer Chemother Pharmacol 1999;43(6):471–8.

15. Lipshultz SE, Colan SD, Gelber RD, Perez-Atayde AR, Sallan SE, Sanders SP. Late cardiac effects of doxorubicin therapy for acute lymphoblastic leukemia in childhood. N Engl J Med 1991;324(12):808–15.

16. Steinherz LJ, Steinherz PG, Tan CT, Heller G, Murphy ML. Cardiac toxicity 4 to 20 years after completing anthracycline therapy. JAMA 1991;266(12):1672–7.

17. Drug news. Anthracycline cardiotoxicity uncovered. Drug Ther 1991;Dec:57.

18. Fahey J. Cardiovascular function in children with acquired and congenital heart disease. Curr Opin Cardiol 1992;7:111–15.

19. Mather FJ, Simon RM, Clark GM, Von Hoff DD. Cardiotoxicity in patients treated with mitoxantrone: Southwest Oncology Group phase II studies. Cancer Treat Rep 1987;71(6):609–13.

20. McQuillan PJ, Morgan BA, Ramwell J. Adriamycin cardiomyopathy. Fatal outcome of general anaesthesia in a child with adriamycin cardiomyopathy. Anaesthesia 1988;43(4):301–4.

21. Coukell AJ, Faulds D. Epirubicin. An updated review of its pharmacodynamic and pharmacokinetic properties and therapeutic efficacy in the management of breast cancer. Drugs 1997;53(3):453–82.

22. Camaggi CM, Comparsi R, Strocchi E, Testoni F, Angelelli B, Pannuti F. Epirubicin and doxorubicin comparative metabolism and pharmacokinetics. A cross-over study. Cancer Chemother Pharmacol 1988;21(3):221–8.

23. Lahtinen R, Kuikka J, Nousiainen T, Uusitupa M, Lansimies E. Cardiotoxicity of epirubicin and doxorubicin: a double-blind randomized study. Eur J Haematol 1991;46(5):301–5.

24. Plosker GL, Faulds D. Epirubicin. A review of its pharmacodynamic and pharmacokinetic properties, and therapeutic use in cancer chemotherapy. Drugs 1993;45(5):788–856.

25. Torti FM, Bristow MM, Lum BL, Carter SK, Howes AE, Aston DA, Brown BW Jr, Hannigan JF Jr, Meyers FJ, Mitchell EP, et al. Cardiotoxicity of epirubicin and doxorubicin: assessment by endomyocardial biopsy. Cancer Res 1986;46(7):3722–7.

26. Booser DJ, Hortobagyi GN. Anthracycline antibiotics in cancer therapy. Focus on drug resistance. Drugs 1994;47(2):223–58.

27. Buckley MM, Lamb HM. Oral idarubicin. A review of its pharmacological properties and clinical efficacy in the treatment of haematological malignancies and advanced breast cancer. Drugs Aging 1997;11(1):61–86.

28. Petti MC, Mandelli F. Idarubicin in acute leukemias: experience of the Italian Cooperative Group GIMEMA. Semin Oncol 1989;16(1 Suppl 2):10–15.

29. Ota K. Clinical review of aclacinomycin A in Japan. Drugs Exp Clin Res 1985;11(1):17–21.

30. Wilke A, Hesse H, Gorg C, Maisch B. Elevation of the pacing threshold: a side effect in a patient with pacemaker undergoing therapy with doxorubicin and vincristine. Oncology 1999;56(2):110–11.

31. Lai KH, Tsai YT, Lee SD, Ng WW, Teng HC, Tam TN, Lo GH, Lin HC, Lin HJ, Wu JC, et al. Phase II study of mitoxantrone in unresectable primary hepatocellular carcinoma following hepatitis B infection. Cancer Chemother Pharmacol 1989;23(1):54–6.

32. Wassmuth R, Lentzsch S, Erdbruegger U, Schulz-Menger J, Doerken B, Dietz R, Friedrich MG. Subclinical cardiotoxic effects of anthracyclines as assessed by magnetic resonance imaging—a pilot study. Am Heart J 2001;141(6):1007–13.

33. Zambetti M, Moliterni A, Materazzo C, Stefanelli M, Cipriani S, Valagussa P, Bonadonna G, Gianni L. Long-term cardiac sequelae in operable breast cancer patients given adjuvant chemotherapy with or without doxorubicin and breast irradiation. J Clin Oncol 2001;19(1):37–43.

34. Dey HM, Kassamali H. Radionuclide evaluation of doxorubicin cardiotoxicity: the need for cautious interpretation. Clin Nucl Med 1988;13(8):565–8.

35. Solymar L, Marky I, Mellander L, Sabel KG. Echocardiographic findings in children treated for malignancy with chemotherapy including adriamycin. Pediatr Hematol Oncol 1988;5(3):209–16.

36. Nakamura K, Miyake T, Kawamura T, Maekawa I. [Prospective monitoring of adriamycin cardiotoxicity with systolic time intervals.] Nippon Gan Chiryo Gakkai Shi 1988;23(8):1633–7.

37. Schwartz CL, Hobbie WL, Truesdell S, Constine LC, Clark EB. Corrected QT interval prolongation in anthracycline-treated survivors of childhood cancer. J Clin Oncol 1993;11(10):1906–10.

38. Vici P, Ferraironi A, Di Lauro L, Carpano S, Conti F, Belli F, Paoletti G, Maini CL, Lopez M. Dexrazoxane cardioprotection in advanced breast cancer patients undergoing high-dose epirubicin treatment. Clin Ter 1998;149(921):15–20.

39. Rowan RA, Masek MA, Billingham ME. Ultrastructural morphometric analysis of endomyocardial biopsies. Idiopathic dilated cardiomyopathy, anthracycline cardiotoxicity, and normal myocardium. Am J Cardiovasc Pathol 1988;2(2):137–44.

40. Weesner KM, Bledsoe M, Chauvenet A, Wofford M. Exercise echocardiography in the detection of anthracycline cardiotoxicity. Cancer 1991;68(2):435–8.

41. Suzuki T, Hayashi D, Yamazaki T, Mizuno T, Kanda Y, Komuro I, Kurabayashi M, Yamaoki K, Mitani K, Hirai H, Nagai R, Yazaki Y. Elevated B-type natriuretic peptide levels after anthracycline administration. Am Heart J 1998;136(2):362–3.

42. Nony P, Guastalla JP, Rebattu P, Landais P, Lievre M, Bontemps L, Itti R, Beaune J, Andre-Fouet X, Janier M. In vivo measurement of myocardial oxidative metabolism and blood flow does not show changes in cancer patients undergoing doxorubicin therapy. Cancer Chemother Pharmacol 2000;45(5):375–80.

43. Cassidy J, Merrick MV, Smyth JF, Leonard RC. Cardiotoxicity of mitozantrone assessed by stress and resting nuclear ventriculography. Eur J Cancer Clin Oncol 1988;24(5):935–8.

44. Brusamolino E, Bertini M, Guidi S, Vitolo U, Inverardi D, Merante S, Colombo A, Resegotti L, Bernasconi C, Ferrini PR, et al. CHOP versus CNOP (N = mitoxantrone) in non-Hodgkin's lymphoma: an interim report comparing efficacy and toxicity. Haematologica 1988;73(3):217–22.

45. Saini J, Rich MW, Lyss AP. Reversibility of severe left ventricular dysfunction due to doxorubicin cardiotoxicity. Report of three cases. Ann Intern Med 1987;106(6):814–16.

46. Moreb JS, Oblon DJ. Outcome of clinical congestive heart failure induced by anthracycline chemotherapy. Cancer 1992;70(11):2637–41.

47. Ferrari S, Figus E, Cagnano R, Iantorno D, Bacci G. The role of corrected QT interval in the cardiologic follow-up of young patients treated with Adriamycin. J Chemother 1996;8(3):232–6.

48. Goenen M, Baele P, Lintermans J, Lecomte C, Col J, Ponlot R, Schoevardts JC, Chalant C. Orthotopic heart transplantation eleven years after left pneumonectomy. J Heart Transplant 1988;7(4):309–11.

49. Puccio CA, Feldman EJ, Arlin ZA. Amsacrine is safe in patients with ventricular ectopy. Am J Hematol 1988;28(3):197–8.

50. Weiss RB, Grillo-Lopez AJ, Marsoni S, Posada JG Jr, Hess F, Ross BJ. Amsacrine-associated cardiotoxicity: an analysis of 82 cases. J Clin Oncol 1986;4(6):918–28.

51. Curran CF, Luce JK. Ocular adverse reactions associated with adriamycin (doxorubicin). Am J Ophthalmol 1989;108(6):709–11.

52. Curran CF, Luce JK. Accidental acute exposure to doxorubicin. Cancer Nurs 1989;12(6):329–31.

53. Abraham R, Basser RL, Green MD. A risk-benefit assessment of anthracycline antibiotics in antineoplastic therapy. Drug Saf 1996;15(6):406–29.

54. Zuckerman KS. Efficacy of intensive, high-dose anthracycline-based therapy in intermediate- and high-grade non-Hodgkin's lymphomas. Semin Oncol 1994;21(1 Suppl 1): 59–64.

55. Lissoni A, Cormio G, Colombo N, Gabriele A, Landoni F, Zanetta G, Mangioni C. High-dose epirubicin in patients with advanced or recurrent uterine sarcoma. Int J Gynaecol Cancer 1997;7:241–4.

56. Bastholt L, Dalmark M, Gjedde SB, Pfeiffer P, Pedersen D, Sandberg E, Kjaer M, Mouridsen HT, Rose C, Nielsen OS, Jakobsen P, Bentzen SM. Dose–response relationship of epirubicin in the treatment of postmenopausal patients with metastatic breast cancer: a randomized study of epirubicin at four different dose levels performed by the Danish Breast Cancer Cooperative Group. J Clin Oncol 1996;14(4):1146–55.

57. Dobbs NA, Twelves CJ. Anthracycline doses in patients with liver dysfunction: do UK oncologists follow current recommendations? Br J Cancer 1998;77(7):1145–8.

58. Scinto AF, Ferraresi V, Campioni N, Tonachella R, Piarulli L, Sacchi I, Giannarelli D, Cognetti F. Accelerated chemotherapy with high-dose epirubicin and cyclophosphamide plus r-met-HUG-CSF in locally advanced and metastatic breast cancer. Ann Oncol 1995;6(7):665–71.

59. Hansen F, Stenbygaard L, Skovsgaard T. Effect of granulocyte-macrophage colony-stimulating factor (GM-CSF) on hematologic toxicity induced by high-dose chemotherapy in patients with metastatic breast cancer. Acta Oncol 1995;34(7):919–24.

60. Chevallier B, Chollet P, Merrouche Y, Roche H, Fumoleau P, Kerbrat P, Genot JY, Fargeot P, Olivier JP, Fizames C, et al. Lenograstim prevents morbidity from intensive induction chemotherapy in the treatment of inflammatory breast cancer. J Clin Oncol 1995;13(7):1564–71.

61. Lawton PA, Spittle MF, Ostrowski MJ, Young T, Madden F, Folkes A, Hill BT, MacRae K. A comparison of doxorubicin, epirubicin and mitozantrone as single agents in advanced breast carcinoma. Clin Oncol (R Coll Radiol) 1993;5(2):80–4.

62. Pedersen-Bjergaard J, Sigsgaard TC, Nielsen D, Gjedde SB, Philip P, Hansen M, Larsen SO, Rorth M, Mouridsen H, Dombernowsky P. Acute monocytic or myelomonocytic leukemia with balanced chromosome translocations to band 11q23 after therapy with 4-epi-doxorubicin and cisplatin or cyclophosphamide for breast cancer J Clin Oncol 1992;10(9):1444–51.

63. Shepherd L, Ottaway J, Myles J, Levine M. Therapy-related leukemia associated with high-dose 4-epi-doxorubicin and cyclophosphamide used as adjuvant chemotherapy for breast cancer. J Clin Oncol 1994;12(11):2514–15.

64. Coombes RC, Bliss JM, Wils J, Morvan F, Espie M, Amadori D, Gambrosier P, Richards M, Aapro M, Villar-Grimalt A, McArdle C, Perez-Lopez FR, Vassilopoulos P, Ferreira EP, Chilvers CE, Coombes G, Woods EM, Marty M. Adjuvant cyclophosphamide, methotrexate, and fluorouracil versus fluorouracil, epirubicin, and cyclophosphamide chemotherapy in premenopausal women with axillary node-positive operable breast cancer: results of a randomized trial. The International Collaborative Cancer Group. J Clin Oncol 1996;14(1):35–45.

65. Marty M. Epirubicin and the risk of leukemia: not substantiated? International Collaborative Cancer Group Steering Committee. J Clin Oncol 1993;11(7):1431–3.

66. Ragaz J, Yun J, Spinelli J. Analysis of incidence of secondary acute myelogenous leukemias (2nd AML) in breast cancer patients (BCP) treated with adjuvant therapy (AT)-association with therapeutic regimens. (Abstract no. 147). Proc Am Soc Clin Oncol 1995;14:112.

67. Carter C, Winfield DA. Factor X deficiency during treatment of relapsed acute myeloid leukaemia with amsacrine. Clin Lab Haematol 1988;10(2):225–8.

68. Zuckerman KS, Case DC Jr, Gams RA, Prasthofer EF. Chemotherapy of intermediate- and high-grade non-Hodgkin's lymphomas with an intensive epirubicin-containing regimen. Blood 1993;82(12):3564–73.

69. Focan C, Andrien JM, Closon MT, Dicato M, Driesschaert P, Focan-Henrard D, Lemaire M, Lobelle JP, Longree L, Ries F. Dose–response relationship of epirubicin-based first-line chemotherapy for advanced breast cancer: a prospective randomized trial. J Clin Oncol 1993;11(7):1253–63.

70. Bissett D, Paul J, Wishart G, Jodrell D, Machan MA, Harnett A, Canney P, George WD, Kaye S. Epirubicin chemotherapy and advanced breast cancer after adjuvant CMF chemotherapy. Clin Oncol (R Coll Radiol) 1995;7(1):12–15.

71. Bertelli G, Gozza A, Forno GB, Vidili MG, Silvestro S, Venturini M, Del Mastro L, Garrone O, Rosso R, Dini D. Topical dimethylsulfoxide for the prevention of soft tissue injury after extravasation of vesicant cytotoxic drugs: a prospective clinical study. J Clin Oncol 1995;13(11):2851–5.

72. Langer SW, Sehested M, Jensen PB. Treatment of anthracycline extravasation with dexrazoxane. Clin Cancer Res 2000;6(9):3680–6.

73. Jensen JN, Lock-Andersen J, Langer SW, Mejer J. Dexrazoxane—a promising antidote in the treatment of accidental extravasation of anthracyclines. Scand J Plast Reconstr Surg Hand Surg 2003;37(3):174–5.

74. Langer SW, Sehested M, Jensen PB. Protection against anthracycline induced extravasation injuries with dexrazoxane: Elucidation of the possible mechanism. Proc Am Soc Clin Oncol 2000;38:492.

75. El-Saghir N, Otrock Z, Mufarrij A, Abou-Mourad Y, Salem Z, Shamseddine A, Abbas J. Dexrazoxane for anthracycline extravasation and GM-CSF for skin ulceration and wound healing. Lancet Oncol 2004;5(5):320–1.

76. Bos AM, van der Graaf WT, Willemse PH. A new conservative approach to extravasation of anthracyclines with dimethylsulfoxide and dexrazoxane. Acta Oncol 2001;40(4):541–2.

77. Perry MC. Complications of chemotherapy. In: Moosa AR, Schimpff SC, Robson MC, editors. Comprehensive Textbook of Oncology. 2nd ed. Baltimore, Maryland: Williams and Wilkins, 1991:1706–19.

78. Ventura MT, Dagnello M, Di Corato R, Tursi A. Allergic contact dermatitis due to epirubicin. Contact Dermatitis 1999;40(6):339.

79. Bronchud MH, Howell A, Crowther D, Hopwood P, Souza L, Dexter TM. The use of granulocyte colony-stimulating factor to increase the intensity of treatment with doxorubicin in patients with advanced breast and ovarian cancer. Br J Cancer 1989;60(1):121–5.

80. Green M. Dose-intensive chemotherapy with cytokine support. Semin Oncol 1994;21(1 Suppl):1–6.

81. Lotem M, Hubert A, Lyass O, Goldenhersh MA, Ingber A, Peretz T, Gabizon A. Skin toxic effects of polyethylene glycol-coated liposomal doxorubicin. Arch Dermatol 2000;136(12):1475–80.

82. Speechly-Dick ME, Owen ER. Mitozantrone-induced onycholysis. Lancet 1988;1(8577):113.

83. Hansen SW, Nissen NI, Hansen MM, Hou-Jensen K, Pedersen-Bjergaard J. High activity of mitoxantrone in previously untreated low-grade lymphomas. Cancer Chemother Pharmacol 1988;22(1):77–9.

84. Burg G, Bieber T, Langecker P. Lokalisierte neutrophile ekkrine Hidradenitis unter Mitroxantron: eine typische Zytostatikanebenwirkung. [Localized neutrophilic eccrine hydradenitis in mitoxantrone therapy: a typical side-effect of cytostatic drugs.] Hautarzt 1988;39(4):233–6.

85. Nikula E, Kiviniitty K, Leisti J, Taskinen PJ. Chromosome aberrations in lymphocytes of nurses handling cytostatic agents. Scand J Work Environ Health 1984;10(2):71–4.

86. Aubier F, Patte C, de Vathaire F, Tournade MF, Oberlin O, Sakiroglu O, Lemerle J. Fertilité masculine après chimiotherapie dans l'enfance. [Male fertility after chemotherapy during childhood.] Ann Endocrinol (Paris) 1995;56(2):141–2.

87. Wils JA, Bliss JM, Marty M, Coombes G, Fontaine C, Morvan F, Olmos T, Perez-Lopez FR, Vassilopoulos P, Woods E, Coombes RC. Epirubicin plus tamoxifen versus tamoxifen alone in node-positive postmenopausal patients with breast cancer: a randomized trial of the International Collaborative Cancer Group. J Clin Oncol 1999;17(7):1988–98.

88. Turchi JJ, Villasis C. Anthracyclines in the treatment of malignancy in pregnancy. Cancer 1988;61(3):435–40.

89. Gessini L, Jandolo B, Pollera C, et al. Neuropatia da cisplatino: un nuovo tipo di polineuropatia assonale ascendente progressiva. Riv Neurobiol 1987;33:75.

90. Benjamin RS, Wiernik PH, Bachur NR. Adriamycin chemotherapy—efficacy, safety, and pharmacologic basis of an intermittent single high-dosage schedule. Cancer 1974;33(1):19–27.

91. Camaggi CM, Strocchi E, Tamassia V, Martoni A, Giovannini M, Lafelice G, Canova N, Marraro D, Martini A, Pannuti F. Pharmacokinetic studies of 4′-epi-doxorubicin in cancer patients with normal and impaired renal function and with hepatic metastases. Cancer Treat Rep 1982;66(10):1819–24.

92. Twelves CJ, Dobbs NA, Michael Y, Summers LA, Gregory W, Harper PG, Rubens RD, Richards MA. Clinical pharmacokinetics of epirubicin: the importance of liver biochemistry tests. Br J Cancer 1992;66(4):765–9.

93. Onrust SV, Wiseman LR, Goa KL. Epirubicin: a review of its intravesical use in superficial bladder cancer. Drugs Aging 1999;15(4):307–33.

94. Masuno T, Kishimoto S, Ogura T, Honma T, Niitani H, Fukuoka M, Ogawa N. A comparative trial of LC9018 plus doxorubicin and doxorubicin alone for the treatment of malignant pleural effusion secondary to lung cancer. Cancer 1991;68(7):1495–500.

95. Sugarbaker PH, Sweatman TW, Graves T, Cunliffe W, Israel M. Early postoperative intraperitoneal adriamycin. Pharmacological studies and a preliminary report. Reg Cancer Treat 1991;4:127–31.

96. Walker-Renard PB, Vaughan LM, Sahn SA. Chemical pleurodesis for malignant pleural effusions. Ann Intern Med 1994;120(1):56–64.

97. Oosterlinck W, Kurth KH, Schroder F, Bultinck J, Hammond B, Sylvester R. A prospective European Organization for Research and Treatment of Cancer Genitourinary Group randomized trial comparing transurethral resection followed by a single intravesical instillation of epirubicin or water in single stage Ta, T1 papillary carcinoma of the bladder. J Urol 1993;149(4):749–52.

98. Cumming JA, Kirk D, Newling DW, Hargreave TB, Whelan P. A multi-centre phase two study of intravesical epirubicin in the treatment of superficial bladder tumour. Eur Urol 1990;17(1):20–2.

99. Okamura K, Murase T, Obata K, Ohshima S, Ono Y, Sakata T, Hasegawa Y, Shimoji T, Miyake K. A randomized trial of early intravesical instillation of epirubicin in superficial bladder cancer. The Nagoya University Urological Oncology Group. Cancer Chemother Pharmacol 1994;35(Suppl):S31–5.

100. Bono AV, Hall RR, Denis L, Lovisolo JA, Sylvester R. Chemoresection in Ta-T1 bladder cancer. Members of the EORTC Genito-Urinary Group. Eur Urol 1996;29(4):385–90.

101. Lukkarinen O, Paul C, Hellstrom P, Kontturi M, Nurmi M, Puntala P, Ottelin J, Tammela T, Tidefeldt U. Intravesical epirubicin with and without verapamil for the prophylaxis of superficial bladder tumours. Scand J Urol Nephrol 1991;25(1):25–8.

102. Bono AV, Lovisolo JA, Saredi G. Conservative treatment of primary T1G3 bladder carcinoma: results from a phase II trial. Br J Urol 1997;80(Suppl 2):117.

103. Melekos MD, Dauaher H, Fokaefs E, Barbalias G. Intravesical instillations of 4-epi-doxorubicin (epirubicin) in the prophylactic treatment of superficial bladder cancer: results of a controlled prospective study. J Urol 1992;147(2):371–5.

104. Ali-el-Dein B, el-Baz M, Aly AN, Shamaa S, Ashamallah A. Intravesical epirubicin versus doxorubicin for superficial bladder tumors (stages pTa and pT1): a randomized prospective study. J Urol 1997;158(1):68–74.

105. Kurth K, Vijgh WJ, ten Kate F, Bogdanowicz JF, Carpentier PJ, Van Reyswoud I. Phase 1/2 study of intravesical epirubicin in patients with carcinoma in situ of the bladder. J Urol 1991;146(6):1508–13.

106. Hermenegildo Caudevilla M, Climente Marti M, Polo i Peris A, Poveda Andres JL, Gasso Matoses M. Fatal adverse reaction after intravesical administration of epirubicin. Farm Hosp 1996;20:395–6.

107. Michelena Hernandez L, Iruin Sanz A, Martinez Lopez de Castro N, Sarobe Carricas M, Oderiz Mendioroz N, Vivanco Arana M, Alfaro Basarte J. Systemic reaction due to intravesical epirubicin. Farm Hosp 1996;20:393–4.

108. Melekos MD, Zarakovitis IE, Fokaefs ED, Dandinis K, Chionis H, Bouropoulos C, Dauaher H. Intravesical bacillus Calmette-Guérin versus epirubicin in the prophylaxis of recurrent and/or multiple superficial bladder tumours. Oncology 1996;53(4):281–8.

109. Gohji K, Hara I, Taguchi I, Ueno K, Yamada Y, Eto H, Arakawa S, Kamidono S, Obe S, Ogawa T, et al. Long-term results of a randomised study of intravesical instillation of epirubicin and doxorubicin as a prophylaxis against superficial bladder recurrence. Nishinihon J Urol 1997;59:785–91.

110. Schon G, Merkle W. Epirubicin vs doxorubicin for the treatment of superficial bladder cancer: a randomised study (Abstract no P1.13). Urologe A 1998;(Suppl 1):S18.

111. Shuin T, Kubota Y, Noguchi S, Hosaka M, Miura T, Kondo I, Fukushima S, Ishizuka E, Furuhata A, Moriyama M, et al. A phase II study of prophylactic intravesical chemotherapy with 4′-epirubicin in recurrent superficial bladder cancer: comparison of 4′-epirubicin and adriamycin. Cancer Chemother Pharmacol 1994;35(Suppl):S52–6.

112. Eto H, Oka Y, Ueno K, Nakamura I, Yoshimura K, Arakawa S, Kamidono S, Obe S, Ogawa T, Hamami G,

et al. Comparison of the prophylactic usefulness of epirubicin and doxorubicin in the treatment of superficial bladder cancer by intravesical instillation: a multicenter randomized trial. Kobe University Urological Oncology Group. Cancer Chemother Pharmacol 1994;35(Suppl):S46–51.

113. Onrust SV, Lamb HM. Valrubicin. Drugs Aging 1999;15(1):69–75.

114. De Renzo A, Santoro LF, Notaro R, Pane F, Buonaiuto MR, Luciano L, Rotoli B. Acute promyelocytic leukemia after treatment for non-Hodgkin's lymphoma with drugs targeting topoisomerase II. Am J Hematol 1999;60(4):300–4.

115. Martin M, Lluch A, Ojeda B, Barnabas A, Colomer R, Massuti B, Benito D. Paclitaxel plus doxorubicin in metastatic breast cancer: preliminary analysis of cardiotoxicity. Semin Oncol 1997;24(5 Suppl 17):S17–26–17–30.

116. Rischin D, Smith J, Millward M, Lewis C, Boyer M, Richardson G, Toner G, Gurney H, McKendrick J. A phase II trial of paclitaxel and epirubicin in advanced breast cancer. Br J Cancer 2000;83(4):438–42.

117. Lalisang RI, Voest EE, Wils JA, Nortier JW, Erdkamp FL, Hillen HF, Wals J, Schouten HC, Blijham GH. Dose-dense epirubicin and paclitaxel with G-CSF: a study of decreasing intervals in metastatic breast cancer. Br J Cancer 2000;82(12):1914–19.

118. Salminen E, Bergman M, Huhtala S, Jekunen A, Ekholm E. Docetaxel, a promising novel chemotherapeutic agent in advanced breast cancer. Anticancer Res 2000;20(5C):3663–8.

119. Cobleigh MA, Vogel CL, Tripathy D, Robert NJ, Scholl S, Fehrenbacher L, Wolter JM, Paton V, Shak S, Lieberman G, Slamon DJ. Multinational study of the efficacy and safety of humanized anti-HER2 monoclonal antibody in women who have HER2-overexpressing metastatic breast cancer that has progressed after chemotherapy for metastatic disease. J Clin Oncol 1999;17(9):2639–48.

120. Slamon DJ, Leyland-Jones B, Shak S, Fuchs H, Paton V, Bajamonde A, Fleming T, Eiermann W, Wolter J, Pegram M, Baselga J, Norton L. Use of chemotherapy plus a monoclonal antibody against HER2 for metastatic breast cancer that overexpresses HER2. N Engl J Med 2001;344(11):783–92.

121. Slamon D, Leyland-Jones B, Shak S, Paton V, Bajamonde A, Flemiong T, Eirmann W, Wolter J, Baselga J, Norton L. Addition of Herceptin (humanized anti-HER2 antibody) to first line chemotherapy for HER2 overexpressing metastatic breast cancer (HER2+/MBC) markedly increases anticancer activity: a randomised, multinational, controlled phase III trial (Abstract 377). Proc Am Soc Clin Oncol 1998;17:98a.

122. Gianni L. Tolerability in patients receiving trastuzumab with or without chemotherapy. Ann Oncol 2001;12(Suppl 1):S63–8.

123. Budman DR, Berry DA, Cirrincione CT, Henderson IC, Wood WC, Weiss RB, Ferree CR, Muss HB, Green MR, Norton L, Frei E 3rd. Dose and dose intensity as determinants of outcome in the adjuvant treatment of breast cancer. The Cancer and Leukemia Group B. J Natl Cancer Inst 1998;90(16):1205–11.

124. Thor AD, Berry DA, Budman DR, Muss HB, Kute T, Henderson IC, Barcos M, Cirrincione C, Edgerton S, Allred C, Norton L, Liu ET. erbB-2, p53, and efficacy of adjuvant therapy in lymph node-positive breast cancer. J Natl Cancer Inst 1998;90(18):1346–60.

125. Smith I. Future directions in the adjuvant treatment of breast cancer: the role of trastuzumab. Ann Oncol 2001;12(Suppl 1):S75–9.

Anthracyclines—liposomal formulations

See also Anthracyclines and cytostatic and immunosuppressant drugs

General Information

Liposomes are microscopic particles composed of a lipid bilayer membrane enclosing active drug in a central aqueous compartment (1). The aim of liposomal encapsulation of a drug is to alter its pharmacokinetics, thus improving efficacy and/or reducing toxicity (2). Current formulations of liposomal formulations of anthracyclines are as follows:

- pegylated liposomal doxorubicin (Caelyx/Doxil)
- liposomal doxorubicin (Myocet)
- liposomal daunorubicin (DaunoXome).

Sterically stabilized liposomal doxorubicin (pegylated liposomal doxorubicin; Caelyx/Doxil) is coated with polyethylene glycol (3), which results in so-called "stealth liposomes." In liposomal daunorubicin the liposome consists of a lipid bilayer of distearoylphosphatidylcholine and cholesterol in a 2:1 molar ratio (4). Both formulations have a hydrophilic outer layer, which attracts a coating of water around the liposomal shell. This increases the circulation time by making the formulation virtually invisible to the reticuloendothelial system.

The second liposome system (Myocet) was designed to preserve the antitumor effects of doxorubicin but with reduced cardiotoxicity. This type of liposome is readily recognized and phagocytosed by the mononuclear phagocyte system. In animals most of the injected cytotoxic agent is rapidly taken up by phagocytes, minimizing exposure of normal tissues, and thus diminishing some acute and chronic adverse effects (5,6). The doxorubicin is then released by the phagocytes in a controlled fashion, similar to a slow infusion.

Pharmacokinetics

The differences between liposomal doxorubicin and liposomal daunorubicin are due to the differences in their liposomal packaging.

Pegylated liposomal doxorubicin (Caelyx/Doxil) and liposomal daunorubicin (DaunoXome) produce lower peak plasma concentrations and longer circulation times than free drug (7).

Liposomal doxorubicin in Myocet has systemic availability, metabolism, and excretion similar to that of conventional doxorubicin, but at a slower rate (8). In dogs, the plasma concentrations of doxorubicin from Myocet were 1000-fold greater than conventional doxorubicin at 6 hours, but the difference diminished at 24 hours (9). This distinguishes Myocet from Doxil, which persists in the circulation for significantly longer.

Caelyx has linear pharmacokinetics and its disposition occurs in two phases, the first relatively short (5 hours) and the second prolonged (55 hours). Unlike free doxorubicin, most of the pegylated liposomal doxorubicin is confined to the vascular fluid volume, and its blood clearance depends on the liposomal carrier. Liposomal daunorubicin acts similarly to Caelyx, but produces a lower AUC and has a higher clearance and a shorter terminal half-life (10).

Pegylated liposomes (diameter about 70–100 nm) and liposomal daunorubicin (diameter 45 nm) are small enough to pass intact through defective blood vessels that supply tumors. This, rather than any particular affinity for tumor cells, is the reason for their accumulation in tumor tissue (2). Caelyx provides a greater concentration of doxorubicin in Kaposi's sarcoma tumors than in normal skin.

Organs and Systems

Cardiovascular

The incidence of cardiotoxicity in anthracycline-treated patients has been related to the peak plasma drug concentration (11,12). One of the aims in developing pegylated liposomal doxorubicin was to reduce plasma concentrations of free doxorubicin and restrict myocardial penetration, to minimize cardiotoxicity. Preclinical data suggested that the liposomal formulation was indeed less cardiotoxic than the free drug: about 50% more pegylated liposomal doxorubicin than free doxorubicin can be given to rabbits without producing the same frequency of cardiotoxicity (13).

Cardiac adverse events that have been considered probably or possibly related to pegylated liposomal doxorubicin have been reported in 3–9% of patients (14–16). These include hypotension, pericardial effusion, thrombophlebitis, heart failure, and tachycardia (14,15).

Left ventricular failure has been reported in a few patients, particularly those who received high cumulative lifetime doses of pegylated liposomal doxorubicin (over 550 mg/m^2) (14,15). However, cumulative doses of 450 mg/m^2 or more and 550 mg/m^2 have been administered without significant reduction in ejection fraction or the development of cardiac failure (17,18). To date, no or minimal cardiotoxicity has been observed in patients with AIDS-related Kaposi's sarcoma who received pegylated liposomal doxorubicin in high cumulative doses (19).

Both peak and overall concentrations of doxorubicin in myocardial tissue are reduced by 30–40% after Myocet relative to conventional doxorubicin (9). This reduced myocardial exposure resulted in a significant reduction in cardiotoxicity, assessed both functionally and histologically (5,6). Compared with free doxorubicin 75 mg/m^2 given 3-weekly, Myocet 75 mg/m^2 caused significantly less congestive cardiac failure (1 versus 6%) (20). However, a high dose of Myocet (135 mg/m^2, median cumulative dose 405 mg/m^2) caused a significant increase in cardiac toxicity: 38% of patients had a protocol-defined cardiac event, including 13% who developed congestive heart failure (21).

In one study there was a significant (over 20%) reduction in the shortening fraction with liposomal daunorubicin measured by echocardiography (22). In contrast, in another study there was no significant fall in cardiac function, even after cumulative doses of liposomal daunorubicin over 1000 mg/m^2 (23).

Women with metastatic breast cancer were randomized to receive either liposomal doxorubicin (Myocet) 75 mg/m^2 ($n = 108$) or conventional doxorubicin 75 mg/m^2 ($n = 116$) (24). The liposomal formulation was less cardiotoxic than the conventional one, and the cumulative doses before the onset of cardiotoxicity were 780 versus 570 mg/m^2 respectively; the liposomal formulation provided comparable antitumor activity. In another study the authors tried to define the cumulative toxic intravenous dose of daunorubicin (DaunoXome) and concluded that it may be 750–900 mg/m^2 or even higher (exceeding 1000 mg/m^2) (25).

Respiratory

Acute dyspnea, low back pain, and/or pain at the site of tumor have been described, beginning within 1–5 minutes of the start of infusion of pegylated liposomal doxorubicin (26). Three of 35 patients were described as suffering acute dyspnea, two with back pain and two with abdominal pain. In each case the symptoms resolved within 5–15 minutes of stopping the infusion, which was restarted without adverse effects. The mechanism of these symptoms was unclear. However, because the dyspnea was reminiscent of that seen in hemodialysis neutropenia, complete blood counts were obtained from four patients about 2 minutes after the onset of symptoms. All four had relative neutropenia (neutrophil counts of 3–46% of pretreatment), which resolved by the end of the infusion. In vitro, pegylated liposomal doxorubicin, in concentrations predicted to be present in the plasma during the start of treatment, stimulates neutrophil adhesion to human umbilical vein endothelial cells (26). Thus, pegylated liposomal doxorubicin may cause transient sequestration of neutrophils in the pulmonary circulation, resulting in reduced lung compliance and associated dyspnea.

Hematologic

In a phase I dose-finding study of pegylated liposomal doxorubicin, myelosuppression was not a major problem with the doses tested (20–80 mg/m^2, re-dosing every 3–4 weeks). Median nadir white cell and platelet counts were well above 2×10^9/l and 100×10^9/l respectively. In the occasional patient in whom profound granulocytopenia developed there was quick recovery of the cell counts within less than 7 days. Neutropenic fever was documented in only one patient at the top dose of 80 mg/m^2 (17). There was no significant indication of cumulative myelosuppression. Treatment-related anemia was generally mild and blood transfusions were not required. However, two patients with head and neck malignancies and extensive pretreatment were given erythropoietin to maintain hemoglobin concentrations above 9.0 g/dl (17).

Pooled data from 12 phase I or II studies, in 308 patients with solid tumors who received pegylated liposomal doxorubicin in doses of 10–80 mg/m^2, showed that there was neutropenia (neutrophil count below 1×10^9/l) in 50%, anemia in 19%, and thrombocytopenia in 9.2% (27).

Of 71 patients with metastatic breast cancer treated with pegylated liposomal doxorubicin in doses of 45–60 mg/m^2 given 3- or 4-weekly, grade 3/4 neutropenia occurred in 10% and thrombocytopenia in 1% (27).

If pegylated liposomal doxorubicin and liposomal daunorubicin are used to treat AIDS-related Kaposi's sarcoma, one has to consider additional factors that affect the white cell count. In patients with HIV/AIDS, myelosuppression was the most frequent dose-limiting adverse effect of liposomal anthracyclines (22,23). In one study of 30 patients with Kaposi's sarcoma given liposomal daunorubicin 40 mg/m^2, 53% developed granulocytopenia (white cell count below 1×10^9/l); 17% had a hemoglobin concentration below 8.0 g/dl, but none had thrombocytopenia (22).

In another study in 53 patients with AIDS-related Kaposi's sarcoma given pegylated liposomal doxorubicin 20 mg/m^2 every 3 weeks, 21 had leukopenia and three had thrombocytopenia (28).

At doses of 20 mg/m^2 liposomal doxorubicin, combined tolerability data from 705 patients with AIDS-related Kaposi's sarcoma showed that neutropenia (below 1×10^9/l) and anemia were the most common adverse events, affecting 50 and 19% of patients respectively (14).

In summary, myelosuppression after treatment with pegylated liposomal doxorubicin does not appear to be a major problem in patients with solid tumors and relatively intact immunological systems, but is the dose-limiting adverse effect in immunocompromised patients with HIV/AIDS.

High-dose Myocet (135 mg/m^2) caused significant hematological toxicity, namely grade 4 neutropenia in 98% and thrombocytopenia in 46 of 52 patients (21). However, Myocet 75 mg/m^2 3-weekly caused less hematological toxicity than conventional doxorubicin (20).

Gastrointestinal

Stomatitis and pharyngitis have been confirmed, along with hand–foot syndrome, as dose-limiting adverse effects of pegylated liposomal anthracyclines (17). Stomatitis was dose-limiting at high single doses over 70 mg/m^2. Similarly, 12 of 35 patients who received pegylated liposomal doxorubicin 50 mg/m^2 every 3 weeks for advanced ovarian carcinoma required dose reduction (to 40 mg/m^2) or treatment delay (to 4 weeks) because of mucositis (18). Stomatitis and mucositis are dose-dependent (29). In the treatment of Kaposi's sarcoma in patients with HIV/ AIDS, mucositis and stomatitis are rarely problematic and are not dose-limiting. Presumably this is because significantly lower doses of pegylated liposomal doxorubicin are used in these patients.

Nausea and vomiting have been reported but appear to be mild and infrequent adverse effects of pegylated liposomal anthracyclines and liposomal daunorubicin (23,30). In most patients pegylated liposomal doxorubicin can be given without prophylactic antiemetics. In one study there was only mild nausea and vomiting in eight of 53 patients who had not received prophylactic antiemetics (28). Further reviews in patients with AIDS-related Kaposi's sarcoma have reported nausea and vomiting in 17 and 8% of patients respectively (29). Pooled data from 12 phase I and II studies in patients with solid tumors showed that 3.6% of patients had had grade 3/4 nausea or vomiting (27). Diarrhea has similarly been recognized as a mild and infrequent adverse effect of pegylated liposomal doxorubicin (three of 53 patients) (28).

Myocet (75 mg/m^2) causes significantly less vomiting (11 versus 23%) than conventional free doxorubicin (75 mg/m^2) (20). It also leads to lower peak-free doxorubicin

concentrations in the gastrointestinal mucosa compared with conventional doxorubicin, and less gastrointestinal toxicity (5). However, high-dose Myocet (135 mg/m^2) caused grade 4 mucositis in 10 of 52 patients (21).

Liver

The authors of a case report suggested that pegylated liposomal doxorubicin was the probable cause of hepatic failure in a patient who, 2 weeks after treatment with pegylated liposomal doxorubicin 10 mg/m^2 (cumulative dose 20 mg/m^2) (15), developed jaundice and ascites (31). Despite withdrawal of other potentially hepatotoxic drugs, the patient died of hepatorenal failure 12 weeks later. This may have been an idiosyncratic effect augmented by hepatitis B viral infection (15,32), as there have been no other reports of hepatorenal failure (14,33).

Skin

Skin toxicity, manifesting primarily as palmar–plantar erythrodysesthesia or hand–foot syndrome, is one of the principal dose-limiting adverse effects of pegylated liposomal anthracyclines (for example Caelyx 50 mg/m^2 given every 4 weeks) and may warrant dosage modification, depending on the severity of the symptoms (17,18). In pooled tolerability data, grade 3/4 hand–foot syndrome was reported in 54 (17.5%) of 308 patients (27). The median time to the development of grade 3/4 hand–foot syndrome was 51 days, corresponding to the second or third cycle of treatment (27). Myocet, even when given in a high dose (135 mg/m^2), was not associated with the hand–foot syndrome characteristic of pegylated liposomal doxorubicin (20,21). This was presumed to be due to differences in the liposomal formulation. Pegylated liposomes circulate for prolonged periods and may undergo some eccrine excretion, particularly in cases of hyperhidrosis, whereas with Myocet the liposome is phagocytosed by the reticuloendothelial system and the active drug is then slowly released into the circulation, similar to a slow infusion. Severe forms of hand–foot syndrome may need acute intervention with oral dexamethasone and topical dimethylsulfoxide; oral vitamin B$_6$ has not been proven to be useful.

Conjunctivitis and skin pigmentation have been reported but are mild (23,27,28).

Unlike extravasation of conventional doxorubicin, which can cause severe local inflammation and tissue damage, extravasation of liposomal doxorubicin was associated with only mild transient irritation at the infusion site in the eight documented cases (34,35).

Four cases of extravasation of liposomal daunorubicin have been reported and were associated with only mild irritation and transient erythema and swelling, similar to pegylated liposomal doxorubicin (36).

In 60 patients receiving polyethylene glycol-coated liposomal doxorubicin (Doxil) 35–70 mg/m^2 by infusion over 1–2 hours there were four patterns of skin eruption: hand–foot syndrome (40%), a diffuse follicular rash (10%), an intertrigo-like eruption (8%), and new melanotic macules (0.5%) (37).

Hair

Alopecia can occur during treatment with doxorubicin (38). It is generally mild during treatment with Caelyx and occurs in 6–9% of patients. The incidence of alopecia with single-agent Myocet is higher.

Immunologic

Acute hypersensitivity reactions have been reported with the first infusion of pegylated liposomal doxorubicin (14,15). The symptoms included flushing, shortness of breath, facial swelling, headache, chills, back pain, tightness in the chest and throat, and hypotension. Similar reactions have been reported after the intravenous administration of colloid imaging agents and unloaded liposomes.

Acute reactions to infusion have been observed on first exposure to the drug in six of 56 patients treated with pegylated doxorubicin 20–60 mg/m^2 (17). The reactions developed at 3–25 minutes after the start of the infusion and were characterized by flushing, sensation of choking, back pain, and in one instance hypotension. All the symptoms disappeared shortly after discontinuation of the infusion. Three patients were re-treated successfully using premedication (hydrocortisone, cimetidine, and diphenhydramine) and a slower infusion rate (initial rate 1 mg/minute). Similarly, acute onset symptoms of dyspnea, back pain, and tumor site pain have been reported in other studies (26). Since this reaction generally improves on rechallenge with or without premedication, it has been termed pseudoallergic.

Long-Term Effects

Tumorigenicity

Two patients with acute promyelocytic leukemia developed therapy-related myelodysplasia 2.0–2.5 years after complete remission and then acute myeloid leukemia; both had received anthracyclines (39). In both cases the cytogenetic changes that usually occur after the use of alkylating agents were observed. There has only been one previous similar report after successful therapy with anthracyclines, but these observations suggest that anthracyclines can cause acute myeloid leukemia similar to that caused by alkylating agents.

A flare phenomenon is a well-documented effect of hormonal therapies and/or hormone-responsive tumors. A prostate-specific antigen flare occurred in four of 28 patients who received liposomal doxorubicin (Caelyx) for symptomatic androgen-independent prostate cancer (40).

Second-Generation Effects

Teratogenicity

Pegylated liposomal doxorubicin is embryotoxic in rats and embryotoxic and abortifacient in rabbits. Teratogenicity cannot therefore be ruled out, but there is no reported experience in pregnant women. Equally, it is not known if the drug is excreted into human breast milk, so breastfeeding should be discontinued before the administration of pegylated liposomal doxorubicin.

Susceptibility Factors

Since Caelyx has activity in Kaposi's sarcoma, many studies have been performed in patients with HIV/AIDS. Thus, assessment of the tolerability of Caelyx and Doxil has been complicated by underlying immune suppression, neutropenia, and co-morbidity commonly present in patients with HIV/AIDS. This has led to a difference in the dose-limiting adverse effects in patients with solid tumors compared to those with Kaposi's sarcoma. Tolerance differs in patients with HIV/AIDS (standard dose 20 mg/m^2 Caelyx every 3 weeks) and those with solid tumors (standard dose 50 mg/m^2 every 4 weeks).

Drug Administration

Drug administration route

Pegylated liposomal doxorubicin has been given to three patients via a catheter located in the hepatic artery (41). No severe adverse effects, such as nausea, vomiting, stomatitis, alopecia, or cardiotoxicity, were observed. There was mild leukopenia (2.8 × 10^9/l) in one patient; neither anemia nor thrombocytopenia were reported.

Drug overdose

Acute overdose with pegylated liposomal doxorubicin worsens the toxic effects of mucositis, leukopenia, and thrombocytopenia. There have been no reports of overdose of liposomal daunorubicin, but the primary anticipated toxic effect would be myelosuppression.

Drug–Drug Interactions

General

No formal drug interaction studies have been conducted with pegylated liposomal doxorubicin, liposomal daunorubicin, or Myocet. Caution should be exercised when using drugs known to interact with doxorubicin or daunorubicin. Equally, caution should be exercised when giving any other cytotoxic drugs, especially myelotoxic agents, at the same time.

References

1. Kim S. Liposomes as carriers of cancer chemotherapy. Current status and future prospects. Drugs 1993;46(4):618–38.
2. Gabizon AA. Liposomal anthracyclines. Hematol Oncol Clin North Am 1994;8(2):431–50.
3. Verrill M. Anthracyclines in breast cancer: therapy and issues of toxicity. Breast 2001;(Suppl 2):S8–15.
4. Forssen EA, Ross ME. DaunoXome treatment of solid tumours: preclinical and clinical investigations. J Liposome Res 1994;4:481–512.
5. Kanter PM, Bullard GA, Pilkiewicz FG, Mayer LD, Cullis PR, Pavelic ZP. Preclinical toxicology study of liposome encapsulated doxorubicin (TLC D-99): comparison with doxorubicin and empty liposomes in mice and dogs. In Vivo 1993;7(1):85–95.
6. Kanter PM, Bullard GA, Ginsberg RA, Pilkiewicz FG, Mayer LD, Cullis PR, Pavelic ZP. Comparison of the

cardiotoxic effects of liposomal doxorubicin (TLC D-99) versus free doxorubicin in beagle dogs. In Vivo 1993;7(1):17–26.

7. Schuller J, Czejka M, Bandak S, Borow D, Pietrzak C, Marei I, Schernthaner G. Comparison of pharmacokinetics (PK) of free and liposome encapsulated doxorubicin in advanced cancer patients. Onkologie 1995;18(Suppl 2):184.

8. Batist G, Ramakrishnan G, Rao CS, Chandrasekharan A, Gutheil J, Guthrie T, Shah P, Khojasteh A, Nair MK, Hoelzer K, Tkaczuk K, Park YC, Lee LW. Reduced cardiotoxicity and preserved antitumor efficacy of liposome-encapsulated doxorubicin and cyclophosphamide compared with conventional doxorubicin and cyclophosphamide in a randomized, multicenter trial of metastatic breast cancer. J Clin Oncol 2001;19(5):1444–54.

9. Kanter PM, Klaich G, Bullard GA, King JM, Pavelic ZP. Preclinical toxicology study of liposome encapsulated doxorubicin (TLC D-99) given intraperitoneally to dogs. In Vivo 1994;8(6):975–82.

10. Sparano JA, Winer EP. Liposomal anthracyclines for breast cancer. Semin Oncol 2001;28(4 Suppl 12):32–40.

11. Legha SS, Benjamin RS, Mackay B, Ewer M, Wallace S, Valdivieso M, Rasmussen SL, Blumenschein GR, Freireich EJ. Reduction of doxorubicin cardiotoxicity by prolonged continuous intravenous infusion. Ann Intern Med 1982;96(2):133–9.

12. Workman P. Infusional anthracyclines: is slower better? If so, why? Ann Oncol 1992;3(8):591–4.

13. Working PK, Dayan AD. Pharmacological–toxicological expert report. CAELYX. (Stealth liposomal doxorubicin HCl.) Hum Exp Toxicol 1996;15(9):751–85

14. Dezube BJ. Safety assessment: Doxil (doxorubicin HCl liposome injection) in refractory AIDS-related Kaposi's sarcoma. Doxil Clinical Series, Vol. 1, No. 2. Menlo Park, California: SEQUUS Pharmaceuticals Inc, 1996.

15. Goebel FD, Goldstein D, Goos M, Jablonowski H, Stewart JS. Efficacy and safety of Stealth liposomal doxorubicin in AIDS-related Kaposi's sarcoma. The International SL-DOX Study Group. Br J Cancer 1996;73(8):989–94.

16. Harrison M, Tomlinson D, Stewart S. Liposomal-entrapped doxorubicin: an active agent in AIDS-related Kaposi's sarcoma. J Clin Oncol 1995;13(4):914–20.

17. Uziely B, Jeffers S, Isacson R, Kutsch K, Wei-Tsao D, Yehoshua Z, Libson E, Muggia FM, Gabizon A. Liposomal doxorubicin: antitumor activity and unique toxicities during two complementary phase I studies. J Clin Oncol 1995;13(7):1777–85.

18. Muggia FM, Hainsworth JD, Jeffers S, Miller P, Groshen S, Tan M, Roman L, Uziely B, Muderspach L, Garcia A, Burnett A, Greco FA, Morrow CP, Paradiso LJ, Liang LJ. Phase II study of liposomal doxorubicin in refractory ovarian cancer: antitumor activity and toxicity modification by liposomal encapsulation. J Clin Oncol 1997;15(3):987–93.

19. Gabizon A, Martin F. Polyethylene glycol-coated (pegylated) liposomal doxorubicin. Rationale for use in solid tumours. Drugs 1997;54(Suppl 4):15–21.

20. Harris L, Winer E, Batist G, Rovira D, Navari R, Lee L; the TLC D-99 Study Group. Phase III study of TLC D-99 (liposome encapsulated doxorubicin) vs. free doxorubicin in patients with metastatic breast cancer (Abstract 26). Proc Am Soc Clin Oncol 1998;17:A474.

21. Shapiro CL, Ervin T, Welles L, Azarnia N, Keating J, Hayes DF. Phase II trial of high-dose liposome-encapsulated doxorubicin with granulocyte colony-stimulating factor in metastatic breast cancer. TLC D-99 Study Group. J Clin Oncol 1999;17(5):1435–41.

22. Girard PM, Bouchaud O, Goetschel A, Mukwaya G, Eestermans G, Ross M, Rozenbaum W, Saimot AG. Phase II study of liposomal encapsulated daunorubicin in the treatment of AIDS-associated mucocutaneous Kaposi's sarcoma. AIDS 1996;10(7):753–7.

23. Gill PS, Espina BM, Muggia F, Cabriales S, Tulpule A, Esplin JA, Liebman HA, Forssen E, Ross ME, Levine AM. Phase I/II clinical and pharmacokinetic evaluation of liposomal daunorubicin. J Clin Oncol 1995;13(4):996–1003.

24. Harris L, Batist G, Belt R, Rovira D, Navari R, Azarnia N, Welles L, Winer E; TLC D-99 Study Group. Liposome-encapsulated doxorubicin compared with conventional doxorubicin in a randomized multicenter trial as first-line therapy of metastatic breast carcinoma. Cancer 2002;94(1):25–36.

25. Fassas A, Buffels R, Anagnostopoulos A, Gacos E, Vadikolia C, Haloudis P, Kaloyannidis P. Safety and early efficacy assessment of liposomal daunorubicin (DaunoXome) in adults with refractory or relapsed acute myeloblastic leukaemia: a phase I–II study. Br J Haematol 2002;116(2):308–15.

26. Skubitz KM, Skubitz AP. Mechanism of transient dyspnea induced by pegylated-liposomal doxorubicin (Doxil). Anticancer Drugs 1998;9(1):45–50.

27. SEQUUS Pharmaceuticals Inc. Doxil safety report (07 Apr 1997). Menlo Park, California, USA.

28. Northfelt DW, Dezube BJ, Thommes JA, Levine R, Von Roenn JH, Dosik GM, Rios A, Krown SE, DuMond C, Mamelok RD. Efficacy of pegylated-liposomal doxorubicin in the treatment of AIDS-related Kaposi's sarcoma after failure of standard chemotherapy. J Clin Oncol 1997;15(2):653–9.

29. Alberts DS, Garcia DJ. A safety review of pegylated liposomal doxorubicin in the treatment of various malignancies. Oncology 1997;11(Suppl 11):54–62.

30. Ranson MR, Carmichael J, O'Byrne K, Stewart S, Smith D, Howell A. Treatment of advanced breast cancer with sterically stabilized liposomal doxorubicin: results of a multicenter phase II trial. J Clin Oncol 1997;15(10):3185–91.

31. Hengge UR, Brockmeyer NH, Rasshofer R, Goos M. Fatal hepatic failure with liposomal doxorubicin. Lancet 1993;341(8841):383–4.

32. Coker RJ, James ND, Stewart JS. Hepatic toxicity of liposomal encapsulated doxorubicin. Lancet 1993;341(8847):756.

33. Stewart S, Jablonowski H, Goebel FD, Arasteh K, Spittle M, Rios A, Aboulafia D, Galleshaw J, Dezube BJ. Randomized comparative trial of pegylated liposomal doxorubicin versus bleomycin and vincristine in the treatment of AIDS-related Kaposi's sarcoma. International Pegylated Liposomal Doxorubicin Study Group. J Clin Oncol 1998;16(2):683–91.

34. Madhavan S, Northfelt DW. Lack of vesicant injury following extravasation of liposomal doxorubicin. J Natl Cancer Inst 1995;87(20):1556–7.

35. Madhavan S, Northfelt DW. Lack of vesicant injury following extravasation of liposomal doxorubicin. Breast Cancer Res Treat 1996;37(Suppl):77.

36. Cabriales S, Bresnahan J, Testa D, Espina BM, Scadden DT, Ross M, Gill PS. Extravasation of liposomal daunorubicin in patients with AIDS-associated Kaposi's sarcoma: a report of four cases. Oncol Nurs Forum 1998;25(1):67–70.

37. Lotem M, Hubert A, Lyass O, Goldenhersh MA, Ingber A, Peretz T, Gabizon A. Skin toxic effects of polyethylene glycol-coated liposomal doxorubicin. Arch Dermatol 2000;136(12):1475–80.

38. Dean JC, Griffith KS, Cetas TC, Mackel CL, Jones SE, Salmon SE. Scalp hypothermia: a comparison of ice packs and the Kold Kap in the prevention of doxorubicin-induced alopecia. J Clin Oncol 1983;1(1):33–7.

39. Zompi S, Legrand O, Bouscary D, Blanc CM, Picard F, Casadevall N, Dreyfus F, Marie JP, Viguie F. Therapy-related acute myeloid leukaemia after successful therapy for acute promyelocytic leukaemia with t(15;17): a report of two cases and a review of the literature. Br J Haematol 2000;110(3):610–13.
40. Fossa SD, Vaage S, Letocha H, Iversen J, Risberg T, Johannessen DC, Paus E, Smedsrud T; Norwegian Urological Cancer Group. Liposomal doxorubicin (Caelyx) in symptomatic androgen-independent prostate cancer (AIPC)—delayed response and flare phenomenon should be considered. Scand J Urol Nephrol 2002;36(1):34–9.
41. Konno H, Maruo Y, Matsuda I, Nakamura S, Baba S. Intra-arterial liposomal adriamycin for metastatic adenocarcinoma of the liver. Eur Surg Res 1995;27(5):301–6.

Anthrax vaccine

See also Vaccines

General Information

Inactivated anthrax vaccine is mainly used for protection against occupational anthrax exposure. A complete vaccine series consists of three 0.5-ml subcutaneous doses at 2-week intervals, followed by three additional doses 6, 12, and 18 months after the first dose. Mild local reactions occur in 30% of vaccinees, including local erythema and tenderness, which occurs within 24 hours and begins to subside within 48 hours. The reactions tend to increase in severity by the fifth injection. Systemic reactions are rare and usually characterized by malaise and lassitude, chills, and fever (1).

Until recently, there has been little research into anthrax vaccines, other than that carried out for anti-bacteriological warfare purposes by the military. Currently, three human vaccines against *Bacillus anthracis* (produced in Russia, the UK, and the USA) are commercially available. The results of two field trials of two vaccines produced in Russia and the USA have been analysed (2). The US killed vaccine was 93% effective in preventing cases of anthrax, and the Russian live attenuated vaccine afforded 75% protection when given by scarification and 84% when a jet-gun was used. The rates of local reactions (erythema, induration, and edema) and systemic reactions (fever, malaise, arthralgia, rash, headache) after the US vaccine were 5.75 and 0.4% respectively, compared with 0.54% local reactions and no systemic reactions after placebo. Adverse effects data on the Russian vaccine were not presented.

In the search for new vaccines against anthrax, manufacturers have aimed for better quality purified protective antigen vaccines with better adjuvants, vaccines made through recombinant gene technology, and mutant vaccines with altered protective antigens.

In a study by the Advisory Group of Medical Countermeasures of the UK Ministry of Defence only mild discomfort at the injection site was reported after the administration of a total of 55 000 doses of anthrax vaccine (3).

References

1. Centers for Disease Control and Prevention (CDC). Use of anthrax vaccine in response to terrorism: supplemental recommendations of the Advisory Committee on Immunization Practices. MMWR Morb Mortal Wkly Rep 2002;51(45):1024–6.
2. Demicheli V, Rivetti D, Deeks JJ, Jefferson T, Pratt M. The effectiveness and safety of vaccines against human anthrax: a systematic review. Vaccine 1998;16(9–10):880–4.
3. Blain P, Lightfoot N, Bannister B. Practicalities of warfare required service personnel to be vaccinated against anthrax. BMJ 1998;317(7165):1077–8.

Antianginal drugs

See also Individual agents

General Information

Drugs that are used in the treatment of angina pectoris include agents from the following groups:

- Nitric oxide donors
- Beta-blockers
- Calcium channel blockers
- Potassium channel activators.

New agents, such as L-carnitine and trimetazidine, are also being studied (1).

Safety factors that govern the choice of antianginal drug

Insights into the epidemiology, physiology, cellular biology, molecular biology, and treatment of ischemic heart disease have shown that there are three major modifiable risk factors (hypertension, hypercholesterolemia, smoking) that are the main targets of our preventive strategies. However, evidence that intervention is beneficial has been considerably strengthened.

Hypertension

In high-risk elderly people, treatment of hypertension prevents coronary events (2,3). In the Hypertension Optimal Treatment (HOT) study, which included middle-aged and elderly subjects, good blood pressure control resulted in improved outcome, the optimal blood pressure in non-diabetic subjects being about 138/82 mmHg (4). The target blood pressure was achievable but most patients required more than one drug. A further finding was that low-dose aspirin was beneficial in high-risk subjects. The HOT study found particular benefits of rigorous blood pressure lowering in diabetic subjects, findings that were confirmed by the UK Prospective Diabetes Study (UKPDS) (5), which did not find an advantage in macrovascular complications with angiotensin converting enzyme inhibitors compared with beta-blockers (6). The CAPPP study similarly showed no benefit of captopril over other drugs (7). This originally led to the advice that drugs other than diuretics and beta-blockers should be used infrequently (8); however, subsequent recommendations for the choice of initial therapy have been increasingly based on indications for other conditions that often co-exist with hypertension (9). The Syst-Eur study of systolic hypertension gave further prominence to isolated systolic hypertension as a treatable risk factor and provided some reassuring data on the efficacy of calcium antagonists (10). Despite rather depressing news about inadequate blood pressure control in the UK (11) and USA (12), the increased use of antihypertensive drugs appears to have resulted in less left ventricular hypertrophy (13). This may account in part for the considerable fall in mortality from cardiovascular disease observed since the late 1960s.

Hypercholesterolemia

The landmark 4S study of cholesterol-lowering therapy has convincingly shown the effectiveness of treating patients with high serum cholesterol concentrations and ischemic heart disease (14). This has largely been confirmed by subsequent studies (15–17), and the beneficial effects of lowering serum cholesterol have been extended to primary prevention (18,19). Currently, statins are recommended in all those over the age of 55 years and/ or in those with pre-existing cardiovascular disease (20). Statins reduce cardiac events if begun early after acute coronary syndromes (21) and may also be indicated in any patient with aortic stenosis, regardless of severity (22).

Smoking

The risks of smoking have been highlighted (23). Evidence has emerged that changing from high-tar to low-tar cigarettes is ineffective in reducing myocardial infarction (24), and the antismoking lobby has become more vocal (25,26). The role of cigarette smoking as a major factor in myocardial infarction has been further emphasized by a study of the survivors of the ISIS studies (27). Smoking increased the risk of a non-fatal myocardial infarction five-, three-, and two-fold in the age ranges 30–49, 50–59, and 70–79 respectively. In addition, the results of this study suggested that enforcement of a European Union upper limit of cigarette tar of 12 mg will result in only a modest reduction in myocardial infarction. Preventing adolescents from smoking seems to be the only strategy, as few adults start smoking after the age of 18 (28). Passive smoking (29) and cigar smoking (30) may be associated with coronary disease, making this initiative even more important. The US ruling in July 1995 that nicotine is an addictive substance (31) was a monumental advance in fighting smoking, since cigarettes are considered to be nicotine delivery systems. If the FDA gains legal jurisdiction in regulating tobacco, active steps will be taken to reduce smoking among children.

The roles of these modifiable risks have thus become more important, and other risks interventions, such as dietary antioxidants (32) and physical activity (33), have also been highlighted. In addition, observational studies have implicated hyperhomocysteinemia as a powerful risk factor for premature atherosclerotic coronary artery disease (34). Whether or not treating this risk factor is beneficial in reducing cardiac events is currently being tested (35). In the USA, grain is already enriched with folic acid (140 μg/100 g) (36), and this has resulted in reduced homocysteine concentrations in the middle-aged and older population from the Framingham Offspring Study cohort (37).

In recent years, potassium channel activators have been added to the antianginal armamentarium. In addition, the line between antianginal drugs and drugs used to prevent angina has become somewhat blurred. Aspirin has now become a mainstay drug in the treatment and prevention of ischemic heart disease (38), and another antiplatelet drug, clopidogrel, has also been licensed for this indication. Lipid-lowering drugs have also been advocated for both primary and secondary prevention, and the role of beta-blockers in the secondary prevention of myocardial infarction has been extended into the treatment of systolic heart failure. The angiotensin-converting-enzyme (ACE) inhibitor enalapril has gained a licence for the prevention of coronary ischemic events in patients with left ventricular dysfunction, following the Studies of Left Ventricular Dysfunction Trials (39). More recently, evidence on lisinopril and trandolapril has suggested that these drugs prolong the lives of subjects who have a myocardial infarction, either uncomplicated or complicated by impaired ventricular function (40). The benefits of ACE inhibitors in secondary prevention are now beyond doubt, and are especially marked in diabetic patients (41).

Our view of drug therapy has subtly changed with these findings. The physician's role was to use drugs to relieve the symptoms of angina. Nowadays, drugs must not only relieve symptoms but also, when possible, improve life expectancy (20). We are also more concerned with the quality of symptomatic relief. The notion of "well-being" has become important and has been assessed in "quality-of-life" comparisons of different agents (42). Subtle effects that individually might not be detected have been highlighted in such studies and can modify our view of a drug's adverse effects profile. As the subtle adverse effects of drugs become more important, serious drug toxicity becomes even more unacceptable.

Other susceptibility factors

The roles of other modifiable susceptibility factors have become more important, and other interventions, such as dietary antioxidants (32) and physical activity (33), have also been highlighted in the past. However, a meta-analysis of the effect of vitamin E supplements has suggested that doses over 400 IU/day can increase the risk of death from any cause (43).

Pharmacoeconomics

A further consideration, the economic evaluation of drugs, has become an issue, although not without criticism (44). In its most rigorous form the cost of drug therapy is measured against the aggregate number of years of improved health that such therapy might be expected to bring (45). These so-called "quality-adjusted life years" (QUALYs) are reduced if a drug has an adverse effect, so that the net benefit of a drug that prolongs life but makes that life miserable may well be a negative number of QUALYs. Such studies have put a price-tag on mild adverse events as well as on beneficial effects. In time we may pay increasing attention to the price of adverse effects when choosing a drug.

The drug treatment of angina is time-consuming, empirical, and often relatively unrewarding. Drug treatment simply palliates the underlying disease, and no symptomatic treatment improves survival or prevents myocardial infarction. This is in contrast to surgical intervention, which, in good hands, prolongs survival (46) and improves its quality. The three main comparisons of coronary surgery with medical therapy (47–49) are now out of date, since both medical therapy and surgical techniques have improved considerably since they were completed. However, long-term medical therapy is now more often being reserved for patients who for one reason or another are unsuitable for surgery or percutaneous coronary angioplasty, which, at least for single-vessel disease, is superior to antianginal drug treatment (50) but may be equivalent to lipid-lowering therapy (51). Preventive therapy must now be the dominant strategy.

References

1. Chierchia SL, Fragasso G. Metabolic management of ischaemic heart disease. Eur Heart J 1993;14(Suppl G):2–5.

2. Dahlof B, Lindholm LH, Hansson L, Schersten B, Ekbom T, Wester PO. Morbidity and mortality in the Swedish Trial in Old Patients with Hypertension (STOP-Hypertension). Lancet 1991;338(8778):1281–5.

3. SHEP Cooperative Research Group. Prevention of stroke by antihypertensive drug treatment in older persons with isolated systolic hypertension. Final results of the Systolic Hypertension in the Elderly Program (SHEP). JAMA 1991;265(24):3255–64.

4. Hansson L, Zanchetti A, Carruthers SG, Dahlof B, Elmfeldt D, Julius S, Menard J, Rahn KH, Wedel H, Westerling S. Effects of intensive blood-pressure lowering and low-dose aspirin in patients with hypertension: principal results of the Hypertension Optimal Treatment (HOT) randomised trial. HOT Study Group. Lancet 1998;351(9118):1755–62.

5. UK Prospective Diabetes Study Group. Tight blood pressure control and risk of macrovascular and microvascular complications in type 2 diabetes: UKPDS 38. BMJ 1998;317(7160):703–13.

6. UKPDS 39. UK Prospective Diabetes Study Group. Efficacy of atenolol and captopril in reducing risk of macrovascular and microvascular complications in type 2 diabetes. BMJ 1998;317(7160):713–20.

7. Hansson L, Lindholm LH, Niskanen L, Lanke J, Hedner T, Niklason A, Luomanmaki K, Dahlof B, de Faire U, Morlin C, Karlberg BE, Wester PO, Bjorck JE. Effect of angiotensin-converting-enzyme inhibition compared with conventional therapy on cardiovascular morbidity and mortality in hypertension: the Captopril Prevention Project (CAPPP) randomised trial. Lancet 1999;353(9153):611–16.

8. Cutler J. Which drug for treatment of hypertension? Lancet 1999;353(9153):604–5.

9. European Society of Hypertension-European Society of Cardiology Guidelines Committee. 2003 European Society of Hypertension–European Society of Cardiology guidelines for the management of arterial hypertension. J Hypertens 2003;21(6):1011–53.

10. Staessen JA, Fagard R, Thijs L, Celis H, Arabidze GG, Birkenhager WH, Bulpitt CJ, de Leeuw PW, Dollery CT, Fletcher AE, Forette F, Leonetti G, Nachev C, O'Brien ET, Rosenfeld J, Rodicio JL, Tuomilehto J, Zanchetti A. Randomised double-blind comparison of placebo and active treatment for older patients with isolated systolic hypertension. The Systolic Hypertension in Europe (Syst-Eur) Trial Investigators. Lancet 1997;350(9080):757–64.

11. Colhoun HM, Dong W, Poulter NR. Blood pressure screening, management and control in England: results from the health survey for England 1994. J Hypertens 1998;16(6):747–52.

12. Berlowitz DR, Ash AS, Hickey EC, Friedman RH, Glickman M, Kader B, Moskowitz MA. Inadequate management of blood pressure in a hypertensive population. N Engl J Med 1998;339(27):1957–63.

13. Mosterd A, D'Agostino RB, Silbershatz H, Sytkowski PA, Kannel WB, Grobbee DE, Levy D. Trends in the prevalence of hypertension, antihypertensive therapy, and left ventricular hypertrophy from 1950 to 1989. N Engl J Med 1999;340(16):1221–7.

14. Scandinavian Simvastatin Survival Study Group. Randomized trial of cholesterol lowering in 4444 patients with coronary heart disease: the Scandinavian Simvastatin Survival Study (4S). Lancet 1994;344:1383.

15. Byington RP, Jukema JW, Salonen JT, Pitt B, Bruschke AV, Hoen H, Furberg CD, Mancini GB. Reduction in cardiovascular events during pravastatin therapy. Pooled analysis of clinical events of the Pravastatin Atherosclerosis Intervention Program. Circulation 1995;92(9):2419–25.

16. Sacks FM, Pfeffer MA, Moye LA, Rouleau JL, Rutherford JD, Cole TG, Brown L, Warnica JW, Arnold JM, Wun CC, Davis BR, Braunwald E. The effect of pravastatin on coronary events after myocardial infarction in patients with average cholesterol levels. Cholesterol and Recurrent Events Trial investigators. N Engl J Med 1996;335(14):1001–9.

17. The Long-Term Intervention with Pravastatin in Ischaemic Disease (LIPID) Study Group. Prevention of cardiovascular events and death with pravastatin in patients with coronary heart disease and a broad range of initial cholesterol levels. N Engl J Med 1998;339(19):1349–57.

18. Shepherd J, Cobbe SM, Ford I, Isles CG, Lorimer AR, MacFarlane PW, McKillop JH, Packard CJ. Prevention of coronary heart disease with pravastatin in men with hypercholesterolemia. West of Scotland Coronary Prevention Study Group. N Engl J Med 1995;333(20):1301–7.

19. Downs JR, Clearfield M, Weis S, Whitney E, Shapiro DR, Beere PA, Langendorfer A, Stein EA, Kruyer W, Gotto AM Jr. Primary prevention of acute coronary events with lovastatin in men and women with average cholesterol levels: results of AFCAPS/TexCAPS. Air Force/Texas Coronary Atherosclerosis Prevention Study. JAMA 1998;279(20):1615–22.

20. Wald NJ, Law MR. A strategy to reduce cardiovascular disease by more than 80%. BMJ 2003;326(7404):1419.

21. Cannon CP, Braunwald E, McCabe CH, Rader DJ, Rouleau JL, Belder R, Joyal SV, Hill KA, Pfeffer MA, Skene AM, for the Pravastatin or Atorvastatin Evaluation and Infection Therapy–Thrombolysis in Myocardial Infarction 22 Investigators. Intensive versus moderate lipid lowering with statins after acute coronary syndromes. N Engl J Med 2004;350(15):1495–504.

22. Rosenhek R, Rader F, Loho N, Gabriel H, Heger M, Klaar U, Schemper M, Binder T, Maurer G, Baumgartner H. Statins but not angiotensin-converting enzyme inhibitors delay progression of aortic stenosis. Circulation 2004;110(10):1291–5.

23. Bartecchi CE, MacKenzie TD, Schrier RW. The human costs of tobacco use (1) N Engl J Med 1994;330(13):907–12

24. Negri E, Franzosi MG, La Vecchia C, Santoro L, Nobili A, Tognoni G. Tar yield of cigarettes and risk of acute myocardial infarction. GISSI-EFRIM Investigators. BMJ 1993;306(6892):1567–70.

25. Vickers A. Why cigarette advertising should be banned. BMJ 1992;304(6836):1195–6.

26. Anonymous. Enlightenment on the road to death. Lancet 1994;343(8906):1109–10.

27. Parish S, Collins R, Peto R, Youngman L, Barton J, Jayne K, Clarke R, Appleby P, Lyon V, Cederholm-Williams S, et al. Cigarette smoking, tar yields, and non-fatal myocardial infarction: 14,000 cases and 32,000 controls in the United Kingdom. The International Studies of Infarct Survival (ISIS) Collaborators. BMJ 1995;311(7003):471–7.

28. McNeill AD, Jarvis MJ, Stapleton JA, Russell MA, Eiser JR, Gammage P, Gray EM. Prospective study of factors predicting uptake of smoking in adolescents. J Epidemiol Community Health 1989;43(1):72–8.

29. He J, Vupputuri S, Allen K, Prerost MR, Hughes J, Whelton PK. Passive smoking and the risk of coronary heart disease—a meta-analysis of epidemiologic studies. N Engl J Med 1999;340(12):920–6.

30. Iribarren C, Tekawa IS, Sidney S, Friedman GD. Effect of cigar smoking on the risk of cardiovascular disease, chronic obstructive pulmonary disease, and cancer in men. N Engl J Med 1999;340(23):1773–80.

31. Roberts J. Nicotine is addictive, rules FDA. BMJ 1995;311(6999):211.

32. Steinberg D. Antioxidant vitamins and coronary heart disease. N Engl J Med 1993;328(20):1487–9.

33. Lakka TA, Venalainen JM, Rauramaa R, Salonen R, Tuomilehto J, Salonen JT. Relation of leisure-time physical activity and cardiorespiratory fitness to the risk of acute myocardial infarction. N Engl J Med 1994;330(22):1549–54.

34. Boushey CJ, Beresford SA, Omenn GS, Motulsky AG. A quantitative assessment of plasma homocysteine as a risk factor for vascular disease. Probable benefits of increasing folic acid intakes. JAMA 1995;274(13):1049–57.

35. Homocysteine Lowering Trialists' Collaboration. Lowering blood homocysteine with folic acid based supplements: meta-analysis of randomised trials. BMJ 1998;316(7135):894–8.

36. Oakley GP Jr, Johnston RB Jr. Balancing benefits and harms in public health prevention programmes mandated by governments. BMJ 2004;329(7456):41–3.

37. Jacques PF, Selhub J, Bostom AG, Wilson PW, Rosenberg IH. The effect of folic acid fortification on plasma folate and total homocysteine concentrations. N Engl J Med 1999;340(19):1449–54.

38. Willard JE, Lange RA, Hillis LD. The use of aspirin in ischemic heart disease. N Engl J Med 1992;327(3):175–81.

39. Yusuf S, Pepine CJ, Garces C, Pouleur H, Salem D, Kostis J, Benedict C, Rousseau M, Bourassa M, Pitt B. Effect of enalapril on myocardial infarction and unstable angina in patients with low ejection fractions. Lancet 1992;340(8829):1173–8.

40. Torp-Pedersen C, Kober L. Effect of ACE inhibitor trandolapril on life expectancy of patients with reduced left-ventricular function after acute myocardial infarction. TRACE Study Group. Trandolapril Cardiac Evaluation. Lancet 1999;354(9172):9–12.

41. MacDonald TM, Butler R, Newton RW, Morris AD. Which drugs benefit diabetic patients for secondary prevention of myocardial infarction? DARTS/MEMO Collaboration. Diabet Med 1998;15(4):282–9.

42. Fitzpatrick R, Fletcher A, Gore S, Jones D, Spiegelhalter D, Cox D. Quality of life measures in health care. I: Applications and issues in assessment. BMJ 1992;305(6861):1074–7.

43. Miller ER 3rd, Pastor-Barriuso R, Dalal D, Riemersma RA, Appel LJ, Guallar E. Meta-analysis: high-dosage vitamin E supplementation may increase all-cause mortality. Ann Intern Med 2005;142(1):37–46.

44. Menard J. Oil and water? Economic advantage and biomedical progress do not mix well in a government guidelines committee. Am J Hypertens 1994;7(10 Pt 1):877–85.

45. Fletcher A. Pressure to treat and pressure to cost: a review of cost-effectiveness analysis. J Hypertens 1991;9(3):193–8.

46. Myers WO, Davis K, Foster ED, Maynard C, Kaiser GC. Surgical survival in the Coronary Artery Surgery Study. (CASS) registry. Ann Thorac Surg 1985;40(3):245–60.

47. Detre K, Murphy ML, Hultgren H. Effect of coronary bypass surgery on longevity in high and low risk patients. Report from the V.A. Cooperative Coronary Surgery Study. Lancet 1977;2(8051):1243–5.

48. European Coronary Surgery Study Group. Long-term results of prospective randomised study of coronary artery bypass surgery in stable angina pectoris. Lancet 1982;2(8309):1173–80.

49. CASS Principal Investigators and their Associates. Coronary artery surgery study (CASS): a randomised trial of coronary artery bypass surgery. Survival data. Circulation 1983;68:939.

50. Parisi AF, Folland ED, Hartigan P. A comparison of angioplasty with medical therapy in the treatment of single-vessel coronary artery disease. Veterans Affairs ACME Investigators. N Engl J Med 1992;326(1):10–16.

51. Pitt B, Waters D, Brown WV, van Boven AJ, Schwartz L, Title LM, Eisenberg D, Shurzinske L, McCormick LS. Aggressive lipid-lowering therapy compared with angioplasty in stable coronary artery disease. Atorvastatin versus Revascularization Treatment Investigators. N Engl J Med 1999;341(2):70–6.

Anti-CD4 monoclonal antibodies

See also Monoclonal antibodies

General Information

Anti-CD4 monoclonal antibodies are used to treat various autoimmune diseases, such as rheumatoid arthritis, asthma, and psoriasis (1–3). Keliximab (rINN) (IDEC CE9.1) is a human-cynomolgus monkey chimeric (primatized) antibody with specificity for human and chimpanzee CD4. Clenoliximab (rINN) is an immunoglobulin G4 derivative of keliximab. These antibodies induce a more than 80% down-regulation of CD4 molecules on the surface of T lymphocytes.

Observational studies

In an open, dose-escalating study, 24 patients were allocated to five consecutive daily doses of a humanized IgG1 anti-CD4 monoclonal antibody (4162W94) (4). There was at least one predefined infusion-related adverse effect (for example fever, chills/rigors, headache, nausea, vomiting, diarrhea, dyspnea, or hypotension) in 17 patients. Most of these events were mild or moderate in intensity, occurred on the first day of dosing, and resolved within 8 hours. In some patients the adverse events were associated with the appearance of TNF alfa in the plasma during the 3 hours after the start of antibody infusion, suggesting that they resulted from cytokine release. There was systolic hypotension, defined as a systolic pressure below 90 mmHg and a fall of at least 20 mmHg, in one patient who was given 10 mg. There were non-specific skin rashes in one patient in each of the groups who were given 10, 30, and 100 mg and in three of those given 300 mg. There were three serious adverse events: fatal rupture of an aortic aneurysm, thought to be unrelated to the drug, an episode of severe reversible airways obstruction in a patient with asthma, and an episode of unexplained collapse, presumed to be vasovagal, followed by full recovery several hours after the end of the first infusion. No opportunistic or other infections were reported.

Placebo-controlled studies

In a placebo-controlled study in 48 patients with active rheumatoid arthritis, CD4 blockade produced clinical benefit (5). Adverse events were reported in 97% of the patients, compared with 73% of those given placebo. In both groups most of the events were mild to moderate. Serious adverse events were reported in five patients who received anti-CD4; syncope/vasovagal attacks ($n = 3$), back pain ($n = 1$), abdominal pain/rectal bleeding ($n = 1$). Skin rashes occurred in 62% of the patients who received the antibody. In five cases a skin biopsy was performed, and showed a cellular infiltration centered on the blood vessels, suggesting a drug-induced vasculitis.

In a randomized, dose-ranging, placebo-controlled study of keliximab in chronic severe asthma, there were no serious adverse effects related to treatment (1).

References

1. Kon OM, Sihra BS, Loh LC, Barkans J, Compton CH, Barnes NC, Larche M, Kay AB. The effects of an anti-CD4 monoclonal antibody, keliximab, on peripheral blood CD4+ T cells in asthma. Eur Respir J 2001;18(1):45–52.
2. Hepburn TW, Totoritis MC, Davis CB. Antibody-mediated stripping of CD4 from lymphocyte cell surface in patients with rheumatoid arthritis. Rheumatology (Oxford) 2003;42(1):54–61.
3. Skov L, Kragballe K, Zachariae C, Obitz ER, Holm EA, Jemec GB, Solvsten H, Ibsen HH, Knudsen L, Jensen P, Petersen JH, Menne T, Baadsgaard O. HuMax-CD4: a fully human monoclonal anti-CD4 antibody for the treatment of psoriasis vulgaris. Arch Dermatol 2003;139(11):1433–9.
4. Choy EH, Connolly DJ, Rapson N, Jeal S, Brown JC, Kingsley GH, Panayi GS, Johnston JM. Pharmacokinetic, pharmacodynamic and clinical effects of a humanized IgG1 anti-CD4 monoclonal antibody in the peripheral blood and synovial fluid of rheumatoid arthritis patients. Rheumatology (Oxford) 2000;39(10):1139–46.
5. Choy EH, Panayi GS, Emery P, Madden S, Breedveld FC, Kraan MC, Kalden JR, Rascu A, Brown JC, Rapson N, Johnston JM. Repeat-cycle study of high-dose intravenous 4162W94 anti-CD4 humanized monoclonal antibody in rheumatoid arthritis. A randomized placebo-controlled trial. Rheumatology (Oxford) 2002;41(10):1142–8.

Anticholinergic drugs

See also Individual agents

General Information

There are many anticholinergic drugs, some structurally related to atropine, others quaternary ammonium compounds or tertiary amines. Although many of these products are claimed to have superior efficacy, specificity, or tolerance, few have ever been critically compared with others. The so-called freedom from adverse effects claimed for many of these compounds can often be traced to uncritical clinical work, the use of ineffective doses, or mere lack of activity of the compound.

General adverse effects

An indication of what may be expected in the way of adverse reactions can be obtained by fitting a drug into its structural class (see Table 1), since the pattern of effects of drugs in each class is generally very similar. The drugs closely related to atropine have the full range

Table 1 General classification of anticholinergic drugs (rINNs except where stated)

Atropine and closely related agents
  Atropine
  Hyoscine (BAN)
  Ipratropium
  Oxitropium
  Tiotropium
Synthetic quaternary ammonium compounds
  Clidinium
  Emepronium bromide
  Isopropamide
  Mepenzolate
  Methanthelinium (pINN)
  Oxyphenonium
  Poldine (pINN)
  Propantheline
Tertiary amines used in visceral disorders
  Adiphenine
  Dicycloverine
  Oxyphencyclimine
  Piperidolate
Drugs with primarily anticholinergic effects used mainly in Parkinson's disease
Tertiary amines related to diphenhydramine
  Chlorphenoxamine
  Orphenadrine
Trihexyphenidyl-related compounds
  Biperiden
  Procyclidine
  Trihexyphenidyl (benzhexol)
Compounds related to both atropine and diphenhydramine
  Benzatropine
  Etybenzatropine
Compounds used topically for pupillary mydriasis
  Cyclopentolate
  Eucatropine
  Homatropine
  Tropicamide

of antinicotinic and antimuscarinic activity of atropine itself. Of the synthetic compounds used in visceral disorders, the quaternary compounds are fully ionized in the pH range found in body fluids and are therefore less lipid-soluble than the corresponding tertiary amines. This means that they penetrate physiological barriers less readily; less drug is absorbed in the intestine, less enters the cerebrospinal fluid and aqueous humor, and less enters cells. Consequently, these drugs tend to be relatively less active by mouth and to have fewer effects on the brain and the eye than the tertiary amines. Of the latter, some have little antimuscarinic activity and indeed probably very little useful activity at all; they may have some specific relaxant effect on smooth muscle, but it seems to be of little clinical significance.

Of the drugs in this class used largely in parkinsonism, the tertiary amines related to diphenhydramine have some antihistaminic activity, as one would expect; some of these drugs are also related to atropine. The derivatives of trihexyphenidyl (benzhexol) are also pharmacologically closely similar: for example, they have some excitatory effects if given in sufficient doses.

The unwanted peripheral effects of all atropine-like drugs include flushing of the skin, dryness of the mucous membranes with fever, tachycardia, reduced salivary secretion and dryness of the mouth, drying up of the gastrointestinal secretions and decreased gastric acidity, and reduced muscle tone in the gut and constipation. Bladder tone and frequency of micturition are reduced and acute urinary retention is a risk, especially in older men with prostatic hyperplasia. Nasal, bronchial, and lacrimal secretions are reduced.

Herbal sources of anticholinergic drugs

Tropane alkaloids, such as hyoscyamine and/or scopolamine, occur in the solanaceous plants *Atropa belladonna*, *Datura stramonium*, *Hyoscyamus niger*, and *Mandragora officinarum*. These alkaloids are powerful anticholinergic agents and can elicit peripheral symptoms (for example blurred vision, dry mouth) as well as central effects (for example drowsiness, delirium). They can potentiate the effects of anticholinergic medicaments.

Organs and Systems

Cardiovascular

The potential dysrhythmogenic effect of anticholinergic drugs has been examined retrospectively in nearly 4000 patients taking flavoxate, oxybutynin, and hyoscyamine between 1991 and 1995, compared with over 10 000 patients who had no exposure to these drugs (1). All the patients were over 65 years old and they were reasonably matched for co-morbidities, although not surprisingly more women than men were taking the antispasmodic drugs (75% women in the treated group versus 67% in the control population). The encouraging conclusion was that there was no evidence that these drugs promote ventricular dysrhythmias or sudden death. However, the authors noted that more detailed analysis of these data is

needed and that it may also be advisable to consider data from newer drugs.

Nervous system

Orofacial dyskinesia, though familiar with dopaminergic drugs, can apparently also occur with some anticholinergic drugs; for example, it has been described with trihexyphenidyl in a patient who did not have this reaction with levodopa (SEDA-18, 160).

Sensory systems

Anticholinergic drugs cause passive pupillary dilatation by paralysing the iridal sphincter, suppress accommodation by paralysing the ciliary muscle, and increase the vascular permeability of the iris and ciliary bodies. They are used topically for diagnostic and refractive purposes, and in combination with other drugs as part of the treatment of several serious ocular conditions, including inflammatory states. Topically applied drugs can cause local adverse effects in the eye (SEDA-23, 504) and systemic effects if sufficient drug is absorbed.

All anticholinergic drugs can cause acute closed-angle glaucoma in patients with an anatomical predisposition. They also cause photophobia and disturbances of accommodation leading to difficulties in reading and driving.

Psychological, psychiatric

Anticholinergic drugs can cause vivid and sometimes exotic hallucinations and this has led to their misuse. Plants containing atropine and related substances were used in witches' brews in the Middle Ages to conjure up the devil, but even synthetic tertiary amines given in eye-drops and depot plasters containing atropine (SEDA-13, 114) have caused hallucinations. Postoperative confusion in elderly patients has been clearly correlated with drugs that have anticholinergic properties (SEDA-13, 114), and the use of anticholinergic drugs for the treatment of Parkinson's disease has long been associated with neuropsychiatric adverse effects. Cyclopentolate is a short-acting cycloplegic with a rapid onset (and considerable intensity) of action, which particularly in children has been reported to cause hallucinations and psychotic episodes (2). It has been suggested that a partial structural affinity of the side-chain to some hallucinogens aggravates the problems associated with cyclopentolate.

Anticholinergic drugs can impair short-term memory. The effects in non-demented patients are reversible, receding within a few weeks of withdrawing treatment (3). Comparisons of dopaminergic drugs with anticholinergic drugs in healthy volunteers have shown that anticholinergic drugs caused significant impairment of memory function, more confusion, and dysphoria (SEDA-13, 115).

Immunologic

Allergic reactions to local application in the eye can occur, usually in the form of contact dermatitis and conjunctival redness and are more common with hyoscine than with atropine, although contact dermatitis is less likely (4).

Long-Term Effects

Drug dependence

Patients taking long-term anticholinergic drugs can develop dependence (SEDA-15, 136).

Susceptibility Factors

Anticholinergic drugs clearly may cause problems in patients with closed-angle glaucoma (or a narrow angle between the iris and cornea), paralytic ileus, pyloric stenosis, or urinary retention. Because of their effects on temperature control they may be undesirable in patients with pyrexia (especially children) and during very hot weather.

Drug Administration

Drug overdose

The clinical effects of overdosage with atropine-like drugs, as recorded in a series of 119 patients, are presented in Table 2 (5). Infrequent manifestations (less than 10% of cases) included seizures, convulsions, vomiting, rash, urinary retention, abdominal distress, paralytic ileus, and constipation. Death, when it occurs, is due primarily to the effects on the central nervous system; a stage of excitement is followed by drowsiness, stupor, and coma, with generalized central depression.

Table 2 Clinical manifestations of anticholinergic drug intoxication in 71 adults and 48 children

Adverse effect	Adults (%)	Children (%)
Pupils widely dilated and poorly reactive	79	88
Flushed face, dry mucous membranes	55	90
Tachycardia (>100)	44	65
Incoherence, confusion, or disorientation	66	56
Restlessness, hyperactivity, or agitation	39	58
Auditory or visual hallucinations	52	27
Ataxia or motor incoordination	35	48
Carphology	37	44
Hyper-reflexia, twitching, or increased muscle tone	25	35
Apprehension, fear, or paranoia	23	14
Somnolence or coma	34	16
"Toxic delirium"	14	40
Giddiness; labile or inappropriate affect	18	13
Dysarthria or slurred speech	14	14
Fever (>100°F)	18	25
Thirst or dry mouth	18	14
Blindness or blurred vision	20	13
Retrograde amnesia	18	13

Drug–Drug Interactions

Other anticholinergic drugs

Some antidepressants, neuroleptic drugs, antihistamines, antispasmodics, and antidysrhythmic drugs have anticholinergic activity, as do some herbal remedies (see the section on Herbal sources of anticholinergic drugs in this monograph). The combined use of such drugs can lead to inadvertent anticholinergic overdosage.

References

1. Wang PS, Levin R, Zhao SZ, Avorn J. Urinary antispasmodic use and the risks of ventricular arrhythmia and sudden death in older patients. J Am Geriatr Soc 2002;50(1):117–24.
2. Khurana AK, Ahluwalia BK, Rajan C, Vohra AK. Acute psychosis associated with topical cyclopentolate hydrochloride. Am J Ophthalmol 1988;105(1):91.
3. van Herwaarden G, Berger HJ, Horstink MW. Short-term memory in Parkinson's disease after withdrawal of long-term anticholinergic therapy. Clin Neuropharmacol 1993;16(5):438–43.
4. Havener WH. Ocular Pharmacology. 4th ed. St Louis: CV Mosby, 1978.
5. Hooper PL, Harrelson LK, Johnson GE. Pseudohemoptysis from isoetharine. N Engl J Med 1983;308(26):1602.

Anticoagulant proteins

General Information

There are several endogenous anticoagulants proteins, antithrombin III, protein C, and protein S. Severe sepsis and septic shock are associated with activation of the coagulation system and depletion of these endogenous anticoagulants. Anticoagulant proteins prevent microthrombus formation, thereby reducing the risk of multiorgan failure.

Antithrombin III

Antithrombin III is a plasma alpha$_2$-glycoprotein that accounts for most of the antithrombin activity in plasma and also inhibits other proteolytic enzymes. Hereditary or acquired antithrombin III deficiency results in thromboembolism. The effectiveness of treatment with antithrombin III, prepared as a concentrate from human plasma, is still a matter of dispute (1,2). Apart from vasodilatation, leading to a reduction in blood pressure, remarkably few adverse effects have been noted (2,3). The fall in blood pressure seems to be related to the rate of the infusion.

High doses of antithrombin III, given to patients with severe sepsis, increased the risk of hemorrhage, particularly when it was given concomitantly with heparin, while there was no treatment benefit (4).

Protein C

The protein C pathway serves as a natural defence mechanism against thrombosis. Patients with severe sepsis have a very low concentration of activated protein C compared with healthy individuals. Protein C is available as either a concentrate prepared from human plasma or as recombinant human activated protein C (drotrecogin alfa). The latter increased the risk of bleeding in patients with severe sepsis (5).

Organs and Systems

Cardiovascular

In a phase III trial of drotrecogin alfa, hypertension (2.6 versus 0.6% with placebo) was one of the most frequent adverse effects (6).

Psychological, psychiatric

In a phase III trial, hallucinations occurred in 1.1% of patients treated with drotrecogin alfa versus 0.1% in the placebo group (6).

Hematologic

The predominant adverse effect of activated protein C is bleeding. In a phase III trial, in which 1690 patients with severe sepsis were treated with drotrecogin alfa or placebo, serious bleeding episodes occurred in 3.5% of patients treated with drotrecogin alfa, compared with 2.0% of those treated with placebo (7–9). It has been suggested that the risk of bleeding can be minimized by withholding drotrecogin alfa immediately after major surgery; when surgery must be performed during the treatment period, drotrecogin alfa should be temporarily withdrawn (10,11).

Drotrecogin alfa should be used with care in patients receiving heparin, thrombolytic drugs, oral anticoagulants, glycoprotein IIb-IIIa inhibitors, and aspirin or other antiplatelet drugs (6).

Immunologic

In two of 370 patients treated with drotrecogin alfa during a phase III trial, antibodies to activated protein C were found, but these were not inhibitory; no cases of neutralizing antibodies have been found (7).

Because activated drotrecogin alfa reduces inflammation, it is theoretically possible that there is an increased risk of infection. However, a phase III trial did not show an increased rate of infection in the drotrecogin alfa-treated patients compared with placebo (6).

References

1. Lechner K, Kyrle PA. Antithrombin III concentrates—are they clinically useful? Thromb Haemost 1995;73(3):340–8.
2. Menache D, O'Malley JP, Schorr JB, Wagner B, Williams C, Alving BM, Ballard JO, Goodnight SH, Hathaway WE, Hultin MB, et al. Evaluation of the safety, recovery, half-life, and clinical efficacy of antithrombin III (human) in patients with hereditary antithrombin III deficiency. Cooperative Study Group. Blood 1990;75(1):33–9.
3. Gromnica-Ihle E, Ziemer S. Treatment with AT III concentrates in hereditary and acquired AT III deficiency. Folia Haematol Int Mag Klin Morphol Blutforsch 1988;115(3):307–13.
4. Warren BL, Eid A, Singer P, Pillay SS, Carl P, Novak I, Chalupa P, Atherstone A, Penzes I, Kubler A, Knaub S, Keinecke HO, Heinrichs H, Schindel F, Juers M, Bone RC, Opal SM; KyberSept Trial Study Group. Caring for the critically ill patient. High-dose antithrombin III in severe sepsis: a randomized controlled trial. JAMA 2001;286(15):1869–78.
5. Bernard GR, Vincent JL, Laterre PF, LaRosa SP, Dhainaut JF, Lopez-Rodriguez A, Steingrub JS, Garber GE, Helterbrand JD, Ely EW, Fisher CJ Jr; Recombinant Human Protein C Worldwide Evaluation in Severe Sepsis (PROWESS) Study Group. Efficacy and safety of recombinant human activated protein C for severe sepsis. N Engl J Med 2001;344(10):699–709.
6. Olsen KM, Martin SJ. Pharmacokinetics and clinical use of drotrecogin alfa (activated) in patients with severe sepsis. Pharmacotherapy 2002;22(12 Pt 2):S196–205.
7. Schein RM, Kinasewitz GT. Risk-benefit analysis for drotrecogin alfa (activated). Am J Surg 2002;184(Suppl 6A):S25–38.
8. Dhainaut JF. Introduction: rationale for using drotrecogin alfa (activated) in patients with severe sepsis. Am J Surg 2002;184(Suppl 6A):S5–10.
9. Levi M, De Jonge E, van der Poll T. Recombinant human activated protein C (Xigris). Int J Clin Pract 2002;56(7):542–5.
10. Laterre PF, Heiselman D. Management of patients with severe sepsis, treated by drotrecogin alfa (activated). Am J Surg 2002;184(Suppl 6A):S39–46.
11. Vincent JL, de Carvalho FB, De Backer D. Management of septic shock. Ann Med 2002;34(7–8):606–13.

Antidepressants, second-generation

See also Individual agents

General Information

The newer antidepressants that have followed the monoamine oxidase inhibitors and tricyclic antidepressants are listed in Table 1. Most of them are covered in separate monographs. They have a wide variety of chemical structures and pharmacological profiles, and are categorized as "second generation" antidepressants purely for convenience. Although these drugs are widely considered to be as effective as each other and as any of the older compounds, they have different adverse effects profiles. No new antidepressant has proven to be sufficiently free of adverse effects to establish itself as a routine first line compound; some share similar adverse effects profiles with the tricyclic compounds, while others have novel or unexpected adverse effects. Complete categorization of each compound will rest on wide-scale general use beyond the artificial confines of clinical trials. This also includes the experience that accumulates from cases of overdosage, which cannot be anticipated before a new drug is released. The selective serotonin reuptake inhibitors are dealt with as a separate group, since they have many class-specific adverse effects.

Table 1 Second-generation antidepressants (rINNs except where stated)

Compound	Structure	Comments
Amfebutamone (bupropion)	Aminoketone	Modulates dopaminergic function Increased risk of seizures in high doses
Maprotiline	Tetracyclic	Strong inhibitory effect on noradrenaline uptake Skin rashes (3%) Increased incidence of seizures in overdose Similar adverse effects profile to tricyclic compounds
Mianserin (pINN)	Tetracyclic	Sedative profile Increased incidence of agranulocytosis Possibly safer in overdose Fewer cardiac effects
Milnacipran	Tetracyclic	Inhibitor of serotonin and noradrenaline reuptake
Mirtazapine	Piperazinoazepine	Noradrenergic and specific serotonergic antidepressant (NaSSA); similar to mianserin
Nefazodone	Phenylpiperazine	Weak serotonin reuptake inhibitor Blocks 5-HT$_2$ receptors Chemically related to trazodone
Reboxetine	Morpholine	Selective noradrenaline reuptake inhibitor (NRI or NARI)
Trazodone	Triazolopyridine	Weak effect on serotonin uptake Blocks 5-HT$_2$ receptors Fewer peripheral anticholinergic properties Sedative profile
Tryptophan	Amino acid	Precursor of serotonin Eosinophilia-myalgia syndrome
Venlafaxine	Bicyclic; cyclohexanol	Serotonin and noradrenaline uptake inhibitor Nausea, sexual dysfunction, and cardiovascular adverse effects
Viloxazine	Bicyclic	Fewer anticholinergic or sedative effects and weight gain Causes nausea, vomiting, and weight loss Can precipitate migraine

Antidysrhythmic drugs

See also Individual agents

General Information

Classification

Drugs used in dysrhythmias can be classified in different ways, the usual classification being according to their effects on the cardiac action potential (1), as shown in Table 1.

Antidysrhythmic drugs with Class I activity reduce the rate of the fast inward sodium current during Phase I of the action potential and increase the duration of the effective refractory period expressed as a proportion of the total action potential duration. The action potential duration is itself affected in different ways by subgroups of the Class I drugs:

- class Ia drugs, of which quinidine is the prototype, prolong the action potential;
- class Ib drugs, of which lidocaine is the prototype, shorten the action potential;
- class Ic drugs, of which flecainide is the prototype, do not alter action potential duration.

The beta-adrenoceptor antagonists (class II) and bretylium inhibit the effect of catecholamines on the action potential.

Antidysrhythmic drugs with class III activity prolong the total action potential duration. These drugs act by effects on potassium channels, altering the rate of repolarization.

Antidysrhythmic drugs with class IV activity prolong total action potential duration by prolonging the plateau phase (phase III) of the action potential via calcium channel blockade.

Other classifications of antidysrhythmic drugs have been proposed, but the most useful clinical classification

Table 1 Electrophysiological classification of antidysrhythmic drugs

Class I	Ia	Ib	Ic
	Quinidine	Lidocaine	Flecainide
	Procainamide	Aprindine	Encainide
	Disopyramide	Mexiletine	Lorcainide
		Phenytoin	Propafenone
		Tocainide	(also has class II activity)
Class II	Beta-adrenoceptor antagonists Bretylium		
Class III	Amiodarone Sotalol (d-sotalol; l-sotalol has class II activity)		
Class IV	Verapamil		

relates to the sites of action of the antidysrhythmic drugs on the various cardiac tissues, as shown in Table 2.

General adverse effects

There have been many reviews of the pharmacology, clinical pharmacology, pharmacokinetics, and adverse effects and interactions of antidysrhythmic drugs (2–13).

The patterns of adverse effects of the antidysrhythmic drugs depend on three features:

1. All antidysrhythmic drugs have effects on the cardiac conducting tissues and can all therefore cause cardiac dysrhythmias.
2. All antidysrhythmic drugs have a negative inotropic effect on the heart, and can result in heart failure. However, the degree of negative inotropy varies from drug to drug; for example, it is less marked with drugs such as lidocaine and phenytoin and very marked with the beta-adrenoceptor antagonists, verapamil, and class 1a drugs.
3. Each antidysrhythmic drug has its own non-cardiac effects, which can result in adverse effects. These are summarized in Table 3.

Table 2 Classification of antidysrhythmic drugs by their actions in different parts of the heart

Sinus node	Anomalous pathways	Atria	Ventricles	Atrioventricular node
Class Ic	Class Ia	Class Ia	Class Ia	Class Ic
Class II	Class Ic	Class Ic	Class Ib	Class II
Class IV	Class III	Class III	Class Ic	Class III
				Class IV

Table 3 Non-cardiac adverse effects of some antidysrhythmic drugs

Drug	Common non-cardiac adverse effects
Acecainide	Gastrointestinal and nervous system effects
Adenosine	Flushing, dyspnea
Ajmaline derivatives	Liver damage; agranulocytosis; nervous system effects
Amiodarone	Corneal microdeposits; altered thyroid function; lipofuscin deposition in skin, lungs, liver, nerves, muscles
Aprindine	Agranulocytosis; nervous system effects; liver damage
Cibenzoline	Gastrointestinal and nervous system effects; hypoglycemia
Disopyramide	Anticholinergic effects
Dofetilide	Nervous system effects
Encainide	Nervous system effects
Flecainide	Nervous system effects
Lidocaine	Nervous system effects
Lorcainide	Nervous system effects
Mexiletine	Nervous system effects
Moracizine	Nervous system effects
Procainamide	Lupus-like syndrome; neutropenia
Propafenone	Nervous system effects
Quinidine	Anticholinergic effects; hypersusceptibility reactions
Tocainide	Nervous system effects

Clinical studies

The efficacy of a large range of antidysrhythmic drugs in converting atrial fibrillation to sinus rhythm acutely and in maintaining it during long-term treatment has been the subject of a systematic review (14). Adverse effects were too sporadically reported to be suitable for proper review. The efficacy results are summarized in Table 4.

There is some doubt about whether conversion to sinus rhythm produces a better long-term outcome than rate control. Five randomized controlled comparisons of rhythm control versus rate control, mostly in patients with persistent atrial fibrillation ($n = 5175$ in all), have all suggested that there are no major differences in beneficial outcomes between the two strategies (15,16), although there were fewer adverse drug reactions in patients randomized to rate control in three of the studies and in all the studies rate control was associated with fewer hospital admissions. Furthermore, in an analysis of cost-effectiveness, rate control plus warfarin was much cheaper than rhythm control in preventing thromboembolism, largely because of the use of expensive modern antidysrhythmic drugs for the latter (17). Although these results suggest that rate control might be preferable to rhythm control, they do not give any information about patients in whom sinus rhythm is established permanently after pharmacological or physical conversion, since many of the patients in whom rhythm control is used as a strategy will actually have paroxysmal atrial fibrillation.

Organs and Systems

Cardiovascular

Cardiac dysrhythmias

Antidysrhythmic drugs can themselves cause cardiac dysrhythmias, their major adverse effect. The risk of antidysrhythmic-induced cardiac dysrhythmias (prodysrhythmic effects) has been estimated at about 11–13% in non-invasive studies (18,19) and at up to 20% in invasive electrophysiological studies. However, the risk varies from drug to drug and is particularly low with class III drugs. In one study the quoted risks of dysrhythmias were: flecainide 30%, quinidine 18%, propafenone 7%, sotalol 6%, and amiodarone 0% (20). However, amiodarone does cause dysrhythmias, especially when the QT_c interval is over 600 ms.

The prodysrhythmic effects of antidysrhythmic drugs have been extensively reviewed (21–36).

Dysrhythmias secondary to antidysrhythmic drugs are arbitrarily defined as either early (within 30 days of starting treatment) or late (22,23). A lack of early dysrhythmias in response to antidysrhythmic drugs does not predict the risk of late dysrhythmias (24).

Ventricular dysrhythmias due to drugs may be either monomorphic or polymorphic. The class Ia drugs are particularly likely to cause polymorphic dysrhythmias, as is amiodarone (although to a lesser extent). In contrast, the class Ic drugs are more likely to cause monomorphic dysrhythmias (25).

Class Ic antidysrhythmic drugs have been reported to cause the characteristic electrocardiographic changes of Brugada syndrome, which consists of right bundle branch block, persistent ST segment elevation, and sudden

Table 4 The results of a systematic review of the efficacy of antidysrhythmic drugs in converting atrial fibrillation to sinus rhythm and maintaining it

Drug	Number of subjects	Efficacy in converting AF to sinus rhythm (odds ratio versus other drugs[1])	Efficacy in maintaining sinus rhythm (odds ratio versus other drugs[1])	Ventricular dysrhythmias[2] (%)	Other dysrhythmias[3] (%)	Drug withdrawal or dosage reduction (%)
Amiodarone	108	5.7		0–15	0–9	
Disopyramide	30	7.0	3.4	0	0	0–55
Dofetilide/ibutilide	530	29.0		3–9		
Flecainide	169	25.0	3.1	0–2	0–12	0–20
Propafenone	1168	4.6	3.7	0–3	0–17	0–55
Quinidine	200	2.9	4.1	0–12	0–28	0–58
Sotalol	34	0.4	7.1	0–1	2–44	4–44

[1] Digoxin, diltiazem, or verapamil
[2] Ventricular fibrillation, polymorphic ventricular tachycardia, torsade de pointes
[3] Symptomatic bradycardia, junctional rhythm, non-sustained and/or monomorphic ventricular tachycardia

cardiac death, in two patients (37). Class Ia drugs did not cause the same effect.

The prodysrhythmic effects of antidysrhythmic drugs have been reviewed in discussions of the pharmacological conversion of atrial fibrillation (38) and the relative benefits of rate control in atrial fibrillation or maintaining sinus rhythm after cardioversion (39).

Mechanisms
There are four major mechanisms whereby antidysrhythmic drugs cause dysrhythmias (21):

1. Worsening of a pre-existing dysrhythmia. For example, ventricular extra beats can be converted to ventricular tachycardia or the ventricular rate in atrial flutter can be accelerated when slowing of the atrial rate results in the conduction of an increased number of atrial impulses through the AV node.
2. The induction of heart block or suppression of an escape mechanism. For example, slowing of conduction through the AV node can impair a mechanism that allows the conducting system to escape a re-entry mechanism.
3. The uncovering of a hidden mechanism of dysrhythmia. For example, antidysrhythmic drugs can cause early or delayed afterdepolarizations, which can result in dysrhythmias.
4. The induction of a new mechanism of dysrhythmia. For example, a patient in whom myocardial ischemia has predisposed to dysrhythmias may be more at risk when an antidysrhythmic drug alters conduction.

Combinations of these different mechanisms are also possible.

The prodysrhythmic effects of antidysrhythmic drugs have been reviewed, with regard to mechanisms at the cellular level (40) and molecular level (41). As far as the cellular mechanisms are concerned, the antidysrhythmic drugs have been divided into three classes (which do not overlap with the classes specified in the electrophysiological classification).

1. Group 1 drugs have fast-onset kinetics and the block saturates at rapid rates (about 300 beats/minute).
2. Group 2 drugs have slow-onset kinetics and the block saturates at rapid rates.
3. Group 3 drugs have slow-onset kinetics and there is saturation of frequency-dependent block at slow heart rates (about 100 beats/minute).

The fast-onset kinetics of the Group 1 drugs makes them the least likely to cause dysrhythmias. Group 2 drugs, which include encainide, flecainide, procainamide, and quinidine, are the most likely to cause dysrhythmias, because of their slow-onset kinetics. Although this also applies to the Group 3 drugs, which include propafenone and disopyramide, block is less likely to occur during faster heart rates and serious dysrhythmias are therefore less likely during exercise.

The most common mechanism of dysrhythmias at the molecular level is by inhibition of the potassium channels known as IK_r, which are encoded by the human ether-a-go-go-related gene (HERG). The antidysrhythmic drugs that affect these channels include almokalant, amiodarone, azimilide, bretylium, dofetilide, ibutilide, sematilide, D-sotalol, and tedisamil (all drugs with Class III actions) and bepridil, disopyramide, prenylamine, procainamide, propafenone, quinidine, and terodiline (all drugs with Class I actions). Other drugs that affect these channels but are not used to treat cardiac dysrhythmias include astemizole and terfenadine (antihistamines), cisapride, erythromycin, haloperidol, sertindole, and thioridazine.

Susceptibility factors
There are no good predictors of the occurrence of dysrhythmias, but there are several susceptibility factors (26,27), including a history of sustained tachydysrhythmias, poor left ventricular function, and myocardial ischemia. Potassium depletion and prolongation of the QT interval are particularly important, and these particularly predispose to polymorphous ventricular dysrhythmias (for example torsade de pointes). Altered metabolism of antidysrhythmic drugs (for example liver disease, polymorphic acetylation or hydroxylation, and drug interactions) can also contribute.

The prodysrhythmic effects of antidysrhythmic drugs have been reviewed in the context of whether patients who are to be given class I or class III antidysrhythmic drugs should first be admitted to hospital for observation in the hope of identifying those who are most likely to develop dysrhythmias (20). The risk of sudden death in patients taking amiodarone was significantly increased in those who had had a prior bout of torsade de pointes. The risk of sotalol-induced torsade de pointes was higher in patients with pre-existing heart failure. Women are at a greater risk of prodysrhythmic drug effects (SEDA-18, 199). The highest risk was in women with heart failure who took more than 320 mg/day (22%); the corresponding figure in men was 8%. The authors delineated certain subgroups that they considered to be at specific risk of dysrhythmias, listing drugs that should be avoided in those subjects. They recommended avoiding drugs of classes Ia and III in women without coronary artery disease, drugs of class Ic in men with coronary artery disease, and drugs of classes Ia, Ic, and III in men with congestive heart failure and women with coronary artery disease.

Factors that predict atrial flutter with 1:1 conduction as a prodysrhythmic effect of class I antidysrhythmic drugs (cibenzoline, disopyramide, flecainide, propafenone, and quinidine) have been studied in 24 patients (aged 46–78 years) with 1:1 atrial flutter and in 100 controls (42). Underlying heart disease was present in nine patients. There was a short PR interval (PR < 0.13 ms) with normal P wave duration in leads V5 and V6 in nine of the 26 patients and only seven of the 100 controls. Signal-averaged electrocardiography showed pseudofusion between the P wave and QRS complex in 19 of the 26 patients and only 11 of the 100 controls. There was rapid atrioventricular nodal conduction (a short AH interval or second-degree atrioventricular block during atrial pacing at over 200 minute) in 19 of the 23 patients. Pseudofusion of the P wave and QRS complex had a sensitivity of 100% and a specificity of 89% for the prediction of an atrial prodysrhythmic effect of class I antidysrhythmic drugs.

Reducing the risk
The methods for minimizing the risks of prodysrhythmic effects of antidysrhythmic drugs (43) are as follows:

- Care in choosing those who are likely to benefit from antidysrhythmic drug therapy.
- Identification and correction, if possible, of impaired pump function and ischemic damage.
- Correction of electrolyte abnormalities.
- Exercise testing before and during the early stages of drug therapy: widening of the QRS complex during exercise predicts a high risk of ventricular tachycardia as does prolongation of the QT interval.
- Instruction of patients about the signs and symptoms that can occur with dysrhythmias.
- Monitoring renal and hepatic function in order to predict reduced drug elimination.
- Avoiding drug interactions or changing the dosage of the antidysrhythmic drug in anticipation of a change in its disposition secondary to an interaction.

Measurement of the concentrations of antidysrhythmic drugs and their metabolites in the plasma can be useful in recognizing the need for changing dosage requirements when cardiac, hepatic, or renal dysfunction occurs, in maintaining serum drug or metabolite concentrations within optimal ranges, and for predicting dosage changes required when interacting drugs are added (28). However, in most hospitals plasma drug concentration measurement is not routinely available for these drugs.

Another strategy for reducing the risk of prodysrhythmias is to use combinations of different classes of antidysrhythmic drugs in lower dosages than those used in monotherapy.

Torsade de pointes can be prevented by withholding antidysrhythmic drug therapy from patients who have pre-existing prolongation of the QT interval, and by correction of low serum potassium and magnesium concentrations before therapy. During therapy patients at risk should have frequent monitoring of the electrocardiogram and serum electrolytes.

The prodysrhythmic risks of using antidysrhythmic drugs have been mentioned in the context of a set of guidelines on the management of patients with atrial fibrillation (44,45). The recommended drugs for maintaining sinus rhythm after cardioversion vary depending on the presence of different risk factors for dysrhythmias:

- heart failure: amiodarone and dofetilide;
- coronary artery disease: sotalol and amiodarone;
- hypertensive heart disease: propafenone and flecainide.

Management
The management of drug-induced cardiac dysrhythmias includes withdrawal of the drug and the administration of potassium if necessary to maintain the serum potassium concentration at over 4.5 mmol/l and magnesium sulfate (SEDA-23, 196). Magnesium sulfate is given intravenously on a dose of 2 g over 2–3 minutes, followed by continuous intravenous infusion at a rate of 2–4 mg/minute; if the dysrhythmia recurs, another bolus of 2 g should be given and the infusion rate increased to 6–8 mg/minute; rarely, a third bolus of 2 g may be required (46). If magnesium is ineffective, cardiac pacing should be tried.

There is some anecdotal evidence that atrioventricular nodal blockade with verapamil or a beta-blocker can also be effective. However, in two cases the addition of a beta-blocker (either atenolol or metoprolol) to treatment with class I antidysrhythmic drugs (cibenzoline in one case and flecainide in the other) did not prevent the occurrence of atrial flutter with a 1:1 response (47). However, the author suggested that in these cases, although the beta-blockers had not suppressed the dysrhythmia, they had at least improved the patient's tolerance of it. In both cases the uses of class I antidysrhythmic drugs was contraindicated by virtue of structural damage, in the first case due to mitral valvular disease and in the second due to an ischemic cardiomyopathy.

Adverse hemodynamic effects of antidysrhythmic drugs
Many antidysrhythmic drugs have negative inotropic effects (48–50). This means that such drugs should be avoided in patients with a history of heart failure, a low left ventricular ejection fraction, or a cardiomyopathy. The general risk of induction or a worsening of heart failure is up to about 5%, but those who have risk factors have a risk of up to 10%. The negative inotropic effects are most marked with drugs of classes Ia, Ic, II, and IV. For drugs with class I activity there is a strong relation between their negative inotropic effect and the extent to which they block the inward sodium current (50). Thus, class Ib drugs that are associated with a short recovery time of sodium channels have a smaller negative inotropic effect than class Ia drugs, which in turn have less of an effect than class Ic drugs. However, the overall hemodynamic effects of antidysrhythmic drugs depend not only on their negative inotropic effects on the heart, but also on their effects on the peripheral circulation (51). Thus, although all drugs with class I activity have similar negative inotropic effects on the heart, disopyramide has large hemodynamic effects (because it increases

Table 5 Some important drug–drug interactions with antidysrhythmic drugs

Object drug(s)	Precipitant drug(s)	Result of interaction
Adenosine	Dipyridamole	Increased effect
Adenosine	Theophylline	Reduced effect
Anticholinergic drugs	Disopyramide, quinidine	Potentiation
Antihypertensive drugs	Bretylium	Severe hypotension
Beta-adrenoceptor antagonists	Propafenone	Potentiation
Class I drugs	Beta-adrenoceptor antagonists	Negative inotropy
Class I drugs	Class I drugs	Potentiation
Class I drugs	Drugs that cause potassium depletion	Prodysrhythmic effects
Digoxin	Amiodarone, quinidine, verapamil	Digoxin toxicity
Disopyramide	Enzyme-inducing drugs	Increased metabolism
Neuromuscular blockers	Quinidine	Potentiation
Procainamide	Cimetidine, trimethoprim	Reduced metabolism
Quinidine	Enzyme-inducing drugs	Increased metabolism
Theophylline	Mexiletine	Cardiac dysrhythmias
Verapamil	Beta-adrenoceptor antagonists	Negative inotropy/bradycardia/asystole
Warfarin	Amiodarone, quinidine	Warfarin toxicity

peripheral resistance) and its hemodynamic effect is therefore greater than that of mexiletine, for example. Similarly the adverse hemodynamic effects of encainide and tocainide are greater than those of procainamide (52).

Death

Sudden death due to antidysrhythmic drugs has been reported in several trials in patients who have had ventricular dysrhythmias after myocardial infarction. The drugs that have been incriminated include disopyramide, encainide, flecainide, mexiletine, moracizine, procainamide, and quinidine (53–59). The class III drug d-sotalol has also been associated with an increased risk of mortality in such patients (60). This increase in mortality is thought to be due to an increased risk of cardiac dysrhythmias, perhaps as a consequence of rate-dependent conduction block and preferential slowing of conduction in the ischemic areas. Cardiac dysrhythmias of this sort may also occur through slowing of the rate of conduction around non-conducting ischemic or infracted areas in the heart.

Susceptibility Factors

Age

The safety of antidysrhythmic drugs in children has not been thoroughly studied. However, the risk of prolongation of the QT interval seems to be considerably less than that in adults (61), although it has been reported with quinidine, disopyramide, amiodarone, sotalol, and diphemanil.

Drug Administration

Drug overdose

The use of techniques of circulatory support (extracorporeal oxygenation and intra-aortic balloon pump) in seven cases of overdose with antidysrhythmic drugs (disopyramide, flecainide, prajmaline, and quinidine) has been reviewed (62).

Drug–Drug Interactions

General

Some important drug–drug interactions with antidysrhythmic drugs are summarized in Table 5.

References

1. Vaughan Williams EM. A classification of antiarrhythmic actions reassessed after a decade of new drugs. J Clin Pharmacol 1984;24(4):129–47.
2. Mason DT, DeMaria AN, Amsterdam EA, Zelis R, Massumi RA. Antiarrhythmic agents. Drugs 1973;5(4):261–317.
3. Winkle RA, Glantz SA, Harrison DC. Pharmacologic therapy of ventricular arrhythmias. Am J Cardiol 1975;36(5):629–50.
4. Singh BN. Side effects of antiarrhythmic drugs. Pharmacol Ther 1977;2:151.
5. Harrison DC, Meffin PJ, Winkle RA. Clinical pharmacokinetics of antiarrhythmic drugs. Prog Cardiovasc Dis 1977;20(3):217–42.
6. Anderson JL, Harrison DC, Meffin PJ, Winkle RA. Antiarrhythmic drugs: clinical pharmacology and therapeutic uses. Drugs 1978;15(4):271–309.
7. Zipes DP, Troup PJ. New antiarrhythmic agents: amiodarone, aprindine, disopyramide, ethmozin, mexiletine, tocainide, verapamil. Am J Cardiol 1978;41(6):1005–24.
8. Nattel S, Zipes DP. Clinical pharmacology of old and new antiarrhythmic drugs. Cardiovasc Clin 1980;11(1):221–48.
9. Schwartz JB, Keefe D, Harrison DC. Adverse effects of antiarrhythmic drugs. Drugs 1981;21(1):23–45.
10. Keefe DL, Kates RE, Harrison DC. New antiarrhythmic drugs: their place in therapy. Drugs 1981;22(5):363–400.
11. Kowey PR, Marinchak RA, Rials SJ, Bharucha DB. Intravenous antiarrhythmic therapy in the acute control of in-hospital destabilizing ventricular tachycardia and fibrillation. Am J Cardiol 1999;84(9A):R46–51.
12. Lip GYH, Kamath S. Adverse reactions of drugs used to treat arrhythmia. Adverse Drug React Bull 2000;201:767–70.
13. Wooten JM, Earnest J, Reyes J. Review of common adverse effects of selected antiarrhythmic drugs. Crit Care Nurs Q 2000;22(4):23–38.

14. Miller MR, McNamara RL, Segal JB, Kim N, Robinson KA, Goodman SN, Powe NR, Bass EB. Efficacy of agents for pharmacologic conversion of atrial fibrillation and subsequent maintenance of sinus rhythm: a meta-analysis of clinical trials. J Fam Pract 2000;49(11):1033–46.

15. Gronefeld G, Hohnloser SH. Rhythm or rate control in atrial fibrillation: insights from the randomized controlled trials. J Cardiovasc Pharmacol Ther 2003;8(Suppl 1):S39–44.

16. Wyse DG. Rhythm versus rate control trials in atrial fibrillation. J Cardiovasc Electrophysiol 2003;14(Suppl 9):S35–9.

17. The Research Group for Antiarrhythmic Drug Therapy. Cost-Effectiveness of antiarrhythmic drugs for prevention of thromboembolism in patients with paroxysmal atrial fibrillation. Jpn Circ J 2001;65(9):765–8.

18. Rinkenberger RL, Prystowsky EN, Jackman WM, Naccarelli GV, Heger JJ, Zipes DP. Drug conversion of nonsustained ventricular tachycardia to sustained ventricular tachycardia during serial electrophysiologic studies: identification of drugs that exacerbate tachycardia and potential mechanisms. Am Heart J 1982;103(2):177–84.

19. Velebit V, Podrid P, Lown B, Cohen BH, Graboys TB. Aggravation and provocation of ventricular arrhythmias by antiarrhythmic drugs. Circulation 1982;65(5):886–94.

20. Thibault B, Nattel S. Optimal management with Class I and Class III antiarrhythmic drugs should be done in the outpatient setting: protagonist. J Cardiovasc Electrophysiol 1999;10(3):472–81.

21. Wellens HJ, Smeets JL, Vos M, Gorgels AP. Antiarrhythmic drug treatment: need for continuous vigilance. Br Heart J 1992;67(1):25–33.

22. Morganroth J. Early and late proarrhythmia from antiarrhythmic drug therapy. Cardiovasc Drugs Ther 1992;6(1):11–14.

23. Morganroth J. Proarrhythmic effects of antiarrhythmic drugs: evolving concepts. Am Heart J 1992;123(4 Pt 2):1137–9.

24. Hilleman DE, Mohiuddin SM, Gannon JM. Adverse reactions during acute and chronic class I antiarrhythmic therapy. Curr Ther Res 1992;51:730–8.

25. Hilleman DE, Larsen KE. Proarrhythmic effects of antiarrhythmic drugs. PT 1991;June:520–4.

26. Libersa C, Caron J, Guedon-Moreau L, Adamantidis M, Nisse C. Adverse cardiovascular effects of anti-arrhythmia drugs. Part I: Proarrhythmic effects. Therapie 1992;47(3):193–8.

27. Podrid PJ, Fogel RI. Aggravation of arrhythmia by antiarrhythmic drugs, and the important role of underlying ischemia. Am J Cardiol 1992;70(1):100–2.

28. Follath F. Clinical pharmacology of antiarrhythmic drugs: variability of metabolism and dose requirements. J Cardiovasc Pharmacol 1991;17(Suppl 6):S74–6.

29. Cowan JC, Coulshed DS, Zaman AG. Antiarrhythmic therapy and survival following myocardial infarction. J Cardiovasc Pharmacol 1991;18(Suppl 2):S92–8.

30. Friedman L, Schron E, Yusuf S. Risk-benefit assessment of antiarrhythmic drugs. An epidemiological perspective. Drug Saf 1991;6(5):323–31.

31. Furberg CD, Yusuf S. Antiarrhythmics and VPD suppression. Circulation 1991;84(2):928–30.

32. Luderitz B. Möglichkeiten und Grenzen der Arrhythmiebehandlung. [Possibilities and limitations of treatment for arrhythmia.] Z Gesamte Inn Med 1991;46(12):425–30.

33. Podrid PJ. Safety and toxicity of antiarrhythmic drug therapy: benefit versus risk. J Cardiovasc Pharmacol 1991;17(Suppl 6):S65–73.

34. Zimmermann M. Antiarrhythmic therapy for ventricular arrhythmias. J Cardiovasc Pharmacol 1991;17(Suppl 6):S59–64.

35. Fauchier JP, Babuty D, Fauchier L, Rouesnel P, Cosnay P. Les effets proarythmiques des antiarythmiques. [Proarrhythmic effects of antiarrhythmic drugs.] Arch Mal Coeur Vaiss 1992;85(6):891–7.

36. Leenhardt A, Coumel P, Slama R. Torsade de pointes. J Cardiovasc Electrophysiol 1992;3:281–92.

37. Fujiki A, Usui M, Nagasawa H, Mizumaki K, Hayashi H, Inoue H. ST segment elevation in the right precordial leads induced with class IC antiarrhythmic drugs: insight into the mechanism of Brugada syndrome. J Cardiovasc Electrophysiol 1999;10(2):214–18.

38. Boriani G. New options for pharmacological conversion of atrial fibrillation. Card Electrophysiol Rev 2001;5:195–200.

39. Donahue TP, Conti JB. Atrial fibrillation: rate control versus maintenance of sinus rhythm. Curr Opin Cardiol 2001;16(1):46–53.

40. Chaudhry GM, Haffajee CI. Antiarrhythmic agents and proarrhythmia. Crit Care Med 2000;28(Suppl 10):N158–64.

41. Witchel HJ, Hancox JC. Familial and acquired long QT syndrome and the cardiac rapid delayed rectifier potassium current. Clin Exp Pharmacol Physiol 2000;27(10):753–66.

42. Brembilla-Perrot B, Houriez P, Beurrier D, Claudon O, Terrier de la Chaise A, Louis P. Predictors of atrial flutter with 1:1 conduction in patients treated with class I antiarrhythmic drugs for atrial tachyarrhythmias. Int J Cardiol 2001;80(1):7–15.

43. Feldman AM, Bristow MR, Parmley WW, Carson PE, Pepine CJ, Gilbert EM, Strobeck JE, Hendrix GH, Powers ER, Bain RP, et al. Effects of vesnarinone on morbidity and mortality in patients with heart failure. Vesnarinone Study Group. N Engl J Med 1993;329(3):149–55.

44. Fuster V, Rydèn LE, Asinger RW, Cannom DS, Crijns HJ, Frye RL, Halperin JL, Kay GN, Klein WW, Levy S, McNamara RL, Prystowsky EN, Wann LS, Wyse DG, Gibbons RJ, Antman EM, Alpert JS, Faxon DP, Fuster V, Gregoratos G, Hiratzka LF, Jacobs AK, Russell RO, Smith SC Jr, Klein WW, Alonso-Garcia A, Blomstrom-Lundqvist C, de Backer G, Flather M, Hradec J, Oto A, Parkhomenko A, Silber S, Torbicki A. American College of Cardiology/American Heart Association Task Force on Practice Guidelines; European Society of Cardiology Committee for Practice Guidelines and Policy Conferences (Committee to Develop Guidelines for the Management of Patients with Atrial Fibrillation); North American Society of Pacing and Electrophysiology. ACC/AHA/ESC Guidelines for the Management of Patients with Atrial Fibrillation: Executive Summary. A Report of the American College of Cardiology/American Heart Association Task Force on Practice Guidelines and the European Society of Cardiology Committee for Practice Guidelines and Policy Conferences (Committee to Develop Guidelines for the Management of Patients with Atrial Fibrillation) Developed in Collaboration with the North American Society of Pacing and Electrophysiology. Circulation 2001;104(17):2118–50.

45. Fuster V, Ryden LE, Asinger RW, Cannom DS, Crijns HJ, Frye RL, Halperin JL, Kay GN, Klein WW, Levy S, McNamara RL, Prystowsky EN, Wann LS, Wyse DG. American College of Cardiology; American Heart Association; European Society of Cardiology; North American Society of Pacing and Electrophysiology. ACC/AHA/ESC Guidelines for the Management of Patients with Atrial Fibrillation. A report of the American College of Cardiology/American Heart Association Task Force on Practice Guidelines and the European Society of Cardiology Committee for Practice Guidelines and Policy Conferences (Committee to Develop Guidelines for the Management of Patients with Atrial Fibrillation) developed in collaboration with the

North American Society of Pacing and Electrophysiology. Eur Heart J 2001;22(20):1852–923.

46. Banai S, Tzivoni D. Drug therapy for torsade de pointes. J Cardiovasc Electrophysiol 1993;4(2):206–10.

47. Brembilla-Perrot B, Houriez P, Claudon O, Yassine M, Suty-Selton C, Vancon AC, Abo el Makarem Y, Makarem E, Courtelour JM. Les effets proarythmiques supraventricularires des antiarythmiques de classe IC sont-ils prévenus par l'association avec des bétabloquants? [Can the supraventricular proarrhythmic effects of class 1C antiarrhythmic drugs be prevented with the association of beta blockers?] Ann Cardiol Angeiol (Paris) 2000;49(8):439–42.

48. Scholz H. Antiarrhythmischer und Kardiodepressive Wirkungen antiarrhythmischer Substanzen. [Anti-arrhythmic and cardiodepressive effects of anti-arrhythmia agents.] Z Kardiol 1988;77(Suppl 5):113–19.

49. Luderitz B, Manz M. Hämodynamic bei ventrikularen Rhythmusstörungen und bei ihrer Behandlung. [Hemodynamics in ventricular arrhythmias and in their treatment.] Z Kardiol 1988;77(Suppl 5):143–9.

50. Schlepper M. Cardiodepressive effects of antiarrhythmic drugs. Eur Heart J 1989;10(Suppl E):73–80.

51. Seipel L, Hoffmeister HM. Hemodynamic effects of antiarrhythmic drugs: negative inotropy versus influence on peripheral circulation. Am J Cardiol 1989;64(20):J37–40.

52. Hammermeister KE. Adverse hemodynamic effects of antiarrhythmic drugs in congestive heart failure. Circulation 1990;81(3):1151–3.

53. The Cardiac Arrhythmia Suppression Trial (CAST) Investigators. Preliminary report: effect of encainide and flecainide on mortality in a randomized trial of arrhythmia suppression after myocardial infarction. N Engl J Med 1989;321(6):406–12.

54. The Cardiac Arrhythmia Suppression Trial II Investigators. Effect of the antiarrhythmic agent moricizine on survival after myocardial infarction. N Engl J Med 1992;327(4):227–33.

55. Impact Research Group. International mexiletine and placebo antiarrhythmic coronary trial: I. Report on arrhythmia and other findings. J Am Coll Cardiol 1984;4(6):1148–63.

56. Coplen SE, Antman EM, Berlin JA, Hewitt P, Chalmers TC. Efficacy and safety of quinidine therapy for maintenance of sinus rhythm after cardioversion. A meta-analysis of randomized control trials. Circulation 1990;82(4):1106–16. Erratum in: Circulation 1991;83(2):714.

57. Flaker GC, Blackshear JL, McBride R, Kronmal RA, Halperin JL, Hart RG. Antiarrhythmic drug therapy and cardiac mortality in atrial fibrillation. The Stroke Prevention in Atrial Fibrillation Investigators. J Am Coll Cardiol 1992;20(3):527–32.

58. Nattel S, Hadjis T, Talajic M. The treatment of atrial fibrillation. An evaluation of drug therapy, electrical modalities and therapeutic considerations. Drugs 1994;48(3):345–71.

59. Moosvi AR, Goldstein S, VanderBrug Medendorp S, Landis JR, Wolfe RA, Leighton R, Ritter G, Vasu CM, Acheson A. Effect of empiric antiarrhythmic therapy in resuscitated out-of-hospital cardiac arrest victims with coronary artery disease. Am J Cardiol 1990;65(18):1192–7.

60. Waldo AL, Camm AJ, deRuyter H, Friedman PL, MacNeil DJ, Pauls JF, Pitt B, Pratt CM, Schwartz PJ, Veltri EP. Effect of d-sotalol on mortality in patients with left ventricular dysfunction after recent and remote myocardial infarction. The SWORD Investigators. Survival With Oral d-Sotalol. Lancet 1996;348(9019):7–12. Erratum in: Lancet 1996;348(9024):416.

61. Villain E. Les syndromes de QT long chez l'enfant. [Long QT syndromes in children.] Arch Fr Pediatr 1993;50(3):241–7.

62. Bosquet C, Jaeger A. Exceptional treatments in toxic circulatory and respiratory failures. Reanim Urgences 2001; 10:402–11.

Antiepileptic drugs

See also Individual agents

General Information

Over 15 drugs are licensed worldwide for the treatment of epilepsy and are the subject of separate monographs. Some of them can be grouped into classes (carbamazepine and its analogue oxcarbazepine, barbiturates, hydantoins, benzodiazepines, and succinimides), while others (for example valproate, felbamate, gabapentin, levetiracetam, lamotrigine, tiagabine, topiramate, vigabatrin, and zonisamide) stand on their own. Individual drugs differ in their spectra of activity and in adverse effects profiles. For adverse effects that occur with all drugs, frequency and severity vary from one agent to another: for example, sedation is more common with barbiturates and benzodiazepines, ataxia and diplopia are more common with phenytoin and carbamazepine, and aplastic anemia is more common with felbamate. Certain adverse effects are related to specific properties shared only by certain drugs: for example, renal stones can occur with drugs causing carbonic anhydrase inhibition (acetazolamide, topiramate, zonisamide), whereas reduced efficacy of oral contraceptives can occur with inducers of isozymes that metabolize these steroids (carbamazepine, oxcarbazepine, phenytoin, barbiturates, felbamate, and topiramate).

The clinical pharmacology and adverse effects of some new antiepileptic drugs (ganaxolone, levetiracetam, losigamone, pregabalin, remacemide, rufinamide, stiripentol, and zonisamide) have been reviewed (1).

The uses and adverse effects of antiepileptic drugs in the treatment of painful peripheral neuropathy have been reviewed (2).

Clinical studies

Efficacy and tolerability data from double-blind, placebo-controlled add-on trials of new antiepileptic drugs in patients with refractory partial epilepsy have been reviewed (3). Although there were differences in adverse events profiles among the various drugs, the review identified major methodological problems, which hamper comparisons across studies and drugs. These included variability in the use of COSTART terminology, marked differences in the occurrence of specific adverse events in the placebo groups (an indication of heterogeneous evaluation procedures), and the use of non-optimal dosages or non-optimal titration schedules in many trials (3).

In a multicenter, randomized, double-blind comparison of diazepam (0.15 mg/kg followed by phenytoin 18 mg/kg), lorazepam (0.1 mg/kg), phenobarbital (15 mg/kg), and phenytoin (18 mg/kg) in 518 patients with generalized convulsive status epilepticus, lorazepam was more effective than phenytoin and at least as effective as phenobarbital or diazepam plus phenytoin (4). Drug-related adverse effects did not differ significantly among treatments and included hypoventilation (up to 17%), hypotension (up to 59%), and cardiac rhythm disturbances (up to 9%).

Comparisons of different antiepileptic drugs

Quality of life
The effects of carbamazepine and lamotrigine on health-related quality of life have been compared for 1 year in 260 patients with newly diagnosed epilepsy randomized to 48 weeks of treatment (5). Patients taking carbamazepine had significantly worse quality of life at week 4 but not later. They also had more cognitive adverse effects in general and more changes in energy and affect during the first 4 weeks of treatment.

Cost-effectiveness
The cost-effectiveness of four antiepileptic drugs used to treat newly diagnosed adult epilepsy has been studied by cost minimization analysis in 12 European countries (6). The analysis took account of each drug's adverse effects and tolerability profiles. Lamotrigine incurred higher costs than carbamazepine, phenytoin, and valproate, whose costs were similar.

Withdrawal of therapy
Gabapentin, lamotrigine, topiramate, and vigabatrin have been compared using Kaplan–Meier survival analysis in 61 patients to see how long they chose to keep taking each drug and, if they stopped, why they stopped (7). The results are shown in Table 1. Lamotrigine seemed to be the best tolerated of the four drugs and topiramate the least. These results have been mirrored by those of two larger retrospective studies (8,9).

Gabapentin and vigabatrin as first-line add-on treatments have been compared in 102 patients with partial epilepsy (10). The improvement rate was 48% with gabapentin and 56% with vigabatrin. There were seven withdrawals in each group because of adverse events. Of the serious adverse events only one was thought to be drug-related—depression and weight gain in a patient taking vigabatrin.

General adverse reactions
The use of antiepileptic drugs (gabapentin, lamotrigine, and topiramate) as mood stabilizers has been reviewed (11). The authors concluded that the benefit : harm ratios of these drugs have not been well enough established for their routine use in bipolar disorder.

Carbamazepine and valproic acid have been compared in a randomized study in 30 patients (12). Significantly more patients taking carbamazepine reported adverse events, including nausea and vomiting, dizziness, lethargy, and ataxia and tremors.

In a comparison of carbamazepine and lamotrigine for trigeminal neuralgia in 18 patients with multiple sclerosis, lamotrigine was more effective (13). After withdrawal of carbamazepine, drowsiness resolved in 16 patients; cerebellar signs improved partially in five patients and completely in two; brainstem signs improved partially in four patients and completely in 3; ambulation improved in 11. In one patient taking lamotrigine a skin rash forced withdrawal.

General adverse reactions

The most important adverse effects of antiepileptic drugs affect the central nervous system and include sedation, fatigue, dizziness, cognitive dysfunction, ataxia, dysarthria, nystagmus, and headache. These effects are often dose-related; they are more prominent with multiple drug therapy and they are usually reversible after dosage adjustment. Behavioral disturbances are relatively common, especially in children and in patients with pre-existing mental handicap. Exacerbation of seizures and psychiatric reactions are not uncommon. Hepatotoxic reactions have especially been reported with felbamate, valproate, carbamazepine, and phenytoin. Endocrine and metabolic changes occur with most drugs, but their clinical relevance is usually limited. Carbamazepine, phenytoin, barbiturates, and to a lesser extent felbamate, topiramate, and oxcarbazepine, are enzyme inducers, whereas felbamate and valproate are enzyme inhibitors. These effects cause significant drug interactions. Most anticonvulsants precipitate attacks in patients with acute intermittent porphyria.

Hypersusceptibility reactions
Hypersusceptibility reactions can involve any system, but they most often affect the skin, leading to drug withdrawal in up to 20% of patients. Aplastic anemia and hepatotoxicity have drastically curtailed the use of felbamate.

Table 1   Persistence with therapy with different antiepileptic drugs in different studies

	Gabapentin	Lamotrigine	Tiagabine	Topiramate	Vigabatrin
Number (Datta and Crawford; 8)	36	37	—	28	26
Median time to 50% drop out (months)	13	>43	—	9.5	29
Withdrawn owing to lack of efficacy (%)	58	24	—	25	62
Number (Lhatoo et al. 9)	146	122	88	70	37
Withdrawn owing to lack of efficacy (%)	25	16	30	30	46
Withdrawn owing to adverse effects (%)	16	15	26	42	16
Number (Lindberger et al. 10)	158	424	—	393	—
Withdrawn owing to lack of efficacy (%)	39	34	—	19	—
Withdrawn owing to adverse effects (%)	37	22	—	40	—

Tumorigenesis

Pseudolymphoma and a condition resembling malignant lymphoma occur very rarely with phenytoin. There is no evidence of a significant increase in the incidence of other tumors.

Second-generation effects

The use of older antiepileptic drugs in pregnancy is associated with a two- to three-fold increase in the risk of fetal malformations, including facial clefts and cardiac defects. Neural tube defects, including spina bifida, are seen in 2–3% of offspring exposed to valproate and in 1% of those exposed to carbamazepine. There is some evidence that fetal exposure to barbiturates and possibly phenytoin can cause impaired postnatal mental development, but in most studies it has been difficult to discriminate the effects of drugs from those of genetic and environmental factors. There are insufficient data to assess fetal risks after exposure to the newer drugs.

Organs and Systems

Cardiovascular

Cardiac dysrhythmias induced by anticonvulsants are rare and occur mainly in patients other than those known to be at high risk of sudden death (14). Phenytoin has been rarely associated with bradydysrhythmias, almost exclusively after intravenous dosing, and some of these have been fatal. Hypotension can also complicate intravenous phenytoin. Carbamazepine can depress cardiac conduction, mostly in elderly or otherwise predisposed patients. Third-degree atrioventricular block occurred in one patient with pre-existing right bundle branch block treated with topiramate, but a cause-and-effect relation was uncertain (SEDA-21, 76).

Respiratory

Respiratory adverse effects are extremely rare, apart from respiratory depression associated with high-dose benzodiazepines or drug overdose.

Nervous system

Most major anticonvulsants can cause cerebellovestibular and oculomotor symptoms (ataxia, dysarthria, dizziness, fatigue, tremor, diplopia, blurred vision, and nystagmus), alterations in cognitive function, and disorders of mood and behavior. Less common effects include parkinsonism (almost exclusively with valproate), exacerbation of seizures, headache, dyskinesias, and dystonias. Neurophysiological evidence of peripheral neuropathy may be common, but neuropathic symptoms are relatively rare. Monoplegia, Babinski reflexes, restless legs syndrome, and retinal/optic nerve disorders are very rare (except for vigabatrin-induced asymptomatic visual field defects, which are relatively common). Neurological adverse effects are usually dose-dependent and more prominent in patients on multiple drug therapy, although it has been suggested that neurotoxicity relates more to total drug load (in terms of sum of defined daily doses for each drug) than to the actual number of drugs taken (SEDA-22, 81).

In some cases, seizure exacerbation occurs as a manifestation of drug intoxication, and is reversible on dosage reduction or elimination of unnecessary polypharmacy (15). In other cases, seizure exacerbation reflects an adverse reaction to a given drug in specific seizure types or syndromes. Carbamazepine in particular can precipitate or exacerbate a variety of seizures, most notably absence, atonic, or myoclonic seizures, especially in children with generalized epilepsies characterized by bursts of diffuse and bilaterally synchronous spike-and-wave EEG activity. Aggravation of seizures has also been reported with phenytoin and vigabatrin, particularly in children with generalized epilepsies. Gabapentin has been implicated in precipitating myoclonic jerks, while benzodiazepines occasionally trigger tonic seizures, particularly when they are given intravenously to patients with Lennox–Gastaut syndrome. Evidence that ethosuximide predisposes to tonic-clonic seizures remains inconclusive.

Experimental or clinical evidence of polyneuropathy, sometimes with paresthesia, has been found in up to 50% of patients treated chronically with carbamazepine, phenytoin, phenobarbital, and/or valproate (SEDA-18, 61), but it is usually not associated with troublesome symptoms.

The risk of aggravating juvenile myoclonic epilepsy with carbamazepine and phenytoin has been assessed in a retrospective study of 170 patients, of whom 40 had taken carbamazepine or phenytoin (16). There was aggravation of seizures in 23 patients, 6 benefited, and there was no effect in the other 11. Of the 28 patients who used carbamazepine, 19 had aggravated symptoms, including myoclonic status in 2. Of the 16 patients who used phenytoin, 6 had aggravated symptoms, including one in association with phenobarbital. Vigabatrin was given in only one case, in association with carbamazepine, and provoked mixed absence and myoclonic status.

Antiepileptic drugs have sometimes been associated with a paradoxical increase in seizures. The evidence for this comes from isolated reports and clinical impressions. Somerville asked five pharmaceutical companies responsible for the development of new antiepileptic drugs to provide data concerning increases in seizure frequency during randomized, placebo-controlled, add-on trials in patients with uncontrolled partial seizures (17). Seizure frequency in individual patients taking the active drug or placebo was compared with the baseline pretreatment seizure frequency. More than 40% of the patients in trials of tiagabine, topiramate, and levetiracetam had an increase in seizures while taking a placebo. Increased seizure frequency was no more likely to occur when they were taking any of the three drugs than when they were taking placebo. A doubling or more of seizure frequency was significantly less likely to occur with topiramate or levetiracetam than with placebo, but more likely with tiagabine. There was some evidence of a dose–response effect with tiagabine, but a negative effect with topiramate (aggravation less likely with increasing dose). Unfortunately, the author did not obtain data on gabapentin and lamotrigine. Thus, aggravation of seizures in patients using some of the new antiepileptic drugs occurs no more often than with placebo and probably represents spontaneous fluctuation of seizure frequency.

Retrospective studies have suggested that antiepileptic drugs can be associated with peripheral nerve dysfunction. This has been studied prospectively in 81 patients (aged 13–67 years) without polyneuropathy who took sodium valproate ($n = 44$) or carbamazepine ($n = 37$) as monotherapy in standard daily doses (18). After 2 years one patient had clinical signs of polyneuropathy and six patients had symptoms of polyneuropathy, but electrophysiology did not show significant changes or trends. Only one patient had abnormal electrophysiological findings, which were only subclinical, and eight patients had abnormal values at two subsequent visits. There were no consistent patterns, and the data were unaffected when the drugs were examined separately or when patients were grouped according to whether or not they had symptoms of polyneuropathy. The authors concluded that previously untreated young to middle-aged patients who take valproic acid or carbamazepine for 2 years are not at risk of polyneuropathy.

Sensory systems

Visual field defects associated with various antiepileptic drugs (carbamazepine, diazepam, gabapentin, phenytoin, tiagabine, and vigabatrin) have been reviewed (19). The true frequency is unknown, but in a retrospective study in 158 patients with partial epilepsy visual field defects were detected in 21 (13%); 13 patients had concentric visual field constriction without subjective spontaneous manifestations. Of these 13 patients, 9 were taking vigabatrin.

Visual-evoked potentials and brainstem auditory-evoked potentials have been measured in 58 children and adolescents taking carbamazepine, phenobarbital, or sodium valproate monotherapy and 50 sex- and age-matched controls (20). After 1 year the patients taking carbamazepine had significantly prolonged visual-evoked P100 latencies compared with both baseline and control values; they also had significantly prolonged peak latencies of auditory waves I-III-V and interpeak interval I-V. Those taking sodium valproate had significantly prolonged visual-evoked P100 latencies. In contrast, children taking phenobarbital had no changes.

In 100 epileptic patients aged 8–18 years taking carbamazepine or valproate in modified-release formulations either alone or with added vigabatrin interpeak latencies of I-III and III-V of brainstem-evoked potentials were significantly delayed and N75/P100 and P100/N145 amplitudes in the visual-evoked potentials were reduced (21). However, the addition of vigabatrin did not worsen the effects caused by the other two drugs alone.

Psychological, psychiatric

Behavioral and psychiatric disturbances are not uncommon (22). Although epilepsy is itself associated with an increased risk of such disturbances, drugs play an important role. Phenobarbital-induced behavioral disturbances, especially hyperkinesia, are especially common in children, with an incidence of 20–50% and need for

drug withdrawal in 20–30% of cases, whereas it is unclear whether and to what extent adults are affected.

Psychiatric effects
Among older drugs, valproic acid and carbamazepine are least likely to cause adverse psychiatric effects, though valproate rarely causes encephalopathy and reversible pseudodementia. Phenytoin has been implicated in psychiatric adverse effects with or without other signs of toxicity, and at serum concentrations above or below the upper limit of the target range, but the actual incidence of these reactions is unknown. Benzodiazepines can cause paradoxical excitation, particularly in children and in anxious patients, and several other psychiatric symptoms can complicate the benzodiazepine withdrawal syndrome. Psychiatric or behavioral disorders have been reported with ethosuximide, but the lack of systematic studies prevents assessment of incidence and cause-and-effect relation. Among newer drugs, vigabatrin has been implicated most commonly in psychiatric adverse effects. With gabapentin, lamotrigine, and levetiracetam aggressiveness or hyperactivity can occur, especially in patients with previous behavioral problems or learning disability. Adverse psychiatric reactions to lamotrigine are uncommon, whereas with topiramate, felbamate, and other new drugs information is still insufficient.

Overall, the problem of drug-induced psychiatric disorders can be minimized by avoiding unnecessarily large dosages and drug combinations and by careful monitoring of the clinical response. In patients with a previous history of psychiatric disorders, carbamazepine and valproate are the first-line drugs, and are least likely to cause behavioral disturbances. The ideal management of such disturbances is withdrawal of the offending agent. When continuation of treatment is necessary for seizure control, psychosocial intervention and psychotropic medication can be useful.

In a retrospective study of 89 patients who developed psychiatric symptoms during treatment with tiagabine, topiramate, or vigabatrin, the psychiatric problem was either an affective or a psychotic disorder (not including affective psychoses) (23). All but one of the patients had complex partial seizures with or without secondary generalization. More than half were taking polytherapy. Nearly two-thirds had a previous psychiatric history, and there was a strong association between the type of previous psychiatric illness and the type of emerging psychiatric problem. Patients taking vigabatrin had an earlier onset of epilepsy and more neurological abnormalities than those taking topiramate.

Patients with chronic epilepsy have a higher likelihood of psychosis than the healthy population (24,25). Psychosis is especially frequent in patients with temporal lobe epilepsy (26). Antiepileptic drugs have been reported to precipitate psychosis, although the literature is confounded by the inclusion of affective and confusional psychoses in this category. Moreover, the purported association has mostly been made through isolated case reports or small non-controlled case series. In fact, most antiepileptic drugs have been associated with psychosis: phenytoin and phenobarbital (27), carbamazepine and valproate (28), felbamate (29), gaba-pentin (30), levetiracetam (31), topiramate (32), vigaba-trin (33), and zonisamide (34). There have been no reports of psychosis associated with lamotrigine.

A retrospective chart review of 44 consecutive patients with epilepsy who had psychotic symptoms with clear consciousness has shown the difficulties in associating psychosis with drug effects (35). These patients were divided into two groups based on the presence or absence of changes in their drug regimen before the onset of the first episode of psychosis. In 27 patients the first episode of psychosis was unrelated to changes in their antiepileptic drug regimen, and in 23 of them the psychosis was temporally related to changes in seizure frequency. In 17 patients the first episode of psychosis developed in association with changes in their antiepileptic drug treatment, and in 12 of them the psychosis was temporally related to seizure attenua-tion or aggravation. This study therefore highlights the fact that psychosis can occur in relation to changes in seizure frequency, sometimes due to lack of effect of the new medication or to concomitant withdrawal of an efficacious medication.

Withdrawal of anticonvulsants with favorable mood stabilization properties, such as carbamazepine, has often been associated with acute psychosis (36,37). Moreover, the phenomenon of "forced normalization," by which complete seizure freedom in a patient with previous refractory epilepsy can lead to a psychotic state, may also contribute to the apparent association between drugs and psychosis (38).

Information from double-blind studies of psychosis as an adverse event is relatively scarce. A double-blind, randomized, add-on, placebo-controlled trial with carba-mazepine showed that there was no increase in chronic psychotic symptoms in patients with suspected temporal lobe seizures (39).

The relation between psychosis and tiagabine has been assessed in an analysis of data from two multi-center, double-blind, randomized, placebo-controlled trials of add-on tiagabine therapy (32 or 56 mg/day) in 554 adolescents and adults with complex partial seizures during 8–12 weeks (40). There were psychotic symptoms (hallucinations) in 3 (0.8%) of 356 patients taking tia-gabine and none of the 198 taking placebo, a non-sig-nificant difference. Thus, it appears that tiagabine does not increase the risk of psychosis, but the result is inconclusive.

An analysis of double-blind, placebo-controlled trials of vigabatrin as add-on therapy for treatment-refractory partial epilepsy showed that compared with placebo patients taking vigabatrin had a significantly higher inci-dence of events coded as psychosis (2.5% versus 0.3%) (17). There were no significant differences between treat-ment groups for aggressive reaction, manic symptoms, agitation, emotional lability, anxiety, or suicide attempts. In an open trial of topiramate, psychosis was seen in 30/1001 (3%) of the patients, and was severe enough to require withdrawal in eight (41).

Should certain antiepileptic drugs be contraindicated in patients with active psychosis? Unfortunately there is not enough solid information to answer this question. Undoubtedly, anticonvulsants that are less likely to cause psychosis (lamotrigine, carbamazepine, oxcarbaze-pine, valproate) should be preferred (42,43). However, patients with psychoses have been successfully treated even with drugs that are believed to be associated with psychosis, such as vigabatrin. For example, in a prospec-tive study in 10 patients with psychosis and epilepsy to whom vigabatrin was added, there was no aggravation of the psychiatric disorder (44).

Cognitive effects

The appropriate methods and timing in assessing cognitive and behavioral adverse events during drug development programs have been thoroughly reviewed (45).

The authors of a critical review focusing on pediatric data concluded that adverse effects on learning and behavior may have been over-rated (46). Because of methodological flaws, many early studies could not dis-criminate between effects of drugs and the influence of heredity, brain damage, seizures, and psychosocial fac-tors. In fact, the majority of children taking antiepileptic drugs do not experience major cognitive or behavioral effects from these medications. In some patients, how-ever, drugs do produce detrimental effects, barbiturates and benzodiazepines being among those most com-monly implicated (47). At least with some agents, such as gabapentin, behavioral adverse effects occur mainly in children with pre-existing learning disability. As to phenytoin, carbamazepine, and valproate which are the drugs most commonly recommended for first-line use, recent investigations have failed to show major differ-ences in cognitive effects between these agents, although in some studies, patients taking phenytoin tended to have lower motor and information process-ing speeds (SED-13, 140) (48,49) (SEDA-19, 72) (SEDA-20, 64).

Endocrine

Although most anticonvulsants interfere with endocrine function, epilepsy may do so itself, and it is difficult to differentiate the effects of drugs from those of the disease. In any case, symptoms of endocrine dysfunction are less common than biochemical abnormalities.

Growth hormone

Normal growth hormone concentrations are found in carbamazepine-treated patients (50). Growth hormone secretion in response to levodopa stimulation was not affected by carbamazepine or phenobarbital, whereas phenytoin and anticonvulsant polytherapy caused an increase in growth hormone concentration, and valproate a fall at varying times after the administration of levodopa (51). Pubertal growth arrest has been described in a 12-year-old girl who had taken valproate for 18 months (SED-13, 152).

Adrenal–pituitary axis

Neither phenytoin, valproate, carbamazepine, nor pheno-barbital altered the circadian ACTH/cortisol rhythm in epileptic patients (51). In some studies, phenytoin and carbamazepine were associated with increased serum concentrations of unbound cortisol (52), but cortisol concentrations were unaffected in other studies (50) and Cushing's syndrome has not been described with these drugs. Valproate can depress ACTH concentrations by inhibiting corticotrophin-releasing factor, and it has been used to treat Nelson's syndrome (53). Serum concentrations of progesterone and cortisol and the excretion of 17-hydroxycorticosteroids have been reported to be lower in untreated patients with epilepsy and to be further reduced by phenytoin (54).

Sex hormones
Carbamazepine, phenobarbital, phenytoin, and anticonvulsant polytherapy increased both basal and stimulated concentrations of prolactin, whereas valproate did not (51). However, in other studies, prolactin was unchanged (50). In boys, phenobarbital lowered baseline LH and FSH concentrations and their response to releasing hormone; baseline prolactin concentration was raised in comparison with healthy children, and the response of prolactin concentrations to stimulation was impaired (55).

Serum concentrations of bound testosterone are increased by phenytoin, carbamazepine, phenobarbital, and primidone owing to increased synthesis of the specific transport protein, sex hormone-binding globulin (SHBG), but concentrations of unbound testosterone, dehydroepiandrosterone sulfate, and 17-α-hydroxyprogesterone and the free androgen index may be reduced (50,56–58). Increased FSH in 31% of carbamazepine-treated men may reflect impairment of spermatogenesis, whereas lower concentrations of inhibin B (in 12% of men) and testosterone/LH ratio (in 50%) indicate impaired function of Sertoli cells and Leydig cells respectively (50). Sexual activity was reduced, while mean plasma concentrations of LH, FSH, PRL, and SHBG were raised in 27 epileptic patients taking phenytoin, primidone, phenobarbital, or combinations of these (59). The often-reported reduction in sexual activity and occasional reports of impotence may be related to the reduction in unbound testosterone caused by enzyme induction. Valproate has been recommended for patients with dysfunctional libido or impotence, because it apparently does not reduce unbound hormone concentrations (60).

In an assessment of the effects of antiepileptic drugs on male sexual function, men taking carbamazepine had higher plasma concentrations of SHBG and lower concentrations of dehydroepiandrosterone compared with controls (61). Patients taking phenytoin had higher total testosterone concentrations and lower dehydroepiandrosterone concentrations. Patients taking carbamazepine and phenytoin also had a lower free androgen index, but free (unbound) testosterone, a more reliable index of active androgen concentrations, did not differ from that of controls. Patients taking valproate showed no differences in hormone concentrations compared with controls. Sexual experience scales showed that treated men embraced a stricter sexual morality than untreated controls, and expressed greater satisfaction with their marriages. Most of the hormonal changes could be explained by enzyme induction, and there was no evidence of hyposexuality in this population.

Reproductive endocrine disorders and sexual dysfunction have often been attributed to epilepsy itself, but antiepileptic drugs can cause various alterations in endocrine functions. Reproductive endocrine function was prospectively evaluated in 90 men taking valproate ($n = 21$), carbamazepine ($n = 40$), or oxcarbazepine ($n = 29$) as monotherapy for epilepsy, and in 25 healthy controls (62). There were increased serum androgen concentrations in 60% of those who took valproate. Carbamazepine had an opposite effect: men had mean low serum concentrations of dehydroepiandrosterone and a high SHBG concentration. Moreover, 18% of men taking carbamazepine for epilepsy reported reduced libido, impaired potency, or both. Low daily doses of oxcarbazepine (under 900 mg/day) did not have any effects on serum concentrations of reproductive hormones, but men taking high doses of oxcarbazepine (over 900 mg/day) had increased serum testosterone, gonadotropin, and SHBG concentrations. Serum insulin concentrations were high in all patients. Thus, the three antiepileptic drugs affected the serum concentrations of reproductive endocrine hormones in men with epilepsy, but in different ways. Valproate directly affects steroid synthesis or metabolism. Oxcarbazepine and carbamazepine differ in their effects, despite their close structural homology: oxcarbazepine does not reduce the activity of androgens, whereas carbamazepine does. The relevance of these hormonal changes to reproductive or sexual function remains to be demonstrated.

In another study changes in reproductive hormones associated with valproate or carbamazepine were prospectively analysed in 17 women and 22 men with recently diagnosed epilepsy (63). There were no clinical signs of hormonal disorders or weight gain during follow-up at 1 and 3 months. Valproate and carbamazepine caused alterations in reproductive hormonal function during the first month of treatment, and these changes were stable or progressive during the next 2 months. Serum testosterone concentrations increased in half of the women taking valproate; mean serum concentrations of gonadotropins and SHBG also increased, but the concentrations of serum dehydroepiandrosterone sulfate fell. On the other hand, in men after 3 months of valproate treatment, serum FSH concentrations were low and serum progesterone and dehydroepiandrosterone sulfate concentrations were high. Carbamazepine increased serum concentrations of SHBG and dehydroepiandrosterone sulfate, while the free androgen index fell. Thus, valproate was associated with increased serum androgen concentrations, but the profiles of hormonal changes were different in men and women. On the other hand, carbamazepine was associated with reduced sex steroid function in both sexes. Although these results are of interest, the study was not randomized and a large number of statistical comparisons were performed, so that no firm conclusions can be drawn.

Thyroid hormones
Total and free (unbound) thyroxine can be reduced by phenytoin and carbamazepine, but free triiodothyronine is normal or only slightly reduced. Thyroid-stimulating hormone is normal or only slightly altered and patients remain clinically euthyroid (50,64). Reductions in the concentrations of some thyroid hormones are probably related to enzyme induction; the concentrations return to

normal after substituting carbamazepine with oxcarbazepine, a less potent enzyme inducer (65). Hypothyroidism has been rarely described in patients taking phenytoin or carbamazepine (66). In contrast to earlier reports, there were no changes in thyroid hormones during treatment with valproate in a later study (67).

Serum thyroid hormones have been compared in 148 healthy children and 141 children with epilepsy who had been taking carbamazepine ($n = 61$), valproate ($n = 51$), or phenobarbital ($n = 29$) for at least 1 year (68). In all the groups mean thyroxine and free thyroxine concentrations were lower than in controls, and those taking carbamazepine and valproate also had lower concentrations of triiodothyronine and thyroid-binding globulin and increased mean TSH concentrations. There was subclinical hypothyroidism, defined as a TSH concentration greater than two standard deviations above the control mean, in 26% of the children taking valproate, 8.2% of those taking carbamazepine, 7.1% of those taking phenobarbital, and 3.6% of controls. However, the magnitude of the TSH increase was usually small and the children were clinically euthyroid.

The effects of antiepileptic drugs on thyroid function have also been studied in an open prospective study in 90 men with epilepsy (40 taking carbamazepine, 29 taking oxcarbazepine, and 21 taking valproate monotherapy) and 25 control subjects (69). Serum thyroxine and/or free thyroxine concentrations were below the reference ranges in 45% of men taking carbamazepine and 24% of men taking oxcarbazepine. Thyroid peroxidase and/or thyroglobulin concentrations were increased in 13% of those taking carbamazepine, 17% of those taking oxcarbazepine, and 6% of controls, but these changes were not associated with altered serum thyroid hormone concentrations. Serum triiodothyronine and thyrotropin (TRH) concentrations in those taking carbamazepine or oxcarbazepine were normal. In men taking valproate, the concentrations of thyroid hormones, thyrotropin, and antithyroid antibodies were normal. Thus, low serum thyroid hormone concentrations appear to be frequent in men taking carbamazepine or oxcarbazepine and are probably not due to liver enzyme induction or activation of immunological mechanisms. The clinical significance of these changes is uncertain: serum TSH was not affected and all the patients were clinically euthyroid. Similar results have been obtained in a retrospective study in 37 children taking valproate or carbamazepine (70).

Metabolism

Phenytoin rarely causes hyperglycemia, and the blood glucose concentration can increase in phenytoin intoxication (SED-13, 139) (71). A reduction in the insulin response to glucose has been noted with therapeutic doses of phenytoin, but glucose intolerance does not arise, probably owing to increased sensitivity to insulin.

Changes in body weight associated with anticonvulsants have been reviewed (72), including the effects of the antiepileptic drugs that have been most commonly associated with this adverse effect (valproic acid, carbamazepine, vigabatrin, and gabapentin) (73). Unlike most anticonvulsants, topiramate, felbamate, and zonisamide can cause weight loss.

Preliminary evidence suggests that certain idiosyncratic reactions to anticonvulsants are mediated by reduced free radical scavenging activity, as indicated by lower selenium concentrations and a higher lipid peroxide index in affected patients (SEDA-19, 62).

Serum lipids
Phenytoin increases high-density lipoprotein (HDL) cholesterol (74), and may also increase total cholesterol and serum triglyceride concentrations (SED-13, 143) (75). In a 5-year prospective study with carbamazepine, there was a persistent rise in total cholesterol and HDL cholesterol, whereas triglycerides and low-density lipoprotein (LDL) cholesterol increased only transiently (76). In a more recent study, total cholesterol fell when 12 patients were switched from carbamazepine to oxcarbazepine, but HDL cholesterol and triglycerides were unchanged (77). In a comparison of 101 epileptic patients with matched controls, valproate was associated with lower total and LDL cholesterol, whereas carbamazepine was associated with higher HDL cholesterol and apolipoprotein A concentrations and phenobarbital with higher concentrations of total and HDL cholesterol and apolipoproteins A and B. The ratio of total to HDL cholesterol was reduced with valproate and carbamazepine but not with phenobarbital (78).

The clinical relevance of these findings is uncertain. The increased HDL cholesterol seen with some drugs might confer some protection against atherosclerosis and coronary heart disease (SEDA-18, 63).

Porphyrin metabolism
Enzyme inducers, such as phenytoin, carbamazepine, and barbiturates, can precipitate attacks in patients with acute intermittent porphyria.

- A patient with uncontrolled posttraumatic epilepsy and acute intermittent porphyria was given phenytoin, carbamazepine, and clonazepam on successive occasions (79). Phenytoin and carbamazepine caused significant increases in porphobilinogen excretion and acute attacks of porphyria. In contrast, clonazepam caused no increase in porphobilinogen excretion.

Valproate (SED-12, 134) (80,81), ethosuximide (82), and some benzodiazepines (83) have also been implicated in the precipitation of acute attacks of porphyria, although valproate is considered safe for patients with porphyria cutanea tarda (SED-13, 150) (84).

Neither vigabatrin nor gabapentin caused porphyrin accumulation in chicken embryo cultured liver cells, whereas felbamate, lamotrigine, and tiagabine were porphyrinogenic in this model (85). For gabapentin, safety in porphyrias has been confirmed in preliminary clinical observations (SEDA-19, 70) (SEDA-20, 62).

Amino acids
Compared with healthy controls, 51 patients with epilepsy taking a variety of antiepileptic drugs (mostly carbamazepine) had higher mean plasma concentrations of homocysteine (86). This effect, which could be related to reductions in the concentrations of folate and vitamin B6, was likely to be drug-induced, but a causative role

of the underlying disease could not be excluded. Although homocysteine is an experimental convulsant and a risk factor for atherosclerosis, the clinical relevance of these findings is uncertain.

Phenytoin can reduce blood and CSF thiamine concentrations (87).

Hyperammonemia and carnitine deficiency are adverse effects of valproate, although carnitine deficiency can also be caused by other anticonvulsants (88).

Concentrations of lipoprotein(a) were measured in 51 patients taking long-term carbamazepine, phenobarbital, phenytoin, or valproate and 51 age- and sex-matched controls (89). Lipoprotein(a) concentrations were above 450 µg/ml in 11 patients compared with only 4 controls, and the mean serum lipoprotein(a) concentrations were 330 and 169 µg/ml respectively. The epileptic patients also had a thicker intima media of the common carotid artery. These results suggest that patients taking antiepileptic drugs may be at a higher risk of atherosclerosis.

Electrolyte balance

Phenytoin inhibits the release of antidiuretic hormone (ADH), but this effect is generally clinically unimportant (SED-13, 138) (90). In contrast, both carbamazepine and, to a greater extent, its analogue oxcarbazepine produce significant dose-dependent antidiuretic effects. This is mediated by an action on hypothalamic osmoreceptors or by increased renal sensitivity to ADH, and it can cause hyponatremia and hypo-osmolality. The incidence of hyponatremia ranges from 0% to 42% in patients taking carbamazepine, and from 23% to 73% in those taking oxcarbazepine (22,91). Factors that increase the risk are high dosage (and high serum drug concentrations), old age, a history of severe head trauma or polydipsia, and possibly concomitant intake of diuretics and various psychotropic drugs. Hyponatremia is usually mild and asymptomatic, but occasionally it can cause fatigue, lethargy, drowsiness, confusion, vomiting, and neurological abnormalities, including an increased susceptibility to seizures (91,92). Demeclocycline has been used in the management of carbamazepine-induced hyponatremia (93), but a reduction in drug dosage (or no action in asymptomatic cases) is usually sufficient.

Mineral balance

Alterations in mineral balance occur in a significant proportion of patients taking antiepileptic drugs. Reductions in serum calcium and phosphate and an increase in serum alkaline phosphatase occur in up to 50% of patients treated with enzyme-inducing anticonvulsants, and there can be clinical or biochemical evidence of rickets and osteomalacia. Phenytoin is most often implicated, but similar disturbances have been reported with carbamazepine and barbiturates. The pathogenesis of these changes may involve enhanced conversion of vitamin D to inactive metabolites, but there may be other mechanisms, such as antagonism of the action of 1,25-dihydroxycholecalciferol on bone (SED-13, 139) (94). Serum calcium, phosphate, and alkaline phosphatase should be checked periodically in patients at increased risk of osteomalacia, such as those with a low intake of vitamin D, inactivity, or lack of exposure to sunlight (95). Treatment with colecalciferol may be useful in patients with evidence of vitamin D deficiency (SEDA-16, 70).

Immunoreactive parathyroid hormone concentrations may be increased by anticonvulsants, while bone mineral content is reduced. Hypocalcemia and osteopenia can occur, despite normal serum concentrations of active vitamin D metabolites, suggesting that they may be independent of drug effects on vitamin D metabolism. Bone biopsies have shown increased osteoid but normal calcification front formation, accelerated rate of mineralization, and reduced mineralization lag time, suggesting increased skeletal turnover rather than osteomalacia (96). The risk of age-related fractures in drug-treated epileptic patients is not greatly increased (97).

Valproate has not been commonly implicated in the disturbances described above. In one study, after correction for age and sex, children taking valproate had 14 and 10% reductions in bone mineral density at the axial and appendicular sites respectively; however, the significance of these findings is uncertain (SEDA-20, 69).

Transient osteosclerosis of the long bones was reported in a 15-year-old boy taking valproate with severe pain in the extremities; it disappeared after drug withdrawal (SED-13, 150) (98).

Acid–base balance

Acetazolamide, sultiame, and topiramate inhibit carbonic anhydrase and occasionally produce biochemical or clinical manifestations of acidosis.

Hematologic

Chronic treatment with phenobarbital, phenytoin, and carbamazepine is associated with reduced serum folate concentrations. Although megaloblastic anemia is rare, macrocytic changes in red cells are common in these patients. The fact that serum folate is not reduced by valproate and zonisamide, which do not induce liver enzymes, is consistent with the hypothesis that enzyme induction plays a role in the pathogenesis of folate deficiency (99).

Blood dyscrasias, ranging from mild leukopenia to fatal aplastic anemia, can occur with most anticonvulsants, but severe hematological reactions are extremely rare, except for felbamate. Thrombocytopenia, platelet dysfunction, and altered coagulation are not uncommon in patients taking valproate, but severe hemorrhagic complications are rare. Newborns of mothers treated with enzyme-inducing anticonvulsants are at risk of serious hemorrhage during the first few days of life and should receive vitamin K prophylactically.

The combination of lamotrigine with valproate has been reported to have caused the production of lupus anticoagulant (100).

- A 5-year-old boy with generalized absence seizures, who had had a moderate reduction in fibrinogen and prolonged partial thromboplastin time while taking valproate was given add-on lamotrigine (2 mg/kg). His seizures disappeared, but the partial thromboplastin time increased and tests for lupus anticoagulant and IgG anticardiolipin antibodies became positive. Serum autoantibody screen and rheumatoid factor were negative. The lupus anticoagulant disappeared after valproate was withdrawn.

The authors suggested that lamotrigine may have exacerbated a mild immune response initially induced by valproate, without clinical evidence of systemic disease.

In a large cohort study of the occurrence of bleeding complications in neonates exposed to maternal enzyme-inducing antiepileptic drugs in utero in 662 pregnancies in women with epilepsy, 463 had been exposed to carbamazepine, 212 to phenytoin, 44 to phenobarbital, 11 to primidone, and 7 to oxcarbazepine (101). Another 1324 "non-epileptic" pregnancies (1334 neonates) were matched for maternal age, parity, number of fetuses, and delivery date. None of the mothers had received vitamin K1 during pregnancy, but all the infants received vitamin K1 1 mg intramuscularly at birth. There were bleeding complications in five (0.7%) of the neonates exposed to maternal enzyme-inducing antiepileptic drugs and in five (0.4%) of the control subjects. Logistic regression analysis showed that bleeding was associated with premature birth and alcohol abuse, but not with exposure to enzyme-inducing antiepileptic drugs. These results contradict the widely held view, based on anecdotal evidence, that maternal enzyme-inducing antiepileptic drugs increase the risk of bleeding in the offspring. Thus, antenatal administration of vitamin K to mothers treated with enzyme-induced drugs may not be needed in most cases. However, prophylaxis may be worth considering when premature delivery is imminent in a woman who uses anticonvulsants. It is worth noting that the findings described in this article are only relevant to patients taking carbamazepine or phenytoin monotherapy. Therefore, extrapolation to individuals on polytherapy or to those taking other enzyme-inducing drugs is not possible.

Gastrointestinal

Nausea, vomiting, diarrhea, and changes in appetite can occur with all anticonvulsants, although they are usually transient and rarely require withdrawal. Felbamate and to a lesser extent valproate are the anticonvulsants that most often cause gastrointestinal adverse effects.

Liver

Virtually all of the major antiepileptic drugs can cause hepatotoxicity, although a fatal outcome is rare. Liver enzymes are increased up to three times the normal limit in up to 40% of patients treated with major antiepileptic drugs, without any additional evidence of overt hepatic disease. Repeated indiscriminate monitoring of liver function tests is not indicated in patients taking most antiepileptic drugs, and greater attention should be focused on the recognition of high-risk groups and supply of information about symptoms of incipient hepatic failure (102,103).

With phenytoin, carbamazepine, phenobarbital, primidone, and lamotrigine, hepatotoxicity usually occurs as part of a hypersensitivity reaction, with skin rashes and fever in the early weeks of treatment. More rarely, hepatic disease can develop after many years without signs of hypersensitivity. Once hepatotoxicity develops, mortality rates are 10–38% with phenytoin and about 25% with carbamazepine (104). Elderly patients may be at higher risk (105).

Fatal valproate hepatotoxicity may occur with greater frequency in children under the age of 2 years who are receiving multiple drug therapy and have additional handicaps (106).

Atrium, a proprietary mixture of phenobarbital, febarbamate, and difebarbamate, has caused several cases of hepatotoxicity, at least one of which was ascribed to the carbamates, because the patient had earlier tolerated phenobarbital (SEDA-18, 74). Atrium-induced hepatitis might be facilitated by defective CYP2C19 activity (SEDA-19, 77).

Pancreas

Pancreatitis is a rare adverse effect of valproate and can occur in isolation or in association with liver toxicity. In a review of the patients of 366 physicians, 23% of patients taking valproic acid had asymptomatic increases in serum amylase activity but there were only 39 cases of valproate-associated pancreatitis (107). Pancreatitis usually presented with epigastric pain, nausea, and vomiting, and was more common in patients aged under 20 years and with mental retardation. In most cases the pancreatitis started within the first 3 months of treatment, but in 18% the onset was after 2 years.

Pancreatitis with other antiepileptic drugs is extremely rare.

Urinary tract

Drugs that inhibit carbonic anhydrase (acetazolamide, topiramate, and zonisamide) are associated with a small risk (up to 1.5%) of nephrolithiasis. Increased excretion of N-acetyl-beta-glucosaminidase, a marker of renal tubular integrity, has been reported with valproate and carbamazepine, but it is probably not clinically significant (SEDA-18, 60).

Skin

All major anticonvulsants have adverse effects on the skin, ranging from a mild maculopapular rash to life-threatening Stevens–Johnson syndrome or Lyell's syndrome (toxic epidermal necrolysis), severe forms of erythema multiforme.

Mild adverse skin reactions to antiepileptic drugs include morbilliform rashes, fixed drug eruptions, bullous reactions, lichenoid-type reactions, urticaria (excluding angioedema), alopecia, pigmentation changes, and photosensitivity (108). There have been reports of positive rechallenge in some patients with exanthems, bullous eruptions, lichenoid-type reactions, and mild urticaria. Mild skin rashes during the first few weeks of treatment are among the most common causes of early withdrawal of carbamazepine, phenytoin, oxcarbazepine, barbiturates, and lamotrigine. Corticosteroids may suppress mild carbamazepine-induced eruptions, allowing continuation of treatment in a few patients.

Anticonvulsants are among the most important causative agents of serious and potentially fatal skin reactions. The management of severe reactions of any type is controversial, but referral to a burns center is recommended. Essential supportive care includes fluids and nutrition management. Prophylactic antibacterial drugs are not recommended. Plasmapheresis has been recommended for emergency treatment of anticonvulsant-induced toxic epidermal necrolysis (SED-13, 141) (109). Most authors advise against the use of corticosteroids, as they increase the risk of infection and sepsis.

Several reports have suggested that patients with brain tumors who undergo radiation therapy while taking phenytoin may be at increased risk of developing Stevens–Johnson syndrome. A 47-year-old black man (110) and four other patients, including one who died (111), were seen in a 24-month period in one department. A review of 20 similar reported cases showed no relation to the dosage of phenytoin or radiation, or to the histological type of the tumor (110). Isolated reports have also implicated carbamazepine and phenobarbital in causing Stevens–Johnson syndrome in patients undergoing radiation therapy. In a 53-year-old man taking phenobarbital, eruptions were limited to the sites of radiation, which were multiple (112). Conversely, a retrospective review of 289 brain tumor patients treated with cranial radiation and anticonvulsant drugs did not identify an increased incidence of severe skin rashes (113). Only one patient with Stevens–Johnson syndrome was found in this series, although the incidence of milder skin rashes was higher than expected (18 versus 5–10%). In three patients who had toxic epidermal necrolysis after taking phenytoin or carbamazepine there was an increase in CD3+CLA+ cells, paralleling the severity of the disease in both peripheral blood and skin, tending to normalize as the condition improved (114). E selectin was detected in endothelial vessels in parallel with CLA expression on lymphocytes. There was overexpression of TNF-alpha, interferon gamma, and interleukin-2 in peripheral monocytes. These results suggest an important role for T cells in the production of drug-induced toxic epidermal necrolysis.

A psoriasiform eruption has been reported in a 28-year-old woman taking carbamazepine and valproate (115). Rechallenge was not attempted, and the association with either of these drugs was not clear.

Cross-reactivity in skin reactions is relatively common, especially with anticonvulsants with an aromatic ring (116). Valproate, clonazepam, or clobazam may be safer alternatives in patients who have had a rash from aromatic anticonvulsants. However, in a 41-year-old man a fixed drug eruption that occurred after phenytoin and carbamazepine also occurred after valproate (SEDA-22, 83).

Acne can complicate treatment with phenytoin and other enzyme-inducing anticonvulsants.

Hirsutism and gingival hyperplasia are important adverse effects of phenytoin and represent a relative contraindication to first-line use of this drug in young women.

Alopecia is not uncommon with valproate, and it can also occasionally occur with phenytoin, carbamazepine, vigabatrin, and gabapentin.

Musculoskeletal

Barbiturates can cause various connective tissue disorders, including Dupuytren's contracture and frozen shoulder.

Phenytoin in young children can cause acromegalic facial features.

Osteoporosis
Epilepsy and osteoporosis are very common and frequently overlap. Nevertheless, the prevalence of low bone density appears to be disproportionately higher in patients with epilepsy, and patients with epilepsy have an excessive risk of fractures. A meta-analysis of 94 cohort studies and 72 case-control studies has shown that anticonvulsant treatment is highly associated with fractures (relative risk over 2) (117). Other risk factors were low body weight, weight loss, physical inactivity, consumption of corticosteroids, primary hyperparathyroidism, type 1 diabetes mellitus, anorexia nervosa, gastrectomy, pernicious anemia, and age over 70 years.

Bone mineral density has been measured in 59 patients and 55 age- and sex-matched controls (118). Bone mineral density in the lumbar spine (L2-4) and femurs was lower in the patients, significantly so in the former case. This reduction depended on the duration of therapy. Excretion of pyridinoline cross-links was markedly increased and 25-hydroxycholecalciferol and 1,25-dihydroxycholecalciferol were significantly reduced. The proliferation rate of human osteoblast-like cells was increased by phenytoin in low doses.

Bone metabolism has been assessed in 27 children aged 3–17 years taking long-term valproate and lamotrigine (119). Valproate and lamotrigine were associated with short stature, low bone mineral density, and reduced bone formation. The effect was larger when the two drugs were used together.

The effects on bone metabolism of carbamazepine, valproate, or phenobarbital as monotherapy have been analysed in a case-control study in 118 ambulatory children with epilepsy and corresponding controls (120). Patients taking carbamazepine or phenobarbital had significantly raised alkaline phosphatase and bone and liver isoenzyme activities compared with controls. Although the authors concluded that children who take anticonvulsants may have their bone metabolism affected, this conclusion was based on abnormal values of a surrogate marker for bone disease.

There has been a prospective study of bone mineral density in patients with epilepsy (121). Femoral neck bone mineral density was analysed by dual-energy X-ray absorptiometry in 81 men with epilepsy. Bone mineral density was more than one standard deviation below normal in 47%, indicating an increased risk of fractures (122). Age and duration of therapy were the most significant risk factors associated with a low bone mineral density. Vitamin D deficiency was not a significant risk factor. Longitudinal analysis showed that only those in the youngest age group (25–44 years) had significant reductions in bone mineral density (1.8% annualized loss) while taking anticonvulsants. There was no evidence that a specific type of antiepileptic drug was more causally related to bone loss, although most patients were taking phenytoin or carbamazepine.

Markers of collagen and bone turnover in 60 children and adolescents with epilepsy taking carbamazepine monotherapy were measured at different pubertal stages after 2 years of treatment (123). Compared with age-matched healthy children, there was an increase in several markers of bone turnover. In particular, there was a nearly 10-fold increase in postpubertal patients of N-telopeptides of type I collagen excretion, indicating increased bone resorption due to excessive osteoclastic activity. These data suggest that carbamazepine can cause increased bone turnover independent of pubertal age.

Predisposing factors for bone disease
In patients with epilepsy, several factors can influence bone health, including poor mobility and anticonvulsant drug treatment. Limitations to physical activity that result from neurological deficits or cerebral palsy underlying symptomatic epilepsies clearly constitute a risk factor for osteoporosis (124). Of 117 children with moderate to severe cerebral palsy, 77% had osteopenia, but the rate was 97% among those who were unable to stand and were over 9 years old; fractures occurred in 26% of the children who were over 10 years old (125). Similarly, adults with neurodevelopmental disorders residing in long-term care facilities have a high rate of both low bone mass and skeletal fractures, especially with concomitant use of anticonvulsant drugs (126). Reduced activity and participation in sports, because of frequent seizures, might also have an impact on bone mineralization.

Certain antiepileptic drugs (carbamazepine, phenytoin, phenobarbital, primidone) are inducers of cytochrome P450 isozymes and increase the breakdown of vitamin D (118,127). Although low vitamin D has been thought to be the cause of low bone density and osteomalacia, a reduction in bone density in the absence of vitamin D deficiency has been also found in children taking either enzyme-inducing agents (123,127) or valproate (128). Moreover, there is recent evidence that although subjects taking enzyme-inducing drugs tend to have lower bone mineral density than those taking non-inducers (clonazepam, ethosuximide, gabapentin, lamotrigine, topiramate, and valproic acid), this is not necessarily due to low vitamin D concentrations. In fact, even though 50% of patients with epilepsy have low vitamin D concentrations, there is no good correlation with bone mineral density (127).

Pathophysiology
The drug-related mechanisms that cause bone loss in patients with epilepsy are not completely understood. Although low vitamin D concentrations may play a part, a direct increase in the proliferation rate of human osteoblast-like cells (observed with phenytoin) might lead to impairment of bone formation (118).

Consequences
Low bone density leads to an increased risk of fractures. There was a 30% increased risk of non-seizure-related fractures in 348 non-institutionalized patients with epilepsy compared with a large control population (129). For non-seizure-related fractures the crude fracture rate was 1.6 fractures per 100 patient-years of observation; a similar rate (1.4) has been found in men with epilepsy (122). In addition, in children with epilepsy, treatment with valproic acid and/or lamotrigine for more than 2 years is associated with short stature, possibly in relation to a low bone mass and reduced bone formation (119).

Assessment
The results of multiple investigations suggest that patients with epilepsy and certain risk factors should be assessed for mineral loss: these include those taking enzyme-inducing agents or long-term treatment (especially polytherapy), those with low or lack of physical activity, postmenopausal women, and elderly people (118,127). Assessment should be done with dual-energy X-ray absorptiometry scanning of the hip (121) and measurement of several biochemical markers (serum total calcium, phosphate, alkaline phosphatase, gamma-glutamyltranspeptidase, aspartate transaminase, 25-hydroxycolecalciferol, and 1,25-dihydroxycolecalciferol). Patients with abnormal findings should have parathyroid hormone and sex hormone concentrations assayed or be referred to an endocrinologist for further assessment.

Despite increasing evidence of bone disease in patients with epilepsy, few pediatric (41%) and adult (28%) neurologists routinely evaluate it (130). A recent survey among neurologists showed that of those who detect bone disease through diagnostic testing, only 40% of pediatric and 37% of adult neurologists prescribed calcium or vitamin D, and about half referred patients to specialists (130). Under 10% of neurologists prescribed prophylactic calcium or vitamin D for patients taking anticonvulsants. This also reflects the fact that evidence about the indications for evaluating and treating bone disorders in patients with epilepsy is currently scarce.

Treatment
Calcium and vitamin D supplementation alone, although necessary to meet normal nutritional guidelines, may be inadequate in preventing bone loss in epilepsy. Bone loss associated with other chronic diseases and other bone-depleting medications has prompted a search for more aggressive therapy. Osteoporosis can be effectively treated with bisphosphonates, which disrupt osteoclastic bone resorption by causing apoptosis of osteoclasts. Oral bisphosphonates are typically administered daily. Third-generation intravenous agents, such as zoledronic acid, can be just as effective when administered once a year. However, there is not currently enough information to support the use of bisphosphonates in patients at risk who are taking antiepileptic drugs.

However, potential therapeutic interventions require randomized prospective studies. Variables that might be addressed in such trials include: the impact of monotherapy and polytherapy on the attainment of peak bone mass in adolescence and adulthood; bone health in women; characterization of the impact of limitations in physical activity on bone density in patients with epilepsy who have cerebral palsy or those with developmental disabilities or mental retardation; the effects of newer antiepileptic drugs on bone metabolism; standardization of the workup for bone disease in patients with epilepsy; and the effectiveness of the current recommendations for supplementation with calcium and vitamin D.

Sexual function

See the section on Endocrine in this monograph.

Reproductive system

The risk of anovulatory cycles and its association with epilepsy syndrome and anticonvulsants has been assessed in a cross-sectional cohort study in women with epilepsy and non-epileptic controls (131). There were 59 patients with localization-related epilepsy and 35 with idiopathic generalized epilepsy. They were treated with monotherapy and followed for 6 months or more. Anovulatory cycles occurred in 11% of cycles in controls, 14% of cycles in women with focal epilepsy, and 27% of cycles in women with idiopathic generalized epilepsy. Anovulatory cycles were more frequent in women taking valproate: 38% had at least one anovulatory cycle in contrast to 11% of women not taking valproate. Predictors of ovulatory failure included generalized idiopathic epilepsy syndrome, use of valproate currently or within 3 years, high concentrations of unbound testosterone, and fewer numbers of luteinizing hormone pulses, but not polycystic-like ovaries. However, the cross-sectional design of the study did not allow firm conclusions to be drawn, especially since previous antiepileptic drug exposure was not controlled.

The incidence of polycystic ovary syndrome in women taking antiepileptic drugs has been studied in a prospective cohort analysis of premenopausal women (aged 20–53 years) with focal epilepsy (132). Of 93 women, 38 were taking one antiepileptic drug (18 valproate, 20 carbamazepine), 36 were taking more than one drug, and 19 were taking no medications. Polycystic ovary syndrome was identified in two of the 19 patients taking no medication, four of the 38 patients taking monotherapy, and one of the patients taking more than one antiepileptic drug. The incidence of polycystic ovary syndrome in patients taking valproate monotherapy (11%) was similar to that in those taking carbamazepine (10%) and those not taking antiepileptic drugs (11%). These results suggest that polycystic ovary syndrome in women with focal epilepsy is not related to valproate or carbamazepine.

Women with valproate-associated obesity have high insulin concentrations and low concentrations of insulin-like growth factor-binding protein 1. These abnormalities might play a role in the pathogenesis of hyperandrogenism and polycystic ovaries in these women (133).

Immunologic

The anticonvulsant hypersensitivity syndrome is a potentially fatal reaction to arene oxide-producing anticonvulsants, such as phenytoin, carbamazepine, and phenobarbital (14,134). It occurs in 1 : 1000 to 1 : 10 000 exposures and its main manifestations include fever, rash, and lymphadenopathy, accompanied by multisystem abnormalities. Cross-reactivity among drugs is as high as 70–80%. The reaction may be genetically determined, and siblings of affected patients may be at increased risk. Management includes rapid withdrawal of the offending agent and care of conjunctival and skin lesions; the use of steroids is controversial, as is the value of cyclophosphamide and intravenous immunoglobulin

(135). Early identification is essential for proper management, and it has been suggested that Bayesian analysis, especially when coupled with a lymphocyte toxicity assay, can improve the differential diagnosis (SEDA-19, 62).

- Within 5 days of being switched to valproate after developing a rash ascribed to carbamazepine, a 55-year-old man developed anticonvulsant hypersensitivity syndrome (maculopapular rash, fever, hepatitis, and eosinophilia) and ocular manifestations consistent with bilateral anterior uveitis (136).

Although mild conjunctivitis is common in the anticonvulsant hypersensitivity syndrome, uveitis has not been reported before in this context.

Death

A nested case-control study showed that the risk of sudden unexpected death in epilepsy (SUDEP) increases with increasing number of seizures, increasing numbers of drugs taken (with a relative risk of 9.89 for polytherapy with three drugs compared with monotherapy), and a high frequency of dosage changes (137). However, these data do not necessarily implicate a role of antiepileptic drugs in the pathogenesis of SUDEP: it is possible that polytherapy and frequent dosage changes are surrogate markers for the severity of the disease. On the other hand, a possible implication of carbamazepine in SUDEP was suggested in a separate survey by the observation that 11 of 14 patients who died suddenly (79%) were taking carbamazepine, while only 38% of patients in the same clinic were taking it (138). The effects of carbamazepine on heart function were discussed as a possible mechanism, but no comment was made on the possibility that the characteristics of patients taking carbamazepine may differ from those of patients taking other drugs.

Another study implicated nitrazepam as a possible cause of increased mortality (139). Among 294 assessable children who took nitrazepam, 62 continued treatment at the last time of follow-up. There were 1.98 deaths/100 patient-years during nitrazepam treatment compared with 0.58 deaths/100 patient-years after nitrazepam withdrawal (RR=3.4). The increase in risk occurred virtually entirely in younger children: among those aged under 3.4 years, the death rate per 100 patient-years was 3.98 on nitrazepam compared with 0.26 off nitrazepam (RR=15). Causes of death differed on and off nitrazepam. Of fourteen deaths during nitrazepam treatment, seven were sudden, six were due to pneumonia, and one was due to cystinosis: nine patients had at least one contributing factor, such as dysphagia, gastroesophageal reflux, or recurrent aspiration. In the off-nitrazepam period, there were two sudden deaths and one death each caused by status epilepticus, head trauma, and shunt complication; only one patient had a contributing factor (gastroesophageal reflux). These findings were interpreted as evidence that nitrazepam increases the risk of death in young children, possibly owing to its ability to increase secretions and to cause drooling, eating difficulties, and aspiration pneumonia (140,141). Although the data suggest a role of nitrazepam in these deaths, only incomplete information was given about the distribution of other risk factors (seizure disorder, associated morbidity) in children who continued nitrazepam therapy. Nitrazepam should be used with caution in young children, especially those with difficulties in swallowing, aspiration pneumonia, or gastroesophageal reflux.

The risk of sudden death associated with antiepileptic drugs has been assessed in a retrospective case-control study in 6880 patients with epilepsy, from whom 57 cases of sudden death and 171 controls (living with the patients with epilepsy) were selected (142). Polytherapy, frequent dosage changes, and high carbamazepine concentrations were identified as risk factors for sudden death, all pointing to risks associated with unstable severe epilepsy. Because the study was retrospective it is difficult to know whether antiepileptic drugs in themselves are associated with sudden death, of if the higher risk is a result of uncontrolled seizures.

Long-Term Effects

Drug withdrawal

Although it has been suggested that worsening of seizures after withdrawal of non-benzodiazepine anticonvulsants may reflect loss of efficacy rather than an abstinence phenomenon (143), rapid drug withdrawal can still result in dangerous loss of seizure control and status epilepticus.

Psychiatric pathology can also occur after rapid drug withdrawal. Of 32 patients withdrawn from all anticonvulsants before a drug trial, 12 developed moderate to severe psychopathology (especially anxiety and depression) and 9 dropped out because of psychiatric symptoms (144). These findings reinforce ethical concerns about some trial designs involving withdrawal of pre-existing therapy.

Epileptic negative myoclonus status (almost continuous lapses in muscle tone associated with epileptiform discharges and interfering with postural control and motor coordination) rarely occurs after rapid withdrawal of clobazam or valproate (145).

Nausea and vomiting have been listed as withdrawal effects of anticonvulsants (146).

Tumorigenicity

Pseudolymphoma and a condition resembling malignant lymphoma occur very rarely with phenytoin (SED-13, 142). There is no evidence of a significant increase in the incidence of other tumors. There have also been reports of pseudolymphoma with other antiepileptic drugs, including carbamazepine (147–149), lamotrigine (150), phenobarbital (151), and valproic acid (151).

Second-Generation Effects

Teratogenicity

The incidence of major congenital anomalies among babies born to epileptic women is about 6–8%, compared with 2–4% in the general population. Although the disease itself and social and environmental factors may play

a role, these abnormalities are related to a large extent to the effects of antiepileptic drugs (152–154).

None of the major anticonvulsants (phenytoin, carbamazepine, valproate, and phenobarbital) is free from teratogenic potential, and there is no pattern of malformations that is specific for a given drug. However, facial clefts and congenital heart defects are somewhat more common with phenytoin and barbiturates, whereas neural tube defects are more common with valproic acid (23% risk) and carbamazepine (0.5–1% risk) (SEDA-16, 72). The risk of congenital anomalies increases with increasing dosages and the number of drugs taken by the mother (SED-12, 123); with valproate, neural tube defects have also been linked to high peak serum drug concentrations. There is preliminary evidence that certain drug combinations, particularly those that include valproic acid, may be more harmful than others. In one study, the combination of phenytoin, phenobarbital, carbamazepine, and valproate was associated with the highest risk (155). In a much smaller study, the risk and severity of meningomyelocele and dysmorphic features associated with valproate seemed to be greater where a benzodiazepine had also been taken (SEDA-18, 61).

In addition to major malformations, a number of mostly craniofacial dysmorphic features, notably growth retardation, microcephaly, and mental retardation have been described as comprising a fetal antiepileptic drug syndrome. This syndrome, originally ascribed only to hydantoins and at one time known as the fetal hydantoin syndrome, has been observed in children exposed to phenytoin, barbiturates, carbamazepine, and valproate. A broad range of signs is observed in at most 5–10% of children exposed to these drugs in utero, but individual signs (for example hypertelorism) are seen in as many as 52% and digital hypoplasia in 23%. Few results from controlled studies are available, and selection criteria and methods of ascertainment are very variable. In one study the association between prenatal phenytoin exposure and digital hypoplasia or hypertelorism was confirmed, but at the age of 5.5 years none of the exposed children had all of the main characteristics of the hydantoin syndrome. The risk of developmental disturbances seemed to be lower than the 7–11% risk of the fetal hydantoin syndrome reported earlier (SED-13, 136) (156).

The rate of congenital malformations in the offspring of 517 mothers exposed to antiepileptic drugs during pregnancy has been examined in a prospective single-center study (157). The overall malformation rate was 9.7%. Malformations were classified as structurally severe (5.3%), structurally mild (2.2%), chromosomal genetic (0.4%), and deformities (1.8%). The malformation rate after exposure to polytherapy (9.6%, $n = 114$) was not higher than after exposure to monotherapy (10.5%, $n = 313$). Among monotherapy exposures, the rates for structural abnormalities were 16% with valproate ($n = 44$), 8.6% with primidone ($n = 35$), 7.1% with carbamazepine ($n = 113$), 4.8% with phenobarbital ($n = 83$), and only 3.2% with phenytoin ($n = 31$). There were no malformations in the offspring of 25 untreated patients. Among women exposed to valproate, the mothers of malformed babies took significantly higher dosages in the first trimester than mothers of non-malformed babies (1712 versus 1008 mg/day). These data confirm that exposure to antiepileptic drugs is associated with an increased risk of fetal malformations, and that the risk may be especially high with high-dose valproate. However, these subgroup analyses should be interpreted cautiously, especially because the numbers were small and the confidence intervals were not calculated.

In a retrospective Dutch study, the rate of major congenital anomalies among 1411 children born of mothers who had taken antiepileptic drugs during the first trimester of pregnancy was 3.7% compared with 1.5% among 2000 children born of matched controls not exposed to anticonvulsants (158). Among monotherapies with a denominator higher than 50, the relative risk (RR) was increased significantly only for carbamazepine (RR = 2.6) and valproate (RR = 4.1); for valproate there was a relation with dose. Although the risk was not increased in offspring exposed to phenobarbital monotherapy, it increased significantly (RR = 2.6) when those exposed to phenobarbital plus caffeine were combined with those who were exposed to phenobarbital alone. Caffeine intake was also associated with an increased risk among exposures to phenobarbital in combination with other anticonvulsants. Among other polytherapies, there was an increased risk for combinations that included clonazepam and for the combination of carbamazepine with valproate. Cautious interpretation of these data is required, because of the retrospective design and the small sample sizes in the subgroup analyses.

The teratogenic effects of antiepileptic drugs have been assessed through the use of a surveillance system (MADRE) in infants with malformations (159). Exposure was defined by the use of antiepileptic drugs during the first trimester of pregnancy. Of 8005 cases of malformations, 299 infants had been exposed in utero to antiepileptic drugs. Of those exposed to monotherapy, 46 were exposed to carbamazepine, 10 to methylphenobarbital, 65 to phenobarbital, 24 to phenytoin, 80 to valproic acid, and 16 to other antiepileptic drugs. The following associations were found:

(a) carbamazepine: cardiac malformations;
(b) methylphenobarbital: oral clefts and cardiac malformations;
(c) phenobarbital: oral clefts and cardiac malformations;
(d) valproate: spina bifida, cardiac malformations, hypospadias, porencephaly, and other specified anomalies of the brain, anomalies of the face, coarctation of the aorta, and limb reduction defects.

Three groups of infants born to 128 049 women were identified at time of delivery: those exposed to anticonvulsant drugs, those unexposed to anticonvulsant drugs but with a maternal history of seizures, and those unexposed to anticonvulsant drugs with no maternal history of seizures (controls) (160). The aim was to determine whether the major malformations associated with antiepileptic drugs are related to maternal epilepsy or exposure to anticonvulsant drugs. The infants were examined systematically for major malformations, signs of hypoplasia of the midface and fingers, microcephaly, and small body size. The combined frequency of anticonvulsant embryopathy was higher in 223 infants exposed to one anticonvulsant drug than in 508 controls (21 versus 8.5%; OR=2.8; 95% CI=1.1, 9.7). The frequency of anticonvulsant embryopathy was also higher in 93 infants exposed to two or more anticonvulsant drugs than in controls (28 versus 8.5%; OR=4.2; 95% CI=1.1, 5.1). The 98 infants whose mothers had a history of epilepsy but took no anticonvulsant drugs during the pregnancy did not have a higher frequency of malformations than the control infants. Thus, fetal malformations in women with epilepsy are associated with the drugs rather than the epilepsy.

The developmental outcome in children of women exposed to antiepileptic drugs has been assessed in a retrospective survey that included 150 women on monotherapy, 74 on polytherapy, and 176 not exposed to any antiepileptic drugs (161). The odds ratio of additional educational needs in children exposed to antiepileptic drugs in utero compared with those not exposed was 1.49 (95% CI=0.83, 2.67). Those exposed to valproate monotherapy had an odds ratio of 3.4 (95% CI=1.63, 7.10), significantly higher than in those exposed to carbamazepine (OR=0.26; 95% CI=0.06, 1.15). Although the authors concluded that valproate during pregnancy impairs development in children exposed in utero, the fact that this was a retrospective study means that firm conclusions are not possible.

In a prospective study of electroencephalograms, intelligence tests (Wechsler), and neurological findings (Touwen) in 67 school-age and adolescent children born to mothers with epilepsy (risk group) and in 49 controls, focal electroencephalographic changes were more common in the offspring of mothers with primary generalized epilepsy, and pathological electroencephalograms were overall more common after maternal exposure to phenobarbital or primidone (162). The prevalence of minor neurological dysfunction was also increased in the risk group, especially in the offspring of mothers who had been exposed to polytherapy. Intelligence scores were lower after maternal exposure to polytherapies in which one of the drugs was phenytoin or primidone, but socioeconomic influences also affected the scores. Higher maternal dosages of primidone were associated with lower IQ scores in the children. This study has reinforced the evidence that antenatal exposure to anticonvulsants can adversely affect postnatal intellectual development. However, it is always difficult to control for confounders, such as hereditary and social and family factors. It is also possible that prenatal drug exposure affects neural vulnerability to external influences.

A case-control study in 116 children born to epileptic women has suggested that for subjects without inherited factors the risk of developmental disorders is related to antenatal exposure to polypharmacy (OR=4.8, 95% CI=1.3, 18) and valproate monotherapy (OR = 9.4, 95% CI = 1.7, 50) (163). The findings were presented in abstract form, precluding close scrutiny of methodological aspects.

The possibility has been raised that a child who is seemingly normal at birth might later show impaired physical and/or mental development as a result of prenatal exposure to the effects of seizures or drugs. In one study, there was a correlation between seizures during pregnancy and impaired cognitive ability and psychomotor function in the child (SEDA-16, 70). In another study there were delays in height and weight gain in the offspring of epileptic mothers after the first month, but weight at 5.5 years of age was not affected (SED-13, 137). There was a reduction in mean head circumference without obvious intellectual impairment in children exposed to monotherapy with carbamazepine and barbiturates, but a low parental mean head circumference was a major confounding factor. In another study (164), children exposed to phenytoin in utero had lower language development scores and mean global IQ scores 10 points lower than matched controls exposed to non-teratogens; in contrast, children exposed prenatally to carbamazepine did not differ from controls. However, the validity of the statistical analysis and the comparability of groups in this study have been questioned.

Barbiturates have been most often implicated in detrimental effects on postnatal mental development. In two double-blind studies in 114 adult men exposed prenatally to phenobarbital, verbal intelligence scores were about 0.5 standard deviations lower than predicted from data in 153 matched controls (165). An exposure period that included the last trimester of pregnancy was most detrimental. Lower socioeconomic status and being the offspring of an unwanted pregnancy increased the magnitude of impairment, suggesting that adverse drug effects are magnified by interactions with environmental conditions.

Overall, the available evidence suggests that the incidence of mental deficiency in children of epileptic mothers is similar to that in the general population, although general intelligence may be lower and specific forms of cognitive dysfunction somewhat more frequent, owing to a combination of factors such as prenatal exposure to certain drugs, genetic influences, and postnatal environment.

Mechanisms

The mechanisms responsible for abnormal embryonic and fetal development in women taking antiepileptic drugs are unclear. There may be an interaction between the drugs and the underlying disease, and research has also focused on drug-induced folate or pantothenic acid deficiency, altered retinoid metabolism (SEDA-20, 59), and tissue damage caused by reactive metabolites or by embryonic hypoxia/reoxygenation. There is evidence that a genetic defect in arene oxide detoxification can increase the risk of birth defects, and epoxide hydrolase might prove useful in identifying probands at greater risk (SED-13, 137) (166).

Of the newer anticonvulsants, lamotrigine, gabapentin, tiagabine, and vigabatrin have little or no teratogenic potential in animals, whereas oxcarbazepine and topiramate are teratogenic in rodents. However, animal studies are not necessarily applicable to humans and clinical data are still insufficient to assess the effects of newer drugs on the development of the human fetus (153).

Management

Current guidelines stress the need for expert counseling, preferably before conception. Comprehensive management should include review of genetic risks, advice about contraception and interactions with oral contraceptives, information on teratogenic risks and methods for prenatal diagnosis, and integrated care by the family doctor, epileptologist, gynecologist, geneticist, and pediatrician (52,167).

Whenever possible, therapy should be optimized before pregnancy. Withdrawal of anticonvulsants can be considered after 2–5 years of seizure freedom, when other prognostic factors indicate little risk for recurrence; in that event, withdrawal should be completed at least 6 months before planning conception. In all other patients, the goal is the minimal drug load associated with acceptable seizure control. This involves selecting the most effective medication, preferably as monotherapy, at the lowest effective dosage. Control of tonic-clonic seizures before pregnancy is especially important. If possible, valproate should be avoided, especially in women with a family history of neural tube defects and in those who may object to early termination of pregnancy if a severe fetal defect should be diagnosed prenatally. If valproate is used, it should be given in two or three divided daily doses, preferably as a modified-release formulation, to minimize fluctuations in serum drug concentrations. Tobacco and alcohol should be avoided (52,167). Folate supplementation has been recommended in all women with epilepsy who plan to become pregnant and should be continued until the twelfth week of gestation. Although there is no consensus about optimal dosage, 0.4 mg/day of folic acid is a reasonable option; a larger dose (4 mg/day) is preferable if the woman has previously given birth to a child with a neural tube defect. Some authors also recommend 4 mg/day in women taking valproate or carbamazepine (168).

Because seizures themselves can adversely affect fetal outcome, and because in most patients any serious teratogenic effect will have occurred by the time pregnancy is diagnosed, changes in drug therapy during pregnancy are not recommended unless they are required by a change in the clinical response. If seizure frequency increases during pregnancy, possible non-compliance and changes in plasma drug concentration need to be considered.

Prenatal diagnosis with ultrasound at weeks 18–20 can assist in the early diagnosis of anomalies such as cleft palate, heart defects, and neural tube defects. In many patients, prenatal assessment of fetal development can be based on a combination of maternal serum alpha-fetoprotein (as screening for neural tube defect) and malformation-directed ultrasonography. Although amniocentesis at week 15–16 for alpha-fetoprotein determination can be considered for patients at high risk of neural tube defect, it carries a small risk of abortion and its use has fallen with advances in ultrasonography (including transvaginal ultrasonography).

Fetotoxicity

Contrary to early reports, which were affected by selection bias, later studies suggested that neither epilepsy nor prenatal exposure to antiepileptic drugs is associated with an increased risk of spontaneous abortion or other obstetric complications (169).

Prenatal exposure to enzyme-inducing anticonvulsants entails a risk of serious neonatal hemorrhage in the first few days after birth. To reduce the risk, some authorities recommend that pregnant women taking enzyme-inducing drugs be given vitamin K (20 mg/day) during the last month of pregnancy. Intramuscular vitamin K (1 mg) should be given to the neonate immediately after birth. The value of additional vitamin K orally for the first 3 months of life is controversial (168).

After delivery, the maternal response to drug treatment and, if appropriate, serum drug concentrations should be monitored, because the disposition of anticonvulsants can change. The neonate should be monitored for potential residual effects of transplacentally acquired anticonvulsants and, in the case of barbiturates and benzodiazepines, withdrawal symptoms such as irritability and feeding difficulties.

Lactation

Most anticonvulsants are excreted in the breast milk in limited amounts, and their use is not generally a contraindication to breastfeeding. Barbiturates, ethosuximide, lamotrigine, and to a lesser extent carbamazepine and benzodiazepines can reach appreciable serum concentrations in breast-fed infants, who should be carefully observed.

Susceptibility Factors

Age

Children
Febrile seizures are the most common seizure disorder in childhood, occurring in 2–5% of children, but there is no unanimity regarding the need for long-term antiepileptic drug therapy. A subcommittee of the American Academy of Pediatrics has recently concluded that there are no long-term adverse effects of simple febrile seizures, and that although there is evidence that continuous antiepileptic therapy with phenobarbital or valproate and intermittent therapy with diazepam are effective in reducing the risk of recurrence, the potential adverse effects associated with antiepileptic drugs outweigh the relatively minor risks associated with simple febrile seizures (170). They recommended that long-term treatment is not indicated.

Renal disease

Renally eliminated drugs should be used in reduced dosages in patients with renal insufficiency.

Hepatic disease

Anticonvulsants that are metabolized should be used cautiously in patients with severe hepatic disease.

Other features of the patient

Most antiepileptic drugs are contraindicated in acute intermittent porphyrias.

Case reports have suggested that the risk of serious skin reactions to phenytoin is increased in patients with brain tumors undergoing cranial irradiation, but the incidence of these reactions is unknown (113). In a retrospective study of 289 patients with brain tumors, rash occurred in 18% of exposures to antiepileptic drugs, including 22% of exposures to phenytoin, compared with an expected rate of 5–10%. Most of the rashes occurred before the start of irradiation therapy. Only one patient developed erythema multiforme. These data suggest that the risk of serious skin reactions in patients with brain tumors is actually low, even though there was an increased frequency of milder rashes. Irradiation did not appear to contribute to the risk. However, it is possible that earlier publications about the risk of serious reactions resulted in the use of lower initial dosages or earlier withdrawal of medication, before the onset of more severe manifestations. The fact that skin rashes were more common in patients with glioma than metastatic disease could be related to the effects of underlying treatments (or disease) on immune function.

Of 65 consecutive patients with malignant glioma started on anticonvulsants (mostly phenytoin), a skin rash developed in 26%; other toxic effects occurred in 14% of patients, including three who developed an encephalopathy sufficient to require hospitalization (SEDA-20, 58).

Drug Administration

Drug formulations

The rationale and use of modified-release formulations of antiepileptic drugs (carbamazepine, valproic acid, and tiagabine) have been reviewed (171). The authors concluded that modified-release formulations afford the advantages of better patient compliance, fewer adverse effects, and less fluctuation in plasma concentrations, making monitoring of drug concentrations easier. They concluded that these advantages should lead to better seizure control and improved quality of life.

Drug overdose

Accidental or deliberate overdose with anticonvulsants is common and can cause serious morbidity, even though deaths are relatively rare (172–174). Clinical manifestations vary from drug to drug, and they tend to affect mainly the central nervous system, with signs ranging from impaired consciousness to motor and coordination disturbances and seizures (for a review, see SEDA-22, 84). Metabolic, cardiac, and respiratory disturbances are seen with individual drugs. Except for flumazenil in benzodiazepine overdose, there are no specific antidotes, and management is primarily supportive. Gastric lavage is indicated within 1 hour of a major overdose with most anticonvulsants. Oral activated charcoal and hemoperfusion can be useful in individual cases of overdose with phenytoin, carbamazepine, valproate, barbiturates, and some other drugs (SEDA-22, 84). In cases of valproate overdose, naloxone has been sometimes beneficial, and carnitine supplementation has been recommended (88).

Drug–Drug Interactions

General

The interactions of anticonvulsants are summarized in Table 2, Table 3, and Table 4. Phenytoin, carbamazepine, and barbiturates are enzyme inducers and can reduce the

Table 2 Interactions of antiepileptic drugs

Interfering drug(s) (precipitant drug(s))	Affected drug(s) (object drug(s))	Implications/comments	Mechanism
Carbamazepine	Phenytoin	Interaction inconsistent and usually of limited clinical significance	Induction and inhibition of phenytoin metabolism
Carbamazepine Phenobarbital Phenytoin Primidone	Ethosuximide Felbamate Lamotrigine Tiagabide Topiramate Valproate Zonisamide Clobazam Clonazepam Diazepam	Reduced effect of the object drug, usually compensated by the effect of the added drug; risk of toxicity when interfering drug is discontinued	Induction of metabolism of the object drug
Carbamazepine Phenytoin	Primidone	Signs of toxicity possible after addition of phenytoin owing to concomitant increase in plasma phenobarbital concentrations in some patients	Induction of primidone metabolism; phenytoin may inhibit the clearance of metabolically derived phenobarbital
Clobazam	Carbamazepine Primidone Valproate Phenytoin	Interaction inconsistent, usually of little clinical significance	Inhibition of metabolism of the object drug
Clobazam	Phenytoin Primidone	Interaction inconsistent, usually of no clinical significance	Unknown
Diazepam	Phenytoin	Interaction inconsistent, usually of no clinical significance	Inhibition of phenytoin metabolism
Ethosuximide	Valproate	Fall in valproate concentrations inconsistent; therapeutic synergism common	Therapeutic synergism due to pharmacodynamic interaction
Felbamate	Clonazepam Diazepam Phenobarbital Phenytoin Valproate	High risk of toxicity with phenytoin, phenobarbital, and valproate	Inhibition of metabolism of the affected drug
Felbamate	Carbamazepine	Risk of toxicity due to concomitant rise in carbamazepine epoxide concentration and pharmacodynamic interaction	Induction of carbamazepine metabolism, possible inhibition of epoxide hydrolase and pharmacodynamic interaction
Gabapentin	Felbamate	Interaction poorly documented; relevance doubtful	Perhaps reduced renal clearance of felbamate
Gamma-vinyl GABA	Phenytoin Phenobarbital Felbamate	Interaction inconsistent and usually of little clinical relevance	Unknown
Oxcarbazepine	Lamotrigine	Interaction less marked than that caused by carbamazepine	Induction of lamotrigine metabolism
Phenobarbital	Phenytoin	Interaction inconsistent and usually of little clinical significance	Induction and inhibition of phenytoin metabolism
Phenobarbital Phenytoin Primidone	Carbamazepine	Reduced effect of carbamazepine usually compensated by the action of the added drug; risk of carbamazepine toxicity when interfering drug is withdrawn	Induction of carbamazepine metabolism
Phenytoin	Phenobarbital	Interaction inconsistent and usually of limited clinical significance	Inhibition of phenobarbital metabolism
Tiagabide	Valproate	Effect of low magnitude, probably clinically irrelevant	Unknown
Topiramate	Phenytoin	Interaction inconsistent, usually of little clinical significance	Inhibition of phenytoin metabolism

Continued

Table 2 _Continued_

Interfering drug (precipitant drug(s))	Affected drug(s) (object drug(s))	Implications/comments	Mechanism
Valproate	Carbamazepine epoxide Diazepam Felbamate Lamotrigine Phenobarbital	Risk of toxicity, particularly with phenobarbital including primidone-derived phenobarbital and lamotrigine	Inhibition of metabolism of the affected drug. Valproate also displaces diazepam from protein binding sites, affecting relation between total diazepam concentration and effect
Valproate	Ethosuximide	Increase in ethosuximide concentration inconsistent; synergistic therapeutic effect common	Inhibition of ethosuximide metabolism; therapeutic synergism due to pharmacodynamic interaction
Valproate	Lamotrigine	Risk of toxicity; therapeutic synergism possible	Inhibition of lamotrigine metabolism and pharmacodynamic interaction
Valproate	Phenytoin	Total serum phenytoin concentration underestimates the unbound phenytoin concentration; toxicity can occur in some patients	Displacement of phenytoin from plasma proteins, sometimes associated with inhibition of phenytoin metabolism
Valproate	Tiagabine	Interaction described in vivo remains to be clarified	Valproate displaces tiagabine from plasma binding sites in vitro
Valproate	Topiramate	Effect of low magnitude, clinically irrelevant	Unknown

Table 3 Interactions in which the serum concentration of an antiepileptic drug is modified by drugs used for other conditions

Interfering drug (precipitant drug(s))	Affected drug(s) (object drug(s))	Implications/comments	Mechanism
Analgesics			
Azapropazone	Phenytoin	Risk of phenytoin toxicity; altered relation between total phenytoin concentration and effect	Displacement from plasma proteins and inhibition of phenytoin metabolism
Bromfenac	Phenytoin	Probably of little clinical significance	Inhibition of phenytoin metabolism
Dextropropoxyphene	Carbamazepine Phenobarbital Phenytoin	Risk of toxicity, particularly with carbamazepine	Inhibition of metabolism of the affected drugs
Ibuprofen	Phenytoin	Interaction probably of little or no clinical significance	Displacement from plasma protein binding sites
Naproxen	Valproate	Interaction of little or no clinical significance	Displacement from plasma protein binding sites
Paracetamol	Lamotrigine	Interaction probably of little or no clinical significance	Unknown
Phenylbutazone	Phenytoin Valproate	Risk of toxicity, particularly with phenytoin; altered relation between total concentration and effect	Displacement from plasma protein binding sites and inhibition of metabolism of the affected drugs
Salicylic acid	Phenytoin Valproate	Altered relation between total anticonvulsant concentration and effect[a]	Displacement from plasma protein binding sites
Tenidap sodium	Phenytoin	Interaction poorly documented	Displacement from plasma protein binding sites
Antineoplastic drugs			
Bleomycin	Phenytoin	Reduced effect of phenytoin; interaction poorly documented	Unknown
Carboplatin	Phenytoin	Reduced effect of phenytoin; interaction poorly documented	Unknown
Carmustine	Phenytoin	Reduced effect of phenytoin; interaction poorly documented	Unknown
Cisplatin	Carbamazepine Phenytoin Valproate	Reduced effect of phenytoin; interaction poorly documented	Unknown
Methotrexate	Phenytoin Valproate	Reduced effect of phenytoin; interaction poorly documented	Unknown

Continued

Table 3   *Continued*

Interfering drug (precipitant drug(s))	Affected drug(s) (object drug(s))	Implications/comments	Mechanism
Vinblastine	Phenytoin	Reduced effect of phenytoin; interaction poorly documented	Unknown
Vincristine	Phenytoin	Reduced effect of phenytoin; interaction poorly documented	Unknown
Tegafur uracil	Phenytoin	Risk of phenytoin toxicity	Unknown
Antimicrobial drugs			
Aciclovir	Phenytoin Valproate	Reduced effect of the object drug; poorly documented	Unknown
Ceftriaxone	Phenytoin	Risk of toxicity; altered relation between total phenytoin concentration and effect	Displacement of phenytoin from binding sites and possible inhibition phenytoin metabolism
Chloramphenicol	Phenobarbital Phenytoin Primidone	Risk of toxicity of the object drugs	Inhibition of metabolism of the object drugs
Ciprofloxacin	Phenytoin	Reduced effect of phenytoin	Unknown
Fluconazole	Phenytoin	Risk of phenytoin toxicity	Inhibition of phenytoin metabolism
Isoniazid	Carbamazepine Diazepam Ethosuximide Phenobarbital Phenytoin Primidone Valproate	High risk of toxicity, especially with carbamazepine and phenytoin	Inhibition of metabolism of the object drugs
Ketoconazole	Carbamazepine Zonisamide	Risk of toxicity of the affected drugs	Inhibition of metabolism of the affected drugs
Erythromycin	Carbamazepine Phenytoin Valproate	Risk of toxicity; particularly with carbamazepine	Inhibition of metabolism of the affected drugs
Other macrolides (clarithromycin, flurithromycin, josamycin, ponsinomycin, triacetyloleandomycin)	Carbamazepine	High risk of carbamazepine toxicity	Inhibition of carbamazepine metabolism
Mefloquine	Valproate	Reduced effect of valproate; interaction poorly documented	Unknown
Metronidazole	Carbamazepine Phenytoin	Risk of toxicity; effect on phenytoin inconsistent	Inhibition of metabolism of the object drugs
Miconazole	Phenytoin Zonisamide	Risk of toxicity of the object drugs	Inhibition of metabolism of the object drugs
Nafcillin	Phenytoin	Altered relation between total phenytoin concentration and effect	Displacement of phenytoin from binding sites
Nitrofurantoin	Phenytoin	Reduced effect of phenytoin; interaction poorly documented	Unknown
Oxacillin	Phenytoin	Reduced effect of phenytoin; interaction poorly documented	Unknown
Panipenem-betamipron	Valproate	Reduced effect of valproate; interaction poorly documented	Unknown
Quinine	Carbamazepine Phenobarbital	Enhanced effect of the object drugs	Inhibition of metabolism of the object drugs
Rifampicin	Diazepam Ethosuximide Phenobarbital Phenytoin Valproate	Reduced effect of the object drugs	Induction of metabolism of the object drugs
Sulfadiazine	Phenytoin	Risk of phenytoin toxicity	Inhibition of phenytoin metabolism
Sulfafurazole	Phenytoin	Risk of phenytoin toxicity	Inhibition of phenytoin metabolism
Sulfamethoxazole	Phenytoin	Risk of phenytoin toxicity	Inhibition of phenytoin metabolism
Sulfamethoxazole + trimethoprim (co-trimoxazole)	Phenytoin	Risk of phenytoin toxicity	Inhibition of phenytoin metabolism

Continued

Table 3 *Continued*

Interfering drug (precipitant drug(s))	Affected drug(s) (object drug(s))	Implications/comments	Mechanism
Sulfamethoxypyridazine	Phenytoin	Risk of phenytoin toxicity	Inhibition of phenytoin metabolism
Sulfametizole	Phenytoin	Risk of phenytoin toxicity	Inhibition of phenytoin metabolism
Sulfaphenazole	Phenytoin	Risk of phenytoin toxicity	Inhibition of phenytoin metabolism
Trimethoprim	Phenytoin	Enhanced effect of phenytoin	Inhibition of phenytoin metabolism
Antiulcer agents			
Antacids	Gabapentin Phenobarbital Phenytoin	Reduced effect of the object drugs	Reduced absorption of the object drugs
Cimetidine	Carbamazepine Clobazam Clonazepam Diazepam Phenytoin Valproate	Risk of toxicity, particularly with phenytoin	Inhibition of metabolism of the object drugs
Omeprazole	Diazepam Phenytoin	Risk of toxicity of the object drugs	Inhibition of metabolism of the object drugs
Ranitidine	Phenytoin	Inconsistent, probably of little clinical significance	Unknown
Sucralfate	Phenytoin	Reduced effect of phenytoin	Reduced absorption of phenytoin
Cardiovascular			
Amiodarone	Clonazepam Phenytoin	Risk of toxicity of the object drugs	Inhibition of metabolism of the object drugs
Bishydroxycoumarin	Phenytoin	Risk of phenytoin toxicity	Inhibition of phenytoin metabolism
Dicoumarol	Phenobarbital Phenytoin	Risk of toxicity, particularly with phenytoin	Inhibition of metabolism of the object drugs
Diltiazem	Carbamazepine Phenytoin	Risk of toxicity, especially with carbamazepine	Inhibition of metabolism of the object drugs
Guanfacine	Valproate	Enhanced effect of valproate; interaction poorly documented	Unknown
Phenprocoumon	Phenytoin	Risk of phenytoin toxicity	Inhibition of phenytoin metabolism
Sulfinpyrazone	Phenytoin	Risk of phenytoin toxicity	Inhibition of phenytoin metabolism
Ticlopidine	Phenytoin	Risk of phenytoin toxicity	Inhibition of phenytoin metabolism
Verapamil	Carbamazepine Phenytoin	High risk of carbamazepine toxicity; interaction with phenytoin inconsistent	Inhibition of metabolism of the object drugs
Verapamil	10-monohydroxy–carbazepine	Interaction probably of limited clinical significance	Unknown
Psychotropic drugs			
Amitriptyline	Phenytoin	Risk of phenytoin toxicity; interaction poorly documented	Inhibition of phenytoin metabolism
Chlorpromazine	Phenobarbital Phenytoin Valproate	Probably of little clinical relevance; for phenytoin, a fall in concentration has also been reported	Inhibition of metabolism of the object drugs
Ethanol	Clobazam Diazepam Phenytoin	Risk of toxicity of the object drugs; chronic ethanol can reduce serum phenytoin concentrations	Inhibition of metabolism; induction of phenytoin metabolism by chronic ethanol
Fluoxetine	Carbamazepine Diazepam Phenytoin Valproate	Risk of toxicity of the object drugs; with carbamazepine and valproate, interaction inconsistent	Inhibition of metabolism of the object drugs
Fluvoxamine	Carbamazepine Diazepam Phenytoin	Risk of toxicity of the affected drugs; with carbamazepine, interaction inconsistent	Inhibition of metabolism of the object drugs
Haloperidol	Carbamazepine	Risk of carbamazepine toxicity	Inhibition of metabolism of the object drugs
Imipramine	Phenytoin	Risk of phenytoin toxicity; interaction inconsistent	Inhibition of phenytoin metabolism
Loxapine	Carbamazepine	Risk of carbamazepine toxicity; interaction poorly documented	Unknown
Mesoridazine	Phenytoin	Reduced effect of phenytoin; interaction poorly documented	Unknown
Methylphenidate	Phenytoin Primidone	Risk of toxicity of the affected drugs; interaction inconsistent	Inhibition of metabolism of the object drugs

Continued

Table 3 *Continued*

Interfering drug (precipitant drug(s))	Affected drug(s) (object drug(s))	Implications/comments	Mechanism
Nefazodone	Carbamazepine	Risk of carbamazepine toxicity; interaction poorly documented	Inhibition of Carbamazepine metabolism
Sertraline	Carbamazepine Diazepam Lamotrigine Phenytoin	Risk of toxicity of the object drugs	Inhibition of metabolism of the object drugs
Thioridazine	Phenobarbital Phenytoin	Probably of little clinical relevance; an increase in serum phenytoin has also been described	Unknown
Trazodone	Phenytoin	Risk of phenytoin toxicity	Inhibition of phenytoin metabolism
Valnoctamide	Carbamazepine	Risk of carbamazepine toxicity	Inhibition of epoxide hydrolase
Viloxazine	Carbamazepine Phenytoin Oxcarbazepine	Risk of phenytoin and carbamazepine toxicity; interaction with oxcarbazepine probably of little clinical significance	Inhibition of metabolism of the object drugs
Miscellaneous			
Acetazolamide	Phenobarbital	Interaction probably of little clinical significance	Unknown
Acetazolamide	Primidone	Interaction probably of little clinical significance	Possibly reduced absorption of primidone
Activated charcoal	Carbamazepine Lamotrigine Phenobarbital Phenytoin Valproate	With some drugs can be exploited to reduce drug concentrations in overdose	Sequestration in the gastrointestinal tract
Allopurinol	Phenytoin	Risk of phenytoin toxicity	Inhibition of phenytoin metabolism
Aminophylline	Carbamazepine	Reduced effect of carbamazepine; interaction poorly documented	Unknown
Caffeine	Carbamazepine	Reduced effect of carbamazepine; interaction poorly documented	Unknown
Calcium carbide	Phenytoin	Risk of phenytoin toxicity	Inhibition of phenytoin metabolism
Chlorphenamine	Phenytoin	Risk of phenytoin toxicity	Inhibition of phenytoin metabolism
Colestyramine	Valproate	Interaction probably of little clinical significance	Reduced absorption of valproate
Danazol	Carbamazepine	Risk of carbamazepine toxicity	Inhibition of carbamazepine metabolism
Dexamethasone	Phenytoin	Interaction inconsistent	Unknown
Diazoxide	Phenytoin	Altered relation between total phenytoin concentration and effect	Displacement from plasma protein binding sites
Disulfiram	Diazepam Phenytoin	Risk of toxicity, particularly with phenytoin	Inhibition of metabolism of the object drugs
Enteral feeding formulas (some)	Phenytoin	Reduced effect of phenytoin	Reduced absorption of Phenytoin
Folic acid	Phenobarbital Phenytoin	Reduced effect of the object drug	Accelerated metabolism of the object drugs
Grapefruit juice	Carbamazepine Phenytoin unbound fraction	Risk of carbamazepine toxicity	Inhibition of carbamazepine metabolism
Halofenate	Phenytoin unbound fraction	Altered relation between total phenytoin concentration and effect	Displacement from plasma protein binding sites
Influenza vaccine	Carbamazepine Phenobarbital Phenytoin	Risk of toxicity of the affected drugs; effect on phenytoin inconsistent	Inhibition of metabolism of the object drugs
Nicotinamide	Carbamazepine Primidone	Risk of toxicity of the object drugs	Inhibition of metabolism of the object drugs
Fenyramidol	Phenytoin	Risk of phenytoin toxicity; interaction poorly documented	Unknown
Tacrolimus	Phenytoin	Risk of phenytoin toxicity	Unknown
Tamoxifen	Phenytoin	Risk of phenytoin toxicity	Unknown
Theophylline	Phenytoin	Reduced effect of phenytoin; interaction poorly documented	Unknown

Continued

Table 3 *Continued*

Interfering drug (precipitant drug(s))	Affected drug(s) (object drug(s))	Implications/comments	Mechanism
Tolbutamide	Phenytoin	Risk of toxicity; altered relation between total phenytoin concentration and effect	Displacement from plasma protein binding sites and possibly inhibition of phenytoin metabolism

*Inconclusive evidence suggests that salicylic acid can potentiate valproate toxicity (mechanism unclear). Sulfafurazole, sulfamethoxypyridazine, possibly other sulfonamides, and sulfinpyrazone displace phenytoin from plasma protein binding sites with different affinities; total phenytoin concentrations may underestimate the concentration of unbound (pharmacologically active) drug.

Table 4 Drugs that inhibit the metabolism of antiepileptic drugs and cause intoxication

Analgesics
Bromfenac
Codeine
Dextropropoxyphene
Methadone
Paracetamol
Pethidine
Phenazone
Phenylbutazone

Anticoagulants
Dicoumarol[1]
Warfarin

Antineoplastic drugs
Aminocamptothecin
Busulfan
Cyclophosphamide
Etoposide
Ifosfamide
Methotrexate[2]
Teniposide
Topotecan
Vincristine

Antimicrobial drugs
Chloramphenicol
Delavirdine
Doxycycline
Griseofulvin[3]
Indinavir
Itraconazole
Ketoconazole
Mebendazole
Metronidazole
Misonidazole
Nelfinavir
Praziquantel
Ritonavir
Saquinavir

Cardiovascular drugs
Alprenolol
Amiodarone
Digitoxin[4]
Digoxin[5]
Disopyramide
Felodipine
Flunarizine
Lidocaine
Metoprolol
Mexiletine
Nifedipine
Nimodipine
Nisoldipine
Propranolol
Quinidine
Timolol

Glucocorticoids
Dexamethasone
Fludrocortisone
Methylprednisolone
Prednisolone
Prednisone

Immunosuppressants
Ciclosporin[6]
Tacrolimus

Neuromuscular blockers[7]
Atracurium
Metocurine
Oxacurium
Pancuronium
Pipecuronium
Rocuronium
Vecuronium

Oral contraceptives[8]

Psychotropic drugs
Alprazolam
Amfebutamone
Amitriptyline
Amoxapine
Bromperidol
Chlorpromazine
Citalopram
Clozapine
Desipramine
Doxepin
Haloperidol
Imipramine
Mesoridazine
Mianserin
Midazolam
Nefazodone
Nortriptyline
Olanzapine
Paroxetine
Protriptyline
Thioridazine[9]
Trazodone
Valnoctamide
Zotepine

Miscellaneous
Chenodeoxycholic acid
Cimetidine
Ethanol
Etretinate
Fentanyl
Folic acid
Furosemide[10]
Metyrapone
Omeprazole
Psoralens
Theophylline
Thyroxine
Tirilazad
Vitamin D analogues

[1] In addition to enzyme induction, phenobarbital can reduce dicoumarol absorption.
[2] Interaction seen only with phenytoin and mediated by displacement from plasma protein binding sites; no reduction in methotrexate activity is expected; the relation between total methotrexate concentration and effect can be altered.
[3] Some anticonvulsants can reduce griseofulvin absorption.
[4] The evidence is conflicting.
[5] In addition to enzyme induction, phenytoin can reduce digoxin absorption.
[6] With phenytoin, reduced absorption can contribute to the fall in ciclosporin concentrations.
[7] A pharmacodynamic interaction may contribute to the reduced effect of neuromuscular blocking drugs.
[8] Carbamazepine, phenytoin, phenobarbital and primidone, felbamate, oxcarbazepine, and topiramate stimulate the metabolism of oral contraceptive steroids.
[9] The concentration of the active metabolite mesoridazine falls more markedly.
[10] Phenytoin and phenobarbital reduce furosemide absorption.

serum concentrations and clinical effects of other anticonvulsants (valproate, carbamazepine itself, including autoinduction, ethosuximide, felbamate, lamotrigine, topiramate, tiagabine, zonisamide, benzodiazepines) and a large number of other drugs that are metabolized by inducible enzymes. Examples of affected agents include oral anticoagulants, glucocorticoids, dihydropyridine calcium channel blockers and other cardioactive drugs, neuroleptic drugs, antimicrobial drugs including antiretroviral drugs, and steroid oral contraceptives. The efficacy of the contraceptive pill can also be reduced by the weaker inducers of CYP3A4, oxcarbazepine, felbamate, and topiramate.

On the other hand, felbamate and to a lesser extent valproate inhibit a range of liver enzymes and can increase the concentration of several drugs, leading to potentiation of their effects.

Similarly, drugs given for the treatment of associated disorders may inhibit the metabolism of anticonvulsants and precipitate signs of intoxication (Table 3). Examples include the increase in serum phenytoin concentrations by isoniazid and the increase in serum carbamazepine concentrations by verapamil, diltiazem, and most macrolide antibiotics (175–179).

Plasma protein binding interactions are usually clinically unimportant, but they should be recognized, because they alter the relation between serum drug concentration and the clinical response: if displacement occurs, therapeutic and toxic effects are reached at a total drug concentration lower than usual. For example, valproic acid and salicylate displace phenytoin from plasma proteins; this usually results in a fall in total phenytoin concentration without any change in the concentration of unbound (pharmacologically active) phenytoin.

Pharmacodynamic interactions also occur. In particular, the adverse effects of any drug can be increased by other drugs with similar properties. One example is the reciprocal potentiation of the neurotoxic effects of carbamazepine and lamotrigine in patients taking a combination of these drugs (180). Some drugs (for example ciclosporin, clozapine) have a proconvulsant effect and can reduce the efficacy of antiepileptic drugs.

Cisatracurium

The effect of cisatracurium on the onset, duration, and speed of recovery from neuromuscular blockade has been studied in 24 patients taking antiepileptic drugs and 14 controls (181). The onset and duration of neuromuscular blockade were not different among the groups, but the speed of recovery was significantly faster in those taking antiepileptic drugs.

Steroid neuromuscular blockers

Patients taking carbamazepine or phenytoin are resistant to steroid neuromuscular blocking drugs (181).

Diagnosis of Adverse Drug Reactions

The routine drug management of epilepsy by community health nurses without prior training in epilepsy management has been evaluated by neurologists in Zimbabwe (182). Of 114 patients (aged 8–56 years, 84% with generalized seizures), 40% had been seizure-free for at least 6 months;

72% took phenobarbital, 36% took carbamazepine, and 20% took phenytoin; 68% took monotherapy. Specialist interventions were required in 60% of consultations. Serum drug concentrations were measured in 38 patients; 58% were below the target range and 16% were above. Increased dosage was required in 29% of patients and dosage reduction or withdrawal in 18%. In several cases drug withdrawal was undertaken to convert polytherapy to monotherapy.

The use of serum antiepileptic drug concentrations has been reviewed (183). The authors suggested that there is still no evidence that specific target drug concentrations are valid in determining appropriate therapy.

References

1. Willmore LJ. Clinical pharmacology of new antiepileptic drugs. Neurology 2000;55(11 Suppl 3):S17–24.
2. Politsky JM. Painful diabetic neuropathy: treatment with modern anticonvulsants. Mature Med Can 2000;3:60–3.
3. Cramer JA, Fisher R, Ben-Menachem E, French J, Mattson RH. New antiepileptic drugs: comparison of key clinical trials. Epilepsia 1999;40(5):590–600.
4. Treiman DM, Meyers PD, Walton NY, Collins JF, Colling C, Rowan AJ, Handforth A, Faught E, Calabrese VP, Uthman BM, Ramsay RE, Mamdani MB. A comparison of four treatments for generalized convulsive status epilepticus. Veterans Affairs Status Epilepticus Cooperative Study Group. N Engl J Med 1998;339(12):792–8.
5. Gillham R, Kane K, Bryant-Comstock L, Brodie MJ. A double-blind comparison of lamotrigine and carbamazepine in newly diagnosed epilepsy with health-related quality of life as an outcome measure. Seizure 2000;9(6):375–9.
6. Heaney DC, Shorvon SD, Sander JW, Boon P, Komarek V, Marusic P, Dravet C, Perucca E, Majkowski J, Lima JL, Arroyo S, Tomson T, Ried S, van Donselaar C, Eskazan E, Peeters P, Carita P, Tjong-a-Hung I, Myon E, Taieb C. Cost minimization analysis of antiepileptic drugs in newly diagnosed epilepsy in 12 European countries. Epilepsia 2000;41(Suppl 5):S37–44.
7. Collins TL, Petroff OA, Mattson RH. A comparison of four new antiepileptic medications. Seizure 2000;9(4):291–3.
8. Datta PK, Crawford PM. Refractory epilepsy: treatment with new antiepileptic drugs. Seizure 2000;9(1):51–7.
9. Lhatoo SD, Wong IC, Polizzi G, Sander JW. Long-term retention rates of lamotrigine, gabapentin, and topiramate in chronic epilepsy. Epilepsia 2000;41(12):1592–6.
10. Lindberger M, Alenius M, Frisen L, Johannessen SI, Larsson S, Malmgren K, Tomson T. Gabapentin versus vigabatrin as first add-on for patients with partial seizures that failed to respond to monotherapy: a randomized, double-blind, dose titration study. GREAT Study Investigators Group. Gabapentin Refractory Epilepsy Add-on Treatment. Epilepsia 2000;41(10):1289–95.
11. Ghaemi SN, Gaughan S. Novel anticonvulsants: a new generation of mood stabilizers? Harv Rev Psychiatry 2000;8(1):1–7.
12. Vasudev K, Goswami U, Kohli K. Carbamazepine and valproate monotherapy: feasibility, relative safety and efficacy, and therapeutic drug monitoring in manic disorder. Psychopharmacology (Berl) 2000;150(1):15–23.
13. Leandri M, Lundardi G, Inglese M, Messmer-Uccelli M, Mancardi GL, Gottlieb A, Solaro C. Lamotrigine in trigeminal neuralgia secondary to multiple sclerosis. J Neurol 2000;247(7):556–8.
14. Tomson T, Kenneback G. Arrhythmia, heart rate variability, and antiepileptic drugs. Epilepsia 1997;38(Suppl 11):S48–51.

15. Perucca E, Gram L, Avanzini G, Dulac O. Antiepileptic drugs as a cause of worsening seizures. Epilepsia 1998;39(1):5–17.

16. Genton P, Gelisse P, Thomas P, Dravet C. Do carbamazepine and phenytoin aggravate juvenile myoclonic epilepsy? Neurology 2000;55(8):1106–9.

17. Somerville ER. Aggravation of partial seizures by antiepileptic drugs: is there evidence from clinical trials? Neurology 2002;59(1):79–83.

18. Bogliun G, Di Viesti P, Monticelli LM, Beghi E, Zarrelli M, Simone P, Airoldi L, Frattola L. Anticonvulsants and peripheral nerve function results of prospective monitoring in patients with newly diagnosed epilepsy. Clin Drug Invest 2000;20:173–80.

19. Stefan H, Bernatik J, Knorr HLJ. Visual field constriction and antiepileptic drug treatment. Neurol Psychiatry Brain Res 2000;7:185–90.

20. Verrotti A, Trotta D, Cutarella R, Pascarella R, Morgese G, Chiarelli F. Effects of antiepileptic drugs on evoked potentials in epileptic children. Pediatr Neurol 2000;23(5):397–402.

21. Zgorzalewicz M, Galas-Zgorzalewicz B. Visual and auditory evoked potentials during long-term vigabatrin treatment in children and adolescents with epilepsy. Clin Neurophysiol 2000;111(12):2150–4.

22. Wong I, Tavernor S, Tavernor R. Psychiatric adverse effects of anticonvulsant drugs: incidence and therapeutic implications. CNS Drugs 1997;8:492–509.

23. Trimble MR, Rusch N, Betts T, Crawford PM. Psychiatric symptoms after therapy with new antiepileptic drugs: psychopathological and seizure related variables. Seizure 2000;9(4):249–54.

24. Adachi N, Onuma T, Hara T, Matsuura M, Okubo Y, Kato M, Oana Y. Frequency and age-related variables in interictal psychoses in localization-related epilepsies. Epilepsy Res 2002;48(1–2):25–31.

25. Bredkjaer SR, Mortensen PB, Parnas J. Epilepsy and nonorganic non-affective psychosis. National epidemiologic study. Br J Psychiatry 1998;172:235–8.

26. Kanemoto K, Tsuji T, Kawasaki J. Reexamination of interictal psychoses based on DSM IV psychosis classification and international epilepsy classification. Epilepsia 2001;42(1):98–103.

27. Iivanainen M, Savolainen H. Side effects of phenobarbital and phenytoin during long-term treatment of epilepsy. Acta Neurol Scand Suppl 1983;97:49–67.

28. McKee RJ, Larkin JG, Brodie MJ. Acute psychosis with carbamazepine and sodium valproate. Lancet 1989;1(8630):167.

29. McConnell H, Snyder PJ, Duffy JD, Weilburg J, Valeriano J, Brillman J, Cress K, Cavalier J. Neuropsychiatric side effects related to treatment with felbamate. J Neuropsychiatry Clin Neurosci 1996;8(3):341–6.

30. Jablonowski K, Margolese HC, Chouinard G. Gabapentin-induced paradoxical exacerbation of psychosis in a patient with schizophrenia. Can J Psychiatry 2002;47(10):975–6.

31. Kossoff EH, Bergey GK, Freeman JM, Vining EP. Levetiracetam psychosis in children with epilepsy. Epilepsia 2001;42(12):1611–13.

32. Stella F, Caetano D, Cendes F, Guerreiro CA. Acute psychotic disorders induced by topiramate: report of two cases. Arq Neuropsiquiatr 2002;60(2-A):285–7.

33. Sander JW, Hart YM, Trimble MR, Shorvon SD. Vigabatrin and psychosis. J Neurol Neurosurg Psychiatry 1991;54(5):435–9.

34. Miyamoto T, Kohsaka M, Koyama T. Psychotic episodes during zonisamide treatment. Seizure 2000;9(1):65–70.

35. Matsuura M. Epileptic psychoses and anticonvulsant drug treatment. J Neurol Neurosurg Psychiatry 1999;67(2):231–3.

36. Darbar D, Connachie AM, Jones AM, Newton RW. Acute psychosis associated with abrupt withdrawal of carbamazepine following intoxication. Br J Clin Pract 1996;50(6):350–1.

37. Heh CW, Sramek J, Herrera J, Costa J. Exacerbation of psychosis after discontinuation of carbamazepine treatment. Am J Psychiatry 1988;145(7):878–9.

38. Wolf P. Acute behavioral symptomatology at disappearance of epileptiform EEG abnormality. Paradoxical or "forced" normalization. Adv Neurol 1991;55:127–42.

39. Neppe VM. Carbamazepine as adjunctive treatment in nonepileptic chronic inpatients with EEG temporal lobe abnormalities. J Clin Psychiatry 1983;44(9):326–31.

40. Sackellares JC, Krauss G, Sommerville KW, Deaton R. Occurrence of psychosis in patients with epilepsy randomized to tiagabine or placebo treatment. Epilepsia 2002;43(4):394–8.

41. Shorvon SD. Safety of topiramate: adverse events and relationships to dosing. Epilepsia 1996;37(Suppl 2):S18–22.

42. Dietrich DE, Kropp S, Emrich HM. Oxcarbazepine in affective and schizoaffective disorders. Pharmacopsychiatry 2001;34(6):242–50.

43. Besag FM. Behavioural effects of the new anticonvulsants. Drug Saf 2001;24(7):513–36.

44. Veggiotti P, De Agostini G, Muzio C, Termine C, Baldi PL, Ferrari Ginevra O, Lanzi G. Vigabatrin use in psychotic epileptic patients: report of a prospective pilot study. Acta Neurol Scand 1999;99(3):142–6.

45. Aldenkamp AP. Cognitive and behavioural assessment in clinical trials: when should they be done? Epilepsy Res 2001;45(1–3):155–7.

46. Bourgeois BF. Antiepileptic drugs, learning, and behavior in childhood epilepsy. Epilepsia 1998;39(9):913–21.

47. Smith DB, Mattson RH, Cramer JA, Collins JF, Novelly RA, Craft B. Results of a nationwide Veterans Administration Cooperative Study comparing the efficacy and toxicity of carbamazepine, phenobarbital, phenytoin, and primidone. Epilepsia 1987;28(Suppl 3):S50–8.

48. Aldenkamp AP, Alpherts WC, Diepman L, van't Slot B, Overweg J, Vermeulen J. Cognitive side-effects of phenytoin compared with carbamazepine in patients with localization-related epilepsy. Epilepsy Res 1994;19(1):37–43.

49. Pulliainen V, Jokelainen M. Comparing the cognitive effects of phenytoin and carbamazepine in long-term monotherapy: a two-year follow-up. Epilepsia 1995;36(12):1195–202.

50. Stoffel-Wagner B, Bauer J, Flugel D, Brennemann W, Klingmuller D, Elger CE. Serum sex hormones are altered in patients with chronic temporal lobe epilepsy receiving anticonvulsant medication. Epilepsia 1998;39(11):1164–73.

51. Franceschi M, Perego L, Cavagnini F, Cattaneo AG, Invitti C, Caviezel F, Strambi LF, Smirne S. Effects of long-term antiepileptic therapy on the hypothalamic–pituitary axis in man. Epilepsia 1984;25(1):46–52.

52. Luhdorf K. Endocrine function and antiepileptic treatment. Acta Neurol Scand Suppl 1983;94:15–19.

53. Elias AN, Gwinup G. Sodium valproate and Nelson's syndrome. Lancet 1981;2(8240):252–3.

54. Ostrowska Z, Buntner B, Rosciszewska D, Guz I. Adrenal cortex hormones in male epileptic patients before and during a 2-year phenytoin treatment. J Neurol Neurosurg Psychiatry 1988;51(3):374–8.

55. Masala A, Meloni T, Alagna S, Rovasio PP, Mele G, Franca V. Pituitary responsiveness to gonadotrophin-releasing and thyrotrophin-releasing hormones in children receiving phenobarbitone. BMJ 1980;281(6249):1175–7.

56. Victor A, Lundberg PO, Johansson ED. Induction of sex hormone binding globulin by phenytoin. BMJ 1977;2(6092):934–5.

57. Dana-Haeri J, Oxley J, Richens A. Reduction of free testosterone by antiepileptic drugs. BMJ (Clin Res Ed) 1982;284(6309):85–6.

58. Isojarvi JI, Repo M, Pakarinen AJ, Lukkarinen O, Myllyla VV. Carbamazepine, phenytoin, sex hormones, and sexual function in men with epilepsy. Epilepsia 1995;36(4):366–70.
59. Toone BK, Wheeler M, Fenwick PB. Sex hormone changes in male epileptics. Clin Endocrinol (Oxf) 1980;12(4):391–5.
60. Macphee GJ, Larkin JG, Butler E, Beastall GH, Brodie MJ. Circulating hormones and pituitary responsiveness in young epileptic men receiving long-term antiepileptic medication. Epilepsia 1988;29(4):468–75.
61. Duncan S, Blacklaw J, Beastall GH, Brodie MJ. Antiepileptic drug therapy and sexual function in men with epilepsy. Epilepsia 1999;40(2):197–204.
62. Rattya J, Turkka J, Pakarinen AJ, Knip M, Kotila MA, Lukkarinen O, Myllyla VV, Isojarvi JI. Reproductive effects of valproate, carbamazepine, and oxcarbazepine in men with epilepsy. Neurology 2001;56(1):31–6.
63. Rattya J, Pakarinen AJ, Knip M, Repo-Outakoski M, Myllyla VV, Isojarvi JI. Early hormonal changes during valproate or carbamazepine treatment: a 3-month study. Neurology 2001;57(3):440–4.
64. Tiihonen M, Liewendahl K, Waltimo O, Ojala M, Valimaki M. Thyroid status of patients receiving long-term anticonvulsant therapy assessed by peripheral parameters: a placebo-controlled thyroxine therapy trial. Epilepsia 1995;36(11):1118–25.
65. Isojarvi JI, Airaksinen KE, Mustonen JN, Pakarinen AJ, Rautio A, Pelkonen O, Myllyla VV. Thyroid and myocardial function after replacement of carbamazepine by oxcarbazepine. Epilepsia 1995;36(8):810–16.
66. Aanerud S, Strandjord RE. Hypothyroidism induced by anti-epileptic therapy. Acta Neurol Scand 1980;61(5):330–2.
67. Isojarvi JI, Pakarinen AJ, Ylipalosaari PJ, Myllyla VV. Serum hormones in male epileptic patients receiving anticonvulsant medication. Arch Neurol 1990;47(6):670–6.
68. Eiris-Punal J, Del Rio-Garma M, Del Rio-Garma MC, Lojo-Rocamonde S, Novo-Rodriguez I, Castro-Gago M. Long-term treatment of children with epilepsy with valproate or carbamazepine may cause subclinical hypothyroidism. Epilepsia 1999;40(12):1761–6.
69. Isojarvi JI, Turkka J, Pakarinen AJ, Kotila M, Rattya J, Myllyla VV. Thyroid function in men taking carbamazepine, oxcarbazepine, or valproate for epilepsy. Epilepsia 2001;42(7):930–4.
70. Verrotti A, Basciani F, Morresi S, Morgese G, Chiarelli F. Thyroid hormones in epileptic children receiving carbamazepine and valproic acid. Pediatr Neurol 2001;25(1):43–6.
71. Carter BL, Small RE, Mandel MD, Starkman MT. Phenytoin-induced hyperglycemia. Am J Hosp Pharm 1981;38(10):1508–12.
72. Dean JC, Penry JK. Weight gain patterns in patients with epilepsy: comparison of antiepileptic drugs. Epilepsia 1995;36:72.
73. Jallon P, Picard F. Bodyweight gain and anticonvulsants: a comparative review. Drug Saf 2001;24(13):969–78.
74. Nikkila EA, Kaste M, Ehnholm C, Viikari J. Elevation of high-density lipoprotein in epileptic patients treated with phenytoin. Acta Med Scand 1978;204(6):517–20.
75. al-Rubeaan K, Ryan EA. Phenytoin-induced insulin insensitivity. Diabet Med 1991;8(10):968–70.
76. Isojarvi JI, Pakarinen AJ, Myllyla VV. Serum lipid levels during carbamazepine medication. A prospective study. Arch Neurol 1993;50(6):590–3.
77. Isojarvi JI, Pakarinen AJ, Rautio A, Pelkonen O, Myllyla VV. Liver enzyme induction and serum lipid levels after replacement of carbamazepine with oxcarbazepine. Epilepsia 1994;35(6):1217–20.
78. Calandre EP, Rodriquez-Lopez C, Blazquez A, Cano D. Serum lipids, lipoproteins and apolipoproteins A and B in epileptic patients treated with valproic acid, carbamazepine or phenobarbital. Acta Neurol Scand 1991;83(4):250–3.
79. Larson AW, Wasserstrom WR, Felsher BF, Chih JC. Posttraumatic epilepsy and acute intermittent porphyria: effects of phenytoin, carbamazepine, and clonazepam. Neurology 1978;28(8):824–8.
80. Isobe T, Horimatsu T, Fujita T, Miyazaki K, Sugiyama T. Adult T cell lymphoma following diphenylhydantoin therapy. Nippon Ketsueki Gakkai Zasshi 1980;43(4):711–14.
81. Norohna MJ, Bevan PLT. A literature review on unwanted effects during treatment with Epilim. In: Legg NJ, editor. Clinical and Pharmacological Aspects of Sodium Valproate (Epilim) in the Treatment of Epilepsy. Tunbridge Wells, UK: MCS, 1976:61.
82. Reynolds NC Jr, Miska RM. Safety of anticonvulsants in hepatic porphyrias. Neurology 1981;31(4):480–4.
83. Rassiat E, Ragonnet D, Barriere E, Soupison A, Bernard P. Porphyrie aiguë intermittente revelée par une réaction paradoxale a une benzodiazepine. [Acute intermittent porphyria revealed by a paradoxical reaction to a benzodiazepine.] Gastroenterol Clin Biol 2001;25(8–9):832.
84. D'Alessandro R, Rocchi E, Cristina E, Cassanelli M, Benassi G, Pizzino D, Baldrati A, Baruzzi A. Safety of valproate in porphyria cutanea tarda. Epilepsia 1988;29(2):159–62.
85. Krauss GL, Hahn M, Gildemeister OS, Lambrecht RW, Pepe JA, Donohue SE, Bonkowsky HL. Porphyrinogenicity of new anticonvulsants in a liver cell culture model. Epilepsia 1996;37(Suppl 5):204.
86. Schwaninger M, Ringleb P, Winter R, Kohl B, Fiehn W, Rieser PA, Walter-Sack I. Elevated plasma concentrations of homocysteine antiepileptic drug treatment. Epilepsia 1999;40(3):345–50.
87. Botez MI, Joyal C, Maag U, Bachevalier J. Cerebrospinal fluid and blood thiamine concentrations in phenytoin-treated epileptics. Can J Neurol Sci 1982;9(1):37–9.
88. De Vivo DC, Bohan TP, Coulter DL, Dreifuss FE, Greenwood RS, Nordli DR Jr, Shields WD, Stafstrom CE, Tein I. L-carnitine supplementation in childhood epilepsy: current perspectives. Epilepsia 1998;39(11):1216–25.
89. Schwaninger M, Ringleb P, Annecke A, Winter R, Kohl B, Werle E, Fiehn W, Rieser PA, Walter-Sack I. Elevated plasma concentrations of lipoprotein(a) in medicated epileptic patients. J Neurol 2000;247(9):687–90.
90. Fichman MP, Kleeman CR, Bethune JE. Inhibition of antidiuretic hormone secretion by diphenylhydantoin. Arch Neurol 1970;22(1):45–53.
91. Huuskonen UEJ, Isojarvi JIT. Antiepileptic drugs and serum sodium. Epilepsia 1997;38(Suppl 8):89–90.
92. Van Amelsvoort T, Bakshi R, Devaux CB, Schwabe S. Hyponatremia associated with carbamazepine oxcarbazepine therapy: a review. Epilepsia 1994;35(1):181–8.
93. Brewerton TD, Jackson CW. Prophylaxis of carbamazepine-induced hyponatremia by demeclocycline in six patients. J Clin Psychiatry 1994;55(6):249–51.
94. Hoikka V, Savolainen K, Alhava M, Sivenius J, Karjalainen P, Repo A. Osteomalacia in institutionalised epileptic patients on long term anticonvulsant therapy. Arch Dis Child 1981;56:446.
95. Morijiri Y, Sato T. Factors causing rickets in institutionalised handicapped children on anticonvulsant therapy. Arch Dis Child 1981;56(6):446–9.
96. Weinstein RS, Bryce GF, Sappington LJ, King DW, Gallagher BB. Decreased serum ionized calcium and normal vitamin D metabolite levels with anticonvulsant drug treatment. J Clin Endocrinol Metab 1984;58(6):1003–9.
97. Annegers JF, Melton LJ 3rd, Sun CA, Hauser WA. Risk of age-related fractures in patients with unprovoked seizures. Epilepsia 1989;30(3):348–55.

98. John G. Transient osteosclerosis associated with sodium valproate. Dev Med Child Neurol 1981;23(2):234–6.

99. Kishi T, Fujita N, Eguchi T, Ueda K. Mechanism for reduction of serum folate by antiepileptic drugs during prolonged therapy. J Neurol Sci 1997;145(1):109–12.

100. Echaniz-Laguna A, Thiriaux A, Ruolt-Olivesi I, Marescaux C, Hirsch E. Lupus anticoagulant induced by the combination of valproate and lamotrigine. Epilepsia 1999;40(11):1661–3.

101. Kaaja E, Kaaja R, Matila R, Hiilesmaa V. Enzyme-inducing antiepileptic drugs in pregnancy and the risk of bleeding in the neonate. Neurology 2002;58(4):549–53.

102. Schmidt D, Siemes H. Role of liver function tests in monitoring anticonvulsant use. CNS Drugs 1998;10:321–8.

103. Dreifuss FE, Langer DH, Moline KA, Maxwell JE. Valproic acid hepatic fatalities. II. US experience since 1984. Neurology 1989;39(2 Pt 1):201–7.

104. Faheem AD, Brightwell DR, Burton GC, Struss A. Respiratory dyskinesia and dysarthria from prolonged neuroleptic use: tardive dyskinesia? Am J Psychiatry 1982;139(4):517–18.

105. Simpson GM, Pi EH, Sramek JJ Jr, Adverse effects of antipsychotic agents. Drugs 1981;21(2):138–51.

106. Portnoy RA. Hyperkinetic dysarthria as an early indicator of impending tardive dyskinesia. J Speech Hear Disord 1979;44(2):214–19.

107. Asconape JJ, Penry JK, Dreifuss FE, Riela A, Mirza W. Valproate-associated pancreatitis. Epilepsia 1993;34(1):177–83.

108. Ruble J, Matsuo H. Anticonvulsant-induced cutaneous reactions. Incidence, mechanisms and management. CNS Drugs 1999;12:215–36.

109. Kamanabroo D, Schmitz-Landgraf W, Czarnetzki BM. Plasmapheresis in severe drug-induced toxic epidermal necrolysis. Arch Dermatol 1985;121(12):1548–9.

110. Micali G, Linthicum K, Han N, West DP. Increased risk of erythema multiforme major with combination anticonvulsant and radiation therapies. Pharmacotherapy 1999;19(2):223–7.

111. Khafaga YM, Jamshed A, Allam AA, Mourad WA, Ezzat A, Al Eisa A, Gray AJ, Schultz H. Stevens–Johnson syndrome in patients on phenytoin and cranial radiotherapy. Acta Oncol 1999;38(1):111–16.

112. Duncan KO, Tigelaar RE, Bolognia JL. Stevens–Johnson syndrome limited to multiple sites of radiation therapy in a patient receiving phenobarbital. J Am Acad Dermatol 1999;40(3):493–6.

113. Mamon HJ, Wen PY, Burns AC, Loeffler JS. Allergic skin reactions to anticonvulsant medications in patients receiving cranial radiation therapy. Epilepsia 1999;40(3):341–4.

114. Leyva L, Torres MJ, Posadas S, Blanca M, Besso G, O'Valle F, del Moral RG, Santamar LF, Juarez C. Anticonvulsant-induced toxic epidermal necrolysis: monitoring the immunologic response. J Allergy Clin Immunol 2000;105(1 Pt 1):157–65.

115. Brenner S, Golan H, Lerman Y. Psoriasiform eruption and anticonvulsant drugs. Acta Derm Venereol 2000;80(5):382.

116. Hyson C, Sadler M. Cross sensitivity of skin rashes with antiepileptic drugs. Can J Neurol Sci 1997;24(3):245–9.

117. Espallargues M, Sampietro-Colom L, Estrada MD, Sola M, del Rio L, Setoain J, Granados A. Identifying bone-mass-related risk factors for fracture to guide bone densitometry measurements: a systematic review of the literature. Osteoporos Int 2001;12(10):811–22.

118. Feldkamp J, Becker A, Witte OW, Scharff D, Scherbaum WA. Long-term anticonvulsant therapy leads to low bone mineral density—evidence for direct drug effects of phenytoin and carbamazepine on human osteoblast-like cells. Exp Clin Endocrinol Diabetes 2000;108(1):37–43.

119. Guo CY, Ronen GM, Atkinson SA. Long-term valproate and lamotrigine treatment may be a marker for reduced growth and bone mass in children with epilepsy. Epilepsia 2001;42(9):1141–7.

120. Voudris K, Moustaki M, Zeis PM, Dimou S, Vagiakou E, Tsagris B, Skardoutsou A. Alkaline phosphatase and its isoenzyme activity for the evaluation of bone metabolism in children receiving anticonvulsant monotherapy. Seizure 2002;11(6):377–80.

121. Andress DL, Ozuna J, Tirschwell D, Grande L, Johnson M, Jacobson AF, Spain W. Antiepileptic drug-induced bone loss in young male patients who have seizures. Arch Neurol 2002;59(5):781–6.

122. Karlsson MK, Johnell O, Nilsson BE, Sernbo I, Obrant KJ. Bone mineral mass in hip fracture patients. Bone 1993;14(2):161–5.

123. Verrotti A, Greco R, Latini G, Morgese G, Chiarelli F. Increased bone turnover in prepubertal, pubertal, and postpubertal patients receiving carbamazepine. Epilepsia 2002;43(12):1488–92.

124. King W, Levin R, Schmidt R, Oestreich A, Heubi JE. Prevalence of reduced bone mass in children and adults with spastic quadriplegia. Dev Med Child Neurol 2003;45(1):12–16.

125. Henderson RC, Lark RK, Gurka MJ, Worley G, Fung EB, Conaway M, Stallings VA, Stevenson RD. Bone density and metabolism in children and adolescents with moderate to severe cerebral palsy. Pediatrics 2002;110(1 Pt 1):e5.

126. Ray JG, Papaioannou A, Ioannidis G, Adachi JD. Anticonvulsant drug use and low bone mass in adults with neurodevelopmental disorders. QJM 2002;95(4):219–23.

127. Farhat G, Yamout B, Mikati MA, Demirjian S, Sawaya R, El-Hajj Fuleihan G. Effect of antiepileptic drugs on bone density in ambulatory patients. Neurology 2002;58(9):1348–53.

128. Sheth RD, Wesolowski CA, Jacob JC, Penney S, Hobbs GR, Riggs JE, Bodensteiner JB. Effect of carbamazepine and valproate on bone mineral density. J Pediatr 1995;127(2):256–62.

129. Vestergaard P, Tigaran S, Rejnmark L, Tigaran C, Dam M, Mosekilde L. Fracture risk is increased in epilepsy. Acta Neurol Scand 1999;99(5):269–75.

130. Valmadrid C, Voorhees C, Litt B, Schneyer CR. Practice patterns of neurologists regarding bone and mineral effects of antiepileptic drug therapy. Arch Neurol 2001;58(9):1369–74.

131. Morrell MJ, Giudice L, Flynn KL, Seale CG, Paulson AJ, Done S, Flaster E, Ferin M, Sauer MV. Predictors of ovulatory failure in women with epilepsy. Ann Neurol 2002;52(6):704–11.

132. Bauer J, Jarre A, Klingmuller D, Elger CE. Polycystic ovary syndrome in patients with focal epilepsy: a study in 93 women. Epilepsy Res 2000;41(2):163–7.

133. Isojarvi JI, Laatikainen TJ, Knip M, Pakarinen AJ, Juntunen KT, Myllyla VV. Obesity and endocrine disorders in women taking valproate for epilepsy. Ann Neurol 1996;39(5):579–84.

134. Schlienger RG, Shear NH. Antiepileptic drug hypersensitivity syndrome. Epilepsia 1998;39(Suppl 7):S3–7.

135. Griebel ML. Acute management of hypersensitivity reactions and seizures. Epilepsia 1998;39(Suppl 7):S17–21.

136. Ciernik IF, Thiel M, Widmer U. Anterior uveitis and the anticonvulsant hypersensitivity syndrome. Arch Intern Med 1998;158(2):192.

137. Nilsson L, Farahmand BY, Persson PG, Thiblin I, Tomson T. Risk factors for sudden unexpected death in epilepsy: a case-control study. Lancet 1999;353(9156):888–93.

138. Timmings PL. Sudden unexpected death in epilepsy: is carbamazepine implicated? Seizure 1998;7(4):289–91.

139. Rintahaka PJ, Nakagawa JA, Shewmon DA, Kyyronen P, Shields WD. Incidence of death in patients with intractable epilepsy during nitrazepam treatment. Epilepsia 1999;40(4):492–6.

140. Murphy JV, Sawasky F, Marquardt KM, Harris DJ. Deaths in young children receiving nitrazepam. J Pediatr 1987;111(1):145–7.

141. Wyllie E, Wyllie R, Cruse RP, Rothner AD, Erenberg G. The mechanism of nitrazepam-induced drooling and aspiration. N Engl J Med 1986;314(1):35–8.

142. Nilsson L, Bergman U, Diwan V, Farahmand BY, Persson PG, Tomson T. Antiepileptic drug therapy and its management in sudden unexpected death in epilepsy: a case-control study. Epilepsia 2001;42(5):667–73.

143. Duncan JS, Shorvon SD, Trimble MR. Withdrawal symptoms from phenytoin, carbamazepine and sodium valproate. J Neurol Neurosurg Psychiatry 1988;51(7):924–8.

144. Ketter TA, Malow BA, Flamini R, White SR, Post RM, Theodore WH. Anticonvulsant withdrawal-emergent psychopathology. Neurology 1994;44(1):55–61.

145. Gambardella A, Aguglia U, Oliveri RL, Russo C, Zappia M, Quattrone A. Negative myoclonic status due to antiepileptic drug tapering: report of three cases. Epilepsia 1997;38(7):819–23.

146. Bare M. Nausea/vomiting associated with antiepileptic drug withdrawal. Epilepsia 1998;39(Suppl 6):160–1.

147. Cogrel O, Beylot-Barry M, Vergier B, Dubus P, Doutre MS, Merlio JP, Beylot C. Sodium valproate-induced cutaneous pseudolymphoma followed by recurrence with carbamazepine. Br J Dermatol 2001;144(6):1235–8.

148. Saeki H, Etoh T, Toda K, Mihm MC, Jr. Pseudolymphoma syndrome due to carbamazepine. J Dermatol 1999;26(5):329–31.

149. Sinnige HA, Boender CA, Kuypers EW, Ruitenberg HM. Carbamazepine-induced pseudolymphoma and immune dysregulation. J Intern Med 1990;227(5):355–8.

150. Pathak P, McLachlan RS. Drug-induced pseudolymphoma secondary to lamotrigine. Neurology 1998;50(5):1509–10.

151. Knowles SR, Shapiro LE, Shear NH. Anticonvulsant hypersensitivity syndrome: incidence, prevention and management. Drug Saf 1999;21(6):489–501.

152. Steegers-Theunissen RP, Renier WO, Borm GF, Thomas CM, Merkus HM, Op de Coul DA, De Jong PA, van Geijn HP, Wouters M, Eskes TK. Factors influencing the risk of abnormal pregnancy outcome in epileptic women: a multi-centre prospective study. Epilepsy Res 1994;18(3):261–9.

153. Lindhout D, Omtzigt JG. Teratogenic effects of antiepileptic drugs: implications for the management of epilepsy in women of childbearing age. Epilepsia 1994;35(Suppl 4):S19–28.

154. Waters CH, Belai Y, Gott PS, Shen P, De Giorgio CM. Outcomes of pregnancy associated with antiepileptic drugs. Arch Neurol 1994;51(3):250–3.

155. Samren EB, van Duijn CM, Koch S, Hiilesmaa VK, Klepel H, Bardy AH, Mannagetta GB, Deichl AW, Gaily E, Granstrom ML, Meinardi H, Grobbee DE, Hofman A, Janz D, Lindhout D. Maternal use of antiepileptic drugs and the risk of major congenital malformations: a joint European prospective study of human teratogenesis associated with maternal epilepsy. Epilepsia 1997;38(9):981–90.

156. Gaily E, Granstrom ML, Hiilesmaa V, Bardy A. Minor anomalies in offspring of epileptic mothers. J Pediatr 1988;112(4):520–9.

157. Canger R, Battino D, Canevini MP, Fumarola C, Guidolin L, Vignoli A, Mamoli D, Palmieri C, Molteni F, Granata T, Hassibi P, Zamperini P, Pardi G, Avanzini G. Malformations in offspring of women with epilepsy: a prospective study. Epilepsia 1999;40(9):1231–6.

158. Samren EB, van Duijn CM, Christiaens GC, Hofman A, Lindhout D. Antiepileptic drug regimens and major congenital abnormalities in the offspring. Ann Neurol 1999;46(5):739–46.

159. Arpino C, Brescianini S, Robert E, Castilla EE, Cocchi G, Cornel MC, de Vigan C, Lancaster PA, Merlob P, Sumiyoshi Y, Zampino G, Renzi C, Rosano A, Mastroiacovo P. Teratogenic effects of antiepileptic drugs: use of an International Database on Malformations and Drug Exposure (MADRE). Epilepsia 2000;41(11):1436–43.

160. Holmes LB, Harvey EA, Coull BA, Huntington KB, Khoshbin S, Hayes AM, Ryan LM. The teratogenicity of anticonvulsant drugs. N Engl J Med 2001;344(15):1132–8.

161. Adab N, Jacoby A, Smith D, Chadwick D. Additional educational needs in children born to mothers with epilepsy. J Neurol Neurosurg Psychiatry 2001;70(1):15–21.

162. Koch S, Titze K, Zimmermann RB, Schroder M, Lehmkuhl U, Rauh H. Long-term neuropsychological consequences of maternal epilepsy and anticonvulsant treatment during pregnancy for school-age children and adolescents. Epilepsia 1999;40(9):1237–43.

163. Ohtsuka Y, Silver K, Lopes-Cendes I, Andermann E, Tsuda T. Effect of antiepileptic drugs on psychomotor development in offspring of epileptic mothers. Epilepsia 1999;40(Suppl 2):296.

164. Scolnik D, Nulman I, Rovet J, Gladstone D, Czuchta D, Gardner HA, Gladstone R, Ashby P, Weksberg R, Einarson T, et al. Neurodevelopment of children exposed in utero to phenytoin carbamazepine monotherapy. JAMA 1994;271(10):767–70.

165. Reinisch JM, Sanders SA, Mortensen EL, Rubin DB. In utero exposure to phenobarbital and intelligence deficits in adult men. JAMA 1995;274(19):1518–25.

166. Buehler BA, Delimont D, van Waes M, Finnell RH. Prenatal prediction of risk of the fetal hydantoin syndrome. N Engl J Med 1990;322(22):1567–72.

167. Zahn CA, Morrell MJ, Collins SD, Labiner DM, Yerby MS. Management issues for women with epilepsy: a review of the literature. Neurology 1998;51(4):949–56.

168. Tomson T, Gram L, Sillampaa M, Johannessen S. Recommendations for the management and care of pregnant women with epilepsy. In: Tomson T, Gram L, Sillampaa M, Johannessen SI, editors. Epilepsy and Pregnancy. Wrightson Biomedical Publishing, 1997:201–8.

169. Annegers JF, Baumgartner KB, Hauser WA, Kurland LT. Epilepsy, antiepileptic drugs, and the risk of spontaneous abortion. Epilepsia 1988;29(4):451–8.

170. Baumann RJ, Duffner PK. Treatment of children with simple febrile seizures: the AAP practice parameter. American Academy for Pediatrics. Pediatr Neurol 2000;23(1):11–17.

171. Collins RJ, Garnett WR. Extended release formulations of anticonvulsant medications clinical pharmacokinetics and therapeutic advantages. CNS Drugs 2000;14:203–12.

172. Jones AL, Proudfoot AT. Features and management of poisoning with modern drugs used to treat epilepsy. QJM 1998;91(5):325–32.

173. Bridge TA, Norton RL, Robertson WO. Pediatric carbamazepine overdoses. Pediatr Emerg Care 1994;10(5):260–3.

174. Spiller HA, Bosse GM. Management of anticonvulsant overdose. CNS Drugs 1996;6:113–29.

175. Perucca E, Bialer M. The clinical pharmacokinetics of the newer antiepileptic drugs. Focus on topiramate, zonisamide and tiagabine. Clin Pharmacokinet 1996;31(1):29–46.

176. Perucca E. The new generation of antiepileptic drugs: advantages and disadvantages. Br J Clin Pharmacol 1996;42(5):531–43.

177. Perucca E. Pharmacokinetic interactions with antiepileptic drugs. Clin Pharmacokinet 1982;7(1):57–84.

178. Patsalos PN, Duncan JS. Antiepileptic drugs. A review of clinically significant drug interactions. Drug Saf 1993;9(3):156–84.

179. Spina E, Pisani F, Perucca E. Clinically significant pharmacokinetic drug interactions with carbamazepine. An update. Clin Pharmacokinet 1996;31(3):198–214.

180. Besag FM, Berry DJ, Pool F, Newbery JE, Subel B. Carbamazepine toxicity with lamotrigine: pharmacokinetic or pharmacodynamic interaction? Epilepsia 1998;39(2):183–7.

181. Koenig MH, Edwards LT. Cisatracurium-induced neuromuscular blockade in anticonvulsant treated neurosurgical patients. J Neurosurg Anesthesiol 2000;12(4):314–18.

182. Adamolekun B, Mielke J, Ball D, Mundanda T. An evaluation of the management of epilepsy by primary health care nurses in Chitungwiza, Zimbabwe. Epilepsy Res 2000;39(3):177–81.

183. Snodgrass SR, Parks BR. Anticonvulsant blood levels: historical review with a pediatric focus. J Child Neurol 2000;15(11):734–46.

Antifungal azoles

See also Individual agents

General Information

The antifungal azoles are a class of synthetic compounds that have one or more azole rings and a more or less complex side chain attached to one of the nitrogen atoms. They are either imidazole or triazole derivatives. The imidazoles miconazole and ketoconazole were the first azoles developed for systemic treatment of human mycoses. However, severe adverse effects associated with the drug carrier (in the case of miconazole) and erratic absorption and significant interference with cytochrome P450 isozymes (in the case of ketoconazole) have limited their usefulness (1). However, the subsequently developed triazoles fluconazole, itraconazole, and voriconazole have become useful additions to the antifungal armamentarium. They have a wider spectrum of activity and greater target specificity and are generally well tolerated (1,2). Other azoles for topical use are reviewed in the monograph on Antifungal azoles and other drugs for topical use.

The azoles act by inhibiting the fungal enzyme lanosterol 14-α-demethylase, which is involved in the synthesis of ergosterol from lanosterol or 24-methylenedihydrolanosterol in the fungal cell membrane. The consequent inhibition of ergosterol synthesis originates from binding of the unsubstituted nitrogen (N-3 or N-4) of the imidazole or triazole moiety to the heme iron and from binding of their N-1 substituent to the apoprotein of a cytochrome P-450 (P-450(14)DM) of the endoplasmic reticulum (3). This inhibition interrupts the conversion of lanosterol to ergosterol, which alters cell membrane function. Itraconazole has the highest affinity for the cytochrome and is about three and ten times more active in vitro than miconazole and fluconazole, respectively (4). They also inhibit the uptake of triglycerides and phospholipids through the cell membrane.

Drug–Drug Interactions

General

Drug interactions with the antifungal azoles are common for several reasons:

- they are substrates of CYP3A4, but also interact with the heme moiety of CYP3A, resulting in non-competitive inhibition of oxidative metabolism of many CYP3A substrates; to a lesser extent they also inhibit other CYP450 isoforms;
- although fluconazole undergoes minimal CYP-mediated metabolism, it nevertheless inhibits CYP3A4 in vitro, albeit much more weakly than other azoles (5,6); however, fluconazole also inhibits several other CYP isoforms in vitro and interacts with enzymes involved in glucuronidation (7);
- interaction of antifungal azoles and other CYP3A substrates can also result from inhibition of P-glycoprotein-mediated efflux; P-glycoprotein is extensively co-localized and exhibits overlapping substrate specificity with CYP3A (7); in a cell line in which human P-glycoprotein was overexpressed, itraconazole and ketoconazole inhibited P-glycoprotein function, with 50% inhibitory concentrations of about 2 and 6 µmol/l respectively; however, fluconazole had no effect (8).
- the systemic availability of the antifungal azoles depends in part on an acidic gastric environment and the activity of intestinal CYP3A4 and P-glycoprotein.

For details of interactions with individual antifungal azoles, see individual monographs (fluconazole, itraconazole, ketoconazole, miconazole, and voriconazole).

References

1. Groll AH, Piscitelli SC, Walsh TJ. Clinical pharmacology of systemic antifungal agents: a comprehensive review of agents in clinical use, current investigational compounds, and putative targets for antifungal drug development. Adv Pharmacol 1998;44:343–500.

2. Hoffman HL, Ernst EJ, Klepser ME. Novel triazole antifungal agents. Expert Opin Investig Drugs 2000;9(3):593–605.

3. Vanden Bossche H, Marichal P, Gorrens J, Coene MC, Willemsens G, Bellens D, Roels I, Moereels H, Janssen PA. Biochemical approaches to selective antifungal activity. Focus on azole antifungals. Mycoses 1989;32(Suppl 1):35–52.

4. Vanden Bossche H, Marichal P, Gorrens J, Coene MC. Biochemical basis for the activity and selectivity of oral antifungal drugs. Br J Clin Pract Suppl 1990;71:41–6.

5. Francis P, Walsh TJ. Evolving role of flucytosine in immunocompromised patients: new insights into safety, pharmacokinetics, and antifungal therapy. Clin Infect Dis 1992;15(6):1003–18.

6. Azon-Masoliver A, Vilaplana J. Fluconazole-induced toxic epidermal necrolysis in a patient with human immunodeficiency virus infection. Dermatology 1993;187(4):268–9.

7. Gubbins PO, McConnell SA, Penzak SR. Antifungal Agents. In: Piscitelli SC, Rodvold KA, editors. Drug Interactions in Infectious Diseases. Totowa, NJ: Humana Press Inc, 2001:185–217.

8. Wang EJ, Lew K, Casciano CN, Clement RP, Johnson WW. Interaction of common azole antifungals with P glycoprotein. Antimicrob Agents Chemother 2002;46(1):160–5.

Antifungal azoles and other drugs for topical use

See also Antifungal azoles

General Information

All the topically used azoles can cause local irritation, burning, and, if used intravaginally, burning, swelling, and discomfort during micturition. There is cross-sensitivity between econazole, enilconazole, miconazole, and probably all other phenethylimidazoles.

Contact allergy to topical imidazoles is rare, considering how commonly they are used. The imidazole derivatives most often reported to be allergens are miconazole, econazole, tioconazole, and isoconazole. As far as cross-reactivity is concerned, in one review, there were statistically significant associations between miconazole, econazole, and isoconazole; between sulconazole, miconazole, and econazole; and between isoconazole and tioconazole (1).

Of 3049 outpatients who were patch-tested for contact dermatitis at the Department of Dermatology, Nippon Medical School Hospital from January 1984 to August 1994, 218 were patch-tested with topical antimycotic agents (2). There were 66 positive tests with imidazole derivatives, of whom 35 were allergic to the active ingredients: 16 were allergic to sulconazole, 11 to croconazole, 3 to tioconazole, 3 to miconazole, 1 to bifonazole, and 1 to clotrimazole. Exposure to croconazole occurred after a significantly shorter time with less drug than with sulconazole. Of the 35 patients who were allergic to an imidazole, 21 cross-reacted to other imidazoles.

Azoles

Bifonazole

Bifonazole has a broad spectrum of activity in vitro against dermatophytes, moulds, yeasts, dimorphic fungi, and some Gram-positive bacteria. It has been used in a strength of 1% in creams, gels, solutions, and powders, applied once a day to treat superficial fungal infections of the skin, such as dermatophytoses, cutaneous candidiasis, and pityriasis versicolor (3). In a multicenter, double-blind, randomized, parallel-group comparison with flutrimazole cream 1% in the treatment of dermatomycoses in 449 patients the overall incidence of adverse effects (mainly mild local effects such as irritation or a burning sensation) was 5% (4).

Clotrimazole

Clotrimazole was the first oral azole. While it was effective in deep mycoses, its limited absorption and induction of liver microsomal enzymes after a few days, leading to accelerated metabolism of the compound, as well as its toxicity, preclude its use for systemic therapy. Clotrimazole is therefore currently only used for topical therapy of mucocutaneous candidiasis.

Comparisons of fluconazole 200 mg/day with clotrimazole 10 mg 5 times/day in the prevention of thrush in patients with AIDS showed little difference in the occurrence of undesirable effects and abnormalities in laboratory measurements but less efficacy of clotrimazole (5,6).

Local problems can occur, including hypersensitivity reactions (1). In one case of contact allergy, patch-testing was positive with clotrimazole (5% in petroleum), itraconazole (1% in ether), and croconazole (1% in ether) (7). The authors reviewed the possible cross-reactions between the subgroups of imidazoles.

- A 71-year-old woman had a severe exacerbation of vulval dermatitis for which she had been using Canesten (clotrimazole) cream (8). There was a positive patch-test reaction with clotrimazole (1% in petrolatum) and patch tests with the other constituents of Canesten were negative.

Topical vaginal administration of even relatively high doses of clotrimazole did not result in systemic toxicity (9).

Croconazole

In one case of contact allergy, patch-testing was positive with clotrimazole (5% in petroleum), itraconazole (1% in ether), and croconazole (1% in ether) (7). The authors reviewed the possible cross-reactions between the subgroups of imidazoles.

Econazole

Econazole is used topically on the skin and also intravaginally, after which about 3–7% is absorbed. It can cause pruritus (10) and vaginal burning (11).

Enilconazole

Enilconazole is used in 10% solution/cream. Contact dermatitis has been reported (12,13).

Isoconazole

Isoconazole is mainly used for vaginal infections with *Candida albicans*. Contact dermatitis has been reported (14), including an unusual case with a papulo-pustular reaction (15).

Itraconazole

In one case of contact allergy, patch-testing was positive with clotrimazole (5% in petroleum), itraconazole (1% in ether), and croconazole (1% in ether) (7). The authors reviewed the possible cross-reactions between the subgroups of imidazoles.

Lanoconazole (latoconazole)

Used in a 1% cream, lanoconazole is effective against *Tinea*, and is more active than clotrimazole or bifonazole. Several cases of contact dermatitis have been reported (16–20).

Miconazole

See the monograph on Miconazole.

Nimorazole

Nimorazole is believed to be active against *Trichomonas vaginalis*. No specific adverse effects have been described after local use.

Ornidazole

Complaints of dizziness (21), mild gastrointestinal symptoms (22), and headache (23) during treatment with intravaginal ornidazole have been reported, since ornidazole is relatively well absorbed after rectal and vaginal administration (23).

Terconazole

Terconazole is prepared in creams and ovules for intravaginal use. Besides local irritation it causes systemic reactions. Headache was reported in over a quarter of patients. Other effects include hypotension, fever, and chills. Terconazole is absorbed to a greater extent than other topical azoles (SED-12, 684).

Tioconazole

Tioconazole is mainly used for vaginal or inguinal *Candida* infections. It has fewer local adverse effects than some of the older imidazoles. Local irritation, burning, rash, erythema, and pruritus have been reported. In a few women there was marked burning on micturition; these women all had signs of vaginal epithelial atrophy (SED-12, 684) (24).

Other topical antifungal drugs

5-Bromo-4-chlorosalicylamide (multifungin)

5-Bromo-4-chlorosalicylamide is one of a group of local antiseptics and fungistatics that can cause photosensitization (25). There is cross-sensitization with bithionol, fenticlor, and tribromosalicylanide.

Buclosamide (N-butyl-4-chlorosalicylamide)

Photocontact dermatitis has been described with buclosamide (25). There is cross-reactivity with a number of other drugs, notably oral hypoglycemic drugs, diuretics, and sulfonamides. Because of these reactions, buclosamide is not recommended for topical use.

Captan (Orthocide-406)

Captan is one of the older fungicides. It is used for pityriasis versicolor and is included in some soaps and cosmetics to provide bactericidal and fungicidal effects. It is allergenic. It is carcinogenic in mice, and in several countries control agencies have taken steps to prohibit its use in cosmetics and non-drug products (SEDA-13, 236).

Ciclopirox

Ciclopirox, a substituted pyridone unrelated to the imidazoles, is effective against a wide variety of dermatophytes, yeasts, actinomycetes, molds, and other fungi. Ciclopirox olamine is generally well tolerated locally, and reactions occur in only 1–4% of cases (SEDA-12, 684).

Clodantoin

Contact dermatitis has been rarely reported with clodantoin.

Fluonilide (4-fluoro-3′,5′-thiocarbanilide)

Contact dermatitis has been reported with fluonilide (26).

Gentian violet

Gentian violet (27) was at one time the treatment of choice for vaginal and oral candidiasis but is now obsolete. The main problem is staining and the messiness of the application, since the purple-colored fluid has to be brushed on to the skin.

Hachimycin (trichomycin)

Contact dermatitis has been reported with hachimycin.

KP-363

KP-363, a benzylamine derivative, is used in creams and solutions in concentrations of 0.1 and 0.6%. It is reported to cause less irritation than bifonazole and tolciclate (SEDA-14, 235).

Naftitine

Naftitine is one of a series of allylamine antifungal agents, derived from heterocyclic spironaphthalenes. It is usually sold in the form of a 1% cream for topical treatment of dermatomycoses, dermatophytes, and yeasts. It is claimed to be more effective than the imidazoles. Local irritation and a burning sensation, if they occur, are only mild (SED-12, 684) (28), (SEDA-16, 297).

Natamycin (pimaricin)

No cases of contact dermatitis were described in industrial workers in frequent contact with natamycin (29).

In the Hungarian Case–Control Surveillance of Congenital Abnormalities between 1980 and 1996, of 38 151 pregnant women who delivered infants without any defects (controls) and 22 843 who had fetuses or neonates with congenital abnormalities, 62 (0.27%) and 98 (0.26%) were treated with vaginal natamycin in the two groups respectively (crude OR = 1.1; 95% CI = 0.8, 1.5). There was thus no evidence of a teratogenic effect of natamycin.

Nifuratel

Contact dermatitis, with facial edema and a generalized erythema, has been described in the partner of a woman treated with nifuratel vaginal suppositories (SED-11, 578) (30).

Niphimycin

Niphimycin, an antimycotic antibiotic derived from *Actinomyces hygroscopicus*, is effective against both dermatomycosis and onychomycosis, with a 16–26% success rate in the latter. Tolerance is reportedly good, but there is a notable lack of recent data (SEDA-12, 236).

Nystatin

See the monograph on Nystatin.

Pecilocin (Variotin)

Skin irritation has been reported in 2–6.5% of patients treated with pecilocin. Contact dermatitis has been described in a few cases (31,32). Of 44 patients treated with pecilocin who were patch-tested with pecilocin, 7 were allergic to it; in three of them the skin disease had been caused or exacerbated by pecilocin (33).

Pyrrolnitrin (Miutrin, 3-chloro-4-(3-chloro-2-nitrophenyl) pyrrole)

Contact dermatitis with pyrrolnitrin and cross-reactivity with dinitrochlorobenzene has been reported in one case (34).

Salicylic acid 3% with benzoic acid 6% (Whitfield's ointment)

Whitfield's ointment, used for *Trichophyton rubrum*, has a keratolytic effect, and local irritation can occur (SED-12, 685) (35).

Sulbentine (dibenzthion)

Photoallergic contact dermatitis has been described with sulbentine, probably through a breakdown product, benzylisothiocyanate (36).

Tolciclate

Tolciclate, a thiocarbamate, is active against most common dermatophytes. Contact dermatitis has been reported (37).

Tolnaftate

Tolerance of tolnaftate is good. Local erythema has been described, as has allergic dermatitis (38).

References

1. Dooms-Goossens A, Matura M, Drieghe J, Degreef H. Contact allergy to imidazoles used as antimycotic agents. Contact Dermatitis 1995;33(2):73–7.
2. Yoneyama E. [Allergic contact dermatitis due to topical imidazole antimycotics. The sensitizing ability of active ingredients and cross-sensitivity.] Nippon Ika Daigaku Zasshi 1996;63(5):356–64.
3. Lackner TE, Clissold SP. Bifonazole. A review of its antimicrobial activity and therapeutic use in superficial mycoses. Drugs 1989;38(2):204–25.
4. Alomar A, Videla S, Delgadillo J, Gich I, Izquierdo I, Forn J. Flutrimazole 1% dermal cream in the treatment of dermatomycoses: a multicentre, double-blind, randomized, comparative clinical trial with bifonazole 1% cream. Efficacy of flutrimazole 1% dermal cream in dermatomycoses. Catalan Flutrimazole Study Group. Dermatology 1995;190(4):295–300.
5. Powderly WG, Finkelstein D, Feinberg J, Frame P, He W, van der Horst C, Koletar SL, Eyster ME, Carey J, Waskin H, et al. A randomized trial comparing fluconazole with clotrimazole troches for the prevention of fungal infections in patients with advanced human immunodeficiency virus infection. NIAID AIDS Clinical Trials Group. N Engl J Med 1995;332(11):700–5.
6. Koletar SL, Russell JA, Fass RJ, Plouffe JF. Comparison of oral fluconazole and clotrimazole troches as treatment for oral candidiasis in patients infected with human immunodeficiency virus. Antimicrob Agents Chemother 1990;34(11):2267–8.
7. Erdmann S, Hertl M, Merk HF. Contact dermatitis from clotrimazole with positive patch-test reactions also to croconazole and itraconazole. Contact Dermatitis 1999;40(1):47–8.
8. Cooper SM, Shaw S. Contact allergy to clotrimazole: an unusual allergen. Contact Dermatitis 1999;41(3):168.
9. Wolfson N, Riley J, Samuels B, Singh JM. Clinical toxicology of clotrimazole when administered vaginally. Clin Toxicol 1981;18(1):41–5.
10. Grigoriu D, Grigoriu A. Double-blind comparison of the efficacy, toleration and safety of tioconazole base 1% and econazole nitrate 1% creams in the treatment of patients with fungal infections of the skin or erythrasma. Dermatologica 1983;166(Suppl 1):8–13.
11. Gouveia DC, Jones da Silva C. Oxiconazole in the treatment of vaginal candidiasis: single dose versus 3-day treatment with econazole. Pharmatherapeutica 1984;3(10):682–5.
12. Piebenga WP, van der Walle HB. Allergic contact dermatitis from 1-[2-(2,4-dichlorophenyl)-2-(2-propenyloxy) ethyl]-1H-imidazole in a water-based metalworking fluid. Contact Dermatitis 2003;48(5):285–6.
13. van Hecke E, de Vos L. Contact sensitivity to enilconazole. Contact Dermatitis 1983;9(2):144.
14. Frenzel UH, Gutekunst A. Contact dermatitis to isoconazole nitrate. Contact Dermatitis 1983;9(1):74.
15. Lazarov A, Ingber A. Pustular allergic contact dermatitis to isoconazole nitrate. Am J Contact Dermat 1997;8(4):229–30.
16. Soga F, Katoh N, Kishimoto S. Contact dermatitis due to lanoconazole, cetyl alcohol and diethyl sebacate in lanoconazole cream. Contact Dermatitis 2004;50(1):49–50.
17. Umebayashi Y, Ito S. Allergic contact dermatitis due to both lanoconazole and neticonazole ointments. Contact Dermatitis 2001;44(1):48–9.
18. Taniguchi S, Kono T. Allergic contact dermatitis due to lanoconazole with no cross-reactivity to other imidazoles. Dermatology 1998;196(3):366.
19. Tanaka N, Kawada A, Hiruma M, Tajima S, Ishibashi A. Contact dermatitis from lanoconazole. Contact Dermatitis 1996;35(4):256–7.
20. Nakano R, Miyoshi H, Kanzaki T. Allergic contact dermatitis from lanoconazole. Contact Dermatitis 1996;35(1):63.
21. Erkkola R, Jarvinen H. Single dose of ornidazole in the treatment of bacterial vaginosis. Ann Chir Gynaecol Suppl 1987;202:94–6.
22. Fugere P, Verschelden G, Caron M. Single oral dose of ornidazole in women with vaginal trichomoniasis. Obstet Gynecol 1983;62(4):502–5.
23. Andersson KE. Pharmacokinetics of nitroimidazoles. Spectrum of adverse reactions. Scand J Infect Dis Suppl 1981;26:60–7.
24. Uyanwah PO. An open non-comparative evaluation of single-dose tioconazole (6%), vaginal ointment in vaginal candidosis. Curr Ther Res 1986;39:30.
25. Burry JN. Photoallergies to Fenticlor and Multifungin. Arch Dermatol 1967;95(3):287–91.
26. van Hecke E. Contact allergy to the topical antimycotic fluoro-4-dichloro-3′5′-thiocarbanilid. Dermatologica 1969;138(6):480–2.
27. Docampo R, Moreno SN. The metabolism and mode of action of gentian violet. Drug Metab Rev 1990;22(2–3):161–78.
28. Ganzinger U, Stutz A, Petranyi G, Stephen A. Allylamines: topical and oral treatment of dermatomycoses with a new class of antifungal agents. Acta Dermatol Venereol Suppl (Stockh) 1986;121:155–60.
29. Raab WP. Natamycin (Pimaricin). Its Properties and Possibilities in Medicine. Stuttgart: Georg Thieme Verlag, 1972.
30. Bedello PG, Goitre M, Cane D, Fogliano MR. Contact dermatitis from nifuratel. Contact Dermatitis 1983;9(2):166.
31. Sundararajan V. Variotin sensitivity. Contact Dermatitis Newslett 1970;8:188.
32. Groen J, Bleumink E, Nater JP. Variotin sensitivity. Contact Dermatitis Newslett 1973;15:456.
33. Norgaard O. Pecilocinum–Allergie. [Pecilocin allergy.] Hautarzt 1977;28(1):35–6.
34. Meneghini CL, Angelini G. Contact dermatitis from pyrrolnitrin (an antimycotic agent). Contact Dermatitis 1975;1(5):288–92.
35. Odom R. A practical review of antifungals. Mod Med Can 1987;42:GP54.
36. Wurbach VG, Schubert H. Untersuchungen über die Afungin Allergie. [Studies on Afungin hypersensitivity..] Dermatol Monatsschr 1976;162(4):317–22.

37. Veraldi S, Schianchi-Veraldi R. Allergic contact dermatitis from tolciclate. Contact Dermatitis 1991;24(4):315.
38. Gellin GA, Maibach HI, Wachs GN. Contact allergy to tolnaftate. Arch Dermatol 1972;106(5):715–16.

Antihistamines

See also Individual agents

General Information

Histamine is both a local hormone and a neurotransmitter in the central nervous system. It is synthesized in neurons and mast cells. There are H_1, H_2, and H_3 receptors in the central nervous system, but they differ in their localization, biochemical machinery, functions, and affinities for histamine; they are particularly important in maintaining a state of arousal or awareness (1).

The early antihistamines, H_1 histamine receptor antagonists, bore some structural resemblance to histamine and, like histamine, contained an ethylamine group. However, the structures of the many antihistamines that are available are disparate, and the traditional classification according to chemical structure (ethanolamine, ethylenediamine, alkylamine, piperazine, and phenothiazine) is outdated, since the second-generation antihistamines, such as terfenadine and astemizole, do not readily fit into the old classification system (2).

Antihistamines act as competitive antagonists of histamine at H_1 histamine receptors, thus inhibiting H_1 receptor-mediated reactions, such as vasodilatation, sneezing, and itching. Histamine release from mast cells and basophils makes a major contribution to the allergic response, and antihistamines are widely used in the treatment of certain symptoms of allergic disease.

The new second-generation antihistamines are more selective H_1 histamine receptor antagonists, and many of them have additional anti-allergic properties in vivo, for example they reduce the release of inflammatory mediators or inhibit the recruitment of inflammatory cells (3–7). They also enter the brain less well and are therefore less likely to cause central adverse effects.

The H_1 histamine receptor antagonists were discovered by Bovet and Staub at the Institut Pasteur in 1937 (8). Although the first antihistamine was too weak and toxic for clinical use, its discovery resulted in an enormous amount of research and led in 1942 to the development of the first antihistamine to be used in the treatment of allergic diseases phenbenzamine (Antegan) (9). Within a few years, three other antihistamines became available and are still in use today: mepyramine (pyrilamine) maleate (10), diphenhydramine (11), and tripelennamine (12). Despite their pronounced adverse effects, these were the first really useful drugs for the symptomatic relief of allergic disorders. During the last 25 years several compounds with greater potency, longer durations of action, and minimal sedative effects have emerged, the so-called second-generation H_1 antihistamines, as opposed to the older, or classic, first-generation antihistamines. Two papers have confirmed the safety of the second-generation antihistamines; in particular, loratadine, fexofenadine, norastemizole, and descarboxyloratadine (desloratadine) were shown not to have sedative effects (13,14).

Spontaneous reports of suspected adverse effects of antihistamines have been analysed (15). The drugs were divided into two groups, sedative and non-sedative. Adverse reactions profiles were broadly similar in the two groups.

First-generation antihistamines

Besides interacting with H_1 histamine receptors, the first-generation antihistamines also have affinity for 5-HT receptors, alpha-adrenoceptors, and muscarinic receptors. They also reduce cyclic GMP concentrations, increase atrioventricular nodal conduction, and inhibit activation of airway vagal afferent nerves. First-generation H_1 receptor antagonists easily cross the blood–brain barrier, and their consequent well-documented sedative and anticholinergic effects, together with short half-lives, greatly limit their use in the treatment of allergic symptoms. However, despite these deficiencies, first-generation drugs are still widely used, mainly as over-the-counter products, often in combination with other drugs. The incidence of adverse effects, especially sedation and antimuscarinic effects, with the first-generation antihistamines is very high, perhaps up to 50%. Although these adverse effects are rarely serious, and often disappear with continued therapy, they are often so troublesome that medication must be withdrawn.

Second-generation antihistamines

The second-generation antihistamines include acrivastine, astemizole, azelastine, carebastine, cetirizine, ebastine, loratadine, mizolastine, and terfenadine. They are used orally and some of them can be given by local application to the nose and eyes (2,16). They are relatively free from anticholinergic, antiserotonergic, and alpha-adrenergic activity. They cause markedly less sedation, perhaps because they penetrate the central nervous system less well than the first-generation antihistamines, being relatively hydrophilic (17–19).

Second-generation antihistamines have proved to be important therapeutic tools in the treatment of atopic disease, including both seasonal and perennial allergic rhinitis, urticaria, and atopic dermatitis (20). Several studies have shown that the use of second-generation antihistamines as adjunctive therapy can benefit patients whose allergic asthma co-exists with allergic rhinitis (21).

There are several novel antihistamines that are either metabolites or enantiomers of existing drugs. The aim has been to develop antihistamines with improved potency, onset and duration of action, and greater predictability and safety. Drugs of this kind that have received regulatory approval and are effective in several allergic conditions include desloratadine, fexofenadine, levocabastine, and levocetirizine. These have been developed in response to widespread concerns about the potential for cardiotoxicity and the impact of drug–drug interactions associated with some earlier second-generation H_1 receptor antagonists. Furthermore, the potential for sedation by some of the newer antihistamines still remains an issue for many. This is important, as many patients using antihistamines want to remain alert and active and may also use other medications.

Organs and Systems

Cardiovascular

Tachycardia and hypertension have long been known as problems arising incidentally reported with various classic antihistamines (SEDA-22, 176).

Prolonged QT interval and ventricular dysrhythmias

DoTS classification
  Dose-relation: toxic effect
  Time-course: time-independent
  Susceptibility factors: genetic (long QT syndrome); altered physiology (hypokalemia); drug interactions (metabolism inhibitors; drugs that prolong the QT interval); diseases (liver disease; cardiac disease with prolongation of QT interval)

Several antihistamines can cause ventricular dysrhythmias of the torsade de pointes type (22), first reported with astemizole (23) and later with terfenadine (24). Astemizole and terfenadine both have a dose-dependent effect on cardiac repolarization and cause prolongation of the QT interval, which can lead to ventricular dysrhythmias (such as torsade de pointes), syncope, and cardiac arrest. Reported cases relate preponderantly to overdosage, especially in children (SEDA-12, 142) (SEDA-14, 135) (SEDA-14, 137) (SEDA-17, 196) (23–25). Terfenadine and astemizole have been described as having dysrhythmogenic actions, and deaths have been described (26,27). The effects of some antihistamines on the QT interval are listed in Table 1.

With a few exceptions, antihistamines are rapidly and completely absorbed after oral administration; peak plasma concentrations are reached after 1–4 hours and are highly variable, owing to differences in tissue distribution and metabolism (20). Many of the second-generation antihistamines (for example astemizole, ebastine, loratadine, and terfenadine) undergo extensive first-pass metabolism to pharmacologically active metabolites; as a common feature, the reaction is primarily supported by CYP3A4. Under normal circumstances this extensive metabolism leads to low or undetectable plasma concentrations of the parent drug. However, sometimes metabolism of the parent compound can be compromised. Accumulation of unmetabolized astemizole or terfenadine can result in blockade of cardiac potassium channels in the ventricular myocytes that regulate the duration of the action potential; consequent prolongation of the QT interval can result in potentially life-threatening ventricular tachycardia (28).

Dysrhythmias can also occur with therapeutic doses of these and other antihistamines, if certain other susceptibility factors are present:

- impaired hepatic metabolism due to liver disease;
- simultaneous treatment with drugs that are inhibitors of the cytochrome P450 enzyme CYP3A4 (for example macrolide antibiotics, antifungal azoles, or grapefruit juice), leading to increased plasma concentrations thereby raising the risk of cardiotoxic effects (29) (SEDA-17, 196);

- pre-existing QT prolongation caused by congenital long QT syndrome, other heart disease, or treatment with antidysrhythmic drugs, such as class I antidysrhythmic drugs, amiodarone, or sotalol;
- electrolyte imbalance; in particular, hypokalemia predisposes to Dysrhythmias.

Terfenadine is especially likely to cause torsade de pointes in patients in whom these risk factors are present (SEDA-19, 176) (SEDA-21, 176). Ventricular dysrhythmias can also occur after overdosage of antihistamines that prolong the QT interval.

The mechanism responsible for dysrhythmias has been identified as blockade of HERG potassium channels (30). The dysrhythmogenic potential of antihistamines has been evaluated in vitro using cloned human potassium channels or guinea-pig heart muscle cells, and using an in vivo guinea-pig model. Studies in humans, including the assessment of drug interactions, are considered more reliable. Investigations in human volunteers have shown that there are no significant electrocardiographic changes with azelastine, cetirizine, fexofenadine, and loratadine even at several times the therapeutic doses, which shows that cardiotoxicity is not a class effect (31) (SEDA-19, 172). Mizolastine also appears to cause no cardiac problems in humans (32). Large doses of ebastine have shown cardiac effects in guinea pigs, but QT prolongation has not occurred in human studies with up to three times therapeutic doses (33). Slight QT prolongation was seen on further increased doses to 100 mg/day and when subjects were given erythromycin or ketoconazole, but the effect was less than the effect of terfenadine and was not considered clinically relevant (33). The active metabolite of ebastine, carebastine, had no effect on the QT interval, even in large doses.

The absolute risk of antihistamine-induced dysrhythmias is low in the general population. In an epidemiological study using a general practice database, the crude incidence of ventricular dysrhythmias was 1.9 per 10 000 person-years, corresponding to a relative risk of 4.2 for all antihistamines compared with non-use. Astemizole presented the highest relative risk, whereas terfenadine was in the range of other non-sedating antihistamines. Older age was associated with greater risk. The absolute risk in this study was one case per 5300 person-years of use (34).

In the USA, terfenadine was withdrawn from the market in 1998, and in other countries terfenadine has been moved from over-the-counter to prescription-only, with only 60 mg tablets available. The active metabolite of terfenadine, fexofenadine, is marketed as an alternative. For astemizole this option was not available, since the main metabolite (desmethylastemizole) is also cardiotoxic and has a half-life of 10 days; astemizole was therefore withdrawn from the market worldwide in June 1999.

Although it is widely believed that cardiotoxicity of antihistamines is limited to second-generation compounds, both hydroxyzine and diphenhydramine can block potassium channels. Caution should therefore be exercised in prescribing first-generation antihistamines for patients with a predisposition to cardiac dysrhythmias. For example, therapeutic doses of diphenhydramine caused prolongation of the QT interval in healthy volunteers and in patients undergoing angioplasty (35), and one cannot exclude the possibility that first-generation drugs that modulate

Table 1 The sedative, anticholinergic, and QT prolonging effects of antihistamines (all rINNs, except where stated)

Drug	Sedative effect	Anticholinergic effect	QT interval prolongation
Acrivastine	+	−	−
Alimemazine (trifluomeprazine, trimeprazine)	++++	+++	
Antazoline			
Astemizole	−		+++
Azelastine			−
Betahistine	+	++	
Brompheniramine	+	++	
Carebastine			−
Cetirizine	±	±	−
Chlorphenamine (chlorpheniramine)	++	±	−
Cinnarizine	+	+	−
Clemastine	+	+	±
Cyclizine	++	++	
Cyproheptadine	++	++	
Desloratadine	−	+	−
Dexbrompheniramine			
Dexchlorpheniramine			
Dimenhydrinate	+++	+++	
Dimetindene			
Diphenhydramine	+++	++	+
Diphenylpyraline			
Doxylamine	+		
Ebastine	−		−
Emedastine			
Fexofenadine	−	−	−
Flunarizine			
Hydroxyzine	+	−	±
Ketotifen	+		−
Levocabastine			
Levocetirizine	−		−
Loratadine	−	±	−
Mebhydrolin			
Meclozine (pINN)			
Mepyramine	++	+	
Mequitazine	+		+
Methapyrilene			
Mizolastine	−	−	−
Oxatomide			
Phenindamine			
Pheniramine			
Promethazine	++++	+++	
Terfenadine	±	+	+++
Thiazinamium			
Tripelennamine			
Triprolidine	++		

potassium channels may in some circumstances cause dysrhythmias (36). All antihistamines should be screened for cardiotoxicity, as some patients may be poor metabolizers or may be susceptible to plasma concentrations near to the usual therapeutic range. Useful information may be obtained from pharmacokinetic studies using potential inhibitors (see under Drug–Drug Interactions).

The single- and multiple-dose pharmacokinetics of ebastine (10 mg) have been determined in elderly and young healthy subjects using 24-hour Holter monitoring (37). There were no clinically relevant effects.

The incidence of ventricular dysrhythmias associated with non-sedating antihistamines (including cetirizine) has also been assessed using the UK-based General Practice Research Database (34). There were 18 cases over the period 1992–96. Astemizole was associated with the highest relative risk. The risk associated with terfenadine was no different from that with other non-sedating antihistamines, and there was no single case of ventricular dysrhythmia with the concomitant use of P450 inhibitors and terfenadine.

In a comparison of the dysrhythmogenic potential of a series of second-generation antihistamines, the antihistamines were given intravenously and electrocardiographic and cardiovascular parameters (blood pressure and heart rate) were measured. The lowest dose that produced significant prolongation of the QT_c interval was compared with the dose required to inhibit by 50% the peripheral bronchospasm elicited by histamine 10 micrograms/kg intravenously. Astemizole, ebastine, and terfenadine produced pronounced dose-dependent QT_c interval prolongation. In contrast, terfenadine carboxylate, norastemizole, and carebastine, the major metabolites of terfenadine, astemizole, and ebastine, and cetirizine had no effects (38).

Respiratory

Phenothiazine derivatives can aggravate asthma. The use of the first-generation antihistamines in asthma was hampered by induction of coughing when inhaled and by their sedative properties when given orally. Furthermore, the desiccating and thickening effect on the airway mucus is undesirable. However, the American Academy of Allergy and Immunology (39) has stated that antihistamines are not contraindicated in patients with asthma, unless there have been previous adverse reactions (SEDA-14, 135).

The effect of the second-generation antihistamines in treating asthma has been investigated. They have a moderate, bronchodilatory effect and an effect on exercise-induced asthma, hyperventilation, and cold-air breathing, and to a varying degree give some protection against the early and late responses to allergen (2) (SEDA-14, 135).

Antihistamines are not first-choice drugs in asthma, however, and although they can contribute to the relief of seasonal asthma symptoms and accompanying allergic rhinitis, the results of a meta-analysis do not support the general use of antihistamines in adult asthmatics (40).

Ear, nose, throat

When used for the treatment of colds and allergic upper airways disorders, antihistamines (alone or in combination with decongestants) can reduce mucociliary motility in the middle ear, thus contributing to the development of otitis media (41).

Nervous system

The sedative and anticholinergic effects of antihistamines, when known, are summarized in Table 1.

Antihistamines and drowsiness

Central nervous depression causing sedation is the most common adverse effect of the first-generation antihistamines (SEDA-21, 171) (42). The sedative effect of antihistamines is evaluated using psychometric tests, tests of driving performance, and subjective scoring or visual analogue scales, but results from studies using healthy volunteers cannot necessarily be extrapolated to patients, one difficulty being that the treated disease can itself cause sedation (43). The drowsiness has been attributed to inhibition of histamine *N*-methyltransferase and to blockade of central histamine receptors, together with actions on other receptors, in particular 5-HT receptors (2,17,19,44). Daytime drowsiness can be a problem, above all when driving or operating machinery. As with many other nervous system depressants, this effect may abate or disappear after several days of use, but co-medication with certain other agents or a short period of withdrawal of therapy may reactivate the sedative effect.

The signal characteristic of the second-generation antihistamines is their freedom from sedation (2,16). The relative lack of sedative properties in the second-generation antihistamines has been ascribed to their relative hydrophilicity. Little is known about intracerebral concentrations of antihistamines and their metabolites, but positron emission tomography has shown that the first-generation antihistamine chlorphenamine occupied a larger fraction of brain histamine H_1 receptors than terfenadine (SEDA-20, 164). Differential affinity for, or different actions on, central and peripheral H_1 receptors (SEDA-21, 171) could also explain variations in sedative effect, but differences in receptor binding have only been shown for loratadine in vitro (45).

The nervous system depressant effects of fexofenadine (46,47), loratadine (48), and mizolastine (49) appear to be no greater than those seen with placebo. However, the generality of the claim that second-generation antihistamines are free of sedative effects has been challenged (50). The issue is complicated by evidence that sedation in allergic disease (and subsequent impairment in performance and learning) can be a consequence of the condition itself, as opposed to being wholly due to antihistamines (20). This raises concerns about the purported risk-free sedation profiles of certain antihistamines, given that they are often based on objective studies in healthy volunteers (42). Another issue is the tendency of patients with allergies to self-medicate, titrating their antihistamine dosage upwards to achieve relief of symptoms; neurological impairment does in fact occur if the doses of cetirizine, loratadine, or mizolastine are increased sufficiently (20). Thus, it is more correct to describe the second-generation antihistamines as having minimal sedative effects when taken in recommended doses. A grouping of the antihistamines into those with marked, moderate, and very low sedative effect is possible. However, the dividing lines are not sharp and classification often depends on how many studies are taken into account, since results are not consistent.

The designs of protocols used in comparisons between sedative and non-sedative compounds have been questioned. They may not accurately reflect the clinical use of each drug, and the data may be misused in advice to prescribers, even though the reason a comparator was included was merely to provide an active control. Extrapolation of the results of cognitive studies in healthy volunteers to patients may be inappropriate, as a drug that is sedative in a healthy volunteer may well not be perceived to be sedative by a patient with allergic symptoms, although caution must be taken in relying on subjective assessments of performance and drowsiness. Patients with mild to moderate allergic rhinitis complain of sleep difficulties, and many who take a sedative can function reasonably well during the next day without further medication. Duration of treatment can also play a part, and certain investigations may have been too brief; in some patients, sedation is induced by the drug only after some weeks of treatment (SEDA-12, 142). Such discrepancies could explain why, despite all the investigations with positive results, some studies report sedation in 30% of the patients (SED-11, 317) (SEDA-9, 149) (SEDA-10, 135).

It is likely that the controversy will be settled by accepting the relative merits of each drug, and that sedative drugs will continue to be prescribed, at least for overnight ingestion and for some skin conditions.

There is the special case of the use of antihistamines by individuals whose work may compromise their own safety or the safety of others, for example transport workers. Indeed, much of the support for second-generation drugs arises from safety considerations. Nevertheless, it is sometimes suggested that recommendations for the use of antihistamines by those involved in skilled activities should be based on studies of the patients themselves carrying out their day-to-day work, for example airline pilots with allergic rhinitis operating aircraft. This is an argument that lacks careful thought. In occupational medicine it is essential that controlled studies in healthy volunteers are used to establish whether an antihistamine has sedative properties, and then to choose the drug that is least likely to impair performance or cause drowsiness.

Observational studies
Antihistamines are effective and safe in preventing the symptoms of a mosquito bite; ebastine and loratadine did not cause sedation in such cases (51,52).

Comparative studies
The frequency of sedation due to acrivastine, cetirizine, fexofenadine, and loratadine has been investigated in four prescription-event monitoring studies in 43 363 patients in general practice in the UK (53). Prescriptions were obtained for each cohort in the immediate postmarketing period. Sedation and drowsiness were the main outcome measures. The odds ratios (adjusted for age and sex) for the incidences of sedation compared with loratadine were: 0.63 (95% CI = 0.36, 1.11) for fexofenadine, 2.79 (1.69, 4.58) for acrivastine, and 3.53 (2.07, 5.42) for cetirizine. There was no increased risk of accident or injury with any of the four drugs.

The effects of diphenhydramine, fexofenadine, and alcohol on driving performance have been studied in a randomized, placebo-controlled trial in the Iowa driving simulator (54). Participants had significantly better coherence after alcohol or fexofenadine than after diphenhydramine. Lane holding (steering instability and crossing the center line) was impaired after alcohol and diphenhydramine compared with fexofenadine. Mean response time to the blocking vehicle was slowest after alcohol (2.21 seconds) compared with fexofenadine (1.95 seconds). Self-reported drowsiness did not predict lack of coherence and was weakly associated with minimum following distance, steering instability, and left-lane excursion. In conclusion, the participants performed similarly when they took fexofenadine or placebo. After alcohol they performed the primary task well but not the secondary tasks, resulting in poorer driving performance. After diphenhydramine, driving performance was poorest, suggesting that diphenhydramine had a greater impact on driving than alcohol did. Drowsiness ratings were not a good predictor of impairment, suggesting that drivers cannot use drowsiness to indicate when they should not drive. Non-sedating antihistamines should therefore be preferred over sedating antihistamines in patients who drive (55).

Mequitazine has a low propensity to cause drowsiness, comparable to that of cetirizine and loratadine; it therefore differs from truly sedative antihistamines, such as dexchlorpheniramine, which cause drowsiness and fatigue in patients with atopy to a degree that is measurably different from placebo (56).

Although allergic rhinitis is not usually severe, it affects school learning performance and work productivity (57). The effects of loratadine and cetirizine on somnolence and motivation during the working day have been compared in 60 patients with allergic rhinitis in a parallel-group, double-blind study (58). Somnolence scores were similar in the two groups at baseline and at the time of dosing (0800 hours). However, cetirizine caused significantly more somnolence at 1000 hours, 1200 hours, and 1500 hours. The scores of motivation to perform activities were similar in the two groups at baseline and 0800 hours. The patients taking loratadine were relatively more motivated at 1000 hours, 1200 hours, and 1500 hours.

In a comparison of the effects over 7 days of a modified-release formulation of brompheniramine (12 mg bd) and loratadine (10 mg od), physicians' and patients' assessments were better for brompheniramine than for loratadine, but somnolence and dizziness were reported less often by those who took loratadine, although occurrences were claimed to be less frequent with brompheniramine as treatment continued (59).

The authors of a report of a comparison of the effectiveness of ebastine (10 and 20 mg) and loratadine (10 mg) for perennial allergic rhinitis claimed that ebastine provided greater symptomatic relief than loratadine, but with a similar low incidence of central effects and headache (60).

In a comparison of the incidence of drowsiness between cinnarizine (25 mg tds for 7 days, 25 mg bd for 15 days, and 25 mg daily for 15 days) and prochlorperazine (5 mg tds for 7 days, 5 mg bd for 15 days, and 5 mg od for 15 days), drowsiness was observed less often in those taking prochlorperazine (61).

In a comparison of diphenhydramine, chlorphenamine, cetirizine, loratadine, and placebo in 15 healthy elderly subjects, there were no significant differences between the first- and second-generation antihistamines (62). In another study, even the first-generation sedative drug chlorphenamine failed to cause significant sedation in a group of children (63).

In a comparison of astemizole, terfenadine, and triprolidine (positive control), only triprolidine caused reduced performance and motor incoordination (64).

In a comparison of the effects of acrivastine, terfenadine, and diphenhydramine on driving performance, there was a dose-dependent effect of acrivastine, with severely affected driving in doses of 16 and 24 mg (SEDA-19, 170). Terfenadine in doses of 60–180 mg did not affect driving performance.

In a comparison of cetirizine and loratadine, cetirizine 10 mg had acute sedative effects and impaired driving performance (65), whereas loratadine had no sedating potential; furthermore, there was an additive effect of alcohol and cetirizine but not alcohol and loratadine. However, in a study using a driving simulator cetirizine 10 mg did not affect driving ability (66). In other studies cetirizine 20 mg caused significant sedation, while in one study there was a dose-dependent sedative effect with 10 mg and 20 mg but not 5 mg (67). Pooling the available data (SEDA-16, 163) shows that cetirizine is little more sedative than loratadine and terfenadine.

In a comparison of ebastine and triprolidine, only those taking triprolidine had impairment of several parameters of car driving performance (SEDA-18, 182).

The effects of loratadine 10, 20, and 40 mg on tests of visuomotor coordination, dynamic visual acuity, short-term memory, digit symbol substitution, and subjective assessments of mood have been studied (68). Triprolidine was used as an active control and impaired performance on all the tasks presented. Loratadine 40 mg caused a significant impairment of the Digit Symbol Substitution Test and the Dynamic Visual Acuity Test, but the 10 and 20 mg doses were without effect. Loratadine did not affect objective sleepiness, as measured by Multiple Sleep Latency Test (69). In other studies of loratadine in the normal 10 mg dose the sedation rate was no different from placebo (SEDA-12, 143) (SEDA-14, 136).

In a comparison of the initial and 5-day steady-state effects of loratadine, diphenhydramine, and placebo, using a number of psychometric tests, there was no detectable effect of loratadine compared with placebo, whereas diphenhydramine clearly reduced performance (70).

Anticholinergic effects

The marked anticholinergic properties of the first-generation antihistamines can cause dryness of the oral and respiratory mucosae. Other antimuscarinic effects are less common, but nasal stuffiness, blurring of vision, urinary retention, and constipation can all occur.

Nervous system stimulation is less frequent than nervous system depression, but when it occurs it causes insomnia, irritability, and tremor; nightmares, and hallucinations. In overt intoxication, these effects may be related to anticholinergic effects. In an analysis of 113 200 admissions to a pediatric hospital there were only two patients with excitation, insomnia, visual hallucinations, and seizures, followed by coma (71).

Antidopaminergic effects

Antidopaminergic effects of antihistamine drugs can cause extrapyramidal symptoms, including neuroleptic malignant syndrome (SEDA-19, 173) (SEDA-22, 178) (72). Prolonged use of antihistamine-containing decongestants can cause facial dyskinesias, including blepharospasm, swallowing difficulties, and dysarthria. As patients with these effects have often been taking combination products containing antihistamines, proper evaluation of interactions is needed before final assessment is possible. As a dyskinesia can be unilateral, a neurological disorder should be excluded before thinking about an adverse effect (SEDA-1, 144).

The prognosis of drug-induced parkinsonism has been discussed (73,74). Negrotri and Calzetti (73) considered that the results of Martí-Massó and Poza (74) were overoptimistic. This they ascribed to uncertainty in the collection of their data, which may not have provided adequate evidence of the course of clinical recovery, although differences in cumulative dosages and concurrent use of other drugs could also have been involved. The differences in prognosis may be attributable to the fact that the patients studied by Martí-Massó and Poza (34) were diagnosed earlier, were less severely affected, and had a good prognosis. Cinnarizine-induced extrapyramidal signs have tended to be associated with old age and prolonged treatment. However, cinnarizine-induced akathisia, parkinsonism, and depression have been reported in a 25-year-old patient after only 11 days of treatment (75).

Sensory systems

A questionnaire showed that women taking antihistamines and/or cold formulations had a tone average 9 dB higher than those not taking such medication (76). Audiography showed differences in threshold of 6.4 and 12.8 dB at 500 and 1000 Hz respectively. The medications involved were primarily meclozine for dizziness and terfenadine for allergy.

Psychological, psychiatric

In healthy volunteers promethazine caused impaired cognitive function and psychomotor performance (77). The test battery consisted of critical flicker fusion, choice reaction time, compensatory tracking task, and assessment of subjective sedation. Cetirizine and loratadine at all doses tested were not significantly different from placebo in any of the tests used.

School performance in 63 children aged 8–10 years was not impaired by short-term diphenhydramine or loratadine (78).

Comparative studies

The effects of ebastine 10 mg on cognitive impairment have been assessed in 20 healthy volunteers who performed six types of attention-demanding cognitive tasks, together with objective measurements of reaction times and accuracy (79). Ebastine was compared with placebo and a positive control, chlorphenamine (chlorphenamine, 2 mg and 6 mg). Compared with placebo, ebastine had no effect on any objective cognitive test nor any effect on subjective sleepiness. In contrast, chlorphenamine significantly increased reaction times, decreased accuracy in cognitive tasks, and increased subjective sleepiness. The effect of chlorphenamine increased with plasma concentration.

In a double-blind, placebo-controlled, randomized trial of the effects of levocetirizine 5 mg and diphenhydramine 50 mg on objective measurements (a word-learning test, the Sternberg Memory Scanning Test, a tracking test, and a divided attention test that measured both tracking and memory scanning simultaneously) in 48 healthy volunteers (24 men and 24 women). Levocetirizine had no effect, while diphenhydramine significantly affected divided attention and tracking after acute administration (80). However, on day 4 the effects of diphenhydramine did not reach significance, suggesting a degree of tolerance to this first-generation drug.

The effects of levocetirizine on cognitive function have been assessed in two comprehensive and well-controlled studies. The first analysed the effects of single and multiple doses of levocetirizine on measures of nervous system activity, using integrated measures of cognitive and psychometric performance. In a three-way crossover design, 19 healthy men took either levocetirizine 5 mg, diphenhydramine 50 mg (positive control), or placebo once-daily on five consecutive days. Critical flicker fusion tests were performed on days 1 and 5 at baseline and up to 24 hours after drug administration. The primary outcome was that, in contrast to diphenhydramine, levocetirizine did not have any deleterious effect on any cognitive or psychometric function compared with placebo (81). In a double-blind, crossover study levocetirizine 5 mg once-daily for 4 days was compared with cetirizine 10 mg, loratadine 10 mg, promethazine 30 mg, and placebo in terms of CNS inhibitory effects in 20 healthy volunteers (82). With the exception of promethazine none of the drugs had disruptive or sedative effects on objective measurements in a comprehensive battery of psychomotor and cognitive tests.

Metabolism

Appetite stimulation and resulting weight gain is a well-known feature of cyproheptadine, but astemizole also causes weight gain in approximately 3% of patients within weeks of treatment (16,83). Cetirizine also has been reported to cause weight gain (about 2.8%) when it is used for a prolonged time (SEDA-17, 200). Increased body weight occurred in three participants in a trial of azelastine (SEDA-21, 172).

In a double-blind, randomized, placebo-controlled study of the effect of cetirizine, clemastine, and loratadine for 7 days on blood glucose concentration in patients with allergic rhinitis, cetirizine produced a significant increase in postprandial blood glucose and a small rise in fasting blood glucose; clemastine caused a small fall in fasting and a small rise in postprandial blood glucose (84). The mechanisms of these effects are not known.

Hematologic

Blood dyscrasias are infrequent with antihistamines, but agranulocytosis, hemolytic anemia, and thrombocytopenia have been described. Thrombocytopenia has been attributed to antazoline (85), agranulocytosis to chlorphenamine (SEDA-16, 162) and mebhydrolin (86), and aplastic anemia to chlorphenamine (87).

Gastrointestinal

Antihistamines do not commonly cause gastrointestinal effects, but nausea, vomiting, gastric pain, diarrhea, or constipation can occur (88).

Liver

Repeated reports of changes in liver function may reflect coincidence, in view of the widespread use of these drugs. Occasionally, however, hepatitis (89) or cholestatic jaundice seems to have occurred.

Skin

Although antihistamines are often used in the treatment of allergic conditions, topical use often produces skin sensitization and subsequent contact dermatitis (90,91). This effect occurs more often with the use of ethylenediamines and phenothiazines; the latter also produce photoallergic cutaneous reactions (92). A photoallergic contact dermatitis followed by a persistent light reaction was attributed to topical dioxopromethazine hydrochloride incorporated into a gel in a woman with periocular pruritus (93). Photosensitivity in sun-exposed areas where she had not applied the formulation persisted for up to 500 days, with a reduced minimal erythema dose (MED) for UVA together with abnormal delayed infiltrated reactions to UVB in repeated phototests.

Cross-reactions between phenothiazine tranquillizers and first-generation antihistamines are possible, as well as reactions between antihistamines and ethylenediamine present in some creams and ointments. As local sensitization is quite common, topical use of antihistamines is not recommended. Despite these disadvantages they are still available in many countries as over-the-counter products. Topical antihistamines in sufficient doses can also cause systemic adverse effects.

Subacute cutaneous lupus-like dermatitis has been associated with cinnarizine and brompheniramine (94,95).

Long-Term Effects

Drug abuse

Some antihistamines, for example tripellenamine (often used in combination with pentazocine), have a particular abuse potential and are used by drug addicts. Psychiatric disturbances, dysphoria, depression, confusion, and hallucinations can occur while under the influence of an antihistamine or during drug withdrawal. Chronic parenteral abuse can cause skin lesions, muscular fibrosis, and vasculitis.

Drug withdrawal

Since dyskinesia can occur after withdrawal of phenothiazine neuroleptic drugs, it is not unlikely that the same problem may follow termination of prolonged antihistamine therapy.

Tumorigenicity

Tumor-inducing effects have been reported in animal studies on methapyrilene; the significance of this finding is not clear (SEDA-4, 171). An association between antihistamine exposure and accelerated tumor growth seen in experimental animal models has found no support in an epidemiological study (96).

Second-Generation Effects

Teratogenicity

Teratogenic effects have not been proven in humans, although some piperazine derivatives have teratogenic effects in laboratory animals. Some studies have suggested an association between palate malformation and antihistamines (97–99).

Teratogenic activity has been attributed to doxylamine, a constituent of many combinations with vitamin B6 and antispasmodic agents, and used in the treatment of hyperemesis gravidarum. However, extensive studies and reviews have suggested that the incidence of malformations is not higher in children whose mothers have taken formulations containing antihistamines as a group, and in particular the combination of doxylamine/pyridoxine with or without dicycloverine (100–102).

A meta-analysis of 24 controlled studies of the association between antihistamines and major congenital malformations (more than 200 000 participating women) did not show an increased risk of malformations (103). Experience with the first-generation antihistamines is more comprehensive than with the second-generation compounds, and in a recent review it was concluded that some of the first-generation drugs can be used for allergic rhinitis in pregnancy (104). Some authors advise avoiding brompheniramine because of a supposed association with birth defects (SEDA-21, 172).

Studies with various antihistamines (105,106) have failed to provide evidence of teratogenicity. However, the samples may not have been large enough to provide adequate statistical power or to establish the true incidence of individual malformations. In study of the effect of treatment with diazepam and promethazine during pregnancy carried out in the late 1980s (minimal doses for the whole pregnancy 50 mg and 250 mg respectively), children of both sexes in the diazepam group had lower birth weights, but normal body weights at 8 months of age; there were no changes in body weight in the promethazine group (107). The incidence of major malformations with terfenadine (mean dose 30–120 mg/day) has been estimated prospectively. Rates of major malformations did not differ from matched controls amongst those exposed during the first trimester. However, birth weight was lower in babies exposed to terfenadine, but not when babies below 2500 g were compared. These findings emphasize the general value of continued studies on antihistamines during pregnancy; the findings with terfenadine may be equally applicable to its metabolite fexofenadine (108).

Cleft palate is seen more often in infants whose mothers have used antihistamines for the treatment of hyperemesis gravidarum (4.44 per 1000 births) than in infants of mothers without hyperemesis gravidarum and not treated with antihistamines (0.78 per 1000) (98). However, children of mothers suffering from hyperemesis gravidarum but not treated also showed a high incidence of cleft palate (3.14 per 1000). It is likely that cleft palate could be a consequence of the maternal condition rather than of drug teratogenicity.

Lactation

There have been no specific reports of harm resulting from the use of antihistamines during lactation, although there have been few studies. Triprolidine and loratadine would reach a breastfed infant in low concentrations (109).

Susceptibility Factors

Hepatic disease

Because sedation can lead to hepatic encephalopathy in patients with hepatic failure, sedative antihistamines should be avoided in such patients. In addition, some antihistamines are themselves hepatotoxic.

Other features of the patient

In view of their anticholinergic effects antihistamines should be avoided in cases of glaucoma and prostatism.

Antihistamines can be dangerous to drivers and people operating machinery, primarily because of their sedative effects but also because of blurring of vision.

Drug Administration

Drug overdose

- A 48-year-old woman was found dead after taking guaifenesin, diphenhydramine, and chlorphenamine, with heart blood concentrations of 27, 8.5, and 0.2 mg/l respectively (110).

Drug–Drug Interactions

Anticholinergic drugs

Drugs with anticholinergic effects (including phenothiazines, tricyclic antidepressants, quinidine, and disopyramide) will have their effects increased by antihistamines.

Cytochrome P450 isozymes

Several of the non-sedating antihistamines (astemizole, ebastine, loratadine, and terfenadine, but not cetirizine, desloratadine, fexofenadine, levocetirizine, or norastemizole) are metabolized by the cytochrome P450 isozyme CYP3A4 (SEDA-21, 177) (111). Concomitant treatment with drugs that inhibit this metabolic pathway (such as ketoconazole, itraconazole, erythromycin, clarithromycin) lead to increased plasma concentrations of the unmetabolized drug. Currently, only astemizole and terfenadine have been associated with cardiac adverse effects caused by such interactions. Terfenadine given with grapefruit juice, which also inhibits CYP3A4, resulted in higher plasma concentrations, but not QT interval prolongation (112).

Pooled human liver microsomes have been used to determine whether loratadine, desloratadine, and 3-hydroxydesloratadine are inhibitors of CYP1A2, CYP2C9, CYP2C19, CYP2D6, and CYP3A4 (113). Loratadine did not inhibit CYP1A2 or CYP3A4 at concentrations up to 3829 ng/ml, about 815 times greater than the expected maximal human plasma concentration (mean 4.7 ng/ml) after the recommended dose of 10 mg/day. Loratadine inhibited CYP2C19 and CYP2D6 with IC_{50} values of about 0.76 µmol/l (291 ng/ml) and 8.1 µmol/l (3100 ng/ml) respectively, about 60 and 660 times the expected loratadine therapeutic concentrations. Neither desloratadine nor 3-hydroxydesloratadine inhibited CYP1A2, CYP2C9, CYP2C19, CYP2D6, or CYP3A4 by more than 25% at concentrations of about 3000 ng/ml. These results suggest that loratadine and its active metabolites desloratadine and 3-hydroxydesloratadine are unlikely to affect the pharmacokinetics of co-administered drugs that are metabolized by these five cytochrome P450 enzymes.

Drugs acting on the brain

Drugs that have effects on the brain (hypnotics, sedatives, narcotic analgesics, neuroleptic drugs, alcohol, lithium, anticonvulsants) will interact with antihistamines, especially the first-generation drugs. The second-generation antihistamines have not yet been proven to interact with drugs such as alcohol or diazepam (114–117).

Histamine

The unwanted effects of histamine injections can be partially blocked by H_1 histamine receptor antagonists, which were once used to prevent systemic adverse effects of histamine when it was used to stimulate gastric acid secretion, which is mediated by H_2 receptors.

Meglumine

When diphenhydramine was mixed with meglumine iodipamide to prevent an allergic reaction to the latter, a precipitate was formed. These two drugs should be regarded as incompatible for in vitro mixing.

Pseudoephedrine

Combinations with decongestants such as pseudoephedrine have been advocated for upper respiratory conditions, but pseudoephedrine can cause additional adverse effects, such as nervousness and raised blood pressure (118,119).

Stimulants

To counteract the sedative effects of the classic antihistamines, combinations with stimulants, such as pemoline and prolintane, have been tried. The efficacy of such combinations has not been proven, but additional adverse effects such as irritability (120) and hallucinations (121) have been observed.

D-Tubocurarine chloride

Tubocurarine can cause release of histamine by direct mast cell degranulation which can result in systemic effects, such as cutaneous flushing, local wheal and flare formation, hypotension, and occasionally bronchospasm. Preoperative oral terfenadine 60 mg + ranitidine 150 mg attenuated the reduction in blood pressure but not cutaneous flushing after the administration of tubocurarine and morphine in 60 women undergoing elective gynaecological surgery in a placebo-controlled study (122).

Interference with Diagnostic Tests

Skin testing

Since antihistamines inhibit the cutaneous response to histamine and allergens, they should be withdrawn (usually for a week, astemizole for up to 8 weeks) before skin testing for allergy is undertaken.

References

1. Nicholson AN, Pascoe PA, Stone BM. Histaminergic systems and sleep. Studies in man with H1 and H2 antagonists. Neuropharmacology 1985;24(3):245–50.
2. Simons FE, Simons KJ. Second-generation H1-receptor antagonists. Ann Allergy 1991;66(1):5–16, 19.
3. Temple DM, McCluskey M. Loratadine, an antihistamine, blocks antigen- and ionophore-induced leukotriene release from human lung in vitro. Prostaglandins 1988;35(4):549–54.
4. Little MM, Wood DR, Casale TB. Azelastine inhibits stimulated histamine release from human lung tissue in vitro but does not alter cyclic nucleotide content. Agents Actions 1989;28(1–2):16–21.
5. Charlesworth EN, Kagey-Sobotka A, Norman PS, Lichtenstein LM. Effect of cetirizine on mast cell-mediator release and cellular traffic during the cutaneous late-phase reaction. J Allergy Clin Immunol 1989;83(5):905–12.
6. Michel L, De Vos C, Rihoux JP, Burtin C, Benveniste J, Dubertret L. Inhibitory effect of oral cetirizine on in vivo antigen-induced histamine and PAF-acether release and eosinophil recruitment in human skin. J Allergy Clin Immunol 1988;82(1):101–9.
7. Leprevost C, Capron M, De Vos C, Tomassini M, Capron A. Inhibition of eosinophil chemotaxis by a new antiallergic compound (cetirizine). Int Arch Allergy Appl Immunol 1988;87(1):9–13.
8. Staub A, Bovet D. Actions de la thymoethyl-diethylamine (929F) et des éthers phénoliques sur le choc anaphylactique du cobaye. CR Soc Biol 1937;128:818–25.
9. Halpern B. Les antihistaminiques de synthèse: essai de chimiothérapie des états allergiques. Arch Int Pharmacodyn Ther 1942;68:339–45.
10. Bovet D, Horclois R, Walthert F. Propriétés antihistaminiques de la N-p-méthoxybenzyl-N-diméthylaminoéthyl alpha aminopyridine. CR Soc Biol 1944;138:99–108.
11. Lowe E, MacMillan R, Katser M. The antihistamine properties of Benadryl, beta-dimethyl-aminoethyl benzhydryl ether hydrochloride. J Pharmacol Exp Ther 1946;86:229.
12. Yonkman F, Chess D, Mathieson D, Hansen N. Pharmacodynamic studies of an new antihistamine agent, N′-pyridyl-N-benzyl-N-dimethylethylene diamine HCl, pyribenzamine HCl. J Pharmacol Exp Ther 1946;87:256.
13. Ellis A, Day J. Second- and third-generation antihistamines. Dermatol Rev 2000;13:327–36.
14. Van Cauwenberge P, Juniper EF. Comparison of the efficacy, safety and quality of life provided by fexofenadine hydrochloride 120 mg, loratadine 10 mg and placebo administered once daily for the treatment of seasonal allergic rhinitis. Clin Exp Allergy 2000;30(6):891–9.
15. Routledge PA, Lindquist M, Edwards IR. Spontaneous reporting of suspected adverse reactions to antihistamines: a national and international perspective. Clin Exp Allergy 1999;29(Suppl 3):240–6.
16. Kunkel G. Antihistamines reassessed. Clin Exp Allergy 1990;20:1.
17. Simons FE. H1-receptor antagonists: clinical pharmacology and therapeutics. J Allergy Clin Immunol 1989;84(6 Pt 1):845–61.
18. Trzeciakowski JP, Levi R. Antihistamines. In: Middleton E, Reed CE, Ellis EF, editors. Allergy. Principles and Practice. 2nd ed. St. Louis: Mosby, 1983.
19. Druce H. Impairment of function by antihistamines. Ann Allergy 1990;64(5):403–5.
20. Walsh GM, Annunziato L, Frossard N, Knol K, Levander S, Nicolas JM, Taglialatela M, Tharp MD, Tillement JP, Timmerman H. New insights into the second generation antihistamines. Drugs 2001;61(2):207–36.
21. Walsh GM. Second-generation antihistamines in asthma therapy: is there a protective effect? Am J Respir Med 2002;1(1):27–34.
22. Honig P, Baraniuk JN. Adverse effects of H1-receptor antagonists in the cardiovascular system. In: Simons FER, editor. Histamine and H1-receptor Antagonists in Allergic Disease. New York: Marcel Dekker Inc, 1996:383–412.

23. Simons FE, Kesselman MS, Giddins NG, Pelech AN, Simons KJ. Astemizole-induced torsade de pointes. Lancet 1988;2(8611):624.

24. Davies AJ, Harindra V, McEwan A, Ghose RR. Cardiotoxic effect with convulsions in terfenadine overdose. BMJ 1989;298(6669):325.

25. Craft TM. Torsade de pointes after astemizole overdose. BMJ (Clin Res Ed) 1986;292(6521):660.

26. Passalacqua G, Bousquet J, Bachert C, Church MK, Bindsley-Jensen C, Nagy L, Szemere P, Davies RJ, Durham SR, Horak F, Kontou-Fili K, Malling HJ, van Cauwenberge P, Canonica GW. The clinical safety of H1-receptor antagonists. An EAACI position paper. Allergy 1996;51(10):666–75.

27. Barbey JT, Anderson M, Ciprandi G, Frew AJ, Morad M, Priori SG, Ongini E, Affrime MB. Cardiovascular safety of second-generation antihistamines. Am J Rhinol 1999;13(3):235–43.

28. Woosley RL. Cardiac actions of antihistamines. Annu Rev Pharmacol Toxicol 1996;36:233–52.

29. Monahan BP, Ferguson CL, Killeavy ES, Lloyd BK, Troy J, Cantilena LR Jr. Torsades de pointes occurring in association with terfenadine use. JAMA 1990;264(21):2788–90.

30. Taglialatela M, Castaldo P, Pannaccione A, Giorgio G, Genovese A, Marone G, Annunziato L. Cardiac ion channels and antihistamines: possible mechanisms of cardiotoxicity. Clin Exp Allergy 1999;29(Suppl 3):182–9.

31. DuBuske LM. Second-generation antihistamines: the risk of ventricular arrhythmias. Clin Ther 1999;21(2):281–95.

32. Chaufour S, Caplain H, Lilienthal N, L'heritier C, Deschamps C, Dubruc C, Rosenzweig P. Study of cardiac repolarization in healthy volunteers performed with mizolastine, a new H1-receptor antagonist. Br J Clin Pharmacol 1999;47(5):515–20.

33. Moss AJ, Chaikin P, Garcia JD, Gillen M, Roberts DJ, Morganroth J. A review of the cardiac systemic side-effects of antihistamines: ebastine. Clin Exp Allergy 1999;29(Suppl 3):200–5.

34. de Abajo FJ, Rodriguez LA. Risk of ventricular arrhythmias associated with nonsedating antihistamine drugs. Br J Clin Pharmacol 1999;47(3):307–13.

35. Khalifa M, Drolet B, Daleau P, Lefez C, Gilbert M, Plante S, O'Hara GE, Gleeton O, Hamelin BA, Turgeon J. Block of potassium currents in guinea pig ventricular myocytes and lengthening of cardiac repolarization in man by the histamine H1 receptor antagonist diphenhydramine. J Pharmacol Exp Ther 1999;288(2):858–65.

36. Taglialatela M, Timmerman H, Annunziato L. Cardiotoxic potential and CNS effects of first-generation antihistamines. Trends Pharmacol Sci 2000;21(2):52–6.

37. Huang MY, Argenti D, Wilson J, Garcia J, Heald D. Pharmacokinetics and electrocardiographic effect of ebastine in young versus elderly healthy subjects. Am J Ther 1998;5(3):153–8.

38. Hey JA, del Prado M, Sherwood J, Kreutner W, Egan RW. Comparative analysis of the cardiotoxicity proclivities of second generation antihistamines in an experimental model predictive of adverse clinical ECG effects. Arzneimittelforschung 1996;46(2):153–8.

39. Sly RM, Kemp JP. The use of antihistamines in patients with asthma. J Allergy Clin Immunol 1988;82:101.

40. Van Ganse E, Kaufman L, Derde MP, Yernault JC, Delaunois L, Vincken W. Effects of antihistamines in adult asthma: a meta-analysis of clinical trials. Eur Respir J 1997;10(10):2216–24.

41. Peerless SA, Noiman AH. Etiology of otitis media with effusion: antihistamines—decongestants. Laryngoscope 1980;90(11 Pt 1):1852–64.

42. Meltzer EIO, Welch MJ. Adverse effects of H1-receptor antagonists in the central nervous system. In: Simons FER, editor. Histamine and H1-receptor Antagonists in Allergic disease. Clin Allergy Immunol Series. New York: Marcel Dekker Inc, 1996:357–81.

43. Spaeth J, Klimek L, Mosges R. Sedation in allergic rhinitis is caused by the condition and not by antihistamine treatment. Allergy 1996;51(12):893–906.

44. Trzeciakowski JP, Mendelsohn N, Levi R. Antihistamines. In: Middleton E, Reed CE, Ellis EF, Adkinson NF, Yuninger JW, editors. Allergy Principles and Practice. 3rd ed. St Louis: C.V. Mosby Company, 1988:715.

45. Ahn HS, Barnett A. Selective displacement of [^{3}H] mepyramine from peripheral vs. central nervous system receptors by loratadine, a non-sedating antihistamine. Eur J Pharmacol 1986;127(1–2):153–5.

46. Hindmarch I, Shamsi Z, Stanley N, Fairweather DB. A double-blind, placebo-controlled investigation of the effects of fexofenadine, loratadine and promethazine on cognitive and psychomotor function. Br J Clin Pharmacol 1999;48(2):200–6.

47. Nicholson AN, Stone BM, Turner C, Mills SL. Antihistamines and aircrew: usefulness of fexofenadine. Aviat Space Environ Med 2000;71(1):2–6.

48. Kay GG, Harris AG. Loratadine: a non-sedating antihistamine. Review of its effects on cognition, psychomotor performance, mood and sedation. Clin Exp Allergy 1999;29(Suppl 3):147–50.

49. Rosenzweig P, Patat A. Lack of behavioural toxicity of mizolastine: a review of the clinical pharmacology studies. Clin Exp Allergy 1999;29(Suppl 3):156–62.

50. Aelony Y. First-generation vs second-generation antihistamines. Arch Intern Med 1998;158(17):1949–50.

51. Karppinen A, Kautiainen H, Reunala T, Petman L, Reunala T, Brummer-Korvenkontio H. Loratadine in the treatment of mosquito-bite-sensitive children. Allergy 2000;55(7):668–71.

52. Karppinen A, Petman L, Jekunen A, Kautiainen H, Vaalasti A, Reunala T. Treatment of mosquito bites with ebastine: a field trial. Acta Derm Venereol 2000;80(2):114–16.

53. Mann RD, Pearce GL, Dunn N, Shakir S. Sedation with "non-sedating" antihistamines: four prescription-event monitoring studies in general practice. BMJ 2000;320(7243):1184–6.

54. Weiler JM, Bloomfield JR, Woodworth GG, Grant AR, Layton TA, Brown TL, McKenzie DR, Baker TW, Watson GS. Effects of fexofenadine, diphenhydramine, and alcohol on driving performance. A randomized, placebo-controlled trial in the Iowa driving simulator. Ann Intern Med 2000;132(5):354–63.

55. Hennessy S, Strom BL. Nonsedating antihistamines should be preferred over sedating antihistamines in patients who drive. Ann Intern Med 2000;132(5):405–7.

56. Didier A, Doussau-Thuron S, Murris-Espin M. Comparative analysis of the sedative effects of mequitazine and other antihistaminic drugs: review of the literature. Curr Ther Res Clin Exp 2000;61:770–80.

57. Bousquet J, et al. Allergic rhinitis and its impact on asthma. J Allergy Clin Immunol 2001;118:315.

58. Salmun LM, Gates D, Scharf M, Greiding L, Ramon F, Heithoff K. Loratadine versus cetirizine: assessment of somnolence and motivation during the workday. Clin Ther 2000;22(5):573–82.

59. Druce HM, Thoden WR, Mure P, Furey SA, Lockhart EA, Xie T, Galant S, Prenner BM, Weinstein S, Ziering R, Brandon ML. Brompheniramine, loratadine, and placebo in allergic rhinitis: a placebo-controlled comparative clinical trial. J Clin Pharmacol 1998;38(4):382–9.

60. Davies RJ. Efficacy and tolerability comparison of ebastine 10 and 20 mg with loratadine 10 mg. A double-blind, randomised study in patients with perennial allergic rhinitis. Clin Drug Invest 1998;16:413–20.

61. Singh AK, Chattiverdi VN. Prochlorperazine versus cinnarizine in cases of vertigo. Indian J Otolaryngol Head Neck Surg 1998;50:392–7.

62. Simons FE, Fraser TG, Maher J, Pillay N, Simons KJ. Central nervous system effects of H1-receptor antagonists in the elderly. Ann Allergy Asthma Immunol 1999;82(2):157–60.

63. Feldman W, Shanon A, Leiken L, Ham-pong A, Peterson R. Central nervous system side-effects of antihistamines in schoolchildren. Rhinol Suppl 1992;13:13–19.

64. Nicholson AN, Stone BM. Performance studies with the H1-histamine receptor antagonists, astemizole and terfenadine. Br J Clin Pharmacol 1982;13(2):199–202.

65. Ramaekers JG, Uiterwijk MM, O'Hanlon JF. Effects of loratadine and cetirizine on actual driving and psychometric test performance, and EEG during driving. Eur J Clin Pharmacol 1992;42(4):363–9.

66. Gengo FM, Gabos C, Mechtler L. Quantitative effects of cetirizine and diphenhydramine on mental performance measured using an automobile driving simulator. Ann Allergy 1990;64(6):520–6.

67. Seidel WF, Cohen S, Bliwise NG, Dement WC. Cetirizine effects on objective measures of daytime sleepiness and performance. Ann Allergy 1987;59(6 Pt 2):58–62.

68. Bradley CM, Nicholson AN. Studies on the central effects of the H1-antagonist, loratadine. Eur J Clin Pharmacol 1987;32(4):419–21.

69. Roth T, Roehrs T, Koshorek G, Sicklesteel J, Zorick F. Sedative effects of antihistamines. J Allergy Clin Immunol 1987;80(1):94–8.

70. Kay GG, Berman B, Mockoviak SH, Morris CE, Reeves D, Starbuck V, Sukenik E, Harris AG. Initial and steady-state effects of diphenhydramine and loratadine on sedation, cognition, mood, and psychomotor performance. Arch Intern Med 1997;157(20):2350–6.

71. Reyes-Jacang A, Wenzl JE. Antihistamine toxicity in children. Clin Pediatr (Phila) 1969;8(5):297–9.

72. Chan-Tack KM. Neuroleptic malignant syndrome due to promethazine. South Med J 1999;92(10):1017–18.

73. Negrotti A, Calzetti S. Cinnarizine-induced parkinsonism: ten years later. Mov Disord 1999;14(3):534–5.

74. Marti-Masso JF, Poza JJ. Reply. Mov Disord 1999;14:534–5.

75. Stucchi-Portocarrero S, Vega-Dienstmaier JM, Saavedra JE, Sagastegui A. Acatisia, parkinsonismo y depresion inducidos por cinaricina: descripcion de un caso. [Akathisia, parkinsonism and depression induced by cinnarizine: a case report.] Rev Neurol 1999;28(9):876–8.

76. Lee FS, Matthews LJ, Mills JH, Dubno JR, Adkins WY. Gender-specific effects of medicinal drugs on hearing levels of older persons. Otolaryngol Head Neck Surg 1998;118(2):221–7.

77. Shamsi Z, Kimber S, Hindmarch I. An investigation into the effects of cetirizine on cognitive function and psychomotor performance in healthy volunteers. Eur J Clin Pharmacol 2001;56(12):865–71.

78. Bender BG, McCormick DR, Milgrom H. Children's school performance is not impaired by short-term administration of diphenhydramine or loratadine. J Pediatr 2001;138(5):656–60.

79. Tagawa M, Kano M, Okamura N, Higuchi M, Matsuda M, Mizuki Y, Arai H, Fujii T, Komemushi S, Itoh M, Sasaki H, Watanabe T, Yanai K. Differential cognitive effects of ebastine and (+)-chlorpheniramine in healthy subjects: correlation between cognitive impairment and plasma drug concentration. Br J Clin Pharmacol 2002;53(3):296–304.

80. Verster JC, Volkerts ER, van Oosterwijck AW, Aarab M, Bijtjes SI, De Weert AM, Eijken EJ, Verbaten MN. Acute and subchronic effects of levocetirizine and diphenhydramine on memory functioning, psychomotor performance, and mood. J Allergy Clin Immunol 2003;111(3):623–7.

81. Gandon JM, Allain H. Lack of effect of single and repeated doses of levocetirizine, a new antihistamine drug, on cognitive and psychomotor functions in healthy volunteers. Br J Clin Pharmacol 2002;54(1):51–8.

82. Hindmarch I, Johnson S, Meadows R, Kirkpatrick T, Shamsi Z. The acute and sub-chronic effects of levocetirizine, cetirizine, loratadine, promethazine and placebo on cognitive function, psychomotor performance, and weal and flare. Curr Med Res Opin 2001;17(4):241–55.

83. Richards DM, Brogden RN, Heel RC, Speight TM, Avery GS. Astemizole. A review of its pharmacodynamic properties and therapeutic efficacy. Drugs 1984;28(1):38–61.

84. Lal A. Effect of a few histamine1-antagonists on blood glucose in patients of allergic rhinitis. Indian J Otolaryngol Head Neck Surg 2000;52:193–5.

85. Lanng Nielsen J, Dahl R, Kissmeyer-Nielsen F. Immune thrombocytopenia due to antazoline (Antistina). Allergy 1981;36(7):517–19.

86. Committee on Safety of Medicines. Mebhydrolin (Fabahistin) and white cell depression. Curr Probl Dec 1981;7:1.

87. Kanoh T, Jingami H, Uchino H. Aplastic anaemia after prolonged treatment with chlorpheniramine. Lancet 1977;1(8010):546–7.

88. Feinberg SM, Malkil S, Feinberg AK. The Antihistamines. Chicago, Ill: Yearbook Medical Publishers Inc, 1950.

89. De Parades V, Roulot D, Neyrolles N, Rautureau J, Coste T. Hépatite cytolotique au cours de l'administration d'oxatomide. [Acute cytolytic hepatitis during administration of oxatomide.] Gastroenterol Clin Biol 1994;18(3):294.

90. Yaffe J, Bierman W, Cann M, et al. Antihistamines in topical preparations. Pediatrics 1973;51(2):299–301.

91. Epstein E. Contact dermatitis in children. Pediatr Clin North Am 1971;18(3):839–52.

92. Bigby M, Stern RS, Arndt KA. Allergic cutaneous reactions to drugs. Prim Care 1989;16(3):713–27.

93. Schauder S. Dioxopromethazine-induced photoallergic contact dermatitis followed by persistent light reaction. Am J Contact Dermat 1998;9(3):182–7.

94. Crowson AN, Magro CM. Lichenoid and subacute cutaneous lupus erythematosus-like dermatitis associated with antihistamine therapy. J Cutan Pathol 1999;26(2):95–9.

95. Toll A, Campo-Pisa P, Gonzalez-Castro J, Campo-Voegeli A, Azon A, Iranzo P, Lecha M, Herrero C. Subacute cutaneous lupus erythematosus associated with cinnarizine and thiethylperazine therapy. Lupus 1998;7(5):364–6.

96. Meltzer EO, Storms WW, Pierson WE, Cummins LH, Orgel HA, Perhach JL, Hemsworth GR. Efficacy of azelastine in perennial allergic rhinitis: clinical and rhinomanometric evaluation. J Allergy Clin Immunol 1988;82(3 Pt 1):447–55.

97. Saxen I. Cleft palate and maternal diphenhydramine intake. Lancet 1974;1(7854):407–8.

98. McBride WG. An aetiological study of drug ingestion by women who gave birth to babies with cleft palate. Aust NZ J Obstet Gynaecol 1969;9(2):103–4.

99. Sadusk JF Jr, Palmisano PA. Teratogenic effect of meclizine, cyclizine, and chlorcyclizine. JAMA 1965;194(9):987–9.

100. Henderson IWD. Congenital deformities associated with Bendectin. Can Med Assoc J 1977;117(7):721–2.

101. Bishai R, Mazzotta P, Atanackovic G, Levichek Z, Pole M, Magee LA, Koren G. Critical appraisal of drug therapy for nausea and vomiting of pregnancy: II. Efficacy and safety of diclectin (doxylamine-B6). Can J Clin Pharmacol 2000;7(3):138–43.

102. Mazzotta P, Magee LA. A risk-benefit assessment of pharmacological and nonpharmacological treatments for nausea and vomiting of pregnancy. Drugs 2000;59(4):781–800.

103. Seto A, Einarson T, Koren G. Pregnancy outcome following first trimester exposure to antihistamines: meta-analysis. Am J Perinatol 1997;14(3):119–24.

104. Mazzotta P, Loebstein R, Koren G. Treating allergic rhinitis in pregnancy. Safety considerations. Drug Saf 1999;20(4):361–75.

105. Einarson A, Bailey B, Jung G, Spizzirri D, Baillie M, Koren G. Prospective controlled study of hydroxyzine and cetirizine in pregnancy. Ann Allergy Asthma Immunol 1997;78(2):183–6.

106. Mazzotta P, Koren G. Nonsedating antihistamines in pregnancy. Can Fam Physician 1997;43:1509–11.

107. Czeizel AE, Szegal BA, Joffe JM, Racz J. The effect of diazepam and promethazine treatment during pregnancy on the somatic development of human offspring. Neurotoxicol Teratol 1999;21(2):157–67.

108. Loebstein R, Lalkin A, Addis A, Costa A, Lalkin I, Bonati M, Koren G. Pregnancy outcome after gestational exposure to terfenadine: a multicenter, prospective controlled study. J Allergy Clin Immunol 1999;104(5):953–6.

109. Mitchell JL. Use of cough and cold preparations during breastfeeding. J Hum Lact 1999;15(4):347–9.

110. Wogoman H, Steinberg M, Jenkins AJ. Acute intoxication with guaifenesin, diphenhydramine, and chlorpheniramine. Am J Forensic Med Pathol 1999;20(2):199–202.

111. Renwick AG. The metabolism of antihistamines and drug interactions: the role of cytochrome P450 enzymes. Clin Exp Allergy 1999;29(Suppl 3):116–24.

112. Rau SE, Bend JR, Arnold MO, Tran LT, Spence JD, Bailey DG. Grapefruit juice–terfenadine single-dose interaction: magnitude, mechanism, and relevance. Clin Pharmacol Ther 1997;61(4):401–9.

113. Barecki ME, Casciano CN, Johnson WW, Clement RP. In vitro characterization of the inhibition profile of loratadine, desloratadine, and 3-OH-desloratadine for five human cytochrome P-450 enzymes. Drug Metab Dispos 2001;29(9):1173–5.

114. Bhatti JZ, Hindmarch I. The effects of terfenadine with and without alcohol on an aspect of car driving performance. Clin Exp Allergy 1989;19(6):609–11.

115. Moser L, Huther KJ, Koch-Weser J, Lundt PV. Effects of terfenadine and diphenhydramine alone or in combination with diazepam or alcohol on psychomotor performance and subjective feelings. Eur J Clin Pharmacol 1978;14(6):417–23.

116. Rombaut N, Heykants J, Vanden Bussche G. Potential of interaction between the H1-antagonist astemizole and other drugs. Ann Allergy 1986;57(5):321–4.

117. Doms M, Vanhulle G, Baelde Y, Coulie P, Dupont P, Rihoux JP. Lack of potentiation by cetirizine of alcohol-induced psychomotor disturbances. Eur J Clin Pharmacol 1988;34(6):619–23.

118. Falliers CJ, Redding MA. Controlled comparison of a new antihistamine–decongestant combination to its individual components. Ann Allergy 1980;45(2):75–80.

119. Tarasido JC. Azatadine maleate/pseudoephedrine sulfate repetabs versus placebo in the treatment of severe seasonal allergic rhinitis. J Int Med Res 1980;8(6):391–4.

120. Newlands WJ. The effect of pemoline on antihistamine-induced drowsiness. Practitioner 1980;224(1349):1199–201.

121. Paya B, Guisado JA, Vaz FJ, Crespo-Facorro B. Visual hallucinations induced by the combination of prolintane and diphenhydramine. Pharmacopsychiatry 2002;35(1):24–5.

122. Treuren BC, Galletly DC, Robinson BJ, Short TG, Ure RW. The influence of the H1 and H2 receptor antagonists, terfenadine and ranitidine on the hypotensive and gastric pH effects of the histamine releasing drugs, morphine and tubocurarine. Anaesthesia 1993;48(9):758–62.

Antimony and antimonials

General Information

Antimony is a brittle, bluish-white, metallic element (symbol Sb; atomic no 51). The symbol Sb comes from the Latin word stibium.

Antimony is found in such minerals as dyscrasite, jamesonite, kermesite, pyrargyrite, stephanite, tetrahedrite, and zinkenite.

The Arabic word for antimony stibnite or antimony trisulfate was kohl, from which the word alcohol ultimately derives (1). Antimonious ores were sometimes confused with lead ores, and alquifou was the name of a Cornish lead ore that looked like antimony and was used by potters to give a green glaze to earthenware. The word that the Quechua Indians of Peru use for antimony is surúcht, which gives soroche, a synonym for mountain sickness, which antimony was thought to cause.

Antimony salts have in the past found many uses in medicine, and antimony compounds, especially pentavalent ones, are still used to treat *Schistosoma japonicum* infestation and leishmaniasis (2). Antimony is also used as an emetic. Attention is being paid to the anticancer potential of antimony compounds (3,4). As with many other metals, occupational and environmental exposure is possible and can act additively with medical exposure.

Common adverse effects of antimony treatment include anorexia, nausea, vomiting, muscle ache, headache, lethargy, and bone and joint pain.

Antimony has been suggested to be a causal factor in sudden infant death syndrome, since fungal transformation of fire retardants containing antimony in cot mattresses will lead to the formation of stibine (SbH_3). However, the involvement of stibine in cot death is most unlikely (5,6).

Salts of antimony

Meglumine antimoniate

Meglumine antimoniate is a pentavalent antimonial chemically similar to sodium stibogluconate and is considered to have similar efficacy and toxicity. Meglutamine antimoniate solution contains pentavalent antimony 8.5% and stibogluconate 10%.

Sodium stibogluconate

Sodium stibogluconate is a pentavalent antimonial that contains pentavalent antimony 10%.

Stibocaptate

Stibocaptate is a trivalent antimony compound, whose toxic effects, especially its acute adverse effects, are similar to those of the pentavalent compounds.

Uses

Antimony salts have in the past found many uses in medicine, and antimony compounds, especially pentavalent ones, are still used to treat *Schistosoma japonicum* infestation and leishmaniasis (2). The standard treatment of most South American cutaneous leishmaniasis is systemic, because of the propensity of the parasites to spread to mucous membranes. The drugs in common use remain parenteral, and are fairly toxic. Sodium stibogluconate, in a dose of 20 mg/kg for 30 days, remains the gold standard, with liposomal amphotericin a possible alternative. Both drugs are also the preferred choice for all strains of visceral leishmaniasis. Stibogluconate achieves a cure in certain cases (7,8) and is reasonably safe, although transient pancreatitis, musculoskeletal pains, and loss of appetite have been reported. Primary unresponsiveness (cure not obtained by the first course of treatment) is being increasingly reported (9) and is a particular problem in the Bihar region of North-East India, where a report documented primary unresponsiveness in 33% of cases (10). The new treatment options for visceral leishmaniasis have been reviewed (11).

Antimony is also used as an emetic. Attention is being paid to the anticancer potential of antimony compounds (3,4). As with many other metals, occupational and environmental exposure is possible and can act additively with medical exposure.

Pharmacokinetics

Antimony is excreted in the urine. Peak concentrations are seen at about 1–2 hours after an intramuscular injection of meglumine antimonate. Serum concentrations fall to about 10% of peak concentrations after about 8 hours. There is some accumulation of antimony during continued treatment. On a weight for weight basis children require a higher dose and tolerate antimony better. Toxicity is more likely in patients with impaired renal function, as would be expected for a drug that is mainly excreted in the urine.

Observational studies

The characteristics of 111 consecutive patients with visceral leishmaniasis in Sicily have been described (12). They were given intramuscular meglumine antimoniate (560 mg/m^2 of pentavalent antimony), generally for 21 days. There were adverse effects in 16 patients, including rash ($n = 3$) and dry cough ($n = 13$). All the adverse effects bar one (a severe urticarial rash) were transient and self-limiting and did not require drug withdrawal.

Comparative studies

In a prospective, open trial, conventional treatment with sodium stibogluconate ($n = 69$) was compared with meglumine antimoniate ($n = 58$) for cutaneous *Leishmania braziliensis* (13). The trial was too small and of too short a duration to compare efficacy reliably, but

significantly fewer patients on meglumine antimoniate developed the myalgia/arthralgia, headache, and abdominal pain that are the most common adverse effects of the drug, and that tend to increase as treatment continues. About 30% developed significant adverse effects early in treatment and 70% late when stibogluconate was used, whereas 12% had early and 45% late adverse effects for antimoniate. Unfortunately, QT intervals were not monitored; a fatal dysrhythmia, usually preceded by increased QT dispersion, is the complication of sodium stibogluconate therapy most likely to lead to death.

There has been a further comparison of meglumine antimoniate ($n = 47$) and sodium stibogluconate ($n = 64$) (14). The trial was too small to examine the efficacy of the two drugs, but there were more adverse events with sodium stibogluconate, with a greater proportion with raised transaminase and amylase activities. There were no differences in electrocardiographic abnormalities between the two groups.

Allopurinol

Allopurinol and meglumine antimoniate (Glucantime™) have been evaluated in a randomized, controlled trial in 150 patients with cutaneous leishmaniasis (15). They received oral allopurinol (15 mg/kg/day) for 3 weeks, or intramuscular meglumine antimoniate (30 mg/kg/day, corresponding to 8 mg/kg/day of pentavalent antimony, for 2 weeks), or combined therapy. There were a few adverse effects in those who used allopurinol: nausea, heartburn ($n = 3$), and mild increases in transaminases ($n = 2$). These symptoms subsided on drug withdrawal.

In an open study, 72 patients each received meglumine antimoniate (60 mg/kg/day) or allopurinol (20 mg/kg/day) plus low-dose meglumine antimoniate (30 mg/kg/day) for 20 days, and each was followed for 30 days after the end of treatment (16). Only six patients in the combined treatment group complained of mild abdominal pain and nausea; however, one patient who received meglumine antimoniate developed a skin eruption. Generalized muscle pain and weakness occurred in four patients.

Paromomycin

In patients with visceral leishmaniasis, paromomycin (12 or 18 mg/kg/d) plus a standard dose of sodium stibogluconate for 21 days was statistically more effective than sodium stibogluconate alone in producing a final cure (17). In an open, randomized comparison of sodium stibogluconate either alone ($n = 50$) or in combination with two regimens of paromomycin ($n = 52$ and $n = 48$), there was improved parasitological cure in both groups given combination therapy (18). There were no differences in adverse events or biochemical and hematological measurements between any of the treatment arms. There was one serious adverse event (myocarditis) in the sodium stibogluconate monotherapy group. It should be noted that there were insufficient auditory examinations performed to assess any ototoxic effects of paromomycin.

Placebo-controlled studies

A randomized, double-blind, placebo-controlled study of sodium stibogluconate for 10 and 20 days has been conducted in 38 US military personnel with cutaneous leishmaniasis; 19 received sodium stibogluconate for 10 days (and placebo for 10 days), and 19 received sodium stibogluconate for 20 days (19). Treatment withdrawal was necessary as a result of pancreatitis in seven patients (four in the 10-day treatment group and three in the 20-day group), and this occurred during the first 10 days of therapy in all seven patients. Myalgia occurred in 8 patients in the 10-day group and in 13 patients in the 20-day group. Patients in the 20-day group had myalgia on significantly more days than those in the 10-day group. Increases in amylase, lipase, and transaminases and falls in white blood cell count, hematocrit, and platelet count also differed significantly between the two groups.

General adverse effects

Common adverse effects of antimony treatment include anorexia, nausea, vomiting, muscle ache, headache, lethargy, and bone and joint pain.

Common adverse effects of meglumine antimonate are anorexia, nausea, vomiting, malaise, myalgia, headache, and lethargy. Muscle, bone, and joint pains have been described (SEDA-12, 710) (SEDA-13, 838) (20). Cardiac toxicity and electrocardiographic changes are dose-related. The general condition of the patient with visceral leishmaniasis probably plays a crucial role in these and other adverse effects. Malnutrition is common, the immune status often severely impaired, and patients are susceptible to intercurrent infections (SEDA-12, 710).

In 96 patients with visceral, mucosal, or viscerotropic leishmaniasis, who were given sodium stibogluconate 20 mg/kg/day for 20–28 days, adverse effects were common and necessitated withdrawal of treatment in 28% of cases. They included arthralgias and myalgias (58%), pancreatitis (97%), increased transaminases (67%), headache (22%), bone marrow suppression (44%), and rash (9%) (8). Arthralgias are more likely to represent reactions to the tissue of the dead or dying parasite than true allergies to the drug.

In 53 patients with dermal leishmaniasis after kala-azar, who were given sodium stibogluconate 20 mg/kg/day intramuscularly, adverse effects were changes in electrocardiographic ST segments and T waves (7%), arthralgias (11%), allergic rashes (7%), swelling at the site of injection (5%), neuralgia (4%), and a metallic taste (6%) (21).

Organs and Systems

Cardiovascular

Electrocardiographic changes are common in patients taking antimony salts; in one group there was an incidence of 7%. The most common changes are ST segment changes, T wave inversion, and a prolonged QT interval. The role of conduction disturbances in cases of cardiac failure and sudden death is not known. Cases of sudden death have been seen early in treatment after a second injection (SEDA-13, 838) (SEDA-16, 311).

Changes in the electrocardiogram depend on the cumulative dose of antimony, and sudden death can occur rarely (22).

- A 4-year-old boy with visceral leishmaniasis was given intravenous sodium stibogluconate 20 mg/kg/day

(1200 mg/day) and oral allopurinol 16 mg/kg/day (100 mg tds). On day 3 he reported chest pain and a persistent cough. Electrocardiography was unremarkable. The drugs were withdrawn and 3 days later he developed a petechial rash on the legs. Sepsis and other causes of petechial rashes were ruled out. Three days after treatment was discontinued he developed ventricular fibrillation and died.

The authors suggested that patients taking antimony compounds should be observed cautiously for signs of cardiological and hematological changes.

Myocarditis with electrocardiographic changes has been well described, but the risk of dysrhythmias is usually small. There have been reports of severe cardiotoxicity, leading in some cases to death (23,24). This may largely be due to changes in physicochemical properties of the drug; one cluster of cases was associated with a high-osmolarity lot of sodium stibogluconate (23).

Because of concerns regarding the cardiac adverse effects of antimonials, it is good practice to admit patients for the duration of therapy whenever practicable. This may mean admitting otherwise fit young patients for several weeks for treatment of a non-healing ulcer. To address the safety of outpatient management, a recent small study of 13 marines in the UK showed that they could be safely managed as outpatients with daily stibogluconate injections, provided there was close monitoring of electrocardiograms and blood tests to provide early warning of bone marrow toxicity (25). Three patients developed minor electrocardiographic changes and one developed thrombocytopenia. All these adverse effects resolved when treatment was withdrawn. Patients with a predisposition to dysrhythmias (such as some with ischemic heart disease) are best treated with pentavalent antimonials as inpatients to identify and manage adverse effects early when resources allow.

The cardiac toxicity of antimony has been explored in cultured myocytes (26,27). Potassium antimony tartrate disrupted calcium handling, leading to a progressive increase in the resting or diastolic internal calcium concentration and eventual cessation of beating activity and cell death. An interaction with thiol homeostasis is also involved. Reduced cellular ATP concentrations paralleled toxicity but appeared to be secondary to other cellular changes initiated by exposure to antimony.

Even the normal dose of sodium stibogluconate can lead to both cardiotoxicity and hemotoxicity, because of its cumulative effects.

- Fatal accumulation of sodium stibogluconate occurred in a 4-year-old boy with visceral leishmaniasis treated with intravenous sodium stibogluconate 20 mg/kg (1200 mg/day) and oral allopurinol 16 mg/kg/day (100 mg tds) (22). On day 3 he reported chest pain and persistent cough, and the drugs were withdrawn. Three days later he developed a petechial rash on the legs and died with ventricular fibrillation.

Respiratory

Antimonate ore caused chronic bronchitis in 16 of 100 miners exposed (28). The chronic bronchitis was characterized by a mild slow course with ventilation disturbances. There were no cases of pneumoconiosis.

Nervous system

Headaches are common during treatment with antimony. Generalized neuralgia was reported in one study, with an incidence of 4% (SEDA-13, 838) (SEDA-16, 311).

Peripheral sensory neuropathy has been described after the use of sodium stibogluconate for cutaneous leishmaniasis (SEDA-21, 300).

Sensory systems

A metallic taste due to antimonials is uncommon but probably under-reported (SEDA-16, 311).

Hematologic

Autoimmune hemolytic anemia has been described with meglumine antimoniate (29).

Thrombocytopenia has been reported in a patient with *Leishmania donovani* infection and AIDS after stibogluconate therapy for 7 days (SEDA-13, 838). There have been two further reports, one involving a patient with cutaneous leishmaniasis (occurring after 19 days of treatment), the second a man with kala-azar (who became thombocytopenic 11 days after starting therapy); in kala-azar a low platelet count is common and the count normally rises with treatment (SEDA-18, 294).

Gastrointestinal

Anorexia, nausea, and vomiting are common with antimonials (30).

Liver

Hepatotoxicity has been described, but the disease itself may play an overriding role. In 16 patients with mucosal leishmaniasis treated with meglumine antimoniate 20 mg/kg intravenously for 28 days, there were raised liver enzyme in conjunction with electrocardiographic abnormalities and/or musculoskeletal complaints in three subjects (SEDA-16, 311).

Pancreas

Pancreatitis has occasionally been reported with antimonials. In 1993, four cases were described in three reports; two of the patients were immunocompromised. One was asymptomatic, while the other three complained of abdominal pain. Rechallenge with half of the standard dose was carried out in one case and resulted in a renewed increase of serum amylase activity.

Acute pancreatitis developed during treatment with meglumine antimoniate for visceral leishmaniasis in a young boy (31).

- A 2-year-old boy with a history of intermittent high-grade fever, sweating, and abdominal distension developed visceral leishmaniasis. He was given meglumine antimoniate (Glucantime®, Rhone Poulenc, France) 5 mg/kg/day, and the dose was doubled every other day to reach 20 mg/kg/day. Two days after he had reached the full dose, his temperature returned to normal, his general condition improved, and his liver and spleen began to shrink. However, the serum amylase increased to 254 U/l. Because he was asymptomatic, treatment with meglumine antimoniate was continued. However, on day 10 he complained of vomiting and abdominal pain with rebound tenderness. Acute pancreatitis was confirmed by serum amylase and lipase values up to 1557 and 320 U/l respectively and by ultrasound findings of dilatation and edema of the pancreatic ducts. Meglumine antimoniate was withdrawn and the pancreatitis was managed conservatively. Two days later his fever increased and the spleen and liver began to enlarge. He was given allopurinol (20 mg/kg/day) and ketoconazole (5 mg/kg/day) and became afebrile; the spleen and liver began to shrink, his pancytopenia improved, and the albumin:globulin ratio and serum amylase and lipase activities returned to normal. The acute pancreatitis resolved uneventfully.

The mechanism and frequency of this adverse effect are unknown. It has been suggested that immunocompromised patients may be at a higher risk (SEDA-18, 294), but pancreatitis is in any case seen more often in patients with AIDS, irrespective of drug treatment.

Urinary tract

- Septic shock with oliguria developed soon after the first intramuscular administration of meglumine antimoniate 20 mg/kg (equivalent to 510 mg of antimony) to a patient with visceral leishmaniasis and normal renal function (32). Creatinine clearance fell to 23 ml/min. Treatment was withdrawn, and antimony urinary excretion was measured. After the initial dose, 500 mg of antimony was recovered in the urine over 8 days (98% of the dose); 66% was eliminated within the first 48 hours. Nine days after the dose, meglumine antimoniate was reintroduced in a dosage of 11.7 mg/kg (equivalent to 300 mg of antimony) every 48 hours, with good tolerance. At that time creatinine clearance had returned to 88 ml/min. By day 14 of therapy the dosage interval was reduced to 24 hours and from day 17 to day 31 the dosage was increased to 16.6 mg/kg/day (equivalent to 425 mg of antimony). The patient eventually completely recovered, with normal renal function. Although there are no specific guidelines for dosage adjustment in renal insufficiency, monitoring antimony urinary excretion indicates that the kidneys are the almost exclusive route of elimination.

Musculoskeletal

Arthralgia is a common complaint during treatment with pentavalent antimonials and is usually dose-related (30). Muscle pain and bone pain have also been described.

- A palindromic arthropathy with effusion and pancreatitis occurred in association with stibogluconate treatment for kala-azar in a 30-year-old man on hemodialysis for chronic renal insufficiency (SEDA-16, 311).

Immunologic

As an industrial and environmental toxin, antimony trioxide can cause disturbances of immune homeostasis.

Workers in antimony trioxide manufacture had reduced serum concentrations of cytokines (interleukin 2, gamma interferon) and immunoglobulin (IgG1, IgE) (33).

Death

Antimony has been suggested to be a causal factor in sudden infant death syndrome, since fungal transformation of fire retardants containing antimony in cot mattresses will lead to the formation of stibine (SbH_3). However, the involvement of stibine in cot death is most unlikely (5,6).

Sudden death has been reported during the use of stibocaptate (SEDA-11, 599) (34).

Long-Term Effects

Drug tolerance

The treatment of cutaneous leishmaniasis has been reviewed, including the use of pentavalent antimonials (35). Antimony-resistant strains continue to emerge (36), leading to the use of higher dosages of antimonials or combinations of antimonials with other compounds, such as paromomycin or gamma interferon (37).

Drug–Drug Interactions

Amiodarone

A pharmacodynamic interaction has been described between amiodarone and meglumine antimoniate, both of which prolong the QT interval; the interaction resulted in torsade de pointes (38).

- A 73-year-old man with visceral leishmaniasis was given meglumine antimoniate intramuscularly 75 mg/kg/day. At that time his QT_c interval was normal at 0.42 seconds. Three weeks later his QT_c interval was prolonged to 0.64 seconds and he was given metildigoxin 0.4 mg and amiodarone 450 mg intravenously over 8.25 hours; 12 hours later he had a cardiac arrest with torsade de pointes, which was cardioverted by two direct shocks of 300 J and lidocaine 100 mg in two bolus injections. Because he had frequent episodes of paroxysmal atrial fibrillation, he was given amiodarone 100 mg over the next 40 hours, and developed recurrent self-limiting episodes of torsade de pointes associated with QT_c interval prolongation, which responded to intravenous magnesium 1500 mg. After withdrawal of amiodarone there was no recurrence and a week later the QT_c interval was 0.48 seconds. The plasma potassium concentration was not abnormal in this case.

In view of this report it is probably wise to avoid co-administration of antimonials and amiodarone.

Amphotericin

Amphotericin can worsen stibogluconate-induced cardiotoxicity; a gap of at least 10 days between sodium stibogluconate and amphotericin is recommended (24).

References

1. Aronson JK. Here's mud in your eye. BMJ 1996;312:373.
2. Croft SL, Yardley V. Chemotherapy of leishmaniasis. Curr Pharm Des 2002;8(4):319–42.
3. Yi T, Pathak MK, Lindner DJ, Ketterer ME, Farver C, Borden EC. Anticancer activity of sodium stibogluconate in synergy with IFNs. J Immunol 2002;169(10):5978–85.
4. Tiekink ER. Antimony and bismuth compounds in oncology. Crit Rev Oncol Hematol 2002;42(3):217–24.
5. Gates PN, Pridham JB, Webber JA. Sudden infant death syndrome and volatile antimony compounds. Lancet 1995;345(8946):386–7.
6. De Wolff FA. Antimony and health. BMJ 1995;310(6989):1216–17.
7. Karki P, Koirala S, Parija SC, Hansdak SG, Das ML. A thirty day course of sodium stibogluconate for treatment of kala-azar in Nepal. Southeast Asian J Trop Med Public Health 1998;29(1):154–8.
8. Aronson NE, Wortmann GW, Johnson SC, Jackson JE, Gasser RA Jr, Magill AJ, Endy TP, Coyne PE, Grogl M, Benson PM, Beard JS, Tally JD, Gambel JM, Kreutzer RD, Oster CN. Safety and efficacy of intravenous sodium stibogluconate in the treatment of leishmaniasis: recent U.S. military experience. Clin Infect Dis 1998;27(6):1457–64.
9. Khalil EA, el Hassan AM, Zijlstra EE, Hashim FA, Ibrahim ME, Ghalib HW, Ali MS. Treatment of visceral leishmaniasis with sodium stibogluconate in Sudan: management of those who do not respond. Ann Trop Med Parasitol 1998;92(2):151–8.
10. Thakur CP, Sinha GP, Pandey AK, Kumar N, Kumar P, Hassan SM, Narain S, Roy RK. Do the diminishing efficacy and increasing toxicity of sodium stibogluconate in the treatment of visceral leishmaniasis in Bihar, India, justify its continued use as a first-line drug? An observational study of 80 cases. Ann Trop Med Parasitol 1998;92(5):561–9.
11. Murray HW. Treatment of visceral leishmaniasis (kala-azar): a decade of progress and future approaches. Int J Infect Dis 2000;4(3):158–77.
12. Cascio A, Colomba C, Antinori S, Orobello M, Paterson D, Titone L. Pediatric visceral leishmaniasis in Western Sicily, Italy: a retrospective analysis of 111 cases. Eur J Clin Microbiol Infect Dis 2002;21(4):277–82.
13. Saldanha AC, Romero GA, Merchan-Hamann E, Magalhaes AV, Macedo V de O. Estudo comparativo entre estibogluconato de sodio BP 88R e antimoniato de meglumina no tratamento da leishmaniose cutanea: I. Eficacia e seguranca. [A comparative study between sodium stibogluconate BP 88R and meglumine antimoniate in the treatment of cutaneous leishmaniasis. I. The efficacy and safety.] Rev Soc Bras Med Trop 1999;32(4):383–7.
14. Saldanha AC, Romero GA, Guerra C, Merchan-Hamann E, Macedo V de O. Estudo comparativo entre estibogluconato de sodio BP 88 e antimoniato de meglumina no tratamento da leishmaniose cutanea. II. Toxicidade bioquimica e cardiaca. [Comparative study between sodium stibogluconate BP 88 and meglumine antimoniate in cutaneous leishmaniasis treatment. II. Biochemical and cardiac toxicity.] Rev Soc Bras Med Trop 2000; 33(4):383–8.
15. Esfandiarpour I, Alavi A. Evaluating the efficacy of allopurinol and meglumine antimoniate (Glucantime) in the treatment of cutaneous leishmaniasis. Int J Dermatol 2002;41(8):521–4.
16. Momeni AZ, Reiszadae MR, Aminjavaheri M. Treatment of cutaneous leishmaniasis with a combination of allopurinol and low-dose meglumine antimoniate. Int J Dermatol 2002;41(7):441–3.

17. Krause PJ, Lepore T, Sikand VK, Gadbaw J Jr, Burke G, Telford SR 3rd, Brassard P, Pearl D, Azlanzadeh J, Christianson D, McGrath D, Spielman A. Atovaquone and azithromycin for the treatment of babesiosis. N Engl J Med 2000;343(20):1454–8.

18. Thakur CP, Kanyok TP, Pandey AK, Sinha GP, Zaniewski AE, Houlihan HH, Olliaro P. A prospective randomized, comparative, open-label trial of the safety and efficacy of paromomycin (aminosidine) plus sodium stibogluconate versus sodium stibogluconate alone for the treatment of visceral leishmaniasis. Trans R Soc Trop Med Hyg 2000;94(4):429–31.

19. Wortmann G, Miller RS, Oster C, Jackson J, Aronson N. A randomized, double-blind study of the efficacy of a 10- or 20-day course of sodium stibogluconate for treatment of cutaneous leishmaniasis in United States military personnel. Clin Infect Dis 2002;35(3):261–7.

20. Castro C, Sampaio RN, Marsden PD. Severe arthralgia, not related to dose, associated with pentavalent antimonial therapy for mucosal leishmaniasis. Trans R Soc Trop Med Hyg 1990;84(3):362.

21. Thakur CP, Kumar K. Efficacy of prolonged therapy with stibogluconate in post kala-azar dermal leishmaniasis. Indian J Med Res 1990;91:144–8.

22. Cesur S, Bahar K, Erekul S. Death from cumulative sodium stibogluconate toxicity on kala-azar. Clin Microbiol Infect 2002;8(9):606.

23. Sundar S, Sinha PR, Agrawal NK, Srivastava R, Rainey PM, Berman JD, Murray HW, Singh VP. A cluster of cases of severe cardiotoxicity among kala-azar patients treated with a high-osmolarity lot of sodium antimony gluconate. Am J Trop Med Hyg 1998; 59(1):139–43.

24. Thakur CP. Sodium antimony gluconate, amphotericin, and myocardial damage. Lancet 1998;351(9120):1928–9.

25. Seaton RA, Morrison J, Man I, Watson J, Nathwani D. Outpatient parenteral antimicrobial therapy—a viable option for the management of cutaneous leishmaniasis. QJM 1999;92(11):659–67.

26. Wey HE, Richards D, Tirmenstein MA, Mathias PI, Toraason M. The role of intracellular calcium in antimony-induced toxicity in cultured cardiac myocytes. Toxicol Appl Pharmacol 1997;145(1):202–10.

27. Tirmenstein MA, Mathias PI, Snawder JE, Wey HE, Toraason M. Antimony-induced alterations in thiol homeostasis and adenine nucleotide status in cultured cardiac myocytes. Toxicology 1997;119(3):203–11.

28. Lobanova EA, Ivanova LA, Pavlova TA, Prosina II. Kliniko-patogeneticheskie osobennosti pri vozdeistvii anti-monitovykh rud na organizm rabotaiushchikh. [Clinical and pathogenetic features of exposure of workers to antimonate ore.] Med Tr Prom Ekol 1996;(4):12–15.

29. De Pablos Gallego JM, Cabrera Torres A, Almagro M, De Puerta S, Lopez Garrido P, Gomez Morales M, Esquivias JJ. Kala-azar y anemia hemolitica autoimmune; a propósito de un caso de evolución fatal por hepatotoxicidad del antimonato de N-metilglucamina. [Kala-azar and autoimmune hemolytic anemia. Apropos of a fatally developing case caused by hepatotoxicity from N-methylglucamine antimonate.] Rev Clin Esp 1982; 164(6):417–20.

30. Arfaa F, Tohidi E, Ardelan A. Treatment of urinary bilharziasis in a small focus with sodium antimony dimer-captosuccinate (astiban). Am J Trop Med Hyg 1967;16(3):300–29.

31. Kuyucu N, Kara C, Bakirtac A, Tezic T. Successful treatment of visceral leishmaniasis with allopurinol plus ketoconazole in an infant who developed pancreatitis caused by meglumine antimoniate. Pediatr Infect Dis J 2001;20(4):455–7.

32. Hantson P, Luyasu S, Haufroid V, Lambert M. Antimony excretion in a patient with renal impairment during meglumine antimoniate therapy. Pharmacotherapy 2000; 20(9):1141–3.

33. Kim HA, Heo Y, Oh SY, Lee KJ, Lawrence DA. Altered serum cytokine and immunoglobulin levels in the workers exposed to antimony. Hum Exp Toxicol 1999;18(10):607–13.

34. Rees PH, Kager PA, Ogada T, Eeftinck Schattenkerk JK. The treatment of kala-azar: a review with comments drawn from experience in Kenya. Trop Geogr Med 1985;37(1):37–46.

35. Moskowitz PF, Kurban AK. Treatment of cutaneous leishmaniasis: retrospectives and advances for the 21st century. Clin Dermatol 1999;17(3):305–15.

36. Lira R, Sundar S, Makharia A, Kenney R, Gam A, Saraiva E, Sacks D. Evidence that the high incidence of treatment failures in Indian kala-azar is due to the emergence of antimony-resistant strains of *Leishmania donovani*. J Infect Dis 1999;180(2):564–7.

37. Aggarwal P, Handa R, Singh S, Wali JP. Kala-azar—new developments in diagnosis and treatment. Indian J Pediatr 1999;66(1):63–71.

38. Segura I, Garcia-Bolao I. Meglumine antimoniate, amiodarone and torsades de pointes: a case report. Resuscitation 1999;42(1):65–8.

Antituberculosis drugs

See also Individual agents

General Information

Antituberculosis drugs are classified as first-line and second-line.

First-line drugs

- ethambutol
- isoniazid
- pyrazinamide
- rifampicin
- streptomycin

Second-line drugs

- capreomycin
- clofazimine
- cycloserine
- ethionamide and propionamide
- fluoroquinolones
- kanamycin
- *para*-aminosalicylic acid
- rifabutin
- thiacetazone

As a rule, a regimen of two, three, or four of the five first-line antituberculosis drugs (isoniazid, rifampicin, pyrazinamide, ethambutol, and streptomycin) is used in tuberculosis (1). The 6-month short-course regimen consists of isoniazid, rifampicin, and pyrazinamide for 2 months, followed by isoniazid and rifampicin for 4 months (1). It may be advisable to include ethambutol in the initial phase when isoniazid resistance is suspected or if the prevalence of primary resistance to isoniazid is over 4% in new cases. A 9-month regimen consisting of isoniazid and rifampicin is also highly successful (1). Treatment should always include at least two drugs to which the mycobacteria are susceptible.

Careful monitoring and the addition of pyridoxine to isoniazid have reduced the number of adverse drug effects in tuberculosis. Awareness of potentially severe hepatotoxic reactions is vital, because hepatic failure may be a devastating and often fatal condition. Fulminant hepatic failure caused by rifampicin, isoniazid, or both has been described (2).

Treatment problems that can arise are mainly of two types: adverse reactions (collateral, toxic, or hypersusceptibility reactions), and initial or acquired resistance of *Mycobacterium tuberculosis*, *Mycobacterium bovis*, or non-tuberculous mycobacteria to one or more of the antituberculosis drugs. The latter probably only occurs when the patient has not taken the full combination or the full doses of the drugs all the time. Combination formulations are thus particularly useful. Multidrug-resistant tuberculosis, defined as resistance against at least isoniazid and rifampicin, is the most clinically relevant form of resistance to treatment worldwide.

Observational studies

An increasing number of patients with multidrug-resistant tuberculosis are being treated with second-line drugs worldwide, often in places with poor resources. The number of drugs used is large (4–7) and treatment is prolonged (1–2 years). There is justifiable concern over patients' tolerance of such regimens and their adverse effects, which determine adherence to treatment. Treatment has to be individualized according to the WHO guidelines for a DOTS-plus strategy.

It is therefore encouraging to read a report from Lima, Peru, where 60 patients from a shanty town tolerated a median of eight antituberculosis drugs fairly well for a median duration of 20 months (3). All received a parenteral aminoglycoside daily for 6 months, cycloserine, and a fluoroquinolone, and most also took *para*-aminosalicylic acid and ethionamide. Of 60 patients, 23 took clofazimine, 23 pyrazinamide, 25 isoniazid, and 3 rifampicin. Commonly encountered adverse effects included dermatological effects, including bronzing of the skin (many of these patients were taking clofazimine and fluoroquinolones), depression, anxiety, and peripheral neuropathy. All complained of mild gastritis. There were no cases of serious hepatic or renal toxicity. This may have been because only a few patients took rifampicin. Absence of eighth nerve toxicity was striking, and can be attributed to close monitoring of patients by physicians with experience of DOTS-plus regimens.

In a similar report from Turkey, adverse reactions to drugs led to withdrawal of one or more drugs in 62 of 158 patients (39%) (4). Outcomes were favorable and cultures became negative in 95% of the patients within 2 months.

General adverse reactions

Adverse reactions are often due to the combined effects of two or more drugs used simultaneously (5). Hypersusceptibility reactions can occur even to more than one agent. The incidence of adverse reactions to drugs used in the treatment of tuberculosis is higher in elderly patients, who are more likely to have intercurrent illnesses and a lower lean body mass than younger patients. In two studies from Hong Kong in patients being treated for tuberculosis with rifampicin, the incidence of adverse reactions was higher with regimens containing rifampicin; furthermore, patients taking rifampicin had a higher steady-state plasma concentration of isoniazid (1,6).

Some simple rules about which drugs are more likely to cause which reactions reflect the principle that the most probable causative agent (or agents) must be stopped.

Nervous and sensory systems

Ethambutol is the most likely drug to cause visual disturbances. Isoniazid is associated with polyneuritis and reactions of the central nervous system. Streptomycin can cause eighth nerve toxicity.

Liver

Hepatotoxicity is consistently the most common serious adverse reaction in patients taking antituberculosis drugs. Hepatic necrosis is the most important adverse effect of first-line antituberculosis drug therapy (2). Asymptomatic rises in transaminases are common and are not by themselves justification for withdrawing medication, since they settle spontaneously in most patients while treatment continues. All patients taking antituberculosis drugs should be told to report all new illnesses, especially when associated with vomiting. Hepatitis B carriers were no more likely to react adversely to antituberculosis drugs than non-carriers (7).

If liver damage occurs, isoniazid is probably an important factor and it should be stopped before rifampicin or pyrazinamide (8). Prediction of hepatotoxicity is possible (9). In a case-control study of 60 patients in India, conducted in order to identify features predicting hepatotoxicity, the body mass index was significantly lower (17.2 kg/m^2) in patients who experienced hepatotoxicity than in controls (19.5 kg/m^2) (10).

Urinary tract

In cases of renal insufficiency, streptomycin and ethambutol or second-line antituberculosis drugs with renal toxicity should be immediately withdrawn.

Skin

Adverse reactions to all types of medication are more common in HIV-positive individuals; skin reactions are especially frequent and often severe. Thiacetazone is well recognized as a cause of severe reactions, some of them fatal, but even in combination antituberculosis drug regimens that exclude thiacetazone, the incidence of adverse skin reactions is much higher in HIV-positive than HIV-negative patients: 23% against 1% in one study from Cameroon (11).

Immunologic

In allergic reactions, the drug most probably responsible can be difficult to identify, since the same kind of reaction can occur independently of the chemical nature of the drug. For evaluation of allergic drug reactions, the analysis of time relations (duration of exposure, reaction time, drug-free interval before re-exposure) is extremely important. Particularly in allergic reactions to rifampicin, intermittent treatment or re-exposure after a drug free-interval favors sensitization and occurrence. Depending on the severity of the adverse effects, one, two, or all drugs must be stopped until the adverse reaction has completely disappeared. The use of second-line antituberculosis drugs may sometimes be necessary. In patients with drug fever or common rashes, specific desensitization may be attempted, at least with isoniazid (12). In more severe reactions, with anaphylactic shock, agranulocytosis, thrombocytopenia, toxic epidermal necrolysis, or Stevens–Johnson syndrome, specific desensitization should not be considered and the drug should be discarded from the combination.

Organs and Systems

Liver

Hepatotoxicity is the most important adverse effect of antituberculosis drug therapy. Isoniazid, rifampicin, and pyrazinamide are the main culprits. There is wide variability in the risk of hepatotoxic reactions reported from different parts of the world or in different populations (for example African-American women in the postpartum period) (SEDA-24, 353).

Risks
The risks of hepatotoxicity differ with different antituberculosis drug combinations.

Rifampicin plus isoniazid
There are mild to moderate increases in liver transaminases during treatment with rifampicin plus isoniazid in most patients. However, biochemical hepatitis is diagnosed when transaminase activities increase to more than four times the upper limit of the reference ranges on two occasions at least 1 week apart, or more than five times on any single occasion. This calls for withdrawal of all potentially hepatotoxic drugs (rifampicin, isoniazid, and pyrazinamide) until the enzymes return to the reference ranges. During this period, streptomycin plus ethambutol, with or without cycloserine and a fluoroquinolone, is recommended in seriously ill patients.

Hepatotoxicity is generally considered to be rare among children who receive antituberculosis drugs. However, a report from Japan has suggested that this might not be the case, at least in Asia (13). The authors noted high activities of transaminases, more than five times the upper end of the reference range, in eight of 99 children aged 0–16 years who received various combinations of drugs, including rifampicin and isoniazid; 18 children were excluded because of baseline abnormalities in liver function. Age under 5 years and pyrazinamide in the drug regimen were risk factors for hepatotoxicity. There have been few other reports of the risk of hepatotoxicity in children.

Pyrazinamide plus rifampicin
There is continuing concern about the hepatotoxicity of the combination of pyrazinamide with rifampicin for the treatment of latent pulmonary tuberculosis. Among 148 who were given the combination for 2 months, grade 3 hepatotoxicity (transaminases more than 5–20 times the upper limit of the reference range) and grade 4 hepatotoxicity (transaminases more than 20 times the upper limit of the reference range) were reported in 10 and four patients respectively (14). The risk of hepatotoxicity was associated with female sex (OR = 4.1; 95% CI = 1.2, 14) and presumed recent infection (OR = 14.3; 95% CI = 1.8, 115). The investigators recommended caution in using the combination of pyrazinamide with rifampicin in populations in whom its safety has not been established.

Others consider that this combination is useful for high-risk, traditionally non-adherent patients, such as alcoholics and the homeless, but have also emphasized the need for careful monitoring for toxicity (15). This suggestion is based on the presumption that the combination regimen, although toxic, is more likely to be completed by high-risk patients than 6 months of isoniazid alone. However, others observed similar completion rates for the two regimens in a multicenter study (61% and 57%) (16), and the safety and cost-effectiveness of this combination in the treatment of latent tuberculosis has been questioned (17).

Two cases of severe and fatal hepatitis have been reported to the CDC from New York and Georgia among patients taking rifampicin and pyrazinamide for latent tuberculosis (18). Between February and August 2001, another 21 patients had severe hepatotoxicity following treatment with rifampicin plus pyrazinamide for 2 months for latent tuberculosis, as reported to the CDC; five died of fulminant hepatic failure, two of whom had recovered from isoniazid-induced hepatitis (19). This report led to revision of previous guidelines of the American Thoracic Society. According to the revised guidelines, isoniazid for 9 months is the preferred treatment for latent tuberculosis infection in HIV-negative subjects, followed by isoniazid for 6 months or rifampicin for 4 months. Rifampicin plus pyrazinamide for 2 months can be used with caution in these patients, especially if they are taking other medications that are associated with liver injury, and those who drink a lot of alcohol. This combination is not recommended for those with underlying liver disease or who have had isoniazid-associated liver damage. Liver function tests should be measured at baseline and at 2-weekly intervals thereafter for 6 weeks. Only two non-fatal cases of severe liver injury have been reported to the CDC since the publication of revised guidelines as of November 2002 (20).

Susceptibility factors
Acetylator status and other genetic factors, old age, pre-existing hepatic dysfunction, alcoholism, co-infection with hepatitis virus, and malnutrition are important potential susceptibility factors for the development of liver damage in patients taking antituberculosis drugs (21), but there have been inconsistent findings with regard to some of these risk factors in different studies.

Genetic factors
The issue of hepatic dysfunction and acetylator status during treatment with isoniazid plus rifampicin has been re-examined in 77 Japanese patients with pulmonary

tuberculosis (22). There was a marked increase in the risk of hepatotoxicity amongst slow acetylator NAT2* genotypes (a combination of mutant alleles) compared with the rapid acetylator genotype (homozygous NAT2*4). Using Taylor's series analysis it can be calculated that the relative risk was 28 (95% CI = 4.1, 192). Despite a small sample size (seven slow acetylator genotypes, 42 intermediate, and 28 rapid) the relative risk was highly significant, which is not surprising if all seven of the slow acetylators and only one of the 28 rapid acetylators developed hepatotoxicity.

A unique feature of this study was the determination of acetylator status by genotyping rather than phenotyping. There is generally good concordance between the two methods, but in the presence of hepatic dysfunction the phenotype assessment may not reflect the genotype. Furthermore, 42 of the 77 patients were assigned to the intermediate acetylator genotype, based on heterozygosity for NAT2*4 and a mutant allele. However, phenotyping by estimation of concentrations of metabolites of the commonly used probes does not consistently result in identification of intermediate acetylators. The Japanese are mostly fast acetylators (~90%) compared with Caucasians or Indians (40–50%). It is unlikely, however, that the observed association between slow acetylator genotype and the high risk of hepatic dysfunction was affected by any of these considerations. The dose of isoniazid was rather large (~8 mg/kg/day) and this may have increased the risk of hepatotoxicity. Furthermore, hepatotoxicity was defined as an increase in transaminases to one and a half times the top of the reference range. This degree of hepatic dysfunction is not uncommon in patients taking antituberculosis drugs, and is no indication for withdrawal or modification of treatment. It is not possible to assess the risk of severe hepatotoxicity during treatment, owing to lack of detailed information in the published report.

A case-control study has suggested that there is also an increased risk of antituberculosis drug-induced hepatotoxicity in individuals with a glutathione-S-transferase M1 "null" mutation (23). Reduced glutathione transferase activity could theoretically predispose individuals to adverse effects of toxic metabolites and xenobiotics. These observations need to be confirmed.

Old age
Old age and the presence of hepatic dysfunction on baseline evaluation are the most consistent predictors of hepatotoxicity during antituberculosis therapy. The association between hepatotoxicity and hepatitis C virus and HIV seropositivity has been reviewed (SEDA-23, 324). A report from Hong Kong has suggested that the risk is much greater in hepatitis B virus carriers taking antituberculosis drugs (24). Even after excluding patients who had raised baseline alanine transaminase activity or with HbeAg seroconversion during the phase of hepatic dysfunction, the risk of hepatotoxicity was still significantly higher in hepatitis B carriers taking antituberculosis drugs compared with non-carriers (26% versus 8.8%). These observations are of considerable importance in regions of the world in which the prevalence of hepatitis B infection as well as tuberculosis is high, such as South-East Asia and sub-Saharan Africa.

Liver transplantation
Enhanced hepatotoxicity of conventional antituberculosis regimens has been reported in recipients of orthotopic liver transplants, which is not unexpected, because of bouts of organ rejection (25). The authors recommended ofloxacin for these patients on the basis of favorable outcome in six cases. A conventional antituberculosis induction regimen was used initially until hepatotoxicity developed in all six patients. Thereafter they were treated with a combination of ofloxacin and ethambutol, with apparent cure in all. It should be noted that most of the patients took isoniazid + rifampicin for almost 2 months, which is the usual period when hepatotoxic reactions occur. Perhaps one should evaluate substitution of rifampicin with ofloxacin from the very beginning in order to minimize hepatotoxicity, as well as interference with ciclosporin leading to graft rejection noted in an earlier study (26).

Prevention
One of the most important predictors of hepatotoxicity during antituberculosis drug therapy is an abnormal liver function test at baseline. It is reasonable to avoid potentially hepatotoxic drugs in the management of patients with pre-existing liver disease.

The use of ofloxacin instead of rifampicin in antituberculosis drug regimens for patients with underlying chronic liver disease has been reported to be associated with a significantly lower risk of hepatotoxicity (27). Similar observations have been reported among carriers of hepatitis B and liver transplant recipients by other investigators.

Management
There are four issues related to the management of patients who develop hepatotoxicity during treatment with antituberculosis drugs:

1. what the preferred treatment regimen should be for patients with significantly abnormal liver functions at baseline;
2. when treatment should be stopped/modified if hepatic dysfunction develops;
3. what antituberculosis treatment, if any, should be used until liver function improves;
4. what a safe regimen is for re-treatment of these patients.

Several herbal products have been claimed to mitigate drug-induced hepatitis caused by antituberculosis agents. However, few of them have undergone rigorous randomized controlled trials.

- Glycyrrhizin is widely used in Japan for the treatment of chronic hepatitis, but in a non-randomized trial in 24 patients who developed drug-induced hepatitis while undergoing antituberculosis chemotherapy, there was no difference in the time required for recovery between the patients who were treated with or without intravenous glycyrrhizin 40 ml/day (28).
- *Moringa oleifera*, commonly known as "drumstick," has been mentioned in the treatment of various illnesses in Indian folk medicine, and an ethanolic extract of the

leaves had a hepatoprotective effect in a rat model of antituberculosis drug-induced liver injury (29).

- Russian investigators have reported a hepatoprotective effect of a plant product "Galstena" in a rat model and have extended their observations to a clinical trial, with favorable results; however, few data were given in this report (30).

It cannot be denied that there is a need for continuing research in this area, but it is necessary to undertake well-conducted scientific studies before claims of hepatoprotective effects of herbal products can be accepted.

There is a lack of consensus on the best re-treatment protocol for patients who develop hepatotoxicity during treatment with standard antituberculosis agents. Investigators from Turkey have reported a high risk of recurrence of hepatitis (in six of 25 patients) on re-introduction of all drugs in full doses after recovery from hepatitis (31). This risk was less when rifampicin and isoniazid were re-introduced sequentially in increasing doses and when pyrazinamide was replaced by streptomycin.

Long-Term Effects

Drug tolerance

Primary and secondary bacterial resistance to antituberculosis drugs represents a major problem. This can be demonstrated by resistance tests, if available. When testing is not done, primary or secondary resistance can only be suspected when drug treatment fails. The incidence of bacterial resistance varies enormously from country to country and from population to population. In Tanzania (32), where the WHO and the International Union Against Tuberculosis and Lung Diseases (IUATLD) has developed antituberculosis programs, primary resistance to isoniazid and/or streptomycin is found in 10% of cases (33). In contrast, South-East Asian and African patients harbor resistant bacteria markedly more often (SED-10, 572); resistance tests therefore remain mandatory for good epidemiological and therapeutic control. Recent reports from the WHO drug resistance surveillance network have allowed an overview of the current situation worldwide and facilitate the choice of medication according to the origin of the patients (34).

Multidrug-resistant tuberculosis generally results from inadequate therapy or lack of compliance with therapy. A strain of mycobacteria is called resistant when it is insensitive to one of the first-line drugs. It is called multiresistant when it is insensitive to both isoniazid and rifampicin. In this case other antituberculosis drugs may also be ineffective (35). In practice, at least two second-line antituberculosis drugs, selected on the basis of individual drug susceptibility, are given in combination with a fluoroquinolone (36).

Drug malabsorption may contribute to the emergence of acquired drug resistance. It has been described in HIV-infected patients with advanced disease (37), and also in immunocompetent patients (38). Thus, in addition to the use of directly observed therapy to ensure compliance, it is advisable to monitor antimycobacterial drug concentrations routinely in such patients. Practical proposals for the choice of antituberculosis drugs in special circumstances, including drug resistance, have been made (39).

Susceptibility Factors

Age

Increasing age predisposes to hepatotoxicity from antituberculosis drugs. Workers from Florida have reported a five-fold increase in the likelihood of drug-induced hepatotoxicity in patients who are hepatitis C-positive and a four-fold increase in patients who are HIV-positive, compared with seronegative patients treated for tuberculosis (40). In all, 134 patients taking antituberculosis drugs were monitored for drug-induced hepatotoxicity, defined as an increase in aspartate transaminase and/or alanine transaminase activity from normal to at least three times normal and/or an increase in bilirubin above normal. Of the 22 patients who developed drug-induced hepatotoxicity, only six developed drug-induced hepatotoxicity on re-introduction of treatment after an interval in which the abnormalities had resolved. Four of the six had liver biopsies, which showed active inflammation, attributed (at least in part) to hepatitis C. These were then treated with interferon alfa, with improvement of liver chemistry. On improvement, antituberculosis drug therapy was successfully re-introduced in the form of isoniazid and rifabutin, the latter being considered to be less hepatotoxic than rifampicin.

References

1. Bass JB Jr, Farer LS, Hopewell PC, O'Brien R, Jacobs RF, Ruben F, Snider DE Jr, Thornton G. Treatment of tuberculosis and tuberculosis infection in adults and children. American Thoracic Society and The Centers for Disease Control and Prevention. Am J Respir Crit Care Med 1994;149(5):1359–74.
2. Mitchell I, Wendon J, Fitt S, Williams R. Anti-tuberculous therapy and acute liver failure. Lancet 1995;345(8949):555–6.
3. Furin JJ, Mitnick CD, Shin SS, Bayona J, Becerra MC, Singler JM, Alcantara F, Castanieda C, Sanchez E, Acha J, Farmer PE, Kim JY. Occurrence of serious adverse effects in patients receiving community-based therapy for multidrug-resistant tuberculosis. Int J Tuberc Lung Dis 2001;5(7):648–55.
4. Tahaoglu K, Torun T, Sevim T, Atac G, Kir A, Karasulu L, Ozmen I, Kapakli N. The treatment of multidrug-resistant tuberculosis in Turkey. N Engl J Med 2001;345(3):170–4.
5. Ormerod LP, Horsfield N. Frequency and type of reactions to antituberculosis drugs: observation in routine treatment. Tubercle Lung Dis 1966;77:37.
6. Combs DL, O'Brien RJ, Geiter LJ. USPHS Tuberculosis Short-Course Chemotherapy Trial 21: effectiveness, toxicity, and acceptability. The report of final results. Ann Intern Med 1990;112(6):397–406.
7. Hwang SJ, Wu JC, Lee CN, Yen FS, Lu CL, Lin TP, Lee SD. A prospective clinical study of isoniazid–rifampicin–pyrazinamide–induced liver injury in an area endemic for hepatitis B. J Gastroenterol Hepatol 1997;12(1):87–91.
8. Schaberg T, Rebhan K, Lode H. Risk factors for side-effects of isoniazid, rifampin and pyrazinamide in patients hospitalized for pulmonary tuberculosis. Eur Respir J 1996;9(10):2026–30.
9. Dossing M, Wilcke JT, Askgaard DS, Nybo B. Liver injury during antituberculosis treatment: an 11-year study. Tuber Lung Dis 1996;77(4):335–40.
10. Singh J, Arora A, Garg PK, Thakur VS, Pande JN, Tandon RK. Antituberculosis treatment-induced hepatotoxicity: role of predictive factors. Postgrad Med J 1995;71(836):359–62.
11. Kuaban C, Bercion R, Koulla-Shiro S. HIV seroprevalence rate and incidence of adverse skin reactions in adults with pulmonary tuberculosis receiving thiacetazone free

anti-tuberculosis treatment in Yaounde, Cameroon. East Afr Med J 1997;74(8):474–7.

12. Hoigne R. Allergische Erkrankungen. In: Stucki P, Hess T, editors. Hadorn, Lehrbuch der Therapie. 7th ed. Berne-Stuttgart-Vienna: Verlag Hans Huber, 1983:155.

13. Ohkawa K, Hashiguchi M, Ohno K, Kiuchi C, Takahashi S, Kondo S, Echizen H, Ogata H. Risk factors for antituberculous chemotherapy-induced hepatotoxicity in Japanese pediatric patients. Clin Pharmacol Ther 2002;72(2):220–6.

14. Lee AM, Mennone JZ, Jones RC, Paul WS. Risk factors for hepatotoxicity associated with rifampin and pyrazinamide for the treatment of latent tuberculosis infection: experience from three public health tuberculosis clinics. Int J Tuberc Lung Dis 2002;6(11):995–1000.

15. Stout JE, Engemann JJ, Cheng AC, Fortenberry ER, Hamilton CD. Safety of 2 months of rifampin and pyrazinamide for treatment of latent tuberculosis. Am J Respir Crit Care Med 2003;167(6):824–7.

16. Jasmer RM, Saukkonen JJ, Blumberg HM, Daley CL, Bernardo J, Vittinghoff E, King MD, Kawamura LM, Hopewell PC; Short-Course Rifampin and Pyrazinamide for Tuberculosis Infection (SCRIPT) Study Investigators. Short-course rifampin and pyrazinamide compared with isoniazid for latent tuberculosis infection: a multicenter clinical trial. Ann Intern Med 2002;137(8):640–7.

17. Jasmer RM, Daley CL. Rifampin and pyrazinamide for treatment of latent tuberculosis infection: is it safe? Am J Respir Crit Care Med 2003;167(6):809–10.

18. Centers for Disease Control and Prevention (CDC). Fatal and severe hepatitis associated with rifampin and pyrazinamide for the treatment of latent tuberculosis infection—New York and Georgia, 2000. MMWR Morb Mortal Wkly Rep 2001;50(15):289–91.

19. Centers for Disease Control and Prevention (CDC). Update: fatal and severe liver injuries associated with rifampin and pyrazinamide for latent tuberculosis infection, and revisions in American Thoracic Society/CDC recommendations—United States, 2001. MMWR Morb Mortal Wkly Rep 2001;50(34):733–5.

20. Centers for Disease Control and Prevention (CDC). Update: fatal and severe liver injuries associated with rifampin and pyrazinamide treatment for latent tuberculosis infection. MMWR Morb Mortal Wkly Rep 2002;51(44):998–9.

21. Pande JN, Singh SP, Khilnani GC, Khilnani S, Tandon RK. Risk factors for hepatotoxicity from antituberculosis drugs: a case-control study. Thorax 1996;51(2):132–6.

22. Ohno M, Yamaguchi I, Yamamoto I, Fukuda T, Yokota S, Maekura R, Ito M, Yamamoto Y, Ogura T, Maeda K, Komuta K, Igarashi T, Azuma J. Slow N-acetyltransferase 2 genotype affects the incidence of isoniazid and rifampicin-induced hepatotoxicity. Int J Tuberc Lung Dis 2000;4(3):256–61.

23. Roy B, Chowdhury A, Kundu S, Santra A, Dey B, Chakraborty M, Majumder PP. Increased risk of antituberculosis drug-induced hepatotoxicity in individuals with glutathione S-transferase M1 'null' mutation. J Gastroenterol Hepatol 2001;16(9):1033–7.

24. Wong WM, Wu PC, Yuen MF, Cheng CC, Yew WW, Wong PC, Tam CM, Leung CC, Lai CL. Antituberculosis drug-related liver dysfunction in chronic hepatitis B infection. Hepatology 2000;31(1):201–6.

25. Meyers BR, Papanicolaou GA, Sheiner P, Emre S, Miller C. Tuberculosis in orthotopic liver transplant patients: increased toxicity of recommended agents; cure of disseminated infection with nonconventional regimens. Transplantation 2000;69(1):64–9.

26. Aguado JM, Herrero JA, Gavalda J, Torre-Cisneros J, Blanes M, Rufi G, Moreno A, Gurgui M, Hayek M, Lumbreras C, Cantarell C. Clinical presentation and outcome of tuberculosis in kidney, liver, and heart transplant recipients in Spain. Spanish Transplantation Infection Study Group, GESITRA. Transplantation 1997; 63(9):1278–86.

27. Saigal S, Agarwal SR, Nandeesh HP, Sarin SK. Safety of an ofloxacin-based antitubercular regimen for the treatment of tuberculosis in patients with underlying chronic liver disease: a preliminary report. J Gastroenterol Hepatol 2001;16(9):1028–32.

28. Miyazawa N, Takahashi H, Yoshiike Y, Ogura T, Watanuki Y, Sato M, Kakemizu N, Yamakawa Y, U CH, Goto H, Odagiri S. [Effect of glycyrrhizin on anti-tuberculosis drug-induced hepatitis.] Kekkaku 2003;78(1):15–9.

29. Pari L, Kumar NA. Hepatoprotective activity of *Moringa oleifera* on antitubercular drug-induced liver damage in rats. J Med Food 2002;5(3):171–7.

30. Katikova OIu, Asanov BM, Vize-Khripunova MA, Burba EN, Ruzov VI. [Use of the plant hepatoprotector *Galstena* tuberculostatics-induced hepatic lesions: experimental and clinical study.] Probl Tuberk 2002;(4):32–6.

31. Tahaoglu K, Atac G, Sevim T, Tarun T, Yazicioglu O, Horzum G, Gemci I, Ongel A, Kapakli N, Aksoy E. The management of anti-tuberculosis drug-induced hepatotoxicity. Int J Tuberc Lung Dis 2001;5(1):65–9.

32. Tanzanian/British Medical Research Council Collaborative Study. Tuberculosis in Tanzania—a national survey of newly notified cases. Tubercle 1985;66(3):161–78.

33. Glassroth J, Robins AG, Snider DE Jr. Tuberculosis in the 1980s. N Engl J Med 1980;302(26):1441–50.

34. WHO Global Tuberculosis Programme, Geneva. Anti-tuberculosis drug resistance in the world. The WHO/IUATLD Global Project on Anti-tuberculosis Drug Resistance Surveillance, 1994–1997.

35. Yew WW, Chau CH. Drug-resistant tuberculosis in the 1990s. Eur Respir J 1995;8(7):1184–92.

36. Iseman MD. Treatment of multidrug-resistant tuberculosis. N Engl J Med 1993;329(11):784–91.

37. Peloquin CA, MacPhee AA, Berning SE. Malabsorption of antimycobacterial medications. N Engl J Med 1993; 329(15):1122–3.

38. Turner M, McGowan C, Nardell E, Haskal R. Serum drug levels in tuberculosis patients. Am J Respir Crit Care Med 1994;149:A102.

39. Des Prez RM, Heim CR. Mycobacterium tuberculosis. In: Mandell GL, Douglas RG Jr, Bennett JE, editors. Principles and Practice of Infectious Diseases. 3rd ed. New York: Churchill Livingstone, 1990:1877.

40. Ungo JR, Jones D, Ashkin D, Hollender ES, Bernstein D, Albanese AP, Pitchenik AE. Antituberculosis drug-induced hepatotoxicity. The role of hepatitis C virus and the human immunodeficiency virus. Am J Respir Crit Care Med 1998;157(6 Pt 1):1871–6.

Antrafenine

See also Non-steroidal anti-inflammatory drugs

General Information

Antrafenine closely resembles glafenine and floctafenine (SED-9, 153) (SEDA-7, 116) (SEDA-11, 96) (1). The same adverse effects must be expected and some have been described, for example nephrotoxicity (SEDA-4, 69) (2). Gastrotoxicity is claimed to be less than with aspirin (3), again no doubt merely because it is a weak anti-inflammatory drug.

References

1. Neuman M. Antrafenine. Drugs of Today 1978;14:56.
2. Leguy P, Herve JP, Garre M, Youinou P, Leroy JP. Nephropathie aiguë tubulo-interstitielle après ingestion d'antrafénine de mécanisme apparemment non immuno-allergique. [Acute tubulo-interstitial nephropathy following ingestion of antrafenine with an apparently non-immuno-allergic mechanism.] Nouv Presse Méd 1981;10(16):1336.
3. Bressot C, Dechavanne M, Ville D, Meunier PJ. Effet antalgique et pertes sanguines fécales induites par l'antraféinine. [Analgesic effect and fecal blood loss induced by antrafenine. A double-blind comparison with aspirin.] Rev Rhum Mal Osteoartic 1981;48(7–9):601–4.

Apiaceae

See also Herbal medicines

General Information

The genera in the family of Apiaceae (formerly Umbelliferae) (Table 1) include a variety of spices and vegetables, such as angelica, anise, carrot, celery, chervil, coriander, cumin, dill, fennel, parsley, and parsnip.

Food allergy to spices accounts for 2% of all cases of food allergies but 6.4% of cases in adults. Prick tests to native spices in 589 patients with food allergies showed frequent sensitization to the Apiaceae coriander, caraway, fennel, and celery (32% of prick tests in children, 23% of prick tests in adults) (1). There were 10 cases of allergy related to the mugwort-celery-spices syndrome: coriander ($n = 1$), caraway ($n = 2$), fennel ($n = 3$), garlic ($n = 3$), and onion ($n = 1$).

Scratch tests with powdered commercial spices in 70 patients with positive skin tests to birch and/or mugwort pollens and celery were positive to aniseed, fennel, coriander, and cumin, all Apiaceae, in more than 24 patients (2). Spices from unrelated families (red pepper, white pepper, ginger, nutmeg, cinnamon) elicited positive immediate skin test reactions in only three of 11 patients. Specific serum IgE to spices (determined in 41 patients with a positive RAST to celery) up to class 3 was found, especially in patients with celery-mugwort or celery-birch-mugwort association. The celery-birch association pattern was linked to positive reactions (RAST classes 1,2) with spices from the Apiaceae family only.

Ammi majus and Ammi visnaga

Ammi majus is also known as bishop's weed or large bullwort, and *Ammi visnaga* as toothpick weed. They have numerous active ingredients, including ammirin, angenomalin, kellactone, majurin, and marmesin, furanocoumarins (psoralen, bergapten, isopimpinellin, imperatorin, umbelliprenin, xanthotoxin), and flavonol triglycosides (kaempferol, isorhamnetin). In modern times they have been used to treat vitiligo, since they contain psoralens, and have several different pharmacological effects in experimental animals, including hypoglycemic effects (3), antischistosomal effects (4), and inhibition of nephrolithiasis (5).

Table 1   The genera of Apiaceae

Aciphylla (fierce Spaniard)	*Levisticum* (levisticum)
Aegopodium (goutweed)	*Ligusticum* (licorice-root)
Aethusa (aethusa)	*Lilaeopsis* (grasswort)
Aletes (Indian parsley)	*Limnosciadium* (dogshade)
Ammi (ammi)	*Lomatium* (desert parsley)
Ammoselinum (sand parsley)	*Musineon* (wild parsley)
Anethum (dill)	*Myrrhis* (myrrhis)
Angelica (angelica)	*Neoparrya* (neoparrya)
Anthriscus (chervil)	*Oenanthe* (water dropwort)
Apiastrum (apiastrum)	*Oreonana* (mountain parsley)
Apium (celery)	*Oreoxis* (oreoxis)
Arracacia (arracacia)	*Orogenia* (Indian potato)
Berula (water parsnip)	*Osmorhiza* (sweetroot)
Bifora (bishop)	*Oxypolis* (cowbane)
Bowlesia (bowlesia)	*Pastinaca* (parsnip)
Bupleurum (bupleurum)	*Perideridia* (yampah)
Carum (carum)	*Petroselinum* (parsley)
Caucalis (burr parsley)	*Peucedanum* (peucedanum)
Centella (centella)	*Pimpinella* (burnet saxifrage)
Chaerophyllum (chervil)	*Podistera* (podistera)
Cicuta (water hemlock)	*Polytaenia* (hairy moss)
Cnidium (snow parsley)	*Pseudocymopterus* (false spring parsley)
Conioselinum (hemlock parsley)	*Pteryxia* (wavewing)
Conium (poison hemlock)	*Ptilimnium* (mock bishop weed)
Coriandrum (coriander)	*Sanicula* (sanicle)
Cryptotaenia (honewort)	*Scandix* (scandix)
Cuminum (cumin)	*Selinum* (selinum)
Cyclospermum (marsh parsley)	*Seseli* (seseli)
Cymopterus (spring parsley)	*Shoshonea* (shoshonea)
	Sium (waterparsnip)
Cynosciadium (cynosciadium)	
Daucosma (daucosma)	*Smyrnium* (smyrnium)
Daucus (wild carrot)	*Spermolepis* (scaleseed)
Dorema (dorema)	*Sphenosciadium* (sphenosciadium)
Erigenia (erigenia)	*Taenidia* (taenidia)
Eryngium (eryngo)	*Tauschia* (umbrellawort)
Eurytaenia (spreadwing)	*Thaspium* (meadowparsnip)
Falcaria (falcaria)	*Tilingia* (tilingia)
Ferula (asafetida)	*Tordylium* (tordylium)
Foeniculum (fennel)	*Torilis* (hedge parsley)
Glehnia (silvertop)	*Trachyspermum* (Ajowan caraway)
Harbouria (harbouria)	*Trepocarpus* (trepocarpus)
Heracleum (cow parsnip)	*Turgenia* (false carrot)
Hydrocotyle (hydrocotyle)	*Yabea* (yabea)
	Zizia (zizia)

Adverse effects

Injudicious use of the fruit of *A. majus* in combination with skin exposure to the sun can cause severe phototoxic dermatitis, owing to the presence of psoralens (6).

- IgE-mediated rhinitis and contact urticaria were caused by exposure to bishop's weed in a 31-year-old atopic female florist (7). A skin prick test with bishop's weed flowers gave an 8 mm wheal, and the bishop's weed-specific serum IgE concentration was 9.7 PRU/ml (RAST class 3).

Prolonged use or overdosing of the fruit of *A. visnaga* can cause nausea, dizziness, constipation, loss of appetite, headache, pruritus, and sleeping disorders.

Angelica sinensis

Angelica sinensis, known in China as "dong quai" or "dang gui," contains antioxidants (8), inhibits the growth of cancer cells in vitro (9) and stimulates immune function in experimental animals (10). It has been used to treat amenorrhea (11) and menopausal hot flushes (12), and to reduce pulmonary hypertension in patients with chronic obstructive pulmonary disease (13).

Adverse effects
Angelica sinensis can cause hypertension (14).

- A 32-year-old woman, 3 weeks post-partum, developed acute headache, weakness, light-headedness, and vomiting. Her blood pressure was 195/85 mmHg. She had taken dong quai for postpartum weakness and said that she had not been taking any other medicines. Her 3-week-old son's blood pressure was raised to 115/69. Dong quai medication of the mother and breast-feeding of the child were discontinued and the blood pressure normalized in both patients within 48 hours.

Conium maculatum

Conium maculatum (hemlock) contains the poisonous piperidine alkaloid, coniine, and related alkaloids, *N*-methyl-coniine, conhydrine, pseudoconhydrine, and gamma-coniceine. It has well-established teratogenic activity in certain animal species.

Adverse effects
The symptoms of hemlock poisoning are effects on the nervous system (stimulation followed by paralysis of motor nerve endings and nervous system stimulation and later depression), vomiting, trembling, difficulty in movement, an initially slow and weak and later a rapid pulse, rapid respiration, salivation, urination, nausea, convulsions, coma, and death (15).

Coriandrum sativum

Coriandrum sativum (coriander) has traditionally been used as a stimulant, aromatic, and carminative, and to disguise the taste of purgatives. In experimental animals it has hypolipidemic effects (16) and hypoglycemic effects (17).

Adverse effects
Respiratory
Occupational asthma has been attributed to various spices from botanically unrelated species, including coriander.

- A 27-year-old man developed rhinitis and asthma symptoms 1 year after starting to prepare a certain kind of sausage (18). He had positive immediate skin prick tests with paprika, coriander, and mace, and specific IgE antibodies to all three. He had immediate asthmatic reactions to bronchial inhalation of extracts from paprika, coriander, and mace, with maximum falls in FEV_1 of 26, 40, and 31% respectively, but no late asthmatic reactions.

Endocrine
Adrenal insufficiency has been attributed to *C. sativum* (19).

- A 28-year-old woman took an extract of *C. sativum* for 7 days to augment lactation while breastfeeding. She developed severe stomach pain and diarrhea and 15 days later resented with dark skin, depression, dehydration, and amenorrhea. A diagnosis of adrenal dysfunction was made, the herbal remedy was withdrawn, and she was treated with dexamethasone, prednisolone, and an oral contraceptive. Her symptoms resolved within 10 days.

Skin
Contact dermatitis from coriander has been described (20).

Immunologic
An anaphylactic reaction has been described in a patient who was sensitized to coriander (21).

Ferula assa-foetida

Ferula assa-foetida (asafetida) contains coumarin sesquiterpenoids, such as fukanefuromarins and kamolonol, which inhibit the production of nitric oxide and relax smooth muscle.

Adverse effects
Methemoglobinemia occurred in a 5-week-old infant treated with a gum asafetida formulation (22).
Asafetida may enhance the activity of warfarin (23).

References

1. Moneret-Vautrin DA, Morisset M, Lemerdy P, Croizier A, Kanny G. Food allergy and IgE sensitization caused by spices: CICBAA data (based on 589 cases of food allergy). Allerg Immunol (Paris) 2002;34(4):135–40.
2. Stager J, Wuthrich B, Johansson SG. Spice allergy in celery-sensitive patients. Allergy 1991;46(6):475–8.
3. Jouad H, Maghrani M, Eddouks M. Hypoglycemic effect of aqueous extract of *Ammi visnaga* in normal and streptozotocin-induced diabetic rats. J Herb Pharmacother 2002;2(4):19–29.
4. Abdulla WA, Kadry H, Mahran SG, el-Raziky EH, el-Nakib S. Preliminary studies on the anti-schistosomal effect of *Ammi majus* L Egypt J Bilharz 1978;4(1):19–26.
5. Khan ZA, Assiri AM, Al-Afghani HM, Maghrabi TM. Inhibition of oxalate nephrolithiasis with *Ammi visnaga* (Al-Khillah). Int Urol Nephrol 2001;33(4):605–8.
6. Ossenkoppele PM, van der Sluis WG, van Vloten WA. Fototoxische dermatitis door het gebruik van de *Ammi majus*-vrucht bij vitiligo. [Phototoxic dermatitis following the use of *Ammi majus* fruit for vitiligo.] Ned Tijdschr Geneeskd 1991;135(11):478–80.
7. Kiistala R, Makinen-Kiljunen S, Heikkinen K, Rinne J, Haahtela T. Occupational allergic rhinitis and contact urticaria caused by bishop's weed (*Ammi majus*). Allergy 1999;54(6):635–9.
8. Wu SJ, Ng LT, Lin CC. Antioxidant activities of some common ingredients of traditional chinese medicine, *Angelica sinensis*, *Lycium barbarum* and *Poria cocos*. Phytother Res 2004;18(12):1008–12.
9. Cheng YL, Chang WL, Lee SC, Liu YG, Chen CJ, Lin SZ, Tsai NM, Yu DS, Yen CY, Harn HJ. Acetone extract of *Angelica sinensis* inhibits proliferation of human cancer cells via inducing cell cycle arrest and apoptosis. Life Sci 2004;75(13):1579–94.
10. Wang J, Xia XY, Peng RX, Chen X. [Activation of the immunologic function of rat Kupffer cells by the

polysaccharides of *Angelica sinensis*.] Yao Xue Xue Bao 2004;39(3):168–71.

11. He ZP, Wang DZ, Shi LY, Wang ZQ. Treating amenorrhea in vital energy-deficient patients with *Angelica sinensis-astragalus* membranaceus menstruation-regulating decoction. J Tradit Chin Med 1986;6(3):187–90.

12. Kupfersztain C, Rotem C, Fagot R, Kaplan B. The immediate effect of natural plant extract, *Angelica sinensis* and *Matricaria chamomilla* (Climex) for the treatment of hot flushes during menopause. A preliminary report. Clin Exp Obstet Gynecol 2003;30(4):203–6.

13. Xu JY, Li BX, Cheng SY. [Short-term effects of *Angelica sinensis* and nifedipine on chronic obstructive pulmonary disease in patients with pulmonary hypertension.] Zhongguo Zhong Xi Yi Jie He Za Zhi 1992;12(12):716–18, 707.

14. Nambiar S, Schwartz RH, Constantino A. Hypertension in mother and baby linked to ingestion of Chinese herbal medicine. West J Med 1999;171(3):152.

15. Vetter J. Poison hemlock (*Conium maculatum* L.). Food Chem Toxicol 2004;42(9):1373–82.

16. Lal AA, Kumar T, Murthy PB, Pillai KS. Hypolipidemic effect of *Coriandrum sativum* L. in triton-induced hyperlipidemic rats. Indian J Exp Biol 2004;42(9):909–12.

17. Gray AM, Flatt PR. Insulin-releasing and insulin-like activity of the traditional anti-diabetic plant *Coriandrum sativum* (coriander). Br J Nutr 1999;81(3):203–9.

18. Sastre J, Olmo M, Novalvos A, Ibanez D, Lahoz C. Occupational asthma due to different spices. Allergy 1996;51(2):117–20.

19. Zabihi E, Abdollahi M. Endocrinotoxicity induced by *Coriandrum sativa*: a case report. WHO Drug Inf 2002;16:15.

20. Kanerva L, Soini M. Occupational protein contact dermatitis from coriander. Contact Dermatitis 2001;45(6):354–5.

21. Manzanedo L, Blanco J, Fuentes M, Caballero ML, Moneo I. Anaphylactic reaction in a patient sensitized to coriander seed. Allergy 2004;59(3):362–3.

22. Kelly KJ, Neu J, Camitta BM, Honig GR. Methemoglobinemia in an infant treated with the folk remedy glycerited asafoetida. Pediatrics 1984;73(5):717–19.

23. Heck AM, DeWitt BA, Lukes AL. Potential interactions between alternative therapies and warfarin. Am J Health Syst Pharm 2000;57(13):1221–7.

Apocynaceae

See also Herbal medicines

General Information

The genera in the family of Apocynaceae (Table 1) include dogbane, oleander, and periwinkle.

Rauwolfia serpentina

The root of *Rauwolfia serpentina* (snakeroot) contains numerous alkaloids, of which reserpine and rescinnamine are said to be the most active as hypotensive agents (1).

Adverse effects

Inexpert use of *R. serpentina* can lead to serious toxicity, including symptoms such as hypotension, sedation, depression, and potentiation of other central depressants.

Table 1 The genera of Apocynaceae

Adenium (desert rose)
Allamanda (allamanda)
Alstonia (alstonia)
Alyxia (alyxia)
Amsonia (blue star)
Anechites (anechites)
Angadenia (pineland golden trumpet)
Apocynum (dogbane)
Carissa (carissa)
Catharanthus (periwinkle)
Cycladenia (waxy dogbane)
Dyera (dyera)
Echites (echites)
Fernaldia (fernaldia)
Forsteronia (forsteronia)
Funtumia (funtumia)
Hancornia (hancornia)
Haplophyton (haplophyton)
Holarrhena (holarrhena)
Landolphia (landolphia)
Lepinia
Macrosiphonia (rock trumpet)
Nerium (oleander)
Ochrosia (yellow wood)
Pentalinon (pentalinon)
Plumeria (plumeria)
Prestonia (prestonia)
Pteralyxia (pteralyxia)
Rauvolfia (devil's pepper)
Rhabdadenia (rhabdadenia)
Saba (saba)
Strophanthus (strophanthus)
Tabernaemontana (milkwood)
Thevetia (thevetia)
Trachelospermum (trachelospermum)
Vallesia (vallesia)
Vinca (periwinkle)

Reference

1. Cieri UR. Determination of reserpine and rescinnamine in *Rauwolfia serpentina* powders and tablets: collaborative study. J AOAC Int 1998;81(2):373–80.

Apomorphine

General Information

Apomorphine, a very potent non-selective dopamine agonist, which acts on both D_1 and D_2 receptors, has been used with some success in Parkinson's disease, particularly in patients with severe long-term adverse effects of levodopa. Because of first-pass metabolism it has to be used subcutaneously, sublingually, or intranasally. Its adverse effects resemble those of levodopa.

Yawning, somnolence, nausea, and vomiting can all result from the use of apomorphine; they respond to naloxone.

Local reactions to subcutaneous infusion of apomorphine in the nose and throat include swelling of the nose and lips, stomatitis, and buccal mucosal ulceration.

Persistent nodules cause major problems in about 10% of patients after 3 or more years. One solution is to give the drug intravenously using an indwelling cannula. Six patients, who had responded well to subcutaneous apomorphine before nodules developed, had such cannulae inserted (1). The apomorphine was given at a mean rate of 9.0 mg/hour to a total mean dose of 257 mg/day, very similar to the subcutaneous dosage. The intravenous therapy virtually abolished "off" periods, reduced oral antiparkinsonian drug dosages by 59%, and produced a marked (but unquantified) reduction in dyskinesias and an improved quality of life. However, there were major problems. Two patients receiving high doses of apomorphine (450 and 290 mg/day, in the latter case a deliberate overdose) developed thromboembolic complications, following crystal formation, in one case to the right lung and in the other with obstruction to the superior vena cava. Both required surgical intervention. Both recovered fully, but the authors understandably commented that this therapeutic approach still needs further development.

Organs and Systems

Nervous system

A paradoxical akinetic response has been reported in a middle-aged man, probably with nigrostriatal degeneration, who became both immobile and mute 15 minutes after taking 4 mg of apomorphine; the effect was seen again on rechallenge with doses as low as 2 mg (2). The mechanism was not clear.

Psychological, psychiatric

Four men with Parkinson's disease underwent long-term treatment with apomorphine and developed dose-related psychosexual disorders (3).

Sexual function

There have been reports that apomorphine causes penile erections in both Parkinsonian and healthy men (4–6).

References

1. Manson AJ, Hanagasi H, Turner K, Patsalos PN, Carey P, Ratnaraj N, Lees AJ. Intravenous apomorphine therapy in Parkinson's disease: clinical and pharmacokinetic observations. Brain 2001;124(Pt 2):331–40.
2. Jenkins JR, Pearce JM. Paradoxical akinetic response to apomorphine in parkinsonism. J Neurol Neurosurg Psychiatry 1992;55(5):414–15.
3. Courty E, Durif F, Zenut M, Courty P, Lavarenne J. Psychiatric and sexual disorders induced by apomorphine in Parkinson's disease. Clin Neuropharmacol 1997;20(2):140–7.
4. Heaton JP. Apomorphine: an update of clinical trial results. Int J Impot Res 2000;12(Suppl 4):S67–73.
5. O'Sullivan JD, Hughes AJ. Apomorphine-induced penile erections in Parkinson's disease. Mov Disord 1999;14(4):701–2.
6. Lal S, Ackman D, Thavundayil JX, Kiely ME, Etienne P. Effect of apomorphine, a dopamine receptor agonist, on penile tumescence in normal subjects. Prog Neuropsychopharmacol Biol Psychiatry 1984;8(4–6):695–9.

Aprindine

See also Antidysrhythmic drugs

General Information

The pharmacology, clinical pharmacology, clinical uses, efficacy, and adverse effects of aprindine have been extensively reviewed (1–5).

The adverse effects of aprindine most commonly affect the central nervous system. However, other less common but serious and potentially fatal adverse effects (neutropenia and liver damage) occur, and these limit its usefulness.

Aprindine is metabolized by CYP2D6, and one would therefore expect interactions with drugs that inhibit this isozyme or are metabolized by it.

Comparative studies

In a comparison of oral aprindine and propafenone in 32 patients (25 men and 7 women, aged 43–82) with paroxysmal or persistent atrial fibrillation, aprindine was effective in five of 29 and propafenone in six of 28; adverse effects were not reported (6).

There has been a multicenter, randomized, placebo-controlled, double-blind comparison of aprindine and digoxin in the prevention of atrial fibrillation and its recurrence in 141 patients with symptomatic paroxysmal or persistent atrial fibrillation who had converted to sinus rhythm (7). They were randomized in equal numbers to aprindine 40 mg/day, digoxin 0.25 mg/day, or placebo and followed every 2 weeks for 6 months. After 6 months the Kaplan–Meier estimates of the numbers of patients who had no recurrences with aprindine, digoxin, and placebo were 33, 29, and 22% respectively. The rates of adverse events were similar in the three groups. This suggests that aprindine has a very small beneficial effect in preventing relapse of symptomatic atrial fibrillation after conversion to sinus rhythm. Furthermore, recurrence occurred later with aprindine than with placebo or digoxin (about 60% recurrence at 115 days compared with 30 days).

Organs and Systems

Respiratory

Pneumonitis has been attributed to aprindine (SEDA-16, 179).

Nervous system

Aprindine can cause adverse effects in the central nervous system (SEDA-1, 156).

Hematologic

The incidence of leukopenia has been estimated at about 2 cases per 1000 patient-years (8).

Liver

Aprindine can cause liver damage (9).

References

1. Zipes DP, Troup PJ. New antiarrhythmic agents: amiodarone, aprindine, disopyramide, ethmozin, mexiletine, tocainide, verapamil. Am J Cardiol 1978;41(6):1005–24.
2. Schwartz JB, Keefe D, Harrison DC. Adverse effects of antiarrhythmic drugs. Drugs 1981;21(1):23–45.
3. Danilo P Jr. Aprindine. Am Heart J 1979;97(1):119–24.
4. Zipes DP, Elharrar V, Gilmour RF Jr, Heger JJ, Prystowsky EN. Studies with aprindine. Am Heart J 1980;100(6 Pt 2):1055–62.
5. Kodama I, Ogawa S, Inoue H, Kasanuki H, Kato T, Mitamura H, Hiraoka M, Sugimoto T. Profiles of aprindine, cibenzoline, pilsicainide and pirmenol in the framework of the Sicilian Gambit. The Guideline Committee for Clinical Use of Antiarrhythmic Drugs in Japan (Working Group of Arrhythmias of the Japanese Society of Electrocardiology). Jpn Circ J 1999;63(1):1–12.
6. Shibata N, Shirato K, Manaka M, Sugimoto C. Comparison of aprindine and propafenone for the treatment of atrial fibrillation. Ther Res 2001;22:794–6.
7. Atarashi H, Inoue H, Fukunami M, Sugi K, Hamada C, Origasa H; Sinus Rhythm Maintenance in Atrial Fibrillation Randomized Trial (SMART) Investigators. Double-blind placebo-controlled trial of aprindine and digoxin for the prevention of symptomatic atrial fibrillation. Circ J 2002;66(6):553–6.
8. Ibanez L, Juan J, Perez E, Carne X, Laporte JR. Agranulocytosis associated with aprindine and other antiarrhythmic drugs: an epidemiological approach. Eur Heart J 1991;12(5):639–41.
9. Elewaut A, Van Durme JP, Goethals L, Kauffman JM, Mussche M, Elinck W, Roels H, Bogaert M, Barbier F. Aprindine-induced liver injury. Acta Gastroenterol Belg 1977;40(5–6):236–43.

Aprotinin

General Information

Aprotinin is a fibrinolytic agent, a naturally occurring serine protease inhibitor derived from bovine lung. It is a polypeptide of 58 amino acids, with a molecular weight of 6512, which inhibits the action of several serine proteases, including trypsin, chymotrypsin, plasmin, and kallikrein. It is extracted on a commercial basis from bovine lung. By inhibiting kallikrein, aprotinin inhibits the formation of activated factor XII indirectly. It thus inhibits the initiation of both coagulation and fibrinolysis induced by the contact of blood with a foreign surface. It does not affect platelet function. In cardiac surgery, aprotinin reduces the risk of bleeding (1,2).

Aprotinin is not effective after oral administration, but is administered intravenously as a loading dose followed by a continuous infusion. Its activity is expressed as kallikrein inactivation units (KIU). The conventional (Munich) dose regimen consists of an initial 2×10^6 KIU bolus, a similar initial dose to prime the bypass machine, and then 0.5×10^6 KIU/ hour by continuous infusion thereafter. The half-life of aprotinin is about 2 hours. Plasma concentrations of 125 KIU/ml are necessary to inhibit plasmin, but a higher concentration of 300–500 KIU/ml is needed to inhibit kallikrein.

During normal fibrinolysis, inactive circulating plasminogen binds to fibrin through an active site that binds lysine. The bound plasminogen is then converted to plasmin by activators (such as tissue plasminogen activator, t-PA) and converted to plasmin, which breaks down the fibrin. Aminocaproic acid (EACA, 6-aminohexanoic acid, Amicar®) and tranexamic acid (Cyklokapron®) are structural analogues of lysine, which bind irreversibly to the lysine-binding sites on plasminogen, inhibiting binding to fibrin and thus the whole process of fibrinolysis (3,4). These agents inhibit the natural degradation of fibrin and so stabilize clots.

Uses

Aprotinin is widely used to inhibit fibrinolysis during cardiac surgery and orthotopic liver transplantation, and reduces the risk of bleeding (1,2). In addition, it is added as a constituent of several commercial formulations of fibrin sealants ("fibrin glues"), such as Quixil. The use of aprotinin in cardiopulmonary bypass surgery was pioneered by Royston, an anesthesiologist in London, who found that it reduced blood loss after both primary and repeat operations (5). It is also effective in operations normally characterized by particularly large blood losses, such as those in patients taking aspirin (6) and patients undergoing cardiac transplantation (7). It is also used to control blood loss in the setting of orthotopic liver transplantation (8,9), where accelerated fibrinolysis is an important component in the abnormalities of hemostasis, which can contribute to perioperative bleeding. Aprotinin is of value in controlling hemorrhage associated with hyperplasminemia (which can, for example, occur after thrombolytic therapy or in association with promyelocytic leukemia). A combination of aprotinin with tranexamic acid can prevent or delay rebleeding after rupture of an intracerebral aneurysm. Clinical trials have not confirmed any benefit from the use of aprotinin in acute pancreatitis.

General adverse effects

Some adverse reactions are associated with all antifibrinolytic agents, reflecting their effect on clot stability. Dissolution of extravascular blood clots may be resistant to physiological fibrinolysis. These drugs should not be used to treat hematuria due to blood loss from the upper urinary tract, as this can provoke painful clot retention and even renal insufficiency associated with bilateral ureteric obstruction (10,11).

Caution should be exercised in the administration of antifibrinolytic agents in disseminated intravascular coagulation (12,13).

Organs and Systems

Cardiovascular

The issue of whether the use of aprotinin is associated with an increased risk of vein graft thrombosis in cardiac bypass surgery has not been resolved (14,15). The use of aprotinin was not associated with an increased rate of early occlusion of saphenous vein or internal mammary artery grafts in controlled studies with coronary angiography (16–19).

In a randomized, placebo-controlled, multicenter study of aprotinin in coronary artery bypass surgery, there was no increase in mortality or the incidence of myocardial infarction (20).

There was no evidence of an increased risk of venous thromboembolism in patients receiving aprotinin in a small study after hip replacement (21).

Psychological, psychiatric

Psychotic reactions, including delirium, hallucinations, and confusion, have also been reported in patients given aprotinin, but it is possible that the symptoms were due to underlying pancreatitis (22).

Hematologic

It has been postulated that aprotinin potentiates a prothrombotic state (2). However, in randomized, controlled studies, there were no significant differences between aprotinin and placebo (2).

Disseminated intravascular coagulation can be aggravated by aprotinin, particularly in elderly people (13).

Urinary tract

Aprotinin has a high affinity for renal tissue; 80–90% is stored in the proximal tubule cells after 4 hours and is excreted over 12–24 hours (2). It has been hypothesized that aprotinin causes reversible overload of tubular reabsorption, resulting in transient renal dysfunction (2). It has also been postulated that aprotinin has a direct toxic effect on the proximal tubule cells or alters intrarenal blood flow, through inhibition of renin and kallikrein activity (2).

Immunologic

As might be expected with a bovine protein, allergic reactions can occur, and repeated exposure can even result in anaphylactic reactions. In view of this, some have advocated a strategy of using aprotinin only if excessive bleeding is a problem after surgery (23).

- An aphylactic reaction has been described after the use of fibrin glue as a sealant after mastectomy, probably due to the presence of bovine aprotinin (24).

In one study of 248 patients undergoing cardiac surgery, seven had allergic reactions, ranging from skin flushing to severe circulatory depression (25). Most of the reactions occurred when aprotinin was given a second time within 6 months after the first exposure. However, anaphylaxis has been documented after primary exposure (26). The reported incidence of anaphylactic reactions in other studies has ranged from 0.3 to 0.6% after a single exposure, rising to almost 5% with prior aprotinin exposure (1).

Up to 1980, 32 cases of non-fatal shock attributed to aprotinin had been reported to the Japanese Ministry of Health and Welfare, most concerning patients treated for pancreatitis (27). Although these patients survived, fatal anaphylaxis has been reported (28). Other apparently allergic reactions reported include erythema, urticaria, bronchospasm, nausea and vomiting, diarrhea, muscle pains, and blood pressure changes (29). A case of allergic pancreatitis attributed to aprotinin has also been reported (30).

There is evidence that severe allergic reactions to aprotinin are mediated by IgE, and preoperative screening for the presence of aprotinin-specific IgE antibodies can be of value in identifying patients at risk (31,32).

The sera of 150 patients who had undergone cardiac surgery and were receiving aprotinin for the first time have been studied before and after the operation. At 3.5 months after surgery, the prevalence of aprotinin-specific IgG antibodies was 33% (15/45) after local, 28% (13/46) after intravenous, and 69% (41/59) after combined exposure (33). The authors concluded that local administration of aprotinin induces a specific immune response and reinforces that of intravenous exposure; they therefore recommended that any exposure in a patient should be documented.

Allergic reactions, including anaphylaxis, can occur on re-exposure to aprotinin. The incidence rates of aprotinin-related reactions are 2.7% in re-exposed adults (5/183) and 1.2% in children (3/354), with an overall incidence of 1.8% (8/437). The following advice has been given to reduce the risk and severity of these reactions (1,2):

- give a test dose of aprotinin
- delay the first bolus injection until the surgeon starts the procedure
- give an antihistamine before re-exposure
- avoid re-exposure within the first 6 months after the last exposure.

Infection risk

Inevitably, concern has recently been expressed about the possibility of transmission of the prion believed to be responsible for bovine spongiform encephalopathy (BSE) and new variant Creutzfeldt-Jakob disease. However, the manufacturers of aprotinin have stated that the bovine lungs used as the source of aprotinin are collected in countries in South America (principally Uruguay) in which no cases of transmissible spongiform encephalopathy have been recorded. There is no evidence that any patient with new variant Creutzfeldt-Jakob disease has received aprotinin. Furthermore, in vitro experiments involving spiking of material with mouse-associated scrapie agent have demonstrated an 18-log reduction of the added prions during the manufacturing process (34).

Second-Generation Effects

Teratogenicity

There is no evidence from animal studies and clinical experience of teratogenicity or other adverse effects of aprotinin (35).

Drug–Drug Interactions

Suxamethonium

Aprotinin slightly reduces plasma cholinesterase activity and would be expected to prolong the action of suxamethonium in combination with other factors. However, re-paralysis has been reported when aprotinin was used after operations during which suxamethonium had been given alone or in combination with normal doses of D-tubocurarine (36).

References

1. Dietrich W. Incidence of hypersensitivity reactions. Ann Thorac Surg 1998;65(Suppl 6):S60–4.
2. Faught C, Wells P, Fergusson D, Laupacis A. Adverse effects of methods for minimizing perioperative allogeneic transfusion: a critical review of the literature. Transfus Med Rev 1998;12(3):206–25.
3. Astedt B. Clinical pharmacology of tranexamic acid. Scand J Gastroenterol Suppl 1987;137:22–5.
4. Hoylaerts M, Lijnen HR, Collen D. Studies on the mechanism of the antifibrinolytic action of tranexamic acid. Biochim Biophys Acta 1981;673(1):75–85.
5. Royston D, Bidstrup BP, Taylor KM, Sapsford RN. Effect of aprotinin on need for blood transfusion after repeat open-heart surgery. Lancet 1987;2(8571):1289–91.
6. Murkin JM, Lux J, Shannon NA, Guiraudon GM, Menkis AH, McKenzie FN, Novick RJ. Aprotinin significantly decreases bleeding and transfusion requirements in patients receiving aspirin and undergoing cardiac operations. J Thorac Cardiovasc Surg 1994;107(2):554–61.
7. Prendergast TW, Furukawa S, Beyer AJ 3rd, Eisen HJ, McClurken JB, Jeevanandam V. Defining the role of aprotinin in heart transplantation. Ann Thorac Surg 1996;62(3):670–4.
8. Neuhaus P, Bechstein WO, Lefebre B, Blumhardt G, Slama K. Effect of aprotinin on intraoperative bleeding and fibrinolysis in liver transplantation. Lancet 1989;2(8668):924–5.
9. Mallett SV, Cox D, Burroughs AK, Rolles K. Aprotinin and reduction of blood loss and transfusion requirements in orthotopic liver transplantation. Lancet 1990;336(8719):886–7.
10. van Itterbeek H, Vermylen J, Verstraete M. High obstruction of urine flow as a complication of the treatment with fibrinolysis inhibitors of haematuria in haemophiliacs. Acta Haematol 1968;39(4):237–42.
11. Fernandez Lucas M, Liano F, Navarro JF, Sastre JL, Quereda C, Ortuno J. Acute renal failure secondary to antifibrinolytic therapy. Nephron 1995;69(4):478–9.
12. Giles AR. Disseminated intravascular coagulation. In: Bloom AL, Forbes CD, Thomas DP, Tuddenham EGSD, editors. Haemostasis and Thrombosis. 3rd ed. Edinburgh: Churchill Livingstone, 1994.
13. Saffitz JE, Stahl DJ, Sundt TM, Wareing TH, Kouchoukos NT. Disseminated intravascular coagulation after administration of aprotinin in combination with deep hypothermic circulatory arrest. Am J Cardiol 1993;72(14):1080–2.
14. Westaby S, Katsumata T. Aprotinin and vein graft occlusion—the controversy continues. J Thorac Cardiovasc Surg 1998;116(5):731–3.
15. Bevan DH. Cardiac bypass haemostasis: putting blood through the mill. Br J Haematol 1999;104(2):208–19.
16. Lemmer JH Jr, Stanford W, Bonney SL, Breen JF, Chomka EV, Eldredge WJ, Holt WW, Karp RB, Laub GW, Lipton MJ, et al. Aprotinin for coronary bypass operations: efficacy, safety, and influence on early saphenous vein graft patency. A multicenter, randomized, double-blind, placebo-controlled study. J Thorac Cardiovasc Surg 1994;107(2):543–51.
17. Havel M, Grabenwoger F, Schneider J, Laufer G, Wollenek G, Owen A, Simon P, Teufelsbauer H, Wolner E. Aprotinin does not decrease early graft patency after coronary artery bypass grafting despite reducing postoperative bleeding and use of donated blood. J Thorac Cardiovasc Surg 1994;107(3):807–10.
18. Kalangos A, Tayyareci G, Pretre R, Di Dio P, Sezerman O. Influence of aprotinin on early graft thrombosis in patients undergoing myocardial revascularization. Eur J Cardiothorac Surg 1994;8(12):651–6.
19. Lass M, Simic O, Ostermeyer J. Re-graft patency and clinical efficacy of aprotinin in elective bypass surgery. Cardiovasc Surg 1997;5(6):604–7.
20. Levy JH, Pifarre R, Schaff HV, Horrow JC, Albus R, Spiess B, Rosengart TK, Murray J, Clark RE, Smith P. A multicenter, double-blind, placebo-controlled trial of aprotinin for reducing blood loss and the requirement for donor-blood transfusion in patients undergoing repeat coronary artery bypass grafting. Circulation 1995;92(8):2236–44.
21. Hayes A, Murphy DB, McCarroll M. The efficacy of single-dose aprotinin 2 million KIU in reducing blood loss and its impact on the incidence of deep venous thrombosis in patients undergoing total hip replacement surgery. J Clin Anesth 1996;8(5):357–60.
22. Vonk J. Ervaringen met Trasylol bij de behandeling van acute pancreatitis. Ned Tijdschr Geneeskd 1965;109:1510.
23. Cicek S, Demirkilic U, Ozal E, Kuralay E, Bingol H, Tatar H, Ozturk OY. Postoperative use of aprotinin in cardiac operations: an alternative to its prophylactic use. J Thorac Cardiovasc Surg 1996;112(6):1462–7.
24. Kon NF, Masumo H, Nakajima S, Tozawa R, Kimura M, Maeda S. [Anaphylactic reaction to aprotinin following topical use of biological tissue sealant.] Masui 1994;43(10):1606–10.
25. Dietrich W, Spath P, Ebell A, Richter JA. Prevalence of anaphylactic reactions to aprotinin: analysis of two hundred forty-eight reexposures to aprotinin in heart operations. J Thorac Cardiovasc Surg 1997;113(1):194–201.
26. Cohen DM, Norberto J, Cartabuke R, Ryu G. Severe anaphylactic reaction after primary exposure to aprotinin. Ann Thorac Surg 1999;67(3):837–8.
27. Japanese Ministry of Health and Welfare. Information on adverse reaction to drugs. Japan Med Gaz 1980;April 20:10.
28. Proud G, Chamberlain J. Anaphylactic reaction to aprotinin. Lancet 1976;2(7975):48–9.
29. Robert S, Wagner BK, Boulanger M, Richer M. Aprotinin. Ann Pharmacother 1996;30(4):372–80.
30. Siegel M, Werner M. Allergische Pankreatitis bei einer Sensibilisierung gegen den Kallikrein-Trypsin-Inaktivator. [Allergic pancreatitis caused by sensitization to the kallikrein–trypsin inactivator.] Dtsch Med Wochenschr 1965;90(39):1712–16.
31. Wuthrich B, Schmid P, Schmid ER, Tornic M, Johansson SG. IgE-mediated anaphylactic reaction to aprotinin during anaesthesia. Lancet 1992;340(8812):173–4.
32. Scheule AM, Beierlein W, Arnold S, Eckstein FS, Albes JM, Ziemer G. The significance of preformed aprotinin-specific antibodies in cardiosurgical patients. Anesth Analg 2000;90(2):262–6.
33. Scheule AM, Beierlein W, Wendel HP, Jurmann MJ, Eckstein FS, Ziemer G. Aprotinin in fibrin tissue adhesives induces specific antibody response and increases antibody response of high-dose intravenous application. J Thorac Cardiovasc Surg 1999;118(2):348–53.

34. Golker CF, Whiteman MD, Gugel KH, Gilles R, Stadler P, Kovatch RM, Lister D, Wisher MH, Calcagni C, Hubner GE. Reduction of the infectivity of scrapie agent as a model for BSE in the manufacturing process of Trasylol. Biologicals 1996;24(2):103–11.

35. Briggs GG, Freeman RK, Jaffe SJ. Drugs in Pregnancy and Lactation. 5th ed. Baltimore: Williams and Wilkins.

36. Chasapakis G, Dimas C. Possible interaction between muscle relaxants and the kallikrein–trypsin inactivator "Trasylol". Report of three cases. Br J Anaesth 1966;38(10):838–9.

Araliaceae

See also Herbal medicines

General Information

The genera in the family of Araliaceae (Table 1) include aralia, ginseng, and ivy.

Ginseng

Ginseng is an ambiguous vernacular term, which can refer to *Panax* species such as *Panax ginseng* (Asian ginseng) and *Panax quinquefolius* (American ginseng), *Eleutherococcus senticosus* (Siberian ginseng), *Pfaffia paniculata* (Brazilian ginseng), or unidentified material (for example Rumanian ginseng).

Asian ginseng (*P. ginseng*) contains a wide variety of flavonoids, saponins, steroids, sesquiterpenoids, and triterpenoids. These include ginsenolides and ginsenosides, protopanaxadiol, panaxadiol, panaxatriol, and panasinsene.

The botanical quality of ginseng preparations is problematic (1). For instance, when a case of neonatal androgenization was associated with maternal use of Siberian ginseng tablets during pregnancy, botanical analysis showed that the incriminated material almost certainly came from *Periploca sepium* (Chinese silk vine) (2).

Brazilian ginseng (*P. glomerata*) has been found to be contaminated with cadmium and mercury (3).

Table 1   The genera of Araliaceae

Aralia (spikenard, angelica)
Cheirodendron (cheirodendron)
Dendropanax (dendropanax)
Eleutherococcus (ginseng)
Fatsia (fatsia)
Hedera (ivy)
Kalopanax (castor aralia)
Meryta (meryta)
Munroidendron (munroidendron)
Oplopanax (oplopanax)
Panax (ginseng)
Polyscias (aralia)
Pseudopanax (pseudopanax)
Reynoldsia (reynoldsia)
Schefflera (schefflera)
Tetraplasandra (tetraplasandra)
Tetrapanax (tetrapanax)

There is no good evidence that ginseng confers benefit for any indication (4).

Adverse effects

The various adverse effects that have been attributed to ginseng formulations include hypertension, pressure headaches, dizziness, estrogen-like effects, vaginal bleeding, and mastalgia. Prolonged use has been associated with a "ginseng abuse syndrome" including symptoms like hypertension, edema, morning diarrhea, skin eruptions, insomnia, depression, and amenorrhea. However, most reports are difficult to interpret, because of the absence of a control group, the simultaneous use of other agents, insufficient information about dosage, and lack of botanical authentication (1).

The authors of a review of the adverse effects associated with *P. ginseng* concluded that it is generally safe but at high doses can cause insomnia, headache, diarrhea, and cardiovascular and endocrine disorders (5). Inappropriate use and suboptimal formulations were deemed to be the most likely reason for adverse effects of ginseng. The authors of a systematic review reached similar conclusions and showed that serious adverse effects of ginseng seem to be true rarities (6).

Cardiovascular

The WHO database contains seven cases from five countries of ginseng intake followed by arterial hypertension (7). In five of them no other medication was noted. In four cases the outcome was mentioned, which was invariably full recovery without sequelae after withdrawal of ginseng.

Nervous system

- A 56-year-old woman with previous affective disorder had an episode of mania while taking ginseng (8). She was treated with neuroleptic drugs and benzodiazepines and ginseng was withdrawn. She made a rapid full recovery.

Ginseng has also been associated with a case of cerebral arteritis (9).

Psychiatric

A woman with prior episodes of depression had a manic episode several days after starting to take *P. ginseng* (10).

Skin

Stevens–Johnson syndrome occurred in a 27-year-old man who was a regular user of *P. ginseng* (11).

Musculoskeletal

Aggravation of muscle injury has been attributed to ginseng (SED-13, 1461) (12).

Drug interactions

- A 74-year-old man had increased serum digoxin concentrations without signs of toxicity while taking Siberian ginseng (13). Common causes of increased serum digoxin were ruled out, and the association with ginseng use was confirmed by dechallenge and rechallenge. The rise in serum digoxin concentration could have been due to cardiac glycosides contained in *Periploca sepium*, a common substitute for *E. senticosus* (14).

Diuretic resistance has been reported in a patient consuming a formulation containing germanium and ginseng (species unspecified) (15).

Interactions of antidepressants with herbal medicines have been reported (16). Ginseng has been reported to cause mania, tremor, and headache when used in combination with conventional monoamine oxidase inhibitors.

In one case the concomitant use of *P. ginseng* and warfarin resulted in loss of anticoagulant activity (17). However, in an open, crossover, randomized study in 12 healthy men ginseng did not affect the pharmacokinetics or pharmacodynamics of *S*-warfarin or *R*-warfarin (18).

References

1. Cui J, Garle M, Eneroth P, Bjorkhem I. What do commercial ginseng preparations contain? Lancet 1994;344(8915):134.
2. Awang DV. Maternal use of ginseng and neonatal androgenization. JAMA 1991;266(3):363.
3. Caldas ED, Machado LL. Cadmium, mercury and lead in medicinal herbs in Brazil. Food Chem Toxicol 2004;42(4):599–603.
4. Vogler BK, Pittler MH, Ernst E. The efficacy of ginseng. A systematic review of randomised clinical trials. Eur J Clin Pharmacol 1999;55(8):567–75.
5. Xie JT, Mehendale SR, Maleckar SA, Yuan CS. Is ginseng free from adverse effects? Oriental Pharm Exp Med 2002;2:80–6.
6. Coon JT, Ernst E. *Panax ginseng*: a systematic review of adverse effects and drug interactions. Drug Saf 2002;25(5):323–44.
7. Anonymous. Ginseng—hypertension. WHO SIGNAL, 2002.
8. Vazquez I, Aguera-Ortiz LF. Herbal products and serious side effects: a case of ginseng-induced manic episode. Acta Psychiatr Scand 2002;105(1):76–8.
9. Ryu SJ, Chien YY. Ginseng-associated cerebral arteritis. Neurology 1995;45(4):829–30.
10. Gonzalez-Seijo JC, Ramos YM, Lastra I. Manic episode and ginseng: report of a possible case. J Clin Psychopharmacol 1995;15(6):447–8.
11. Dega H, Laporte JL, Frances C, Herson S, Chosidow O. Ginseng as a cause for Stevens–Johnson syndrome? Lancet 1996;347(9011):1344.
12. Anonymous. Ginseng—muskelskada? Inf Socialstyr Läkemedelsavd 1988;4:114.
13. McRae S. Elevated serum digoxin levels in a patient taking digoxin and Siberian ginseng. CMAJ 1996;155(3):293–5.
14. Awang DVC. Siberian ginseng toxicity may be case of mistaken identity. Can Med Assoc J 1996;155:1237.
15. Becker BN, Greene J, Evanson J, Chidsey G, Stone WJ. Ginseng-induced diuretic resistance. JAMA 1996;276(8):606–7.
16. Fugh-Berman A. Herb–drug interactions. Lancet 2000;355(9198):134–8.
17. Janetzky K, Morreale AP. Probable interaction between warfarin and ginseng. Am J Health Syst Pharm 1997;54(6):692–3.
18. Jiang X, Williams KM, Liauw WS, Ammit AJ, Roufogalis BD, Duke CC, Day RO, McLachlan AJ. Effect of St John's wort and ginseng on the pharmacokinetics and pharmacodynamics of warfarin in healthy subjects. Br J Clin Pharmacol 2004;57(5):592–9.

Arecaceae

See also Herbal medicines

General Information

The genera in the family of Arecaceae (Table 1) include various types of palm.

Areca catechu

Areca catechu (areca, betel) contains piperidine alkaloids, such as guvacine, guvacoline, and isoguvacine, and pyridine alkaloids, such as arecaidine, arecolidine, and arecoline.

Many of the world's population (more than 200 million people worldwide) chew betel nut quid, a combination of areca nut, betel pepper leaf (from *Piper betle*), lime paste, and tobacco leaf. The major alkaloid of the areca nut, arecoline, can produce cholinergic adverse effects (such as bronchoconstriction) (1) as well as antagonism of anticholinergic agents (2). The lime in the betel quid causes hydrolysis of arecoline to arecaidine, a central nervous system stimulant, which accounts, together with the essential oil of the betel pepper, for the euphoric effects of chewing betel quid.

Adverse effects

Glycemia and anthropometric risk markers for type 2 diabetes were examined in relation to betel usage. Of 993 supposedly healthy Bangladeshis 12% had diabetes. A further 145 of 187 subjects at risk of diabetes (spot glucose over 6.5 mmol/l less than 2 hours after food or over 4.5 mmol/l more than 2 hours after food) had a second blood glucose sample taken; 61 were confirmed as being at risk, and had an oral glucose tolerance test; nine new diabetics were identified. Spot blood

Table 1 The genera of Arecaceae

Acoelorraphe (palm)
Acrocomia (acrocomia)
Aiphanes (aiphanes)
Archontophoenix (archontophoenix)
Calyptronoma (manac)
Caryota (fishtail palm)
Chamaedorea (chamaedorea)
Coccothrinax (silver palm)
Cocos (coconut palm)
Dypsis (butterfly palm)
Elaeis (oil palm)
Gaussia (gaussia)
Livistona (livistona)
Phoenix (date palm)
Prestoea (prestoea)
Pritchardia (pritchardia)
Pseudophoenix (pseudophoenix)
Ptychosperma (ptychosperma)
Rhapidophyllum (rhapidophyllum)
Roystonea (royal palm)
Sabal (palmetto)
Serenoa (serenoa)
Thrinax (thatch palm)
Washingtonia (fan palm)

glucose values fell with time after eating and increased independently with waist size and age. Waist size was strongly related to use of betel, and was independent of other factors such as age. The authors suggested that betel chewing may contribute to the risk of type 2 diabetes mellitus (3).

The saliva of betel nut chewers contains nitrosamines derived from areca nut alkaloids (4), and the use of areca nuts has been widely implicated in the development of oral cancers.

Serenoa repens

S. repens (American dwarf palm tree, cabbage palm, sabal, saw palmetto) has mainly been used to treat benign prostatic hyperplasia. In placebo-controlled and comparative studies its efficacy in benign prostatic hyperplasia and lower urinary tract symptoms has been demonstrated (5). Numerous mechanisms of action have been proposed, including an antiandrogenic action, an anti-inflammatory effect, and an antiproliferative influence through inhibition of growth factors.

A systematic review and meta-analysis of randomized trials of *S. repens* in men with benign prostatic hyperplasia showed that saw palmetto extracts improve urinary symptoms and flow measures to a greater extent than placebo, and similar improvements in urinary symptoms and flow measures to the 5-alpha-reductase inhibitor finasteride with fewer adverse effects (6).

Adverse effects
Hematologic

- A 53-year-old man, who had self-medicated with a saw palmetto supplement for benign prostatic hyperplasia, had profuse bleeding (estimated blood loss 2 liters) after resection of a meningioma and required 4 units of packed erythrocytes, 3 units of platelets, and 3 units of fresh frozen plasma (7). Postoperatively his bleeding time was 21 minutes (reference range 2–10 minutes), but all other coagulation tests were normal. He made an uneventful recovery.

The authors concluded that the cyclo-oxygenase inhibitory activity of saw palmetto had caused platelet dysfunction, which had resulted in abnormal bleeding.

References

1. Taylor RF, al-Jarad N, John LM, Conroy DM, Barnes NC. Betel-nut chewing and asthma. Lancet 1992;339(8802):1134–6.
2. Deahl M. Betel nut-induced extrapyramidal syndrome: an unusual drug interaction. Mov Disord 1989;4(4):330–2.
3. Mannan N, Boucher BJ, Evans SJ. Increased waist size and weight in relation to consumption of *Areca catechu* (betel-nut); a risk factor for increased glycaemia in Asians in east London. Br J Nutr 2000;83(3):267–75.
4. Pickwell SM, Schimelpfening S, Palinkas LA. "Betelmania." Betel quid chewing by Cambodian women in the United States and its potential health effects. West J Med 1994;160(4):326–30.
5. Buck AC. Is there a scientific basis for the therapeutic effects of *Serenoa repens* in benign prostatic hyperplasia? Mechanisms of action. J Urol 2004;172(5 Pt 1):1792–9.
6. Wilt T, Ishani A. *Serenoa repens* for treatment of benign prostatic hyperplasia (Cochrane Review). In: The Cochrane Library. Oxford: Update Software, 1999:1.
7. Cheema P, El-Mefty O, Jazieh AR. Intraoperative haemorrhage associated with the use of extract of saw palmetto herb: a case report and review of literature. J Intern Med 2001;250(2):167–9.

Aristolochiaceae

See also Herbal medicines

General Information

The family of Aristolochiaceae contains three genera:

1. *Aristolochia* (dutchman's pipe)
2. *Asarum* (wild ginger)
3. *Hexastylis* (heartleaf).

Aristolochia species

Plants belonging to the genus of *Aristolochia* are rich in aristolochic acids and aristolactams.

In the UK, the long-term (2 and 6 years) use of *Aristolochia* species in Chinese herbal mixtures, taken as an oral medication or herbal tea, resulted in Chinese-herb nephropathy with end-stage renal insufficiency (1). In reaction to these reports, the erstwhile Medicines Control Agency banned all *Aristolochia* species for medicinal use in the UK.

In June 2001, the FDA issued a nationwide alert, recalling 13 "Treasure of the East" herbal products containing aristolochic acid. Before this alert, the FDA had issued several warnings:

- On 4 April 2001 a "Dear Health Professional" letter was sent, drawing attention to serious renal disease associated with the use of aristolochic acid-containing dietary supplements or "traditional medicines." Health professionals were urged to review patients who had had unexplained renal disease, especially those with urothelial tract tumors and interstitial nephritis with end-stage renal insufficiency, to determine if such products had been used.
- On 9 April 2001 a letter was sent to industry associations, detailing the reported cases of renal disease associated with aristolochic acid.
- On 11 April 2001 the FDA cautioned consumers to immediately discontinue any dietary supplements or "traditional medicines" that contain aristolochic acid, including products with "Aristolochia," "Bragantia," or "Asarum" listed as their ingredients.

In a related action, Health Canada first issued a warning on aristolochic acid in November 1999 that this ingredient posed a Class I Health Hazard with a potential to cause serious health effects or death (2) and warned consumers not to use the pediatric product Tao Chih Pien. This Chinese product, sold in the form of tablets, is said to be a diuretic and a laxative. It is not labeled to contain aristolochic acid. However, the Chinese labeling says that it contains Mu Tong, a traditional term used to describe numerous herbs, including aristolochia; subsequent product analysis showed that Tao Chih Pien does indeed contain aristolochic acid. Health Canada advised individuals in possession of this product not to consume it and to return it to the place of purchase. It also issued a Customs Alert for the product to prevent the importation and sale of Tao Chih Pien and advised Canadians not to consume Longdan or Lung Tan Xi Gan products, since they may also contain aristolochic acid.

The product Longdan Qiegan Wan ("Wetness Heat" Pill) was removed from the Australian Register of Therapeutic Goods following the detection of aristolochic acid by laboratory testing by the Therapeutic Goods Administration (3).

In 2002 the Medicines Safety Authority of the Ministry of Health in New Zealand (Medsafe) ordered the withdrawal of several traditional Chinese medicines sold as herbal remedies (4). The products included Guan Xin Su He capsules, Long Dan Xie Gan Wan Pills, and Zhiyuan Xinqinkeli sachets.

In 2004 the UK's Medicines and Healthcare products Regulatory Agency, with the co-operation of Customs and Excise, seized a potentially illegal consignment of 90 000 traditional Chinese medicine tablets, Jingzhi Kesou Tanchuan, which reportedly contained *Aristolochia*.

In December 2004 the Hong Kong authorities warned the public not to take the product Shen yi Qian Lie Hui Chin, as laboratory tests showed that it contained aristolochic acid.

Adverse effects
Several review articles have covered the toxicology of *Aristolochia* (5–8).

Liver
Hepatitis has been attributed to *Aristolochia* (9).

- A 49-year-old woman developed signs of hepatitis. All the usual causes were ruled out. The history revealed that she had recently started to use a Chinese herbal tea to treat her eczema. Examination of the herbal mixture showed that it contained *Aristolochia debilis* root and seven other medicinal plants.

Like *Aristolochia fangchi*, *A. debilis* contains the highly toxic aristolochic acid and was therefore the likely cause of the toxic hepatitis.

Urinary tract
Aristolochic acid is a potent carcinogen and can cause serious kidney damage, "Chinese herb nephropathy," which can be fatal (10). Renal fibrosis has also been reported (11).

Numerous reports from many countries have confirmed that plants from the *Aristolochia* species are the cause of the nephropathy (12,13), and the toxic agent has been confirmed to be aristolochic acid (14).

- A 46-year-old Chinese woman, living in Belgium and China, developed subacute renal insufficiency (15). Her creatinine concentration had increased from 80 µmol/l (November 1998) to 327 µmol/l (January 2000). During the preceding 6 months she had taken a patent medicine

bought in China "for waste discharging and youth keeping." The package insert did not list any herbs of the *Aristolochia* species. Kidney biopsy showed extensive hypocellular interstitial fibrosis, tubular atrophy, and glomerulosclerosis. Analysis of the Chinese medicine demonstrated the presence of aristolochic acid. She required hemodialysis in June 2000 and received a renal transplant 4 months later.

- A 58-year-old Japanese woman with CREST syndrome (calcinosis, Raynaud's syndrome, esophageal sclerosis, sclerodactyly, and telangiectasia) developed progressive renal dysfunction (16). Renal biopsy showed changes typical of Chinese herb nephropathy. Analyses of Chinese herbs she had taken for several years demonstrated the presence of aristolochic acid. Oral prednisolone improved her renal function and anemia.
- A 59-year-old man developed renal insufficiency after self-medication for 5 years with a Chinese herbal remedy to treat his hepatitis (17). Renal biopsy showed signs characteristic of Chinese herb nephropathy. Analysis of the remedy proved the presence of aristolochic acids I and II.

In Belgium, an outbreak of nephropathy in about 70 individuals was attributed to a slimming formulation that supposedly included the Chinese herbs *Stephania tetrandra* and *Magnolia officinalis*. However, analysis showed that the root of *S. tetrandra* (Chinese name Fangji) had in all probability been substituted or contaminated with the root of *Aristolochia fangchi* (Chinese name Guang fangji) (18,19). The nephropathy was characterized by extensive interstitial fibrosis with atrophy and loss of the tubules (20). At least one patient had evidence suggestive of urothelial malignancies (21). The same remedy was apparently also distributed in France, and two cases have been reported from Toulouse and one possible case from Nice (22).

Subsequently, Belgian nephrologists re-investigated 71 patients who were originally affected by this syndrome (23). Using multiple regression analysis, they showed that the original dose of *Aristolochia* was the only significant predictor of progression of renal insufficiency. The risk of end-stage renal insufficiency in these patients increased linearly with the dose of *Aristolochia*.

In Japan two cases of Chinese herb nephropathy were associated with chronic use of *Aristolochia manchuriensis* (Kan-mokutsu) (24). The diagnosis was confirmed by renal biopsy and the toxic constituents were identified as aristolochic acids I, II, and D.

Taiwanese authors have reported 12 cases of suspected Chinese herb nephropathy, confirmed by renal biopsy (25). Renal function deteriorated rapidly in most patients, despite withdrawal of the Aristolochia. Seven patients underwent dialysis and the rest had slowly progressive renal insufficiency. One patient was subsequently found to have a bladder carcinoma. Other cases have been reported from mainland China (26) and Taiwan (27).

Because of fear of malignancies the Belgian researchers who first described the condition have advocated prophylactic removal of the kidneys and ureters in patients with Chinese herb nephropathy. Of 39 patients who agreed to this, 18 (46%) had urothelial carcinoma, 19 of the others had mild to moderate urothelial dysplasia, and only two had normal urothelium (28). All tissue samples contained aristolochic acid-related DNA in adducts. The original dose of *Aristolochia* correlated positively with the risk of urothelial carcinoma.

Animal experiments have shed more light on Chinese herb nephropathy (29). Salt-depleted male Wistar rats were regularly injected with two different doses of aristolochic acid or with vehicle only for 35 days. The histological signs of Chinese herb nephropathy were demonstrated only in animals that received the high dose of 10 mg/kg. The authors presented this as an animal model for studying the pathophysiology of Chinese herb nephropathy.

Tumorigenicity
Aristolochic acid I and aristolochic acid II are mutagenic in several test systems. A mixture of these two compounds was so highly carcinogenic in rats that even homeopathic *Aristolochia* dilutions have been banned from the German market. The closely related aristolactam I and aristolactam II have not been submitted to carcinogenicity testing, but these compounds similarly show mutagenic activity in bacteria.

When 19 kidneys and urethras removed from 10 patients with Chinese herb nephropathy who required kidney transplantation were examined histologically, there were conclusive signs of neoplasms in 40% (30).

One patient who had a urothelial malignancy 6 years after the onset of Chinese herb nephropathy later developed a breast carcinoma that metastasised to the liver (31). The urothelial malignancy contained aristolochic acid-DNA adducts and mutations in the p53 gene, and the same mis-sense mutation in codon 245 of exon 7 of p53 was found in DNA from the breast and liver tumors. However, DNA extracted from the urothelial tumor also showed a mutation in codon 139 of exon 5, which was not present in the breast and liver.

Asarum heterotropoides

The Chinese herbal medicine Xu xin (32) is made from the leaves and aerial parts of *Asarum heterotropoides*. It is used for the symptomatic relief of colds, headaches, and other pains.

Adverse effects
The volatile oil of Xu xin causes the following adverse effects: vomiting, sweating, dyspnea, restlessness, fever, palpitation, and nervous system depression. Death can result from respiratory paralysis at high doses.

References

1. Lord GM, Tagore R, Cook T, Gower P, Pusey CD. Nephropathy caused by Chinese herbs in the UK. Lancet 1999;354(9177):481–2.
2. Anonymous. Aristolochic acid. Warnings on more products containing aristolochic acid. WHO Pharmaceuticals Newslett 2002;3:1.
3. Anonymous. *Aristolochia*. More products cancelled WHO Pharmaceuticals Newslett 2002;1:1.
4. Anonymous. Traditional medicines. Several Chinese medicines withdrawn due to presence of prescription and pharmacy-only components. WHO Pharmaceuticals Newslett 2003;1:2–3.
5. Chen JK. Nephropathy associated with the use of *Aristolochia*. Herbal Gram 2000;48:44–5.
6. Pokhrel PK, Ergil KV. Aristolochic acid: a toxicological review. Clin Acupunct Orient Med 2000;1:161–6.
7. Hammes MG. Anmerkungen zu *Aristolochia*—eine Recherche in chinesischen Originaltexten. Dtsch Z Akupunkt 2000;3:198–200.
8. Wiebrecht A. Über die *Aristolochia*-Nephropathie. Dtsch Z Akupunkt 2000;3:187–97.
9. Levi M, Guchelaar HJ, Woerdenbag HJ, Zhu YP. Acute hepatitis in a patient using a Chinese herbal tea—a case report. Pharm World Sci 1998;20(1):43–4.
10. Anonymous. *Aristolochia*. Alert against products containing aristolochic acid. WHO Pharm Newslett 2001;2/3:1.
11. Anonymous. Aristolochic acid. Warning concerning interstitial renal fibrosis. WHO Newslett 2000;2:1.
12. Xi-wen D, Xiang-rong R, Shen LI. Current situation of Chinese-herbs-induced renal damage and its countermeasures. Chin J Integrative Med 2001;7:162–6.
13. Tamaki K, Okuda S. Chinese herbs nephropathy: a variant form in Japan. Intern Med 2001;40(4):267–8.
14. Lebeau C, Arlt VM, Schmeiser HH, Boom A, Verroust PJ, Devuyst O, Beauwens R. Aristolochic acid impedes endocytosis and induces DNA adducts in proximal tubule cells. Kidney Int 2001;60(4):1332–42.
15. Gillerot G, Jadoul M, Arlt VM, van Ypersele De Strihou C, Schmeiser HH, But PP, Bieler CA, Cosyns JP. Aristolochic acid nephropathy in a Chinese patient: time to abandon the term "Chinese herbs nephropathy?" Am J Kidney Dis 2001;38(5):E26.
16. Nishimagi E, Kawaguchi Y, Terai C, Kajiyama H, Hara M, Kamatani N. Progressive interstitial renal fibrosis due to Chinese herbs in a patient with calcinosis Raynaud esophageal sclerodactyly telangiectasia (CREST) syndrome. Intern Med 2001;40(10):1059–63.
17. Cronin AJ, Maidment G, Cook T, Kite GC, Simmonds MS, Pusey CD, Lord GM. Aristolochic acid as a causative factor in a case of Chinese herbal nephropathy. Nephrol Dial Transplant 2002;17(3):524–5.
18. Vanherweghem JL, Depierreux M, Tielemans C, Abramowicz D, Dratwa M, Jadoul M, Richard C, Vandervelde D, Verbeelen D, Vanhaelen-Fastre R, et al. Rapidly progressive interstitial renal fibrosis in young women: association with slimming regimen including Chinese herbs. Lancet 1993;341(8842):387–91.
19. Vanhaelen M, Vanhaelen-Fastre R, But P, Vanherweghem JL. Identification of aristolochic acid in Chinese herbs. Lancet 1994;343(8890):174.
20. Depierreux M, Van Damme B, Vanden Houte K, Vanherweghem JL. Pathologic aspects of a newly described nephropathy related to the prolonged use of Chinese herbs. Am J Kidney Dis 1994;24(2):172–80.
21. Cosyns JP, Jadoul M, Squifflet JP, Van Cangh PJ, van Ypersele de Strihou C. Urothelial malignancy in nephropathy due to Chinese herbs. Lancet 1994;344(8916):188.
22. Stengel B, Jones E. Insuffisance rénale terminale associée à la consommation d'herbes chinoises en France. [End-stage renal insufficiency associated with Chinese herbal consumption in France.] Nephrologie 1998;19(1):15–20.
23. Martinez MC, Nortier J, Vereerstraeten P, Vanherweghem JL. Progression rate of Chinese herb nephropathy: impact of *Aristolochia fangchi* ingested dose. Nephrol Dial Transplant 2002;17(3):408–12.
24. Tanaka A, Nishida R, Maeda K, Sugawara A, Kuwahara T. Chinese herb nephropathy in Japan presents adult-onset Fanconi syndrome: could different components of aristolochic acids cause a different type of Chinese herb nephropathy? Clin Nephrol 2000;53(4):301–6.

25. Yang CS, Lin CH, Chang SH, Hsu HC. Rapidly progressive fibrosing interstitial nephritis associated with Chinese herbal drugs. Am J Kidney Dis 2000;35(2):313–18.

26. But PP, Ma SC. Chinese-herb nephropathy. Lancet 1999;354(9191):1731–2.

27. Lee CT, Wu MS, Lu K, Hsu KT. Renal tubular acidosis, hypokalemic paralysis, rhabdomyolysis, and acute renal failure—a rare presentation of Chinese herbal nephropathy. Ren Fail 1999;21(2):227–30.

28. Nortier JL, Martinez MC, Schmeiser HH, Arlt VM, Bieler CA, Petein M, Depierreux MF, De Pauw L, Abramowicz D, Vereerstraeten P, Vanherweghem JL. Urothelial carcinoma associated with the use of a Chinese herb (*Aristolochia fangchi*). N Engl J Med 2000;342(23):1686–92.

29. Debelle FD, Nortier JL, De Prez EG, Garbar CH, Vienne AR, Salmon IJ, Deschodt-Lanckman MM, Vanherweghem JL. Aristolochic acids induce chronic renal failure with interstitial fibrosis in salt-depleted rats. J Am Soc Nephrol 2002;13(2):431–6.

30. Cosyns JP, Jadoul M, Squifflet JP, Wese FX, van Ypersele de Strihou C. Urothelial lesions in Chinese-herb nephropathy. Am J Kidney Dis 1999;33(6):1011–17.

31. Lord GM, Hollstein M, Arlt VM, Roufosse C, Pusey CD, Cook T, Schmeiser HH. DNA adducts and p53 mutations in a patient with aristolochic acid-associated nephropathy. Am J Kidney Dis 2004;43(4):e11–17.

32. Drew AK, Whyte IM, Bensoussan A, Dawson AH, Zhu X, Myers SP. Chinese herbal medicine toxicology database: monograph on Herba Asari, "xi xin." J Toxicol Clin Toxicol 2002;40(2):169–72.

Arsenic

General Information

Arsenic is a metallic element (symbol As; atomic no. 33), which exists in several allotropic forms. Various ores contain crystalline forms of arsenic salts: cobaltite contains cobalt arsenic sulfide; mispickel (arsenopyrite) iron arsenic sulfide; orpiment arsenic trisulfide; proustite (ruby silver ore) silver arsenic sulfide; realgar arsenic sulfide; and tennantite copper arsenic sulfide.

Arsenic has a long history of medicinal uses. Thomas Fowler introduced it in the form of potassium arsenite (Fowler's solution) in the late 18th century to treat ague and Sir David Bruce used it in the late 19th century to treat trypanosomiasis. In the early 20th century Paul Ehrlich synthesized and tested a large series of arsenicals, in the hope of finding one that was effective in syphilis, and emerged with arsphenamine (Salvarsan, compound 606). Subsequently other arsenicals were synthesized, such as neoarsphenamine (for syphilis) and tryparsamide and acetarsol (for trypanosomiasis).

In recent times arsenic and arsenicals have been considered obsolete in medicine, because of their limited therapeutic value, multisystem toxicity, and apparent carcinogenic properties (SED-8, 502) (SED-9, 368). However, arsenic compounds have been used to treat various types of leukemia (1–3), including acute promyelocytic leukemia, chronic myelogenous leukemia, and multiple myeloma (4). Arsenic trioxide is effective in acute promyelocytic leukemia, achieving a complete remission rate of 60–90% (5,6). It is particularly used in patients who are resistant to all-trans retinoic acid (7). Arsenic trioxide is also emerging as a therapy for multiple myeloma (8).

Reports continue to be published on incidents related to the use of traditional herbal medications from China and elsewhere that contain arsenic among other toxic substances (9,10).

There are still occasional cases of patients with late effects from obsolete formulations such as Fowler's solution or neoarsphenamine (SEDA-16, 231). As late as 1998 a case of severe chronic poisoning resulting in fatal multiorgan failure including hepatic portal fibrosis and subsequent angiosarcoma was traced back to exposure to arsenical salts used for the treatment of psoriasis many years before (11) (SEDA-22, 243). In some non-Western countries arsenic is apparently still being used in dentistry for devitalization of inflamed pulp and sensitive dentine, and cases have been described in which this has resulted in arsenical necrosis of the jaws, affecting the maxilla or mandible (12). Some exposure to arsenic may still be occurring from traditional remedies of undeclared composition, and as with other metals there may be environmental contact, notably from semiconductor materials.

General adverse effects

Chronic arsenic poisoning is marked by edema of the eyelids and face, mucosal inflammation, pruritus, anorexia, vomiting, and diarrhea. Long-term use of small doses can produce keratinization and dryness of the skin, sometimes with frank dermatitis and pigmentation; alopecia can follow, and basal cell epithelioma is a late effect (13). In the long run, as in the fatal cases noted in the introduction of this monograph, there is serious damage to internal organs.

The adverse effects of arsenic trioxide have been described in a patient with recurrent acute promyelocytic leukemia resistant to all-trans retinoic acid (14).

- A 15-year-old African American girl, with multiple recurrent acute promyelocytic leukemia that had resisted conventional chemotherapy, was given arsenic trioxide (As_2O_3) 10 mg intravenously for 28 days and again for a further 28 days after a 4-week break. She had a complete remission by morphological, cytogenetic, and molecular criteria. About 6 months later she again relapsed and had another course of arsenic trioxide, which produced a morphological, but not a cytogenetic or molecular, remission. Arsenic trioxide was well tolerated. Skin dryness was treated with topical moisturizers. Gastrointestinal upset, including mild nausea without vomiting or cramping pain, occurred only during intravenous therapy. No other toxicity was noted.

In acute promyelocytic leukemia arsenic trioxide can cause a syndrome similar to the retinoic acid syndrome (15), with fever, skin rash, edema, pleural effusion, pericardial effusion, and acute respiratory failure.

- A 37-year-old woman with acute promyelocytic leukemia was treated with all-trans retinoic acid, idarubicin, and cytosine arabinoside, with complete remission after one course. However, she had an episode of retinoic acid syndrome with fever, edema, and pericardial effusion, which resolved after all-*trans* retinoic acid was withdrawn. When her leukemia relapsed she was treated with arsenic trioxide 10 mg/day. Leukocytosis again developed, with symptoms (fever, skin rash, and edema) resembling the retinoic acid syndrome, which was quickly relieved by steroids. She received two courses of arsenic trioxide each for 30 days and her complete blood count returned to normal 2 weeks after the second course of treatment. The bone marrow also reached complete remission.

Organs and Systems

Cardiovascular

Atrioventricular block is very rare after arsenic trioxide treatment for refractory acute promyelocytic leukemia (16).

- A 34-year-old woman with acute promyelocytic leukemia was given arsenic trioxide solution 0.1%, 10 ml/day for 7 days. A generalized skin rash appeared, and her serum transaminases rose. An electrocardiogram was normal. A second course of arsenic trioxide was used about 3 months later. She felt palpitation and mild dyspnea and had complete atrioventricular block. Echocardiography showed a normal left ventricle. A ^{201}thallium myocardial perfusion scan did not show a perfusion defect. Arsenic trioxide was withheld. Sinus rhythm returned 3 days later. Complete atrioventricular block recurred later when arsenic trioxide was re-administered, albeit in a lower dosage for a shorter period of time.

The heart block due to arsenic trioxide in this case was reversible and did not correlate with the patient's leukemic status.

In 19 patients with hematological malignancies given arsenic trioxide 10–20 mg in 500 ml of 5% dextrose/isotonic saline over 3 hours daily for up to 60 days, there were three cases of torsade de pointes (17).

Nervous system

In a case of a rapidly progressive neuropathy with arsenic, a contributory role of thiamine deficiency was implied (18).

- A 46-year-old woman with acute promyelocytic leukemia was given arsenic trioxide 10 mg/day for 28 days. On day 33 she complained of numbness in the legs and on day 37 all four limbs were paralysed and areflexic. Her speech was inaudible and she had bulbar paralysis. Nerve conduction studies showed a generalized reduction in sensory action potentials. Thiamine deficiency was confirmed and she was given parenteral thiamine (100 mg/day). By the next day the power in her arms had dramatically improved and her speech had become audible. Over the next 5 days, she regained full power in the arms. Subsequently she was given arsenic trioxide 5 mg/day for 28 days with oral thiamine, without neurological deterioration this time. The power in her legs continued to improve.

The members of a family in India, in the business of preparing and manufacturing indigenous medicines containing arsenicals, consumed a home-made vitalizer for health which accidentally got contaminated with arsenicals (19).

- A 50-year-old woman developed severe vomiting, abdominal colic, and diarrhea, which persisted for 5–6 days and 2 weeks later developed tingling, numbness, paresthesia, and gradually progressive weakness of all four limbs. She had gross hyperpigmentation of the face, arms, and upper chest, hyperkeratosis of the palms, and transverse white lines (Mees' lines) in the finger nails. She had a symmetrical, predominantly distal, peripheral sensorimotor neuropathy in all four limbs. Meanwhile, her 52-year-old husband and her 28-year-old son developed severe gastrointestinal problems. Her husband died within 48 hours of onset and the son developed severe wasting, weakness, and a sensorimotor flaccid quadriparesis, similar to that of his mother. Two younger sons, aged 22 and 20 years, and an 18-year-old daughter were out of town but returned after the death of their father. They also developed severe diarrhea, vomiting, abdominal pain, and tingling of the hands and feet within 2–3 weeks. Arsenic concentrations were found in the hair and nails, and the concentrations were directly proportional to the severity of the illness. They were given dimercaprol, and 6 months later all had significant clinical improvement.

Arsenic-induced neurotoxicity in a child was caused by the use of an Indian ethnic remedy.

- A 5-year-old child who had been taking Indian ethnic remedies for congenital bilateral retinoblastoma became anorexic and restless, with nausea, fatigue, paresthesia, and progressive weakness of the legs (20). A year later he developed vomiting, cough, hoarseness, and a recurrent fever. Blood tests showed a severe normochromic anemia and a leukopenia with relative and absolute neutropenia. Electromyography showed a moderate distal chronic axonal polyneuropathy. The urinary arsenic concentration was not high (15 µg/g creatinine; reference range below 40 µg/g), but the hair arsenic concentration was 6.6 mg/kg (reference range below 1 mg/kg). Chronic arsenic poisoning was diagnosed. Arsenic (184 mg/g) was found in one of the ethnic remedies.

Hematologic

Leukocytosis has been commonly noted with arsenic trioxide, but this adverse effect usually resolves spontaneously and is generally not treated. However, one death has been reported.

- A 27-year-old woman (21) with acute promyelocytic leukemia was given arsenic trioxide 0.15 mg/kg/day intravenously. Her white cell count was 8.2×10^9/l; after two doses it rose to 15×10^9/l and after three doses to 21×10^9/l. The white blood cell count continued to rise to 101×10^9/l on day 7 and 213×10^9/l on day 8; the platelet count was 61×10^9/l. Arsenic trioxide was withdrawn. Later that day she became confused with slurred speech and right-sided weakness. A CT scan showed a left middle cerebral artery infarct.

Twelve hours later she had a generalized seizure. The white blood cell count was now $292 \times 10^9/l$ and chemotherapy with idarubicin and cytarabine was started. She continued to deteriorate and died on day 15.

Liver

Arsenic salts can cause liver damage (11).

- A 60-year-old man, a heavy drinker, with psoriasis of the palms and soles was treated with arsenical salt derivatives from 1972 to 1982. In 1984 he had an upper gastrointestinal hemorrhage. Only hyperkeratosis and palmar erythema were observed. His liver enzymes were raised. Endoscopy showed an antral ulcer with signs of recent bleeding and grade IV esophageal varices with no evidence of bleeding. Liver biopsy showed preservation of the parenchymal architecture, fibrous expansion of the portal spaces, and minimal lymphocytic infiltration. The diagnosis was portal fibrosis compatible with idiopathic portal hypertension. When he died of multiorgan failure in 1997, autopsy showed a moderately differentiated multifocal hepatic angiosarcoma with bone, gastric, and splenic metastases.

This patient had both idiopathic portal hypertension and hepatic angiosarcoma, in which the common causative factor was the chronic use of arsenical salts for the treatment of psoriasis. In a review of the literature the authors found only five other cases in which both diseases were associated, while exposure to arsenical salts was found in only one of them.

- A 50-year-old man developed upper gastrointestinal bleeding, with no history of alcohol abuse, viral hepatitis, hepatotoxic drugs, or any family history of liver disease (22). He had thalassemia minor and psoriasis, for which he had taken Fowler's solution, 2 ml/day for 5 years. Fowler's solution is a solution of potassium arsenite that contains 10 mg of arsenic trioxide. He had palmar and plantar hyperkeratosis, splenomegaly, and signs of hypovolemia, normal liver function tests, negative viral serological markers and autoantibodies, and high arsenic excretion in the urine. Abdominal ultrasonography and color Doppler showed marked wall thickening of the portal vein and its intrahepatic branches, with signs of portal hypertension and partial splenic vein thrombosis. Endoscopy showed grade III esophageal varices, with signs of recent bleeding. Liver biopsy showed venous wall hyperplasia, with signs of cellular regeneration tending toward a focal nodular pattern and terminal hepatic vein fibrosis. The wedge hepatic pressure was 12 mmHg and the free hepatic venous pressure 5 mmHg; splenoportography confirmed partial obstruction of the splenic vein.

Skin

Human papillomavirus has been implicated as a co-factor in the pathogenesis of arsenic-induced skin tumors (23).

- A 38-year-old Pakistani woman developed verrucose papules on her palms and soles 3 years after she had been treated orally with an herbal solution by a traveling Indian doctor for a period of 12 months for "white

spot disease." She had widespread depigmented macules on the trunk and limbs, suggestive of vitiligo, and multiple hyperkeratotic papules on her palms and soles, some of which were coalescing into large leathery plaques. Histological examination showed compact hyperkeratosis, intermittent columns of parakeratosis, and an akanthotic epidermis with minor nuclear atypicality. Polymerase chain reaction analysis with degenerate primers identified an atypical human papillomavirus; sequencing showed an RX-variant of HPV, type 23. There were no other signs of chronic arsenic intoxication, and clinical, radiographic, and laboratory investigations showed no evidence of an internal malignancy.

Musculoskeletal

The use of arsenical paste in dental medicine can lead to severe toxicity. Severe alveolar bone necrosis has been reported as a result of leakage of an arsenical devitalization paste into the periodontium (24).

- An 18-year-old woman with dental pain had a tooth devitalized with an arsenical paste and soon after developed excruciating pain and denudation of bone. She had slightly inflamed gums and loss of the mesial papillary gingivae. The surrounding bone was exposed to a height of 3–4 mm and the exposed bone had a greyish color. The non-vital tooth was preserved by root canal treatment and flap surgery to remove necrotic bone and the associated root, and 3 months later a definitive cuspal coverage restoration was placed over the tooth. At 1 year the patient reported that the tooth was functional without any problems.

References

1. Rousselot P, Dombret H, Fermand JP. Arsenic derivatives: old drugs for new indications. Hematologie 1998;5(Suppl 2):95–7.
2. Novick SC, Warrell RP Jr. Arsenicals in hematologic cancers. Semin Oncol 2000;27(5):495–501.
3. Zhang TD, Chen GQ, Wang ZG, Wang ZY, Chen SJ, Chen Z. Arsenic trioxide, a therapeutic agent for APL. Oncogene 2001;20(49):7146–53.
4. Chen Z, Chen GQ, Shen ZX, Sun GL, Tong JH, Wang ZY, Chen SJ. Expanding the use of arsenic trioxide: leukemias and beyond. Semin Hematol 2002;39(2 Suppl 1):22–6.
5. Lehmann S, Paul C. Arsenik effektivt vid akut promyelocytleukemi. [Arsenic efficient in acute promyelocytic leukaemia.] Lakartidningen 1999;96(50):5626–8.
6. Haanen C, Vermes I. Arseentrioxide, een nieuw therapeuticum bij de behandeling van acute promyelocytenleukemie in geval van resistentie tegen tretinoine. [Arsenic trioxide, a new drug for the treatment of acute promyelocytic leukemia resistant to tretinoine.] Ned Tijdschr Geneeskd 1999;143(34):1738–41.
7. Lin CP, Huang MJ, Chang IY, Lin WY. Successful treatment of all-trans retinoic acid resistant and chemotherapy naive acute promyelocytic patients with arsenic trioxide—two case reports. Leuk Lymphoma 2000;38(1–2):191–4.
8. Munshi NC. Arsenic trioxide: an emerging therapy for multiple myeloma. Oncologist 2001;6(Suppl 2):17–21.
9. Wong ST, Chan HL, Teo SK. The spectrum of cutaneous and internal malignancies in chronic arsenic toxicity. Singapore Med J 1998;39(4):171–3.

10. Ernst E. Adverse effects of herbal drugs in dermatology. Br J Dermatol 2000;143(5):923–9.
11. Duenas C, Perez-Alvarez JC, Busteros JI, Saez-Royuela F, Martin-Lorente JL, Yuguero L, Lopez-Morante A. Idiopathic portal hypertension and angiosarcoma associated with arsenical salts therapy. J Clin Gastroenterol 1998;26(4):303–5.
12. Bataineh AB, al-Omari MA, Owais AI. Arsenical necrosis of the jaws. Int Endod J 1997;30(4):283–7.
13. Feinsilber D, Cha D, Lemos A, et al. Arsenicismo cronico medicamentoso. Rev Argent Dermatol 1990;71:178–84.
14. Bergstrom SK, Gillan E, Quinn JJ, Altman AJ. Arsenic trioxide in the treatment of a patient with multiply recurrent, ATRA-resistant promyelocytic leukemia: a case report. J Pediatr Hematol Oncol 1998;20(6):545–7.
15. Che-Pin Lin, Huang MJ, Chang IY, Lin WY, Sheu YT. Retinoic acid syndrome induced by arsenic trioxide in treating recurrent all-trans retinoic acid resistant acute promyelocytic leukemia. Leuk Lymphoma 2000;38(1–2):195–8.
16. Huang CH, Chen WJ, Wu CC, Chen YC, Lee YT. Complete atrioventricular block after arsenic trioxide treatment in an acute promyelocytic leukemic patient. Pacing Clin Electrophysiol 1999;22(6 Pt 1):965–7.
17. Unnikrishnan D, Dutcher JP, Varshneya N, Lucariello R, Api M, Garl S, Wiernik PH, Chiaramida S. Torsades de pointes in 3 patients with leukemia treated with arsenic trioxide. Blood 2001;97(5):1514–16.
18. Yip SF, Yeung YM, Tsui EY. Severe neurotoxicity following arsenic therapy for acute promyelocytic leukemia: potentiation by thiamine deficiency. Blood 2002;99(9):3481–2.
19. Jha S, Dhanuka AK, Singh MN. Arsenic poisoning in a family. Neurol India 2002;50(3):364–5.
20. Muzi G, Dell'omo M, Madeo G, Abbritti G, Caroli S. Arsenic poisoning caused by Indian ethnic remedies. J Pediatr 2001;139(1):169.
21. Roberts TF, Sprague K, Schenkein D, Miller KB, Relias V. Hyperleukocytosis during induction therapy with arsenic trioxide for relapsed acute promyelocytic leukemia associated with central nervous system infarction. Blood 2000;96(12):4000–1.
22. Viudez P, Castano G, Sookoian S, Frider B, Alvarez E. Arsenic and portal hypertension. Am J Gastroenterol 2000;95(6):1602–4.
23. Gerdsen R, Stockfleth E, Uerlich M, Fartasch M, Steen KH, Bieber T. Papular palmoplantar hyperkeratosis following chronic medical exposure to arsenic: human papillomavirus as a co-factor in the pathogenesis of arsenical keratosis? Acta Derm Venereol 2000;80(4):292–3.
24. Ozmeric N. Localized alveolar bone necrosis following the use of an arsenical paste: a case report. Int Endod J 2002;35(3):295–9.

Arsenobenzol

General Information

Arsenobenzol has been used to treat syphilis (1,2) and as a topical antiseptic in combination with cortisone and silver colloid (3). Like other compounds with an arsenic base, it can cause gastrointestinal complaints, but also polyneuritis and encephalopathy. Adrenaline prevented the development of encephalopathy and was helpful in treating hemorrhagic encephalopathy (SEDA-11, 597).

References

1. Ebner H, Raab W. Nachbeobachtungen an arsenobenzol-schwermetall-behandelten faellen frischer lues. Hautarzt 1964;15:120–4.
2. Rossberg J. Katamnestische Untersuchungen an Arsenobenzol-Penizillin-Wismut behandelten Syphilitikern. [Catamnestic studies of syphilis patients treated with arsenobenzene-penicillin-bismuth.] Dermatol Wochenschr 1967;153(7):161–4.
3. Sacco S, Barlocco ME. Cortisone-arsenobenzolo-argento colloidale: la piu recente associazione antisettico-antiflogistica in parodontologia e stomatologia. [Cortisone-arsenobenzol-silver colloid: the newest antiseptic and anti-inflammatory combination in periodontology.] Riv Ital Stomatol 1970;25(12):1071–85.

Artemisinin derivatives

General Information

The herb Qinghaosu (*Artemisia annua*) has been known to Chinese medicine for centuries and was used in the treatment of fevers, in particular malaria fever; it is not clear why it did not become more widely used elsewhere. The plant can be grown in locations other than China, and field studies in propagating and growing the plant are being carried out in many parts of the world. In 1979 the Qinghaosu Antimalarial Coordinating Research Group reported their experience with four formulations of qinghaosu in both *Plasmodium vivax* and *Plasmodium falciparum* malaria (SEDA-13, 818) (SEDA-17, 326) (1).

Artemisinin is an antimalarial constituent isolated from Qinghao. It is a sesquiterpene lactone with an endoperoxide bridge, structurally distinct from other classes of antimalarial agents. Several derivatives of the original compound have proved effective in the treatment of *Plasmodium falciparum* malaria and are currently available in a variety of formulations: artesunate (intravenous, rectal, oral), artelinate (oral), artemisinin (intravenous, rectal, oral), dihydroartemisinin (oral), artemether (intravenous, oral, rectal), and artemotil (intravenous). Artemisinic acid (qinghao acid), the precursor of artemisin, is present in the plant in a concentration up to 10 times that of artemisinin. Several semisynthetic derivatives have been developed from dihydroartemisinin (1).

Artemether

Artemether is a methyl ether derivative of dihydroartemisinin. It is dispensed in ampoules for intramuscular injection suspended in groundnut oil and in capsules for oral use. Like artesunate and artemisinin it has been used for both severe and uncomplicated malaria. Artesunate is probably faster-acting than the other two.

Artemotil (arteether)

Artemotil is the ethyl ether derivative of dihydroartemisinin. It was the choice of the WHO for development and was considered less toxic, because one would expect it to be metabolized to ethanol rather than methanol. It is also more lipophilic than artemether, a possible advantage for accumulation in brain tissues. The beta anomer was chosen since it is a crystalline solid and relatively easy to separate from the alpha anomer, which is liquid; it was necessary to choose a single anomer because of the more complex rules for the development of a drug with two anomers in the USA.

Artesunate

Artesunate is a water-soluble hemisuccinate derivative, available in parenteral and oral formulations. The parenteral drug is dispensed as powdered artesunic acid. Neutral aqueous solutions are unstable. Artesunate is effective by the intravenous, intramuscular, and oral routes in a dose of 10 mg/kg given for 5–7 days. The combination with mefloquine is very effective even against highly multiresistant strains of *Plasmodium falciparum*; the combination must be given for at least 3 days.

None of these medications has yet been registered for use in Europe or North America. In recent years there has been a substantial increase in our knowledge of their safety, efficacy, and pharmacokinetics. Higher cure rates are achieved when they are combined with longer-acting antimalarial drugs, such as mefloquine. After years of continued use, the sequential use of artesunate and mefloquine remains an effective treatment in areas of multidrug resistance in South-East Asia and provides an impetus for the evaluation of other artesunate-containing combination regimens for the treatment of uncomplicated malaria, such as artemether + benflumetol (2–6).

Mechanism of action

All three *Artemisia* derivatives are quickly hydrolysed to the active substance dihydroartemisinin. They produce a more rapid clinical and parasitological response than other antimalarial drugs. There are no reports of significant toxicity, and as late as 1994 there was no convincing evidence of specific resistance, but chloroquine-resistant *Plasmodium berghei* is resistant to artemisinin as well. The recrudescence rate is fairly high (1).

The mode of action is not fully known. There is strong evidence that the antimalarial activity of these drugs depends on the generation of free radical intermediates; free radical scavengers, such as ascorbic acid and vitamin E, therefore antagonize the antimalarial activity.

Drug activation by iron and heme may explain why endoperoxides are selectively toxic to malaria parasites. The malaria parasites live in a milieu of heme iron, which the parasite converts into insoluble hemozoin. Chloroquine, which binds heme, antagonizes the antimalarial activity of artemisinin.

Observational studies

Some impression of possible adverse effects in humans can be gained from a primarily pharmacokinetic study, in which artemotil solution in sesame oil was given intramuscularly. The half-life was 25–72 hours. Adverse effects in 23 subjects after the single dose included local pain in two, bitter taste and dryness of the mouth in one, and a mild but slightly itching papular rash that persisted for 14 days in another. There were no biochemical or electrocardiographic changes. Similar adverse effects were seen after 5 days of therapy in 14 of the 27 subjects; there was local pain in three, metallic taste in two, flu-like symptoms in three, and in two a maculopapular rash, which receded within 24 hours. One subject developed shivering, clammy hands and feet, dizziness, headache, nausea, and a metallic taste in the mouth, all lasting for about an hour, but the same reaction occurred after an injection of sesame oil only. Apart from some increase in eosinophil count in all groups, there were no significant hematological changes (7).

In 25 patients with acute uncomplicated *Plasmodium falciparum* malaria treated with artemotil (3.2 mg/kg followed by either 1.6 mg/kg or 0.8 mg/kg), the most frequent adverse events were headache, dizziness, nausea, vomiting, and abdominal pain; two patients complained of mild pain at the site of injection (8).

In a postmarketing surveillance study of artemotil in 300 patients, 294 (98%) were cured, five improved, and one did not show any change (9). The adverse effects were mild headache, nausea, vomiting, and giddiness.

Combination therapy

The artemisinin derivatives are limited by an unacceptable incidence of recrudescence with monotherapy, and they therefore need to be used in combination. A summary of prospective trials that looked specifically for adverse effects showed that artemisinins alone are very well tolerated (10). The same study showed no evidence of adverse interactions of artesunate with mefloquine, with an incidence of adverse effects similar to that expected from malaria and mefloquine (25 mg/kg) together. Reducing doses of mefloquine increases recrudescence rates to unacceptable levels (11). Combinations of artemisinins with quinine, co-trimoxazole, and doxycycline are well tolerated.

Artemether + benflumetol
A large trial of the first fixed-dose combination of an artemisinin derivative likely to be licensed (artemether + benflumetol) had disappointing relapse rates compared with mefloquine monotherapy (6). In the 126 patients who took artemether + benflumetol there were no adverse effects attributed to drug treatment. However, less than 70% of patients were cured at 28 days. Benflumetol may be more effective at higher concentrations (12) but toxicity studies are lacking.

Artesunate + lumefantrine
There has been a meta-analysis of 15 trials from Africa, Europe, and Asia of the use of varying doses of artesunate plus lumefantrine compared with several alternative antimalarial drugs in 1869 patients conducted by the manufacturers Novartis into its clinical safety and tolerability in the treatment of uncomplicated malaria (13). The most common adverse events were gastrointestinal—nausea (6.3%), abdominal pain (12%), vomiting (2.4%), anorexia (13%)—or central nervous—headache (21%) or dizziness (16%). There were 20 serious adverse events with artesunate plus lumefantrine, but only one (hemolytic anemia) was possibly due to artesunate plus lumefantrine. There was no QT prolongation associated with artesunate plus lumefantrine.

Artesunate + mefloquine

Artesunate has been combined with mefloquine in areas with a high prevalence of multiresistant *Plasmodium falciparum* in Thailand and the Thai-Burmese border. In a study reported in 1992 in 127 patients who were followed for 28 days, group A took artesunate 100 mg immediately and then 50 mg every 12 hours for 5 days (total 600 mg), group M took mefloquine 750 mg and another 500 mg 6 hours later, and group AM took first artesunate and then the two doses of mefloquine (14). Fever and parasite clearance time were significantly shorter in the two groups treated with artesunate. Table 1 gives the results and adverse effects. The combination of artesunate with mefloquine was more effective than either drug alone. However, the trial design was such that the patients who took both drugs were in fact treated twice, so the findings did not prove synergism between the two drugs.

In a second Thai study, 652 adults and children were treated with artesunate plus mefloquine (15). A single dose of artesunate 4 mg/kg plus mefloquine 25 mg/kg gave a rapid response but did not improve cure rate. Artesunate given for 3 days in a total dose of 10 mg/kg plus mefloquine was 98% effective. The incidence of vomiting was significantly reduced by giving the mefloquine on day 2 of the treatment. There were no adverse effects attributed to artesunate.

Artesunate plus pyrimethamine + sulfadoxine

In Irian Jaya, a randomized, controlled trial ($n = 105$; 88 children) of oral artesunate (4 mg/kg od for 3 days) with pyrimethamine (1.25 mg/kg) + sulfadoxine or pyrimethamine + sulfadoxine alone (same dose) showed reduced gametocyte carriage and reduced treatment failure rates (RR = 0.3; 95% CI = 0.1, 1.3) in the combination group (16). Self-limiting adverse events of combination treatment were mild diarrhea (2.1%), rashes (4.3%), and itching (2.1%).

In a double-blind, randomized, placebo-controlled trial in Gambian children with uncomplicated falciparum malaria treated with pyrimethamine + sulfadoxine (25/500 mg; $n = 600$) or pyrimethamine + sulfadoxine combined with two regimens of oral artesunate (4 mg/kg, $n = 200$ or 4 mg/kg od for 3 days, $n = 200$), there were mild adverse events, such as headache, anorexia, nausea, vomiting, abdominal pain, and diarrhea, in a high proportion of children (56%) (17). Combination treatment with

artesunate was associated with more rapid parasite clearance and less gametocytemia. Three-dose artesunate conferred no additional benefit over the one-dose regimen.

Artesunate + tetracycline

In a comparison between oral artesunate (700 mg over 5 days) plus tetracycline (250 mg at 6-hour intervals) and quinine (600 mg quinine sulfate at 8-hour intervals) for 7 days, artesunate was more effective and better tolerated in uncomplicated malaria (see Table 2) (18). Convulsions occurred in one case.

Dihydroartemisinin + piperaquine

The novel combination (Artekin™) of dihydroartemisinin and piperaquine has been assessed in 106 patients (76 children and 30 adults) with uncomplicated *Plasmodium falciparum* malaria in Cambodia (19). The respective doses of dihydroartemisinin and piperaquine, which were given at 0, 8, 24, and 32 hours, were 9.1 mg/kg and 74 mg/kg in children and 6.6 and 53 mg/kg in adults. All the patients became aparasitemic within 72 hours. Excluding the results in one child who died on day 4, there was a 97% 28-day cure rate (99% in children and 92% in adults). Patients who had recrudescent infections used low doses of Artekin. Adverse effects, most commonly gastrointestinal complaints, were reported by 22 patients (21%) but did not necessitate premature withdrawal.

Comparative studies

Three large clinical trials (in Kenya, the Gambia, and Vietnam) compared intramuscular artemether with intravenous quinine in severe malaria tropica (SEDA-20, 259). The treatments were similarly efficacious. There were no serious adverse effects.

Placebo-controlled studies

In a double-blind, randomized study in Vietnam ($n = 227$), extending the duration of oral artemisinin monotherapy 500 mg/day from 5 to 7 days did not reduce recrudescence rates (total 23%) (20).

Table 1 Adverse effects of artesunate with or without mefloquine in acute uncomplicated malaria tropica

	Mefloquine	Artesunate	Artesunate + Mefloquine
Total number of patients (M/F)	39/4	38/4	39/3
Number of patients with 18-day follow-up	37	40	39
Number (%) cured at 28 days	30 (81)	35 (88)	39 (100)
Fever clearance time (hours)	70	35	38
Parasite clearance time (hours)	64	36	38
Headache (%)	17 (39)	14 (33)	12 (28)
Dizziness (%)	8 (18)	6 (14)	5 (11)
Nausea (%)	9 (20)	6 (14)	9 (21)
Vomiting (%)	7 (16)	8 (19)	11 (26)
Abdominal pain (%)	1 (2)	2 (4)	1 (2)
Diarrhea (%)	1 (2)	3 (7)	1 (2)
Itching and rash (%)	0	3 (7)	1 (2)

Table 2 Adverse effects in a comparison of artesunate plus tetracycline versus quinine

	Artesunate + Tetracycline	Quinine
Number	31	33
Parasite clearance time (hours)	37 (24–52)	73 (26–135)
Cure rate on day 27 (%)	97	10
Nausea (%)	14 (45)	20 (60)
Dizziness (%)	16 (52)	16 (48)
Vomiting (%)	9 (26)	30 (91)
Tinnitus (%)	0	29 (88)
Convulsions (%)	1 (3)	0
Bradycardia (%)	7 (23)	Not done

General adverse effects

The safety of the peroxide antimalarial drugs has been reviewed (21). In animal studies, high doses of artemotil and artemether have been associated with hemopoietic, cardiac, and nervous system toxicity. Some subclinical neurotoxicity has been reported, with a discrete distribution in the brain stems of rats and dogs after multiple (high) doses (22). Dogs given high doses (15 mg/kg artemether for 28 days) had a progressive syndrome of clinical neurological defects with terminal cardiorespiratory collapse and death. There has been no evidence of neurotoxicity in man, but the human dosage of these ethers is of course lower. Reviews of clinical trials have reaffirmed the high tolerability of the artemisinins (11,23). Adverse effects have been chiefly limited to the GI tract. Most reported adverse events were described as mild and transient and none resulted in withdrawal of treatment.

Organs and Systems

Cardiovascular

Sinus bradycardia and a reversible prolongation of the QT interval have been reported (SEDA-21, 293).

A combination of artemether + lumefantrine (co-artemether, six doses over 3 days) followed by quinine (a 2-hour intravenous infusion of 10 mg/kg, not exceeding 600 mg in total, 2 hours after the last dose of co-artemether) was given to 42 healthy volunteers in a double-blind, parallel, three-group study (14 subjects per group) to examine the electrocardiographic effects of these drugs (24). Co-artemether had no effect on the QT$_c$ interval. The infusion of quinine alone caused transient prolongation of the QT$_c$ interval, and this effect was slightly but significantly greater when quinine was infused after co-artemether. Thus, the inherent risk of QT$_c$ prolongation by intravenous quinine was enhanced by prior administration of co-artemether. Overlapping therapy with co-artemether and intravenous quinine in the treatment of patients with complicated or multidrug-resistant *Plasmodium falciparum* malaria may result in a modest increased risk of QT$_c$ prolongation, but this is far outweighed by the potential therapeutic benefit.

The effects on the QT$_c$ interval of single oral doses of halofantrine 500 mg and artemether 80 mg + lumefantrine 480 mg have been studied in 13 healthy men in a double-blind, randomized, crossover study (25). The length of the QT$_c$ interval correlated positively with halofantrine exposure but was unchanged by co-artemether.

Nervous system

Although in animals several of the artemisinin derivatives have produced a characteristic neurological lesion, there is no good evidence of neurotoxicity in man. A study in mice suggested that intramuscular artemether is significantly more neurotoxic than intramuscular artesunate (26).

In one case, an inadequately treated non-immune subject developed neurological symptoms after relapse and re-treatment; the symptoms were ascribed to artemether (27), although the well-recognized post-malaria neurological syndrome was much more likely, which the authors did not discuss (28).

One man developed ataxia and slurred speech after taking a 5-day course of oral artesunate (SEDA-21, 293).

A study of brain-stem auditory-evoked potentials showed no electrophysiological evidence of brain-stem damage in adults treated with artemisinin derivatives (29).

Neurotoxicity from artemether is related to drug accumulation due to slow and prolonged absorption from intramuscular injection sites. In mice, high doses of intramuscular artemether (50–100 mg/kg/day for 28 days) resulted in an unusual pattern of selective damage to certain brain-stem nuclei, especially those implicated in hearing and balance (30).

Fluid balance

Sodium artesunate inhibits sodium chloride transport in the thick ascending limb of the loop of Henle and therefore has a diuretic effect.

- In two men, aged 16 and 32 years, with falciparum malaria who were given four intravenous doses of sodium artesunate 60 mg, neither of whom had received diuretics or vasoactive drugs, there was a diuresis (6 l/day) accompanied by a natriuresis (31).

Hematologic

A transient dose-dependent reduction in reticulocyte count has been reported in healthy subjects (SEDA-21, 294).

Body temperature

Drug fever has been reported in healthy subjects taking artemether, artesunate, and artemisinin (SEDA-21, 294).

Second-Generation Effects

Pregnancy

Artemisinin derivatives (artesunate and artemether) for the treatment of multidrug-resistant *Plasmodium falciparum* malaria have been evaluated in 83 Karen pregnant women in Thailand; 55 women were treated for recrudescent infection after quinine or mefloquine, 12 for uncomplicated hyperparasitemic episodes, and 16 had not declared their pregnancy when treated (32).

Artesunate and artemether were well tolerated and there was no drug-related adverse effect. Overall, 73 pregnancies resulted in live births, three in abortions and two in still-births; five women were lost to follow-up before delivery. There was no congenital abnormality in any of the neonates, and the 46 children followed for more than 1 year all developed normally.

Artemisinin derivatives have been studied in 461 pregnant women in a prospective cohort study in Thailand over 8 years (33). Oral artesunate monotherapy was associated with a treatment failure rate of 6.6%. Artesunate and artemether were well tolerated. The rates of abortions (including 44 first-trimester exposures), stillbirths, or congenital abnormalities were 4.8%, 1.58%, and 0.8% respectively, and were not significantly different from pregnant controls. These results are reassuring, but further information is needed before the safety of artesunate in pregnancy can be confirmed.

Drug Administration

Drug formulations

When the sesame oil vehicle in beta-artemotil was replaced by Cremophor (polyethoxylated castor oil) the total exposure in rats was 2.7-fold higher, owing to increased systemic availability (34). Anorexia and gastrointestinal toxicity from artemotil in sesame oil were significantly more severe than with artemotil in Cremophor. However, histological examination of the brain showed neurotoxic changes, which were worse with the castor oil formulation.

Drug administration route

A crossover pharmacokinetic study of single-dose rectal artesunate (10 or 20 mg/kg as a suppository) or intravenous artesunate (2.4 mg/kg) in moderate falciparum malaria in 34 Ghanaian children has been reported (35). The intravenous route gave much higher peak concentrations but more rapid elimination of artesunate and its active metabolite dihydroartemisinin than the rectal route. Rectal artesunate had higher systemic availability in the low-dose group than in the high-dose group (58% versus 23%). This is lower than published estimates of the systemic availability of oral artesunate (61–85%) (36). Parasite clearance kinetics were comparable in the two groups. There were no adverse events attributable to the drug. The results of Phase III and Phase IV studies of rectal artesunate as an alternative to parenteral antimalarial drugs in African children are awaited.

Drug–Drug Interactions

Chloroquine

Although an early report suggested antagonism between chloroquine and artemisinin (37), more recent evidence suggests the opposite, that is a synergistic effect between the two (38,39).

Deferoxamine

Co-administration of artemisinin derivatives, such as artesunate, with deferoxamine may be useful in patients with cerebral malaria, because of the combination of rapid parasite clearance by the former and central nervous system protection by the latter. Artesunate has been studied alone and in combination with deferoxamine in a single-blind comparison (40). Adverse effects were generally mild and there were no differences between the two regimens.

Omeprazole

Artemisinin induces its own elimination and that of omeprazole through an increase in CYP2C19 activity and that of another enzyme, as yet to be identified (41).

References

1. Ridley RG, Hudson AT. Chemotherapy of malaria. Curr Opin Infect Dis 1998;11:691–705.
2. von Seidlein L, Jaffar S, Pinder M, Haywood M, Snounou G, Gemperli B, Gathmann I, Royce C, Greenwood B. Treatment of African children with uncomplicated falciparum malaria with a new antimalarial drug, CGP 56697. J Infect Dis 1997;176(4):1113–16.
3. von Seidlein L, Bojang K, Jones P, Jaffar S, Pinder M, Obaro S, Doherty T, Haywood M, Snounou G, Gemperli B, Gathmann I, Royce C, McAdam K, Greenwood B. A randomized controlled trial of artemether/benflumetol, a new antimalarial and pyrimethamine/sulfadoxine in the treatment of uncomplicated falciparum malaria in African children. Am J Trop Med Hyg 1998;58(5):638–44.
4. Hatz C, Abdulla S, Mull R, Schellenberg D, Gathmann I, Kibatala P, Beck HP, Tanner M, Royce C. Efficacy and safety of CGP 56697 (artemether and benflumetol) compared with chloroquine to treat acute falciparum malaria in Tanzanian children aged 1–5 years. Trop Med Int Health 1998;3(6):498–504.
5. van Vugt M, Brockman A, Gemperli B, Luxemburger C, Gathmann I, Royce C, Slight T, Looareesuwan S, White NJ, Nosten F. Randomized comparison of artemether-benflumetol and artesunate-mefloquine in treatment of multidrug-resistant falciparum malaria. Antimicrob Agents Chemother 1998;42(1):135–9.
6. Looareesuwan S, Wilairatana P, Chokejindachai W, Chalermrut K, Wernsdorfer W, Gemperli B, Gathmann I, Royce C. A randomized, double-blind, comparative trial of a new oral combination of artemether and benflumetol (CGP 56697) with mefloquine in the treatment of acute *Plasmodium falciparum* malaria in Thailand Am J Trop Med Hyg 1999;60(2):238–43.
7. Kager PA, Schultz MJ, Zijlstra EE, van den Berg B, van Boxtel CJ. Arteether administration in humans: preliminary studies of pharmacokinetics, safety and tolerance. Trans R Soc Trop Med Hyg 1994;88(Suppl 1):S53–4.
8. Looareesuwan S, Oosterhuis B, Schilizzi BM, Sollie FA, Wilairatana P, Krudsood S, Lugt ChB, Peeters PA, Peggins JO. Dose-finding and efficacy study for i.m. artemotil (beta-arteether) and comparison with i.m. artemether in acute uncomplicated *P. falciparum* malaria. Br J Clin Pharmacol 2002;53(5):492–500.
9. Asthana OP, Srivastava JS, Das Gupta P. Post-marketing surveillance of arteether in malaria. J Assoc Physicians India 2002;50:539–45.
10. Price R, van Vugt M, Phaipun L, Luxemburger C, Simpson J, McGready R, ter Kuile F, Kham A, Chongsuphajaisiddhi T, White NJ, Nosten F. Adverse effects in patients with acute

falciparum malaria treated with artemisinin derivatives. Am J Trop Med Hyg 1999;60(4):547–55.

11. Na-Bangchang K, Tippanangkosol P, Ubalee R, Chaovanakawee S, Saenglertsilapachai S, Karbwang J. Comparative clinical trial of four regimens of dihydroartemisinin–mefloquine in multidrug-resistant falciparum malaria. Trop Med Int Health 1999;4(9):602–10.

12. Ezzet F, Mull R, Karbwang J. Population pharmacokinetics and therapeutic response of CGP 56697 (artemether + benflumetol) in malaria patients. Br J Clin Pharmacol 1998;46(6):553–61.

13. Bakshi R, Hermeling-Fritz I, Gathmann I, Alteri E. An integrated assessment of the clinical safety of artemether–lumefantrine: a new oral fixed-dose combination antimalarial drug. Trans R Soc Trop Med Hyg 2000;94(4):419–24.

14. Looareesuwan S, Viravan C, Vanijanonta S, Wilairatana P, Suntharasamai P, Charoenlarp P, Arnold K, Kyle D, Canfield C, Webster K. Randomised trial of artesunate and mefloquine alone and in sequence for acute uncomplicated falciparum malaria. Lancet 1992;339(8797):821–4.

15. Nosten F, Luxemburger C, ter Kuile FO, Woodrow C, Eh JP, Chongsuphajaisiddhi T, White NJ. Treatment of multidrug-resistant Plasmodium falciparum malaria with 3-day artesunate–mefloquine combination. J Infect Dis 1994;170(4):971–7.

16. Tjitra E, Suprianto S, Currie BJ, Morris PS, Saunders JR, Anstey NM. Therapy of uncomplicated falciparum malaria: a randomized trial comparing artesunate plus sulfadoxine–pyrimethamine versus sulfadoxine-pyrimethamine alone in Irian Jaya, Indonesia. Am J Trop Med Hyg 2001;65(4):309–17.

17. von Seidlein L, Milligan P, Pinder M, Bojang K, Anyalebechi C, Gosling R, Coleman R, Ude JI, Sadiq A, Duraisingh M, Warhurst D, Alloueche A, Targett G, McAdam K, Greenwood B, Walraven G, Olliaro P, Doherty T. Efficacy of artesunate plus pyrimethamine–sulphadoxine for uncomplicated malaria in Gambian children: a double-blind, randomised, controlled trial. Lancet 2000;355(9201):352–7.

18. Karbwang J, Na-Bangchang K, Thanavibul A, Bunnag D, Chongsuphajaisiddhi T, Harinasuta T. Comparison of oral artesunate and quinine plus tetracycline in acute uncomplicated falciparum malaria. Bull World Health Organ 1994;72(2):233–8.

19. Denis MB, Davis TM, Hewitt S, Incardona S, Nimol K, Fandeur T, Poravuth Y, Lim C, Socheat D. Efficacy and safety of dihydroartemisinin-piperaquine (Artekin) in Cambodian children and adults with uncomplicated falciparum malaria. Clin Infect Dis 2002;35(12):1469–76.

20. Giao PT, Binh TQ, Kager PA, Long HP, Van Thang N, Van Nam N, de Vries PJ. Artemisinin for treatment of uncomplicated falciparum malaria: is there a place for monotherapy? Am J Trop Med Hyg 2001;65(6):690–5.

21. Brewer TG, Peggins JO, Grate SJ, Petras JM, Levine BS, Weina PJ, Swearengen J, Heiffer MH, Schuster BG. Neurotoxicity in animals due to arteether and artemether. Trans R Soc Trop Med Hyg 1994;88(Suppl 1):S33–6.

22. Wesche DL, DeCoster MA, Tortella FC, Brewer TG. Neurotoxicity of artemisinin analogues in vitro. Antimicrob Agents Chemother 1994;38(8):1813–19.

23. Ribeiro IR, Olliaro P. Safety of artemisinin and its derivatives. A review of published and unpublished clinical trials. Med Trop (Mars) 1998;58(Suppl 3):50–3.

24. Lefevre G, Carpenter P, Souppart C, Schmidli H, Martin JM, Lane A, Ward C, Amakye D. Interaction trial between artemether–lumefantrine (Riamet) and quinine in healthy subjects. J Clin Pharmacol 2002;42(10):1147–58.

25. Bindschedler M, Lefevre G, Degen P, Sioufi A. Comparison of the cardiac effects of the antimalarials co-artemether and halofantrine in healthy participants. Am J Trop Med Hyg 2002;66(3):293–8.

26. Nontprasert A, Nosten-Bertrand M, Pukrittayakamee S, Vanijanonta S, Angus BJ, White NJ. Assessment of the neurotoxicity of parenteral artemisinin derivatives in mice. Am J Trop Med Hyg 1998;59(4):519–22.

27. Elias Z, Bonnet E, Marchou B, Massip P. Neurotoxicity of artemisinin: possible counseling and treatment of side effects. Clin Infect Dis 1999;28(6):1330–1.

28. White NJ. Neurological dysfunction following malaria: disease- or drug-related? Clin Infect Dis 2000;30(5):836.

29. Van Vugt M, Angus BJ, Price RN, Mann C, Simpson JA, Poletto C, Htoo SE, Looareesuwan S, White NJ, Nosten F. A case-control auditory evaluation of patients treated with artemisinin derivatives for multidrug-resistant Plasmodium falciparum malaria. Am J Trop Med Hyg 2000;62(1):65–9.

30. Nontprasert A, Pukrittayakamee S, Dondorp AM, Clemens R, Looareesuwan S, White NJ. Neuropathologic toxicity of artemisinin derivatives in a mouse model. Am J Trop Med Hyg 2002;67(4):423–9.

31. Seguro AC, Campos SB. Diuretic effect of sodium artesunate in patients with malaria. Am J Trop Med Hyg 2002;67(5):473–4.

32. McGready R, Cho T, Cho JJ, Simpson JA, Luxemburger C, Dubowitz L, Looareesuwan S, White NJ, Nosten F. Artemisinin derivatives in the treatment of falciparum malaria in pregnancy. Trans R Soc Trop Med Hyg 1998;92(4):430–3.

33. McGready R, Cho T, Keo NK, Thwai KL, Villegas L, Looareesuwan S, White NJ, Nosten F. Artemisinin antimalarials in pregnancy: a prospective treatment study of 539 episodes of multidrug-resistant Plasmodium falciparum. Clin Infect Dis 2001;33(12):2009–16.

34. Li QG, Mog SR, Si YZ, Kyle DE, Gettayacamin M, Milhous WK. Neurotoxicity and efficacy of arteether related to its exposure times and exposure levels in rodents. Am J Trop Med Hyg 2002;66(5):516–25.

35. Krishna S, Planche T, Agbenyega T, Woodrow C, Agranoff D, Bedu-Addo G, Owusu-Ofori AK, Appiah JA, Ramanathan S, Mansor SM, Navaratnam V. Bioavailability and preliminary clinical efficacy of intrarectal artesunate in Ghanaian children with moderate malaria. Antimicrob Agents Chemother 2001;45(2):509–16.

36. Newton P, Suputtamongkol Y, Teja-Isavadharm P, Pukrittayakamee S, Navaratnam V, Bates I, White N. Antimalarial bioavailability and disposition of artesunate in acute falciparum malaria. Antimicrob Agents Chemother 2000;44(4):972–7.

37. Stahel E, Druilhe P, Gentilini M. Antagonism of chloroquine with other antimalarials. Trans R Soc Trop Med Hyg 1988;82(2):221.

38. Hallett RL, Sutherland CJ, Alexander N, Ord R, Jawara M, Drakeley CJ, Pinder M, Walraven G, Targett GA, Alloueche A. Combination therapy counteracts the enhanced transmission of drug-resistant malaria parasites to mosquitoes. Antimicrob Agents Chemother 2004;48(10):3940–3.

39. Olliaro PL, Taylor WR. Developing artemisinin based drug combinations for the treatment of drug resistant falciparum malaria: A review. J Postgrad Med 2004;50(1):40–4.

40. Looareesuwan S, Wilairatana P, Vannaphan S, Gordeuk VR, Taylor TE, Meshnick SR, Brittenham GM. Co-administration of desferrioxamine B with artesunate in malaria: an assessment of safety and tolerance. Ann Trop Med Parasitol 1996;90(5):551–4.

41. Svensson US, Ashton M, Trinh NH, Bertilsson L, Dinh XH, Nguyen VH, Nguyen TN, Nguyen DS, Lykkesfeldt J, Le DC. Artemisinin induces omeprazole metabolism in human beings. Clin Pharmacol Ther 1998;64(2):160–7.

Articaine

See also Local anesthetics

General Information

Articaine is an aminoamide that also contains an ester group, which is rapidly hydrolysed by plasma esterases. It is 4-methyl-3([2-(propylamino)propion-amido)]-2-thiophenecarboxylic acid, methyl ester hydrochloride. The thiophene group increases its lipid solubility while the ester group enables it to undergo plasma esterase hydrolysis as well as hepatic enzyme metabolism. Articaine is formulated as a 4% solution with adrenaline. It is the most widely used local anesthetic agent in dentistry in some parts of Europe.

The rapid breakdown of articaine to an inactive metabolite means that it has low systemic toxicity. However, the risk of intravascular injection is high in dentistry, and articaine can cause central nervous system and cardiovascular toxicity. However, articaine is slightly more potent than lidocaine and causes less nervous system toxicity (1).

The safety of articaine has been studied in a series of three randomized trials (2). The adverse effects deemed to be related to articaine were headache, paresthesia/hyperesthesia after injection, infection, and rash. There was one case of mouth ulceration. The overall incidence of adverse effects was comparable to that of lidocaine.

Organs and Systems

Cardiovascular

The incidence of hypotension and headache after spinal anesthesia was similar to that encountered with lidocaine (SED-12, 256) (3).

Nervous system

Four cases of persistent lingual paresthesia or hyperesthesia after inferior dental block with articaine have been reported (4). Although resolution of neurological complications usually occurs within 2 weeks, the authors reported that the symptoms in their cases persisted for 6–18 months and noted that they were aware of another four cases of persistent paresthesia with articaine that had not been formally reported.

Skin

- An 11-year-old boy developed severe dermatomyositis only a few days after injection of articaine in the jaw for tooth extraction; cause and effect were not established (SEDA-10, 105).

References

1. Oertel R, Rahn R, Kirch W. Clinical pharmacokinetics of articaine. Clin Pharmacokinet 1997;33(6):417–25.
2. Malamed SF, Gagnon S, Leblanc D. Articaine hydrochloride: a study of the safety of a new amide local anesthetic. J Am Dent Assoc 2001;132(2):177–85.
3. Kaukinen S, Eerola R, Eerola M, Kaukinen L. A comparison of carticaine and lidocaine in spinal anaesthesia. Ann Clin Res 1978;10(4):191–4.
4. van Eeden SP, Patel MF. Re: prolonged paraesthesia following inferior alveolar nerve block using articaine. Br J Oral Maxillofac Surg 2002;40(6):519–20.

Artificial sweeteners

General Information

Acesulfame

Acesulfame is an artificial sweetener derived from aceto-acetic acid. It is used in a wide range of non-medicinal products (1).

Aspartame

Aspartame is a dipeptide that is used as an artificial sweetener. It is completely hydrolysed in the gastrointestinal tract to methanol, aspartic acid, and phenylalanine (2).

Aspartame appears to be a safe sweetener, and despite numerous studies of its safety during the past three decades, the incidence of serious adverse effects has been difficult to determine in controlled studies. Since one of the metabolic products of aspartame is phenylalanine, excessive use of aspartame should be avoided by patients with phenylketonuria (3–5). Toxicity of another possible metabolic product, methanol, is unlikely, even when aspartame is used in extraordinary amounts (6,7).

Aspartame has reportedly caused angioedema and urticaria (SEDA-21, 526).

Cyclamates

Sodium cyclamate is a potent sweetening agent. It has been subjected to numerous safety and carcinogenicity studies. Animal data led to warning against excessive and indiscriminate use a long time ago, causing the World Health Organization in 1967 to adopt a safety limit of 50 mg/kg. However, in 1982 a joint FAO/WHO expert committee on food additives revised this recommendation to allow for a maximum daily intake of up to 11 mg/kg of sodium or calcium cyclamate (as cyclamic acid) (8). Nevertheless, since in certain climates and populations the amount of cyclamates in soft drinks and other beverages can exceed these limits, more epidemiological data are needed to evaluate, for example, a possible association with cancer of the uropoietic system (9) and with histological and radiological abnormalities of the small intestine and malabsorption (10).

Saccharin

Saccharin and its salts are potent sweeteners, about 300 times as sweet as sucrose. It is used to sweeten foods and beverages.

Sorbitol

Sorbitol, a polyhydric alcohol, is used as a sweetening agent in many oral medicinal liquids. In addition to enhancing the palatability of these liquids, it improves solution stability and reduces crystallization of syrup vehicles (11). It is used as a sweetener in many sugar-free food products and confectioneries. Sorbitol-containing food products are often recommended for patients with diabetes, because sorbitol does not raise blood glucose concentrations or require insulin for its metabolism (12).

Organs and Systems

Cardiovascular

Two patients with Raynaud's phenomenon (13) and one man with fibromyalgia had all used aspartame 6–15 g/day (0.12–0.16 mg/kg/day) as well as a dietary drink containing aspartame, and no other risk factors were identified. All three described regular keyboarding to the extent of 30 hours per week but had used wrist rests, "stretch breaks," and other steps to optimize their work practices. Complete resolution of symptoms occurred over 2 weeks after they had eliminated aspartame from the diet, despite no changes in the intensity of keyboarding or other work practices. Nerve conduction velocities had been within normal limits before the withdrawal of aspartame and were not repeated.

Nervous system

Headaches can follow aspartame ingestion (14). Up to July 1991 the FDA had received over 5000 reports of adverse effects in a passive surveillance program; in this and other studies the main complaints were of neurological symptoms, and headaches accounted for 18–45% of cases (15). It appears that some people are particularly susceptible to headaches caused by aspartame and may want to limit their consumption (16). In a double-blind, crossover study using volunteers with self-identified headaches after aspartame, some were particularly susceptible, and their headaches were attributed to aspartame (17).

Aspartame can alter brain wave activity in epileptic children (18). It has been associated with seizures, but only anecdotally (19).

In three non-obese individuals (two women and one man), it was suspected that heavy use of aspartame was causally related to symptoms of carpal tunnel syndrome (20). All three reported moderate pain and tingling in the hands, especially at night, using a self-administered questionnaire for the assessment of severity of symptoms and functional status (21). Given the ubiquity of aspartame—one manufacturer has stated that it is used in 5000 products—physicians may want to inquire about its use in patients who report symptoms of carpal tunnel syndrome.

Psychological, psychiatric

Aspartame has been associated with mood disturbances, but only anecdotally (19).

Gastrointestinal

Sorbitol is slowly absorbed by passive diffusion in the small intestine. After oral administration, it increases osmotic pressure in the bowel by drawing in water, and is thus an osmotic laxative, sometimes leading to diarrhea (22). Bacterial fermentation of sorbitol in the large bowel is associated with increased flatulence and abdominal cramping. Sorbitol 10 g can cause flatulence and bloating, and 20 g abdominal cramps and diarrhea.

Many healthy individuals are intolerant of sorbitol, and develop abdominal cramping and diarrhea with less than the usual laxative dose (23). It has been suggested that more than 30% of healthy adults, irrespective of ethnic origin, cannot tolerate 10 g of sorbitol (24).

Certain other patients are especially sensitive to the gastrointestinal effects of sorbitol; for example, diabetics can be prone to sorbitol intolerance, because of altered gastrointestinal transit time and motility. Some of them also have a higher consumption of sorbitol-containing dietary foods. Patients on chronic hemodialysis can be predisposed to sorbitol intolerance as a result of carbohydrate malabsorption (25).

Kayexalate (sodium polystyrene sulfonate) in sorbitol is commonly used to treat hyperkalemia in patients with renal insufficiency. Case reports have documented intestinal necrosis after the administration of kayexalate in sorbitol (26,27). In one study, there was an incidence of 1.8%, and the authors concluded that sorbitol-associated complications may not be uncommon postoperatively (28). Furthermore, it has been suggested that some cases of idiopathic colonic ulcers in patients with renal failure are due to the effects of sorbitol. While kayexalate crystals, which are purple, irregular, and jagged, can be an incidental finding and are not known to cause injury, they are a helpful histological clue to the possibility that sorbitol has been administered (29).

Five cases of extensive mucosal necrosis and transmural infarction of the colon have been reported after the use of kayexalate and sorbitol enemas to treat hyperkalemia in uremic patients (30). The authors also studied the effects of kayexalate sorbitol enemas in normal and uremic rats and concluded that sorbitol was responsible for colonic damage and that the injury was potentiated in uremic rats. When sorbitol alone or kayexalate sorbitol were given, extensive transmural necrosis developed in 80% of normal rats and in all the uremic rats.

Following reports of colonic necrosis, the Pharmaceutical Affairs Bureau of Japan has revised the product information for enemas of polystyrene sulfonate cation exchange resin suspension in sorbitol solution for potassium removal (31). Although a causal relation has not been established definitively, the Bureau has decided that sorbitol solution should not be used for enemas of sodium polystyrene sulfonate cation exchange resins.

Immunologic

The role of aspartame in hypersensitivity reactions is controversial, although there have been case reports (32). In a multicenter, randomized, double-blind, placebo-controlled, crossover study, aspartame was more likely than placebo to cause urticaria or angioedema (33).

Aspartame can cause granulomatous septal panniculitis (34).

Lobular panniculitis has been described in a 57-year-old diabetic man who ingested large amounts of aspartame as a sweetener, in soft drinks and other products. He stopped taking aspartame and the tender subcutaneous nodules disappeared (35).

Long-Term Effects

Tumorigenicity

Acesulfame

The studies on the basis of which acesulfame gained approval showed no evidence in animals of mutagenicity, teratogenicity, or adverse reproductive effects; a 2-year toxicology study in beagles showed no untoward adverse effects. The incidence of lymphocytic leukemia was slightly increased in high-dosed female mice, but not beyond the spontaneous variation with this strain. No other evidence of potential carcinogenicity was obtained, and it has been concluded that at the estimated level of exposure, acesulfame and its metabolites are not a health hazard (36).

Aspartame

It has been suggested that aspartame may be linked to the increase in incidence of brain tumors. Brain tumor incidence increases in the USA occurred in two distinct phases, an early modest increase that may have primarily reflected improved diagnostic technology, and a later-sustained increase in the incidence and shift toward greater malignancy that must be explained by some other factor(s) (37). Evidence potentially implicating aspartame includes an early animal study that showed an exceedingly high incidence of brain tumors in aspartame-fed rats compared with no brain tumors in concurrent controls, the finding that aspartame has mutagenic potential, and the close temporal association (aspartame was introduced into US food and beverage markets several years prior to the sharp increase in brain tumor incidence and malignancy). The authors concluded that the carcinogenic potential of aspartame needs to be reassessed.

Saccharin

Saccharin has been considered to be a possible human carcinogen on the basis of animal experiments. This suspicion has now been discredited. There is no evidence that people with diabetes, who consume larger quantities of saccharin than non-diabetics, are at greater risk of developing bladder cancer (38) or other malignancies. However, in the USA, saccharin-containing medicines are required to carry the following warning: "Use of this product may be hazardous to your health. This product contains saccharin which has been determined to cause cancer in laboratory animals" (39).

Susceptibility Factors

Individuals with mood disorders are thought to be particularly sensitive to aspartame, and it has been suggested that its use in such patients should be discouraged (40).

References

1. Anonymous. Acesulfame Fed Regist 1988;53(145):28379.
2. Trefz F, de Sonneville L, Matthis P, Benninger C, Lanz-Englert B, Bickel H. Neuropsychological and biochemical investigations in heterozygotes for phenylketonuria during ingestion of high dose aspartame (a sweetener containing phenylalanine). Hum Genet 1994;93(4):369–74.
3. Council on Scientific Affairs. Aspartame. Review of safety issues. JAMA 1985;254(3):400–2.
4. Stegink LD, Koch R, Blaskovics ME, Filer LJ Jr, Baker GL, McDonnell JE. Plasma phenylalanine levels in phenylketonuric heterozygous and normal adults administered aspartame at 34 mg/kg body weight. Toxicology 1981;20(1):81–90.
5. Stegink LD, Filer LJ Jr, Baker GL. Repeated ingestion of aspartame-sweetened beverage: effect on plasma amino acid concentrations in normal adults. Metabolism 1988;37(3):246–51.
6. Stegink LD, Filer LJ, Baker GL, et al. Aspartame metabolism in human subjects. In: Health and Sugar Substitutes. Proceedings of ERGOB Conference, Geneva 1978:160–5.
7. Shahangian S, Ash KO, Rollins DE. Aspartame not a source of formate toxicity. Clin Chem 1984;30(7):1264–5.
8. FAO/WHO. Evaluation of certain food additives and contaminants. Thirty-seventh report of the Joint FAO/WHO Expert Committee on Food Additives. World Health Organ Tech Rep Ser 1991;806:1–52.
9. Barkin M, Comisarow RH, Taranger LA, Canada A. Three cases of human bladder cancer following high dose cyclamate ingestion. J Urol 1977;118(2):258–9.
10. Derfler K, Meryn S, Herold C, Neuhold N, Mostbeck G, Gangl A. Reversible malabsorption caused by high doses of cyclamate. Am J Med 1988;85(3):446–7.
11. Lutomski DM, Gora ML, Wright SM, Martin JE. Sorbitol content of selected oral liquids. Ann Pharmacother 1993;27(3):269–74.
12. Dills WL Jr. Sugar alcohols as bulk sweeteners. Annu Rev Nutr 1989;9:161–86.
13. Pal B, Keenan J, Misra HN, Moussa K, Morris J. Raynaud's phenomenon in idiopathic carpal tunnel syndrome. Scand J Rheumatol 1996;25(3):143–5.
14. Johns DR. Migraine provoked by aspartame. N Engl J Med 1986;315(7):456.
15. Bradstock MK, Serdula MK, Marks JS, Barnard RJ, Crane NT, Remington PL, Trowbridge FL. Evaluation of reactions to food additives: the aspartame experience. Am J Clin Nutr 1986;43(3):464–9.
16. Blumenthal HJ, Vance DA. Chewing gum headaches. Headache 1997;37(10):665–6.
17. Van den Eeden SK, Koepsell TD, Longstreth WT Jr, van Belle G, Daling JR, McKnight B. Aspartame ingestion and headaches: a randomized crossover trial. Neurology 1994;44(10):1787–93.
18. Camfield PR, Camfield CS, Dooley JM, Gordon K, Jollymore S, Weaver DF. Aspartame exacerbates EEG spike-wave discharge in children with generalized absence epilepsy: a double-blind controlled study. Neurology 1992;42(5):1000–3.
19. Koehler SM, Glaros A. The effect of aspartame on migraine headache. Headache 1988;28(1):10–14.
20. Robbins PI, Raymond L. Aspartame and symptoms of carpal tunnel syndrome. J Occup Environ Med 1999;41(6):418.
21. Levine DW, Simmons BP, Koris MJ, Daltroy LH, Hohl GG, Fossel AH, Katz JN. A self-administered questionnaire for the assessment of severity of symptoms and functional status in carpal tunnel syndrome. J Bone Joint Surg Am 1993;75(11):1585–92.
22. Gatto-Smith AG, Scott RB, Machida HM, Gall DG. Sorbitol as a cryptic cause of diarrhea. Can J Gastroenterol 1988;2:140–2.
23. Badiga MS, Jain NK, Casanova C, Pitchumoni CS. Diarrhea in diabetics: the role of sorbitol. J Am Coll Nutr 1990;9(6):578–82.
24. Jain NK, Patel VP, Pitchumoni CS. Sorbitol intolerance in adults. Prevalence and pathogenesis on two continents. J Clin Gastroenterol 1987;9(3):317–19.

25. Coyne MJ, Rodriguez H. Carbohydrate malabsorption in black and Hispanic dialysis patients. Am J Gastroenterol 1986;81(8):662–5.

26. Gardiner GW. Kayexalate (sodium polystyrene sulphonate) in sorbitol associated with intestinal necrosis in uremic patients. Can J Gastroenterol 1997;11(7):573–7.

27. Wootton FT, Rhodes DF, Lee WM, Fitts CT. Colonic necrosis with kayexalate–sorbitol enemas after renal transplantation. Ann Intern Med 1989;111(11):947–9.

28. Gerstman BB, Kirkman R, Platt R. Intestinal necrosis associated with postoperative orally administered sodium polystyrene sulfonate in sorbitol. Am J Kidney Dis 1992;20(2):159–61.

29. Rashid A, Hamilton SR. Necrosis of the gastrointestinal tract in uremic patients as a result of sodium polystyrene sulfonate (kayexalate) in sorbitol: an underrecognized condition. Am J Surg Pathol 1997;21(1):60–9.

30. Lillemoe KD, Romolo JL, Hamilton SR, Pennington LR, Burdick JF, Williams GM. Intestinal necrosis due to sodium polystyrene (kayexalate) in sorbitol enemas: clinical and experimental support for the hypothesis. Surgery 1987;101(3):267–72.

31. Anonymous. Sorbitol as a solvent for cation exchange resin enemas composed of polystyrene sulfonate-revised data sheet-colonic necrosis. WHO Newslett 1996;5,6:4.

32. Kulczycki A Jr. Aspartame-induced urticaria. Ann Intern Med 1986;104(2):207–8.

33. Geha R, Buckley CE, Greenberger P, Patterson R, Polmar S, Saxon A, Rohr A, Yang W, Drouin M. Aspartame is no more likely than placebo to cause urticaria/angioedema: results of a multicenter, randomized, double-blind, placebo-controlled, crossover study. J Allergy Clin Immunol 1993;92(4):513–20.

34. Novick NL. Aspartame-induced granulomatous panniculitis. Ann Intern Med 1985;102(2):206–7.

35. McCauliffe DP, Poitras K. Aspartame-induced lobular panniculitis. J Am Acad Dermatol 1991;24(2 Pt 1):298–300.

36. FAO/WHO. Evaluation of certain food additives and contaminants. Twenty-sixth report of the Joint FAO/WHO Expert Committee on Food Additives. World Health Organ Tech Rep Ser 1982;683:7–51.

37. Olney JW, Farber NB, Spitznagel E, Robins LN. Increasing brain tumor rates: is there a link to aspartame? J Neuropathol Exp Neurol 1996;55(11):1115–23.

38. Walker AM, Dreyer NA, Friedlander E, Loughlin J, Rothman KJ, Kohn HI. An independent analysis of the National Cancer Institute study on non-nutritive sweeteners and bladder cancer. Am J Public Health 1982;72(4):376–81.

39. US Food and Drug Administration. Saccharin. FDA Talk Paper T87-38, 1 September 1987.

40. Walton RG, Hudak R, Green-Waite RJ. Adverse reactions to aspartame: double-blind challenge in patients from a vulnerable population. Biol Psychiatry 1993;34(1-2):13–17.

Asclepiadaceae

See also Herbal medicines

General Information

The genera in the family of Asclepiadaceae (Table 1) include milkweed and periploca.

Asclepias tuberosa

Asclepias tuberosa (pleurisy root) contains cardenolides such as uzarigenin, coroglaucigenin, and corotoxigenin,

Table 1 The genera of Asclepiadaceae

Araujia (araujia)
Asclepias (milkweed)
Calotropis (calotropis)
Cryptostegia (rubbervine)
Cynanchum (swallow-wort)
Funastrum (twinevine)
Gonolobus (gonolobus)
Hoya (hoya)
Marsdenia (marsdenia)
Matelea (milkvine)
Metaplexis (metaplexis)
Morrenia (morrenia)
Oxypetalum (oxypetalum)
Periploca (periploca)
Stapelia (stapelia)
Xysmalobium (xysmalobium)

the coumarins isorhamnetin, kaempferol, quercetin, and rutin, the steroid sitosterol, and the triterpenoids amyrin, friedelin, and lupeol.

Adverse effects

Because it contains cardenolides, *Asclepias* can have digitalis-like effects and potentiate digitalis toxicity (See monograph on Cardiac glycosides). Interference with assays of plasma digoxin concentrations is also possible (1).

Xysmalobium undulatum

Xysmalobium undulatum (xysmalobium) contains the cardiac glycoside ascleposide. It has been used topically to treat wounds (2). Its adverse effects are likely to be those of other cardiac glycosides (see monograph on Cardiac glycosides).

References

1. Longerich L, Johnson E, Gault MH. Digoxin-like factors in herbal teas. Clin Invest Med 1993;16(3):210–18.
2. Steenkamp V, Mathivha E, Gouws MC, van Rensburg CE. Studies on antibacterial, antioxidant and fibroblast growth stimulation of wound healing remedies from South Africa. J Ethnopharmacol 2004;95(2–3):353–7.

Ascorbic acid (vitamin C)

See also Vitamins

General Information

The Average Requirement of ascorbic acid is 30 mg/day. The Population Reference Intake is 45 mg/day for adults. The Lowest Threshold Intake, for which considerable evidence exists, is 12 mg/day (1). These estimates have been supported by the relevant committee of the European Union. A communication from the US National Academy of Sciences, as part of the revision of US Dietary Reference Intakes, while estimating rather higher average requirements of ascorbic acid than the EU committee, does (100 mg/day) also proposed a "tolerable upper intake level" of less than 1 g of ascorbic acid/day (2). "Normal" plasma ascorbic acid concentrations are 60–80 μmol/l (2).

In spite of the lack of unequivocal evidence of a beneficial effect of large doses of ascorbic acid for preventing or treating the common cold, the use of ascorbic acid for this indication is still widespread.

The adverse effects of high-dose ascorbic acid have been reviewed in the context of its pharmacokinetics (3). Pharmacokinetic analysis shows that there is no justification for the use of megadoses of ascorbic acid (4). The body goes to great lengths to avoid excess accumulation of vitamin C, and has at least three ways of accomplishing this. First, absorption of vitamin C from the gut is highly saturable, ensuring that the amount that is absorbed reaches a maximum at relatively low doses. Secondly, the kidney rapidly excretes vitamin C, because its reabsorption from the renal tubules after filtration by the renal glomerulus is also highly saturable. Virtually all the vitamin C that is absorbed from the gut is thus excreted in the urine. For example, when the daily dose is increased from 200 to 2500 mg (from 1.1 to 14 mmol) the mean steady-state plasma concentration increases only from about 12–15 mg/l (from 68 to 85 mol/l)—no matter how high a dose of vitamin C you take orally there is a limit to the plasma concentration that can be reached. Thirdly, tissue uptake is also saturable. An increase in plasma concentration of vitamin C is not associated with a parallel increase in tissue concentration (5). Indeed, the tissue vitamin C concentration, measured in leukocytes, saturates at 100 mg/day (6) or plasma concentrations of 14 μg/ml (80 mol/l) (5). So no matter how much you take, all you do is increase the concentrations in your urine and gut, and that can cause adverse effects (7). Vitamin C is partly excreted as oxalate, and very high doses can lead to hyperoxaluria and kidney stones (8), particularly after intravenous use and in people with renal insufficiency. Adverse effects in the gut include nausea, abdominal cramps, and diarrhea (9).

General adverse effects

Hot flushes, headache, fatigue, insomnia, nausea, vomiting, and diarrhea have been observed with large doses, but it is difficult to tell to what extent these are real rather than placebo effects. The best evidence of problems caused by high doses relates to stone formation, mainly in patients with chronic renal insufficiency. Certain hematological and metabolic effects have been reported in premature infants; however, these have not been corroborated (10). Several cases of hemolysis have been reported. Respiratory and cutaneous allergies to ascorbic acid have been described (11). Tumor-inducing effects have not been reported.

Organs and Systems

Respiratory

Ascorbic acid 3 g/day for 6 days causes a significant loss of high altitude resistance, persisting for 2 weeks after withdrawal of treatment. High doses may therefore constitute a risk in people who take them under conditions in which the oxygen supply suddenly becomes impaired, and is also undesirable in people with pathological hypoxia, for example due to respiratory diseases (12).

A trial in 868 children showed that in those with high plasma ascorbic acid concentrations, the duration of upper respiratory infection was greater than in those with low concentrations (13). This finding, which contrasted with the optimistic expectations of other workers, requires confirmation.

Metabolism

Dehydroascorbic acid appears to have a diabetogenic effect and ascorbic acid causes increased excretion of glucose. High ascorbic acid concentrations can delay the insulin response to a glucose challenge and prolong postprandial hyperglycemia (14).

An increase in serum cholesterol has been reported in patients with atherosclerosis taking high doses of ascorbic acid (9).

Metal metabolism

Binding of zinc and copper by high doses of ascorbic acid has been reported (9).

Hematologic

Under experimental conditions, ascorbic acid 5 g/day increased the lytic sensitivity of erythrocytes to hydrogen peroxide (15). Similar doses, given with mandelamine or antibiotics, lower urinary pH and have a small effect on blood pH; in patients with sickle-cell anemia such doses can precipitate a crisis (9). The erythrocytes of premature infants can be damaged by ascorbic acid (SEDA-14, 332); reduced glutathione concentrations and increased Heinz-body formation have been seen (16). Possible explanations may be higher glucose consumption and increased glycolytic enzyme activities compared with erythrocytes in adults, accompanied by increased sensitivity to hemolysis (17).

Also at risk of hemolysis are patients with glucose-6-phosphate dehydrogenase deficiency, in whom ascorbic acid can denature hemoglobin and reduce erythrocyte glutathione concentrations; one such case proved fatal (18). This was further demonstrated by reports of hemolytic effects (19); in two young subjects with glucose-6-phosphate dehydrogenase deficiency hemolysis was induced by excessive intake of "fizzy drinks" fortified with ascorbic acid (20).

Gastrointestinal

Nausea, abdominal cramps, and diarrhea are not uncommon (9). In runners taking daily doses of 1 g of ascorbic acid for reduction of musculoskeletal symptoms, mild diarrhea is common (21). Ascorbic acid stones have been found to obstruct the ileocecal valve (22).

Urinary tract

Ascorbic acid 4 g/day increases uric acid clearance in volunteers (23), although it does not reduce protein-bound uric acid in blood. Ascorbic acid 4–12 g/day causes acidification of the urine, which can cause precipitation of urate and cystine and consequently formation of urate stones or cystinuria. Ascorbic acid is excreted largely as oxalate, and hyperoxaluria results when large doses are taken. In patients with pre-existing oxalosis, gram doses of ascorbic acid further increase oxalate excretion (9,24).

Whether this increased oxalate excretion has consequences in terms of stone formation depends very much on the dosage and duration of treatment. In a small study in healthy individuals short-term, high-dose ascorbic acid (4 g in 5 days) did not affect the risk factors associated with calcium oxalate kidney stone formation (8). A prospective study of the association between doses of pyridoxine and ascorbic acid and the risk of symptomatic kidney stones was undertaken in a large cohort of US nurses. Ascorbic acid was not associated with a higher risk of stone formation (25).

In a study to determine the biochemical and physicochemical risks of high doses of ascorbic acid a man with no history of nephrolithiasis took ascorbic acid 2 g qds while following his normal diet (26). The study was planned to last 9 days. However, he developed significant hematuria on the eighth day. Urinary oxalate and ascorbic acid concentrations were increased. The intestinal absorption of ascorbic acid falls from almost 100% at normal doses to 20% at a dose of 5 g/day (27), and the high concentrations of ascorbic acid in this study suggest that, irrespective of the quantity converted to oxalate, at least 35% of the ingested ascorbic acid had been absorbed. The relative supersaturation of oxalate and the Tiselius risk index both increased. Increases in the calcium oxalate relative supersaturation (28) and Tiselius index (29) are powerful physicochemical indicators of increases in the crystal-forming potential of the urine. In this case the increases in both measures were impressively substantiated by scanning electron microscopy, which showed large crystals and crystal aggregates in the urine. The authors suggested that the passage of these crystals caused irritation and epithelial injury manifesting as hematuria.

Oxalate-induced renal damage has been related to excessive doses of ascorbic acid (30).

- A 31-year-old man developed a headache, nausea, and vomiting. He had taken ascorbic acid, 2–2.5 g/day and before the onset of symptoms up to 5 g/day. He had a raised serum creatinine (1000 µmol/l). Renal ultrasound showed increased cortical echogenicity, and a renal biopsy showed acute tubular necrosis and massive oxalate deposition. He was given pyridoxine and two sessions of hemodialysis.

Various forms of renal damage, notably tubulointerstitial nephropathy, have been associated with long-term use of high dosages of ascorbic acid, for example 3 g/day (31).

Skin

Cutaneous allergy has been described with ascorbic acid (11).

Contact dermatitis has been attributed to ascorbic acid in a cosmetic anti-ageing cream (32).

- A 47-year-old woman developed eczema of the face, consisting initially of edematous lesions on the eyelids and then spreading to the rest of the face and the folds of the neck. Patch tests to a cosmetic cream she had used before the start of the eczema (Active C dry skin, La Roche Posay Laboratory) gave positive results (++D2 and D3). Subsequent patch tests with the ingredients showed positive results only to ascorbic acid. Oral provocation tests with ascorbic acid 50–2000 mg were negative. Withdrawal of the cream resulted in complete healing of the eczema without relapse over 6 months.

Musculoskeletal

In animal experiments, high doses of ascorbic acid adversely influenced skeleton stability. In chicks, supplementary ascorbic acid 220 mg/kg in the food increased mobilization of calcium and phosphate from the skeleton, as demonstrated by ^{45}Ca studies and determination of acid phosphatase activity in plasma. Increased ascorbic acid also resulted in increased oxygen consumption and decreased lactic acid production by cultured chick tibiae; in growing swine, large doses (about 1 g/day for 32 days) led to a significant increase in the excretion rate of hydroxyproline, indicating an increased rate of collagen breakdown (SED-8, 803) (33). The relevance of these old findings to humans has never been confirmed.

Immunologic

As noted above, ascorbic acid can sometimes cause immune reactions. Ascorbic acid and citric acid are used as food additives, ascorbic acid (E300) as an acidifier, an antioxidant, and an additive in wheat, and citric acid as an acidifying complex-binding agent. Because additives are widely used in foods, beverages, and drugs, people with allergies or intolerance have to be carefully instructed. Caution must also be taken when scratch tests are performed with these substances (34).

- A 62-year-old man had frequent angioedema, and a scratch test was performed with several food additives. Scratching with 1% ascorbic acid and 1% citric acid in vaseline resulted in a +3 reaction, and 20 minutes later he developed angioedema with swelling of the glottis, reddening of the face and hands, itching, vertigo, tachycardia, and hypotension. He was given a glucocorticoid and an antihistamine and recovered within half an hour.

Second-Generation Effects

Fertility

Earlier evidence that ascorbic acid in gram doses might reduce fertility was disputed; however, a case of sterility apparently due to ascorbic acid has been described (9).

Teratogenicity

Animal teratological evidence is not entirely uniform, but very high doses in rats and mice have been given without deleterious effects on the fetus (35).

Susceptibility Factors

Genetic factors

Patients with idiopathic (genetic) hemochromatosis constitute a risk group with regard to ingestion of large doses of ascorbic acid, which can lead to deterioration in cardiac function (36).

Age

An esophageal stricture, with ulceration, inflammation, and fibrosis, has been reported in an elderly patient who had taken ascorbic acid for 2 months (37). A 500 mg tablet of ascorbic acid dissolves only slowly and is in vitro associated with a shift in saliva pH from 6.2 to 2.8. Since elderly individuals usually have less frequent esophageal contractions, it is not uncommon for this group to have a capsule lodged for a time in the esophagus (SEDA-13, 348) and it is entirely possible that cases like the above are more frequent than previously thought.

Renal disease

The use of ascorbic acid in patients with renal insufficiency should be carefully monitored to avoid accelerated development of secondary oxalosis; hyperoxalemia has been reported to be aggravated by ascorbic acid supplementation in regular hemodialysis patients (38). The pharmacological mechanism has been clarified in animal experiments (SEDA-15, 414) (39).

Other features of the patient

Ascorbic acid has been thought to precipitate widespread tumor hemorrhage and necrosis with disastrous consequences in patients with very rapidly proliferating and widely disseminating tumors. These observations suggest that ascorbic acid should be prescribed with extreme caution for persons with advanced cancer (40).

Drug–Drug Interactions

Amphetamines

Decreased renal tubular reabsorption of amphetamines can be caused by ascorbic acid (40).

Aspirin

Enhanced drug crystalluria with aspirin can be caused by ascorbic acid (40).

Fluphenazine

Ascorbic acid may lower serum fluphenazine concentrations by liver enzyme induction and by interference with absorption (41).

Iron

Ascorbic acid promotes the absorption of iron, a reason for caution in giving high doses to patients with iron overload (SEDA-9, 324). In particular, patients with hemochromatosis, polycythemia, and leukemia who present with marked iron overload should keep their intake of ascorbic acid to a minimum (42). However, ascorbic acid can also interfere with the distribution of iron in the body in these patients. One consequence is that in patients with iron overload who also have scurvy, iron tends to be deposited in the reticuloendothelial system rather than the parenchymal cells, which may reduce the risks of damage to the liver, heart, or endocrine glands. It has conversely been noted that in beta-thalassemia major with iron overload, ascorbic acid can be associated with deterioration in cardiac function (43).

Isoprenaline

Ascorbic acid in large doses (5 g/day) reduces the chronotropic effect of isoprenaline (44).

Oral anticoagulants

The effect of ascorbate in reducing prothrombin time is potentially dangerous during oral anticoagulant therapy. In one patient taking dicoumarol the prothrombin time fell from 19 seconds to normal values after intake of ascorbic acid. A similar effect was noted in a patient with thrombophlebitis given ascorbic acid 16 g/day (9). Earlier data suggested that even doses of 200 mg may have resulted in a slight increase in mortality from thromboembolism in patients in a geriatric unit (45).

Tricyclic antidepressants

Decreased renal tubular reabsorption of tricyclic antidepressants can be caused by ascorbic acid (40).

Vitamin B$_{12}$

Because ascorbic acid in the gastrointestinal tract can reduce the vitamin B$_{12}$ content of food, patients with vitamin B$_{12}$ deficiency should always be questioned about their intake of ascorbic acid (40).

Interference with Diagnostic Tests

Tests for plasma ethinylestradiol concentrations

Plasma ethinylestradiol concentrations increase when it is taken with ascorbic acid. This interaction is of significance in women taking oral contraceptives (SEDA-6, 328).

Tests for urinary glucose

The presence of high concentrations of ascorbic acid in the urine can interfere with tests for urinary glucose. With concentrations as low as 200 µg/ml, tests performed with glucose oxidase paper can be inhibited, giving a false negative result (46).

Ascorbic acid can also result in false positive tests for glucose in urine (Benedict's test, Clinitest) and blood. Any reports of glycosuria or hyperglycemia in patients taking ascorbic acid must therefore be regarded with suspicion unless a specific (for example chromatographic) test for glucose has been performed (9).

Tests for occult blood

There were false negative tests for occult blood after the ingestion of moderately high doses of ascorbic acid (250 mg) (47). Quantities in excess of this are excreted and can affect tests for occult gastric or stool blood (7,48,49). Lack of ascorbic acid can, because of its effect on iron distribution, alter laboratory indices for iron overload, causing the plasma iron or ferritin levels (or the degree of iron excretion after a challenge with deferoxamine) to be considerably less than the degree of severity of iron overload that would normally lead one to expect (50).

Tests for serum enzymes

Ascorbic acid interferes with the autoanalyser determination of serum transaminases and lactic dehydrogenase (7,9). Serum bilirubin concentrations may be reduced by ascorbic acid, so that the presence of liver disease may be masked (9).

References

1. Scientific Committee for Food. Nutrient and energy intakes for the European Community. Directorate-General Industry, Commission of the European Communities. Luxembourg, 1993.
2. Levine M, Rumsey SC, Daruwala R, Park JB, Wang Y. Criteria and recommendations for vitamin C intake. JAMA 1999;281(15):1415–23.
3. Aronson JK. Forbidden fruit. Nat Med 2001;7(1):29–30.
4. Blanchard J, Tozer TN, Rowland M. Pharmacokinetic perspectives on megadoses of ascorbic acid. Am J Clin Nutr 1997;66(5):1165–71.
5. Basu TK, Schorah CJ. Vitamin C in health and disease. Westport, Connecticut: The Avi Publishing Company 1982:61–3.
6. Levine M, Conry-Cantilena C, Wang Y, Welch RW, Washko PW, Dhariwal KR, Park JB, Lazarev A, Graumlich JF, King J, Cantilena LR. Vitamin C pharmacokinetics in healthy volunteers: evidence for a recommended dietary allowance. Proc Natl Acad Sci USA 1996;93(8):3704–9.
7. Meyers DG, Maloley PA, Weeks D. Safety of antioxidant vitamins. Arch Intern Med 1996;156(9):925–35.
8. Auer BL, Auer D, Rodgers AL. The effect of ascorbic acid ingestion on the biochemical and physicochemical risk factors associated with calcium oxalate kidney stone formation. Clin Chem Lab Med 1998;36(3):143–7.
9. Barness LA. Safety considerations with high ascorbic acid dosage. Ann NY Acad Sci 1975;258:523–8.
10. Doyle J, Vreman HJ, Stevenson DK, Brown EJ, Schmidt B, Paes B, Ohlsson A, Boulton J, Kelly E, Gillie P, Lewis N, Merko S, Shaw D, Zipursky A. Does vitamin C cause hemolysis in premature newborn infants? Results of a multicenter double-blind, randomized, controlled trial. J Pediatr 1997;130(1):103–9.
11. Vasal P. A propos de trois allergies réspiratoires et cutanés d'l'acide ascorbique. Rev Fr Allergol 1976;16:103.
12. Schrauzer GN, Ishmael D, Kiefer GW. Some aspects of current vitamin C usage: diminished high-altitude resistance following overdosage. Ann NY Acad Sci 1975;258:377–81.
13. Coulehan JL, Eberhard S, Kapner L, Taylor F, Rogers K, Garry P. Vitamin C and acute illness in Navajo school children. N Engl J Med 1976;295(18):973–7.
14. Johnston CS, Yen MF. Megadose of vitamin C delays insulin response to a glucose challenge in normoglycemic adults. Am J Clin Nutr 1994;60(5):735–8.
15. Mengel CE, Greene HL Jr. Ascorbic acid effects on erythrocytes. Ann Intern Med 1976;84(4):490.
16. Ballin A, Brown EJ, Koren G, Zipursky A. Vitamin C-induced erythrocyte damage in premature infants J Pediatr 1988;113(1 Pt 1):114–20.
17. Petrich C, Goebel U. Vitamin C-induced damage of erythrocytes in neonates. J Pediatr 1989;114(2):341–2.
18. Campbell GD Jr, Steinberg MH, Bower JD. Ascorbic acid-induced hemolysis in G-6-PD deficiency. Ann Intern Med 1975;82(6):810.
19. Rees DC, Kelsey H, Richards JD. Acute haemolysis induced by high dose ascorbic acid in glucose-6-phosphate dehydrogenase deficiency. BMJ 1993;306(6881):841–2.
20. Mehta JB, Singhal SB, Mehta BC. Ascorbic-acid-induced haemolysis in G-6-PD deficiency. Lancet 1990;336(8720):944.
21. Hoyt CJ. Diarrhea from vitamin C. JAMA 1980;244(15):1674.
22. Vickery RE. Unusual complication of excessive ingestion of vitamin C tablets. Int Surg 1973;58(6):422–3.
23. Stein HB, Hasan A, Fox IH. Ascorbic acid-induced uricosuria. A consequency of megavitamin therapy. Ann Intern Med 1976;84(4):385–8.
24. Roth DA, Breitenfield RV. Vitamin C and oxalate stones. JAMA 1977;237(8):768.
25. Curhan GC, Willett WC, Speizer FE, Stampfer MJ. Intake of vitamins B6 and C and the risk of kidney stones in women. J Am Soc Nephrol 1999;10(4):840–5.
26. Auer BL, Auer D, Rodgers AL. Relative hyperoxaluria, crystalluria and haematuria after megadose ingestion of vitamin C. Eur J Clin Invest 1998;28(9):695–700.
27. Marcus R, Coulston AM. The vitamins. In: Goodman Gilman A, Rall TN, Nies AS, Taylor P, editors. The Pharmacological Basis of Therapeutics. 8th ed. New York: Pergamon Press, 1990:1530–52.
28. Werness PG, Brown CM, Smith LH, Finlayson B. EQUIL2: a BASIC computer program for the calculation of urinary saturation. J Urol 1985;134(6):1242–4.
29. Tiselius HG. An improved method for the routine biochemical evaluation of patients with recurrent calcium oxalate stone disease. Clin Chim Acta 1982;122(3):409–18.
30. Mashour S, Turner JF Jr, Merrell R. Acute renal failure, oxalosis, and vitamin C supplementation: a case report and review of the literature. Chest 2000;118(2):561–3.
31. Nakamoto Y, Motohashi S, Kasahara H, Numazawa K. Irreversible tubulointerstitial nephropathy associated with prolonged, massive intake of vitamin C. Nephrol Dial Transplant 1998;13(3):754–6.
32. Belhadjali H, Giordano-Labadie F, Bazex J. Contact dermatitis from vitamin C in a cosmetic anti-aging cream. Contact Dermatitis 2001;45(5):317.
33. Brown RG. Possible problems of large intakes of ascorbic acid. JAMA 1973;224(11):1529–30.
34. Thumm EJ, Jung EG, Bayerl C. Anaphylaktische Reaktion nach Scratchtestung mit Ascorbinsäure (E 300) und Zitronensäure (E 330). Allergologie 2000;23:354–9.
35. Nishimura H, Tanimura T. Clinical Aspects of the Teratogenicity of Drugs. Amsterdam, Oxford: Excerpta Medica, 1976:251.
36. Van der Weyden MB. Vitamin C, desferrioxamine and iron loading anemias. Aust NZ J Med 1984;14(5):593–5.
37. Bonavina L, DeMeester TR, McChesney L, Schwizer W, Albertucci M, Bailey RT. Drug-induced esophageal strictures. Ann Surg 1987;206(2):173–83.
38. Ono K. Secondary hyperoxalemia caused by vitamin C supplementation in regular hemodialysis patients. Clin Nephrol 1986;26(5):239–43.
39. Ono K, Ono H, Ono T, Kikawa K, Oh Y. Effect of vitamin C supplementation on renal oxalate deposits in five-sixths nephrectomized rats. Nephron 1989;51(4):536–9.
40. Sestili MA. Possible adverse health effects of vitamin C and ascorbic acid. Semin Oncol 1983;10(3):299–304.
41. Dysken MW, Cumming RJ, Channon RA, Davis JM. Drug interaction between ascorbic acid and fluphenazine. JAMA 1979;241(19):2008.
42. Hallberg L. Effect of vitamin C on the bioavailability of iron from food. In: Counsell JN, Hornig DH, editors. Vitamin C (Ascorbic Acid). New Jersey: Applied Science Publishers, 1981:49.
43. Cohen A, Cohen IJ, Schwartz E. Scurvy and altered iron stores in thalassemia major. N Engl J Med 1981;304(3):158–60.

44. Hajdu E, Jaranyi B, Matos L. The effect of large oral doses of vitamin C on the chronotropic action of isoprenaline in man. Br J Pharmacol 1979;66(3):460P.
45. Andrews CT, Wilson TS. Vitamin C and thrombotic episodes. Lancet 1973;2(7819):39.
46. Mayson JS, Schumaker O, Nakamura RM. False negative tests for urinary glucose in the presence of ascorbic acid. Am J Clin Pathol 1972;58(3):297–9.
47. Jaffe RM, Kasten B, Young DS, MacLowry JD. False-negative stool occult blood tests caused by ingestion of ascorbic acid (vitamin C). Ann Intern Med 1975;83(6):824–6.
48. Anonymous. Vitamin C verfälscht Bluttests. Klinikarzt 1976;5:515.
49. Gogel HK, Tandberg D, Strickland RG. Substances that interfere with guaiac card tests: implications for gastric aspirate testing. Am J Emerg Med 1989;7(5):474–80.
50. Nienhuis AW. Vitamin C and iron. N Engl J Med 1981;304(3):170–1.

Asparaginase

See also Cytostatic and immunosuppressant drugs

General Information

Asparaginase is an enzyme that acts by breaking down the amino acid L-asparagine to aspartic acid and ammonia. It interferes with the growth of malignant cells that cannot synthesize L-asparagine. Its action is reportedly specific for the G_1 phase of the cell cycle. It is used mainly for the induction of remissions in acute lymphoblastic leukemia.

Nomenclature

Colaspase and crisantaspase are the British Approved Names of asparaginase obtained from cultures of *Escherichia coli* and *Erwinia carotovora* respectively.

Organs and Systems

Nervous system

In a review of 28 central nervous system thrombotic or hemorrhagic events and eight peripheral thromboses related to L-asparaginase, the median time from initial treatment to adverse reaction was 16–17 days (1). Most patients recovered completely, although five cases had residual neurological deficits and one died from superior sagittal sinus thrombosis. Five patients with cerebral thrombosis complicating asparaginase/prednisone/vincristine induction therapy for acute lymphoblastic leukemia were found to have a reduced platelet count after the event and, in three of them, sequential changes in von Willebrand factor multimer pattern (2). The other two patients were only studied at presentation and their multimer pattern was not appreciably different to pooled plasma from seven controls without thromboses. The findings were consistent with thrombotic complications caused by platelet agglutination by plasma Von Willebrand factor.

Metabolism

Asparaginase can reduce insulin production (3) and precipitate diabetic ketoacidosis (4,5).

Hematologic

Thrombosis and hemorrhage are well-recognized complications in 1–2% of patients receiving asparaginase. This is due to a coagulopathy, which has been variously attributed to reduced concentrations of fibrinogen, factors IX, XI, VIII complex, antithrombin III, and plasminogen (6).

In one study, 12 children in complete remission treated with daily asparaginase alone were investigated for platelet and clotting abnormalities (7). Changes in prothrombin time, partial thromboplastin time, and fibrinogen remained close to the reference range, and platelet function was normal. There were reduced concentrations of physiological inhibitors of coagulation (protein C and antithrombin III). Thrombosis was uncommon. These results are consistent with those of another study of asparaginase as a single agent in 14 children with acute lymphoblastic leukemia (8). There was severe deficiency of antithrombin III and protein C, with co-existing hypocoagulability; equilibrium between the two partly explained the lack of thromboembolic phenomena. The hypocoagulability was due to hypofibrinogenemia and reduced concentrations of vitamin K-dependent factors.

Three patients developed bilateral venous sinus thromboses after receiving asparaginase; the diagnosis and follow-up of this complication have been succinctly reviewed (9). In another patient receiving asparaginase, central nervous system thrombosis was associated with a transient acquired type II pattern of von Willebrand's disease (10).

Mouth and teeth

Acute parotitis has been attributed to L–asparaginase in association with hyperglycemia (11).

Liver

Most patients who receive asparaginase develop liver function abnormalities, which can be fatal (12). This adverse effect is of major concern in patients who are also taking other hepatotoxic drugs, such as methotrexate and mercaptopurine. Jaundice and increased serum bilirubin and transaminases occur often, and hepatomegaly and fatty deposits occur occasionally.

Pancreas

Pancreatitis has been reported in up to 16% of children receiving asparaginase for a variety of neoplasms (13). Pseudocyst formation has been described (14).

Immunologic

Asparaginase can cause allergic reactions (15), which increase with the number of doses within a cycle and the number of exposures, irrespective of drug-free intervals. There is a pegylated formulation (PEG-ASNase; Oncaspar™) with a prolonged half-life and different allergenic properties from conventional asparaginase-containing formulations. These claims have been investigated, and the authors concluded that although the hypersensitivity rate was lower, it was still significant; furthermore, there was no cross-sensitivity in previously treated patients (16). There were no allergic reactions to pegylated asparaginase compared with 30% with non-pegylated asparaginase in 70 children with acute lymphoblastic leukemia or non-Hodgkin's lymphoma, and other toxic effects were also less common (17).

References

1. Ott N, Ramsay NK, Priest JR, Lipton M, Pui CH, Steinherz P, Nesbit ME Jr. Sequelae of thrombotic or hemorrhagic complications following L-asparaginase therapy for childhood lymphoblastic leukemia. Am J Pediatr Hematol Oncol 1988;10(3):191–5.
2. Pui CH, Jackson CW, Chesney CM, Abildgaard CF. Involvement of von Willebrand factor in thrombosis following asparaginase–prednisone–vincristine therapy for leukemia. Am J Hematol 1987;25(3):291–8.
3. Meschi F, di Natale B, Rondanini GF, Uderzo C, Jankovic M, Masera G, Chiumello G. Pancreatic endocrine function in leukemic children treated with L-asparaginase. Horm Res 1981;15(4):237–41.
4. Rovira A, Cordido F, Vecilla C, Bernacer M, Valverde I, Herrera Pombo JL. Study of beta-cell function and erythrocyte insulin receptors in a patient with diabetic ketoacidosis associated with L-asparaginase therapy. Acta Paediatr Scand 1986;75(4):670–1.
5. Hsu YJ, Chen YC, Ho CL, Kao WY, Chao TY. Diabetic ketoacidosis and persistent hyperglycemia as long-term complications of L-asparaginase-induced pancreatitis. Zhonghua Yi Xue Za Zhi (Taipei) 2002;65(9):441–5.
6. O'Meara A, Daly M, Hallinan FH. Increased antithrombin III concentration in children with acute lymphatic leukaemia receiving L-asparaginase therapy. Med Pediatr Oncol 1988;16(3):169–74.
7. Homans AC, Rybak ME, Baglini RL, Tiarks C, Steiner ME, Forman EN. Effect of L-asparaginase administration on coagulation and platelet function in children with leukemia. J Clin Oncol 1987;5(5):811–17.
8. Mielot F, Danel P, Boyer C, Coulombel L, Dommergues JP, Tchernia G, Larrieu MJ. Déficits acquis en antithrombine III et en proteine C au cours due traitement par la L-asparaginase. [Acquired deficiencies in antithrombin III and C protein during treatment with L-asparaginase.] Arch Fr Pediatr 1987;44(3):161–5.
9. Schick RM, Jolesz F, Barnes PD, Macklis JD. MR diagnosis of dural venous sinus thrombosis complicating L-asparaginase therapy. Comput Med Imaging Graph 1989;13(4):319–27.
10. Shapiro AD, Clarke SL, Christian JM, Odom LF, Hathaway WE. Thrombosis in children receiving L-asparaginase. Determining patients at risk. Am J Pediatr Hematol Oncol 1993;15(4):400–5.
11. Uysal K, Uguz A, Olgun N, Sarialioglu F, Buyukgebiz A. Hyperglycemia and acute parotitis related to L-asparaginase therapy. J Pediatr Endocrinol Metab 1996;9(6):627–9.
12. Sahoo S, Hart J. Histopathological features of L-asparaginase-induced liver disease. Semin Liver Dis 2003;23(3):295–9.
13. Sadoff J, Hwang S, Rosenfeld D, Ettinger L, Spigland N. Surgical pancreatic complications induced by L-Asparaginase. J Pediatr Surg 1997;32(6):860–3.
14. Bertolone SJ, Fuenfer MM, Groff DB, Patel CC. Delayed pancreatic pseudocyst formations. Long-term complication of L-asparaginase treatment. Cancer 1982;50(12):2964–6.
15. Korholz D, Wahn U, Jurgens H, Wahn V. Allergische Reaktionen unter der Behandlung mit L-Asparaginase. Bedeutung spezifischer IgE-Antikorper. [Allergic reactions in treatment with L-asparaginase. Significance of specific IgE antibodies.] Monatsschr Kinderheilkd 1990;138(1):23–5.
16. Vieira Pinheiro JP, Muller HJ, Schwabe D, Gunkel M, Casimiro da Palma J, Henze G, von Schutz V, Winkelhorst M, Wurthwein G, Boos J. Drug monitoring of low-dose PEG-asparaginase (Oncaspar) in children with relapsed acute lymphoblastic leukaemia. Br J Haematol 2001;113(1):115–19.
17. Muller HJ, Loning L, Horn A, Schwabe D, Gunkel M, Schrappe M, von Schutz V, Henze G, Casimiro da Palma J, Ritter J, Pinheiro JP, Winkelhorst M, Boos J. Pegylated asparaginase (Oncaspar) in children with ALL: drug monitoring in reinduction according to the ALL/NHL-BFM 95 protocols. Br J Haematol 2000;110(2):379–84.

Astemizole

See also Antihistamines

General Information

Astemizole is a second-generation antihistamine that has been withdrawn from the market because of the association with life-threatening cardiac arrhythmias.

Organs and Systems

Cardiovascular

Astemizole is metabolized by CYP3A4 to desmethyl-astemizole and norastemizole, although these metabolites may not be free of the potential to prolong the QT interval.

- A 77-year-old woman with QT interval prolongation and torsade de pointes had been taking astemizole 10 mg/day for 6 months (1). She had markedly raised plasma concentrations of astemizole and was also taking cimetidine.

However, cardiac dysrhythmias in patients taking antihistamines may be related to other factors, and in this case the patient was also taking another antihistamine and had a history of hepatitis.

Nervous system

The incidence of sedation with astemizole has been reported to be similar to placebo in most studies (2–4) (SEDA-14, 136) (SEDA-18, 183).

Skin

PLEVA (pityriasis lichenoides et varioliformis) has been convincingly ascribed to astemizole by reappearance after rechallenge (SEDA-18, 4).

Stevens–Johnson syndrome has been reported with astemizole (SEDA-20, 162).

Drug Administration

Drug overdose

Two cases of overdosage with astemizole (200 mg in a 2-year-old child and 200 mg in a 16-year-old girl) were associated with cardiovascular complications (5). The authors recommended that patients should be observed for at least 24 hours after overdosage with astemizole.

References

1. Ikeda S, Oka H, Matunaga K, Kubo S, Asai S, Miyahara Y, Osaka A, Kohno S. Astemizole-induced torsades de pointes in a patient with vasospastic angina. Jpn Circ J 1998;62(3):225–7.
2. XIVth Congress of the European Academy of Allergology and Clinical immunology. Berlin. Proceedings. Antihistamines reassessed. Clin Exp Allergy 1990;20(Suppl 2):1–54.
3. Richards DM, Brogden RN, Heel RC, Speight TM, Avery GS. Astemizole. A review of its pharmacodynamic properties and therapeutic efficacy. Drugs 1984;28(1):38–61.
4. Barlow JL, Beitman RE, Tsai TH. Terfenadine, safety and tolerance in controlled clinical trials. Arzneimittelforschung 1982;32(9a):1215–17.
5. Bosse GM, Matyunas NJ. Delayed toxidromes. J Emerg Med 1999;17(4):679–90.

Asteraceae

See also Herbal medicines

General Information

The genera in the family of Asteraceae (Table 1) (formerly Compositae) include various types of asters (daisies), arnica, chamomile, goldeneye, marigold, snakeroot, tansy, thistle, and wormwood.

Table 1   The genera of Asteraceae

Acamptopappus (goldenhead)
Acanthospermum (starburr)
Achillea (yarrow)
Achyrachaena (blow wives)
Acmella (spotflower)
Acourtia (desert peony)
Acroptilon (hard heads)
Adenocaulon (trail plant)
Adenostemma (medicine plant)
Adenophyllum (dogweed)
Ageratum (whiteweed)
Ageratina (snakeroot)
Agoseris (agoseris)
Almut aster (alkali marsh aster)
Amberboa (amberboa)
Amblyolepis (amblyolepis)
Amblyopappus (amblyopappus)
Ambrosia (ragweed)
Ampel aster (climbing aster)
Amphipappus (chaffbush)
Amphiachyris (broomweed)
Anacylus (anacylus)
Anaphalis (pearly everlasting)
Ancistrocarphus (nest straw)
Anisocoma (anisocoma)
Antennaria (pussytoes)
Anthemis (chamomile)
Antheropeas (e aster bonnets)
Aphanostephus (doze daisy)

Arctium (burrdock)
Arctotheca (capeweed)
Arctotis (arctotis)
Argyroxiphium (silver sword)
Argyranthemum (dill daisy)
Argyrautia (arhyrautia)
Arnica (arnica)
Arnoglossum (Indian plaintain)
Arnoseris (arnoseris)
Artemisia (sagebrush, wormwood)
Asanthus (brickell bush)
Aster (aster)
Astranthium (western daisy)
Atrichoseris (atrichoseris)
Baccharis (baccharis)
Bahia (bahia)
Baileya (desert marigold)
Balduina (honeycombhead)
Balsamorhiza (balsam root)
Balsamita (balsamita)
Baltimora (baltimora)
Barkleyanthus (willow ragwort)
Bartlettia (bartlettia)
Bartlettina (bartlettina)
Bebbia (sweetbush)
Bellis (bellis)
Benitoa (benitoa)
Berkheya (berkheya)
Berlandiera (green eyes)
Bidens (beggar ticks)
Bigelowia (rayless goldenrod)
Blennosperma (sticky seed)
Blepharipappus (blepharipappus)
Blepharizonia (blepharizonia)
Blumea (false ox tongue)
Boltonia (doll's daisy)
Borrichia (seaside tansy)
Brickellia (brickell bush)
Brickelliastrum (brickell bush)
Buphthalmum (ox eye)
Cacaliopsis (cacaliopsis)
Calendula (marigold)
Callilepis (ox-eye daisy)
Callistephus (callistephus)
Calotis (calotis)
Calycadenia (western rosinweed)
Calycoseris (tackstem)
Calyptocarpus (calyptocarpus)
Canadanthus (mountain aster)
Carduus (plumeless thistle)
Carlina (carline thistle)
Carminatia (carminatia)
Carphephorus (chaffhead)
Carphochaete (bristlehead)
Carthamus (distaff thistle)
Castalis (castalis)
Celmisia (celmisia)
Centaurea (knapweed)
Centipeda (centipeda)
Centratherum (centratherum)
Chaenactis (pin cushion)
Chaetadelpha (skeletonweed)
Chaetopappa (least daisy)
Chamaemelum (dog fennel)
Chamaechaenactis (chamaechaenactis)
Chaptalia (sun bonnets)
Chloracantha (chloracantha)
Chondrilla (chondrilla)

Continued

Table 1 *Continued*

Chromolaena (thoroughwort)
Chrysactinia (chrysactinia)
Chrysoma (chrysoma)
Chrysanthemum (daisy)
Chrysogonum (chrysogonum)
Chrysopsis (golden aster)
Chrysothamnus (rabbit brush)
Cichorium (chicory)
Cineraria (cineraria)
Cirsium (thistle)
Clappia (clapdaisy)
Clibadium (clibadium)
Cnicus (cnicus)
Columbiadoria (columbiadoria)
Condylidium (villalba)
Conoclinium (thoroughwort)
Conyza (horseweed)
Coreocarpus (coreocarpus)
Coreopsis (tickseed)
Corethrogyne (sand aster)
Cosmos (cosmos)
Cotula (waterbuttons)
Crassocephalum (ragleaf)
Crepis (hawksbeard)
Critonia (thoroughwort)
Crocidium (spring gold)
Croptilon (scratch daisy)
Crupina (crupina)
Cyanopsis (knapweed)
Cyanthillium (ironweed)
Cymophora (cymophora)
Cynara (cynara)
Dahlia (dahlia)
Delairea (capeivy)
Dendranthema (arctic daisy)
Dichaetophora (dichaetophora)
Dicoria (twin bugs)
Dicranocarpus (dicranocarpus)
Dimeresia (dimeresia)
Dimorphotheca (cape marigold)
Dittrichia (dittrichia)
Doellingeria (whitetop)
Doronicum (false leopardbane)
Dracopis (coneflower)
Dubautia (dubautia)
Dysodiopsis (dog fennel)
Dyssodia (dyssodia)
Eastwoodia (eastwoodia)
Eatonella (eatonella)
Echinacea (purple coneflower)
Echinops (globe thistle)
Eclipta (eclipta)
Egletes (tropic daisy)
Elephantopus (elephant's foot)
Eleutheranthera (eleutheranthera)
Emilia (tasselflower)
Encelia (brittlebush)
Enceliopsis (sunray)
Engelmannia (Engelmann's daisy)
Enydra (swampwort)
Erechtites (burnweed)
Ericameria (goldenbush)
Erigeron (fleabane)
Eriophyllum (woolly sunflower)
Erlangea (erlangea)
Eucephalus (aster)
Euchiton (euchiton)

Eupatorium (thoroughwort)
Eurybia (aster)
Euryops (euryops)
Euthamia (goldentop)
Evax (pygmy cudweed)
Facelis (trampweed)
Filago (cottonrose)
Fitchia (fitchia)
Flaveria (yellowtops)
Fleischmannia (thoroughwort)
Florestina (florestina)
Flourensia (tarwort)
Flyriella (brickell bush)
Gaillardia (blanket flower)
Galinsoga (gallant-soldier)
Gamochaeta (everlasting)
Garberia (garberia)
Gazania (gazania)
Geraea (desertsunflower)
Gerbera (Transvaal daisy)
Glyptopleura (glyptopleura)
Gnaphalium (cudweed)
Gochnatia (gochnatia)
Grindelia (gumweed)
Guardiola (guardiola)
Guizotia (guizotia)
Gundelia (gundelia)
Gundlachia (gundlachia)
Gutierrezia (snakeweed)
Gymnosperma (gymnosperma)
Gymnostyles (burrweed)
Gynura (gynura)
Haploesthes (false broomweed)
Haplocarpha (onefruit)
Haplopappus (haplopappus)
Hartwrightia (hartwrightia)
Hasteola (false Indian plaintain)
Hazardia (bristleweed)
Hebeclinium (thoroughwort)
Hecastocleis (hecastocleis)
Hedypnois (hedypnois)
Helenium (sneezeweed)
Helianthell (helianthella)
Helianthus (sunflower)
Helichrysum (strawflower)
Heliopsis (heliopsis)
Heliomeris (false goldeneye)
Hemizonia (tarweed)
Hesperevax (dwarf-cudweed)
Hesperomannia (island aster)
Hesperodoria (glowweed)
Heteranthemis (ox eye)
Heterosperma (heterosperma)
Heterotheca (false golden aster)
Hieracium (hawkweed)
Holocarpha (tarweed)
Holozonia (holozonia)
Hulsea (alpinegold)
Hymenoclea (burrobrush)
Hymenopappus (hymenopappus)
Hymenothrix (thimblehead)
Hymenoxys (rubberweed)
Hypochaeris (cat's ear)
Hypochoeris (cat's ear)
Inula (yellowhead)
Ionactis (aster)
Isocarpha (pearlhead)
Isocoma (golden bush)

Continued

Table 1 *Continued*

Iva (marsh elder)
Ixeris (ixeris)
Jamesianthus (jamesianthus)
Jaumea (jaumea)
Jefea (jefea)
Kalimeris (aster)
Koanophyllon (thoroughwort)
Krigia (dwarf dandelion)
Lactuca (lettuce)
Laennecia (laennicia)
Lagascea (lagascea)
Lagenifera (island daisy)
Lagophylla (hareleaf)
Lapsana (nipplewort)
Lapsanastrum (nipplewort)
Lasianthaea (lasianthaea)
Lasiospermum (cocoonhead)
Lasthenia (goldfields)
Launaea (launaea)
Layia (tidy tips)
Leibnitzia (sun bonnets)
Lembertia (lembertia)
Leontodon (hawkbit)
Lepidospartum (broom sage)
Lessingia (lessingia)
Leucanthemum (daisy)
Leucanthemella (leucanthemella)
Liatris (blazing star)
Lindheimera (lindheimera)
Lipochaeta (nehe)
Logfia (cotton rose)
Luina (silverback)
Lygodesmia (skeleton plant)
Machaeranthera (tansy aster)
Madia (tarweed)
Malacothrix (desert dandelion)
Malperia (malperia)
Mantisalca (mantisalca)
Marshallia (Barbara's buttons)
Matricaria (mayweed)
Megalodonta (water marigold)
Melampodium (blackfoot)
Melanthera (squarestem)
Micropus (cottonseed)
Microseris (silver puffs)
Mikania (hemp vine)
Monolopia (monolopia)
Monoptilon (desert star)
Montanoa (montanoa)
Mycelis (mycelis)
Neurolaena (neurolaena)
Nicolletia (hole-in-the-sand plant)
Nothocalais (prairie dandelion)
Oclemena (aster)
Olearia (daisy bush)
Oligoneuron (goldenrod)
Omalotheca (arctic cudweed)
Oncosiphon (oncosiphon)
Onopordum (cotton thistle)
Oonopsis (false goldenweed)
Oreochrysum (goldenrod)
Oreostemma (aster)
Orochaenactis (orochaenactis)
Osmadenia (osmadenia)
Osteospermum (daisy bush)
Packera (ragwort)
Palafoxia (palafox)

Parasenecio (Indian plantain)
Parthenice (parthenice)
Parthenium (feverfew)
Pascalia (Pascalia)
Pectis (cinchweed)
Pentachaeta (pygmy daisy)
Pentzia (pentzia)
Pericome (pericome)
Pericallis (ragwort)
Perityle (rock daisy)
Petasites (butterbur)
Petradoria (rock goldenrod)
Peucephyllum (pygmy cedar)
Phalacroseris (mock dandelion)
Phoebanthus (false sunflower)
Picradeniopsis (bahia)
Picris (ox tongue)
Picrothamnus (bud sagebrush)
Pinaropappus (rock lettuce)
Piptocarpha (ash daisy)
Piptocoma (velvet shrub)
Pityopsis (silk grass)
Platyschkuhria (basin daisy)
Pleurocoronis (pleurocoronis)
Pluchea (camphorweed)
Polymnia (polymnia)
Porophyllum (poreleaf)
Prenanthes (rattlesnake root)
Prenanthella (prenanthella)
Proustia (proustia)
Psacalium (Indianbush)
Psathyrotes (turtleback)
Pseudogynoxys (pseudogynoxys)
Pseudelephantopus (dog's tongue)
Pseudobahia (sunburst)
Pseudoclappia (false clap daisy)
Pseudognaphalium (cudweed)
Psilactis (tansy aster)
Psilocarphus (woolly heads)
Psilostrophe (paper flower)
Pterocaulon (blackroot)
Pulicaria (false fleabane)
Pyrrhopappus (desert chicory)
Pyrrocoma (goldenweed)
Rafinesquia (California chicory)
Raillardella (raillardella)
Raillardiopsis (raillardiopsis)
Rainiera (rainiera)
Ratibida (prairie coneflower)
Rayjacksonia (tansy aster)
Reichardia (bright eye)
Remya (remya)
Rhagadiolus (rhagadiolus)
Rigiopappus (rigiopappus)
Rolandra (yerba de plata)
Roldana (groundsel)
Rudbeckia (coneflower)
Rugelia (Rugel's Indian plantain)
Sachsia (sachsia)
Salmea (bejuco de miel)
Santolina (lavender cotton)
Sanvitalia (creeping zinnia)
Sartwellia (glowwort)
Saussurea (sawwort)
Schkuhria (false threadleaf)
Sclerocarpus (bone bract)
Sclerolepis (bog button)
Scolymus (golden thistle)

Continued

Table 1 *Continued*

Scorzonera (scorzonera)
Senecio (ragwort)
Sericocarpus (whitetop aster)
Serratula (plumeless sawwort)
Shinnersoseris (beaked skeletonweed)
Sigesbeckia (St Paul's wort)
Silphium (rosinweed)
Silybum (milk thistle)
Simsia (bush sunflower)
Smallanthus (smallanthus)
Solidago (goldenrod)
Soliva (burrweed)
Sonchus (sow thistle)
Sphaeromeria (chicken sage)
Sphagneticola (creeping ox eye)
Spilanthes (spilanthes)
Spiracantha (dogwood leaf)
Stebbinsoseris (silver puffs)
Stenotus (mock goldenweed)
Stephanomeria (wire lettuce)
Stevia (candyleaf)
Stokesia (stokesia)
Struchium (struchium)
Stylocline (nest straw)
Symphyotrichum (aster)
Synedrella (synedrella)
Syntrichopappus (Fremont's gold)
Tagetes (marigold)
Tamaulipa (boneset)
Tanacetum (tansy)
Taraxacum (dandelion)
Tephroseris (groundsel)
Tetramolopium (tetramolopium)
Tetraneuris (four-nerve daisy)
Tetradymia (horsebrush)
Tetragonotheca (nerve ray)
Thelesperma (green thread)
Thurovia (thurovia)
Thymophylla (pricklyleaf)
Tithonia (tithonia)
Tolpis (umbrella milkwort)
Tonestus (serpentweed)
Townsendia (Townsend daisy)
Tracyina (Indian headdress)
Tragopogon (goat's beard)
Trichocoronis (bugheal)
Trichoptilium (trichoptilium)
Tridax (tridax)
Tripleurospermum (mayweed)
Tripolium (sea aster)
Trixis (threefold)
Tussilago (coltsfoot)
Uropappus (silver puffs)
Urospermum (urospermum)
Vanclevea (vanclevea)
Varilla (varilla)
Venegasia (venegasia)
Venidium (venidium)
Verbesina (crownbeard)
Vernonia (ironweed)
Viguiera (goldeneye)
Wedelia (creeping ox eye)
Whitneya (whitneya)
Wilkesia (iliau)
Wollastonia (watermeal)
Wyethia (mule-ears)
Xanthisma (sleepy daisy)

Xanthium (cocklebur)
Xanthocephalum (xanthocephalum)
Xylorhiza (woody aster)
Xylothamia (desert goldenrod)
Yermo (desert yellowhead)
Youngia (youngia)
Zinnia (zinnia)

Delayed hypersensitivity reactions to the Asteraceae (Compositae) can arise from sesquiterpene lactones. To detect contact allergy to sesquiterpene lactones, a mixture of lactones (alantolactone, costunolide, and dehydrocostus lactone) is used. However, Compositae contain other sensitizers, such as polyacetylenes and thiophenes. In a prospective study, the lactone mixture was complemented with a mixture of Compositae (containing ether extracts of arnica, German chamomile, yarrow, tansy, and feverfew) to detect contact allergy to Compositae (1). Of 346 patients tested, 15 (4.3%) reacted to the mixture of Compositae, compared with eight of 1076 patients (0.7%) who gave positive results with the lactone mixture, indicating the importance of the addition of Compositae allergens to the lactone mixture. However, the authors warned that patch-testing with these mixtures can cause active sensitization.

- Compositae dermatitis occurred in a 9-year-old boy with a strong personal and family history of atopy. Positive patch test reactions were 2+ for dandelion (*Taraxacum officinale*), false ragweed (*Ambrosia acanthicarpa*), giant ragweed (*Ambrosia trifida*), short ragweed (*Ambrosia artemisifolia*), sagebrush (*Artemisia tridentata*), wild feverfew (*Parthenium hysterophorus*), yarrow (*Achillea millifolium*), and tansy (*Tanacetum vulgare*), and 1+ for *Dahlia* species and English ivy (*Hedera helix*) (2). Patch tests were negative for another 30 plants, including cocklebur (*Xanthium strumarium*), dog fennel (*Anthemis cotula*), fleabane (*Erigeron strigosus*), sneezeweed (*Helenium autumnale*), and feverfew (*Tanacetum parthenium*).

An Austrian study has re-confirmed the importance of testing with not only a mixture of Compositae and a mixture of sesquiterpene lactones, but also with additional plant extracts when there is continuing clinical suspicion of allergy to one of the Compositae (3). By using additional short ether extracts, the authors found two of five patients who had otherwise been overlooked.

Achillea millefolium

Achillea millefolium (yarrow) can cause contact dermatitis (4); a generalized eruption following the drinking of yarrow tea has also been reported (5).

- A female florist from North Germany, who ran a flower shop from 1954 to 1966 had to quit her job because of contact allergy to chrysanthemums and primrose. After a further 12 years she started to suffer occasionally from redness of the pharynx and stomachache after drinking tea prepared from yarrow and camomile. Skin tests were positive to chrysanthemum with cross-reactions to sunflower, arnica, camomile, yarrow, tansy, mugwort, and frullania (a lichen that does not occur in the Northern part of Germany). Patch-testing with primin showed high-grade hypersensitivity to Primula.

A. millefolium contains sesquiterpene lactones, polyacetylenes, coumarins, and flavonoids. Extracts have often been used in cosmetics in concentrations of 0.5–10%. *A. millefolium* was weakly genotoxic in *Drosophila melanogaster*. In provocative testing, patients reacted to a mix of *Compositae* that contained yarrow, as well as to yarrow itself. In clinical use, a formulation containing a 0.1% extract was not a sensitizer and alcoholic extracts of the dried leaves and stalks of the flower were not phototoxic (6). However, positive patch tests to *A. millefolium* have been reported (7).

Anthemis species and Matricaria recutita (chamomile)

Chamomile is the vernacular name of *Anthemis* genus and *Matricaria recutita* (German chamomile, pinhead). The former are more potent skin sensitizers (delayed-type) than the latter, presumably because they can contain a higher concentration of the sesquiterpene lactone, anthecotullid. Cross-sensitivity with related allergenic sesquiterpene lactones in other plants is possible.

Adverse effects
Internal use of chamomile tea has been associated with rare cases of anaphylactic reactions (8) and its use in eyewashes can cause allergic conjunctivitis (9).

Arnica montana

Arnica montana (arnica) contains a variety of terpenoids and has mostly been used in the treatment of sprains and bruises but is also used in cosmetics.

Ingestion of tea prepared from *Arnica montana* flowers can result in gastroenteritis reference.

- A 27-year-old woman presented with a rapidly enlarging necrotic lesion on her face and left leg together with malaise and high fever (10). She reported that she had applied a 1.5% arnica cream to her face before these symptoms had occurred. The diagnosis was Sweet's syndrome elicited by pathergy to arnica. She was treated with prednisolone and her skin lesions disappeared within 3 weeks.

Of 443 individuals who were tested for contact sensitization, 5 had a positive reaction to *A. montana* and 9 to *Calendula officinalis* (marigold); a mixture of the two was positive in 18 cases (3). Sensitization was often accompanied by reactions to nickel, *Myroxylon pereirae* resin, fragrance mix, propolis, and colophon.

Artemisia species

There are about 60 different species of Artemisia, of which the principal are *Artemisia absinthium*, *Artemisia annua*, *Artemisia cina*, and *Artemisia vulgaris*.

Artemisia absinthium

The volatile oil of *A. absinthium* (wormwood), which gives the alcoholic liqueur absinthe its flavor, can damage the nervous system and cause mental deterioration. This toxicity is attributed to thujones (alpha-thujone and beta-thujone), which constitute 0.25–1.32% in the whole herb and 3–12% of the oil. Alcoholic extracts and the essential oil are forbidden in most countries.

Artemisia annua

Artemisia annua, known in China as Qinghaosu, contains artemisinin, which has antimalarial activity. Several derivatives of the original compound have proved effective in the treatment of *Plasmodium falciparum* malaria and are currently available in a variety of formulations: artesunate (intravenous, rectal, oral), artelinate (oral), artemisinin (intravenous, rectal, oral), dihydroartemisinin (oral), artemether (intravenous, oral, rectal), and artemotil (intravenous). Artemisinic acid (qinghao acid), the precursor of artemisin, is present in the plant in a concentration up to 10 times that of artemisinin. Several semisynthetic derivatives have been developed from dihydroartemisinin (11). The artemisinin derivatives are the subject of a separate monograph.

Artemisia cina

Artemisia cina (wormseed) contains the toxic lactone, santonin, which was formerly used as an antihelminthic drug, but has now been superseded by other less toxic compounds.

Artemisia vulgaris

Artemisia vulgaris (common wormwood) contains the toxic lactone, santonin, which was formerly used as an antihelminthic drug, but has now been superseded by other less toxic compounds. Depending on the origin of the plant, 1,8-cineole, camphor, linalool, and thujone may all be major components. Allergic skin reactions (12) and abortive activity have been described.

Calendula officinalis

Calendula officinalis (marigold) contains a variety of carotenoids, saponins, steroids, sesquiterpenoids, and triterpenoids.

Of 443 individuals who were tested for contact sensitization, five had a positive reaction to *A. montana* and nine to *C. officinalis*; a mixture of the two was positive in 18 cases (3). Sensitization was often accompanied by reactions to nickel, *Myroxylon pereirae* resin, fragrance mix, propolis, and colophon.

Callilepis laureola

Callilepis laureola (impila, ox-eye daisy) contains the toxic compound atractyloside and related compounds. The plant is responsible for the deaths of many Zulu people in Natal, who use its roots as a herbal medicine.

Adverse effects
Necropsy records of 50 children who had taken herbal medicines made from *C. laureola* showed typical hepatic and renal tubular necrosis (13). In young Black children the plant causes hypoglycaemia, altered consciousness,

and hepatic and renal dysfunction. This syndrome can be hard to distinguish from Reye's syndrome.

Acute renal insufficiency has been attributed to *C. laureola* (14).

Chrysanthemum vulgaris

Chrysanthemum vulgaris (common tansy) contains essential oils and thujone in such amounts that even normal doses can be neurotoxic (15).

Cynara scolymus

Cynara scolymus (artichoke) contains a variety of flavonoids, phenols, and sesquiterpenoids, including cynarapicrin, cynaratriol, cynarolide, and isoamberboin. It has been used to lower serum cholesterol, with little evidence of efficacy (16).

Adverse effects

Two vegetable warehouse workers developed occupational rhinitis and bronchial asthma by sensitization to *C. scolymus* (17). Skin prick tests to artichoke were positive and IgE specific for artichoke was found. Nasal challenge with artichoke extract triggered a reduction in peak nasal inspiratory flow of 81 and 85%. One patient had a reduction in peak expiratory flow rate of up to 36% after exposure to artichoke in the workplace.

Allergic contact dermatitis (18) and occupational contact urticaria (19) have also been reported.

Echinacea species

Echinacea species (coneflower, black Sampson hedgehog, Indian head, snakeroot, red sunflower, scurvy root) have become increasingly popular, particularly for the prophylaxis and treatment and prevention of cold and flu symptoms. However, the claimed efficacy of *Echinacea* in the common cold has not been confirmed in a randomized, double-blind, placebo-controlled trial (20) or a systematic review (21). *Echinacea* is claimed to have antiseptic and antiviral properties and is under investigation for its immunostimulant action. The active ingredients are glycosides (echinacoside), polysaccharides, alkamides, and flavonoids.

Adverse effects

Between July 1996 and November 1998, the Australian Adverse Drug Reactions Advisory Committee received 37 reports of suspected adverse drug reactions in association with *Echinacea* (22). Over half of these (n = 21) described allergic-like effects, including bronchospasm (n = 9), dyspnea (n = 8), urticaria (n = 5), chest pain (n = 4), and angioedema (n = 3). The 21 patients were aged 3–58 (median 31) years and 12 had a history of asthma (n = 7) and/or allergic rhinitis/conjuctivitis/hayfever (n = 5). *Echinacea* was the only suspected cause in 19 of the 21 cases. The symptoms began at variable times, within 10 minutes of the first dose to a few months, and all but two cases occurred within 3 days of starting treatment. At the time of reporting 17 of the patients had recovered, 2 had not yet recovered, and the outcome was unknown in the other two cases.

Hematologic
Possible leukopenia has been associated with long-term use of *Echinacea* (23).

Skin
Recurrent erythema nodosum has been attributed to *Echinacea*.

- A 41-year-old man, who had taken *Echinacea* intermittently for the previous 18 months, had four episodes of erythema nodosum, preceded by myalgia and arthralgia, fever, headache, and malaise (24). The skin lesions resolved within 2–5 weeks and responded to oral prednisolone. He was advised to discontinue *Echinacea* and 1 year later remained free from further recurrence.

Immunologic
Intravenous administration of *Echinacea* has been associated with severe allergic reactions. Oral ingestion can cause allergic skin and respiratory responses (25).

Five cases of adverse drug reactions have been attributed to oral *Echinacea* extracts (26). Two of the patients had anaphylaxis and one had an acute attack of asthma. The authors also tested 100 atopic subjects and found that 20 of them, who had never before taken *Echinacea*, had positive reactions to skin prick tests.

An anaphylactic reaction to *Echinacea angustifolia* has been reported (27).

- A 37-year-old woman who took various food supplements on an irregular basis self-medicated with 5 ml of an extract of *E. angustifolia*. She had immediate burning of the mouth and throat followed by tightness of the chest, generalized urticaria, and diarrhea. She made a full recovery within 2 hours.

The basis for this anaphylactic reaction was hypersensitivity to *Echinacea*, confirmed by skin prick and RAST testing. However, others have challenged the notion of a causal relation in this case (28). Nevertheless, the author affirmed his belief that *Echinacea* was the causal agent and reported that at that time *Echinacea* accounted for 22 of 266 suspected adverse reactions to complementary medicines reported to the Australian Adverse Drug Reaction Advisory Committee (28).

Sjögren's syndrome has been attributed to *Echinacea* (29).

Teratogenicity
Of 412 pregnant Canadian women who contacted a specialized information service between 1996 and 1998 with concerns about the use of *Echinacea* during pregnancy, 206 had already taken the remedy and the other 206 eventually decided not to use it (30). In the *Echinacea* group, 54% had taken it during the first trimester of pregnancy; 12 babies had malformations, six major and six minor. The figures in the control group were seven and seven respectively. Thus, there was no difference in the incidence of birth defects. However, the study lacked sufficient power to generate reliable data.

Eupatorium species

Several *Eupatorium* species, such as *Eupatorium cannabinum* (hemp agrimony) and *Eupatorium purpureum* (gravel root), have hepatotoxic potential due to the presence of pyrrolizidine alkaloids, which are covered in a separate monograph.

There is no evidence of pyrrolizidine alkaloids in *Eupatorium rugosum* (white snakeroot) but this plant also has poisonous properties, which are attributed to an unstable toxin called tremetol. Transfer from cow's milk to humans can produce a condition known as milk sickness, including trembles, weakness, nausea and vomiting, prostration, delirium, and even death.

Inula helenium

Large doses of the root of *Inula helenium* (elecampane) can cause vomiting, diarrhea, cramps, and paralytic symptoms.

Petasites species

Petasites species have hepatotoxic potential, owing to the presence of pyrrolizidine alkaloids, which are covered in a separate monograph. Extracts of *Petasites hybridus* (blatterdock, bog rhubarb, butterbur, butterdock) contain little in the way of these alkaloids (31). Butterbur has been used to treat allergic rhinitis and asthma and in the prevention of migraine.

Senecio species

Many species of *Senecio*, such as *Senecio jacobaea* (ragwort) and *Senecio longilobus* (thread leaf groundsel), contain hepatotoxic amounts of pyrrolizidine alkaloids (which are covered in a separate monograph). Honey made from *Senecio* plants also contains pyrrolizidine alkaloids (32).

Adverse effects
Veno-occlusive disease has been attributed to *Senecio* after chronic use (33,34).

- Hepatic veno-occlusive disease occurred in a 38-year-old woman who had occasionally consumed "Huamanrripa" (*Senecio tephrosioides*) as a cough remedy for many years (35). She had abdominal pain, jaundice, and anasarca. A hepatic biopsy showed pronounced congestion with a centrilobular predominance, foci of necrosis, and in some areas a reversed lobulation pattern. During the next 13 months she was hospitalized four times with complications of portal hypertension.
- An infant developed hepatic veno-occlusive disease after having been fed a herbal tea known as gordolobo yerba, commonly used as a folk remedy among Mexican-Americans; there was acute hepatocellular disease and portal hypertension, which progressed over 2 months to extensive hepatic fibrosis (36).

In one case hepatic damage due to *Senecio* mimicked Reye's syndrome (37).

Silybum marianum

Silybum marianum (holy thistle, lady's thistle, milk thistle, St. Mary's thistle) has been used to treat liver problems, such as hepatitis, and prostatic cancer. It contains a variety of lignans, including silandrin, silybin, silychristin, silydianin, silymarin, and silymonin.

Adverse effects

- A 57-year-old Australian woman presented with a 2-month history of intermittent episodes of sweating, nausea, colicky abdominal pain, fluid diarrhea, vomiting, weakness, and collapse (38). She was taking ethinylestradiol and amitriptyline and had taken milk thistle for 2 months. A thorough check-up showed no abnormalities. On reflection she realized that all her attacks had invariably occurred after taking the milk thistle. She stopped taking it and had no symptoms until a few weeks later, when she tried another capsule and had the same symptoms.

This idiosyncratic reaction to milk thistle seems to be a rarity. The Australian authorities knew of only two other adverse drug reactions associated with milk thistle.

Immunologic
Anaphylactic shock has been reported after the use of a herbal tea containing an extract of the fruit of the milk thistle (39).

Drug interactions
Milk thistle inhibits CYP3A4 and uridine diphosphoglucuronosyl transferase in human hepatocyte cultures (40).

In 10 healthy subjects silymarin 160 mg tds had no effect on the pharmacokinetics of indinavir 800 mg tds (41). In a similar study silymarin 175 mg tds had no effect on the pharmacokinetics of indinavir 800 mg tds (42).

Tanacetum parthenium

Tanacetum parthenium (feverfew, bachelor's buttons, motherherb) has been used in the prevention of migraine, with some benefit (43), and for rheumatoid arthritis, without (44).

Adverse effects
As *Tanacetum parthenium* is rich in allergenic sesquiterpene lactones, such as parthenolide, it is not surprising that contact dermatitis has been observed (SEDA-11, 426). The most common adverse effect of oral feverfew is mouth ulceration. A more widespread inflammation of the oral mucosa and tongue, swelling of the lips, and loss of taste have also been reported.

Feverfew inhibits platelet aggregation (45), and its concomitant use with anticoagulants such as warfarin is therefore not advised.

Tussilago farfara

Tussilago farfara (coltsfoot) has hepatotoxic potential owing to the presence of pyrrolizidine alkaloids (see separate monograph).

- An 18-month-old boy who had regularly consumed a herbal tea mixture since the 3rd month of life developed veno-occlusive disease with portal hypertension and severe ascites (46). Histology of the liver showed centrilobular sinusoidal congestion with perivenular bleeding and parenchymal necrosis without cirrhosis. The child was given conservative treatment only and recovered completely within 2 months.

The tea contained peppermint and what the mother thought was coltsfoot (*T. farfara*), analysis of which revealed high amounts of pyrrolizidine alkaloids. Seneciphylline and the corresponding *N*-oxide were identified as the major components, and the child had consumed at least 60 µg/kg/day of the toxic pyrrolizidine alkaloid mixture over 15 months. Macroscopic and microscopic analysis of the leaf material indicated that *Adenostyles alliariae* (Alpendost) had been erroneously gathered by the parents in place of coltsfoot. The two plants can easily be confused especially after the flowering period.

References

1. Kanerva L, Estlander T, Alanko K, Jolanki R. Patch test sensitization to Compositae mix, sesquiterpene–lactone mix, Compositae extracts, laurel leaf, chlorophorin, mansonone A, and dimethoxydalbergione. Am J Contact Dermat 2001;12(1):18–24.
2. Guin JD, Skidmore G. Compositae dermatitis in childhood. Arch Dermatol 1987;123(4):500–2.
3. Reider N, Komericki P, Hausen BM, Fritsch P, Aberer W. The seamy side of natural medicines: contact sensitization to arnica (*Arnica montana* L.) and marigold (*Calendula officinalis* L.). Contact Dermatitis 2001;45(5):269–72.
4. Jovanovic M, Poljacki M, Duran V, Vujanovic L, Sente R, Stojanovic S. Contact allergy to Compositae plants in patients with atopic dermatitis. Med Pregl 2004;57(5-6):209–18.
5. Hausen BM, Schulz KH. Polyvalente Kontaktallergie bei einer Floristin. [Polyvalent contact allergy in a florist.] Derm Beruf Umwelt 1978;26(5):175–6.
6. Anonymous. Final report on the safety assessment of yarrow (*Achillea millefolium*) Extract. Int J Toxicol 2001;20(Suppl 2):79–84.
7. Stingeni L, Agea E, Lisi P, Spinozzi F. T lymphocyte cytokine profiles in compositae airborne dermatitis. Br J Dermatol 1999;141(4):689–93.
8. Subiza J, Subiza JL, Hinojosa M, Garcia R, Jerez M, Valdivieso R, Subiza E. Anaphylactic reaction after the ingestion of chamomile tea: a study of cross-reactivity with other composite pollens. J Allergy Clin Immunol 1989;84(3):353–8.
9. Subiza J, Subiza JL, Alonso M, Hinojosa M, Garcia R, Jerez M, Subiza E. Allergic conjunctivitis to chamomile tea. Ann Allergy 1990;65(2):127–32.
10. Delmonte S, Brusati C, Parodi A, Rebora A. Leukemia-related Sweet's syndrome elicited by pathergy to *Arnica*. Dermatology 1998;197(2):195–6.
11. Ridley RG, Hudson AT. Chemotherapy of malaria. Curr Opin Infect Dis 1998;11:691–705.
12. Kurz G, Rapaport MJ. External/internal allergy to plants (*Artemesia*). Contact Dermatitis 1979;5(6):407–8.
13. Watson AR, Coovadia HM, Bhoola KD. The clinical syndrome of impila (*Callilepis laureola*) poisoning in children. S Afr Med J 1979;55(8):290–2.
14. Seedat YK, Hitchcock PJ. Acute renal failure from *Callilepsis laureola*. S Afr Med J 1971;45(30):832–3.
15. Holstege CP, Baylor MR, Rusyniak DE. Absinthe: return of the Green Fairy. Semin Neurol 2002;22(1):89–93.
16. Pittler MH, Thompson CO, Ernst E. Artichoke leaf extract for treating hypercholesterolaemia. Cochrane Database Syst Rev 2002;(3):CD003335.
17. Miralles JC, Garcia-Sells J, Bartolome B, Negro JM. Occupational rhinitis and bronchial asthma due to artichoke (*Cynara scolymus*). Ann Allergy Asthma Immunol 2003;91(1):92–5.
18. Meding B. Allergic contact dermatitis from artichoke, *Cynara scolymus*. Contact Dermatitis 1983;9(4):314.
19. Quirce S, Tabar AI, Olaguibel JM, Cuevas M. Occupational contact urticaria syndrome caused by globe artichoke (*Cynara scolymus*). J Allergy Clin Immunol 1996;97(2):710–11.
20. Yale SH, Liu K. Echinacea purpurea therapy for the treatment of the common cold: a randomized, double-blind, placebo-controlled clinical trial. Arch Intern Med 2004;164(11):1237–41.
21. Melchart D, Linde K, Fischer P, Kaesmayr J. *Echinacea* for preventing and treating the common cold. Cochrane Database Syst Rev 2000;(2):CD000530.
22. Anonymous. *Echinacea*-allergic reactions. WHO Pharm Newslett 1999;5/6:7.
23. Kemp DE, Franco KN. Possible leukopenia associated with long-term use of *Echinacea*. J Am Board Fam Pract 2002;15(5):417–19.
24. Soon SL, Crawford RI. Recurrent erythema nodosum associated with *Echinacea* herbal therapy. J Am Acad Dermatol 2001;44(2):298–9.
25. Anonymous. Wie verträglich sind *Echinacea*-haltige Präparate? Dtsch Arzteblatt 1996;93:2723.
26. Mullins RJ, Heddle R. Adverse reactions associated with echinacea: the Australian experience. Ann Allergy Asthma Immunol 2002;88(1):42–51.
27. Mullins RJ. *Echinacea*-associated anaphylaxis. Med J Aust 1998;168(4):170–1.
28. Myers SP, Wohlmuth H. *Echinacea*-associated anaphylaxis. Med J Aust 1998;168(11):583–4.
29. Logan JL, Ahmed J. Critical hypokalemic renal tubular acidosis due to Sjögren's syndrome: association with the purported immune stimulant *Echinacea*. Clin Rheumatol 2003;22(2):158–9.
30. Gallo M, Sarkar M, Au W, Pietrzak K, Comas B, Smith M, Jaeger TV, Einarson A, Koren G. Pregnancy outcome following gestational exposure to *Echinacea*: a prospective controlled study. Arch Intern Med 2000;160(20):3141–3.
31. Kalin P. Gemeine Pestwurz (*Petasites hybridus*)—Portrait einer Arzneipflanze. [The common butterbur (*Petasites hybridus*)—portrait of a medicinal herb.] Forsch Komplementarmed Klass Naturheilkd 2003;10(Suppl 1): 41–4.
32. Deinzer ML, Thomson PA, Burgett DM, Isaacson DL. Pyrrolizidine alkaloids: their occurrence in honey from tansy ragwort (*Senecio jacobaea* L.). Science 1977;195(4277):497–9.
33. Ortiz Cansado A, Crespo Valades E, Morales Blanco P, Saenz de Santamaria J, Gonzalez Campillejo JM, Ruiz Tellez T. Enfermedad venoclusiva hepatica por ingestion de infusiones de *Senecio vulgaris*. [Veno-occlusive liver disease due to intake of *Senecio vulgaris* tea.] Gastroenterol Hepatol 1995;18(8):413–16.
34. Radal M, Bensaude RJ, Jonville-Bera AP, Monegier Du Sorbier C, Ouhaya F, Metman EH, Autret-Leca E. Maladie veino-occlusive apres ingestion chronique d'une specialite a base de senecon. [Veno-occlusive disease following chronic ingestion of drugs containing senecio.] Therapie 1998;53(5):509–11.
35. Tomioka M, Calvo F, Siguas A, Sanchez L, Nava E, Garcia U, Valdivia M, Reategui E. Enfermedad hepatica veno-oclusiva asociada a la ingestion de huamanrripa (*Senecio tephrosioides*). [Hepatic veno-occlusive disease associated with ingestion of *Senecio tephrosioides*.] Rev Gastroenterol Peru 1995;15(3):299–302.
36. Stillman AS, Huxtable R, Consroe P, Kohnen P, Smith S. Hepatic veno-occlusive disease due to pyrrolizidine (*Senecio*) poisoning in Arizona. Gastroenterology 1977;73(2):349–52.
37. Fox DW, Hart MC, Bergeson PS, Jarrett PB, Stillman AE, Huxtable RJ. Pyrrolizidine (*Senecio*) intoxication mimicking Reye syndrome. J Pediatr 1978;93(6):980–2.
38. Adverse Drug Reactions Advisory Committee. An adverse reaction to the herbal medication milk thistle (*Silybum marianum*). Med J Aust 1999;170(5):218–19.

39. Geier J, Fuchs T, Wahl R. Anaphylaktischer Schock durch einen Mariendistel-Extrakt bei Soforttyp-Allergie auf Kiwi. Allergologie 1990;13:387–8.
40. Venkataramanan R, Ramachandran V, Komoroski BJ, Zhang S, Schiff PL, Strom SC. Milk thistle, a herbal supplement, decreases the activity of CYP3A4 and uridine diphosphoglucuronosyl transferase in human hepatocyte cultures. Drug Metab Dispos 2000;28(11):1270–3.
41. DiCenzo R, Shelton M, Jordan K, Koval C, Forrest A, Reichman R, Morse G. Coadministration of milk thistle and indinavir in healthy subjects. Pharmacotherapy 2003;23(7):866–70.
42. Piscitelli SC, Formentini E, Burstein AH, Alfaro R, Jagannatha S, Falloon J. Effect of milk thistle on the pharmacokinetics of indinavir in healthy volunteers. Pharmacotherapy 2002;22(5):551–6.
43. Pittler MH, Vogler BK, Ernst E. Feverfew for preventing migraine. Cochrane Database Syst Rev 2000;(3):CD002286.
44. Pattrick M, Heptinstall S, Doherty M. Feverfew in rheumatoid arthritis: a double blind, placebo controlled study. Ann Rheum Dis 1989;48(7):547–9.
45. Groenewegen WA, Heptinstall S. A comparison of the effects of an extract of feverfew and parthenolide, a component of feverfew, on human platelet activity in-vitro. J Pharm Pharmacol 1990;42(8):553–7.
46. Sperl W, Stuppner H, Gassner I, Judmaier W, Dietze O, Vogel W. Reversible hepatic veno-occlusive disease in an infant after consumption of pyrrolizidine-containing herbal tea. Eur J Pediatr 1995;154(2):112–16.

Atenolol

See also Beta-adrenoceptor antagonists

General Information

Although atenolol, a hydrophilic cardioselective beta-adrenoceptor antagonist with no partial agonist activity, is generally regarded as one of the safest beta-blockers, severe adverse effects are occasionally reported. These include profound hypotension after a single oral dose (1), organic brain syndrome (2), cholestasis (3), and cutaneous vasculitis (4).

Organs and Systems

Nervous system

Atenolol is hydrophilic, making it less likely to cross the blood–brain barrier. However, nervous system effects are occasionally reported.

- A 54-year-old man developed progressive memory loss after taking atenolol 100 mg/day for 3 years. Four weeks after withdrawal, he completely recovered his memory (5).

References

1. Kholeif M, Isles C. Profound hypotension after atenolol in severe hypertension. BMJ 1989;298(6667):161–2.
2. Arber N. Delirium induced by atenolol. BMJ 1988;297(6655):1048.
3. Schwartz MS, Frank MS, Yanoff A, Morecki R. Atenolol-associated cholestasis. Am J Gastroenterol 1989;84(9):1084–6.
4. Wolf R, Ophir J, Elman M, Krakowski A. Atenolol-induced cutaneous vasculitis. Cutis 1989;43(3):231–3.
5. Ramanathan M. Atenolol induced memory impairment: a case report. Singapore Med J 1996;37(2):218–19.

Atorvastatin

See also HMG Co-A reductase inhibitors

General Information

Atorvastatin is an HMG Co-A reductase inhibitor. Pooled data from 21 completed and 23 continuing trials representing 3000 patient-years have shown that constipation, flatulence, dyspepsia, abdominal pain, headache, and myalgia occur in 1–3% of patients. Under 2% of atorvastatin-treated patients discontinued treatment because of an adverse event (1). Serious events in this review amounted to one patient with pancreatitis and one with cholestatic jaundice (1). There were no differences in adverse effects in 177 patients randomized for 52 weeks to either simvastatin or atorvastatin (2).

Organs and Systems

Nervous system

A peripheral neuropathy has been reported with atorvastatin.

- A 60-year-old woman had painless horizontal diplopia, vertigo, blurry vision, and paresthesia in both arms after taking atorvastatin 10 mg/day (3). Neurological improvement began 2 days after drug withdrawal. Antiacetylcholine receptor antibodies were 10 times the upper limit of the reference range.

Although some features of this patient's external ophthalmoplegia were similar to myasthenia and there was a reversible rise in antiacetylcholine receptor antibody titer, a negative edrophonium test and a negative repetitive stimulation test on electromyography argued against a myasthenia-like drug reaction.

Sensory systems

In 696 patients taking atorvastatin and 235 taking lovastatin for 1 year there were no significant differences in the distribution of lenticular opacities or cortical opacities and spokes between the two drugs (4).

Hematologic

Thrombocytopenia occurred in a 46-year-old man coinciding with atorvastatin treatment; he had already tolerated simvastatin (5).

Pancreas

Pancreatitis has been observed with atorvastatin (6).

Skin

Potentially life-threatening toxic epidermal necrolysis occurred in a 73-year-old moderately obese woman with type 2 diabetes and hypertension after she had taken 40 mg of atorvastatin (7).

- A 59-year-old man developed urticaria while taking atorvastatin for hypercholesterolemia (8). Scratch tests with his medications gave a strong positive reaction only with atorvastatin. Atorvastatin was withdrawn and his urticaria resolved over the next 10 days.

Linear IgA bullous dermatosis (9) and dermographism (10) have been described in patients taking atorvastatin.

Musculoskeletal

In one study of 133 patients there was myalgia in 3% of those taking atorvastatin, but no patient had persistent increases in creatine kinase activity above 10 times the top of the reference range (11).

Immunologic

A hypersensitivity reaction to atorvastatin has been reported.

- Antinuclear and antihistone antibodies developed in a 26-year-old man who was taking atorvastatin (12). He had constitutional symptoms and slight headaches but no definite symptoms of lupus. After some months without medication he became seronegative and asymptomatic.

This case was similar to other previous reports with other statins.

Drug–Drug Interactions

Ciclosporin

Rhabdomyolysis occurred when atorvastatin was combined with ciclosporin for 2 months in a woman with systemic lupus erythematosus and a renal transplant (13).

Terfenadine

Atorvastatin, although a substrate for CYP3A4, does not affect blood terfenadine concentrations to a clinically significant extent (14).

Warfarin

In 12 patients chronically maintained on warfarin, atorvastatin 80 mg/day for 2 weeks reduced mean prothrombin times slightly, but only for the first few days of the 2-week treatment period (15). Thus, atorvastatin had no consistent effect on the anticoagulant activity of warfarin and adjustments in warfarin doses should not be necessary.

References

1. Yee HS, Fong NT. Atorvastatin in the treatment of primary hypercholesterolemia and mixed dyslipidemias. Ann Pharmacother 1998;32(10):1030–43.
2. Dart A, Jerums G, Nicholson G, d'Emden M, Hamilton-Craig I, Tallis G, Best J, West M, Sullivan D, Bracs P, Black D. A multicenter, double-blind, one-year study comparing safety and efficacy of atorvastatin versus simvastatin in patients with hypercholesterolemia. Am J Cardiol 1997;80(1):39–44.
3. Negevesky GJ, Kolsky MP, Laureno R, Yau TH. Reversible atorvastatin-associated external ophthalmoplegia, anti-acetylcholine receptor antibodies, and ataxia. Arch Ophthalmol 2000;118(3):427–8.
4. Reid L, Bakker-Arkema R, Black D. The effect of atorvastatin on the human lens after 52 weeks of treatment. J Cardiovasc Pharmacol Ther 1998;3(1):71–6.
5. Gonzalez-Ponte ML, Gonzalez-Ruiz M, Duvos E, Gutierrez-Iniguez MA, Olalla JI, Conde E. Atorvastatin-induced severe thrombocytopenia. Lancet 1998;352(9136):1284.
6. Belaiche G, Ley G, Slama JL. Pancreatite aiguë associée a la prise d'atorvastatine. [Acute pancreatitis associated with atorvastatine therapy.] Gastroenterol Clin Biol 2000;24(4):471–2.
7. Pfeiffer CM, Kazenoff S, Rothberg HD. Toxic epidermal necrolysis from atorvastatin. JAMA 1998;279(20):1613–14.
8. Anliker MD, Wuthrich B. Chronic urticaria to atorvastatin. Allergy 2002;57(4):366.
9. Konig C, Eickert A, Scharfetter-Kochanek K, Krieg T, Hunzelmann N. Linear IgA bullous dermatosis induced by atorvastatin. J Am Acad Dermatol 2001;44(4):689–92.
10. Adcock BB, Hornsby LB, Jenkins K. Dermographism: an adverse effect of atorvastatin. J Am Board Fam Pract 2001;14(2):148–51.
11. Lea AP, McTavish D. Atorvastatin. A review of its pharmacology and therapeutic potential in the management of hyperlipidaemias. Drugs 1997;53(5):828–47.
12. Jimenez-Alonso J, Jaimez L, Sabio JM, Hidalgo C, Leon L. Atorvastatin-induced reversible positive antinuclear antibodies. Am J Med 2002;112(4):329–30.
13. Maltz HC, Balog DL, Cheigh JS. Rhabdomyolysis associated with concomitant use of atorvastatin and cyclosporine. Ann Pharmacother 1999;33(11):1176–9.
14. Stern RH, Smithers JA, Olson SC. Atorvastatin does not produce a clinically significant effect on the pharmacokinetics of terfenadine. J Clin Pharmacol 1998;38(8):753–7.
15. Stern R, Abel R, Gibson GL, Besserer J. Atorvastatin does not alter the anticoagulant activity of warfarin. J Clin Pharmacol 1997;37(11):1062–4.

Atovaquone

General Information

Atovaquone is a hydroxynaphthaquinone that is effective in the prevention and treatment of murine *Pneumocystis jiroveci* pneumonitis. It also has effects against *Toxoplasma gondii* and *Plasmodium falciparum*. Food increases its absorption. The maximum serum concentration is dose-dependent, but absorption is reduced at doses above 750 mg. The maximum concentration occurs after 4–6 hours, with a second peak 24–96 hours later, suggesting enterohepatic cycling. The half-life is 77 hours.

Observational studies

In a 3-week study with test doses of 100–3000 mg/day, atovaquone was well tolerated. Three patients reported increased appetite; two of these had transient sinus arrhythmia. One of the 24 patients had a transient maculopapular rash that resolved without withdrawal. There were no abnormalities in hematological parameters or renal function. Two patients had slightly raised serum bilirubin concentrations and one each had raised transaminase activities. Two other patients had mildly increased transaminase activities, but both were known to have chronic hepatitis B (SEDA-13, 828).

Comparative studies

Atovaquone 250 mg tds has been compared with co-trimoxazole 320/1600 mg/day for 21 days in the treatment of *P. jiroveci* pneumonia in 408 patients. Therapeutic efficacy was similar, but atovaquone was much better tolerated, with a far lower incidence of rash, liver dysfunction, fever, nausea, and pruritus, and no neutropenia, chills, headache, renal impairment, or thrombocytopenia (1). However, pre-existing diarrhea was associated with an increased mortality in the atovaquone group.

Of 39 patients who had bone marrow transplants and who were randomized to receive either co-trimoxazole or atovaquone as prophylaxis in an open-label trial, eight taking co-trimoxazole withdrew because of presumed drug reactions, although in five of these the reported neutropenia and thrombocytopenia could have been a consequence of transplantation itself or of other drugs (2). None of 16 patients treated with atovaquone withdrew. This rate of reported adverse effects with co-trimoxazole is higher than usually reported in clinical practice with prophylactic dosages.

A study conducted by the AIDS Clinical Trials Group (ACTG) has shown that among patients who cannot tolerate treatment with co-trimoxazole, atovaquone and dapsone are similarly effective in preventing *P. jiroveci* pneumonia. Among patients who did not originally take dapsone, atovaquone was better tolerated and it might be the preferred choice for prophylaxis of *P. jiroveci* pneumonia in this setting (3). Inexplicably the rate of *P. jiroveci* pneumonia showed a greater fall in patients who discontinued the study drugs compared with those who continued to take them.

When atovaquone was compared with intravenous pentamidine in the treatment of mild and moderate *Pneumocystis jiroveci* pneumonia in an open trial, the success rates were similar. However, withdrawal of the original treatment was much more frequent with pentamidine (36%) than atovaquone (4%) (4). However, the authors' conclusion that the two approaches have a similar success rate has been challenged, and their series was small (5,6). Treatment-limited adverse effects occurred in only 7% of patients given atovaquone, compared with 41% given pentamidine. They included cases of rash and an increase in creatinine concentrations; atovaquone (unlike pentamidine) produced no vomiting, nausea, hypotension, leukopenia, acute renal insufficiency, or electrocardiographic abnormalities, but it did cause one case of dementia (4).

Combinations

Atovaquone + azithromycin
Human babesiosis has been traditionally treated with quinine plus clindamycin, a combination that has been compared with atovaquone plus azithromycin in a randomized, multicenter, unblinded study (7). The treatments

were both completely effective. There were considerably fewer adverse events with azithromycin plus atovaquone than with quinine plus clindamycin.

Atovaquone + proguanil
Atovaquone acts synergistically with proguanil, and the combination of these two drugs (Malarone®) is highly efficacious in the treatment of uncomplicated malaria (8), including that against multidrug resistant forms, and in prophylaxis (9). It has not yet been widely marketed, so data on rare adverse effects are currently sparse.

An inpatient study of 79 patients given proguanil + atovaquone compared with 79 patients given mefloquine showed no malaria-independent adverse effects (10). Although there was a significant transient increase in liver enzymes, this was probably of limited clinical importance.

Prophylaxis with either one or two tablets containing atovaquone 250 mg plus proguanil hydrochloride 100 mg (one quarter or one half of the daily treatment dose), taken once-daily for 10 weeks, prevented *P. falciparum* malaria in 100% of semi-immune adults in a highly endemic area of Kenya (11). Children in Gabon taking daily Malarone at approximately one quarter of the treatment dose were similarly protected (12). Gastrointestinal adverse effects, including abdominal pain and vomiting, were relatively common in the initial parasite clearance phase of the pediatric study (when a full treatment course was given) and there was one case of repeated vomiting in the parasite clearance phase of the adult study. In both studies, the regimens were well tolerated in the prophylaxis phase (no difference from placebo). This efficacy and tolerability profile may be applicable to malaria prevention outside Africa. The use of the combination is predicted to reduce the development of resistance to each drug. Furthermore, atovaquone eliminates parasites during the hepatic phase of infection (causal prophylaxis), potentially removing the requirement to continue prophylaxis for several weeks after return from a malarious area, a period when compliance with current regimens is likely to be poor.

Proguanil plus atovaquone has been studied for chemoprophylaxis of malaria in African children (12) and in travelers (13) and is formulated as a combination of proguanil 100 mg plus atovaquone 250 mg for daily dosing. Atovaquone is a hydroxynaphthoquinone that inhibits the electron transport system (bc1 system) of parasites. Proguanil plus atovaquone is active against hepatic stages of *P. falciparum*, making it unnecessary to continue 4 weeks of prophylaxis after return from an endemic region. Current recommendations are that proguanil plus atovaquone should be continued for 1 week after returning from a malaria-endemic region.

In a comparison of proguanil plus atovaquone with proguanil (100 mg/day) plus chloroquine (155 mg base weekly) in travelers, proguanil plus atovaquone was 100% effective in the prevention of malaria (13). Those who took proguanil plus atovaquone ($n = 540$) had significantly fewer adverse events than those who took proguanil plus chloroquine ($n = 543$) (22% versus 28% respectively), particularly less diarrhea, abdominal pain, and vomiting. Only one person who took proguanil plus atovaquone had to discontinue prophylaxis owing to adverse events, as opposed to ten who had to discontinue proguanil plus chloroquine. There have been no other studies of similar size on the use of proguanil plus atovaquone. This combination is becoming established for the prophylaxis of malaria and the results of further phase IV studies are awaited.

The use of proguanil plus atovaquone has been reviewed (14). Neuropsychiatric adverse events were more frequent with mefloquine, whereas other adverse events occurred with similar frequencies as with chloroquine plus proguanil and mefloquine. Proguanil plus atovaquone is contraindicated in severe renal insufficiency. Co-administration of proguanil plus atovaquone with rifampicin is not recommended because of reductions in plasma atovaquone concentrations.

General adverse effects

Mild rashes are fairly common, and more serious rashes, like erythema multiforme, are rare. Gastrointestinal upsets, including abdominal pain, nausea, and diarrhea, are common. Mild nervous system disturbances have been mentioned (SEDA-18, 286) (15). Other adverse effects include fever.

Organs and Systems

Gastrointestinal

In a prospective efficacy trial of atovaquone suspension (750 mg od or 250 mg tds for 1 year) in *P. jiroveci* prophylaxis in 28 liver transplant recipients intolerant of co-trimoxazole, the adverse events reported included diarrhea ($n = 7$) and bloating or abdominal pain ($n = 3$) (16). No patient had developed *P. jiroveci* pneumonia by 37 months. This is a smaller dose than approved for *Pneumocystis* prophylaxis in HIV infection (1500 mg/day). Further studies in recipients of solid organ transplants are needed to confirm the efficacy of this prophylactic dose.

Atovaquone suspension (1500 mg orally bd) plus either pyrimethamine (75 mg/day after a 200 mg loading dose) or sulfadiazine (1500 mg qds), as treatment for acute *Toxoplasma* encephalitis (for 6 weeks) and as maintenance therapy (for 42 weeks), has been studied in a randomized phase II trial in HIV-positive patients (17). There were good responses in 21 of 28 patients who received pyrimethamine and nine of 11 who received sulfadiazine. Of 20 patients in the maintenance phase, only one relapsed. Of 40 eligible patients, 11 discontinued treatment as a result of adverse events, nine because of nausea and vomiting or intolerance of the taste of the atovaquone suspension.

Drug Administration

Drug formulations

Atovaquone suspension (750 mg bd; $n = 34$) or tablets (750 mg tds; $n = 20$) have been retrospectively compared in the treatment of *P. jiroveci* pneumonia in HIV-positive individuals (18). Efficacy was similar (74 and 70% successfully treated). Atovaquone suspension was associated with nausea in one patient and a rash in another.

Drug–Drug Interactions

Zidovudine

The metabolism of the antiviral nucleoside zidovudine to the inactive glucuronide form in vitro was inhibited by atovaquone (19,20).

References

1. Hughes WT, LaFon SW, Scott JD, Masur H. Adverse events associated with trimethoprim–sulfamethoxazole and atovaquone during the treatment of AIDS-related *Pneumocystis carinii* pneumonia. J Infect Dis 1995;171(5):1295–301.
2. Colby C, McAfee S, Sackstein R, Finkelstein D, Fishman J, Spitzer T. A prospective randomized trial comparing the toxicity and safety of atovaquone with trimethoprim/sulfamethoxazole as *Pneumocystis carinii* pneumonia prophylaxis following autologous peripheral blood stem cell transplantation. Bone Marrow Transplant 1999;24(8):897–902.
3. El-Sadr WM, Murphy RL, Yurik TM, Luskin-Hawk R, Cheung TW, Balfour HH Jr, Eng R, Hooton TM, Kerkering TM, Schutz M, van der Horst C, Hafner R. Atovaquone compared with dapsone for the prevention of *Pneumocystis carinii* pneumonia in patients with HIV infection who cannot tolerate trimethoprim, sulfonamides, or both. Community Program for Clinical Research on AIDS and the AIDS Clinical Trials Group. N Engl J Med 1998;339(26):1889–95.
4. Dohn MN, Weinberg WG, Torres RA, Follansbee SE, Caldwell PT, Scott JD, Gathe JC Jr, Haghighat DP, Sampson JH, Spotkov J, Deresinski SC, Meyer RD, Lancaster DJ. Oral atovaquone compared with intravenous pentamidine for *Pneumocystis carinii* pneumonia in patients with AIDS. Atovaquone Study Group. Ann Intern Med 1994;121(3):174–80.
5. Lederman MM, van der Horst C. Atovaquone for *Pneumocystis carinii* pneumonia. Ann Intern Med 1995;122(4):314.
6. Stoeckle M, Tennenberg A. Atovaquone for *Pneumocystis carinii* pneumonia. Ann Intern Med 1995;122(4):314.
7. Krause PJ, Lepore T, Sikand VK, Gadbaw J Jr, Burke G, Telford SR 3rd, Brassard P, Pearl D, Azlanzadeh J, Christianson D, McGrath D, Spielman A. Atovaquone and azithromycin for the treatment of babesiosis. N Engl J Med 2000;343(20):1454–8.
8. Farver DK, Lavin MN. Quinine-induced hepatotoxicity. Ann Pharmacother 1999;33(1):32–4.
9. Kedia RK, Wright AJ. Quinine-mediated disseminated intravascular coagulation. Postgrad Med J 1999;75(885):429–30.
10. Newton P, Keeratithakul D, Teja-Isavadharm P, Pukrittayakamee S, Kyle D, White N. Pharmacokinetics of quinine and 3-hydroxyquinine in severe falciparum malaria with acute renal failure. Trans R Soc Trop Med Hyg 1999;93(1):69–72.
11. Shanks GD, Gordon DM, Klotz FW, Aleman GM, Oloo AJ, Sadie D, Scott TR. Efficacy and safety of atovaquone/proguanil as suppressive prophylaxis for *Plasmodium falciparum* malaria. Clin Infect Dis 1998;27(3):494–9.

12. Lell B, Luckner D, Ndjave M, Scott T, Kremsner PG. Randomised placebo-controlled study of atovaquone plus proguanil for malaria prophylaxis in children. Lancet 1998;351(9104):709–13.
13. Hogh B, Clarke PD, Camus D, Nothdurft HD, Overbosch D, Gunther M, Joubert I, Kain KC, Shaw D, Roskell NS, Chulay JD; Malarone International Study Team. Atovaquone–proguanil versus chloroquine–proguanil for malaria prophylaxis in non-immune travellers: a randomised, double-blind study. Malarone International Study Team. Lancet 2000;356(9245):1888–94.
14. Anonymous. Atovaquone + proguanil for malaria prophylaxis. Drug Ther Bull 2001;39(10):73–5.
15. Masur H. Prevention and treatment of *Pneumocystis* pneumonia. N Engl J Med 1992;327(26):1853–60.
16. Meyers B, Borrego F, Papanicolaou G. Pneumocystis carinii pneumonia prophylaxis with atovaquone in trimethoprim–sulfamethoxazole-intolerant orthotopic liver transplant patients: a preliminary study. Liver Transpl 2001;7(8):750–1.
17. Chirgwin K, Hafner R, Leport C, Remington J, Andersen J, Bosler EM, Roque C, Rajicic N, McAuliffe V, Morlat P, Jayaweera DT, Vilde JL, Luft BJ. Randomized phase II trial of atovaquone with pyrimethamine or sulfadiazine for treatment of toxoplasmic encephalitis in patients with acquired immunodeficiency syndrome: ACTG 237/ANRS 039 Study. AIDS Clinical Trials Group 237/Agence Nationale de Recherche sur le SIDA, Essai 039. Clin Infect Dis 2002;34(9):1243–50.
18. Rosenberg DM, McCarthy W, Slavinsky J, Chan CK, Montaner J, Braun J, Dohn MN, Caldwell PT. Atovaquone suspension for treatment of *Pneumocystis carinii* pneumonia in HIV-infected patients. AIDS 2001;15(2):211–14.
19. Trapnell CB, Klecker RW, Jamis-Dow C, Collins JM. Glucuronidation of 3'-azido-3'-deoxythymidine (zidovudine) by human liver microsomes: relevance to clinical pharmacokinetic interactions with atovaquone, fluconazole, methadone, and valproic acid. Antimicrob Agents Chemother 1998;42(7):1592–6.
20. Lee BL, Tauber MG, Sadler B, Goldstein D, Chambers HF. Atovaquone inhibits the glucuronidation and increases the plasma concentrations of zidovudine. Clin Pharmacol Ther 1996;59(1):14–21.

Atracurium dibesilate

See also Neuromuscular blocking drugs

General Information

Atracurium is a muscle relaxant with approximately one-fifth the potency of pancuronium (initial doses of 0.3–0.6 mg/kg and maintenance doses of 0.2 mg/kg being commonly used), an onset of action of 1.2–4 minutes (depending on the dose and the investigator), a medium duration of effect similar to (or slightly longer than) vecuronium, a rapid spontaneous recovery (slightly longer than vecuronium), and a virtual lack of accumulation. Atracurium-induced neuromuscular block is easily reversed by neostigmine.

In contrast to other non-depolarizing drugs, atracurium is completely broken down at normal blood pH and temperature by Hofmann elimination, principally (although to disputed degrees) by nucleophilic substitution and enzymatic ester hydrolysis (1–4). Four metabolites are known, laudanosine being the main biotransformation product. Of the other metabolites, the acrylate esters might possibly give rise to adverse effects. Acrylates are highly reactive pharmacologically and are potentially toxic, theoretically having the capacity to form immunogens and to alkylate cellular nucleophils (3), but so far no effects have been reported (5,6).

In animal experiments, atracurium in large concentrations, many times those providing complete neuromuscular blockade, causes vagal blockade and changes attributed to histamine release; at high dosages some hypotension is seen, possibly because of histamine release; alkalosis diminishes the neuromuscular block, and acidosis prolongs it (7). In cats, high doses of some of the breakdown products of atracurium produced dose-dependent neuromuscular blockade, hypotension, and autonomic effects (5). However, it was considered that these effects were of no pharmacological significance, in view of the low potencies of these substances and the quantities likely to be found in man. From interaction studies in cats (8) it was concluded that the action of atracurium is enhanced by D-tubocurarine, halothane, gentamicin, neomycin, and polymyxin, and antagonized by adrenaline and transiently by suxamethonium. Pretreatment with suxamethonium did not affect the subsequent block by atracurium in cats. Ciclosporin has also been reported to potentiate atracurium in cats (SEDA-12, 118) (9).

In man, histamine release by atracurium is common. The clinical significance of this is disputed, but it can cause minor transient skin reactions. Systemic effects of histamine release are much rarer than cutaneous manifestations.

Organs and Systems

Cardiovascular

There have been reports of hypotension (SEDA-15, 125) (10–12), attributed to histamine release by atracurium. A large prospective surveillance study involving more than 1800 patients given atracurium showed a 10% incidence of adverse reactions, with moderate hypotension (20–50% decrease) in 3.5% of patients (13). In one study cardiovascular stability was maintained with atracurium up to doses of 0.4 mg/kg (14). However, at higher doses (0.5 and 0.6 mg/kg) arterial pressure fell by 13 and 20% and heart rate increased by 5 and 8% respectively. These effects were maximal at 1–1.5 minutes. Since these cardiovascular effects were associated with facial flushing, it was suggested that they might have resulted from histamine release. In a subsequent study the same investigators linked significant cardiovascular changes to increased plasma histamine concentrations at a dose of atracurium of 0.6 mg/kg (15). Injecting this dose slowly over 75 seconds caused less histamine release and adverse hemodynamic effects (16). However, other investigators found no correlation between histamine plasma concentrations and hemodynamic reactions after atracurium administration (17).

Cardiovascular effects, apart from those resulting from histamine release, appear to be almost entirely limited to bradycardia. From animal studies, vagolytic (7) and ganglion-blocking (18) effects are very unlikely to occur at neuromuscular blocking doses, and these predictions appear to be borne out by investigations in man, cardiovascular effects being reported only at high dosages associated with signs suggestive of histamine release (14,15,19). The bradycardia (20–22) is occasionally severe, but, as with vecuronium, the explanation seems to be that the bradycardic effects of other agents used during anesthesia are not attenuated by atracurium as they are by alcuronium, gallamine, or pancuronium, which have vagolytic (or sympathomimetic) effects. The possibility that bradycardia can be caused by one of the metabolites, such as laudanosine (SEDA-12, 115), which is structurally similar to apomorphine, has yet to be excluded. An animal study has suggested that noradrenaline release from sympathetic nerve terminals can be increased by very large doses of atracurium, probably because of high concentrations of laudanosine (SEDA-14, 117) (23). Clinically, cardiovascular effects from this source would only be expected in circumstances that produced much higher than usual laudanosine concentrations.

Hypoxemia has been incidentally reported (SEDA-15, 125) (24), and most probably resulted from an increase in right-to-left cardiac shunting (in a patient with a ventricular septal defect and pulmonary atresia). Atracurium (0.2 mg/kg) may have produced a fall in systemic vascular resistance, perhaps from histamine release; pancuronium was subsequently given without incident.

Nervous system

The major metabolite of atracurium, laudanosine, can cross the blood–brain barrier (CSF/plasma ratios of 0.3–0.6 are found in dogs) (25) and produce strychnine-like nervous system stimulation, which at high plasma concentrations (around 17 ng/ml) leads to convulsions in dogs (25–27). CSF/plasma ratios of laudanosine in man have been reported to be between 0.01 and 0.14 after a 0.5 mg/kg dose of atracurium in a study in which the highest laudanosine concentration was 14 ng/ml (28). Much higher CSF laudanosine concentrations (mean 202 ng/ml, highest 570 ng/ml) were measured after larger atracurium doses (0.5 mg/kg/hour) during intracranial surgery (SEDA-15, 126) (29).

Patients in whom the blood–brain barrier is not intact, such as during neurosurgical procedures, may be at risk from exposure of the brain to unpredictable concentrations of laudanosine (and other drugs). Two patients had fits but these were not thought to be related to laudanosine (29). Under normal circumstances plasma concentrations in man will be far below those required for significant central nervous stimulation. However, the half-life of laudanosine (25) is considerably longer than that of atracurium (30), so that there is a possibility of laudanosine accumulation if many repeated doses or prolonged infusions of atracurium are given.

Skin

Minor skin reactions lasting 5–30 minutes occur in 10–50% of patients according to various studies and are not usually associated with obvious systemic effects (10,31–34). They are probably due to histamine release. A 42% incidence of cutaneous flushing has been reported in 200 patients; the effect was dose-dependent, being 18% at 0.4 mg/kg, 33% at 0.5 and 0.6 mg/kg, and 73% at 1 mg/kg (35). One patient in this study, in the 1 mg/kg group, developed generalized erythema, hypotension, tachycardia, and bronchospasm.

Immunologic

There have been reports of angioedema (10) and bronchospasm (11,36), attributed to histamine release. A large prospective surveillance study involving more than 1800 patients given atracurium showed a 10% incidence of adverse reactions, with bronchospasm in 0.2% of patients (13).

Extreme sensitivity to an intradermal skin test (0.003 mg), some 24 hours after a severe skin reaction to the intravenous administration of atracurium, has been described (37).

Severe systemic reactions after atracurium administration may be due to antibody-mediated anaphylaxis (38) rather than non-specific histamine liberation. It has been suggested that systemic effects from non-specific histamine release are dose-dependent.

Second-Generation Effects

Fetotoxicity

Placental transfer of atracurium occurs (39). In 46 patients undergoing cesarean section (SEDA-17, 18), while the Apgar scores did not differ between neonates whose mothers had received atracurium (0.3 mg/kg) or tubocurarine (0.3 mg/kg), the neurological and adaptive capacity scores (NACS) at 15 minutes (but not at 2 and 24 hours) after birth were lower after atracurium. The NACS values were normal in 83% of the babies in the tubocurarine group and in 55% of those in the atracurium group. The difference was primarily due to lower scores for active contraction of the neck extensor and flexor muscles. These results cannot be satisfactorily explained by partial curarization in some neonates of the atracurium group because the placental transfer of atracurium was lower in the atracurium group; the umbilical vein concentrations of atracurium after clamping of the umbilical cord being approximately one-tenth of the EC_{50} for block of neuromuscular transmission in neonates.

Susceptibility Factors

Age

It has been recommended that doses also be reduced in small neonates less than 3 days old, particularly if their core temperatures are less than 36°C (40), since the breakdown of atracurium is pH- and temperature-dependent.

In elderly patients atracurium infusion requirements appear not to be reduced and its effects are not prolonged (41), probably because the action of atracurium is independent of routes of elimination that are affected by age.

Other features of the patient

Temperature and pH
The breakdown of atracurium is pH-dependent and temperature-dependent. Alkalosis reduces neuromuscular blockade by atracurium, and acidosis prolongs it.

Hypothermia, during cardiopulmonary bypass, has been reported as reducing atracurium requirements by half (42); pH changes may also have occurred.

Burns

Burns are associated with resistance to atracurium (43), as for several other non-depolarizing neuromuscular blocking agents. The EC_{50} is increased and dose requirements may be increased by up to 2–3 times. The resistance varies with the burn area and the time from injury (SEDA-12, 116), being maximal at 15–40 days in patients repeatedly anesthetized.

Dystrophia myotonica

Patients with dystrophia myotonica may be extremely sensitive to atracurium according to a case report (SEDA-10, 110) (44). Resistance to atracurium and higher than normal concentrations of acetylcholine receptors in muscle biopsies have been reported in a patient with multiple sclerosis (SEDA-13, 105) (45).

Pheochromocytoma

It has been suggested (46) that atracurium is unsuitable for use in patients with a pheochromocytoma, since increases in catecholamine concentrations, which are associated with hypertension and other unwanted cardiovascular effects, occur after the injection of relatively large doses (0.6–0.7 mg/kg). However, in an earlier report catecholamine concentrations did not increase and there were no untoward cardiovascular effects after atracurium (47). Nevertheless, considering atracurium's potential for histamine release (which can secondarily lead to increases in circulating catecholamines), vecuronium or pipecuronium are probably better choices in this condition.

Renal and hepatic insufficiency

Renal and liver dysfunction appear to have little effect on the neuromuscular blocking action of atracurium (30,48,49), although resistance has been reported in end-stage renal insufficiency (37% greater ED_{50} values and shorter duration of bolus doses) (SEDA-13, 103) (50,51).

Laudanosine metabolism may be reduced in liver disease (52), and in renal insufficiency higher plasma concentrations and an apparently delayed elimination of laudanosine have been reported (53). Prolonged infusion of atracurium in intensive care (for 38–219 hours) led to slowly increasing plasma laudanosine concentrations, which appeared to plateau after 2–3 days (54). The maximum plasma laudanosine concentrations in six patients were 1.9–5 µg/ml. There was no evidence of cerebral excitation. Nevertheless, caution is urged in patients with severe hepatic dysfunction (55,56), particularly if associated with renal insufficiency, when repeated bolus doses or an infusion of atracurium are given over a prolonged period.

Drug–Drug Interactions

Aminoglycoside antibiotics

Another interaction that has been reported not to occur in man is potentiation by the aminoglycoside antibiotics,

gentamicin and tobramycin (57). In animals, however, gentamicin was found to enhance atracurium blockade (8), so further investigation is required to clarify this point.

Azathioprine

Azathioprine has been reported to reduce atracurium blockade transiently and to a clinically insignificant extent (50).

Carbamazepine

In contrast to reports on other non-depolarizing neuromuscular blocking agents, resistance to atracurium has not been found in patients taking long-term carbamazepine (SEDA-13, 104) (58).

Diisopropylphenol

The intravenous anesthetic agent, diisopropylphenol, is said to potentiate atracurium (59).

D-Tubocurarine

Small doses of D-tubocurarine (0.05 or 0.1 mg/kg) administered 3 minutes before atracurium potentiated its action synergistically (SEDA-12, 117) (60).

Halothane

From animal experiments (8) it seems likely that drug interactions with atracurium will be similar to those for other non-depolarizing neuromuscular blocking agents. Laudanosine has been reported to increase the MAC for halothane in animals (61).

In man, potentiation and prolongation of the action of atracurium by halothane (62–64) have been reported, as has potentiation after 30 minutes of isoflurane anesthesia (65). Whether the dose of atracurium should be reduced from that used during balanced anesthesia by 20, 30, or 50% when patients are anesthetized with inhalational anesthetics can only be decided in the case of an individual patient if neuromuscular monitoring is available, since many other variables, such as the tissue concentrations of the volatile anesthetic and the response of the individual patient to the neuromuscular blocking drug, will influence the overall blocking effect.

Isoflurane

A synergistic interaction between isoflurane and atracurium (high doses) has been incriminated in the causation of an increased incidence of generalized tonic-clonic seizures after neurosurgical operations (SEDA-15, 125) (66).

Ketamine

Ketamine has been shown to prolong the action of atracurium slightly (67).

Pancuronium

Small doses of pancuronium (0.5 or 1 mg) administered 3 minutes before atracurium potentiated its action synergistically (SEDA-12, 117) (60).

Phenytoin

In contrast to reports about other non-depolarizing neuromuscular blocking agents, resistance to atracurium has not been found in patients taking long-term phenytoin (SEDA-13, 104) (68).

Suxamethonium

Prior administration of suxamethonium potentiates the action of atracurium by about 30% (69).

Tamoxifen

Tamoxifen has been associated with prolonged atracurium block in a patient with breast cancer (SEDA-12, 117) (70).

References

1. Nigrovic V, Auen M, Wajskol A. Enzymatic hydrolysis of atracurium in vivo. Anesthesiology 1985;62(5):606–9.
2. Stiller RL, Cook DR, Chakravorti S. In vitro degradation of atracurium in human plasma. Br J Anaesth 1985;57(11):1085–8.
3. Nigrovic V. New insights into the toxicity of neuromuscular-blocking drugs and their metabolites. Curr Opin Anaesthesiol 1991;4:603.
4. Miller RD, Rupp SM, Fisher DM, Cronnelly R, Fahey MR, Sohn YJ. Clinical pharmacology of vecuronium and atracurium. Anesthesiology 1984;61(4):444–53.
5. Chapple DJ, Clark JS. Pharmacological action of breakdown products of atracurium and related substances. Br J Anaesth 1983;55(Suppl 1):S11–15.
6. Cato AE, Lineberry CG, Macklin AW. Concerning toxicity testing of atracurium. Anesthesiology 1985;62(1):94–5.
7. Hughes R, Chapple DJ. The pharmacology of atracurium: a new competitive neuromuscular blocking agent. Br J Anaesth 1981;53(1):31–44.
8. Chapple DJ, Clark JS, Hughes R. Interaction between atracurium and drugs used in anaesthesia. Br J Anaesth 1983;55(Suppl 1):S17–22.
9. Gramstad L, Gjerlow JA, Hysing ES, Rugstad HE. Interaction of cyclosporin and its solvent, Cremophor, with atracurium and vecuronium. Studies in the cat. Br J Anaesth 1986;58(10):1149–55.
10. Srivastava S. Angioneurotic oedema following atracurium. Br J Anaesth 1984;56(8):932–3.
11. Siler JN, Mager JG Jr, Wyche MQ Jr. Atracurium: hypotension, tachycardia and bronchospasm. Anesthesiology 1985;62(5):645–6.
12. Lynas AG, Clarke RS, Fee JP, Reid JE. Factors that influence cutaneous reactions following administration of thiopentone and atracurium. Anaesthesia 1988;43(10):825–8.
13. Beemer GH, Dennis WL, Platt PR, Bjorksten AR, Carr AB. Adverse reactions to atracurium and alcuronium. A prospective surveillance study. Br J Anaesth 1988;61(6):680–4.
14. Basta SJ, Ali HH, Savarese JJ, Sunder N, Gionfriddo M, Cloutier G, Lineberry C, Cato AE. Clinical pharmacology of atracurium besylate (BW 33A): a new non-depolarizing muscle relaxant. Anesth Analg 1982;61(9):723–9.
15. Basta SJ, Savarese JJ, Ali HH, Moss J, Gionfriddo M. Histamine-releasing potencies of atracurium, dimethyl tubocurarine and tubocurarine. Br J Anaesth 1983;55(Suppl 1):S105–6.
16. Scott RP, Savarese JJ, Ali HH, et al. Atracurium: clinical strategies for preventing histamine release and attenuating the hemodynamic response. Anesthesiology 1984;61:A287.
17. Shorten GD, Goudsouzian NG, Ali HH. Histamine release following atracurium in the elderly. Anaesthesia 1993;48(7):568–71.
18. Healy TE, Palmer JP. In vitro comparison between the neuromuscular and ganglion blocking potency ratios of atracurium and tubocurarine. Br J Anaesth 1982;54(12):1307–11.
19. Guggiari M, Gallais S, Bianchi A, Guillaume A, Viars P. Effets hémodynamiques de l'atracurium chez l'homme. [Hemodynamic effects of atracurium in man.] Ann Fr Anesth Reanim 1985;4(6):484–8.
20. Carter ML. Bradycardia after the use of atracurium. BMJ (Clin Res Ed) 1983;287(6387):247–8.
21. McHutchon A, Lawler PG. Bradycardia following atracurium. Anaesthesia 1983;38(6):597–8.
22. Woolner DF, Gibbs JM, Smeele PQ. Clinical comparison of atracurium and alcuronium in gynaecological surgery. Anaesth Intensive Care 1985;13(1):33–7.
23. Kinjo M, Nagashima H, Vizi ES. Effect of atracurium and laudanosine on the release of ³H-noradrenaline. Br J Anaesth 1989;62(6):683–90.
24. Sudhaman DA. Atracurium and hypoxaemic episodes. Anaesthesia 1990;45(2):166.
25. Hennis PJ, Fahey MR, Canfell PC, Shi WZ, Miller RD. Pharmacology of laudanosine in dogs. Anesthesiology 1984;61:A305.
26. Babel A. Etude comparative de la laudanosine et de la papavérine au point de vue pharmacodynamique. Rev Méd Suisse Romande 1989;19:657.
27. Mercier J, Mercier E. Action de quelques alcaloïdes secondaires de l'opium sur l'électrocorticogramme du chien. [Effect of certain opium alkaloids on electrocorticography in dogs.] C R Seances Soc Biol Fil 1955;149(7-8):760–2.
28. Fahey MR, Canfell PC, Taboada T, Hosobuchi Y, Miller RD. Cerebrospinal fluid concentrations of laudanosine after administration of atracurium. Br J Anaesth 1990;64(1):105–6.
29. Eddleston JM, Harper NJ, Pollard BJ, Edwards D, Gwinnutt CL. Concentrations of atracurium and laudanosine in cerebrospinal fluid and plasma during intracranial surgery. Br J Anaesth 1989;63(5):525–30.
30. Fahey MR, Rupp SM, Fisher DM, Miller RD, Sharma M, Canfell C, Castagnoli K, Hennis PJ. The pharmacokinetics and pharmacodynamics of atracurium in patients with and without renal failure. Anesthesiology 1984;61(6):699–702.
31. Lavery GG, Mirakhur RK. Atracurium besylate in paediatric anaesthesia. Anaesthesia 1984;39(12):1243–6.
32. Mirakhur RK, Lyons SM, Carson IW, Clarke RS, Ferres CJ, Dundee JW. Cutaneous reaction after atracurium. Anaesthesia 1983;38(8):818–19.
33. Watkins J. Histamine release and atracurium. Br J Anaesth 1986;58(Suppl 1):S19–22.
34. Doenicke A, Moss J, Lorenz W, Hoernecke R, Gottardis M. Are hypotension and rash after atracurium really caused by histamine release? Anesth Analg 1994;78(5):967–72.
35. Mirakhur RK, Lavery GG, Clarke RS, Gibson FM, McAteer E. Atracurium in clinical anaesthesia: effect of dosage on onset, duration and conditions for tracheal intubation. Anaesthesia 1985;40(8):801–5.
36. Sale JP. Bronchospasm following the use of atracurium. Anaesthesia 1983;38(5):511–12.
37. Aldrete JA. Allergic reaction after atracurium. Br J Anaesth 1985;57(9):929–30.
38. Kumar AA, Thys J, Van Aken HK, Stevens E, Crul JF. Severe anaphylactic shock after atracurium. Anesth Analg 1993;76(2):423–5.
39. Flynn PJ, Frank M, Hughes R. Use of atracurium in caesarean section. Br J Anaesth 1984;56(6):599–605.

40. Nightingale DA. Use of atracurium in neonatal anaesthesia. Br J Anaesth 1986;58(Suppl 1):S32–6.

41. d'Hollander AA, Luyckx C, Barvais L, De Ville A. Clinical evaluation of atracurium besylate requirement for a stable muscle relaxation during surgery: lack of age-related effects. Anesthesiology 1983;59(3):237–40.

42. Flynn PJ, Hughes R, Walton B. Use of atracurium in cardiac surgery involving cardiopulmonary bypass with induced hypothermia. Br J Anaesth 1984;56(9):967–72.

43. Dwersteg JF, Pavlin EG, Heimbach DM. Patients with burns are resistant to atracurium. Anesthesiology 1986;65(5):517–20.

44. Stirt JA, Stone DJ, Weinberg G, Willson DF, Sternick CS, Sussman MD. Atracurium in a child with myotonic dystrophy. Anesth Analg 1985;64(3):369–70.

45. Brett RS, Schmidt JH, Gage JS, Schartel SA, Poppers PJ. Measurement of acetylcholine receptor concentration in skeletal muscle from a patient with multiple sclerosis and resistance to atracurium. Anesthesiology 1987; 66(6):837–9.

46. Amaranath L, Zanettin GG, Bravo EL, Barnes A, Estafanous FG. Atracurium and pheochromocytoma: a report of three cases. Anesth Analg 1988;67(11):1127–30.

47. Stirt JA, Brown RE Jr, Ross TW Jr, Althaus JS. Atracurium in a patient with pheochromocytoma. Anesth Analg 1985;64(5):547–50.

48. Ward S, Neill EA. Pharmacokinetics of atracurium in acute hepatic failure (with acute renal failure). Br J Anaesth 1983;55(12):1169–72.

49. Hunter JM, Jones RS, Utting JE. Use of atracurium in patients with no renal function. Br J Anaesth 1982;54(12):1251–8.

50. Gramstad L. Atracurium, vecuronium and pancuronium in end-stage renal failure. Dose-response properties and interactions with azathioprine. Br J Anaesth 1987;59(8):995–1003.

51. Vandenbrom RH, Wierda JM, Agoston S. Pharmacokinetics of atracurium and metabolites in normal and renal failure patients. Anesthesiology 1987;67:A606.

52. Sharma M, Fahey MR, Castagnoli K, et al. In vitro metabolic studies of atracurium with rabbit liver preparations. Anesthesiology 1984;61:A304.

53. Fahey MR, Rupp SM, Canfell C, Fisher DM, Miller RD, Sharma M, Castagnoli K, Hennis PJ. Effect of renal failure on laudanosine excretion in man. Br J Anaesth 1985;57(11):1049–51.

54. Yate PM, Flynn PJ, Arnold RW, Weatherly BC, Simmonds RJ, Dopson T. Clinical experience and plasma laudanosine concentrations during the infusion of atracurium in the intensive therapy unit. Br J Anaesth 1987;59(2):211–17.

55. Ward S, Weatherley BC. Pharmacokinetics of atracurium and its metabolites. Br J Anaesth 1986;58(Suppl 1):S6–10.

56. Hughes R. Atracurium: an overview. Br J Anaesth 1986;58(Suppl 1):S2–5.

57. Dupuis JY, Martin R, Tetrault JP. Atracurium and vecuronium interaction with gentamicin and tobramycin. Can J Anaesth 1989;36(4):407–11.

58. Ebrahim Z, Bulkley R, Roth S. Carbamazepine therapy and neuromuscular blockade with atracurium and vecuronium. Anesth Analg 1988;67:555.

59. Robertson EN, Fragen RJ, Booij LH, van Egmond J, Crul JF. Some effects of diisopropyl phenol (ICI 35 868) on the pharmacodynamics of atracurium and vecuronium in anaesthetized man. Br J Anaesth 1983;55(8):723–8.

60. Gerber HR, Romppainen J, Schwinn W. Potentiation of atracurium by pancuronium and D-tubocurarine. Can Anaesth Soc J 1986;33(5):563–70.

61. Shi WZ, Fahey MR, Fisher DM, Miller RD, Canfell C, Eger EI 2nd. Laudanosine (a metabolite of atracurium) increases the minimum alveolar concentration of halothane in rabbits. Anesthesiology 1985;63(6):584–8.

62. Payne JP, Hughes R. Evaluation of atracurium in anaesthetized man. Br J Anaesth 1981;53(1):45–54.

63. Katz RL, Stirt J, Murray AL, Lee C. Neuromuscular effects of atracurium in man. Anesth Analg 1982;61(9):730–4.

64. Stirt JA, Murray AL, Katz RL, Schehl DL, Lee C. Atracurium during halothane anesthesia in humans. Anesth Analg 1983;62(2):207–10.

65. Rupp SM, Fahey MR, Miller RD. Neuromuscular and cardiovascular effects of atracurium during nitrous oxide-fentanyl and nitrous oxide–isoflurane anaesthesia. Br J Anaesth 1983;55(Suppl 1):S67–70.

66. Beemer GH, Dawson PJ, Bjorksten AR, Edwards NE. Early postoperative seizures in neurosurgical patients administered atracurium and isoflurane. Anaesth Intensive Care 1989;17(4):504–9.

67. Toft P, Helbo-Hansen S. Interaction of ketamine with atracurium. Br J Anaesth 1989;62(3):319–20.

68. Ornstein E, Matteo RS, Schwartz AE, Silverberg PA, Young WL, Diaz J. The effect of phenytoin on the magnitude and duration of neuromuscular block following atracurium or vecuronium. Anesthesiology 1987;67(2):191–6.

69. Stirt JA, Katz RL, Murray AL, Schehl DL, Lee C. Modification of atracurium blockade by halothane and by suxamethonium. A review of clinical experience. Br J Anaesth 1983;55(Suppl 1):S71–5.

70. Naguib M, Gyasi HK. Antiestrogenic drugs and atracurium–a possible interaction? Can Anaesth Soc J 1986;33(5):682–3.

Atropine

See also Anticholinergic drugs

General Information

Atropine is an anticholinergic drug that is mainly used today in premedication and occasionally to treat bradycardia in the acute phase of myocardial infarction.

Organs and Systems

Cardiovascular

In a classic study, more than a generation ago, of patients given atropine sulfate intravenously as premedication in a total dose of 1 mg, dysrhythmias occurred in over one-third of the subjects, and in over half of those younger than 20 years.

In adults, atrioventricular dissociation was common and in children atrial rhythm disturbances (1). In volunteers, atropine in doses of 1.6 mg/70 kg/minute causes episodes of nodal rhythm with absent P waves on the electrocardiogram (2); the episodes occurred before the heart rate had increased under the influence of the drug. In healthy men being anesthetized for dental surgery a dose of only 0.4 mg atropine intravenously 5 minutes before induction caused reductions in mean arterial pressure, stroke volume, and total peripheral resistance (3).

Second- or third-degree heart block occurred in three of 23 male heart transplant recipients given intravenous atropine (SEDA-22, 156). The mechanism is unknown but it appears that particular caution is needed when atropine is used in this group of patients.

The use of atropine in myocardial infarction to increase the heart rate succeeds as a rule, but in some patients with second-degree heart block the ventricular rate is slowed by atropine, resulting in bradycardia. In contrast, other patients can have tachycardia, and even ventricular fibrillation has been seen, occasionally even in doses as low as 0.5 mg (4).

Possible precipitation of acute myocardial infarction has been discussed by two American emergency medicine specialists (5).

- A 62-year-old woman developed chest pain and sinus bradycardia (41/minute). She had third-degree heart block and was given atropine 1 mg intravenously. Three minutes later, her chest pain increased and the electrocardiogram now showed an acute inferior myocardial infarction, confirmed by serum markers. Angioplasty recanalized the right coronary artery.

The authors discussed the possibility, suggested by others, that atropine can precipitate acute myocardial infarction in an ischemic setting. They concluded that while this may be true, on the whole the advantages of successfully correcting bradycardia outweigh the risks of this rare complication.

Respiratory

Atropine increases the rate and depth of respiration, probably as a reaction to the increase in the dead space resulting from bronchodilatation (5).

Sensory systems

Transient central blindness has followed an intravenous injection of atropine 0.8 mg in the course of spinal anesthesia; blink reflex and pupillary response to light and accommodation were lost; vision returned slowly after some hours after the instillation of pilocarpine (6).

Psychological, psychiatric

Atropine can cause slight memory impairment, detectable if special studies of mental function are performed (SEDA-13, 115).

Immunologic

Hypersensitivity to atropine is most usually seen in the form of contact dermatitis and conjunctivitis. One case of anaphylactic shock after intravenous injection of atropine has been reported (SEDA-14, 122).

Body temperature

Atropine was thought to have produced hypothermia in a boy aged 14 who was being treated with paracetamol (acetaminophen) and cooling blankets for hyperthermia (7). As atropine can cause hypothermia in animals, a causal relation cannot be excluded, even if a concomitant action with paracetamol is assumed.

Second-Generation Effects

Fetotoxicity

Atropine methylbromide crosses the placenta less readily than atropine; when given close to term, it has much less effect on the fetal heart rate than on the maternal heart rate (8).

Susceptibility Factors

In Down's syndrome, atropine produces an abnormally large degree of pupillary dilatation, probably because of a genetically abnormal response; there is also a much greater acceleration of the heart rate than that produced by atropine in healthy subjects.

In congenital albinism, by contrast, the duration of dilatation of the pupil is much shorter than usual; the response to homatropine, scopolamine, and pilocarpine appears to be normal.

Drug Administration

Drug formulations

A total of 1077 patients continued to take extended-release tolterodine 4 mg/day after participating in a randomized trial, about 78% of those who completed the double-blind phase of the study (9). Of the patients who took open treatment, 71% were still doing so after 12 months. The only significant adverse effect was a dry mouth in 13%, while 3.3% complained of constipation. There was no serious systemic toxicity of any kind and efficacy was judged to be at least equivalent to that of the immediate-release formulation.

Drug administration route

Atropine administered by aerosol has a selective effect on the airways because of its low systemic absorption. Adverse effects are those of atropine and atropine-like drugs, but systemic effects are unlikely after topical administration. Two patients developed the signs and symptoms of angle-closure glaucoma after receiving aerosolized atropine. Patients with shallow anterior chambers or possible prior angle-closure glaucoma are probably at greater risk (10). Atropine methylnitrate, a quaternary ammonium derivative, is more selective than atropine sulfate because it is less readily absorbed.

In a child with regular akinetic seizures, atropine sulfate eye-drops increased the frequency of seizures (11).

Drug overdose

When parasympathicolytic or anticholinergic agents are used to dilate the pupils, it is important to recognize systemic anticholinergic intoxication, because the outcome can be fatal without treatment. In patients who are confused or have difficulty speaking, large fixed pupils, and fever, anticholinergic intoxication has to be considered.

- A 3-year-old boy with amblyopia was vomiting, had difficulty in walking, had fever, was agitated, and had a warm red skin and dilated pupils that did not respond to light (12). An empty bottle of atropine eye-drops was found in his home, and suspected anticholinergic intoxication was confirmed. He made a full recovery following treatment with physostigmine.

It should also be remembered that there are other sources of atropine.

- A 52-year-old woman was confused and had dysarthria and difficulty in walking and swallowing (13). That same day she had eaten berries that she thought were bilberries, but were instead *Atropa belladonna* (deadly nightshade).

Drug–Drug Interactions

Paracetamol

Atropine slows the rate of absorption of paracetamol (14).

References

1. Dauchot P, Gravenstein JS. Effects of atropine on the electrocardiogram in different age groups. Clin Pharmacol Ther 1971;12(2):274–80.
2. Gravenstein JS, Ariet M, Thornby JI. Atropine on the electrocardiogram. Clin Pharmacol Ther 1969;10(5):660–6.
3. Allen GD, Everett GB, Kennedy WF Jr. Cardiorespiratory effects of general anesthesia in outpatients: the influence of atropine. J Oral Surg 1972;30(8):576–80.
4. Lunde P. Ventricular fibrillation after intravenous atropine for treatment of sinus bradycardia. Acta Med Scand 1976;199(5):369–71.
5. Brady WJ, Perron AD. Administration of atropine in the setting of acute myocardial infarction: potentiation of the ischemic process? Am J Emerg Med 2001;19(1):81–3.
6. Gooding JM, Holcomb MC. Transient blindness following intravenous administration of atropine. Anesth Analg 1977;56(6):872–3.
7. Lacouture PG, Lovejoy FH Jr, Mitchell AA. Acute hypothermia associated with atropine. Am J Dis Child 1983;137(3):291–2.
8. De Padua CB, Gravenstein JS. Atropine sulfate vs atropine methyl bromide. Effect on maternal and fetal heart rate. JAMA 1969;208(6):1022–3.
9. Kreder K, Mayne C, Jonas U. Long-term safety, tolerability and efficacy of extended-release tolterodine in the treatment of overactive bladder. Eur Urol 2002;41(6):588–95.
10. Berdy GJ, Berdy SS, Odin LS, Hirst LW. Angle closure glaucoma precipitated by aerosolized atropine. Arch Intern Med 1991;151(8):1658–60.
11. Wright BD. Exacerbation of akinetic seizures by atropine eye drops. Br J Ophthalmol 1992;76(3):179–80.
12. Piepoli M, Villani GQ, Ponikowski P, Wright A, Flather MD, Coats AJ. Overview and meta-analysis of randomised trials of amiodarone in chronic heart failure. Int J Cardiol 1998;66(1):1–10.
13. Jellema K, Groeneveld GJ, van Gijn J. Koorts, grote ogen en verwardheid; het anticholinergisch syndroom. [Fever, large eyes and confusion; the anticholinergic syndrome.] Ned Tijdschr Geneeskd 2002;146(46):2173–6.
14. Wojcicki J, Gawronska-Szklarz B, Kazimierczyk J. Wplyw atropiny na wchlanianie paracetamolu z przewodu pokarmowego ludzi zdrowych. [Effect of atropine on the absorption of paracetamol from the digestive tract of healthy subjects.] Pol Tyg Lek 1977;32(29):1111–13.

Azapropazone

See also Non-steroidal anti-inflammatory drugs

General Information

Azapropazone is structurally related to phenylbutazone and probably shares the same adverse effects: gastrotoxicity, skin reactions, headache, vertigo, edema, and renal impairment. A review of a very large series described azapropazone adverse effects in 1724 patients (18%), causing withdrawal in 3.7%. Surprisingly, however, there were no phenylbutazone-type blood dyscrasias (SED-11, 176) (1). Azapropazone should be prescribed only for patients with active rheumatic diseases who have failed to respond to other NSAIDs (2).

Organs and Systems

Hematologic

Hemolytic anemia has been reported (SEDA-10, 79) (SEDA-12, 83). A high percentage of patients taking azapropazone had a positive direct Coombs' test, but this did not persist after treatment had been stopped for several weeks (SEDA-12, 83). Hemolytic anemia has also been described in combination with pulmonary alveolitis, which suggests an allergic or immune reaction (3). Photosensitivity is often reported: 190 reports of photosensitivity were submitted to several national drug-monitoring centers in Europe in 1985 (SEDA-10, 79) (SEDA-12, 83).

Skin

Photosensitivity is more frequent with azapropazone than with almost any other NSAID (4).

Immunologic

Patients with aspirin intolerance often also react to many other NSAIDs. Azapropazone seems to be a safe alternative in these patients, according a study that showed good tolerance of the drug in patients with aspirin intolerance (5).

Susceptibility Factors

Renal disease

Because of increases in unbound drug and reduced clearance in renal insufficiency, the dosage should be carefully adjusted in patients with renal disease (SEDA-11, 92).

Hepatic disease

Because of increases in the unbound drug and reduced clearance, the dosage should be carefully adjusted in patients with liver disease (SEDA-11, 92).

Drug–Drug Interactions

Oral anticoagulants

Azapropazone has the same pattern of interactions as phenylbutazone with oral anticoagulants (SEDA-2, 98).

Phenytoin

Azapropazone has the same pattern of interactions as phenylbutazone with phenytoin (6,7).

Tolbutamide

Azapropazone has the same pattern of interactions as phenylbutazone with tolbutamide (8).

References

1. Sondervosst M. Azapropazone. Clin Rheum Dis 1979;5:465.
2. Anonymous. CSM recommends azapropazone restriction. Scrip 1994;1957:24.
3. Albbazzaz MK, Harvey JE, Hoffman JN, Siddorn JA. Alveolitis and haemolytic anaemia induced by azapropazone. BMJ (Clin Res Ed) 1986;293(6561):1537–8.
4. Olsson S, Biriell C, Boman G. Photosensitivity during treatment with azapropazone. BMJ (Clin Res Ed) 1985;291(6500):939.
5. Gutgesell C, Fuchs T. Azapropazone in aspirin intolerance. Allergy 1999;54(8):897–8.
6. Geaney DP, Carver JG, Aronson JK, Warlow CP. Interaction of azapropazone with phenytoin. BMJ (Clin Res Ed) 1982;284(6326):1373.
7. Geaney DP, Carver JG, Davies CL, Aronson JK. Pharmacokinetic investigation of the interaction of azapropazone with phenytoin. Br J Clin Pharmacol 1983;15(6):727–34.
8. Andreasen PB, Simonsen K, Brocks K, Dimo B, Bouchelouche P. Hypoglycaemia induced by azapropazone–tolbutamide interaction. Br J Clin Pharmacol 1981;12(4):581–3.

Azathioprine and mercaptopurine

General Information

Azathioprine, a prodrug converted to 6-mercaptopurine, is widely used as a post-transplant immunosuppressant and in various autoimmune or chronic inflammatory disorders, such as rheumatoid arthritis, dermatomyositis, systemic lupus erythematosus, skin diseases, and inflammatory bowel diseases.

Adverse effects usually occur during the first two months of treatment, do not correlate with the daily dose, and result in treatment withdrawal in 14–18% of patients, mainly because of bone marrow suppression, gastrointestinal symptoms, hypersensitivity reactions, and infections (1–3). Immediate or long-term adverse effects are of particular concern outside the field of immunosuppression where other treatment options are frequently available, but in any field of use the adverse effects of these drugs weigh heavily.

Observational studies

In a follow-up study of 157 patients receiving azathioprine or mercaptopurine for Crohn's disease, the long-term risks (mainly hematological toxicity and malignancies) over 4 years of treatment were deemed to outweigh the therapeutic benefit (4). In contrast to these findings, both drugs were considered efficacious and reasonably safe in patients with inflammatory bowel disease, provided that patients are carefully selected and regularly investigated for bone marrow toxicity (5). Similar opinions were expressed regarding renal transplant patients. Conversion from ciclosporin to azathioprine in selected and carefully monitored patients had beneficial effects, by improving renal function, reducing cardiovascular risk factors, and reducing financial costs, without increasing the incidence of chronic rejection and graft loss (6).

Experience in children with juvenile chronic arthritis or chronic inflammatory bowel disease has also accumulated, and the toxicity profile of azathioprine or mercaptopurine appears to be very similar to that previously found in the adult population (SEDA-21, 381) (SEDA-22, 410).

The "azathioprine hypersensitivity syndrome"

The complex of azathioprine-associated multisystemic adverse effects is referred to by the misnomer "azathioprine hypersensitivity syndrome." This well-characterized reaction has been described in numerous case reports and includes various symptoms which can occur separately or concomitantly; they comprise fever and rigors, arthralgia, myalgia, leukocytosis, cutaneous reactions, gastrointestinal disturbances, hypotension, liver injury, pancreatitis, interstitial nephritis, pneumonitis, and pulmonary hemorrhage (SED-13, 1121) (SEDA-20, 341) (SEDA-21, 381) (SEDA-22, 410) (7). Isolated fever and rigors are sometimes observed, and severe renal and cardiac toxicity or leukocytoclastic cutaneous vasculitis are infrequent. Symptoms usually occur within the first 6 weeks of treatment and can mimic sepsis. The initial febrile reaction is often misdiagnosed as infectious, and could be associated with acute exacerbation of the underlying disease, for example myasthenia gravis (SEDA-21, 381) (SEDA-22, 410). Hypersensitivity associated with reversible interstitial nephritis can also be mistaken for an acute rejection episode (8). This syndrome should therefore be promptly recognized to avoid unnecessary and costly investigations, and further recurrence on azathioprine rechallenge.

Organs and Systems

Respiratory

Although azathioprine-associated pulmonary toxicity mostly occurs as part of the azathioprine hypersensitivity reaction, isolated interstitial pneumonitis has been reported in a 13-year-old girl with autoimmune chronic active hepatitis (9).

Acute upper airway edema has been observed after a single dose of azathioprine (10).

- A 57-year-old woman with a history of several drug allergies underwent renal transplantation for end-stage polycystic kidney disease and 1 hour later was given intravenous azathioprine 400 mg. She developed profound hypotension and bradycardia within 30 minutes, reversed by sympathomimetics. Shortly after extubation, she had severe breathing difficulties with loss of consciousness. Laryngoscopy showed massive swelling of the tongue and upper airways. Later, while still taking glucocorticoids, she was rechallenged with azathioprine and had milder hypotension and edema of the airways.

Even if no clear mechanism can account for this adverse effect, positive rechallenge strongly suggested that azathioprine was the culprit.

Hematologic

Hematological toxicity is the most commonly reported severe adverse effect of azathioprine, and is marked by predominant leukopenia, thrombocytopenia, and pancytopenia (SED-13, 1120). In a 27-year survey of 739 patients treated with azathioprine 2 mg/kg for inflammatory bowel disease, dosage reduction or withdrawal of the drug because of bone marrow toxicity was necessary in 37 patients (5%) (11). There was moderate or severe leukopenia in 3.8% of patients; in three patients pancytopenia resulted in severe sepsis or death.

Leukopenia is the most serious adverse effect of azathioprine in patients with inflammatory bowel disease (12). It is variable and unpredictable and occurs 2 weeks to 11 years after the start of treatment (median 9 months); most cases recover 1 month after withdrawal.

Dual therapy with ciclosporin and prednisone has been compared with triple therapy with ciclosporin, prednisone, and azathioprine in a randomized trial in 250 renal transplant patients (13). Patients in the triple therapy group had less frequent severe episodes of acute rejection and more frequent episodes of leukopenia than the double therapy group (28% versus 4%). There were no other differences in the adverse effects profiles, in particular the incidence of infectious complications.

Macrocytic anemia and isolated thrombocytopenia without severe clinical consequences have sometimes been observed. Pure red cell aplasia can occur, but the few relevant reports concern only isolated instances involving renal transplant patients (14,15). The facts in one patient suggested that parvovirus B19 infection resulting from the immunosuppressive effects of azathioprine should also be considered as a possible indirect cause (16). Although blood cell disorders usually occur in the first 4 weeks of treatment, strict and regular surveillance of blood cell counts continuing for as long as treatment is maintained is usually recommended, since delayed hematological toxicity remains possible.

- Immune hemolytic anemia has been reported in a 67-year-old man taking mercaptopurine for chronic myelomonocytic leukemia (17). Serology showed a positive direct antiglobulin test and confirmed the presence of mercaptopurine drug-dependent antibodies. He improved and the direct antiglobulin test was no longer positive 20 days after mercaptopurine withdrawal.

Aplastic anemia due to azathioprine therapy after corneal transplantation has reportedly caused bilateral macular hemorrhage (18).

- A 38-year-old man underwent therapeutic penetrating keratoplasty for non-healing fungal keratitis in his left eye. Although the infection was controlled, he underwent a second corneal transplantation after 2 years. Since there was corneal vascularization in three quadrants, he was given oral azathioprine postoperatively. Four months later he developed gastrointestinal bleeding and a sudden reduction in vision in both eyes. His platelet count was less than 30×10^9/l, his hemoglobin 4.1 g/dl, and a bone marrow aspirate was hypocellular. There were macular hemorrhages in both eyes. The hemorrhages resolved within 2 months.

Gastrointestinal

Gastrointestinal disturbances with nausea, vomiting, and diarrhea are frequent in patients taking azathioprine or mercaptopurine. Diarrhea may be isolated or part of the azathioprine hypersensitivity syndrome. In two patients with azathioprine-induced diarrhea proven by positive rechallenge, the period of sensitization ranged from 1 week to 1 year (19).

In two cases, azathioprine caused severe gastrointestinal symptoms that could have been easily confused with an acute exacerbation of the underlying inflammatory bowel disease (20).

- A 32-year-old man with ulcerative colitis improved with prednisolone, mesalazine, and antibiotics. The dose of prednisolone was reduced and the disease flared up again. He was therefore given azathioprine and an increased dose of prednisolone, with rapid clinical improvement. After 3 weeks, he reported increasing abdominal pain, worse diarrhea, and weight loss of 3 kg. He stopped taking azathioprine and the pain improved. Because of progressive disease and active pancolitis at colonoscopy, he was given high-dose prednisolone, mesalazine, and ciprofloxacin, without improvement. He was therefore given intravenous azathioprine, but developed devastating diarrhea and weight loss of more than 6 kg in 24 hours, his CRP rose from 5 to 305 µg/ml, and he developed hypovolemic shock. He recovered after treatment with parenteral nutrition for 7 days.
- A 50-year-old woman with Crohn's disease and active disease throughout the colon was given prednisolone, mesalazine, and azathioprine 50 mg/day. After 3 weeks, the dose of azathioprine was increased to 100 mg/day, but she developed nausea, severe diarrhea, and abdominal tenderness. The symptoms subsided after azathioprine was withdrawn. She was then given mercaptopurine, without significant adverse effects.

Liver

Although rarely severe, any increase in liver enzyme activity justifies careful and regular monitoring of liver function and the results may be a reason for withdrawing treatment (SED-8, 1118) (21). In a retrospective study, hepatitis was found in 21 (2%) of 1035 renal transplant patients, and it was suggested that hepatitis B or C infection increases the risk of azathioprine hepatotoxicity (22). In 29 cardiac transplant recipients who had had probable azathioprine-induced liver dysfunction, cyclophosphamide was given, with improvement of liver enzyme activities and no increase in the rate of graft rejection or significant changes in the doses of other immunosuppressive drugs (23).

Azathioprine can cause reversible cholestasis (24), perhaps due to bile duct injury (25).

Direct hepatocellular injury with acute cytolytic hepatitis has been reported rarely (SEDA-21, 381).

In one patient, azathioprine-induced lymphoma with massive liver infiltration was the probable cause of fulminant hepatic failure (SEDA-21, 381).

Other histological features that have been described include lesions of the hepatic venous system (peliosis hepatis, sinusoidal dilatation, perivenous fibrosis, and nodular regenerative hyperplasia) and these can be associated with portal hypertension (SEDA-16, 520) (SED-13, 1120) (21). Particularly severe and potentially fatal veno-occlusive liver disease has been reported in patients with renal and allogeneic bone marrow transplants taking chronic treatment (26) (SEDA-12, 386), but complete histological reversal can be observed (SEDA-20, 341).

- In a 33-year-old man azathioprine-induced veno-occlusive disease was treated with a transjugular intrahepatic portosystemic shunt over 26 months, with progressive worsening 15 months after renal transplantation (27).

Four patients with renal transplants developed hepatic veno-occlusive disease after immunosuppression with azathioprine. The diagnosis was based on typical histopathological findings: perivenular fibrosis, trilobular sinusoidal dilatation and congestion, and perisinusoidal fibrosis. The patients presented with severe progressive portal hypertension followed by fulminant liver failure and death. The disease was associated with cytomegalovirus infection, and it was not related to the dose of azathioprine (26). Veno-occlusive liver disease has also been described shortly after liver transplantation (28,29). A history of acute liver rejection affecting the hepatic veins was supposedly a contributing factor in these patients, and the presence of non-inflammatory small hepatic vein lesions was a possible early indicator of hepatotoxicity. Liver biopsy should therefore be considered in liver recipients who have biological features of hepatitis, so that treatment can be withdrawn rapidly if necessary.

Azathioprine allergy can be associated with biochemical hepatitis and a normal liver biopsy, apart form marked lipofuscin deposition (30). These findings, combined with patchy isotope uptake on technetium scintigraphy, are suggestive of focal hepatocellular necrosis.

It has been suggested that there is an increased risk of azathioprine-induced liver damage in renal transplant patients with chronic viral hepatitis (SEDA-20, 341) (SEDA-23, 402).

- Fatal fibrosing cholestatic hepatitis has been reported in a 63-year-old cardiac transplant patient with acquired post-transplant hepatitis C virus infection whose immunosuppressive regimen included azathioprine

(31). Histology showed several features of azathioprine hepatotoxicity, namely veno-subocclusive lesions and nodular regenerative diffuse hyperplasia, suggesting a pathogenic role of azathioprine.

In 79 renal transplant patients with chronic viral hepatitis, azathioprine maintenance treatment ($n = 34$) was associated with a poorer outcome than in 45 patients who discontinued azathioprine (32). Cirrhosis was more frequent in the first group (six versus one), and more patients died with a functioning graft (14 versus two), mostly because of liver dysfunction ($n = 5$) or infection ($n = 6$). These results suggest that azathioprine further accelerates the course of the liver disease in these patients.

- A 50-year-old woman with nodular sclerosis developed azathioprine-induced hepatotoxicity within the first weeks of treatment (33), the usual time-course. Positive rechallenge confirmed the role of azathioprine.

However, delayed occurrence of hepatitis is also possible.

- Canalicular cholestasis with portal fibrosis and ductal proliferation has been reported after 24 years of azathioprine in a 57-year-old woman with myasthenia gravis (34).

An unusual diffuse liver disease with sinusoidal dilatation (SEDA-11, 392) has been described.

Pancreas

Pancreatitis due to azathioprine or mercaptopurine has usually been reported as part of the hypersensitivity syndrome (SEDA-16, 520) (SEDA-20, 341). It has mostly been observed in patients with inflammatory bowel disease, and required withdrawal of treatment in 1.3% of patients with Crohn's disease (3). Pancreatitis was not dose-related within the therapeutic range of doses and often recurred in patients who were rechallenged with either drug (SEDA-20, 341) (35). Fatal hemorrhagic pancreatitis occurred in one patient, but a role of concomitant drugs was also possible (SEDA-20, 341). Pancreatitis or hyperamylasemia were not significantly different in renal transplant patients randomly assigned to receive azathioprine or ciclosporin, and other causative factors were found in most patients with pancreatitis (36).

In a review of definite or probable drug-associated pancreatitis spontaneously reported to the Dutch adverse drug reactions system during 1977–98, azathioprine was the suspected drug in four of 34 patients, two of whom had positive rechallenge (37). Although most of the carefully described reports of azathioprine-induced pancreatitis were found in patients with inflammatory bowel disease, transplant recipients can also suffer this complication.

- Over a year after renal transplantation, a 48-year-old man, who took azathioprine, ciclosporin, and prednisolone, developed acute necrotizing pancreatitis (38). Improvement was obtained after azathioprine withdrawal, but he again took azathioprine and had similar symptoms within 30 hours after a single dose.
- Pancreatitis has been reported after a progressive increase in dose of 6-thioguanine in a 10-year-old infant (39). She had had two previous episodes of pancreatitis after mercaptopurine.

The chemical structure of 6-thioguanine, which results from the metabolism of azathioprine/mercaptopurine, is very similar to that of mercaptopurine. Therefore, a history of previous adverse effects with mercaptopurine should be anticipated in patients considered for 6-thioguanine treatment.

Skin

Rashes or other allergic-type cutaneous reactions are usually noted during the azathioprine hypersensitivity syndrome. Isolated but convincing reports point to the occurrence of vasculitis with microscopic polyarteritis (SEDA-21, 381) and Sweet's syndrome, which recurred after subsequent azathioprine exposure (SEDA-22, 410).

Pellagra with a photosensitivity-like rash and skin peeling syndrome has also been noted (SEDA-21, 381).

Musculoskeletal

Severe myalgia and symmetrical polyarthritis are sometimes reported in patients taking azathioprine. Eight cases of azathioprine-associated arthritis were identified in the WHO Drug Monitoring Database, including six cases with a typical hypersensitivity syndrome and two cases in whom joint involvement was the only reported symptom (40). Rhabdomyolysis has also been reported as a possible feature of the azathioprine hypersensitivity syndrome (SEDA-20, 341).

In two patients with Crohn's disease, azathioprine was suspected to have caused severe gait disorders with an inability to walk (41). Within 1 month of treatment, both had joint pains or diffuse arthralgias that were the presumed cause of pseudoparalysis of the legs. In one patient other causes were carefully ruled out and similar symptoms recurred shortly after azathioprine was re-introduced.

Immunologic

The distinction between relapse of the treated disease, systemic sepsis, and acute azathioprine allergy can be difficult, as has been shown in three patients with vasculitic disorders (42).

Allergic reactions to azathioprine were recorded in 2% of patients with Crohn's disease taking azathioprine (3), and there was no evidence to suggest that the incidence depended on the underlying disease. The more rapid recurrence and/or the severity of symptoms following rechallenge were in keeping with a putative immune-mediated reaction, but no immunological mechanism has been conclusively demonstrated (SED-13, 1121) (43,44). In one patient, progressively rising doses of azathioprine were successfully administered, despite positive skin prick tests (SEDA-21, 382). Anaphylactic shock has been occasionally reported (45). Delayed contact hypersensitivity with a positive patch test was described in a pharmaceutical handler of azathioprine (46).

Allergic reactions to mercaptopurine or azathioprine are well described, but a true immunoallergic reaction has never been convincingly demonstrated. Desensitization has been successfully performed in isolated patients (47), and this has been more extensively addressed in a retrospective analysis of the charts of patients treated for inflammatory bowel disease (48). Of 591 patients observed over a 28-year period, 16 (2.7%) developed allergic reactions, which mostly consisted of fever ($n = 14$), joint pains ($n = 6$), or severe back pain ($n = 5$). Symptoms commonly appeared within 1 month and lasted 5 days on average. All nine patients rechallenged with mercaptopurine had similar but less severe symptoms. Further rechallenge with azathioprine in six of these patients caused symptoms in five of them. Careful desensitization with mercaptopurine or azathioprine was attempted in five patients, and resulted in tolerance and therapeutic success in four. The last patient, who had a previous history of mercaptopurine-induced sepsis-like syndrome with renal insufficiency, had a similar reaction only after one-quarter of the dose of azathioprine. This study suggests that a direct switch from mercaptopurine to the parent drug azathioprine cannot be recommended in patients who developed allergic reactions to mercaptopurine, and that desensitization should not be attempted in patients with previous life-threatening hypersensitivity reactions.

A genetic predisposition is suspected, with a possible association between the hypersensitivity syndrome and the Bw4 and Bw6 phenotypes (SED-13, 1121). Mercaptopurine has sometimes been re-administered safely after a severe hypersensitivity reaction to azathioprine (49), suggesting a major role for the imidazole moiety of azathioprine. However, typical allergic reactions to mercaptopurine can also occur (SEDA-21, 381).

Infection risk

Infections, in particular bacterial and viral (cytomegalovirus, *Herpes simplex* virus, Epstein–Barr virus), and also protozoal and fungal infections, are major causes of morbidity and mortality in the post-transplantation period, whatever the immunosuppressive regimen used (50–52). Based on an analysis of medical and autopsy records, infections were found to be the cause of death in 70% of transplant patients, with bacteria (50%) or fungi (29%) the most common pathogens (53).

The frequency, course, and severity of *Herpes zoster* infection have been retrospectively evaluated in a sample of 550 patients treated with 6-mercaptopurine for inflammatory bowel disease (54). Twelve patients aged 14–73 years developed shingles after an average of 921 days, an incidence that was about two-fold higher than in the general population. Only three patients were still taking glucocorticoids at the time of onset of the shingles, and leukopenia was not associated with the occurrence of the infection. In nine patients, the course of the infection was 7–71 days and was uncomplicated. Two patients had more severe symptoms and suffered from postherpetic neuralgia. The last patient, a 14-year-old boy, had a brief episode of *H. zoster* during initial treatment and had *H. zoster* encephalitis at the age of 23 years, 16 months after 6-mercaptopurine had been restarted. From this report, it appears that 6-mercaptopurine can be restarted after brief discontinuation in patients who are expected to benefit from it.

- Fatal Epstein–Barr virus-associated hemophagocytic syndrome was reported in a young man taking azathioprine and prednisone for Crohn's disease (55).

Donor-specific blood transfusion in the preparation for transplantation was complicated by a higher incidence of cytomegalovirus infection in patients receiving azathioprine (56).

Long-Term Effects

Tumorigenicity

Because of the varied indications for azathioprine and mercaptopurine, it is difficult to determine whether there is an increased incidence of cancer specifically related to prolonged drug exposure. Data from the Cincinnati Transplant Tumor Registry, published in 1993, helped to define comprehensively the characteristics of neoplasms observed in organ transplant recipients (57). Skin and lip cancers were the most common, and non-Hodgkin's lymphomas represent the majority of lymphoproliferative disorders, with an incidence some 30- to 50-fold higher than in controls. An excess of Kaposi's sarcomas, carcinomas of the vulva and perineum, hepatobiliary tumors, and various sarcomas has also been reported. In contrast, the incidence of common neoplasms encountered in the general population is not increased. In renal transplant patients, the actuarial cumulative risk of cancer was 14–18% at 10 years and 40–50% at 20 years (58,59). Skin cancers accounted for about half of the cases. Very similar figures were found in later studies (SEDA-20, 341).

While there is no doubt that the incidence of malignancies is increased in the transplant population, there have been controversies as to which factors (duration of treatment, total dosage, the degree of immunosuppression, or the type of immunosuppressive regimens) are the most relevant in determining risk. Partial or complete regression of lymphoproliferative disorders and Kaposi's sarcomas after reduction of immunosuppressive therapy argues strongly for the role of the degree of immunosuppression (57). The incidence of cancer was also significantly higher in renal transplant patients taking triple therapy regimens compared with dual therapy (60). Similarly, aggressive immunosuppressive therapy may account for the higher incidence of lymphomas in patients with cardiac versus renal allografts.

In a large multicenter study in more than 52 000 kidney or heart transplant patients between 1983 and 1991, the rate of non-Hodgkin's lymphomas in the first post-transplantation year was 0.2% in kidney and 1.2% in heart recipients, and fell substantially thereafter (61). Initial immunosuppression with azathioprine and ciclosporin and prophylactic treatment with antilymphocyte antibodies or muromonab were associated with a significantly increased incidence of non-Hodgkin's lymphomas compared with other immunosuppressive regimens, which confirmed the major role of the level of immunosuppression. Later studies confirmed that immunosuppression per se rather than a single agent is responsible for the increased risk of cancer (SEDA-20, 340). Finally, the most striking difference between conventional and modern immunosuppressive regimens, including ciclosporin, was the average time to the appearance of tumors, in particular skin cancers and lymphomas, which was shorter in ciclosporin-treated patients (62,63). There was

an increased incidence of non-Hodgkin's lymphomas in patients receiving long-term azathioprine and prednisolone for rheumatoid disease, although the latent period was longer than in other patients, perhaps reflecting a different pathogenesis (64).

Multiple factors with complex interactions are involved in the observed pattern and increased incidence of neoplasms. They include severely depressed immunity with an impaired immune surveillance against various carcinogens, the activation of several oncogenic viruses, and a possible mutagenic effect of the drugs. Viruses, such as papillomavirus, cytomegalovirus, and Epstein–Barr virus, are believed to play an important role in the development of several post-transplant cancers. From a theoretical point of view, the use of antiviral drugs active against herpes viruses, which are commonly implicated as co-factors, can be expected to produce a reduction in the incidence of post-transplant lymphoproliferative disorders.

Long-term treatment with azathioprine has been associated with transitional carcinoma of the bladder and non-Hodgkin's lymphoma in a single case (65).

- A 59-year-old man who had had a testicular non-Hodgkin's lymphoma for 9 years, developed diplopia and ptosis due to myasthenia gravis with antibodies to the acetylcholine receptor. He was given pyridostigmine and prednisolone. After 6 months he developed pernicious anemia, and he was given vitamin B_{12} injections. An attempt to reduce the dose of prednisolone failed, and he was therefore given azathioprine and the dose of prednisone was progressively reduced. Two years later he developed a transitional carcinoma of the bladder (pTa g1), which was removed by transurethral resection. Seven years later he developed a swollen tender right testis due to a B cell lymphoma. He tolerated chemotherapy (CHOP) poorly and died 2 months later.

In renal transplant recipients, premalignant dysplastic keratotic lesions increased in frequency by 6.8% per year after the first 3.5 years after transplantation, and were ultimately observed in all 167 patients within 16 years of transplantation (66). No relation with sun exposure or skin type was found. The great majority of these patients were taking prednisolone and azathioprine, but azathioprine was considered as the main causative factor, possibly due to a carcinogenic effect rather than to immunosuppression itself.

Several isolated reports and epidemiological studies have addressed the risk of cancer in non-transplant patients treated with azathioprine. Promptly reversible Epstein–Barr virus-associated lymphomas have been reported as single cases, as have reports of acute myeloid leukemia with 7q deletion, rapidly aggressive squamous cell carcinomas, soft tissue carcinomas, or fatal Merkel cell carcinomas in patients taking long-term azathioprine maintenance (SED-13, 1122) (SEDA-20, 342) (SEDA-21, 382) (SEDA-22, 410). Although epidemiological studies allow a more accurate estimate, conflicting results have emerged and there is as yet no definite evidence that azathioprine actually increases the risk of cancer.

An increased risk of non-Hodgkin's lymphomas, possibly related to treatment duration, has been found in patients with rheumatoid arthritis (67). There was no evidence that azathioprine increased the overall incidence of any cancer in 259 patients with rheumatoid arthritis on immunosuppressive treatment (azathioprine in 223) and matched for age and sex (but not for disease duration and severity) with unexposed patients (68). However, death more often resulted from malignancies in those taking azathioprine.

In cases of inflammatory bowel disease, no overall increased incidence of cancer was noted after a median of 9 years follow-up in 755 patients who had taken less than 2 mg/kg/day of azathioprine over a median period of 12.5 years (69). Only colorectal cancers (mostly adeno-carcinoma) were more frequent, but their incidence was also increased in chronic inflammatory bowel diseases. More specifically, there was no excess of non-Hodgkin's lymphoma, but the power of the study to detect an increased risk of this disorder was low.

Another group of investigators has estimated that the potential long-term risk of malignancies outweighs the therapeutic benefit, but this conclusion was based on the follow-up of only 157 patients treated for Crohn's disease (4).

In 626 patients with inflammatory bowel disease who had taken azathioprine for a mean duration of 27 months (mean follow-up 6.9 years), there was no increased risk of cancer (colorectal or other) (70).

In a case-control study using a database of 1191 patients with multiple sclerosis, 23 cancers (17 solid tumors, two skin tumors, and four hemopoietic cancers) were found. The relative risk of cancer was 1.3 in patients treated for less than 5 years, 2.0 in those treated for 5–10 years, and 4.4 in those treated for more than 10 years; however, none of these later changes was significant (71). Nevertheless, there was a significant association for cumulative dosages in excess of 600 g. Taken together, these results suggest a low risk of cancer in non-transplant patients, but they cannot exclude a possible dose-related increase in risk during long-term treatment.

Skin carcinoma (predominantly squamous-cell carcinoma), cancer of the lip, Kaposi's sarcoma, and carcinoma of the cervix and anus are reported to be more common following azathioprine than in the general population (72).

Mercaptopurine is not considered to be leukemogenic, but this assumption has been disputed in a study of 439 children who received mercaptopurine as part of their maintenance therapy for acute lymphoblastic leukemia (73). Five patients developed secondary myelodysplasia or acute myeloid leukemia 23–53 months after diagnosis, a consequence that was attributed to mercaptopurine. These five patients had significantly lower TPMT activity, and two were classified as heterozygous for TPMT deficiency on genotype analysis. Although the number of evaluable patients was small, the suggestion was that a subset of patients with low TMPT activity might have an increased leukemogenic risk when exposed to mercaptopurine with other cytotoxic agents. Whether these findings can be extrapolated to patients without cancers is not known.

Of 550 patients with inflammatory bowel disease treated for a mean of 8 years, 25 (4.5%) developed a malignancy, with an overall incidence of 2.7 neoplasms per 1000 years of follow-up (74). The numbers of the most commonly observed cancers, such as bowel cancers ($n = 8$), breast cancers ($n = 3$), or single cases of other cancers, did not seem to be higher than expected in the general population or in the inflammatory bowel disease population. Although mercaptopurine was suspected in two cases of testicular carcinoma, two cases of lymphoma, and one case of leukemia, the authors emphasized the small risk of malignancies compared with the beneficial results of mercaptopurine in inflammatory bowel disease.

Second-Generation Effects

Pregnancy

Even though azathioprine is teratogenic in animals, human experience allows no firm conclusions, being limited to single case reports of birth defects after first trimester exposure to azathioprine. More convincingly, there was no evidence of increased risk or of a specific pattern of congenital anomalies among hundreds of infants born to azathioprine-treated transplant patients (75–77), but large series with adequate long-term follow-up are still lacking. The absence of inosinate pyrophosphorylase, an enzyme that converts azathioprine to its active metabolites, in the fetus was suggested to account for these reassuring data. Other potential risks, that is miscarriages or stillbirths, were also within the normal range, and intrauterine growth retardation did not appear to be specifically related to azathioprine use. Potential neonatal consequences of maternal azathioprine maintenance during the whole pregnancy should be borne in mind, in view of isolated reports of immunohematological immunosuppression, pancytopenia, cytomegalovirus infection, and chromosome aberrations. Unfortunately, the extent of this risk has not been carefully evaluated.

Teratogenicity

Maternal azathioprine treatment during pregnancy is clearly teratogenic in animals, but the mechanisms are not known. A large number of reports have described the outcome of pregnancies following the use of immunosuppressant drugs, in particular in renal transplant patients, and hundreds of pregnancies have been analysed (75). The largest experience is that derived from the National Transplantation Pregnancy Registry which has been built up in the USA since 1991 (76). This registry has accumulated data on more than 900 pregnancies, of which 83% followed kidney transplantation. Overall, the immunosuppressant drug regimens commonly used in transplant patients (azathioprine or ciclosporin) do not appear to increase the overall risk of congenital malformations or produce a specific pattern of malformation. Risk factors associated with adverse pregnancy outcomes included a short time interval between transplantation and pregnancy (that is less than 1–2 years), graft dysfunction before or during pregnancy, and hypertension (78).

Possible long-term effects of in utero exposure to immunosuppressants are still seldom investigated. There have been no reports that physical and mental development or renal function are altered. In one study, there were changes in T lymphocyte development in seven children born to mothers who had taken azathioprine or ciclosporin, but immune function assays were normal, suggesting that development of the fetal immune system was not affected (79).

In 27 clinical series, the frequency of congenital anomalies among infants of patients who took azathioprine after renal transplantation ranged from 0 to 11% (80).

The consequences of paternal mercaptopurine exposure on the outcome of pregnancies have been retrospectively studied in 57 men with inflammatory bowel disease: 23 men had fathered 50 pregnancies and had taken mercaptopurine before conception; of these, 13 pregnancies were conceived within 3 months of paternal mercaptopurine use (group 1A) and 37 pregnancies were conceived at least 3 months after paternal mercaptopurine withdrawal (group 1B); the other 34 men, who fathered 90 pregnancies, had not been exposed to mercaptopurine before conception (group II) (81). Of the 140 conceptions, two resulted in congenital anomalies in group 1A, whereas there were no congenital anomalies in the other groups. One child had a missing thumb, and the other had acrania with multiple digital and limb abnormalities. The overall number of complications (spontaneous abortion and congenital anomalies) was significantly higher in group 1A (4/13) compared with both group IB (1/37) and group II (2/90). Although the retrospective nature of this study and the limited number of evaluable patients precluded any definitive conclusion, the observed congenital anomalies were similar to those found in the offspring of female rabbits treated with mercaptopurine during pregnancy, and suggested that paternal mercaptopurine treatment should ideally be discontinued at least 3 months before planned conception.

Whereas neutropenia and immune deficiencies can affect neonates born to transplant patients, the exact role of azathioprine is difficult to establish. A report has suggested that such effects should also be expected in neonates born to patients taking azathioprine for other conditions (82).

- A 27-year-old woman, who took azathioprine (125 mg/day) and mesalazine (3 g/day) during her whole pregnancy, delivered a normal boy who had febrile respiratory distress after 36 hours. Chest X-ray showed interstitial pneumonitis and thymus hypoplasia. There was severe neutropenia (20×10^6/l), lymphopenia (24×10^6/l), and hypogammaglobulinemia. His clinical condition improved over the next 26 days with immunoglobulin treatment and antibiotics, but B lymphocytes and IgM were still undetectable.

Lactation

Very few data on breastfed infants from azathioprine-treated mothers are available. Breastfeeding is not recommended owing to the potential risk of immuno-suppression, growth retardation, and carcinogenesis.

Susceptibility Factors

Genetic factors

The complex metabolism of azathioprine and mercaptopurine is subject to a pharmacogenetic polymorphism that is relevant to the degree of efficacy and toxicity attained in a given individual. Thiopurine methyltransferase (TPMT) is one of the key enzymes regulating the catabolism of thiopurine drugs to inactive products. Owing to an inherited autosomal codominant trait, a significant number of patients have intermediate (11%) to low or undetectable (0.3%) TPMT activity (83). These patients produce larger amounts of the active 6-thioguanine nucleotides and may therefore be unusually sensitive to commonly used dosages and an increased risk of myelotoxicity (SED-13, 1120) (SEDA-21, 381).

Monitoring azathioprine therapy by measuring erythrocyte 6-thioguanine concentrations and TPMT activity is thought to ensure optimal immunosuppressive effects and to reduce the likelihood of hematological toxicity (84,85). Low or completely absent erythrocyte TPMT activity and high concentrations of erythrocyte 6-thioguanine metabolites have been found in patients with severe azathioprine-induced bone marrow toxicity, as compared to those without bone marrow toxicity (86,87). However, intracellular concentrations of thiopurine nucleotides alone did not always correlate with hematological toxicity (88). In patients in whom TPMT deficiency was not clearly demonstrated, low lymphocyte 5'-nucleotidase activity and xanthine oxidase deficiency or other factors have been postulated as possible causes of hemotoxicity, suggesting that bone marrow toxicity is probably multifactorial (87,89,90). Although not all investigators recommend systematic pretreatment screening for purine enzyme activities, evidence of deficiency of purine enzymes could well be sought when early bone marrow toxicity occurs.

In a retrospective analysis of 106 patients with inflammatory bowel disease, to evaluate the importance of thiopurine methyl transferase (TPMT) activity in the management of azathioprine therapy in inflammatory bowel disease, the relation between inherited variations in TPMT enzyme activity and azathioprine toxicity was confirmed (91).

In 3291 patients receiving azathioprine, 10% had a low TPMT activity and 15 (1 in 220 or 0.46%) had no detectable enzymatic activity at all (92), slightly more common than has been reported in other studies (1 in 300). This makes the economics of screening, to avoid myelosuppression in patients receiving azathioprine, attractive.

Of 78 patients treated with azathioprine for systemic lupus erythematosus, 10 developed azathioprine-associated reversible neutropenia (93). Only one of these patients was homozygous for TPMT deficiency, but he had the most severe episode (aplastic anemia).

In one study, 14 of 33 patients with rheumatoid arthritis had severe adverse effects (mostly gastrointestinal toxicity, flu-like reactions or fever, pancytopenia, and hepatotoxicity) within 1–8 weeks after azathioprine was started (94). The adverse effects subsided after withdrawal in all patients, but all eight patients who were rechallenged developed the same adverse effect. A baseline reduction in TPMT activity was significantly associated with the occurrence of these adverse effects in seven of eight patients, with a relative risk of 3.1 (95% CI = 1.6–6.2) compared with patients with high TPMT activity (seven of 25 patients). Another prospective evaluation in 67 patients with rheumatic disorders showed that TPMT genotype analysis is useful in identifying patients at risk of azathioprine toxicity (95). Treatment duration was significantly longer in patients with the wild-type TPMP alleles than in those with mutant alleles, and that was due to the early occurrence of leukopenia in the latter.

In 22 children with renal transplants, high erythrocyte TPMT activity, measured 1 month after transplantation, correlated positively with rejection episodes during the first 3 months, and this was probably due to more rapid azathioprine catabolism (96). As suggested in a study of 180 patients with acute lymphoblastic leukemia, determination of genetic polymorphisms in TMPT can be useful in predicting potential toxicity and in optimizing the determination of an appropriate dose in patients who are homozygous or heterozygous for TMPT deficiency (97).

In 30 heart transplant patients taking azathioprine, the myelosuppressive effects of azathioprine/mercaptopurine were predicted by systematic genotypic screening of thiopurine methyltransferase deficiency (98). However, myelosuppression can also be observed in patients without the thiopurine methyltransferase mutation. Of 41 patients with leukopenia or thrombocytopenia taking azathioprine/mercaptopurine for Crohn's disease, four were classified as low methylators, seven as intermediate methylators, and 30 as high methylators by genotypic analysis (99). Thus, only 27% of the patients had the typical mutations associated with enzyme deficiency and a risk of myelosuppression. The delay in bone marrow toxicity was shorter in the four homozygous patients (median 1 month) than in the others (median 3–4 months). Many other causes, including viral infections, associated drugs, or another azathioprine/mercaptopurine metabolic pathway, were suggested to account for most of the cases of late hemotoxicity. This confirmed that continuous hematological monitoring is required, even in patients with no thiopurine methyltransferase mutations.

Drug–Drug Interactions

Allopurinol

Allopurinol inhibits xanthine oxidase, which is involved in the inactivation of azathioprine and mercaptopurine, and bone marrow suppression is a well-known complication of the concomitant use of allopurinol and azathioprine (SEDA-16, 114) (SEDA-20, 342). A reduction in the dosage of azathioprine or mercaptopurine by at least two-thirds and careful hematological monitoring during the first weeks of the combination has been proposed if combined use with allopurinol is required. However, compliance with these above guidelines was observed in only 58% of 24 patients with heart or lung transplants (100). In addition, although adequate azathioprine dosage reduction reduces the incidence of cytopenias, the risk persists even after the first month of the combination.

Because of the possible risks of reduced immunosuppression if the dose of azathioprine is reduced when allopurinol is given, cyclic urate oxidase can be given instead, as has been shown in six hyperuricemic transplant patients treated with azathioprine (101).

Aminosalicylates

In vitro studies have suggested that sulfasalazine and other aminosalicylates can inhibit TPMT activity, predisposing to an increased risk of bone marrow suppression in patients taking azathioprine or mercaptopurine. This was not clinically substantiated until an extensively investigated case was reported of leukopenia and anemia in a patient treated with both olsalazine and mercaptopurine (SEDA-21, 382). A further inhibiting effect of olsalazine was suggested in this patient, who had a relatively low baseline TPMT activity.

In 16 patients with Crohn's disease taking a stable dose of azathioprine, plus sulfasalazine or mesalazine, mean 6-thioguanine nucleotide concentrations fell significantly over 3 months; withdrawal of the aminosalicylates had no effect on the clinical and biological evolution of Crohn's disease in these patients (102).

Coumarin anticoagulants

Azathioprine or mercaptopurine have been sometimes involved in reduced warfarin and acenocoumarol activity, and increased warfarin dosages may be necessary (103). Similar findings were found in a patient taking maintenance phenprocoumon (SEDA-21, 382).

- Two patients required an approximate three-fold increase in the weekly anticoagulant dosage while taking azathioprine or mercaptopurine (104,105).

A pharmacokinetic interaction is the most likely cause, but the mechanism (impaired absorption or enhanced anticoagulant metabolism) is unknown.

Isotretinoin

The combination of isotretinoin and azathioprine was reported to have a synergistic effect on the occurrence of curly hair in three transplant patients with ciclosporin-induced acne (SEDA-20, 342).

Methotrexate

In 43 patients with rheumatoid arthritis, methotrexate was thought to have increased the risk of the azathioprine-induced hypersensitivity syndrome (106).

References

1. Savolainen HA, Kautiainen H, Isomaki H, Aho K, Verronen P. Azathioprine in patients with juvenile chronic arthritis: a longterm followup study. J Rheumatol 1997;24(12):2444–50.

2. Kirschner BS. Safety of azathioprine and 6-mercaptopurine in pediatric patients with inflammatory bowel disease. Gastroenterology 1998;115(4):813–21.

3. Pearson DC, May GR, Fick GH, Sutherland LR. Azathioprine and 6-mercaptopurine in Crohn disease. A meta-analysis. Ann Intern Med 1995;123(2):132–42.

4. Bouhnik Y, Lemann M, Mary JY, Scemama G, Tai R, Matuchansky C, Modigliani R, Rambaud JC. Long-term follow-up of patients with Crohn's disease treated with azathioprine or 6-mercaptopurine. Lancet 1996;347(8996): 215–19.

5. Sandborn WJ. A review of immune modifier therapy for inflammatory bowel disease: azathioprine, 6-mercaptopurine, cyclosporine, and methotrexate. Am J Gastroenterol 1996;91(3):423–33.

6. Hollander AAMJ, Van der Woude FJ. Efficacy and tolerability of conversion from cyclosporin to azathioprine after

kidney transplantation. A review of the evidence. BioDrugs 1998;9:197–210.

7. Saway PA, Heck LW, Bonner JR, Kirklin JK. Azathioprine hypersensitivity. Case report and review of the literature. Am J Med 1988;84(5):960–4.

8. Parnham AP, Dittmer I, Mathieson PW, McIver A, Dudley C. Acute allergic reactions associated with azathioprine. Lancet 1996;348(9026):542–3.

9. Perreaux F, Zenaty D, Capron F, Trioche P, Odievre M, Labrune P. Azathioprine-induced lung toxicity and efficacy of cyclosporin A in a young girl with type 2 autoimmune hepatitis. J Pediatr Gastroenterol Nutr 2000;31(2):190–2.

10. Jungling AS, Shangraw RE. Massive airway edema after azathioprine. Anesthesiology 2000;92(3):888–90.

11. Connell WR, Kamm MA, Ritchie JK, Lennard-Jones JE. Bone marrow toxicity caused by azathioprine in inflammatory bowel disease: 27 years of experience. Gut 1993;34(8):1081–5.

12. Cunliffe RN, Scott BB. Review article: monitoring for drug side-effects in inflammatory bowel disease. Aliment Pharmacol Ther 2002;16(4):647–62.

13. Amenabar JJ, Gomez-Ullate P, Garcia-Lopez FJ, Aurrecoechea B, Garcia-Erauzkin G, Lampreabe I. A randomized trial comparing cyclosporine and steroids with cyclosporine, azathioprine, and steroids in cadaveric renal transplantation. Transplantation 1998;65(5):653–61.

14. Creemers GJ, van Boven WP, Lowenberg B, van der Heul C. Azathioprine-associated pure red cell aplasia. J Intern Med 1993;233(1):85–7.

15. Pruijt JF, Haanen JB, Hollander AA, den Ottolander GJ. Azathioprine-induced pure red-cell aplasia. Nephrol Dial Transplant 1996;11(7):1371–3.

16. Higashida K, Kobayashi K, Sugita K, Karakida N, Nakagomi Y, Sawanobori E, Sata Y, Aihara M, Amemiya S, Nakazawa S. Pure red blood cell aplasia during azathioprine therapy associated with parvovirus B19 infection. Pediatr Infect Dis J 1997;16(11):1093–5.

17. Pujol M, Fernandez F, Sancho JM, Ribera JM, Milla F, Feliu E. Immune hemolytic anemia induced by 6-mercaptopurine. Transfusion 2000;40(1):75–6.

18. Sudhir RR, Rao SK, Shanmugam MP, Padmanabhan P. Bilateral macular hemorrhage caused by azathioprine-induced aplastic anemia in a corneal graft recipient. Cornea 2002;21(7):712–14.

19. Santiago M. Diarrhoea secondary to azathioprine in two patients with SLE. Lupus 1999;8(7):565.

20. Marbet U, Schmid I. Severe life-threatening diarrhea caused by azathioprine but not by 6-mercaptopurine. Digestion 2001;63(2):139–42.

21. Kowdley KV, Keeffe EB. Hepatotoxicity of transplant immunosuppressive agents. Gastroenterol Clin North Am 1995;24(4):991–1001.

22. Pol S, Cavalcanti R, Carnot F, Legendre C, Driss F, Chaix ML, Thervet E, Chkoff N, Brechot C, Berthelot P, Kreis H. Azathioprine hepatitis in kidney transplant recipients. A predisposing role of chronic viral hepatitis. Transplantation 1996;61(12):1774–6.

23. Wagoner LE, Olsen SL, Bristow MR, O'Connell JB, Taylor DO, Lappe DL, Renlund DG. Cyclophosphamide as an alternative to azathioprine in cardiac transplant recipients with suspected azathioprine-induced hepatotoxicity. Transplantation 1993;56(6):1415–18.

24. Ramalho HJ, Terra EG, Cartapatti E, Barberato JB, Alves VA, Gayotto LC, Abbud-Filho M. Hepatotoxicity of azathioprine in renal transplant recipients. Transplant Proc 1989;21(1 Pt 2):1716–17.

25. Horsmans Y, Rahier J, Geubel AP. Reversible cholestasis with bile duct injury following azathioprine therapy. A case report. Liver 1991;11(2):89–93.

26. Read AE, Wiesner RH, LaBrecque DR, Tifft JG, Mullen KD, Sheer RL, Petrelli M, Ricanati ES, McCullough AJ. Hepatic veno-occlusive disease associated with renal transplantation and azathioprine therapy. Ann Intern Med 1986;104(5):651–5.

27. Azoulay D, Castaing D, Lemoine A, Samuel D, Majno P, Reynes M, Charpentier B, Bismuth H. Successful treatment of severe azathioprine-induced hepatic veno-occlusive disease in a kidney-transplanted patient with transjugular intrahepatic portosystemic shunt. Clin Nephrol 1998;50(2):118–22.

28. Mion F, Cloix P, Boillot O, Gille D, Bouvier R, Paliard P, Berger F. Maladie veino-occlusive après transplantation hépatique. Association d'un rejet aiguë cellulaire et de la toxicité de l'azathioprine. [Veno-occlusive disease after liver transplantation. Association of acute cellular rejection and toxicity of azathioprine.] Gastroenterol Clin Biol 1993;17(11):863–7.

29. Sterneck M, Wiesner R, Ascher N, Roberts J, Ferrell L, Ludwig J, Lake J. Azathioprine hepatotoxicity after liver transplantation. Hepatology 1991;14(5):806–10.

30. Cooper C, Cotton DW, Minihane N, Cawley MI. Azathioprine hypersensitivity manifesting as acute focal hepatocellular necrosis. J R Soc Med 1986;79(3):171–3.

31. Delgado J, Munoz de Bustillo E, Ibarrola C, Colina F, Morales JM, Rodriguez E, Aguado JM, Fuertes A, Gomez MA. Hepatitis C virus-related fibrosing cholestatic hepatitis after cardiac transplantation: is azathioprine a contributory factor? J Heart Lung Transplant 1999;18(6):607–10.

32. David-Neto E, da Fonseca JA, de Paula FJ, Nahas WC, Sabbaga E, Ianhez LE. Is azathioprine harmful to chronic viral hepatitis in renal transplantation? A long-term study on azathioprine withdrawal. Transplant Proc 1999;31(1–2):1149–50.

33. Eaton VS, Casanova JM, Kupa A. Azathioprine hepatotoxicity confirmed by rechallenge. Aust J Hosp Pharm 2000;30:58–9.

34. Muszkat M, Pappo O, Caraco Y, Haviv YS. Hepatocanalicular cholestasis after 24 years of azathioprine administration for myasthenia gravis. Clin Drug Invest 2000;19:75–8.

35. Present DH, Meltzer SJ, Krumholz MP, Wolke A, Korelitz BI. 6-Mercaptopurine in the management of inflammatory bowel disease: short- and long-term toxicity. Ann Intern Med 1989;111(8):641–9.

36. Frick TW, Fryd DS, Goodale RL, Simmons RL, Sutherland DE, Najarian JS. Lack of association between azathioprine and acute pancreatitis in renal transplantation patients. Lancet 1991;337(8735):251–2.

37. Eland IA, van Puijenbroek EP, Sturkenboom MJ, Wilson JH, Stricker BH. Drug-associated acute pancreatitis: twenty-one years of spontaneous reporting in The Netherlands. Am J Gastroenterol 1999;94(9):2417–22.

38. Siwach V, Bansal V, Kumar A, Rao Ch U, Sharma A, Minz M. Post-renal transplant azathioprine-induced pancreatitis. Nephrol Dial Transplant 1999;14(10):2495–8.

39. Bisschop D, Germain ML, Munzer M, Trenque T. Thioguanine, pancréatotoxicité? [Thioguanine, pancreatotoxicity?] Therapie 2001;56(1):67–9.

40. Pillans PI, Tooke AF, Bateman ED, Ainslie GM. Acute polyarthritis associated with azathioprine for interstitial lung disease. Respir Med 1995;89(1):63–4.

41. Bellaiche G, Cosnes J, Nouts A, Ley G, Slama JL. Troubles de la marche secondaires à la prise d'azathioprine chez 2 malades ayant une maladie de Crohn. [Gait disorders secondary to azathioprine treatment in 2 patients with Crohn's disease.] Gastroenterol Clin Biol 1999;23(4):533–4.

42. Stratton JD, Farrington K. Relapse of vasculitis, sepsis, or azathioprine allergy? Nephrol Dial Transplant 1998;13(11):2927–8.

43. Jeurissen ME, Boerbooms AM, van de Putte LB, Kruijsen MW. Azathioprine induced fever, chills, rash, and hepatotoxicity in rheumatoid arthritis. Ann Rheum Dis 1990;49(1):25–7.

44. Meys E, Devogelaer JP, Geubel A, Rahier J, Nagant de Deuxchaisnes C. Fever, hepatitis and acute interstitial nephritis in a patient with rheumatoid arthritis. Concurrent manifestations of azathioprine hypersensitivity. J Rheumatol 1992;19(5):807–9.

45. Jones JJ, Ashworth J. Azathioprine-induced shock in dermatology patients. J Am Acad Dermatol 1993;29(5 Pt 1):795–6.

46. Burden AD, Beck MH. Contact hypersensitivity to azathioprine. Contact Dermatitis 1992;27(5):329–30.

47. Dominguez Ortega J, Robledo T, Martinez-Cocera C, Alonso A, Cimarra M, Chamorro M, Plaza A. Desensitization to azathioprine. J Investig Allergol Clin Immunol 1999;9(5):337–8.

48. Korelitz BI, Zlatanic J, Goel F, Fuller S. Allergic reactions to 6-mercaptopurine during treatment of inflammatory bowel disease. J Clin Gastroenterol 1999;28(4):341–4.

49. Godeau B, Paul M, Autegarden JE, Leynadier F, Astier A, Schaeffer A. Hypersensitivity to azathioprine mimicking gastroenteritis. Absence of recurrence with 6-mercaptopurine. Gastroenterol Clin Biol 1995;19(1):117–19.

50. Garcia VD, Keitel E, Almeida P, Santos AF, Becker M, Goldani JC. Morbidity after renal transplantation: role of bacterial infection. Transplant Proc 1995;27(2):1825–6.

51. Wade JJ, Rolando N, Hayllar K, Philpott-Howard J, Casewell MW, Williams R. Bacterial and fungal infections after liver transplantation: an analysis of 284 patients. Hepatology 1995;21(5):1328–36.

52. Singh N, Yu VL. Infections in organ transplant recipients. Curr Opin Infect Dis 1996;9:223–9.

53. Reis MA, Costa RS, Ferraz AS. Causes of death in renal transplant recipients: a study of 102 autopsies from 1968 to 1991. J R Soc Med 1995;88(1):24–7.

54. Korelitz BI, Fuller SR, Warman JI, Goldberg MD. Shingles during the course of treatment with 6-mercaptopurine for inflammatory bowel disease. Am J Gastroenterol 1999;94(2):424–6.

55. Posthuma EF, Westendorp RG, van der Sluys Veer A, Kluin-Nelemans JC, Kluin PM, Lamers CB. Fatal infectious mononucleosis: a severe complication in the treatment of Crohn's disease with azathioprine. Gut 1995;36(2):311–13.

56. Suassuna JH, Machado RD, Sampaio JC, Leite LL, Villela LH, Ruzany F, Souza ER, Moraes JR. Active cytomegalovirus infection in hemodialysis patients receiving donor-specific blood transfusions under azathioprine coverage. Transplantation 1993;56(6):1552–4.

57. Penn I. Tumors after renal and cardiac transplantation. Hematol Oncol Clin North Am 1993;7(2):431–45.

58. Gaya SB, Rees AJ, Lechler RI, Williams G, Mason PD. Malignant disease in patients with long-term renal transplants. Transplantation 1995;59(12):1705–9.

59. London NJ, Farmery SM, Will EJ, Davison AM, Lodge JP. Risk of neoplasia in renal transplant patients. Lancet 1995;346(8972):403–6.

60. Kehinde EO, Petermann A, Morgan JD, Butt ZA, Donnelly PK, Veitch PS, Bell PR. Triple therapy and incidence of de novo cancer in renal transplant recipients. Br J Surg 1994;81(7):985–6.

61. Opelz G, Henderson R. Incidence of non-Hodgkin lymphoma in kidney and heart transplant recipients. Lancet 1993;342(8886–8887):1514–16.

62. Gruber SA, Gillingham K, Sothern RB, Stephanian E, Matas AJ, Dunn DL. De novo cancer in cyclosporine-treated and non-cyclosporine-treated adult primary renal allograft recipients. Clin Transplant 1994;8(4):388–95.

63. Hiesse C, Kriaa F, Rieu P, Larue JR, Benoit G, Bellamy J, Blanchet P, Charpentier B. Incidence and type of malignancies occurring after renal transplantation in conventionally and cyclosporine-treated recipients: analysis of a 20-year period in 1600 patients. Transplant Proc 1995;27(1):972–4.

64. Pitt PI, Sultan AH, Malone M, Andrews V, Hamilton EB. Association between azathioprine therapy and lymphoma in rheumatoid disease. J R Soc Med 1987;80(7):428–9.

65. Barthelmes L, Thomas KJ, Seale JR. Prostatic involvement of a testicular lymphoma in a patient with myasthenia gravis on long-term azathioprine. Leuk Lymphoma 2002;43(12):2425–6.

66. Taylor AE, Shuster S. Skin cancer after renal transplantation: the causal role of azathioprine. Acta Dermatol Venereol 1992;72(2):115–19.

67. Silman AJ, Petrie J, Hazleman B, Evans SJ. Lymphoproliferative cancer and other malignancy in patients with rheumatoid arthritis treated with azathioprine: a 20 year follow up study. Ann Rheum Dis 1988;47(12):988–92.

68. Jones M, Symmons D, Finn J, Wolfe F. Does exposure to immunosuppressive therapy increase the 10 year malignancy and mortality risks in rheumatoid arthritis? A matched cohort study. Br J Rheumatol 1996;35(8):738–45.

69. Connell WR, Kamm MA, Dickson M, Balkwill AM, Ritchie JK, Lennard-Jones JE. Long-term neoplasia risk after azathioprine treatment in inflammatory bowel disease. Lancet 1994;343(8908):1249–52.

70. Fraser AG, Orchard TR, Robinson EM, Jewell DP. Long-term risk of malignancy after treatment of inflammatory bowel disease with azathioprine. Aliment Pharmacol Ther 2002;16(7):1225–32.

71. Confavreux C, Saddier P, Grimaud J, Moreau T, Adeleine P, Aimard G. Risk of cancer from azathioprine therapy in multiple sclerosis: a case-control study. Neurology 1996;46(6):1607–12.

72. Penn I. Cancers in cyclosporine-treated vs azathioprine-treated patients. Transplant Proc 1996;28(2):876–8.

73. Bo J, Schroder H, Kristinsson J, Madsen B, Szumlanski C, Weinshilboum R, Andersen JB, Schmiegelow K. Possible carcinogenic effect of 6-mercaptopurine on bone marrow stem cells: relation to thiopurine metabolism. Cancer 1999;86(6):1080–6.

74. Korelitz BI, Mirsky FJ, Fleisher MR, Warman JI, Wisch N, Gleim GW. Malignant neoplasms subsequent to treatment of inflammatory bowel disease with 6-mercaptopurine. Am J Gastroenterol 1999;94(11):3248–53.

75. Ramsey-Goldman R, Schilling E. Immunosuppressive drug use during pregnancy. Rheum Dis Clin North Am 1997;23(1):149–67.

76. Armenti VT, Moritz MJ, Davison JM. Drug safety issues in pregnancy following transplantation and immunosuppression: effects and outcomes. Drug Saf 1998;19(3):219–32.

77. Cararach V, Carmona F, Monleon FJ, Andreu J. Pregnancy after renal transplantation: 25 years experience in Spain. Br J Obstet Gynaecol 1993;100(2):122–5.

78. Armenti VT, Ahlswede BA, Moritz MJ, Jarrell BE. National Transplantation Pregnancy Registry: analysis of pregnancy outcomes of female kidney recipients with relation to time interval from transplant to conception. Transplant Proc 1993;25(1 Pt 2):1036–7.

79. Pilarski LM, Yacyshyn BR, Lazarovits AI. Analysis of peripheral blood lymphocyte populations and immune function from children exposed to cyclosporine or to azathioprine in utero. Transplantation 1994;57(1):133–44.

80. Polifka JE, Friedman JM. Teratogen update: azathioprine and 6-mercaptopurine. Teratology 2002;65(5):240–61.

81. Rajapakse RO, Korelitz BI, Zlatanic J, Baiocco PJ, Gleim GW. Outcome of pregnancies when fathers are treated with 6-mercaptopurine for inflammatory bowel disease. Am J Gastroenterol 2000;95(3):684–8.

82. Cissoko H, Jonville-Bera AP, Lenain H, Riviere MF, Saugier J, Casanova JL, Autret-Leca E. Agranulocytose et déficit immunitaire transitoires après expostition fœtale à l'azathioprine et mésalazine. [Agranulocytosis and transitory immune deficiency after fetal exposure to azathioprine and mesalazine.] Arch Pediatr 1999;6(10):1136–7.

83. Cuffari C, Hunt S, Bayless T. Utilisation of erythrocyte 6-thioguanine metabolite levels to optimise azathioprine therapy in patients with inflammatory bowel disease. Gut 2001;48(5):642–6.

84. Bergan S. Optimisation of azathioprine immunosuppression after organ transplantation by pharmacological measurements. BioDrugs 1997;8:446–56.

85. Meggitt SJ, Reynolds NJ. Azathioprine for atopic dermatitis. Clin Exp Dermatol 2001;26(5):369–75.

86. Schutz E, Gummert J, Mohr FW, Armstrong VW, Oellerich M. Azathioprine myelotoxicity related to elevated 6-thioguanine nucleotides in heart transplantation. Transplant Proc 1995;27(1):1298–300.

87. Kerstens PJ, Stolk JN, De Abreu RA, Lambooy LH, van de Putte LB, Boerbooms AA. Azathioprine-related bone marrow toxicity and low activities of purine enzymes in patients with rheumatoid arthritis. Arthritis Rheum 1995;38(1):142–5.

88. Boulieu R, Lenoir A, Bertocchi M, Mornex JF. Intracellular thiopurine nucleotides and azathioprine myelotoxicity in organ transplant patients. Br J Clin Pharmacol 1997;43(1):116–18.

89. Soria-Royer C, Legendre C, Mircheva J, Premel S, Beaune P, Kreis H. Thiopurine-methyl-transferase activity to assess azathioprine myelotoxicity in renal transplant recipients. Lancet 1993;341(8860):1593–4.

90. Serre-Debeauvais F, Bayle F, Amirou M, Bechtel Y, Boujet C, Vialtel P, Bessard G. Hématotoxicité de l'azathioprine à déterminisme génétique aggravé par un déficit en xanthine oxyase chez une transplantée rénale. [Hematotoxicity caused by azathioprine genetically determined and aggravated by xanthine oxidase deficiency in a patient following renal transplantation.] Presse Méd 1995;24(21):987–8.

91. Ansari A, Hassan C, Duley J, Marinaki A, Shobowale-Bakre EM, Seed P, Meenan J, Yim A, Sanderson J. Thiopurine methyltransferase activity and the use of azathioprine in inflammatory bowel disease. Aliment Pharmacol Ther 2002;16(10):1743–50.

92. Holme SA, Duley JA, Sanderson J, Routledge PA, Anstey AV. Erythrocyte thiopurine methyl transferase assessment prior to azathioprine use in the UK. QJM 2002;95(7):439–44.

93. Naughton MA, Battaglia E, O'Brien S, Walport MJ, Botto M. Identification of thiopurine methyltransferase (TPMT) polymorphisms cannot predict myelosuppression in systemic lupus erythematosus patients taking azathioprine. Rheumatology (Oxford) 1999;38(7):640–4.

94. Stolk JN, Boerbooms AM, de Abreu RA, de Koning DG, van Beusekom HJ, Muller WH, van de Putte LB. Reduced thiopurine methyltransferase activity and development of side effects of azathioprine treatment in patients with rheumatoid arthritis. Arthritis Rheum 1998;41(10):1858–66.

95. Black AJ, McLeod HL, Capell HA, Powrie RH, Matowe LK, Pritchard SC, Collie-Duguid ES, Reid DM. Thiopurine methyltransferase genotype predicts therapy-limiting severe toxicity from azathioprine. Ann Intern Med 1998;129(9):716–18.

96. Dervieux T, Medard Y, Baudouin V, Maisin A, Zhang D, Broly F, Loirat C, Jacqz-Aigrain E. Thiopurine methyltransferase activity and its relationship to the occurrence of rejection episodes in paediatric renal transplant recipients treated with azathioprine. Br J Clin Pharmacol 1999;48(6):793–800.

97. Relling MV, Hancock ML, Rivera GK, Sandlund JT, Ribeiro RC, Krynetski EY, Pui CH, Evans WE. Mercaptopurine therapy intolerance and heterozygosity at the thiopurine S-methyltransferase gene locus. J Natl Cancer Inst 1999;91(23):2001–8.

98. Sebbag L, Boucher P, Davelu P, Boissonnat P, Champsaur G, Ninet J, Dureau G, Obadia JF, Vallon JJ, Delaye J. Thiopurine S-methyltransferase gene polymorphism is predictive of azathioprine-induced myelosuppression in heart transplant recipients. Transplantation 2000;69(7):1524–7.

99. Colombel JF, Ferrari N, Debuysere H, Marteau P, Gendre JP, Bonaz B, Soule JC, Modigliani R, Touze Y, Catala P, Libersa C, Broly F. Genotypic analysis of thiopurine S-methyltransferase in patients with Crohn's disease and severe myelosuppression during azathioprine therapy. Gastroenterology 2000;118(6):1025–30.

100. Cummins D, Sekar M, Halil O, Banner N. Myelosuppression associated with azathioprine–allopurinol interaction after heart and lung transplantation. Transplantation 1996;61(11):1661–2.

101. Ippoliti G, Negri M, Campana C, Vigano M. Urate oxidase in hyperuricemic heart transplant recipients treated with azathioprine. Transplantation 1997;63(9):1370–1.

102. Dewit O, Vanheuverzwyn R, Desager JP, Horsmans Y. Interaction between azathioprine and aminosalicylates: an in vivo study in patients with Crohn's disease. Aliment Pharmacol Ther 2002;16(1):79–85.

103. Singleton JD, Conyers L. Warfarin and azathioprine: an important drug interaction. Am J Med 1992;92(2):217.

104. Fernandez MA, Regadera A, Aznar J. Acenocoumarol and 6-mercaptopurine: an important drug interaction. Haematologica 1999;84(7):664–5.

105. Rotenberg M, Levy Y, Shoenfeld Y, Almog S, Ezra D. Effect of azathioprine on the anticoagulant activity of warfarin. Ann Pharmacother 2000;34(1):120–2.

106. Blanco R, Martinez-Taboada VM, Gonzalez-Gay MA, Armona J, Fernandez-Sueiro JL, Gonzalez-Vela MC, Rodriguez-Valverde V. Acute febrile toxic reaction in patients with refractory rheumatoid arthritis who are receiving combined therapy with methotrexate and azathioprine. Arthritis Rheum 1996;39(6):1016–20.

Azelastine

See also Antihistamines

General Information

Azelastine is a second-generation antihistamine, a phthalazinone compound with antiallergic and bronchodilator properties (SEDA-12, 375) (SEDA-15, 155) (SEDA-17, 199) (SEDA-18, 182, 184) (SEDA-19, 171–172) (SEDA-20, 162) (SEDA-21, 172) (SEDA-22, 178). It is available as a nasal spray and in oral form for the treatment of allergic rhinitis and asthma as well as dermatoses. It reduces rhinorrhea, sneezing, and nasal congestion. Azelastine is effective against exercise-induced asthma and allergen challenge in patients with extrinsic asthma. It can inhibit histamine release from mast cells and inhibit histamine- and leukotriene-mediated bronchospasm (1).

Comparative studies

There have been three double-blind, randomized, parallel-group comparisons of the effects of azelastine nasal spray (1.1 mg/day) with combined treatment with oral loratadine (10 mg/day) and budesonide nasal spray (336 µg/day) in 1070 patients with allergic rhinitis unresponsive to monotherapy (2). The primary outcome measure was the percentage of patients who needed additional therapy for rhinitis after 7 days of treatment, and this was 32–46% across the three studies, with no significant difference between the two treatment groups. The most common adverse event with azelastine was a transient after-taste (8% compared with 1% in the combined group) and the most common adverse event for combined treatment was headache (6% compared with 5% in the azelastine group). Rhinitis and somnolence were the other commonly reported adverse events, in 3 and 2% with azelastine, and 1 and 1% in the combined group. The authors concluded that monotherapy with azelastine is as effective and as well tolerated as combination therapy in improving symptoms in moderate to severe allergic rhinitis, and this seems to be a reasonable claim.

Azelastine has been compared with the potent antihistamine cetirizine in the treatment of pruritic dermatoses. Taste disturbance occurred in 9.7% of patients taking azelastine and headaches in 10.4% of patients taking cetirizine (3).

Similar complaints regarding taste or smell were noted in some patients when azelastine nasal spray was used alongside budesonide (4) or ebastine (5) in allergic rhinitis in equieffective doses.

General adverse effects

In controlled studies, azelastine nasal spray produced a high incidence of itching and burning of the nasal mucosa together with taste disturbance and sometimes unpleasant smell. Sedation does not seem to be frequent; in most studies, the frequency of fatigue and drowsiness was not significantly different from placebo. In an open trial in which 119 patients with various types of pruritic dermatoses were treated with oral azelastine, 27 patients reported mild adverse effects such as drowsiness (15 cases, 12.5%) and a bitter after-taste (six cases, 5%). In four patients the treatment was withdrawn because of adverse effects (SEDA-15, 2).

Organs and Systems

Sensory systems

There have been several reports of a bitter taste associated with azelastine nasal spray for the treatment of allergic and non-allergic rhinitis compared with placebo in adults and children (6–8). Azelastine has also been reported to alter taste perception for several hours after ingestion (9).

Azelastine eye drops (0.025 and 0.05%) can produce slight reactions at the site of application and a bitter or unpleasant taste (10).

References

1. Kemp JP, Meltzer EO, Orgel HA, Welch MJ, Bucholtz GA, Middleton E Jr, Spector SL, Newton JJ, Perhach JL Jr. A dose-response study of the bronchodilator action of azelastine in asthma. J Allergy Clin Immunol 1987;79(6):893–9.
2. Berger WE, Fineman SM, Lieberman P, Miles RM. Double-blind trials of azelastine nasal spray monotherapy versus combination therapy with loratadine tablets and beclomethasone nasal spray in patients with seasonal allergic rhinitis. Rhinitis Study Groups. Ann Allergy Asthma Immunol 1999;82(6):535–41.
3. Henz BM, Metzenauer P, O'Keefe E, Zuberbier T. Differential effects of new-generation H$_1$-receptor antagonists in pruritic dermatoses. Allergy 1998;53(2):180–3.
4. Gastpar H, Aurich R, Petzold U, Dorow P, Enzmann H, Gering R, Kochy HP, Philippe A, Renz W, Wendenburg G. Intranasal treatment of perennial allergic rhinitis. Comparison of azelastine nasal spray and budesonide nasal aerosol. Arzneimittelforschung 1993;43(4):475–9.
5. Antepara I, Jauregui I, Basomba A, Cadahia A, Feo F, Garcia JJ, Gonzalo MA, Luna I, Rubio M, Vazquez M. Investigacion de la eficacia y tolerabilidad de azelastina spray nasal versus ebastina comprimidos en pacientes con rinitis alergica estacional. [Investigation of the efficacy and tolerability of azelastine nasal spray versus ebastine tablets in patients with seasonal allergic rhinitis.] Allergol Immunopathol (Madr) 1998;26(1):9–16.
6. Duarte C, Baehre M, Gharakhanian S, Leynadier F; French Azelastine Study Group. Treatment of severe seasonal rhinoconjunctivitis by a combination of azelastine nasal spray and eye drops: a double-blind, double-placebo study. J Investig Allergol Clin Immunol 2001;11(1):34–40.
7. Banov CH, Lieberman P; Vasomotor Rhinitis Study Groups. Efficacy of azelastine nasal spray in the treatment of vasomotor (perennial nonallergic) rhinitis. Ann Allergy Asthma Immunol 2001;86(1):28–35.
8. Fineman SM. Clinical experience with azelastine nasal spray in children: physician survey of case reports. Pediatr Asthma Allergy Immunol 2001;15:49–54.
9. Weiss SR, McFarland BH, Burkhart GA, Ho PT. Cancer recurrences and secondary primary cancers after use of antihistamines or antidepressants. Clin Pharmacol Ther 1998;63(5):594–9.
10. Giede-Tuch C, Westhoff M, Zarth A. Azelastine eye-drops in seasonal allergic conjunctivitis or rhinoconjunctivitis. A double-blind, randomized, placebo-controlled study. Allergy 1998;53(9):857–62.

Azipranone

General Information

Azipranone is a cough suppressant claimed to have effects comparable to those of codeine (1). Limited evidence suggests that its adverse effects are no different from those of placebo (SEDA-9, 157).

Reference

1. Yanaura S, Fujikura H, Hosokawa T, Kitagawa H, Kamei J, Misawa M. Antitussive effect of RU-20201–central and peripheral actions. Jpn J Pharmacol 1984;34(3):289–98.

Azithromycin

See also Macrolide antibiotics

General Information

Observational studies

In 3995 patients who took azithromycin 1.5 g in divided doses over 5 days or who took 1 g as a single dose for urethritis/cervicitis adverse events occurred in 12% (1). In patients over 65 years the rate was 9.3%, and in children under 14 years of age it was 5.4%. The most common adverse effects were gastrointestinal (9.6%); central nervous system and peripheral nervous system effects were reported in 1.3%. Overall, 59% of the adverse events were considered mild, 34% moderate, and only 6% severe, involving mainly the gastrointestinal tract. Adverse events resulted in withdrawal in 0.7% of patients, lower than the rate reported with other macrolides. Treatment-related rises in liver enzymes were uncommon (under 2%), as was leukopenia (1.1–1.5%).

Phase II/III clinical trials in the USA have yielded data on 1928 children aged 6 months to 15 years who took azithromycin for infections that included acute otitis media ($n = 1150$) and streptococcal pharyngitis ($n = 754$) (2). Most took a 5-day course of azithromycin (5–12 mg/kg/day). There were adverse effects in 190 patients (9.9%): diarrhea (3.1%), vomiting (2.5%), abdominal pain (1.9%), loose stools (1%), and rash (2.5%). In three comparisons with co-amoxiclav, the overall incidence of adverse effects was significantly lower with azithromycin (7.7 versus 29%), with withdrawal rates of 0.3 versus 3.6%. However, the incidence of adverse effects was significantly greater with azithromycin than with penicillin V in comparisons in patients with streptococcal pharyngitis (13 versus 6.7%). In conclusion, it appears that the safety and tolerability of azithromycin is similar in children and adults.

In an open study, children with end-stage lung disease or chronic airflow limitation unresponsive to conventional therapy were treated with long-term azithromycin. Seven children (mean age 12 years), all of whom were colonized with *Pseudomonas aeruginosa* and who took azithromycin for more than 3 months, were studied. There was a significant improvement in FVC and FEV_1 (3). The mechanism whereby azithromycin works is unknown, but it may be other than antibacterial. It has been hypothesized that the effect may be due to upregulation of a P glycoprotein, a member of the family of multidrug resistant proteins, since erythromycin upregulates P glycoprotein expression in a monkey model. Multidrug resistance (MDR) is homologous to CFTR, and previous in vitro experiments have shown that the MDR and CFTR genes can complement each other (4). However, direct proof of this hypothesis is lacking at the moment.

Of 42 adult HIV-positive patients with confirmed or presumed acute toxoplasmic encephalitis who received azithromycin 900, 1200, or 1500 mg/day plus pyrimethamine, 28 responded to therapy during the induction period (5). Six patients withdrew during the induction period because of reversible toxic effects (three with raised liver enzymes, two with hearing loss, one with neutropenia). Treatment-terminating adverse events occurred most often among the patients who took 1500 mg/day.

In an open, prospective trial gingival hyperplasia due to ciclosporin was successfully treated with azithromycin 250 mg/day for 5 days in 30 of 35 patients, who reported esthetic satisfaction and disappearance of bleeding and pain (6). There was no change in ciclosporin concentration or renal function after azithromycin.

Comparative studies

The tolerability of azithromycin oral suspension, 10 mg/kg od for 3 days, has been assessed in children in a review of 16 multicenter studies (7). Of 2425 patients, 1213 received azithromycin and 1212 received other drugs. The incidence of treatment-related adverse events was significantly lower in those who took azithromycin, while withdrawal rates were similar. There were significantly fewer gastrointestinal events with azithromycin and their duration was significantly shorter.

Co-amoxiclav

In a multicenter, parallel-group, double-blind trial in 420 evaluable patients aged 6 months to 16 years with community-acquired pneumonia, the therapeutic effect of azithromycin (once-daily for 5 days) was similar to that of co-amoxiclav in children under 5 years and to that of erythromycin tds for 10 days. Treatment-related adverse events occurred in 11% of those given azithromycin and 31% in the comparator group (8).

Azithromycin (500 mg/day for 3 days) has been used to treat acute periapical abscesses (9). Of 150 patients treated with azithromycin 18 reported a total of 26 adverse events. Slightly more (24 out of 153) treated with co-amoxiclav reported 34 adverse events, but this difference did not reach statistical significance. Most of the adverse events (44/60) were gastrointestinal, mostly diarrhea or abdominal pain. There were no significant differences between the two groups in the severity of adverse events or in the number of withdrawals because of adverse events.

Fluoroquinolones

In a multicenter, open, randomized comparison of levofloxacin 500 mg/day orally or intravenously and azithromycin 500 mg/day intravenously for up to 2 days plus ceftriaxone 1 g/day intravenously for 2 days in 236 patients, the most common drug-related adverse events in those given azithromycin were diarrhea (4.2%), vein disorders (2.5%), and pruritus (1.7%) (10).

Other macrolides

The incidence of disseminated MAC infection has increased dramatically with the AIDS epidemic. Treatment regimens for patients with a positive culture for MAC from a sterile site should include two or more drugs, including clarithromycin. Prophylaxis against disseminated MAC should be considered for patients with a CD4 cell count of less than $50 \times 10^6/l$ (11). In a randomized, open trial in 37 patients with HIV-associated disseminated MAC infection, treatment with clarithromycin + ethambutol produced more rapid resolution of bacteremia, and was more effective at sterilization of blood cultures after 16 weeks than azithromycin + ethambutol (12).

Tetracyclines

Compared with tetracycline, azithromycin had a favorable short-term effect on childhood morbidity in a mass trial for trachoma in rural Gambian villages, and adverse effects were limited (13).

Treatment of facial comedonic and papulopustular acne with azithromycin (500 mg/day for 4 days in four cycles every 10 days) may be at least as effective as minocycline (100 mg/day for 6 weeks). Both were well tolerated and mild adverse effects were reported in 10% of patients given azithromycin and 12% of those given minocycline (14).

Placebo-controlled studies

In 169 patients with acute infective rhinitis, azithromycin (500 mg/day for 3 days) resulted in a better cure rate after 11 days than placebo; however, after 25 days the results for both improvement and cure were equal (15).

In a randomized, double-blind, placebo-controlled multicenter trial in 174 HIV-infected patients with CD4 cell counts of under 100×10^6/l, azithromycin (1200 mg once a week) was safe and effective in preventing disseminated MAC infection, death due to MAC infection, and respiratory tract infections (16).

In a triple-masked, randomized, placebo-controlled study in 1867 women, prophylaxis with azithromycin 500 mg 1 hour before IUCD insertion did not affect the rate of IUCD removal, the frequency of medical attention after insertion, or the risk of upper genital tract infection at 90 days (17). Women were at low risk of sexually transmitted disease according to self-reported medical history. Gastrointestinal adverse effects were infrequent (3% azithromycin; 2% placebo). Fewer women taking azithromycin (0.7%) than those taking placebo (1.3%) were treated with antibiotics for pelvic tenderness; however, this difference was not statistically significant. Since cervical infections increase the risk of pelvic infection in women who use IUCDs, generalization of these results may be difficult (18).

In a meta-analysis of randomized, controlled trials of 3–5 days of azithromycin or other antibiotics that are typically given in longer courses for upper respiratory tract infections, there were no significant differences in bacteriological outcomes (19). Azithromycin was withdrawn because of adverse events in only 37 (0.8%) of 4870 patients.

Organs and Systems

Cardiovascular

Torsade de pointes and cardiorespiratory arrest have been reported in a patient with congenital long QT syndrome who took azithromycin (20). In a prospective study of 47 previously healthy people, there was a modest statistically insignificant prolongation of the QT_c interval without clinical consequences after the end of a course of azithromycin 3 g/day for 5 days (21).

Sensory systems

Ears

Azithromycin can cause ototoxicity. In one study, 8 (17%) of 46 HIV-positive patients had probable ($n = 6$) or possible ($n = 2$) ototoxicity with azithromycin (22). The effects were

hearing loss (88%), tinnitus (37%), plugged ears (37%), and vertigo (25%), developing at a mean of 7.6 weeks (1.5–20 weeks) after the start of long-term azithromycin therapy for *Mycobacterium avium* infection. The symptoms resolved in a mean of 4.9 weeks (2–11 weeks) after withdrawal.

Sensorineural hearing loss has been attributed to azithromycin (23).

- A 35-year old Caucasian man with AIDS and multiple opportunistic infections, including *Mycobacterium kansasii* and *Mycobacterium avium* complex (MAC) disease developed moderate to severe primary sensorineural hearing loss after 4–5 months of therapy with oral azithromycin 500 mg/day. Other medications included ethambutol, isoniazid, rifabutin, ciprofloxacin, co-trimoxazole, fluconazole, zidovudine (later switched to stavudine), lamivudine, indinavir, methadone, modified-release oral morphine, pseudoephedrine, diphenhydramine, megestrol acetate, trazodone, sorbitol, salbutamol by metered-dose inhaler and nebulizer, ipratropium, and oral morphine solution as needed. Significant improvement of the hearing impairment was documented 3 weeks after drug withdrawal.

A literature review identified several cases of ototoxicity in HIV-positive patients treated with azithromycin for *M. avium* complex infection. In four series, 14–41% of such patients had some degree of hearing loss. However, some patients were also taking other potentially ototoxic drugs, which may have contributed to the high frequency of hearing loss reported. Hearing loss improved markedly after withdrawal of azithromycin. Hearing loss may be more common and probably more severe with high-dose azithromycin than with high-dose clarithromycin.

- A 47-year-old woman who had a left lung transplantation 3 months earlier and who was taking ticarcillin + -clavulanate and aztreonam for sinusitis, was given co-trimoxazole, ticarcillin + clavulanate, azithromycin (500 mg/day intravenously), and ganciclovir for presumed pneumonia (24). Other drugs included tacrolimus, mycophenolate, prednisone, lansoprazole, diltiazem, itraconazole, warfarin, alendronate, ipratropium bromide, folic acid, and nystatin. The next day, rimantadine and vancomycin were added, and co-trimoxazole was reduced. A neurological examination to assess symptoms of peripheral neuropathy noted no hearing deficit. On day 3, vancomycin, ticarcillin + -clavulanate, and ganciclovir were withdrawn. On the fifth day, mild tinnitus and reduced hearing developed and gradually progressed to complete deafness. After eight doses, azithromycin was withdrawn, and 20 days later her hearing was back to baseline.

Low-dose exposure to azithromycin has been associated with irreversible sensorineural hearing loss in otherwise healthy subjects (25). Even a single oral dose of azithromycin altered the conjunctival bacterial flora of children from a trachoma endemic area (26). However, the clinical significance is not yet clear.

Psychological, psychiatric

Azithromycin can cause delirium (27).

Hematologic

The effects of combining azithromycin and rifabutin have been studied in 50 subjects with or without HIV infection, of whom 19 took azithromycin 1200 mg/day and rifabutin 600 mg/day, and 31 took azithromycin 600 mg/day and rifabutin 300 mg/day (28). Neutropenia was the most common adverse event, in 33 of 50 subjects. Low-grade nausea, diarrhea, fatigue, and headache were also common, and most subjects had more than one type of event. There was no significant pharmacokinetic interaction between the two drugs.

Gastrointestinal

In a review of 12 clinical studies most of the adverse events in those taking azithromycin affected the gastrointestinal system, and were reported in 138 (8.5%) azithromycin-treated patients (29). Abdominal pain, diarrhea, nausea, and vomiting were the most frequently reported gastrointestinal adverse events.

Gastrointestinal symptoms were the most common adverse effects reported in a trial of azithromycin in disseminated *Mycobacterium avium* complex in 62 patients with AIDS (30). Erythromycin is a motilin receptor agonist (31–33). This mechanism may be at least partly responsible for the gastrointestinal adverse effects of macrolides. Azithromycin may act on gastrointestinal motility in a similar way to erythromycin, as it produces a significant increase in postprandial antral motility (34).

Liver

Azithromycin can cause intrahepatic cholestasis (35).

• A 33-year-old woman and a 72-year-old man developed cholestasis after they had taken a 5-day course of azithromycin. The woman was given colestyramine and underwent six courses of plasmapheresis; 2 months later, her total bilirubin and serum transaminases were back to normal (36). After withdrawal of azithromycin, the man's symptoms resolved within 1 month and his liver enzymes returned to normal (37).

Skin

• A 19-year-old man with infectious mononucleosis developed a maculopapular, non-pruritic rash after one dose of azithromycin 500 mg (38).

Immunologic

Occupational allergic contact dermatitis has been attributed to azithromycin (39).

• A 32-year-old pharmaceutical worker had been loading reactors at three different stages of azithromycin synthesis for the past 3 years and had been exposed to airborne powders. He wore overalls and latex gloves. His symptoms had persisted for 1 year in the form of pruritus, erythema, vesicles, and scaling of the face and forearms. A positive patch test and a positive workplace challenge were considered reliable in the diagnosis of occupational allergic contact dermatitis induced by azithromycin. After transfer to another work station that excluded exposure to azithromycin, he had no further work-related symptoms.

Hypersensitivity to azithromycin has been reported (40).

• A 79-year-old man developed fever, mental changes, a rash, acute renal insufficiency, and hepatitis after he had completed a 5-day course of oral azithromycin (500 mg initially then 250 mg/day). With intravenous hydration only, his fever abated and his urinary output and renal and hepatic function returned to normal over the next 4 days. His mental status improved significantly. The skin rash was followed by extensive desquamation.

Azithromycin has been associated with Churg–Strauss syndrome in a patient with atopy (41).

Second-Generation Effects

Pregnancy

In two randomized trials in pregnant women with cervical *Chlamydia trachomatis* infection, women were randomized to oral amoxicillin 500 mg tds for 7 days or oral azithromycin 1 g in a single dose (42,43). The two drugs had similar efficacy. Adverse effects were common in both groups: 40% of those who took azithromycin reported moderate to severe gastrointestinal adverse effects compared with 17% of those who took amoxicillin.

Susceptibility Factors

Renal disease

In eight patients a single 500 mg oral dose of azithromycin was not substantially removed by continuous ambulatory peritoneal dialysis in the absence of peritonitis. Azithromycin cannot be recommended for widespread use in CAPD at present. However, the successful use of azithromycin in treating peritonitis, perhaps because of an intracellular drug transport mechanism, has been reported (44).

Drug–Drug Interactions

Antacids

Owing to interference by antacids, azithromycin should be given at least 1 hour before or 2 hours after antacids. Antacids containing aluminium and magnesium reduce peak serum concentrations, but the total extent of azithromycin absorption is not altered (45).

Antihistamines

The effects of azithromycin 250 mg/day on the pharmacokinetics of desloratadine 5 mg/day and fexofenadine 60 mg bd have been studied in a parallel-group, third-party-blind, multiple-dose, randomized, placebo-controlled study (46). There were small increases (under 15%) in the mean plasma concentrations of desloratadine. In contrast, peak fexofenadine concentrations were increased by 69% and the AUC by 67%. There were no changes in the electrocardiogram.

Carbamazepine

A retrospective analysis of 3995 patients treated with azithromycin did not show any pharmacokinetic interactions in patients who were also taking various other drugs, including carbamazepine (1,45).

Ciclosporin

When azithromycin is used concomitantly with ciclosporin, blood ciclosporin concentrations need to be monitored (47).

Cimetidine

A retrospective analysis of 3995 patients treated with azithromycin did not show any pharmacokinetic interactions in patients who were also taking various other drugs, including cimetidine (1,45).

Cytochrome P450

Azithromycin has a 15-membered ring and does not induce or inhibit cytochrome P450 in rats (48).

Digoxin

When azithromycin is used concomitantly with digoxin, serum digoxin concentrations need to be monitored (47). While data on the effects of azithromycin on the intestinal metabolism of digoxin have not been reported so far, it is likely that it will affect *Eubacterium lentum*, like other macrolides.

Methylprednisolone

A retrospective analysis of 3995 patients treated with azithromycin did not show any pharmacokinetic interactions in patients who were also taking various other drugs, including methylprednisolone (1,45).

Midazolam

In an open, randomized, crossover, pharmacokinetic and pharmacodynamic study in 12 healthy volunteers who took clarithromycin 250 mg bd for 5 days, azithromycin 500 mg/day for 3 days, or no pretreatment, followed by a single dose of midazolam (15 mg), clarithromycin increased the AUC of midazolam by over 3.5 times and the mean duration of sleep from 135 to 281 minutes (49). In contrast, there was no change with azithromycin, suggesting that it is much safer for co-administration with midazolam.

Piroxicam

In 66 patients undergoing oral surgery, treatment with azithromycin impaired the periodontal disposition of piroxicam (50).

Rifamycins

An interaction involving azithromycin with rifabutin, and less commonly rifampicin, was observed in patients with MAC infections (51).

Terfenadine

The potential interaction of azithromycin with terfenadine has been evaluated in a randomized, placebo-controlled study in 24 patients who took terfenadine plus azithromycin or terfenadine plus placebo (52). Azithromycin did not alter the pharmacokinetics of the active carboxylate metabolite of terfenadine or the effect of terfenadine on the QT interval.

Theophylline and other xanthines

A retrospective analysis of 3995 patients treated with azithromycin did not show any pharmacokinetic interactions in patients who were also taking various other drugs, including theophylline (1,45).

In two double-blind, randomized, placebo-controlled studies there was no inhibition of the metabolism of theophylline by azithromycin (53,54). However, there has been a report of reduced theophylline concentrations after withdrawal of azithromycin (55). The authors concluded that the mechanism of interaction was best explained by concomitant induction and inhibition of theophylline metabolism by azithromycin, followed by increased availability of unbound enzyme sites as azithromycin was cleared from the system.

Warfarin

A retrospective analysis of 3995 patients treated with azithromycin did not show any pharmacokinetic interactions in patients who were also taking various other drugs, including warfarin (1,45).

Zidovudine

Zidovudine does not affect azithromycin concentrations and azithromycin does not affect zidovudine concentrations (56).

Food–Drug Interactions

Owing to interference by food (57), azithromycin should be given at least 1 hour before or 2 hours after food.

References

1. Peters DH, Friedel HA, McTavish D. Azithromycin. A review of its antimicrobial activity, pharmacokinetic properties and clinical efficacy. Drugs 1992;44(5):750–99.
2. Hopkins SJ, Williams D. Clinical tolerability and safety of azithromycin in children. Pediatr Infect Dis J 1995;14(Suppl):S67–71.
3. Jaffe A, Francis J, Rosenthal M, Bush A. Long-term azithromycin may improve lung function in children with cystic fibrosis. Lancet 1998;351(9100):420.
4. Altschuler EL. Azithromycin, the multidrug-resistant protein, and cystic fibrosis. Lancet 1998;351(9111):1286.
5. Jacobson JM, Hafner R, Remington J, Farthing C, Holden-Wiltse J, Bosler EM, Harris C, Jayaweera DT, Roque C, Luft BJ; ACTG 156 Study Team. Dose-escalation, phase I/II study of azithromycin and pyrimethamine for the treatment of toxoplasmic encephalitis in AIDS. AIDS 2001;15(5):583–9.
6. Citterio F, Di Pinto A, Borzi MT, Scata MC, Foco M, Pozzetto U, Castagneto M. Azithromycin treatment of

gingival hyperplasia in kidney transplant recipients is effective and safe. Transplant Proc 2001;33(3):2134–5.

7. Treadway G, Reisman A. Tolerability of 3-day, once-daily azithromycin suspension versus standard treatments for community-acquired paediatric infectious diseases. Int J Antimicrob Agents 2001;18(5):427–31.

8. Harris JA, Kolokathis A, Campbell M, Cassell GH, Hammerschlag MR. Safety and efficacy of azithromycin in the treatment of community-acquired pneumonia in children. Pediatr Infect Dis J 1998;17(10):865–71.

9. Adriaenssen CF. Comparison of the efficacy, safety and tolerability of azithromycin and co-amoxiclav in the treatment of acute periapical abscesses. J Int Med Res 1998;26(5):257–65.

10. Frank E, Liu J, Kinasewitz G, Moran GJ, Oross MP, Olson WH, Reichl V, Freitag S, Bahal N, Wiesinger BA, Tennenberg A, Kahn JB. A multicenter, open-label, randomized comparison of levofloxacin and azithromycin plus ceftriaxone in hospitalized adults with moderate to severe community-acquired pneumonia. Clin Ther 2002;24(8):1292–308.

11. Faris MA, Raasch RH, Hopfer RL, Butts JD. Treatment and prophylaxis of disseminated *Mycobacterium avium* complex in HIV-infected individuals. Ann Pharmacother 1998;32(5):564–73.

12. Ward TT, Rimland D, Kauffman C, Huycke M, Evans TG, Heifets L. Randomized, open-label trial of azithromycin plus ethambutol vs. clarithromycin plus ethambutol as therapy for *Mycobacterium avium* complex bacteremia in patients with human immunodeficiency virus infection. Veterans Affairs HIV Research Consortium. Clin Infect Dis 1998;27(5):1278–85.

13. Whitty CJ, Glasgow KW, Sadiq ST, Mabey DC, Bailey R. Impact of community-based mass treatment for trachoma with oral azithromycin on general morbidity in Gambian children. Pediatr Infect Dis J 1999;18(11):955–8.

14. Gruber F, Grubisic-Greblo H, Kastelan M, Brajac I, Lenkovic M, Zamolo G. Azithromycin compared with minocycline in the treatment of acne comedonica and papulo-pustulosa. J Chemother 1998;10(6):469–73.

15. Haye R, Lingaas E, Hoivik HO, Odegard T. Azithromycin versus placebo in acute infectious rhinitis with clinical symptoms but without radiological signs of maxillary sinusitis. Eur J Clin Microbiol Infect Dis 1998;17(5):309–12.

16. Oldfield EC 3rd, Fessel WJ, Dunne MW, Dickinson G, Wallace MR, Byrne W, Chung R, Wagner KF, Paparello SF, Craig DB, Melcher G, Zajdowicz M, Williams RF, Kelly JW, Zelasky M, Heifets LB, Berman JD. Once weekly azithromycin therapy for prevention of *Mycobacterium avium* complex infection in patients with AIDS: a randomized, double-blind, placebo-controlled multicenter trial. Clin Infect Dis 1998;26(3):611–19.

17. Walsh T, Grimes D, Frezieres R, Nelson A, Bernstein L, Coulson A, Bernstein G. Randomised controlled trial of prophylactic antibiotics before insertion of intrauterine devices. IUD Study Group. Lancet 1998;351(9108):1005–8.

18. Coggins C, Sloan NL. Prophylactic antibiotics before insertion of intrauterine devices. Lancet 1998;351(9120):1962–3.

19. Ioannidis JP, Contopoulos-Ioannidis DG, Chew P, Lau J. Meta-analysis of randomized controlled trials on the comparative efficacy and safety of azithromycin against other antibiotics for upper respiratory tract infections. J Antimicrob Chemother 2001;48(5):677–89.

20. Arellano-Rodrigo E, Garcia A, Mont L, Roque M. Torsade de pointes y parada cardiorrespiratoria inducida pot azitromicina en una paciente con sindrome de QT largo congenito. [Torsade de pointes and cardiorespiratory arrest induced by azithromycin in a patient with congenital long QT syndrome.] Med Clin (Barc) 2001;117(3):118–19.

21. Strle F, Maraspin V. Is azithromycin treatment associated with prolongation of the Q-Tc interval? Wien Klin Wochenschr 2002;114(10–11):396–9.

22. Tseng AL, Dolovich L, Salit IE. Azithromycin-related ototoxicity in patients infected with human immunodeficiency virus. Clin Infect Dis 1997;24(1):76–7.

23. Lo SH, Kotabe S, Mitsunaga L. Azithromycin-induced hearing loss. Am J Health Syst Pharm 1999;56(4):380–3.

24. Bizjak ED, Haug MT 3rd, Schilz RJ, Sarodia BD, Dresing JM. Intravenous azithromycin-induced ototoxicity. Pharmacotherapy 1999;19(2):245–8.

25. Mamikoglu B, Mamikoglu O. Irreversible sensorineural hearing loss as a result of azithromycin ototoxicity. A case report. Ann Otol Rhinol Laryngol 2001;110(1):102.

26. Chern KC, Shrestha SK, Cevallos V, Dhami HL, Tiwari P, Chern L, Whitcher JP, Lietman TM. Alterations in the conjunctival bacterial flora following a single dose of azithromycin in a trachoma endemic area. Br J Ophthalmol 1999;83(12):1332–5.

27. Sirois F. Delirium associé à l'azithromycine. [Delirium associated with azithromycin administration.] Can J Psychiatry 2002;47(6):585–6.

28. Hafner R, Bethel J, Standiford HC, Follansbee S, Cohn DL, Polk RE, Mole L, Raasch R, Kumar P, Mushatt D, Drusano G; DATRI 001B Study Group. Tolerance and pharmacokinetic interactions of rifabutin and azithromycin. Antimicrob Agents Chemother 2001;45(5):1572–7.

29. Treadway G, Pontani D, Reisman A. The safety of azithromycin in the treatment of adults with community-acquired respiratory tract infections. Int J Antimicrob Agents 2002;19(3):189–94.

30. Koletar SL, Berry AJ, Cynamon MH, Jacobson J, Currier JS, MacGregor RR, Dunne MW, Williams DJ. Azithromycin as treatment for disseminated *Mycobacterium avium* complex in AIDS patients. Antimicrob Agents Chemother 1999;43(12):2869–72.

31. Lin HC, Sanders SL, Gu YG, Doty JE. Erythromycin accelerates solid emptying at the expense of gastric sieving. Dig Dis Sci 1994;39(1):124–8.

32. Hasler WL, Heldsinger A, Chung OY. Erythromycin contracts rabbit colon myocytes via occupation of motilin receptors. Am J Physiol 1992;262(1 Pt 1):G50–5.

33. Kaufman HS, Ahrendt SA, Pitt HA, Lillemoe KD. The effect of erythromycin on motility of the duodenum, sphincter of Oddi, and gallbladder in the prairie dog. Surgery 1993;114(3):543–8.

34. Sifrim D, Matsuo H, Janssens J, Vantrappen G. Comparison of the effects of midecamycin acetate and azithromycin on gastrointestinal motility in man. Drugs Exp Clin Res 1994;20(3):121–6.

35. Longo G, Valenti C, Gandini G, Ferrara L, Bertesi M, Emilia G. Azithromycin-induced intrahepatic cholestasis. Am J Med 1997;102(2):217–18.

36. Suriawinata A, Min AD. A 33-year-old woman with jaundice after azithromycin use. Semin Liver Dis 2002;22(2):207–10.

37. Chandrupatla S, Demetris AJ, Rabinovitz M. Azithromycin-induced intrahepatic cholestasis. Dig Dis Sci 2002;47(10):2186–8.

38. Dakdouki GK, Obeid KH, Kanj SS. Azithromycin-induced rash in infectious mononucleosis. Scand J Infect Dis 2002;34(12):939–41.

39. Milkovic-Kraus S, Kanceljak-Macan B. Occupational airborne allergic contact dermatitis from azithromycin. Contact Dermatitis 2001;45(3):184.

40. Cascaval RI, Lancaster DJ. Hypersensitivity syndrome associated with azithromycin. Am J Med 2001;110(4):330–1.

41. Hubner C, Dietz A, Stremmel W, Stiehl A, Andrassy H. Macrolide-induced Churg–Strauss syndrome in a patient with atopy. Lancet 1997;350(9077):563.

42. Kacmar J, Cheh E, Montagno A, Peipert JF. A randomized trial of azithromycin versus amoxicillin for the treatment of *Chlamydia trachomatis* in pregnancy. Infect Dis Obstet Gynecol 2001;9(4):197–202.

43. Jacobson GF, Autry AM, Kirby RS, Liverman EM, Motley RU. A randomized controlled trial comparing amoxicillin and azithromycin for the treatment of *Chlamydia trachomatis* in pregnancy. Am J Obstet Gynecol 2001;184(7):1352–4; discussion 1354–6.

44. Kent JR, Almond MK, Dhillon S. Azithromycin: an assessment of its pharmacokinetics and therapeutic potential in CAPD. Perit Dial Int 2001;21(4):372–7.

45. Hopkins S. Clinical toleration and safety of azithromycin. Am J Med 1991;91(3A):S40–5.

46. Gupta S, Banfield C, Kantesaria B, Marino M, Clement R, Affrime M, Batra V. Pharmacokinetic and safety profile of desloratadine and fexofenadine when coadministered with azithromycin: a randomized, placebo-controlled, parallel-group study. Clin Ther 2001;23(3):451–66.

47. Ljutic D, Rumboldt Z. Possible interaction between azithromycin and cyclosporin: a case report. Nephron 1995;70(1):130.

48. Yeates RA, Laufen H, Zimmermann T. Interaction between midazolam and clarithromycin: comparison with azithromycin. Int J Clin Pharmacol Ther 1996;34(9):400–5.

49. Amacher DE, Schomaker SJ, Retsema JA. Comparison of the effects of the new azalide antibiotic, azithromycin, and erythromycin estolate on rat liver cytochrome P-450. Antimicrob Agents Chemother 1991;35(6):1186–90.

50. Malizia T, Batoni G, Ghelardi E, Baschiera F, Graziani F, Blandizzi C, Gabriele M, Campa M, Del Tacca M, Senesi S. Interaction between piroxicam and azithromycin during distribution to human periodontal tissues. J Periodontol 2001;72(9):1151–6.

51. Griffith DE, Brown BA, Girard WM, Wallace RJ Jr. Adverse events associated with high-dose rifabutin in macrolide-containing regimens for the treatment of *Mycobacterium avium* complex lung disease. Clin Infect Dis 1995;21(3):594–8.

52. Harris S, Hilligoss DM, Colangelo PM, Eller M, Okerholm R. Azithromycin and terfenadine: lack of drug interaction. Clin Pharmacol Ther 1995;58(3):310–15.

53. Gardner M, Coates P, Hilligoss D, Henry E. Lack of effect of azithromycin on the pharmacokinetics of theophylline in man. In: Proceedings of the Mediterranean Congress of Chemotherapy, Athens, 1992.

54. Clauzel A, Visier S, Michel F. Efficacy and safety of azithromycin in lower respiratory tract infections. Eur Resp J 1990;3(Suppl 10):89.

55. Pollak PT, Slayter KL. Reduced serum theophylline concentrations after discontinuation of azithromycin: evidence for an unusual interaction. Pharmacotherapy 1997;17(4):827–9.

56. Chave JP, Munafo A, Chatton JY, Dayer P, Glauser MP, Biollaz J. Once-a-week azithromycin in AIDS patients: tolerability, kinetics, and effects on zidovudine disposition. Antimicrob Agents Chemother 1992;36(5):1013–18.

57. Schmidt LE, Dalhoff K. Food–drug interactions. Drugs 2002;62(10):1481–502.

B

Bacille Calmette–Guérin (BCG) vaccine

See also Vaccines

General Information

Bacille Calmette–Guérin (BCG) vaccine is a suspension of living tubercle bacilli of the Calmette–Guérin strain. It is used mainly prophylactically against tuberculosis, but also as a means of stimulating the immune response in malignant disease. There are variations in the characteristics of BCG vaccines, depending on the strain of BCG derived from the original BCG strain and employed for vaccine production. BCG is generally used intradermally, except for instillation in intravesical immunotherapy. The risk of adverse effects after BCG immunization is related to the BCG strain, the dose, the age of the vaccinee, the technique of immunization, and the skill of the vaccinator.

Therapeutic uses of BCG

In addition to its use in preventing tuberculosis, BCG has been used as an immunostimulant or immunomodulator. The degree of safety of this procedure differs with the technique and the purpose for which it is used. In most areas, the use of BCG to counter cancer has proved disappointing, although it is still used to some extent, generally as an adjunct to other forms of treatment (1–7). More encouraging is the use of intravesical instillation of BCG for recurrent superficial transitional cell carcinoma of the bladder, for which it now constitutes the treatment of choice.

BCG immunotherapy in bladder tumors

Intravesical instillation of BCG has been used to treat superficial bladder carcinoma and interstitial cystitis. Many reports have confirmed the efficacy of BCG in the treatment of transitional cell bladder cancers and have delineated its adverse effects (SEDA-12, 273) (SEDA-13, 278) (SEDA-15, 344) (SEDA-16, 375) (SEDA-17, 366) (SEDA-18, 328) (SEDA-20, 287) (SEDA-21, 328) (SEDA-22, 336). The exact mechanism of its antitumor activity is unknown, but live BCG provokes an inflammatory response that includes activation of macrophages, a delayed hypersensitivity reaction, and stimulation of T and B lymphocytes and natural killer cells.

In general, BCG immunotherapy of bladder cancer is considered to be relatively safe. However, it does have adverse effects, including fever, arthritis/arthralgia, bladder irritability, bladder contracture, cytopenias, cystitis, disseminated intravascular coagulation, respiratory failure, epididymitis, hepatitis, loss of bladder capacity, miliary tuberculosis, pneumonitis, polyarthritis, prostatitis, pyelonephritis, pseudotumoral granulomatous renal mass, rhabdomyolysis, renal granulomas, renal insufficiency, skin abscess, tuberculous aneurysm of the aorta and femoral artery, ureteral obstruction, vertebral osteomyelitis, and psoas abscess. A small number of reports of life-threatening adverse effects after BCG instillation have been published, including disseminated BCG infection (8–11), some fatal. These tragic cases illustrate many points of critical importance to all urologists using BCG. BCG should never be given at the same time as tumor resection or transurethral resection of the prostate. The dose of BCG given intravesically corresponds to a potentially lethal intravenous dose. Intravasation as a result of catheterization, tumor resection or biopsy, or cystitis has occurred in two-thirds of the reported cases of systemic BCG infection.

In a review of those observed among 195 patients with bladder cancer treated with various substrains of BCG, there were frequent but mild to moderate local adverse effects, with irritative cystitis leading to frequency and dysuria in 91% of patients and hematuria in 43% (12). Low-grade fever (24%), malaise (24%), and nausea (8%) also occurred. These symptoms usually occurred after two or three instillations and lasted for about 2 days. It has been stated that these frequent adverse effects did not seriously affect the quality of life of patients (13). Additional information was obtained from a multinational retrospective survey in order to cover the whole scope of severe and/or systemic complications associated with BCG immunotherapy, and to propose guidelines for management (14). Among 2602 patients in this survey, more than 95% had no serious adverse effects. Apart from fever higher than 39°C (2.9%) and major hematuria (1%) serious adverse effects comprised granulomatous prostatitis (0.9%), granulomatous pneumonitis and/or hepatitis (0.7%), arthritis and arthralgia (0.5%), epididymo-orchitis (0.4%), life-threatening BCG sepsis (0.4%), skin rashes (0.3%), ureteric obstruction (0.3%), bladder contracture (0.2%), renal abscesses (0.1%), and cytopenias (0.1%). There was no major difference in incidence among the different substrains used. Lowering the dose of BCG in an attempt to reduce the incidence of adverse effects produced somewhat contrasting results, with a reduced incidence of various adverse effects but no significant difference (or an apparently increased incidence) in the case of pollakiuria, hematuria, fever, and headache (SEDA-20, 287) (15).

Other rare complications have been seldom reported, namely cryoglobulinemia with evidence of disseminated BCG infection (16), ruptured mycotic aneurysm of the abdominal aorta (17), bladder wall calcification (18), rhabdomyolysis (19), iritis or conjunctivitis with arthritis or Reiter's syndrome (20,21), and severe acute renal insufficiency due to granulomatous interstitial nephritis, which can occur even in the absence of other systemic complications (22).

In 1990, the US Food and Drug Administration approved the marketing of BCG Live (intravesical) for use in the treatment of primary or relapsed carcinoma in situ of the urinary bladder, with or without associated papillary tumors. BCG is not recommended for treatment of papillary tumors that occur alone. The drug is marketed by Connaught Laboratories as TheraCys and by Organon as TiceBCG. The manufacturers recommend a 6-week induction course of weekly intravesical BCG, usually starting 1–2 weeks after biopsy or after transurethral resection of papillary tumors. Follow-up courses of treatment at 3, 6, 12, and 24 months or monthly for 6–12 months after initial treatment are recommended.

Influence of dosage

The degree of success of different doses of BCG vaccine (100–120 mg, 20–50 mg, or a much smaller dose of 1 mg) in preventing tumor relapse has been described in patients with superficial bladder cancers (23). Adverse reactions were dose-related. The authors considered that endovesical instillation of BCG vaccine 1 mg would be the optimal dosage for prevention of relapse.

In 108 patients with bladder cancer, tumor relapse was prevented by the use of BCG vaccine 1 mg (24). Inguinal lymphadenitis and dysuria have occurred (SEDA-20, 287).

Comparison of BCG strains

In a comparison of 56 patients who received BCG instillations using Berna strain BCG and 32 patients who received Pasteur strain BCG for treatment of superficial bladder cancer, the patients who received Pasteur strain BCG had the highest tumor-free rate but had significantly more toxicity (25). The answer to another difficult question connected with the use of intravesical BCG, that is whether the treatment increases the incidence of second primary malignancies, has been sought (26,27). It was suggested that BCG immunotherapy could accelerate the growth and cause metastatic spread of a growing second primary malignancy that had remained undetected at the start of BCG therapy, and that the time relation between the starting point of second primary tumor development and the starting point of BCG treatment might be crucial in determining whether BCG eradicates the tumor or accelerates its growth. However, in 153 patients there was no evidence that intravesical BCG did increase the incidence of second primary malignancies (26). The matter is therefore still unresolved.

Comparison of different regimens for carcinoma in situ of the bladder

The efficacy and adverse effects of various alternative treatment regimens for carcinoma in situ of the bladder have been compared with those of instillation of BCG in 21 patients. All were treated initially with intravesicular instillations of Keyhole-Limpet Hemocyanin (first course: 20 mg weekly for six weeks; second course: 20 mg monthly for 1 year or bimonthly for 2 subsequent years). Patients who did not respond to two courses were treated with regular instillations of BCG Connaught strain 120 mg. Eleven patients were free from tumor tissue after the first or second course of Keyhole-Limpet Hemocyanin. Ten patients had to have a cystectomy because of persistence or progression of carcinoma after hemocyanin or hemocyanin with subsequent BCG. However, instillations of BCG caused severe dysuria in 60% and fever in 40% of patients, whereas hemocyanin treatment had only minor adverse effects (28). Combined therapy with mitomycin C and BCG was more effective in 28 patients with carcinoma in situ of the bladder than mitomycin alone (29). Compared with

BCG monotherapy there were only a few adverse effects. The success rates were comparable.

Two different methods of treating superficial bladder cancer have also been compared in a randomized, multicenter trial, setting transurethral resection only against transurethral resection plus adjuvant mitomycin C and BCG instillation (30). The rate of progression was comparable in the two groups; at a medium follow-up of 20 months there was a reduction in recurrence rates with the combination therapy. Adverse effects occurred most often during or after BCG instillation. Other investigators have found the same degree of efficacy of the same regimen in reducing the incidence of recurrence of superficial urothelial cancer after transurethral bladder resection in 99 patients (31).

Treatment of adverse effects after intravesical instillation of BCG

The prompt recognition of risk factors for severe complications, namely traumatic catheterization or concurrent cystitis, that increase BCG absorption, and treatment of early adverse effects, is expected to reduce the incidence of severe adverse effects. Severe local and systemic adverse effects can be successfully treated with tuberculostatic drugs for up to 6 months (14).

Severe local and systemic adverse effects of BCG treatment can be treated successfully with tuberculostatic drugs, to most of which BCG is very susceptible, for up to 6 months (32). The effects of isoniazid on the incidence and severity of adverse effects of intravesical BCG therapy have been analysed in patients who received BCG with ($n = 289$) and without ($n = 190$) isoniazid (33). The authors concluded that prophylactic oral administration of isoniazid (300 mg/day with every BCG instillation) caused no reduction in any adverse effect of BCG. In contrast, transient liver function disturbances occurred slightly more often when isoniazid was used. The polymerase chain reaction has been used to monitor BCG in the blood after intravesical BCG instillation (22 patients) as well as after antituberculosis therapy (34). The early and fast diagnosis of BCG in the blood was considered to be potentially valuable in initiating specific early treatment of BCG complications.

General adverse effects of prophylactic BCG immunization

BCG immunization is generally well tolerated. Locally a small papule appears which scales and ultimately leaves a scar; however, abnormal reactions can occur. The most common adverse local reaction, suppurative lymphadenitis, has been reported in 0.1–10% of immunized children under 2 years of age. Faulty immunization technique is the most frequent cause of severe abnormal BCG primary reactions (35). The most serious generalized complications of BCG immunization involve disseminated infection with the BCG bacillus and BCG osteitis. Allergic reactions are unusual, but severe anaphylactic reactions can occur, especially when the product is used as an immunostimulant.

Tuberculin

Mammalian tuberculin purified protein derivative (tuberculin PPD) is the active principle of old tuberculin. A small test dose in a healthy individual, given intracutaneously, is likely to produce only a little local pain and pruritus. If tuberculous infection is present, the local reaction is more marked, with vesiculation, ulceration, and even granuloma annulare or necrosis.

If more than a minimal dose is used in cases of tuberculous infection, a severe and even fatal generalized anaphylactic reaction can develop within about 4 hours of the injection (36).

People who are engaged in manufacturing PPD can easily become sensitized to it, and severe allergic reactions can occur if they later inhale even small quantities (37).

Lymphangitis after tuberculin testing is rare (SED-11, 686).

Acute panuveitis has been reported (38). The episodes developed after each of two tests carried out at intervals of 8 years and responded well to glucocorticoid therapy.

Organs and Systems

Cardiovascular

A mycotic aneurysm, a rare complication of intravesical BCG therapy, has been reported (17).

- A 71-year-old man with bladder carcinoma in situ received six instillations of BCG at weekly intervals followed 3 months later by three booster instillations at weekly intervals. Four months later an inflammatory aortic aneurysm, which had ruptured into a pseudoaneurysm, was diagnosed and excised. *Mycobacterium bovis* was found. After treatment with isoniazid and rifampicin he recovered. There was no sign of tumor in the bladder at cystocopy 8 months after the last BCG instillation.

Respiratory

There have been two reports of micronodular pulmonary infiltrates (BCG pneumonitis) associated with fever, chills, and night sweats following multiple instillations of intravesical BCG (39). Both patients were 71 years old. The reactions, including radiographic infiltrates, resolved spontaneously or after steroid therapy.

Nervous system

There have been two reports of tuberculous meningitis after BCG immunization in immunocompetent individuals, in two French children aged 4.5 and 5 years (40) and in a 22-year-old woman from Cambridge, UK (41).

Polyneuritis has been attributed to BCG immunization (42).

Sensory systems

Responding to the question of whether accidental inoculation of one drop of BCG vaccine into the eye of a health-care worker could be a risk, Pless (personal communication) has reported the case of a urologist who developed a corneal ulcer after a similar accident.

Endogenous endophthalmitis (SEDA-15, 344) and bilateral optic neuritis (43) have been reported after BCG immunization.

Hematologic

Clinical trials in BCG-vaccinated newborns in different countries have variously found a dose–effect relation for the risk of suppurative lymphadenitis:

- Croatia (SED-12, 799)
- French Guyana (SEDA-16, 373)
- Germany (SED-12, 798)
- Hong Kong (SED-12, 799)
- Hungary (SED-12, 798)
- India (SEDA-18, 328)

or a strain-dependent relation:

- Austria (SEDA-16, 374) (SEDA-17, 366)
- Germany (SED-12, 798)
- India (SEDA-18, 328)
- Saudi Arabia (SED-12, 799)
- Togo (SED-12, 799)
- Turkey (SED-12, 799)
- Zaire (SED-12, 799)

Since 1984, WHO's Expanded Programme on Immunization has received many reports from various countries of an increased incidence of suppurative lymphadenitis after BCG immunization. Careful investigations of risk factors have been carried out, particularly in Zimbabwe and Mozambique (1987, 1988). Those studies established a strong association between an increased risk of lymphadenitis within 6 months of immunization and both the use of the Pasteur BCG strain, and programmatic errors, such as poor injection technique, poor technique in reconstituting and mixing the freeze-dried vaccine with diluent, or an incorrectly administered dose of vaccine. The incidence of lymphadenitis was 9.9% with the suspect Pasteur strain versus 0% with two other strains used under the same conditions. Experience gained in other countries has suggested that when Pasteur strain BCG vaccine is administered properly, the rate of lymphadenitis in newborns should not exceed 1%. The increased occurrence of lymphadenitis may require both a reactogenic strain and poor technique (44). A rare case of BCG lymphangitis occurring 11 years and again 18 years after immunization has been reported (45).

Liver

Granulomatous neonatal hepatitis has been reported after BCG immunization (46).

Skin

Since the initial report of lupus vulgaris following BCG immunization in 1946, about 60 cases have been published, mostly following (multiple) revaccination.

The risk of developing lupus vulgaris following primary immunization is extremely low.

- Lupus vulgaris occurred in a 7-year-old girl after only a single BCG immunization (47). She was treated with conventional antituberculosis therapy with an excellent response.
- Six months after BCG vaccination, an 18-year-old man developed lupus vulgaris on his right shoulder (48). He was successfully treated with rifampicin, isoniazid, and ethambutol. He had had lupus vulgaris after BCG vaccination on his left shoulder 8 years before.

Acute febrile neutrophilic dermatosis (49) and eczema vaccinatum (50) have been reported after BCG immunization.

Musculoskeletal

Arthritis and arthralgia are well-known adverse effects of intravesical BCG instillation as part of therapy of bladder cancer (SED-13, 925). The etiology and the different clinical pictures of BCG immunotherapy have been discussed (51). Considering that mycobacteria are potent stimulators of the immune system and especially of T cells, it is not surprising to observe T cell-mediated aseptic arthritis after BCG therapy. The authors suggested that the site of immune stimulation is critical, since intradermal injection produces a clinical presentation similar to reactive arthritis, and intravesical therapy causes a clinical picture identical to Reiter's syndrome.

In a large worldwide analysis of BCG adverse effects (1948–74) co-ordinated by the International Union Against Tuberculosis and Lung Disease (SED-12, 795) there were 272 cases of lesions of bones and joints, including synovial lesions. However, case reports of arthritis after BCG vaccination in healthy individuals are rare. Polyarthritis has been reported in a 33-year-old healthy woman 3 weeks after BCG vaccination (52).

Osteitis

Osteitis occurred in <0.1–30/100 000 vaccinees and has been reported mainly among infants immunized with BCG in the neonatal period in the Scandinavian countries. A retrospective study showed that BCG osteitis was present in Sweden from 1949 onwards. The reported incidence was one per 40 000 in children born between 1960 and 1969 (53,54). In Sweden, the reported incidence of osteitis rose to one per 3000 and one per 4000 for children vaccinated in the neonatal period during 1972–75. Compulsory notification of BCG adverse effects to the Swedish Adverse Drug Reaction Committee was introduced at that time.

The incidence of BCG osteitis correlates closely with the BCG vaccine used. Between 1960 and 1970, when the vaccine based on the Gothenburg strain was prepared in Sweden, the incidence of BCG osteitis was 7.3 per 100 000 vaccinees. There was a significant increase to 37 per 100 000 in the early 1970s, when the vaccine was prepared in Copenhagen using the same Gothenburg strain. Because of the increased incidence, in 1978 the vaccine was replaced by a BCG vaccine made by Glaxo, UK. Since then, the incidence has been similar to that reported in the 1960s (6.4 per 100 000 vaccinees) (55).

Following a report of 10 cases of BCG osteitis in Finland (56), the medical records of 222 children with BCG osteitis registered from 1960 to 1988 in Finland were analysed (55). The most common sites of osteitis were the metaphyses of the long bones; the legs were affected more often (58%) than the arms (14%). There was also osteitis of the sternum (15%) and ribs (11%). With adequate treatment, the prognosis for children with BCG osteitis was good, but six children were left with sequelae, with abnormalities of the limbs in five cases and pronounced cheloid formation in the other.

In Czechoslovakia, BCG osteitis was not diagnosed before 1981. However, from March 1980 onwards another BCG vaccine (Moscow strain) was introduced (57), and after 1981 12 cases of BCG osteitis were diagnosed (58). Most of the cases developed between 7 and 24 months after immunization, but some occurred later. The risk of osteitis rose to 35 per million in the period 1982–85. There were 28 cases of BCG osteomyelitis during the period from 1980 to June 1985, when Russian BCG vaccine containing a higher amount of culturable particles was used, and only 11 cases during the period from July 1985–89, by which time the dose of vaccine had been halved (59). During the last 2 years of the second period there was only one case in each immunized birth cohort. Elsewhere, an infant developed BCG osteomyelitis of the upper spine, a very rare complication described only three times before (60).

Six cases of BCG osteitis in Switzerland occurred in 1980–85 (61). Reports from various countries, for example New Zealand (62) and India (63), have emphasized the increasing knowledge of BCG osteitis. BCG osteitis has never been reported in the UK with use of the Glaxo vaccine. Table 1 shows rates of BCG osteitis in different countries (64).

Sexual function

- Following a 6-week course of intravesical BCG a 65-year-old man with carcinoma of the bladder developed a BCG-derived inflammatory infiltrate of the penis. The induration and lesions resolved after treatment with isoniazid and ethambutol (65).

Immunologic

The incidence of adverse effects after BCG immunization has been extensively investigated by the Committee on Prophylaxis of the International Union Against Tuberculosis and Lung Disease (IUATLD). Retrospective studies including 51 countries worldwide and collecting data from 1948–74, according to organ and system category, have been published (SED-12, 795) (64,66). The IUATLD carried out a second

Table 1 Rates of BCG osteitis in different countries

Country	Number of vaccinees (all age groups) (millions)	BCG osteitis Number	Rate per million vaccinees
Finland	2.79	128	45.9
Sweden	3.42	121	35.4
Denmark	2.28	4	1.75
West Germany	9.03	14	1.55
Norway	2.32	2	0.86
East Germany	8.68	5	0.58
Switzerland	2.17	1	0.46
France	16.2	6	0.37
Austria	2.86	1	0.35
Yugoslavia	17.4	2	0.11
Europe (33 countries)	498	284	0.57
Israel	1.92	3	1.56
Algeria	8.05	2	0.25
Japan	166	2	0.01

(prospective) 6-country study (1979–83) (67), using the classification system already used in the retrospective study. The mean risk of local complications and suppurative lymphadenitis was low: 0.387 per 1000 vaccinees or 0.093 per 1000 with positive bacteriological/histological findings, respectively. There were 21 cases of disseminated BCG infections and allergic manifestations recorded in four countries. The estimated risks of serious disseminated BCG infection were higher than calculated previously (except for bone and joint lesions), but very low when comparing the benefit and risks of BCG immunization, especially in infants (67).

Anaphylactic reactions

Allergy to BCG exceptionally occurs when intravesical BCG is used as an immunoenhancing agent. An anaphylactic reaction has been reported (68).

Three cases of anaphylactic reactions to BCG have been described in young children, one (in a 3-month-old girl) being fatal (69).

An acute shock-like syndrome developed 30 minutes after BCG immunization of a newborn girl.

Non-IgE-mediated anaphylactic (anaphylactoid) reactions suspected to be caused by dextran as used in BCG vaccines have been described (SEDA-16, 375).

Disseminated BCG infection

Dissemination of BCG infection occurs in under 0.1/100 000 vaccinees and is usually associated with severe abnormalities of cellular immunity. Data collected on cases immunized between 1948 and 1974 (from the retrospective IUATLD study) are shown in Table 2 (64,66).

Many authors have provided detailed reports of disseminated BCG infection after BCG immunization at birth in newborns with various underlying immunodeficiency syndromes (severe combined immunodeficiencies, cellular immunodeficiency syndromes, X-linked chronic granulomatous disease or autosomal recessive chronic granulomatous disease) (70–72) and include patients with AIDS. 108 cases of disseminated BCG infection reported worldwide since 1951, including 30 cases of disseminated infection during 1974 to 1994 in France, have been analysed (73,74). Four well-defined immunodeficiency conditions predispose to disseminated BCG infection: severe combined immunodeficiency, chronic granulomatous disease, Di George syndrome, and AIDS. About half the cases of disseminated BCG infection occur in the absence of any well-defined underlying immunological defect. However, there is little doubt that children with idiopathic BCG infection are immunodeficient, and there is good evidence

Table 2 Number of complications recorded until December 1977 in a retrospective study of adverse effects of BCG worldwide among cohorts vaccinated during 1948–74

Adverse effect	Patients in 187 countries ($n = 1\,470\,208\,160$)		Patients in 51 countries in which some cases were recorded in any category ($n = 1\,053\,402\,835$)		Cases proven bacteriologically and/or histologically	
	Number	Rate	Number	Rate	Number	Rate
1 Abnormal BCG primary complex[a]	6602	4.49	6602	6.27	1100	1.04
2 and 3. Disseminated BCG infection: generalized and/or localized lesions (non-fatal and fatal)[b]	1072	0.73	1072	1.02	561	0.53
4. Syndromes or disease clinically associated with BCG immunization[c]	1838	1.25	1838	1.74	7	0.01
All categories	9512	6.47	9512	9.04	1668	1.58

[a] Such cases have often been proven bacteriologically and/or histologically.
[b] Until now, such cases have never been proven either bacteriologically or histologically.
[c] For these seven cases, TB lesions were seen at post-mortem examination, but BCG etiology was doubtful.

that their immunodeficient status is inherited: four pairs of siblings and one pair of cousins were found among 60 children with idiopathic disseminated BCG infection; in addition, among the 50 single-case families, parental consanguinity was found in 7 of 24 families for whom information was available.

There have been reports of disseminated BCG infection in children with chronic granulomatous disease which can result in prolonged and relapsing local complications to BCG immunization (75–77). In a series of autopsies, 26 of 36 children who had been given BCG shortly after birth showed tuberculoid granulomas at various sites. None of the infants had histological evidence of immune deficiency (SEDA-8, 301) (78).

- Recovery from BCG sepsis has been documented in a 7-year-old girl with immunodeficiency (79).
- Two other infants with severe combined immunodeficiency who had developed BCG dissemination after neonatal BCG immunization were treated successfully by bone marrow transplantation and tuberculostatic therapy (80).

However, recovery may not always be complete.

- One girl in her third year, who had been immunized against tuberculosis at birth, developed an abscess of the associated lymph nodes (which were extirpated) and some weeks later developed intestinal BCG dissemination, which appeared to be cured by tuberculostatic treatment. Despite this, at the age of 22 years she developed a left-sided hemiplegia due to aneurysms and thrombosis of cerebral arteries, and 4 years later an oculomotor nerve paralysis was diagnosed. She died at 26 from recurrent intestinal BCG dissemination, which developed at the end of a pregnancy (a healthy premature child was born).

The autopsy confirmed the diagnoses and showed acid-fast bacilli in the adventitia of the basilar artery; the paralysis of the oculomotor nerve was caused by the brain lesion. Defective function of macrophages was suggested as the possible cause of the underlying immunological abnormality (81).

- A 7-week-old infant died under circumstances reminiscent of SIDS; the histopathological examination revealed disseminated BCG infection, no abnormalities of the immune system were detected (82).
- X-ray and CT scan examinations suggested a teratoma in a 1-year-old girl who had received BCG vaccine at birth; however, histology and microbiology revealed the diagnosis of mediastinal BCGitis (83).

Histiocytosis

Cases of fatal histiocytosis have been reported in babies with immune defects immunized with BCG shortly after birth (84).

- One boy who had been immunized shortly after birth developed ipsilateral axillary lymphoma at the age of 6 months. Microscopically the picture was typical of BCG histiocytosis. The child survived. The underlying immunological disturbance was considered to be a temporary derangement of T lymphocyte function (SEDA-8, 300) (85).

Safe immunization with BCG: the WHO view

Taking into account the results of the investigations mentioned above, the WHO made the following recommendations to ensure safe and effective vaccination:

1. Pasteur BCG vaccine should be supplied only to countries using the product without problems. In no case should the vaccine be sent to a country which has been successfully using another product unless the country specifically requests this product.
2. UNICEF supplies of BCG vaccine should specify the doses to be given to infants (0.05 ml), and when possible 0.05 ml syringes should be supplied with the vaccine to reduce the likelihood of too large a dose being given.
3. WHO will supply to country programs a short protocol to assess the incidence of BCG-associated lymphadenitis using a standard case definition. Evidence of a rate greater than 1% would be the basis for investigating the problem and for reviewing the vaccine strain being used.

Additionally it is recommended that training in the technique of BCG immunization should be re-emphasized (44).

Treatment

Erythromycin for a period of 2–4 weeks resolved troublesome post-BCG-lesions in six patients (86). The effect of erythromycin on the atypical mycobacteria was described as early as 1957 (87), but its use for treatment of BCG lesions has not previously been reported. Erythromycin has been used to treat cold abscesses (88).

Neonates with suppurative lymphadenitis have been treated with isoniazid (10 mg/kg/day for 3–9 months) (89). The treatment resulted in complete resolution of the adenitis. There was no significant difference between infants with ruptured nodes and those with intact nodes.

There was no statistical difference between patients who received different forms of treatment for suppurative lymphadenitis: 36 patients received erythromycin, 21 isoniazid, and 21 isoniazid + rifampicin (90). When lymphadenitis developed rapidly (within 2 months), the incidence of spontaneous drainage and suppuration was reported to be significantly higher than in patients with slowly developing processes. Total surgical excision is recommended in these rapidly evolving cases.

Long-Term Effects

Tumorigenicity

The effects of immunization with BCG have been studied extensively (91–94) (SEDA-7, 323) (95,96). On the whole the results are inconclusive, with little good evidence of either preventive or tumor-inducing effects.

Second-Generation Effects

Pregnancy

No harmful effects of BCG vaccine on the fetus have been seen. Nevertheless, it is prudent to avoid immunization of women during pregnancy, unless there is immediate excessive risk of unavoidable exposure to infective tuberculosis (97).

Susceptibility Factors

Disseminated BCG infection is usually associated with severe abnormalities of immunity. BCG for prevention of tuberculosis should therefore not be given to persons with impaired immune responses, such as occur in congenital immunodeficiency, leukemia, lymphoma, generalized malignancy, or AIDS, and when immunological responses have been suppressed by glucocorticoids, alkylating agents, antimetabolites, or radiation (97). The risks are greater in the debilitated or the very young.

Reports on complications after BCG immunization in HIV-positive individuals and patients with AIDS have been published. Disseminated BCGitis has been described (98–101), for example involving the spleen and mediastinal and mesenteric lymph nodes in one case and the liver and the lung in another case (100) or leading to pneumonitis (102). In one case BCG lymphadenitis occurred 30 years after BCG immunization in a 36-year-old patient with AIDS (103). Surgical excision and biopsy revealed a puriform abscess. Pathological examination established the diagnosis of Kaposi's sarcoma; no granulomatous changes were found. BCG was grown. The authors believe that the BCG lymphadenitis was due to a late reactivation of the bacillus.

BCG reactions in HIV-positive and HIV-negative children have been compared in African children. The rates of local adenitis were equal (104,105). These results have been confirmed by a number of other studies, among them one in Haiti. The Haitian investigators found that the risk of complications after BCG vaccination in HIV-infected children is low and that the risk does not outweigh the benefits of BCG vaccination in populations at high risk of tuberculosis during infancy and childhood. Mild or moderate adverse effects occurred in 19 (9.6%) of 166 infants born to HIV-seronegative mothers as compared with 4 (31%) of 13 HIV-infected infants (106).

Organisms of the *Mycobacterium avium* complex (MAC) commonly cause disseminated bacterial infection among patients with AIDS. There is evidence that immunoprophylaxis against MAC infection may be possible. A heat-killed *Mycobacterium vaccae* vaccine was given in a three-dose schedule to 12 HIV-infected adults with CD4 cell counts below $300 \times 10^6/l$ (107). The vaccine was well tolerated and produced detectable immunological responses in 3 of 11 subjects who completed the trial.

The WHO has recommended that individuals with clinical (symptomatic) AIDS or other clinical manifestations of HIV-infection should not receive BCG (108). The Global Advisory Committee on Vaccine Safety has noted that there has been repeated reference to local or disseminated BCG infection several years after BCG immunization in HIV-infected persons (109). However, the Committee has not recommended a change in immunization policy (BCG immunization recommended in asymptomatic HIV-infected persons; not recommended in symptomatic HIV-infected persons), but surveillance for BCG-immunized, HIV-infected persons should be continued for 5–7 years.

References

1. Crispen RG. BCG and cancer. Dev Biol Stand 1986;58(Pt A):371–7.
2. Schult C. Nebenwirkungen der BCG-Immuntherapie bei 511 Patienten mit malignem Melanom. [Side effects of BCG immune therapy in 511 patients with malignant melanoma.] Hautarzt 1984;35(2):78–83.
3. Grigorovich NA, Risina DIa, Nodel'son SE. [Treatment of the complications occurring in BCG vaccine immunotherapy of patients with malignant neoplasms.] Vopr Onkol 1984;30(7):102–6.
4. Hoover HC Jr, Surdyke MG, Dangel RB, Peters LC, Hanna MG Jr. Prospectively randomized trial of adjuvant active-specific immunotherapy for human colorectal cancer. Cancer 1985;55(6):1236–43.
5. Shea CR, Imber MJ, Cropley TG, Cosimi AB, Sober AJ. Granulomatous eruption after BCG vaccine immunotherapy for malignant melanoma. J Am Acad Dermatol 1989;21(5 Pt 2):1119–22.
6. Torisu M, Iwasaki K, Sakata M. Immunotherapy of cancer patients with BCG: summary of ten years experience in Japan. Dev Biol Stand 1986;58(Pt A):451–6.
7. The Ludwig Lung Cancer Study Group (LLCSG). Immunostimulation with intrapleural BCG as adjuvant therapy in resected non-small cell lung cancer. Cancer 1986;58(11):2411–6.
8. Steg A, Leleu C, Debre B, Boccon-Gibod L, Sicard D. Systemic bacillus Calmette–Guerin infection, "BCGitis", in patients treated by intravesical Bacillus Calmette–Guerin therapy for bladder cancer. Eur Urol 1989;16(3):161–4.
9. Deresiewicz RL, Stone RM, Aster JC. Fatal disseminated mycobacterial infection following intravesical bacillus Calmette–Guerin. J Urol 1990;144(6):1331–3.
10. Rawls WH, Lamm DL, Lowe BA, Crawford ED, Sarosdy MF, Montie JE, Grossman HB, Scardino PT. Fatal sepsis following intravesical Bacillus Calmette–Guerin administration for bladder cancer. J Urol 1990;144(6):1328–30.
11. Sakamoto GD, Burden J, Fisher D. Systemic Bacillus–Calmette Guerin infection after transurethral administration for superficial bladder carcinoma. J Urol 1989;142(4):1073–5.
12. Lamm DL, Stogdill VD, Stogdill BJ, Crispen RG. Complications of Bacillus Calmette–Guerin immunotherapy in 1,278 patients with bladder cancer. J Urol 1986;135(2):272–4.
13. Bohle A, Balck F, von Weitersheim J, Jocham D. The quality of life during intravesical Bacillus Calmette–Guerin therapy. J Urol 1996;155(4):1221–6.
14. Lamm DL, van der Meijden PM, Morales A, Brosman SA, Catalona WJ, Herr HW, Soloway MS, Steg A, Debruyne FM. Incidence and treatment of complications of Bacillus Calmette–Guerin intravesical therapy in superficial bladder cancer. J Urol 1992;147(3):596–600.
15. Galvan L, Ayani I, Arrizabalaga MJ, Rodriguez-Sasiain JM. Intravesical BCG therapy of superficial bladder cancer: study of adverse effects. J Clin Pharm Ther 1994;19(2):101–4.
16. Durand JM, Roubicek C, Retornaz F, Cretel E, Payan MJ, Bernard JP, Kaplanski G, Soubeyrand J. Cryoglobulinemia after intravesical administration of Bacille Calmette–Guerin. Clin Infect Dis 1998;26(2):497–8.
17. Damm O, Briheim G, Hagstrom T, Jonsson B, Skau T. Ruptured mycotic aneurysm of the abdominal aorta: a serious complication of intravesical instillation Bacillus Calmette–Guerin therapy. J Urol 1998;159(3):984.
18. Spirnak JP, Lubke WL, Thompson IM, Lopez M. Dystrophic bladder wall calcifications following

intravesical BCG treatment for superficial transitional cell carcinoma of bladder. Urology 1993;42(1):89–92.

19. Armstrong RW. Complications after intravesical instillation of Bacillus Calmette–Guerin: rhabdomyolysis and metastatic infection. J Urol 1991;145(6):1264–6.

20. Nesher G. Syndrome de Reiter après BCG therapie intravésicale. [Reiter syndrome after intravésical BCG therapy.] Rev Rhum Ed Fr 1993;60(12):941.

21. Price GE. Arthritis and iritis after BCG therapy for bladder cancer. J Rheumatol 1994;21(3):564–5.

22. Binaut R, Bridoux F, Provot F, Daniel N, Fleury D, Mougenot B, Vanhille P. Néphrite interstitielle granulomateuse avec insufifsance rénale aiguë, une complication potentielle de la BCG thérapie intravésicale. [Granulomatous interstitial nephritis with acute renal insufficiency, a potential complication of intravesicular bcg therapy.] Nephrologie 1997;18(5):187–91.

23. Corti Ortiz D, Rivera Garay P, Aviles Jasse J, Hidalgo Carmona F, MacMillan Soto G, Coz Canas LF, Vargas Delaunoy R, Susaeta Saenz de San Pedro R. Profilaxis del cancer vesical superficial con 1 mg de BCG endovesical: comparacion con otras dosis. [Prophylaxis of superficial bladder cancer with 1 mg of intravesical BCG: comparison with other doses.] Actas Urol Esp 1993;17(4):239–42.

24. Rivera P, Caffarena E, Cornejo H, Del Pino M, Foneron A, Haemmersli J, Sepulveda M, Ubilla A. Microdosis de vacuna BCG como profilaxis en cancer vesical etapa T1. [Microdoses of BCG vaccine for prophylaxis in bladder cancer stage T1.] Actas Urol Esp 1993;17(4):243–6.

25. Lo Cigno M, Emili E, Iraci F, Soli M, Bercovich E, Rusconi R. Confronto tra BCG Berna e Pasteur F nella profilassi delle recidive neoplastiche superficiali della vescica. Acta Urol Ital 1991;6(Suppl 1):145–8.

26. Guinan P, Brosman S, DeKernion J, Lamm D, Williams R, Richardson C, Reitsma D, Hanna M. Intravesical Bacillus Calmette–Guerin and second primary malignancies. Urology 1989;33(5):380–1.

27. Khanna OP. Intravesical BCG and second primary malignancies. Urology 1989;34(2):113.

28. Jurincic-Winkler C, Metz KA, Beuth J, Sippel J, Klippel KF. Effect of keyhole limpet hemocyanin (KLH) and Bacillus Calmette–Guerin (BCG) instillation on carcinoma in situ of the urinary bladder. Anticancer Res 1995;15(6B):2771–6.

29. Rintala E, Jauhiainen K, Rajala P, Ruutu M, Kaasinen E, Alfthan O, Hansson E, Juusela H, Kanerva K, Korhonen H, Nurmi M, Permi J, Petays P, Tainio H, Talja M, Tuhkanen K, Viitanen J. Alternating mitomycin C and Bacillus Calmette–Guerin instillation therapy for carcinoma in situ of the bladder. The Finnbladder Group. J Urol 1995;154(6):2050–3.

30. Krege S, Giani G, Meyer R, Otto T, Rubben H. A randomized multicenter trial of adjuvant therapy in superficial bladder cancer: transurethral resection only versus transurethral resection plus mitomycin C versus transurethral resection plus Bacillus Calmette–Guerin. Participating Clinics. J Urol 1996;156(3):962–6.

31. Nohales Taurines G, Cortadellas Angel R, Arango Toro O, Bielsa Gali O, Gelabert Mas A. Resultados de un estudio prospectivo de quimioprofilaxis con mitomycina–C y BGG alternades: respuesta completa, indice de recidives y de progresion. [Results of a prospective study of chemoprophylaxis with alternating mitomycin-C and BCG: complete response and recurrence and progression index.] Arch Esp Urol 1996;49(7):689–92.

32. van der Meijden AP. Practical approaches to the prevention and treatment of adverse reactions to BCG. Eur Urol 1995;27(Suppl 1):23–8.

33. Vegt PD, van der Meijden AP, Sylvester R, Brausi M, Holtl W, de Balincourt C, Andriole GL. Does isoniazid reduce side effects of intravesical Bacillus Calmette–Guerin therapy in superficial bladder cancer? Interim results of European Organization for Research and Treatment of Cancer Protocol 30911. J Urol 1997;157(4):1246–9.

34. Tuncer S, Tekin MI, Ozen H, Bilen C, Unal S, Remzi D, Lamm DL. Detection of Bacillus Calmette–Guerin in the blood by the polymerase chain reaction method of treated bladder cancer patients. J Urol 1997;158(6):2109–12.

35. Galazka AM, Lauer BA, Henderson RH, Keja J. Indications and contraindications for vaccines used in the Expanded Programme on Immunization. Bull World Health Organ 1984;62(3):357–66.

36. DiMaio VJ, Froeda RG. Allergic reactions to the tine test. JAMA 1975;233(7):769.

37. Radonic M. Systemic allergic reactions due to occupational inhalation of tuberculin aerosol. Ind Med Surg 1966;35(1):24–6.

38. Burgoyne CF, Verstraeten TC, Friberg TR. Tuberculin skin-test-induced uveitis in the absence of tuberculosis. Graefes Arch Clin Exp Ophthalmol 1991;229(3):232–6.

39. Namen AM, Grosvenor AR, Chin R, Daybell D, Adair N, Woodruff RD, Kavanagh PV, Haponik EF. Pulmonary infiltrates after intravesical Bacille Calmette–Guerin: two cases and review of the literature. Clin Pulm Med 2001;8:177–9.

40. Tardieu M, Truffot-Pernot C, Carriere JP, Dupic Y, Landrieu P. Tuberculous meningitis due to BCG in two previously healthy children. Lancet 1988;1(8583):440–1.

41. Morrison WL, Webb WJ, Aldred J, Rubenstein D. Meningitis after BCG vaccination. Lancet 1988;1(8586):654–5.

42. Katznelson D, Gross S, Sack J. Polyneuritis following BCG re-vaccination. Postgrad Med J 1982;58(682):496–7.

43. Yen MY, Liu JH. Bilateral optic neuritis following Bacille Calmette–Guerin (BCG) vaccination. J Clin Neuroophthalmol 1991;11(4):246–9.

44. Milstien JB, Gibson JJ. Quality control of BCG vaccine by WHO: a review of factors that may influence vaccine effectiveness and safety. Bull World Health Organ 1990;68(1):93–108.

45. Easton PA, Hershfield ES. Lymphadenitis as a late complication of BCG vaccination. Tubercle 1984;65(3):205–8.

46. Simma B, Dietze O, Vogel W, Ellemunter H, Guggenbichler JP. Bacille Calmette–Guerin-associated neonatal hepatitis. Eur J Pediatr 1991;150(6):423–4.

47. Kanwar AJ, Kaur S, Bansal R, Radotra BD, Sharma R. Lupus vulgaris following BCG vaccination. Int J Dermatol 1988;27(7):525–6.

48. Sasmaz R, Altinyazar HC, Tatlican S, Eskioglu F, Yurtsever P. Recurrent lupus vulgaris following repeated BCG (Bacillus Calmette Guerin) vaccination. J Dermatol 2001;28(12):762–4.

49. Radeff B, Harms M. Acute febrile neutrophilic dermatosis (Sweet's syndrome) following BCG vaccination. Acta Derm Venereol 1986;66(4):357–8.

50. Sadeghi E, Kumar PV. Eczema vaccinatum and postvaccinal BCG adenitis—case report. Tubercle 1990;71(2):145–6.

51. Buchs N, Chevrel G, Miossec P. Bacillus Calmette–Guerin induced aseptic arthritis: an experimental model of reactive arthritis. J Rheumatol 1998;25(9):1662–5.

52. Kodali VR, Clague RB. Arthritis after BCG vaccine in a healthy woman. J Intern Med 1998;244(2):183–4.

53. Bottiger M, Romanus V, de Verdier C, Boman G. Osteitis and other complications caused by generalized BCG-itis. Experiences in Sweden. Acta Paediatr Scand 1982;71(3):471–8.

54. Boman G, Sjogren I, Dahlstrom G. A follow-up study of BCG-induced osteo-articular lesions in children. Bull Int Union Tuberc 1984;59:198.

55. Kroger L, Korppi M, Brander E, Kroger H, Wasz-Hockert O, Backman A, Rapola J, Launiala K, Katila ML. Osteitis caused by Bacille Calmette–Guerin vaccination: a retrospective analysis of 222 cases. J Infect Dis 1995;172(2):574–6.

56. Peltola H, Salmi I, Vahvanen V, Ahlqvist J. BCG vaccination as a cause of osteomyelitis and subcutaneous abscess. Arch Dis Child 1984;59(2):157–61.

57. Krepela K, Galliova J, Sejdova E, Hajkova H, Maliniak J. Kostni komplikace po BCG vakcinaci. [Osseous complications after BCG vaccination.] Cesk Pediatr 1985; 40(5): 263–6.

58. Marik I, Kubat R, Slosarek M. BCG osteomyelitis et gonitis u batolete. [BCG osteomyelitis and gonitis in a small child.] Acta Chir Orthop Traumatol Cech 1984;51(6):495–503.

59. Krepela V, Galliova J, Kubec V, Marik J. Vliv snizene davky BCG vakciny na vyskyt kostnich komplikaci po kalmetizaci. [The effect of reduced doses of BCG vaccine on the occurrence of osseous complications after vaccination.] Cesk Pediatr 1992;47(3):134–6.

60. Geissler W, Pumberger W, Wurnig P, Stuhr O. BCG osteomyelitis as a rare cause of mediastinal tumor in a one-year-old child. Eur J Pediatr Surg 1992;2(2):118–21.

61. Hanimann B, Morger R, Baerlocher K, Brunner C, Giger T, Schopfer K. BCG Osteitis in der Schweiz. [BCG osteitis in Switzerland. A report of 6 cases.] Schweiz Med Wochenschr 1987;117(6):193–8.

62. Aftimos S, Nicol R. BCG osteitis: a case report. NZ Med J 1986;99(800):271–3.

63. Kolandaivelu G, Manohar K, Bose JC, Rajagopal P. Osteitis of humerus following BCG vaccination. J Indian Med Assoc 1986;84(6):184–5.

64. Lotte A, Wasz-Hockert O, Poisson N, Dumitrescu N, Verron M, Couvet E. BCG complications. Estimates of the risks among vaccinated subjects and statistical analysis of their main characteristics. Adv Tuberc Res 1984;21:107–93.

65. Latini JM, Wang DS, Forgacs P, Bihrle W 3rd. Tuberculosis of the penis after intravesical Bacillus Calmette–Guerin treatment. J Urol 2000;163(6):1870.

66. Lotte A, Wasz-Hockert O, Poisson N, Dumitrescu N, Verron M, Couvet E. A bibliography of the complications of BCG vaccination. A comprehensive list of the world literature since the introduction of BCG up to July 1982, supplemented by over 100 personal communications. Adv Tuberc Res 1984;21:194–245.

67. Lotte A, Wasz-Hockert O, Poisson N, Engbaek H, Landmann H, Quast U, Andrasofszky B, Lugosi L, Vadasz I, Mihailescu P, et al. Second IUATLD study on complications induced by intradermal BCG-vaccination. Bull Int Union Tuberc Lung Dis 1988;63(2):47–59.

68. Proctor JW, Zidar B, Pomerantz M, Yamamura Y, Eng CP, Woodside D. Anaphylactic reaction to intralesional B.C.G. Lancet 1978;2(8081):162.

69. Tshabalala RT. Anaphylactic reactions to BCG in Swaziland. Lancet 1983;1(8325):653.

70. Gonzalez B, Moreno S, Burdach R, Valenzuela MT, Henriquez A, Ramos MI, Sorensen RU. Clinical presentation of Bacillus Calmette–Guerin infections in patients with immunodeficiency syndromes. Pediatr Infect Dis J 1989;8(4):201–6.

71. Minegishi M, Tsuchiya S, Imaizumi M, Yamaguchi Y, Goto Y, Tamura M, Konno T, Tada K. Successful transplantation of soy bean agglutinin-fractionated, histoincompatible, maternal marrow in a patient with severe combined immunodeficiency and BCG infection. Eur J Pediatr 1985;143(4):291–4.

72. Lin CY, Hsu HC, Hsieh HC. Treatment of progressive Bacillus Calmette–Guerin infection in an immunodeficient infant with a specific bovine thymic extract (thymostimulin). Pediatr Infect Dis 1985;4(4):402–5.

73. Casanova JL, Jouanguy E, Lamhamedi S, Blanche S, Fischer A. Immunological conditions of children with BCG disseminated infection. Lancet 1995;346(8974):581.

74. Casanova JL, Blanche S, Emile JF, Jouanguy E, Lamhamedi S, Altare F, Stephan JL, Bernaudin F, Bordigoni P, Turck D, Lachaux A, Albertini M, Bourrillon A, Dommergues JP, Pocidalo MA, Le Deist F, Gaillard JL, Griscelli C, Fischer A. Idiopathic disseminated Bacillus Calmette–Guerin infection: a French national retrospective study. Pediatrics 1996;98(4 Pt 1):774–8.

75. Hodsagi M, Uhereczky G, Kiraly L, Pinter E. BCG dissemination in chronic granulomatous disease (CGD). Dev Biol Stand 1986;58(Pt A):339–46.

76. Kobayashi Y, Komazawa Y, Kobayashi M, Matsumoto T, Sakura N, Ishikawa K, Usui T. Presumed BCG infection in a boy with chronic granulomatous disease. A report of a case and a review of the literature. Clin Pediatr (Phila) 1984;23(10):586–9.

77. Smith PA, Wittenberg DF. Disseminated BCG infection in a child with chronic granulomatous disease. A case report. S Afr Med J 1984;65(20):821–2.

78. Trevenen CL, Pagtakhan RD. Disseminated tuberculoid lesions in infants following BCG vaccination. Can Med Assoc J 1982;127(6):502–4.

79. Erdos Z, Szabo I. Recovered case of BCG sepsis. Dev Biol Stand 1986;58:319.

80. Heyderman RS, Morgan G, Levinsky RJ, Strobel S. Successful bone marrow transplantation and treatment of BCG infection in two patients with severe combined immunodeficiency. Eur J Pediatr 1991;150(7):477–80.

81. Ehrengut W. BCG-itis während der Kindheit und in der Schwangerschaft. Zugleich ein Beitrag zu einer BCG-bedingten nekrotisierenden zerebralen Arteriitis. [BCG-induced inflammation during childhood and in pregnancy. Additionally a contribution to BCG-induced necrotising cerebral arteriitis.] Klin Padiatr 1990;202(5):303–7.

82. Molz G, Hartmann HP, Griesser HR. Generalisierte BCG-Infektion bei einem 7 Wochen alten, plötzlich gestorbenen Säugling. [Generalized BCG infection associated with the sudden death of a 7-week-old infant.] Pathologe 1986;7(4):216–21.

83. Wolff M, Dopfer R, Hassberg D, Niethammer D. BCGi tis als Ursache eines Mediastinaltumors. [BCGitis as a cause of mediastinal tumor.] Monatsschr Kinderheilkd 1993; 141(5): 409–11.

84. Baum WF, Wessel H, Exadaktylos P, et al. Die BCG-Histiocytose-eine Form der generalisierten BCG-Infektion. Dtsch Gesundheitswes 1983;37:1384.

85. Kunzel W, Frey G, Gunther J, et al. Geheilte BCG-Histiocytose bei isolierter temporärer Störung der T-Lymphocytenfunktion. Dtsch Gesundheitswes 1982;37:1384.

86. Power JT, Stewart IC, Ross JD. Erythromycin in the management of troublesome BCG lesions. Br J Dis Chest 1984;78(2):192–4.

87. Wolinsky E, Smith MM, Steenken W Jr. Drug susceptibilities of 20 atypical as compared with 19 selected strains of mycobacteria. Am Rev Tuberc 1957;76(3):497–502.

88. Singh G, Singh M. Erythromycin for BCG cold abscess. Lancet 1984;2(8409):979.

89. Akenzua GI, Sykes RM. Management of suppurative regional lymphadenitis complicating BCG vaccination in newborns. Niger J Pediatr 1986;13:65.

90. Caglayan S, Yegin O, Kayran K, Timocin N, Kasirga E, Gun M. Is medical therapy effective for regional lymphadenitis following BCG vaccination? Am J Dis Child 1987;141(11):1213–14.

91. Skegg DC. BCG vaccination and the incidence of lymphomas and leukaemia. Int J Cancer 1978;21(1):18–21.

92. Lilienfeld AM, Pedersen E, Dowd JE. Cancer Epidemiology: Methods of Study. Baltimore, MD: Johns Hopkins Press, 1967;72.

93. Snider DE, Comstock GW, Martinez I, Caras GJ. Efficacy of BCG vaccination in prevention of cancer: an update. J Natl Cancer Inst 1978;60(4):785–8.

94. Kendrick MA, Comstock GW. BCG vaccination and the subsequent development of cancer in humans. J Natl Cancer Inst 1981;66(3):431–7.

95. Ambrosch F, Wiedermann G, Krepler P. Studies on the influence of BCG vaccination on infantile leukemia. Dev Biol Stand 1986;58(Pt A):419–24.

96. Haro AS. The effect of BCG-vaccination and tuberculosis on the risk of leukaemia. Dev Biol Stand 1986;58(Pt A):433–49.

97. Immunizations Practices Advisory Committee (ACIP). Recommendations on BCG vaccines. MMWR Morb Mortal Wkly Rep 1979;28(1):241.

98. Ninane J, Grymonprez A, Burtonby G, Francois A, Cornus G. Disseminated BCG in HIV infection. In: Arch Dis Child 1988;63:1268–9.

99. Clements CJ, von Reyn CF, Mann JM. HIV infection and routine childhood immunization: a review. Bull World Health Organ 1987;65(6):905–11.

100. Besnard M, Sauvion S, Offredo C, Gaudelus J, Gaillard JL, Veber F, Blanche S. Bacillus Calmette–Guerin infection after vaccination of human immunodeficiency virus-infected children. Pediatr Infect Dis J 1993;12(12):993–7.

101. Borderon JC, Despert F, Le Touze A, Boscq M, Quentin R, Laugier J. Mesenteric adenitis due to BCG in an 8-year-old girl with AIDS vaccinated at the age of 1 month. Med Mal Infect 1996;26(Special Issue Jun):676–8.

102. von Reyn CF, Clements CJ, Mann JM. Human immunodeficiency virus infection and routine childhood immunisation. Lancet 1987;2(8560):669–72.

103. Reynes J, Perez C, Lamaury I, Janbon F, Bertrand A. Bacille Calmette–Guerin adenitis 30 years after immunization in a patient with AIDS. J Infect Dis 1989;160(4):727.

104. Mvula M, Ryder R, Manzila T, et al. Response to childhood vaccination in African children with HIV infection. In: Abstracts, IV International Conference on AIDS, Stockholm, Sweden, 12–16 June 1988.

105. Embree J, Datta P, Braddick M, et al. Vaccinations of infants of HIV-seropositive mothers. In: Abstracts, IV International Conference on AIDS, Stockholm, Sweden, 12–16 June 1988.

106. O'Brien KL, Ruff AJ, Louis MA, Desormeaux J, Joseph DJ, McBrien M, Coberly J, Boulos R, Halsey NA. Bacillus Calmette–Guerin complications in children born to HIV-1-infected women with a review of the literature. Pediatrics 1995;95(3):414–18.

107. Committee on Immunization. Guide for adult immunization. Philadelphia: American College of Physicians, 1985.

108. Global Advisory Group of the Expanded Programme on Immunization (EPI). Report on the meeting 13–17 October, 1986, New Delhi. Unedited document. WHO/EPI/Geneva/87/1, 1986.

109. Global Advisory Committee on Vaccine Safety, 11–12 June 2003. Wkly Epidemiol Rec 2003;78(32):282–4.

Bacitracin

General Information

Bacitracin has mostly dermatological uses. It can cause allergic reactions of the delayed type. A shock-like picture after local application has occurred in a hypersensitive individual (1). Since bacitracin is nephrotoxic, it should not be given intraperitoneally to patients with renal impairment.

Observational studies

In a randomized study of the effects of a triple antibiotic ointment (polymyxin B + bacitracin + neomycin) and simple gauze-type dressings on scarring of dermabrasion wounds, the ointment was superior to the simple dressing in minimizing scarring; the beneficial effect on pigmentary changes was especially pronounced (2).

Organs and Systems

Sensory systems

Inadvertent injection of bacitracin ointment into the orbit can cause a postoperative orbital compartment syndrome.

- Acute proptosis, chemosis, reduced vision, and ophthalmoplegia occurred after endoscopic sinus surgery in a 73-year-old woman (3). The orbit was tense and the intraocular pressure was 54 mmHg. The presence of bacitracin ointment was established by computed tomography.

Immunologic

Bacitracin is one of the most important clinical allergens (4). Anaphylaxis rarely occurs after topical administration of bacitracin ointment (5,6).

- A 45-year-old man developed a near-fatal anaphylactic reaction after he applied bacitracin ointment to an excoriated area on his foot. He had had a similar, but less severe, episode 4 years earlier. IgE antibodies to bacitracin were positive.
- A 24-year-old man injured in a motorcycle accident was treated with viscous lidocaine and bacitracin zinc ointment for extensive abrasions on the extremities. Five minutes later, he developed symptoms of severe anaphylaxis and required adrenaline, antihistamines, intravenous fluids, and glucocorticoids. Two weeks later, only the prick test to bacitracin zinc ointment was positive.

Anaphylaxis has also been reported after bacitracin nasal packing (7).

- A 48-year-old man underwent uneventful septorhinoplasty, after which his right nostril was packed with 6 ft of vaseline gauze placed in the finger of a latex glove coated with bacitracin ointment. Within seconds, his oxygen saturation fell from 97 to 94% (and increased to 97% with 100% oxygen), but blood pressure and heart rate were unchanged. After the left nostril had been packed, his oxygen saturation fell to 89%, no pulse wave was registered and an electrocardiogram showed a heart rate of 39/minute with first-degree atrioventricular block, and the blood pressure was not obtainable by non-invasive measurement. Cardiopulmonary resuscitation was successful, but the patient remained intubated for 2 days because of concerns about facial and upper airway edema. Later he gave a history of an episode of irritation and swelling after nasal application of polymyxin B and bacitracin ointment 2–3 weeks before surgery. Skin prick testing was positive for bacitracin but negative for latex, polymyxin, cefazolin, and saline.

Cases of anaphylaxis have also been reported after bacitracin irrigation (8,9).

- A 65-year-old man undergoing elective sternal debridement and rewiring was given a prophylactic infusion of vancomycin 1 g preoperatively. Anesthesia was induced with thiopental, suxamethonium, and fentanyl, and maintained with fentanyl, vecuronium, and isoflurane. A few minutes after wound irrigation with bacitracin (about 25 U/ml), his blood pressure fell precipitously, necessitating intravenous fluids and adrenaline. His face and arms were flushed. Afterwards, he reported having had a rash several years before after the use of an over-the-counter ointment composed of polymyxin B, bacitracin, and neomycin.
- A 9-year-old child with a repaired myelomeningocele and congenital hydrocephalus who had undergone four previous shunt revisions in the past had two episodes of anaphylaxis during insertion of the ventriculoperitoneal shunt. The shunt tubing had been soaked in a solution of bacitracin 2500 U/ml. A skin prick test was positive for bacitracin.

Thiomersal, a mercury derivative of thiosalicylic acid, is a preservative used in several types of consumer products, including cosmetics, ophthalmic and otolaryngological medications, and vaccines. In a retrospective study in 574 patients, people who were allergic to thiomersal were more likely to be allergic to bacitracin (10).

Long-Term Effects

Drug resistance

Although there is evidence of acquired resistance to bacitracin in enterococci and staphylococci isolated from animals (11), a review found no evidence that the prevalence of such resistance has increased over time or in relation to the use of bacitracin in man or in animals (in which bacitracin is used as a growth promoter) (12).

Drug Administration

Drug contamination

Commercial bacitracin comprises more than 30 different substances, but the major antibiotic isoforms A and B account for about 60% of the mixture. An impurity has been identified in some but not all bacitracin lots (13). The impurity is a powerful subtilisin-type protease capable of cleaving many proteins, including protein disulfide isomerase, myosin, and a variety of artificial substrates. Investigators using bacitracin are therefore

reminded to determine whether their bacitracin is contaminated by a protease. If it is, careful reinterpretation of the results or retesting with an enzyme-free bacitracin reagent may be warranted.

Interference with Diagnostic Tests

Semen detection

In forensic medicine, the detection of semen may be critical, and identification due to Wood's lamp-induced fluorescence has been suggested to be helpful. In a study to investigate whether semen can be distinguished from other products, none of 41 physicians was able to differentiate semen from other products using a Wood's lamp; however, some ointments and creams that contained bacitracin were mistaken for semen (14).

References

1. Kanof NB. Bacitracin and tyrothricin. Med Clin North Am 1970;54(5):1291–3.
2. Berger RS, Pappert AS, Van Zile PS, Cetnarowski WE. A newly formulated topical triple-antibiotic ointment minimizes scarring. Cutis 2000;65(6):401–4.
3. Castro E, Seeley M, Kosmorsky G, Foster JA. Orbital compartment syndrome caused by intraorbital bacitracin ointment after endoscopic sinus surgery. Am J Ophthalmol 2000;130(3):376–8.
4. Maouad M, Fleischer AB Jr, Sherertz EF, Feldman SR. Significance–prevalence index number: a reinterpretation and enhancement of data from the North American contact dermatitis group. J Am Acad Dermatol 1999;41(4):573–6.
5. Lin FL, Woodmansee D, Patterson R. Near-fatal anaphylaxis to topical bacitracin ointment. J Allergy Clin Immunol 1998;101(1 Pt 1):136–7.
6. Saryan JA, Dammin TC, Bouras AE. Anaphylaxis to topical bacitracin zinc ointment. Am J Emerg Med 1998;16(5):512–13.
7. Gall R, Blakley B, Warrington R, Bell DD. Intraoperative anaphylactic shock from bacitracin nasal packing after septorhinoplasty. Anesthesiology 1999;91(5):1545–7.
8. Blas M, Briesacher KS, Lobato EB. Bacitracin irrigation: a cause of anaphylaxis in the operating room. Anesth Analg 2000;91(4):1027–8.
9. Carver ED, Braude BM, Atkinson AR, Gold M. Anaphylaxis during insertion of a ventriculoperitoneal shunt. Anesthesiology 2000;93(2):578–9.
10. Suneja T, Belsito DV. Thimerosal in the detection of clinically relevant allergic contact reactions. J Am Acad Dermatol 2001;45(1):23–7.
11. Butaye P, Devriese LA, Haesebrouck F. Phenotypic distinction in *Enterococcus faecium* and *Enterococcus faecalis* strains between susceptibility and resistance to growth-enhancing antibiotics. Antimicrob Agents Chemother 1999;43(10):2569–70.
12. Phillips I. The use of bacitracin as a growth promoter in animals produces no risk to human health. J Antimicrob Chemother 1999;44(6):725–8.
13. Rogelj S, Reiter KJ, Kesner L, Li M, Essex D. Enzyme destruction by a protease contaminant in bacitracin. Biochem Biophys Res Commun 2000;273(3):829–32.
14. Santucci KA, Nelson DG, McQuillen KK, Duffy SJ, Linakis JG. Wood's lamp utility in the identification of semen. Pediatrics. 1999;104(6):1342–4.

Baclofen

General Information

Baclofen is a chlorophenyl derivative of gamma-aminobutyric acid (GABA), a naturally occurring inhibitory neurotransmitter in the brain and spinal cord. It is of proven therapeutic value in reducing the severity of flexor or extensor spasms resulting from spinal cord injury or disease. The recommended oral dose is 5 mg tds, which can be carefully increased; however, the total daily dose should not exceed 80 mg (20 mg qds). It is also used for the treatment of intractable hiccups, especially in patients with uremia.

The most commonly reported adverse effects are drowsiness, dizziness, fatigue, confusion, hypotension, and nausea.

Organs and Systems

Nervous system

Altered consciousness is a major adverse effect of baclofen, because of its GABA-mimetic effects. While this reflects global nervous system depression, other adverse effects, such as seizures and dyskinesias, are probably better explained by selective effects on different brain areas. A case of akinetic mutism associated with baclofen might be an example of this (1).

- A 76-year-old man with a history of cognitive decline of unknown origin had severe contractures with increasing pain in his legs. He was given baclofen 10 mg tds, and 2 days later had difficulty following commands. Another 2 days later he could not speak and would not follow commands, although he was alert with his eyes open. He had no spontaneous movements, but would withdraw to painful stimuli. The electroencephalogram showed intermittent, bilateral, symmetrical, sharp waves. Computed tomography and laboratory tests showed no specific abnormalities. Baclofen was withdrawn and he improved over the next 4 days, after which there was no difference to his prebaclofen condition.

The authors explained that akinetic mutism occurs when bilateral frontal lobe or diencephalic–mesencephalic dysfunction interrupts the limbic circuitry. As symptoms were observed immediately after the start of treatment and resolved completely after withdrawal, the condition was probably caused by baclofen. It is not known why baclofen in this case impaired neuronal activity specifically in these areas. The authors found only one previous report describing the case of a 57-year-old woman with end-stage renal insufficiency, who developed akinetic mutism after a single dose of baclofen (2). In this case, the symptoms resolved after dialysis. Therefore, adverse effects of baclofen should be suspected if neuropsychiatric symptoms occur after baclofen treatment has been started. Electroencephalography and computerized tomography may be necessary to exclude other causes.

Because the systemic effects of baclofen can cause a reduced level of consciousness, intrathecal administration via a catheter is widely used to avoid systemic effects.

However, because a continuous infusion is required, implantable pumps containing a very concentrated solution of baclofen are used to avoid frequent refills. Inadvertent subarachnoid bolus administration of a concentrated solution will produce cranial spread of baclofen within the CSF, resulting in cerebral effects. This is most likely to occur when a new catheter or pump is implanted or during surgical revision of a catheter or implantable pump in cases of malfunction. A report of coma after implantation of a baclofen pump in five out of nine consecutive children illustrates this (3). The authors suggested that these children should be monitored in the recovery room for 5 hours postoperatively, in order to cover both the peak effect of any baclofen bolus and the additive effects of other perioperative CNS suppressants, such as opioids, benzodiazepines, or sedative antiemetics. In another report of transient coma after perioperative intrathecal bolus administration it was shown that the management of this complication can require admission to an intensive care unit (4).

Impairment of speech, memory, and mental acuity, associated with an abnormal electroencephalogram, has been described in a young patient taking normal doses (20 mg bd); gradual withdrawal restored the patient and electroencephalogram to normal (SEDA-12, 119) (5). Abnormal electroencephalographic changes have also been reported in a patient with deteriorating multiple sclerosis who developed encephalopathy 48 hours after starting baclofen in low dosage (10 mg tds), but this patient also had renal impairment; withdrawal led to reversal of symptoms in this case (6).

Epilepsy, progressing to status epilepticus, has been ascribed to baclofen (80 mg/day); the fits stopped on gradual withdrawal of the baclofen (7). In contrast to other reports, this patient had no history of seizures.

An elderly patient with a 4-year history of Alzheimer's disease developed chorea 2 weeks after starting a trial of baclofen (SEDA-16, 23). The dosage had been gradually increased to 15 mg tds. The chorea resolved within 24 hours after the baclofen was withdrawn. The authors suggested that the chorea might have resulted from the combination of the GABA-agonist drug and deficient cholinergic function in Alzheimer's disease.

A case of aseptic meningitis after intrathecal administration of baclofen has been reported but, as viral causes could not be ruled out, the causative role of baclofen was unclear (8).

Psychological, psychiatric

Euphoria or depression can occur, and mania has been reported in a patient with schizophrenia (9).

Gastrointestinal

A possible effect of intrathecal baclofen on intestinal motility has been proposed (10). Triggered by two cases of paralytic ileus in patients receiving continuous intrathecal baclofen, the authors reviewed the case notes of 14 patients and summed the days without bowel movements before and after intrathecal baclofen therapy. Intestinal function deteriorated in 10 patients, was unchanged in one, and improved in three. They therefore advised that intestinal activity should be closely observed in patients receiving intrathecal baclofen. However, they felt that treatment could be continued, even in particularly sensitive patients, if prokinetic, laxative, or eubiotic drugs were used to promote peristaltic function.

Liver

Rarely, deterioration in liver function tests (increases in aspartate transaminase and alkaline phosphatase) can occur (SEDA-6, 132).

Musculoskeletal

With regard to its effects on spinal GABA receptors, intrathecal baclofen has been compared with intrathecal fentanyl for postoperative pain treatment in six children (mean age 4.2 years) with cerebral palsy undergoing bilateral dorsal rhizotomy (11). Both intrathecal baclofen and intrathecal fentanyl reduced postoperative pain. However, three of five children had severe muscle weakness after intrathecal baclofen 1–1.5 µg/kg, which prompted the authors to discontinue their study. An accompanying editorial dealt with the possible mechanisms of action of spinal GABA agonists on postoperative pain, suggesting that the effects on sensory processing probably cannot be separated from the changes in motor function (12). Therefore, this report of muscle weakness should not prompt us to close the file on intrathecal baclofen for pain treatment. More experience is needed and different dose regimens should be tested.

Sexual function

Intrathecal baclofen caused a reduction in erection rigidity and duration in eight of nine men. When ejaculation was possible before the start of baclofen treatment it disappeared or was more difficult to obtain during treatment. These effects resolved after withdrawal of baclofen (13).

Body temperature

Febrile reactions after intrathecal baclofen stopped a patient from receiving this treatment for spinal spasticity (14).

- A 33-year-old woman with spasticity caused by a myelopathy after numerous operations on her spine received a single bolus dose of baclofen 50 µg via a lumbar puncture, which resulted in complete resolution of her spasticity for almost 24 hours. However, her temperature increased to 39.0°C within 2 hours after the injection, and she had flu-like symptoms. Influenza was assumed to be the most likely explanation, as a child in her house had influenza at that time. Subsequently, an intrathecal catheter was placed and a baclofen pump implanted. However, her temperature rose again after baclofen administration had been started and the pump was halted. Subsequently, several attempts were made to restart the infusion, followed each time by spikes of fever. In the end, continuous intrathecal baclofen therapy had to be abandoned, and the fever did not recur. Several investigations to identify other causes of fever were mostly negative. However, based on bilateral hilar adenopathy on the chest X-ray and increased concentrations of angiotensin-converting enzyme, sarcoidosis was suspected.

The authors claimed that this was the first report of this problem. Referring to the observation that baclofen injection into the cerebral ventricles can produce fever in rats (15), they assumed that rostral spread of baclofen could have initiated a thermoregulatory response via the chemo-trigger zone in the third ventricle. They suggested that a percutaneous subarachnoid catheter could facilitate the decision to either proceed with or abort surgical catheter or pump implantation when baclofen is associated with fever.

Long-Term Effects

Drug tolerance

Tolerance to intrathecal baclofen developed in three of 23 patients with spinal spasticity (16).

Drug withdrawal

Like many other agents that act at the GABA receptor, abrupt termination of long-term administration of baclofen can result in withdrawal symptoms, even after intrathecal administration (17,18). Patients can present with different symptoms, not all of which would be considered classical of drug withdrawal.

Clinical presentation

Common presenting features are muscular hyperactivity, hyperthermia, metabolic derangements, and rhabdomyolysis when baclofen therapy is abruptly discontinued, and several deaths have occurred (19). Clinicians should be suspicious of baclofen withdrawal if patients taking baclofen present with fever, muscle cramps, and hypotension. A case of brain death due to baclofen withdrawal with severe hypotension and hyperthermia up to 43°C has underscored the need for immediate and aggressive treatment (20).

Sudden withdrawal can cause hallucinations and grand mal convulsions or worsening of pre-existing epilepsy (SED-9, 206) (21,22).

There is a similarity between baclofen withdrawal and the neuroleptic malignant syndrome.

- A 36-year-old man with paraplegia after a spinal cord injury became disoriented (23). He had marked rigidity in both arms and legs, he was sweating and pyrexial (38°C), and his heart rate was 112/minute. His serum creatine kinase was raised at 2668 U/l and rose to 2982 U/l on day 3. At that time, baclofen was restarted. Within 3 days he was fully oriented. Over 2 weeks his creatine kinase activity gradually fell to normal and his temperature settled. It turned out that he had neglected to take any medication for several days before admission.

The authors believed that symptoms in this case resembled the neuroleptic malignant syndrome, based on the combination of muscle rigidity, pyrexia, signs of autonomic disturbance, and altered consciousness. They did not think that the raised serum creatine kinase activity was associated with rhabdomyolysis, stating that there was no evidence from urinalysis to suggest this. Unfortunately, they did not specify whether there was myoglobin in the urine or not. Creatine kinase activities up to 40 000 U/l have been noted during baclofen withdrawal (24), compared with which creatine kinase activity in this case was much lower, suggesting only moderate muscle damage. One might assume that muscle damage after baclofen withdrawal correlates with the duration and intensity of muscular hyperactivity. In addition, prolonged muscular hyperactivity may be expected to be followed by an increase in both body temperature and heart rate, owing to hypermetabolism and sympathetic activation. Sweating will result from sympathetic activation and a thermoregulatory response to hyperthermia and is not necessarily an autonomic disturbance. Disorientation is also an expected symptom of baclofen withdrawal. In conclusion, this patient's combination of symptoms could have been explained by baclofen withdrawal alone. Assuming that disturbances in central dopaminergic systems could have been involved, as in neuroleptic malignant syndrome, is speculative.

This is not the first report of similarities between the neuroleptic malignant syndrome and baclofen withdrawal (18,20,24). In addition, hyperthermia seems to be common in baclofen withdrawal (20).

- A 14-year-old child receiving continuous intrathecal baclofen treatment developed a fever of up to 40°C and painful muscle spasms, attributed to baclofen withdrawal due to failure of the intrathecal catheter. The symptoms resolved promptly after reintroduction of intrathecal baclofen (25).

If intrathecal baclofen has to be interrupted or cannot be restarted immediately, enteral baclofen should be given. However, finding the appropriate dose for this can be difficult and close observation of the patient is required, as illustrated in the following report (26).

- A 34-year-old man who was receiving continuous intrathecal baclofen (700 micrograms/day) for muscle spasticity after a spinal cord injury developed a fever, and infection of the implanted baclofen pump was suspected. The device was removed and he was given replacement therapy with oral baclofen (40 mg tds). He developed a tremor 12 hours after pump removal and his heart rate increased to 120/minute. Another 12 hours later he was somnolent, agitated, and confused, and had visual hallucinations. His blood pressure rose to 198/108 mmHg and his temperature to 40°C. This was followed by atrial fibrillation with a ventricular rate of 170/minute. The dose of oral baclofen was increased to 80 mg tds and he was given intravenous lorazepam 6–8 mg every 4 hours. During the following 24 hours his blood pressure, pulse, and temperature normalized and he recovered fully.

Management

Baclofen should always be withdrawn gradually. If a patient stops taking baclofen, a blood sample for baclofen serum concentration measurement should be taken if possible, to confirm the diagnosis post hoc if hyperthermia occurs. If a patient taking long-term baclofen

presents with similar symptoms, baclofen withdrawal should be considered. If this is not effective and the patient deteriorates, with hyperthermia, increasing creatine kinase activity, and metabolic sequelae, dantrolene can be given.

Dantrolene is life-saving in malignant hyperthermia associated with volatile anesthetics and suxamethonium and is also the drug of choice for the treatment of neuroleptic malignant syndrome. Dantrolene has therefore been suggested as an additional therapeutic option in baclofen withdrawal (18), but there is only limited experience (24). In one case of baclofen withdrawal, dantrolene was given with success (24).

It should be stressed that baclofen withdrawal is a potentially fatal emergency. Because of the risk of rhabdomyolysis, disseminated intravascular coagulation, acute renal insufficiency, and other organ complications, patients should be transferred to the intensive care unit and given parenteral baclofen.

Since it has been hypothesized that the baclofen withdrawal syndrome might have similarities with the serotonin syndrome caused by overdose of serotonin reuptake inhibitors or amphetamines, the serotonin receptor antagonist cyproheptadine has been used in combination with oral baclofen and a benzodiazepine in four patients with baclofen withdrawal syndrome after continuous intrathecal baclofen therapy (27). The authors claimed that their patients improved significantly when cyproheptadine was given. Body temperature fell by at least 1.5°C and heart rate fell from 120–140/minute to under 100/minute. Muscular tone and myoclonus improved. Two patients also reported that itching was less intense. All this was felt to be temporarily related to the repeated administration of cyproheptadine. The authors concluded that cyproheptadine was a useful adjunct for the treatment of baclofen withdrawal syndrome. However, one of their patients suffered severe brain damage during withdrawal and subsequently died of pulmonary complications. This illustrates that early intensive care is required.

Second-Generation Effects

Fetotoxicity

Convulsions have been attributed to withdrawal of baclofen after in utero exposure (28).

- A 7-day-old baby was admitted to hospital with generalized convulsions, which did not respond to phenobarbital, phenytoin, clonazepam, lidocaine, or pyridoxine. A variety of investigations all gave negative results. Electroencephalography 4 days later showed prolonged episodes of epileptic activity. At that time baclofen withdrawal was suspected, as the paraplegic mother had been taking baclofen 20 mg tds throughout pregnancy. The baby was given baclofen 0.25 mg/kg qds and 30 minutes after the first dose the convulsions stopped. The baclofen was then slowly withdrawn over 2 weeks. An MRI scan of the brain on day 17 suggested a hypoxic ischemic insult in the perinatal period, which was considered to have been secondary to convulsions.

As convincingly presented by the authors, baclofen withdrawal was the most likely explanation for the convulsions. In discussing the possible mechanisms of the delayed onset of convulsions the authors assumed that a secondary increase in baclofen serum concentration due to redistribution might have prevented earlier onset of the withdrawal symptoms. This is of course speculative; nothing is known about baclofen pharmacokinetics in neonates. On the other hand, the authors stated that the mother had noted some abnormal movements starting on the second day postpartum, which might have represented the first signs of withdrawal. The half-life of baclofen in adults is 3–6 hours, and adults usually become symptomatic 24–72 hours after baclofen is reduced or withdrawn (20). In conclusion, baclofen withdrawal should be suspected if postnatal convulsions occur after intrauterine exposure. The first priority in such a case is to rule out other causes, such as infections, electrolyte disturbances, and intracranial pathology, and to prevent secondary brain damage due to prolonged convulsions. Baclofen should probably be considered at an early stage, as it might be the most effective anticonvulsant in such cases.

Susceptibility Factors

Renal disease

As 70% of baclofen is excreted unchanged in the urine (29), accumulation and overdosage of baclofen can occur in patients with end-stage renal disease. Confusion, drowsiness, and coma after standard doses have been reported (30). In addition, abdominal pain was a common adverse effect of baclofen in patients with severe renal insufficiency (31). Toxic reactions characterized by a psychotic syndrome and myoclonus have also been reported (32). Patients with severely impaired renal function typically present with altered consciousness after very small doses of baclofen (31). Symptoms of overdose may resolve after hemodialysis (30,31).

- An 82-year-old man with left ventricular dysfunction and gout had worsening renal function (33). He was taking lisinopril, furosemide, naproxen, allopurinol, and baclofen 20 mg tds. As no reason could be found for the use of baclofen the dose was halved and then stopped 10 days later. The next day he had visual hallucinations, confusion, and agitation, and required sedation with diazepam. He was afebrile, with normal inflammatory markers, and a CT scan of the brain showed only cerebral atrophy. Baclofen was reintroduced, with complete resolution of neuropsychiatric symptoms within 48 hours.

Other features of the patient

Generally, patients with a history of seizures, convulsive disorders, or psychiatric disturbances, and also elderly patients with cerebrovascular disease, should be regarded as patients at risk of developing the more serious side effects (SED-9, 206).

Drug Administration

Drug administration route

Intrathecal baclofen is becoming increasingly popular for the treatment of severe spasticity in an attempt to reduce the incidence and severity of systemic adverse effects. However, hypotonia, respiratory depression, and coma can occur. Severe arterial hypotension also has been observed in two of 23 patients (16). Occasionally, nervous system suppression can be severe enough to require mechanical ventilation. Adverse effects have been seen not only with high doses (2000 micrograms/day produced flaccid quadriplegia with total areflexia) (SEDA-12, 119) (34), but also after a single bolus dose of 80 micrograms in a patient known to be very sensitive to the action of baclofen (SEDA-15, 128) (35).

Drugs injected directly into the cerebrospinal fluid have a tendency to produce unpredictable effects, their spread being influenced not only by the volume administered, but also by the concentration of the drug, its specific gravity in relation to that of cerebrospinal fluid, the positioning of the patient (head-up or head-down), and on the speed of injection of bolus doses. Truncal muscle spasms can also increase the spread of drug within the cerebrospinal fluid. All these parameters need to be taken into consideration. Standardization is required as a first step. Rapid bolus injection in particular can produce unexpectedly severe adverse effects.

Drug overdose

Overdose, which may be absolute or relative (due to impaired renal excretion or in elderly patients who develop adverse effects at lower dosages), leads to severe hypotonia, mental confusion and somnolence, respiratory depression, and eventually apnea, bradycardia, cardiac conduction abnormalities, hypotension, and coma. Convulsions can occur and hypertension has been reported. It is possible that during recovery the picture may be complicated by an acute withdrawal syndrome, with agitation, psychosis, tremor and dystonic movements, convulsions, and hallucinations (SEDA-11, 126) (36–40).

Physostigmine is rapidly effective in reversing not only the respiratory depression but also the coma and hypotonia seen in cases of intrathecal baclofen overdosage (SEDA-15, 128) (35). The doses recommended for physostigmine salicylate are 1–2 mg intravenously over 5–10 minutes, which may have to be repeated after 30–40 minutes, as the action of physostigmine is fairly short. However, physostigmine may be ineffective when large doses of baclofen are involved (41), and it also has adverse effects of its own, so that the above dosage guidelines should not be exceeded. In particular, bradycardia and cardiac conduction defects can be worsened (cardiac arrest has been reported in connection with baclofen) and it should not be used in these circumstances, respiratory support and symptomatic treatment being recommended (42).

Phaclofen is a more specific baclofen antagonist (43), but more research is required to ascertain if it can be safely used in the treatment of baclofen overdose.

Drug–Drug Interactions

Tricyclic antidepressants

Tricyclic antidepressants can potentiate the muscle relaxant effects of baclofen, resulting in severe hypotonic weakness (44); the combination has also been incriminated in the causation of short-term memory impairment (SEDA-11, 127) (45).

References

1. Rubin DI, So EL. Reversible akinetic mutism possibly induced by baclofen. Pharmacotherapy 1999;19(4):468–70.
2. Parmar MS. Akinetic mutism after baclofen. Ann Intern Med 1991;115(6):499–500.
3. Anderson KJ, Farmer JP, Brown K. Reversible coma in children after improper baclofen pump insertion. Paediatr Anaesth 2002;12(5):454–60.
4. Lyew MA, Mondy C, Eagle S, Chernich SE. Hemodynamic instability and delayed emergence from general anesthesia associated with inadvertent intrathecal baclofen overdose. Anesthesiology 2003;98(1):265–8.
5. Wainapel SF, Lee L, Riley TL. Reversible electroencephalogram changes associated with administration of baclofen in a quadriplegic patient: case report. Paraplegia 1986;24(2):123–6.
6. Hormes JT, Benarroch EE, Rodriguez M, Klass DW. Periodic sharp waves in baclofen-induced encephalopathy. Arch Neurol 1988;45(7):814–15.
7. Rush JM, Gibberd FB. Baclofen-induced epilepsy. J R Soc Med 1990;83(2):115–16.
8. Naveira FA, Speight KL, Rauck RL, Carpenter RL. Meningitis after injection of intrathecal baclofen. Anesth Analg 1996;82(6):1297–9.
9. Wolf ME, Almy G, Toll M, Mosnaim AD. Mania associated with the use of baclofen. Biol Psychiatry 1982;17(6):757–9.
10. Kofler M, Matzak H, Saltuari L. The impact of intrathecal baclofen on gastrointestinal function. Brain Inj 2002;16(9):825–36.
11. Soliman IE, Park TS, Berkelhamer MC. Transient paralysis after intrathecal bolus of baclofen for the treatment of post-selective dorsal rhizotomy pain in children. Anesth Analg 1999;89(5):1233–5.
12. Yaksh TL. A drug has to do what a drug has to do. Anesth Analg 1999;89(5):1075–7.
13. Denys P, Mane M, Azouvi P, Chartier-Kastler E, Thiebaut JB, Bussel B. Side effects of chronic intrathecal baclofen on erection and ejaculation in patients with spinal cord lesions. Arch Phys Med Rehabil 1998;79(5):494–6.
14. Wu SS, Dolan KA, Michael Ferrante F. Febrile reaction to subarachnoid baclofen administration. Anesthesiology 2002;96(5):1270–2.
15. Zarrindast MR, Oveissi Y. GABA$_A$ and GABA$_B$ receptor sites involvement in rat thermoregulation. Gen Pharmacol 1988;19(2):223–6.
16. Abel NA, Smith RA. Intrathecal baclofen for treatment of intractable spinal spasticity. Arch Phys Med Rehabil 1994;75(1):54–8.
17. Sampathkumar P, Scanlon PD, Plevak DJ. Baclofen withdrawal presenting as multiorgan system failure. Anesth Analg 1998;87(3):562–3.
18. Reeves RK, Stolp-Smith KA, Christopherson MW. Hyperthermia, rhabdomyolysis, and disseminated intravascular coagulation associated with baclofen pump catheter failure. Arch Phys Med Rehabil 1998;79(3):353–6.
19. Coffey RJ, Edgar TS, Francisco GE, Graziani V, Meythaler JM, Ridgely PM, Sadiq SA, Turner MS. Abrupt withdrawal from intrathecal baclofen: recognition and management of a potentially life-threatening syndrome. Arch Phys Med Rehabil 2002;83(6):735–41.
20. Green LB, Nelson VS. Death after acute withdrawal of intrathecal baclofen: case report and literature review. Arch Phys Med Rehabil 1999;80(12):1600–4.
21. Lees AJ, Clarke CRA, Harrison MJ. Hallucinations after sudden withdrawal of baclofen. Lancet 1977;2(8027):44–5.
22. Fromm GH, Terrence CF, Chattha AS, Glass JD. Baclofen in trigeminal neuralgia: its effect on the spinal trigeminal nucleus: a pilot study. Arch Neurol 1980;37(12):768–71.
23. Turner MR, Gainsborough N. Neuroleptic malignant-like syndrome after abrupt withdrawal of baclofen. J Psychopharmacol 2001;15(1):61–3.
24. Khorasani A, Peruzzi WT. Dantrolene treatment for abrupt intrathecal baclofen withdrawal. Anesth Analg 1995;80(5):1054–6.
25. Alden TD, Lytle RA, Park TS, Noetzel MJ, Ojemann JG. Intrathecal baclofen withdrawal: a case report and review of the literature. Childs Nerv Syst 2002;18(9–10):522–5.
26. Greenberg MI, Hendrickson RG. Baclofen withdrawal following removal of an intrathecal baclofen pump despite oral baclofen replacement. J Toxicol Clin Toxicol 2003;41(1):83–5.
27. Meythaler JM, Roper JF, Brunner RC. Cyproheptadine for intrathecal baclofen withdrawal. Arch Phys Med Rehabil 2003;84(5):638–42.
28. Ratnayaka BD, Dhaliwal H, Watkin S. Drug points. Neonatal convulsions after withdrawal of baclofen. BMJ 2001;323(7304):85.
29. Faigle JW, Keberle H, Degen PH. Chemistry and pharmacokinetics of baclofen. In: Feldman RG, Young RR, Koella WP, editors. Spasticity: Disordered Motor Control. Chicago: Year Book, 1980:461–75.
30. Peces R, Navascues RA, Baltar J, Laures AS, Alvarez-Grande J. Baclofen neurotoxicity in chronic haemodialysis patients with hiccups. Nephrol Dial Transplant 1998;13(7):1896–7.
31. Chen KS, Bullard MJ, Chien YY, Lee SY. Baclofen toxicity in patients with severely impaired renal function. Ann Pharmacother 1997;31(11):1315–20.
32. Seyfert S, Kraft D, Wagner K. Baclofen-Dosis bei Haemodialyse und Niereninsuffizienz. [Baclofen toxicity during intermittent renal dialysis.] Nervenarzt 1981;52(10):616–17.
33. O'Rourke F, Steinberg R, Ghosh P, Khan S. Withdrawal of baclofen may cause acute confusion in elderly patients. BMJ 2001;323(7317):870.
34. Romijn JA, van Lieshout JJ, Velis DN. Reversible coma due to intrathecal baclofen. Lancet 1986;2(8508):696.
35. Muller-Schwefe G, Penn RD. Physostigmine in the treatment of intrathecal baclofen overdose. Report of three cases. J Neurosurg 1989;71(2):273–5.
36. Wimmer C. Über Lioresal- (Baclofen-) Intoxikationen— Ein kasuistischer Beitrag. Dtsch Gesundheitsw 1982;37:1500.
37. May CR. Baclofen overdose. Ann Emerg Med 1983;12(3):171–3.
38. White WB. Aggravated CNS depression with urinary retention secondary to baclofen administration. Arch Intern Med 1985;145(9):1717–18.
39. Nugent S, Katz MD, Little TE. Baclofen overdose with cardiac conduction abnormalities: case report and review of the literature. J Toxicol Clin Toxicol 1986;24(4):321–8.
40. Perry HE, Wright RO, Shannon MW, Woolf AD. Baclofen overdose: drug experimentation in a group of adolescents. Pediatrics 1998;101(6):1045–8.
41. Saltuari L, Baumgartner H, Kofler M, Schmutzhard E, Russegger L, Aichner F, Gerstenbrand F. Failure of physostigmine in treatment of acute severe intrathecal baclofen intoxication. N Engl J Med 1990;322(21):1533–4.

42. Penn RD, Kroin JS. Failure of physostigmine in treatment of acute severe intrathecal baclofen intoxication. N Engl J Med 1990;322:1533.
43. Kerr DI, Ong J, Prager RH, Gynther BD, Curtis DR. Phaclofen: a peripheral and central baclofen antagonist. Brain Res 1987;405(1):150–4.
44. Silverglat MJ. Baclofen and tricyclic antidepressants: possible interaction. JAMA 1981;246(15):1659.
45. Sandyk R, Gillman MA. Baclofen-induced memory impairment. Clin Neuropharmacol 1985;8(3):294–5.

Bambuterol

See also Beta$_2$-adrenoceptor agonists

General Information

The efficacy of long-acting beta$_2$-adrenoceptor agonists in patients with chronic obstructive pulmonary disease remains unclear, but their role in treatment regimens, particularly in comparison with oral theophylline, has been reviewed (1).

Bambuterol is a beta$_2$-adrenoceptor agonist, a biscarbamate ester prodrug of terbutaline (SEDA-18, 188) (SEDA-22, 188). It is available as the hydrochloride salt in 10 and 20 mg tablets. It escapes first-pass elimination and is concentrated in lung tissue after absorption from the gastrointestinal tract. It is hydrolysed to terbutaline primarily by an enzyme, butyrylcholinesterase, found in lung tissue. Terbutaline is therefore formed preferentially in the lung, and as a result bambuterol should have a more selective effect than terbutaline. The effect of bambuterol lasts for 24 hours. Peak plasma concentrations of terbutaline occur 4–7 hours after the administration of bambuterol. Maximum therapeutic benefit occurs 1 week after starting treatment.

Except for suppression of plasma butyrylcholinesterase, the adverse effects of bambuterol are those of a beta$_2$-adrenoceptor agonist and are related to the plasma concentration of terbutaline. Plasma butyrylcholinesterase returns to control values about 2 weeks after stopping treatment (SEDA-22, 188).

Placebo-controlled studies

Oral bambuterol 20 mg at night has been compared with inhaled salmeterol 50 µg bd for persistent nocturnal symptoms in 117 asthmatics already taking inhaled corticosteroids in a randomized, double-blind, placebo-controlled trial for 6 weeks (2). The treatments resulted in significant and equivalent improvements in nocturnal and daytime asthma symptoms, peak flow, and the use of short-acting beta-adrenoceptor agonists. Drug-related adverse events included headache (six with bambuterol, two with salmeterol), tremor (three in each group), cramps (two with bambuterol), and palpitation (three with bambuterol, one with salmeterol). Four patients taking bambuterol withdrew owing to possible drug-related adverse effects

(insomnia, headache, flushing, and mental excitation) compared with one patient taking salmeterol (tremor). Bambuterol appears to be a safe and effective alternative to inhaled long-acting beta$_2$-adrenoceptor agonists for poorly controlled nocturnal symptoms in asthma.

Comparative studies

The comparative safety and efficacy of oral bambuterol given once daily and oral terbutaline given three times daily in children with asthma aged 2–12 years has recently been reported in two large similar trials from the same research group. In the first study they reported results from 3 months of treatment in 155 children aged 2–6 years (3); in the second study they reported results from 12 months of treatment in 130 children aged 2–12 years (4). Both were double-blind studies with a 2:1 bambuterol:terbutaline randomization pattern. In both studies, the bambuterol and terbutaline regimens were similarly efficacious in reducing asthma symptoms and improving peak expiratory flow rate. In the 3-month study, the most commonly reported adverse event was restlessness, reported in over 85% of patients in both treatment groups; other adverse events were described as mild to moderate, and overall there was no difference in the safety profile of the two drugs. In the 12-month trial, one subject in each treatment group withdrew because of an adverse event (urticaria and dermatitis). The most commonly reported adverse events attributable to the drugs were headache and tremor, which respectively occurred in 9 and 0% with terbutaline and 6 and 2% with bambuterol. Other adverse events were not described in detail. It seems that oral bambuterol has an efficacy and safety profile similar to that of oral terbutaline, with the advantage of once-daily dosing. The caveat is that inhaled therapy has fewer systemic adverse effects and is the route of choice.

Bambuterol once a day and modified-release salbutamol bd both produced a significant reduction in the severity of nocturnal asthma, but bambuterol caused significantly less tremor (5).

Organs and Systems

Cardiovascular

A retrospective study of prescriptions from three cohort studies suggested a possible adverse effect of oral bambuterol: cardiac failure. A cohort of 12 294 patients who received at least one prescription for nedocromil acted as the control group and was compared with 15 407 patients given inhaled salmeterol and 8098 patients given oral bambuterol. Questionnaires were sent to each prescriber asking for details of significant medical events after the first prescription (prescription event monitoring). From this information, rates and relative risks of non-fatal cardiac failure and ischemic heart disease were calculated. The age- and sex-adjusted relative risk of non-fatal cardiac failure associated with bambuterol was 3.41 (CI = 1.99, 5.86) compared with nedocromil. When salmeterol was compared with nedocromil the relative risk for developing non-fatal cardiac failure was 1.1 (CI = 0.63, 1.91). The adjusted relative risks of non-fatal ischemic heart disease with bambuterol and salmeterol compared with nedocromil were 1.23 (CI = 0.73, 2.08) and 1.07 (CI = 0.69, 1.66) respectively. In the month after the first prescription, the relative risk of non-fatal ischemic heart disease was 3.95 (CI = 1.38, 11.31), when bambuterol was compared with nedocromil. The authors concluded that care should be exercised when prescribing long-acting oral beta$_2$-adrenoceptor agonists for patients at risk of cardiac failure.

This study at best generates the hypothesis that the oral use of a particular beta$_2$-agonist is linked to an increased risk of cardiac disease. However, the study had several flaws. The three cohorts of patients were not strictly comparable: they were not treated concurrently nor were they sufficiently matched for age and diagnosis before prescription of the study drugs. It took nearly 3 years to recruit the patients, who preferred or needed an oral agent. A smaller proportion of patients in this cohort were treated for "asthmatic wheeze"—57 versus 70% in the salmeterol cohort. More of the bambuterol patients were given the drug for other indications, such as dyspnea, bronchitis, cough, chest infection, emphysema, and bronchitis—15 versus 2.8%. The salmeterol cohort consisted mostly of patients who were changing to a longer-acting agent and those using nedocromil were mostly changing from cromoglicate. The bambuterol group was more heterogeneous. Some patients with impending or undiagnosed heart failure may have presented with dyspnea, cough, or wheeze and received bambuterol. During the first month the correct diagnosis would become evident.

A review of the preclinical studies, clinical studies, and postmarketing surveillance data has given no support to the proposed association between bambuterol and cardiac failure. The UK Committee on Safety of Medicines has received no spontaneous reports of cardiac failure due to bambuterol. Data from the WHO database, INTDIS, show no reports of cardiac failure with bambuterol, in contrast to ten reports for salmeterol.

So, there is no evidence that oral beta$_2$-adrenoceptor agonists cause cardiac failure. The epidemiological study proposing the link is inadequate, and the authors themselves have emphasized the need for prospective, randomized trials.

Drug–Drug Interactions

Mivacurium

Bambuterol has been reported to alter the metabolism of mivacurium (6). Bambuterol has a dose-dependent inhibitory effect on plasma cholinesterase activity and prolongs the effects of suxamethonium. Bambuterol 10 mg was given to 28 patients 2 hours before an elective operation requiring general anesthesia. The study was originally designed as a randomized, blinded trial, but was converted to an open study. The patients given bambuterol had a 67–97% fall in plasma cholinesterase activity, leading to reduced clearance of mivacurium. This resulted in a shorter onset and a 3- to 4-fold prolongation of action of the neuromuscular blockade produced by standard doses of mivacurium.

References

1. Cazzola M, Donner CF, Matera MG. Long acting beta(2) agonists and theophylline in stable chronic obstructive pulmonary disease. Thorax 1999;54(8):730–6.
2. Wallaert B, Brun P, Ostinelli J, Murciano D, Champel F, Blaive B, Montane F, Godard P. A comparison of two long-acting beta-agonists, oral bambuterol and inhaled salmeterol, in the treatment of moderate to severe asthmatic patients with nocturnal symptoms. The French Bambuterol Study Group. Respir Med 1999;93(1):33–8.
3. Kuusela AL, Marenk M, Sandahl G, Sanderud J, Nikolajev K, Persson B. Comparative study using oral solutions of bambuterol once daily or terbutaline three times daily in 2–5-year-old children with asthma. Bambuterol Multicentre Study Group. Pediatr Pulmonol 2000;29(3):194–201.
4. Zarkovic JP, Marenk M, Valovirta E, Kuusela AL, Sandahl G, Persson B, Olsson H. One-year safety study with bambuterol once daily and terbutaline three times daily in 2–12-year-old children with asthma. The Bambuterol Multicentre Study Group. Pediatr Pulmonol 2000;29(6):424–9.
5. Gunn SD, Ayres JG, McConchie SM. Comparison of the efficacy, tolerability and patient acceptability of once-daily bambuterol tablets against twice-daily controlled release salbutamol in nocturnal asthma. ACROBATICS Research Group. Eur J Clin Pharmacol 1995;48(1):23–8.
6. Lebeau B, Gence B, Bourdain M, Loria Y. Le Kétotifene dans le traitement préventif de l'asthme. Analyse synthétique de 1791 observations de médecine praticienne. [Preventive treatment of asthma with ketotifen: an analysis of 1791 cases treated in general practice.] Poumon Coeur 1982;38(2):125–9.

Barium sulfate

General Information

Oral barium sulfate is theoretically non-toxic, but constipation and abdominal pain are not uncommon after barium meals or barium enemas (1). The main risk is that collections of barium will remain in the colon; they can persist for 6 weeks or longer in elderly patients or cases of colonic obstruction; barium fecoliths may even have to be removed surgically. Prolonged stasis of barium can occur after a barium enema into the distal loop of a colostomy. Residues in the appendix have caused appendicitis. Toxic dilatation of the colon can be aggravated by barium sulfate.

Organs and Systems

Cardiovascular

Electrocardiographic changes have been recorded during administration of barium enemas and could represent a hazard in cases of cardiac disease (2–4).

Respiratory

Aspiration of barium sulfate into the lungs during barium meal examination can cause significant respiratory embarrassment, particularly in patients with poor respiratory function. It is recommended that water-soluble low-osmolar contrast media, which are less harmful, should be used instead of barium if there is a possibility of aspiration during examination of the upper gastrointestinal tract.

Aspiration of barium sulfate can cause obstruction of the small air passages, compromising respiratory function, and can cause inflammation in the bronchial tree and lung parenchyma (5).

- A 68-year-old woman, with a history of alcohol abuse and a leiomyoma of the stomach, aspirated barium sulfate and became dyspneic and developed hypoxia (PaO_2 46 mmHg). At bronchoscopy the bronchial mucosa was coated with barium and a chest X-ray showed heavy alveolar deposition of barium sulfate distributed over the entire lung, with some predominance in the lower zones. The patient developed a fever (39°C) and a leukocytosis (12×10^9/l) the day after aspiration. She was given cefotiam 2000 mg and metronidazole 500 mg intravenously every 8 hours. The fever resolved within 2 days and *Staphylococcus aureus* was cultured from the bronchial fluid. She was discharged 2 days later, but the chest X-ray continued to show persistent alveolar deposition of the barium sulfate with only a slight improvement compared with the initial X-ray.
- A 60-year-old man with carcinoma of the hypopharynx aspirated barium into both lower lobes. He became hypoxic (PaO_2 64 mmHg) and barium was extracted at bronchoscopy. He was given prophylactic antibiotics (cefotiam 2000 mg and metronidazole 500 mg intravenously every 8 hours for 4 days). A chest X-ray 6 days later showed residual barium deposition in the lower lobes. No further respiratory complications occurred.

The authors recommended that bronchoscopy should be performed early after aspiration to extract barium from the bronchial tree, and that prophylactic antibiotic therapy is important to prevent lung infection.

Gastrointestinal

Perforation

After a barium enema, perforation occurs rarely in children and debilitated adults or when the colon is already weakened by inflammatory, malignant, or parasitic diseases. Perforation can be triggered by manipulations involved in giving the barium enema or can result from hydrostatic pressure. In one case, perforation followed air contrast insufflation for barium enema in a patient in whom the sigmoid colon became trapped in an inguinal hernia.

At least 12 cases of perforation of the colon by barium enema, with four deaths, were reported in a series of publications (SED-12, 1165) (6–8). The incidence of perforation was about 1 in 6000 examinations. Even sterile barium sulfate can cause marked peritoneal irritation, with considerable fluid loss into the peritoneal cavity, but in practice it is usually a mixture of barium and feces that escapes and this, not surprisingly, produces severe peritonitis and dense adhesions. Mortality has been reported to be 58% with conservative treatment, and as high as 47% with surgical intervention (9). Early operation is indicated, and large volumes of intravenous fluids improve the prognosis. Patients who recover can develop fibrogranulomatous reactions and adhesions, which can lead to bowel obstruction or ureteric occlusion.

Perforation can occur elsewhere than in the colon; in one case a duodenal ulcer was apparently made to perforate. In both this and another case of perforation of a sigmoid diverticulum the complication was not immediately recognized, the duodenal perforation only being detected 5 days after administration of the barium meal (SEDA-17, 535).

In air-contrast examinations, colonic perforation can actually precede the administration of the barium enema itself. In such cases it is due to the preparatory insufflation of air if this is conducted with excessive enthusiasm in a high-risk patient (for example an elderly patient with a hitherto unrecognized epigastric hernia) (10).

Extraperitoneal perforation and leakage of barium may cause few immediate symptoms, but delayed endotoxic shock can develop some 12 hours later, often causing death. Bowel infarction can also result. Barium granulomata can occur, causing painful masses, rectal strictures, or ulcers. On proctoscopy, an ulcer with a whitish base can mimic a carcinoma. In one rare case, perforation of a barium enema into a sigmoid abscess was followed by intravasation into the portal venous system (11).

Baroliths

Baroliths are rare complications of barium contrast examinations and are usually seen in colonic diverticula. They are often asymptomatic but may be associated with abdominal pain, appendicitis, and bowel obstruction or perforation. A case of ileal obstruction by a barolith has been reported (12)

- An 83-year-old woman developed postprandial abdominal pain. Physical examination and laboratory tests were normal. She underwent gastroscopy, abdominal ultrasound, small bowel barium meal, and a double-contrast barium enema, all of which were normal, although a moderate amount of barium refluxed into the small bowel during the double-contrast examination. She continued to have postprandial abdominal pain and weight loss. A repeat abdominal X-ray 6 months after the barium enema showed an unremarkable bowel gas pattern without evidence of obstruction. However, there was a 4.5 cm triangular radio-opaque structure in the right lower quadrant, consistent with retained barium, possibly in a diverticulum. A small bowel barium meal showed that the retained barium was intraluminal within a loop of ileum. At laparotomy, a hardened short segment of ileum was resected and histology showed an intraluminal barolith adjacent to a carcinoid tumor.

In this case, narrowing of a loop of ileum secondary to a carcinoid tumor caused interference with the flow of barium and caused the development of a barolith.

Immunologic

Hypersensitivity reactions to products used during barium meal examinations are extremely rare. Barium sulfate is generally regarded as an inert and insoluble compound that is neither absorbed nor metabolized and is eliminated unchanged from the body. However, some studies have shown that very small amounts of barium sulfate can be absorbed from the gastrointestinal tract. Plasma and urine barium concentrations can be increased after oral barium sulfate. In addition, there are many additives in commercially prepared barium products, some of which can cause immune responses. A patient with a history of a severe reaction to barium agents should not receive barium products again (SEDA-22, 503).

Reactions to other constituents of barium sulfate enemas have been recognized (SEDA-18, 441) and could be as common as one in 1000. They vary from urticarial rashes to severe anaphylactic reactions, and can be particularly severe in patients with asthma (13). Hypersensitivity to the latex balloon catheter used in double contrast barium enemas appears to be a common mechanism (14), but hypersensitivity to glucagon, to the preservative methylparabens, or to other additives seems to be responsible in some cases. Insofar as the latex balloon is concerned, thorough washing will remove the allergen responsible for the reaction (15).

Infection risk

Transient bacteremia was recorded in 11.4% of a series of 175 patients who had undergone barium enema examination; it appeared almost at once and lasted up to 15 minutes (16). Although a second study elsewhere failed to confirm these findings, a subsequent fatal case of staphylococcal septicemia in an elderly patient with an immune deficiency suggests that the risks are not merely theoretical (17).

Drug Administration

Drug additives

Tannic acid (up to 1.5%) was at one time added to barium enemas in order to improve the quality of the radiological picture. Tannic acid is hepatotoxic and fulminant liver disease very occasionally resulted. Although it was perhaps avoidable, being apparently associated mainly with higher tannic acid concentrations, mucosal damage, or a prior tannic acid washout of the bowel, the risks have made this technique obsolete.

Drug administration route

Accidental administration of a barium enema into the vagina instead of the rectum can occur and can be very hazardous; in some of these patients there has been fatal rupture of the vagina, with venous intravasation of the barium.

Barium given orally can be inhaled, and if there is incoordination of swallowing, inhalation of thick paste can cause fatal asphyxiation (18); aspiration of barium can also cause fatal pneumonia (19).

Accidental venous intravasation of barium during administration of a barium enema usually has a high immediate mortality, due to barium embolism in the lungs, but it occasionally causes few symptoms. In one intermediate case there was hypotension and evidence of disseminated intravascular coagulation (SEDA-9, 407); the patient recovered after intensive treatment.

Drug overdose

A fatal case of poisoning resulted from the use of barium sulfide, which had been mistaken for barium sulfate (SED-8, 1022) (20). Isolated cases of barium encephalopathy have been attributed to absorption of barium after the use of barium sulfate (SEDA-15, 498).

References

1. Smith HJ, Jones K, Hunter TB. What happens to patients after upper and lower gastrointestinal tract barium studies? Invest Radiol 1988;23(11):822–6.
2. Eastwood GL. ECG abnormalities associated with the barium enema. JAMA 1972;219(6):719–21.
3. Stremple J, Montgomery C. Nonspecific electrocardiographic abnormalities: the EKG during the barium enema procedure. Marquette Med Rev 1961;27:20–4.
4. Yigitbasi O, Sari S, Kiliccioglu B, Nalbantgil I. Recherche par l'ECG dynamique des modificiations cardiaques pouvant survenir pendant l'administration de lavements opaques. Effets protecteurs des bloqueurs des beta-recepteurs. [Dynamic ECG studies on possible cardiac modifications during the course of barium enemas. Protective effect of beta-receptor blockers.] J Radiol Electrol Med Nucl 1978;59(2):125–8.
5. Tamm I, Kortsik C. Severe barium sulfate aspiration into the lung: clinical presentation, prognosis and therapy. Respiration 1999;66(1):81–4.
6. Peterson N, Rohrmann CA Jr, Lennard ES. Diagnosis and treatment of retroperitoneal perforation complicating the double-contrast barium-enema examination. Radiology 1982;144(2):249–52.
7. Han SY, Tishler JM. Perforation of the colon above the peritoneal reflection during the barium-enema examination. Radiology 1982;144(2):253–5.
8. Nelson RL, Abcarian H, Prasad ML. Iatrogenic perforation of the colon and rectum Dis Colon Rectum 1982;25(4):305–308.
9. Zheutlin N, Lasser EC, Rigler LG. Clinical studies on effect of barium in the peritoneal cavity following rupture of the colon. Surgery 1952;32(6):967–79.
10. Rai AM, Johnson S. Epigastric hernia and perforation during air-contrast barium examinations. Am J Roentgenol 1990;155(2):420.
11. Wheatley MJ, Eckhauser FE. Portal venous barium intravasation complicating barium enema examination. Surgery 1991;109(6):788–91.
12. Regan JK, O'Neil HK, Aizenstein RI. Small bowel carcinoid presenting as a barolith. Clin Imaging 1999;23(1):22–5.
13. Stringer DA, Hassall E, Ferguson AC, Cairns R, Nadel H, Sargent M. Hypersensitivity reaction to single contrast barium meal studies in children. Pediatr Radiol 1993;23(8):587–8.
14. Ownby DR, Tomlanovich M, Sammons N, McCullough J. Anaphylaxis associated with latex allergy during barium enema examinations. Am J Roentgenol 1991;156(5):903–8.
15. Anonymous. Literature review: Allergic reactions to barium procedures and latex rubber. London: E-Z-EM Ltd.
16. Le Frock J, Ellis CA, Klainer AS, Weinstein L. Transient bacteremia associated with barium enema. Arch Intern Med 1975;135(6):835–7.
17. Hammer JL. Septicemia following barium enema. South Med J 1977;70(11):1361–3.
18. Lareau DG, Berta JW. Fatal aspiration of thick barium. Radiology 1976;120(2):317.

19. Gray C, Sivaloganathan S, Simpkins KC. Aspiration of high-density barium contrast medium causing acute pulmonary inflammation—report of two fatal cases in elderly women with disordered swallowing. Clin Radiol 1989; 40(4):397–400.
20. Govindiah D, Bhaskar GR. An unusual case of barium poisoning. Antiseptic 1972;69:675.

Barnidipine

See also Calcium channel blockers

General Information

Barnidipine is a dihydropyridine with antihypertensive activity and tolerability similar to that of other calcium antagonists of the same class. The most frequent adverse events are edema, headache, and flushing, but barnidipine does not cause reflex tachycardia (1).

Reference

1. Malhotra HS, Plosker GL. Barnidipine. Drugs 2001;61(7): 989–96.

Basidiomycetes

See also Herbal medicines

General Information

Basidiomycetes are fungi that include mushrooms, puff-balls, and bracket fungi.

Lentinus edodes

Lentinus edodes (shiitake) is an edible mushroom that contains a polysaccharide, lentinan. Its use is occasionally associated with skin reactions (1,2).

Adverse effects

Most adverse effects of *Lentinus edodes* occur in shiitake workers.

Respiratory
Lentinus edodes can cause an interstitial hypersensitivity pneumonitis called mushroom worker's lung, associated with IgG antibodies against shiitake spore antigens; those who cultivate white button mushrooms (*Agaricus*

bisporus) or the oyster mushroom (*Pleurotus* species) have only low titers (3).

Workers at a shiitake farm developed cough and sputum production after a variable period of exposure to shiitake mushrooms (4). All four had abnormal diffusing capacity and three had abnormal spirometry. Chest X-rays showed an interstitial pattern in one case. Pulmonary function tests fell significantly during several days of work, with a more than 20% fall in forced vital capacity and/or maximal mid-expiratory flow. Antigens to shiitake spore antigens, in common with antigens from other cultivated mushrooms (*Agaricus* and *Pleurotus*), were demonstrated by ELISA.

Bronchial asthma has been attributed to shiitake (5).

Skin
Skin reactions due to *Lentinus edodes* are not uncommon (1,2).

- A 42-year-old female shiitake grower developed skin lesions while planting shiitake hyphae into bed logs (6). She complained of repeated eczematous skin lesions during the planting season, from March to July, for 10 years. Each day she handled 7000 pieces of small conic blocks made of beech, with shiitake hyphae attached to their surface, and altogether 300 000 pieces each season. Patch tests with extracts of shiitake hyphae were positive. In contrast, female shiitake growers with skin lesions associated with work other than planting, and without skin lesions, were negative on patch-testing.

Drug interactions
Lentinan inhibits CYP1A (7), but the relevance of this to drug interactions in man is not known.

References

1. Nakamura T, Kobayashi A. Toxikodermie durch den Speisepilz Shiitake (*Lentinus edodes*). [Toxicodermia cause by the edible mushroom shiitake (*Lentinus edodes*).] Hautarzt 1985;36(10):591–3.
2. Nakamura T. Shiitake (*Lentinus edodes*) dermatitis Contact Dermatitis 1992;27(2):65–70.
3. Van Loon PC, Cox AL, Wuisman OP, Burgers SL, Van Griensven LJ. Mushroom worker's lung. Detection of antibodies against shii-take (*Lentinus edodes*) spore antigens in shii-take workers J Occup Med 1992;34(11):1097–101.
4. Sastre J, Ibanez MD, Lopez M, Lehrer SB. Respiratory and immunological reactions among shiitake (*Lentinus edodes*) mushroom workers Clin Exp Allergy 1990;20(1):13–19.
5. Kondo T. [Case of bronchial asthma caused by the spores of *Lentinus edodes* (Berk) Sing.] Arerugi 1969;18(1):81–5.
6. Ueda A, Obama K, Aoyama K, Ueda T, Xu BH, Li Q, Huang J, Kitano T, Inaoka T. Allergic contact dermatitis in shiitake (*Lentinus edodes* (Berk) Sing) growers Contact Dermatitis 1992;26(4):228–33.
7. Okamoto T, Kodoi R, Nonaka Y, Fukuda I, Hashimoto T, Kanazawa K, Mizuno M, Ashida H. Lentinan from shiitake mushroom (*Lentinus edodes*) suppresses expression of cytochrome P450 1A subfamily in the mouse liver Biofactors 2004;21(1–4):407–9.

Basiliximab

See also Monoclonal antibodies

General Information

Basiliximab is a chimeric (human/mouse) anti-interleukin-2 receptor monoclonal antibody used in the prophylaxis of acute renal transplant rejection. It acts by binding the alpha chain of interleukin-2 receptors on activated T lymphocytes. Initially positive results in phase III trials have not been generally confirmed (1,2).

Compared with placebo, basiliximab was not associated with any specific adverse effects in early studies (3). However, severe hypersensitivity reactions can occur and can be associated with the cytokine release syndrome.

Organs and Systems

Respiratory

There have been reports of non-cardiogenic pulmonary edema in three adolescent renal transplant recipients, one of whom died (4).

Immunologic

Basiliximab is composed of murine sequences (30%), which can cause IgE-mediated hypersensitivity reactions. Important warnings have been released by the manufacturers regarding the possible risk of severe hypersensitivity reactions within 24 hours of initial exposure or after re-exposure after several months, based on 17 reports that included cardiac and/or respiratory failure, bronchospasm, urticaria, cytokine release syndrome, and capillary leak syndrome.

- A 42-year-old Hispanic woman, with end-stage renal disease, anemia, hypertension, and a history of an anaphylactic reaction to basiliximab, was scheduled to receive a living donor transplant and received basiliximab uneventfully (5). However, owing to donor infection the procedure was cancelled and rescheduled for 2 weeks later. Within 10 minutes after basiliximab reinduction she developed an anaphylactic reaction. In an attempt to find another induction therapy for this patient, skin testing was performed for daclizumab without response. She therefore received full-dose induction with daclizumab before her organ transplant without adverse effect.
- A child had anaphylactic shock when he received a second course of basiliximab at the time of a second renal transplantation (6). There were antibasiliximab IgE antibodies in the serum, but no IgE reactivity toward a control murine IgG_{2a} monoclonal antibody, suggesting that the IgE response was directed exclusively against basiliximab idiotypes. There was no IgE reactivity against the humanized anti-interleukin-2 receptor monoclonal antibody daclizumab. The patient's basophils harvested months after the

anaphylactic shock produced leukotrienes in vitro on exposure to basiliximab.

Daclizumab, a humanized monoclonal antibody, is composed of only 10% murine antibody sequences and therefore is less immunogenic. These findings suggest that despite the similar compositions of human and mouse antibody protein sequences the IgE responsiveness is significantly different.

Drug–Drug Interactions

Ciclosporin

Basiliximab can inhibit ciclosporin metabolism transiently in children with renal transplants (7). Despite the use of lower daily doses, ciclosporin trough concentrations were significantly higher during the first 10 days after transplantation in 24 children who received basiliximab at days 0 and 4 after transplantation compared with 15 children who did not receive basiliximab. Ciclosporin dosage requirements again increased by 20% to achieve the target blood concentration at days 28–50 after transplantation. It is noteworthy that all seven acute episodes of rejection in the basiliximab group occurred during this period of time. However, these results have been debated, and there were no changes in ciclosporin dosage requirements in 54 children with liver transplants (8).

References

1. Crompton JA, Somerville T, Smith L, Corbett J, Nelson E, Holman J, Shihab FS. Lack of economic benefit with basiliximab induction in living related donor adult renal transplant recipients. Pharmacotherapy 2003;23(4):443–50.
2. Webster AC, Playford EG, Higgins G, Chapman JR, Craig J. Interleukin 2 receptor antagonists for kidney transplant recipients. Cochrane Database Syst Rev 2004;(1):CD003897.
3. Nashan B, Moore R, Amlot P, Schmidt AG, Abeywickrama K, Soulillou JP. Randomised trial of basiliximab versus placebo for control of acute cellular rejection in renal allograft recipients. CHIB 201 International Study Group. Lancet 1997;350(9086):1193–8.
4. Bamgbola FO, Del Rio M, Kaskel FJ, Flynn JT. Non-cardiogenic pulmonary edema during basiliximab induction in three adolescent renal transplant patients. Pediatr Transplant 2003;7(4):315–20.
5. Leonard PA, Woodside KJ, Gugliuzza KK, Sur S, Daller JA. Safe administration of a humanized murine antibody after anaphylaxis to a chimeric murine antibody. Transplantation 2002;74(12):1697–700.
6. Baudouin V, Crusiaux A, Haddad E, Schandene L, Goldman M, Loirat C, Abramowicz D. Anaphylactic shock caused by immunoglobulin E sensitization after retreatment with the chimeric anti-interleukin-2 receptor monoclonal antibody basiliximab. Transplantation 2003; 76(3):459–63.
7. Strehlau J, Pape L, Offner G, Nashan B, Ehrich JH. Interleukin-2 receptor antibody-induced alterations of ciclosporin dose requirements in paediatric transplant recipients. Lancet 2000;356(9238):1327–8.
8. Ganschow R, Grabhorn E, Burdelski M. Basiliximab in paediatric liver-transplant recipients. Lancet 2001; 357(9253):388.

Batanopride

General Information

Batanopride is a substituted benzamide with 5-HT$_3$ receptor antagonist activity. It is claimed to be free of dopaminergic properties. Clinical studies have concentrated on its use in patients suffering severe vomiting as a result of cytostatic therapy, but have run into problems because of poor tolerance at effective doses. The most important dose-limiting adverse effect is severe hypotension (1) but diarrhea and electrocardiographic changes also occur.

Comparative studies

In a randomized, double-blind comparison of intravenous batanopride 0.2–6.0 mg/kg and methylprednisolone 250 mg before cancer chemotherapy in 208 patients, the highest dose of batanopride was associated with a higher complete protection rate than the control group, but also had higher incidences of diarrhea, hypotension, and electrocardiographic abnormalities (2).

Organs and Systems

Cardiovascular

In a double-blind, randomized, crossover comparison of batanopride and metoclopramide in 21 chemotherapy-naive patients who received cisplatin at least 70 mg/m^2, the study was terminated when hypotension was observed after infusion of batanopride at other institutions testing similar drug schedules, although the authors themselves saw no cases of hypotension after treatment with batanopride (3). However, they did note asymptomatic prolongation of the QTc interval, PR interval, and QRS complex.

Susceptibility Factors

Renal disease

In 27 subjects with various degrees of renal function who were given an intravenous infusion of a single dose of batanopride 3.6 mg/kg over 15 minutes, the half-life was significantly prolonged from 2.7 hours in those with normal renal function to 9.9 hours in those with severe renal impairment (creatinine clearance below 30 ml/minute) (4). This was associated with a significant reduction in renal clearance. There were no differences in plasma protein binding or steady-state volume of distribution. There were significantly lower renal clearances of all three of the metabolites of batanopride in those with impaired renal function.

References

1. Herrstedt J, Jeppesen BH, Dombernowsky P. Dose-limiting hypotension with the 5-HT3-antagonist batanopride (BMY-25801). Ann Oncol 1991;2(2):154–5.
2. Rusthoven J, Pater J, Kaizer L, Wilson K, Osoba D, Latreille J, Findlay B, Lofters WS, Warr D, Laberge F, et al. A randomized, double-blinded study comparing six doses of batanopride (BMY-25801) with methylprednisolone in patients receiving moderately emetogenic chemotherapy Ann Oncol 1991;2(9):681–6.
3. Fleming GF, Vokes EE, McEvilly JM, Janisch L, Francher D, Smaldone L. Double-blind, randomized crossover study of metoclopramide and batanopride for prevention of cisplatin-induced emesis. Cancer Chemother Pharmacol 1991;28(3):226–7.
4. St Peter JV, Brady ME, Foote EF, Dandekar KA, Smaldone L, Pykkonen JL, Keane WF, Halstenson CE. The disposition and protein binding of batanopride and its metabolites in subjects with renal impairment. Eur J Clin Pharmacol 1993;45(1):59–63.

Bemetizide

See also Diuretics

General Information

Bemetizide is chemically unrelated to the thiazides, but it shares many of their actions and adverse effects.

Susceptibility Factors

Age

The pharmacokinetics and pharmacodynamics of a fixed combination of bemetizide 25 mg and triamterene 50 mg have been evaluated in 15 elderly patients (aged 70–84 years) and 10 young volunteers (aged 18–30 years) after single doses (on day 1) and multiple doses (at steady state on day 8) (1). Mean plasma concentrations of bemetizide, triamterene, and the active metabolite of triamterene, hydroxytriamterene, were significantly higher in the elderly subjects after single and multiple doses, and urine flow and sodium excretion rates fell in tandem with the accumulation of these drugs. The glomerular filtration rate, which is reduced in elderly people, was further reduced at higher concentrations of bemetizide and triamterene, which may explain why there were limited diuretic and saliuretic effects after multiple doses. This study clearly points to a modulating effect of the degree of renal function on the diuretic actions of these compounds in elderly people.

Drug–Drug Interactions

Triamterene

In 1988 the Federal German Health Authorities issued a warning about fixed combinations of the thiazide bemetizide and triamterene that they could cause allergic vasculitis (2). Thiazides can occasionally cause allergic vasculitis and it is not clear on what basis the combination might be more likely to cause the same problem.

References

1. Muhlberg W, Mutschler E, Hofner A, Spahn-Langguth H, Arnold O. The influence of age on the pharmacokinetics and pharmacodynamics of bemetizide and triamterene: a single and multiple dose study. Arch Gerontol Geriatr 2001;32(3):265–73.
2. Anonymous. Bemetizide/triamterene: warning of allergic vasculitis. WHO Drug Inform 1988;2:148.

Benazepril

See also Angiotensin converting enzyme inhibitors

General Information

Safety data derived from the controlled trials submitted in the benazepril New Drug Application for hypertension have been reviewed (1). In more than 100 trials involving 6000 patients with hypertension or congestive heart failure, the types and incidences of adverse effects were comparable with those of other ACE inhibitors.

Organs and Systems

Pancreas

Benazepril has been associated with pancreatitis (2).

- A 70-year old man with type II diabetes had severe epigastric pain 30 minutes after taking his first dose of 5 mg benazepril and lasting 6–8 hours. The next day he had the same pain, complicated by vomiting. Benazepril was withdrawn and he was unable to eat for 4 days. He later developed severe epigastric pain, nausea, and vomiting 30 minutes after taking a third dose. Laboratory findings confirmed pancreatitis and imaging showed a mildly edematous inflamed pancreas. He improved progressively with bowel rest and pethidine. He was symptom-free 2 months after discharge.

References

1. MacNab M, Mallows S. Safety profile of benazepril in essential hypertension. Clin Cardiol 1991;14(8 Suppl 4):IV33–7.
2. Muchnick JS, Mehta JL. Angiotensin-converting enzyme inhibitor-induced pancreatitis. Clin Cardiol 1999;22(1):50–1.

Benorilate

General Information

Benorilate is an acetylsalicylic ester of paracetamol. It is slowly absorbed unchanged from the gastrointestinal tract but is rapidly hydrolysed to its components, aspirin and paracetamol. Thereafter its effects and kinetics are those of the two moieties. However, the delay in its metabolism reduces the incidence of direct gastric irritation, delays its onset of action, and prolongs its duration of action (1,2).

Drug Administration

Drug overdose

In cases of suspected benorilate overdosage, both salicylate and paracetamol should be assayed.

References

1. Reizenstein P, Doberl A. Relevance of gastrointestinal symptoms and blood loss after long term treatment with a salicylate-paracetamol ester. A new anti-inflammatory agent (benorylate). Rheum and Rehab Suppl 1973;75.
2. Wright V. A review of benorylate – a new antirheumatic drug. Scand J Rheumatol Suppl 1975;(13):5–8.

Benoxaprofen

See also Non-steroidal anti-inflammatory drugs

General Information

Since benoxaprofen, like zomepirac, provided an experience from which several lessons can be learnt, it deserves to be briefly reviewed, even though it was withdrawn 10 years ago. Some newer drugs may have some of its chemical or pharmacological characteristics and, consequently, its problems. Benoxaprofen was originally launched in 1980, with claims of a favorable adverse effects profile and "unique disease-modifying properties" in rheumatoid arthritis. These claims appeared to have been based on the fact that it was a relatively more potent inhibitor of leukotriene production and a less potent inhibitor of prostaglandin synthesis than other NSAIDs. Having passed all preclinical and clinical tests and satisfied the safety requirements set by regulatory authorities in many countries (despite rejection in several on grounds of safety), benoxaprofen was then suspended by the UK Committee on Safety of Medicines in 1982, about 18 months after marketing. Shortly afterwards it was withdrawn worldwide by its manufacturers (1). Benoxaprofen was associated with a very high incidence of adverse effects, prominent effects on the skin and nails and liver reactions, which sometimes proved fatal, particularly in elderly people.

The case led to considerable regulatory and medicolegal discussions in the 10 years after withdrawal. In the USA the company was charged by the Food and Drug Administration with misbranding the drug in press statements and associated materials, which contained a misleading headline implying that the drug was harmless, even though the company was aware of a report of deaths related to the use of benoxaprofen. The company's intense marketing campaign was heavily criticized (SEDA-8) and it was noted that the recommendation of the WHO that drugs likely to be used in elderly people should be investigated in them at an early stage had certainly been disregarded in the premarketing phases. In the UK the company rejected patients' demands to establish a compensation scheme and offered instead a financial settlement that the patients rejected as inadequate. The case shows how some legal systems are inadequate for dealing with mass claims of personal injury due to drugs.

Organs and Systems

Gastrointestinal

The hope of better gastric tolerance of benoxaprofen was not fulfilled, and the incidence of this type of reaction was actually higher in elderly patients.

Liver

Fatal liver damage was observed particularly in the UK and tended to occur in elderly subjects. The complication initially presented as jaundice or raised liver enzymes (including alkaline phosphatase). Surprisingly, biochemical and histological liver changes were not consistent with major hepatocellular damage. There were three reports of primary biliary cirrhosis, but a causal relation was not proven (SEDA-12, 84).

Urinary tract

All types of kidney damage were reported, ranging from a transitory fall in glomerular filtration rate and reversible renal insufficiency (part of multisystem disease with circulating LE cells) to the nephrotic syndrome.

Skin

Cutaneous adverse effects were the most frequent problem and (together with hepatic complications) the most serious: 63% of 300 patients treated for 6 months complained of one or more adverse effects (total 259 reactions); 70% were cutaneous; photosensitivity led to withdrawal in 30% of cases. Multiple subepidermal cysts (milia) on sun-exposed skin areas and onycholysis (13% of patients) were documented. Other skin reactions included rashes, hypertrichosis, erythema multiforme, and Stevens–Johnson syndrome (2). Phototoxicity persisted for many months after withdrawal (SEDA-12, 84); although a later study on persistent photosensitivity as a sequel to benoxaprofen in 42 subjects failed to confirm the link between photosensitivity and the drug (3), this was contrary to the overwhelming experience in the field. In retrospect, it seems likely that one problem was that benoxaprofen had largely been studied during the winter months, whereas in the UK it was launched in the summer.

References

1. Anonymous. Benoxaprofen. BMJ (Clin Res Ed) 1982; 285(6340):459–60.
2. Halsey JP, Cardoe N. Benoxaprofen: side-effect profile in 300 patients. BMJ (Clin Res Ed) 1982;284(6326):1365–8.
3. Frain-Bell W. A study of persistent photosensitivity as a sequel of the prior administration of the drug benoxaprofen. Br J Dermatol 1989;121(5):551–62.

Bentazepam

See also Benzodiazepines

General Information

Bentazepam is a benzodiazepine with properties similar to those of diazepam.

Organs and Systems

Liver

In three cases chronic hepatocellular injury developed with oral bentazepam (1).

Reference

1. Andrade RJ, Lucena MI, Aguilar J, Lazo MD, Camargo R, Moreno P, Garcia-Escano MD, Marquez A, Alcantara R, Alcain G. Chronic liver injury related to use of bentazepam: an unusual instance of benzodiazepine hepatotoxicity. Dig Dis Sci 2000;45(7):1400–4.

Benzalkonium chloride

See also Disinfectants and antiseptics

General Information

Quaternary ammonium compounds are surface-active agents. Some of them precipitate or denature proteins and destroy microorganisms. The most important disinfectants in this group are cationic surface-active agents, such as benzalkonium chloride, benzethonium chloride and methylbenzethonium chloride, and cetylpyridinium chloride; the problems that they cause are similar.

Benzalkonium chloride is composed of a mixture of alkyldimethylbenzylammonium chlorides. The hydrophobic alkyl residues are paraffinic chains with 8–18 carbon atoms. Benzalkonium chloride is used as a preservative in suspensions and solutions for nasal sprays and in eye-drops. Depending on the concentration of the solution, local irritant effects can occur. In nasal sprays it can exacerbate rhinitis (1) and in eye-drops it can cause irritation or keratitis (2).

A total of 125 ophthalmologists in private practice located throughout France examined 919 glaucomatous patients treated with eye-drops which either did or did not contain a preservative; the proportion of patients who experienced discomfort or pain during instillation was 58% for eye-drops containing a preservative and 30% for eye-drops with no preservative (2). Moreover, the proportion of patients presenting at least one symptom of eye irritation (sensation of itching or burning, sensation of a foreign body in the eye, and flow of tears) was greater with preservative-containing eye-drops (53 versus 34%). The experience of discomfort during instillation was more often associated with problems later on. The patient's complaints were correlated with objective signs of conjunctival damage (conjunctival redness, conjunctival follicles), or corneal damage (superficial punctate keratitis). A higher proportion of patients treated with eye-drops containing a preservative had at least one conjunctival sign (52 versus 35%) or superficial punctate keratitis (12 versus 4%). In 164 patients whose treatment was changed from eye-drops containing a preservative to eye-drops with no preservative and who were examined a second time (mean interval between visits 3.3 months) the frequency of all symptoms and objective signs fell by a factor of 3 to 4.

Organs and Systems

Respiratory

An asthmatic patient whose salbutamol formulation was replaced by another containing benzalkonium chloride as an excipient developed bronchospasm as a result (3).

Benzalkonium chloride is used as a preservative in nebulizer solutions and can cause secondary paradoxical bronchoconstriction in patients with bronchial asthma. Although nebulizers containing beta-adrenoceptor agonists may also contain benzalkonium chloride, reports are more common with anticholinergic drugs. This is probably because of the more rapid onset and larger effect of sympathomimetic-induced bronchodilatation compared with anticholinergic drugs (4).

Ear, nose, throat

Benzalkonium chloride accentuated the severity of rhinitis medicamentosa and increased histamine sensitivity in a 30-day study with oxymetazoline nasal spray in healthy volunteers (5,6).

Sensory systems

Benzalkonium chloride is used in eye-drops in concentrations of 0.033 or 0.025%. At a dilution of 1:1000 (0.1%), a drop applied to the human cornea causes mild discomfort that persists for 2 or 3 hours. Slit-lamp examination within 90 seconds shows fine grey clots (epithelial keratitis) in the corneal epithelium. Within 10 minutes, a grey haze can be seen on the corneal surface; superficial desquamation of the conjunctival epithelium can follow. The superficial irritation and disturbances disappear in a day or less.

Patients with glaucoma, dry eyes, infections, or iritis, sometimes use solutions containing benzalkonium chloride often enough and for long enough to cause damage. In these patients, there is a higher incidence of endothelial damage, epithelial edema, and bullous keratopathy, and because of the severity of the disease, additional damage from the medication can be overlooked. This is especially true in patients with defective epithelium or corneal ulcers, in whom the medication can penetrate well and who can be most vulnerable. There have been analogous results in investigations of benzethonium chloride, cetrimonium bromide, cetylpyridinium chloride, decyldodecylbromide, hexadecyl, and tetradecyltrimethylammonium bromide (SEDA-11, 490).

Immunologic

Life-threatening anaphylactic reactions that rarely occur during general anesthesia are mostly due to neuromuscular blockers. They may be due to cross-allergy mediated by drug-specific IgE antibodies to the quaternary ammonium moiety of the neuromuscular blocker molecule, perhaps with a contribution from IgE-independent mechanisms. Quaternary ammonium compounds, such as benzalkonium, in cosmetics and toiletries may play a role in sensitization (7).

Allergic reactions can occur after topical use, but are fairly rare. Allergic contact dermatitis has been reported in some cases. Allergic rhinitis on contact has also been reported.

In a study of the efficacy and acceptability of benzalkonium chloride-containing contraceptives (vaginal sponges, pessaries, and creams) in 56 women, one developed an allergic reaction with edema of the vulva (4). Non-allergic local irritation, itching, and a burning sensation were reported in nine women and nine husbands.

Infection risk

The bactericidal activity of benzalkonium chloride is limited to the Gram-positive and some of the Gram-negative bacteria, but *Pseudomonas* species are especially resistant and can cause severe infection. Too often it is not realized that the disinfectant can be contaminated with active multiplying resistant organisms.

Pseudomonas bacteremia has been attributed to the use of material in open-heart surgery that was stored in accidentally contaminated benzalkonium solutions, and after cardiac catheterization caused by inadequate disinfection of the catheters with benzalkonium solutions. In 1961, about 15 patients were reported with *Pseudomonas* infections caused by cotton pledgets kept in a contaminated aqueous solution used for skin antisepsis before intravenous and intramuscular injection (8). In 1976 there were outbreaks of *Pseudomonas cepacia* infections in two American general hospitals (9) and pseudobacteremia (*Pseudomonas cepacia* or *Enterobacter*) caused by contamination of blood cultures in 79 patients in whom contaminated aqueous benzalkonium solutions were used for skin and antisepsis before venepuncture and due to contamination of the samples (SEDA-11, 490) (10).

References

1. Hillerdal G. Adverse reaction to locally applied preservatives in nose drops. ORL J Otorhinolaryngol Relat Spec 1985;47(5):278–9.
2. Levrat F, Pisella PJ, Baudouin C. Tolérance clinique des collyres antiglaucomateux conservés et non conservés. Résultats d'une enquête inédite en Europe. [Clinical tolerance of antiglaucoma eyedrops with and without a preservative. Results of an unpublished survey in Europe.] J Fr Ophtalmol 1999;22(2):186–91.
3. Ontario Medical Association's Committee on Drugs and Pharmacotherapy. Preservatives: bronchospasm. The Drug Report 1987;24.
4. Meyer U, Gerhard I, Runnebaum B. Benzalkonium-chlorid zur vaginaten Kontrazeption—der Scheidenschwamm. [Benzalkonium chloride for vaginal contraception—the

vaginal sponge.] Geburtshilfe Frauenheilkd 1990;50(7): 542–7.

5. Graf P, Hallen H, Juto JE. Benzalkonium chloride in a decongestant nasal spray aggravates rhinitis medicamentosa in healthy volunteers. Clin Exp Allergy 1995;25(5):395–400.

6. Hallen H, Graf P. Benzalkonium chloride in nasal decongestive sprays has a long-lasting adverse effect on the nasal mucosa of healthy volunteers. Clin Exp Allergy 1995;25(5): 401–5.

7. Weston A, Assem ES. Possible link between anaphylactoid reactions to anaesthetics and chemicals in cosmetics and biocides. Agents Actions 1994;41(Spec No):C138–9.

8. Lee JC, Fialkow PJ. Benzalkonium chloride-source of hospital infection with Gram-negative bacteria. JAMA 1961;177:708–10.

9. Dixon RE, Kaslow RA, Mackel DC, Fulkerson CC, Mallison GF. Aqueous quaternary ammonium antiseptics and disinfectants. Use and misuse. JAMA 1976;236(21): 2415–17.

10. Kaslow RA, Mackel DC, Mallison GF. Nosocomial pseudobacteremia. Positive blood cultures due to contaminated benzalkonium antiseptic. JAMA 1976;236(21):2407–9.

Benzatropine and etybenzatropine

See also Anticholinergic drugs

General Information

Benzatropine and etybenzatropine (ethylbenzatropine) are anticholinergic drugs. They represent attempts to combine atropine-like and antihistaminic effects in single molecules. The dose is determined individually and varies from 0.5 to 6 mg/day for benzatropine and 6 to 30 mg/day for etybenzatropine. Although the adverse reactions are essentially those of the anticholinergic drugs, sedation is very likely to occur and these drugs should not be used in patients who need to drive motor vehicles. Benzatropine has also been reported to cause rash, peripheral numbness, and muscular weakness.

Organs and Systems

Cardiovascular

A paradoxical sinus bradycardia in a psychotic patient was attributed to benzatropine since it abated when benzatropine (but not others) was withdrawn (SEDA-17, 174).

Psychological, psychiatric

Benzatropine can cause slight memory impairment, detectable if special studies of mental function are performed (SEDA-13, 115) (SEDA-15, 137).

Second-Generation Effects

Teratogenicity

There have been two cases of "small left colon" in infants whose mothers had taken various psychotropic drugs,

including benzatropine, late in pregnancy; the causal link was not at all clear (SEDA-6, 142).

Drug–Drug Interactions

Paroxetine

When paroxetine was introduced in a patient taking benzatropine and haloperidol, the circulating concentrations of benzatropine rose and delirium occurred (SEDA-22, 157) (1).

Reference

1. Boudouresques G, Tafani B, Benichou M, Sarlon R. Encéphalopathie myoclonique à la dopamine. [Myoclonal encephalopathy due to dopamine.] Sem Hop 1982;58(46): 2729–30.

Benzbromarone

General Information

Benzbromarone is a benzofuran derivative chemically related to amiodarone. It increases uric acid excretion by non-specifically inhibiting its tubular reabsorption.

It is used in patients with venous disorders to prevent, retard, or reverse varicose degenerative changes in the vessel wall.

Benzbromarone causes diarrhea (3–4% of patients), urate and oxalate stones, urinary sand, renal colic, and allergy in a small number of patients (1). Liver damage, which reverses after withdrawal, has been described (SEDA-18, 108).

Organs and Systems

Liver

After reports of several cases of acute hepatitis (SEDA-16, 205) benzbromarone was withdrawn from the market in several European countries (SEDA-17, 244). Liver damage reportedly reverses after withdrawal (SEDA-18, 108)

Drug–Drug Interactions

Anticoagulants

As benzbromarone is a coumarin derivative, it can potentiate the effects of anticoagulants, which act as vitamin K antagonists.

Reference

1. Masbernard A, Giudicelli CP. Ten years' experience with benzbromarone in the management of gout and hyperuricaemia. S Afr Med J 1981;59(20):701–6.

Benzethonium chloride and methylbenzethonium chloride

See also Disinfectants and antiseptics

General Information

Quaternary ammonium compounds are surface-active agents. Some of them precipitate or denature proteins and destroy microorganisms. The most important disinfectants in this group are cationic surface-active agents, such as benzalkonium chloride, benzethonium chloride and methylbenzethonium chloride, and cetylpyridinium chloride; the problems that they cause are similar.

In an extensive report, the Expert Panel of the American College of Toxicology (1) has concluded that both benzethonium chloride and methylbenzethonium chloride can be regarded as safe when applied to the skin at a concentration of 0.5% or when used around the eye in cosmetics at a maximum concentration of 0.02%. In clinical studies, benzethonium chloride produced mild skin irritation at 5%, but not at lower concentrations. Neither ingredient is considered to be a sensitizer.

Drug Administration

Drug overdose

The Paris Poison Center has received reports on 45 cases of acute accidental poisoning, with 18 deaths (2). All the victims were mentally disturbed patients who had ingested Airsane HP 800, a water-soluble powder packed in a sachet; it contains a mixture of quaternary ammonium compounds and was left in the patients' rooms by hospital workers. Symptoms were corrosive burns of the mouth, pharynx, esophagus, and sometimes of the respiratory tract.

References

1. Anonymous. Final report on the safety assessment of benzethonium chloride and methylbenzethonium chloride. J Am Coll Toxicol 1985;4:65.
2. Chataigner D, Garnier R, Sans S, Efthymiou ML. Intoxication aiguë accidentelle par un désinfectant hospitalier. 45 cas dont 13 d'évolution mortelle. [Acute accidental poisoning with hospital disinfectant. 45 cases of which 13 with fatal outcome.] Presse Méd 1991;20(16):741–3.

Benzimidazoles

See also Individual agents

General Information

The benzimidazoles are a group of compounds that include albendazole, flubendazole, mebendazole, niridazole, triabendazole, and triclabendazole.

The newer broad-spectrum benzimidazoles have a wide spectrum of antihelminthic activity, killing larval and adult cestodes as well as intestinal nematodes, with generally low mammalian toxicity, apart from a potential for teratogenicity and embryotoxicity. The principal members of the group are mebendazole, its fluorine analogue flubendazole, and the better-absorbed albendazole. Mebendazole and albendazole are active orally in a single dose for a wide range of intestinal nematodes and are being used increasingly in the treatment of hydatid disease, in which experience is rapidly advancing. Flubendazole is very poorly absorbed and causes local tissue reactions at the site of injection when given parenterally.

None of the benzimidazoles is known to be safe in pregnancy and animal studies and their spectrum of toxicity suggest that they should be avoided. The absence of reports of harm in human pregnancy does not mean that no harm can occur.

The antihelminthic activity of the benzimidazoles is thought to result from selective blockade of glucose uptake by adult worms lodged in the intestine and their tissue-dwelling larvae, resulting in endogenous depletion of glycogen stores and reduced formation of adenosine triphosphate, which appears to be essential for parasite reproduction and survival. However, benzimidazole antihelminthics may also have antiparasitic activity by binding to free β-tubulin, thereby inhibiting the polymerization of tubulin and microtubule-dependent glucose uptake (1).

Uses

Ankylostomiasis

In 13 British soldiers with cutaneous larva migrans after a 2-week jungle training exercise in Belize the median incubation period was 10 (range 4–38) days; in 12 there were skin lesions on the calves or shins, and only two had foot or ankle lesions (2). Ten received oral thiabendazole, one oral mebendazole, one oral albendazole, and one topical thiabendazole. All those treated with oral thiabendazole complained of unpleasant reactions, predominantly nausea, vomiting, and dizziness. The one patient treated with topical thiabendazole returned with a new lesion 12 months later. He was then treated with systemic albendazole, with rapid resolution of symptoms. A 45-year-old woman developed larva migrans 20 days after lying on a beach in Singapore and was treated with thiabendazole 50 mg/kg in two doses for one day; she had no adverse effects (3).

The treatment of cutaneous larva migrans in 56 Italian patients aged 2–60 years has been retrospectively reviewed (4). All 13 patients treated with cryotherapy reported that it was painful, but none had recurrent disease or scarring. A further six patients were treated with oral thiabendazole 25–50 mg/kg/day for 2 days, and one had both thiabendazole and cryotherapy. In all cases there was regression of itching and skin lesions, but they had nausea, diarrhea, and dizziness while taking oral thiabendazole. No adverse effects were reported in 36 patients who were treated with albendazole 400 mg/day for 3 days (two were also treated with cryotherapy). Despite the low dose, larval migration was stopped in 1–2 days. Although a prompt and definitive cure was achieved in all 56 patients, albendazole was considered the treatment of choice given its minimal adverse effects. Until about 1980, surgery was the only treatment available for larval infections with *Echinococcus granulosus* or *Echinococcus multilocularis*. However, cysts are not always amenable to surgical removal, and operation is associated with the risk of rupture, leading to anaphylactic shock and re-infection; a proportion of cases are in any case not fit enough for surgery. The benzimidazoles have been used in varying high dosages over extended periods, initially to treat inoperable hydatid cysts and before surgery in attempts to sterilize cysts.

Echinococcosis

The epidemiology, clinical presentation, and treatment of alveolar echinococcosis of the liver have been described in French patients followed between 1972 and 1993 (5). From 1982 benzimidazoles were used. Of 117 patients, 72 took either albendazole or mebendazole for 4–134 months. The most common adverse effects were an increase in alanine transaminase activity to more than five times the top of the reference range (in six patients taking albendazole and in three taking mebendazole). Neutropenia (leukocyte count below $1.0 \times 10^9/l$) occurred in two patients taking albendazole. Alopecia occurred in four patients taking mebendazole. Minor adverse effects of albendazole included malaise, anorexia, and digestive intolerance in one patient each. In 13 patients treatment had to be withdrawn because of adverse effects ($n = 10$) or non-adherence to therapy ($n = 3$).

While mebendazole is used in continuous therapy of human alveolar echinococcosis, albendazole has been used in cyclic treatment. One treatment cycle consists of 28 days followed by a washout phase of 14 days without treatment, intended to reduce toxicity. Whether albendazole can also be used on a continuous basis has recently been studied in an open observational study in 35 patients with alveolar echinococcosis (in seven of 35 patients a curative operation was performed) (6). The outcome (lack of progression) was compared with the results obtained with continuous treatment with mebendazole or cyclic albendazole. Albendazole 10–15 mg/kg/day and mebendazole 40–50 mg/kg/day were equally effective. Seven patients were treated with continuous albendazole for an average of 28 (range 13–50) months. All patients taking continuous albendazole had stable or even regressive disease. The continuous dosing regimen was well tolerated without increased toxicity or higher rates of adverse reactions. Therefore, continuous dosing of albendazole is a promising alternative in cases of inoperable or progressive alveolar echinococcosis.

Prolonged cyclic albendazole treatment (for more than 9 years) was safe and effective in a patient with isolated cervical spine echinococcosis in whom surgery was performed without preoperative antihelminthic therapy because of a delay in diagnosis (7).

There have been several studies of the efficacy of albendazole in preventing recurrences of hydatid disease and cyst fluid spillage complications after surgery. In one Turkish study 22 of 36 patients with echinococcosis were treated with albendazole after surgical intervention (8). There was no significant benefit of perioperative albendazole over operation alone, although the recurrence rate of hepatic echinococcosis was lower than in historical controls. In contrast, in another study in 22 patients with hepatic echinococcosis there was a clear benefit of peri- and postoperative cyclic albendazole (12–15 mg/kg/day in four divided doses) (9). There were no cases of secondary hydatid disease or recurrence after a mean follow-up of 20 months. In two cases there were liver function abnormalities, which normalized after withdrawal.

Neurocysticercosis

Cysticercosis is caused by the larval stage of the pork tapeworm *Tenia solium*. Neurocysticercosis is the most severe and common clinical manifestation in humans and probably the most frequent parasitic infection of the central nervous system. *T. solium* is endemic in Latin America, Asia, and sub-Saharan Africa. However, with the advent of computerized neuroradiology and improved serological tests, neurocysticercosis is increasingly being diagnosed throughout the world.

Controversies in the management of neurocysticercosis have been described (10–12). The management of the neurological complications of cysticercosis and in particular the role of antiparasitic drugs are issues of debate. It is commonly believed that the use of antiparasitic drugs and steroids should be individualized, based on the presence of active or inactive disease, the location of the cysts, and the presence or absence of complications such as hydrocephalus.

Some imidazoles have been used to treat parenchymal brain cysticerci. Initially, flubendazole (40 mg/kg for 10 days) was given to 13 patients with neurocysticercosis, with promising results. However, owing to its poor intestinal absorption, the use of flubendazole is limited. Albendazole is usually well absorbed and well tolerated, and albendazole serum concentrations are not significantly affected by glucocorticoids or anticonvulsants. Albendazole was given in daily doses of 15 mg/kg for 30 days. Further studies, however, showed that a treatment course could be shortened from 30 to 8 days without affecting efficacy. Direct comparative trials have shown that albendazole usually destroys 75–90% of parenchymal brain cysts, whereas praziquantel destroys 60–70%. The advantage of albendazole over praziquantel is limited not to its better efficacy, but also to better penetration of the subarachnoid space, allowing destruction of meningeal cysticerci. It also costs less than praziquantel.

References

1. Georgiev VS. Necatoriasis: treatment and developmental therapeutics. Expert Opin Investig Drugs 2000;9(5):1065–78.
2. Green AD, Mason C, Spragg PM. Outbreak of cutaneous larva migrans among British military personnel in Belize. J Travel Med 2001;8(5):267–9.
3. Gourgiotou K, Nicolaidou E, Panagiotopoulos A, Hatziolou JE, Katsambast AD. Treatment of widespread cutaneous larva migrans with thiabendazole. J Eur Acad Dermatol Venereol 2001;15(6):578–80.
4. Albanese G, Venturi C, Galbiati G. Treatment of larva migrans cutanea (creeping eruption): a comparison between albendazole and traditional therapy. Int J Dermatol 2001;40(1):67–71.
5. Bresson-Hadni S, Vuitton DA, Bartholomot B, Heyd B, Godart D, Meyer JP, Hrusovsky S, Becker MC, Mantion G, Lenys D, Miguet JP. A twenty-year history of alveolar echinococcosis: analysis of a series of 117 patients

from eastern France. Eur J Gastroenterol Hepatol 2000;12(3):327–36.

6. Reuter S, Jensen B, Buttenschoen K, Kratzer W, Kern P. Benzimidazoles in the treatment of alveolar echinococcosis: a comparative study and review of the literature. J Antimicrob Chemother 2000;46(3):451–6.

7. Garcia-Vicuna R, Carvajal I, Ortiz-Garcia A, Lopez-Robledillo JC, Laffon A, Sabando P. Primary solitary echinococcosis in cervical spine. Postsurgical successful outcome after long-term albendazole treatment. Spine 2000;25(4):520–3.

8. Mentes A, Yalaz S, Killi R, Altintas N. Radical treatment for hepatic echinococcosis. HPB 2000;2:49–54.

9. Erzurumlu K, Hokelek M, Gonlusen L, Tas K, Amanvermez R. The effect of albendazole on the prevention of secondary hydatidosis. Hepatogastroenterology 2000;47(31):247–50.

10. Di Pentima MC, White AC. Neurocysticercosis: controversies in management. Semin Pediatr Infect Dis 2000;11:261–8.

11. Del Brutto OH. Medical therapy for cysticercosis: indications, risks, and benefits. Rev Ecuat Neurol 2000;9:13–15.

12. Garg RK. Medical management of neurocysticercosis. Neurol India 2001;49(4):329–37.

Benznidazole

General Information

Benznidazole, a nitroimidazole, is used in the treatment of *Trypanosoma cruzi* infections and Chagas' disease, and is recommended for use in urogenital trichomoniasis, all forms of amebiasis, giardiasis, and anaerobic infections. Its adverse effects are similar to those of metronidazole (SEDA-13, 833). Drowsiness, dizziness, headache, and ataxia occur occasionally. With prolonged and/or high doses, transient peripheral neuropathy and epileptiform seizures can be seen. Other frequently mentioned adverse effects are unpleasant taste, furred tongue, nausea, vomiting, and gastrointestinal disturbances. Skin rash and pruritus can occur. One case each of erythema multiforme and of toxic epidermolysis have been reported. Benznidazole causes a disulfiram-like effect with ethanol.

Placebo-controlled studies

In a double-blind, randomized, clinical trial, benznidazole 5 mg/kg/day for 60 days was compared with placebo in children in the indeterminate phase of infection by *Trypanosoma cruzi* (1). In general, treatment was well tolerated. The treated children had a significant reduction in mean titers of antibodies against *T. cruzi* measured by indirect hemagglutination, indirect immunofluorescence, and ELISA. At 4-year follow-up, 62% of the benznidazole-treated children and no placebo-treated child were seronegative for *T. cruzi*. Xenodiagnosis after 48 months was positive in 4.7% of the benznidazole-treated children and in 51% of the placebo-treated children.

General adverse effects

The adverse effects of benznidazole can be classified into three groups (2,3):

1. symptoms of hypersensitivity—dermatitis with skin eruptions (usually occurring at 7–10 days of treatment), generalized edema, fever, lymphadenopathy, and joint and muscle pains;
2. bone marrow suppression, thrombocytopenia, and agranulocytosis being the most severe manifestations;
3. peripheral polyneuropathy, paresthesia, and polyneuritis.

In a Cochrane systematic review the incidence of adverse effects was less than 20% (4). In one study, under 5% of participants complained of a variety of minor symptoms, but rash and pruritus were reported more commonly. In children the drug was well tolerated and there were no severe adverse effects. The only study in adults reported a non-quantified variety of mild adverse effects (skin reactions, peripheral neuropathy, digestive disturbances), but it was said that they were less intense than those seen with nifurtimox.

Long-Term Effects

Mutagenicity

Like metronidazole, benznidazole is mutagenic. In tests for chromosomal aberrations and induction of micronuclei in cultures of peripheral lymphocytes from children with Chagas' disease, there were increases in micronucleated interphase lymphocytes and of chromosomal aberrations after treatment with benznidazole (4).

Drug–Drug Interactions

Disulfiram

Like metronidazole, benznidazole has a disulfiram-like effect if alcohol is taken (5).

References

1. Sosa Estani S, Segura EL, Ruiz AM, Velazquez E, Porcel BM, Yampotis C. Efficacy of chemotherapy with benznidazole in children in the indeterminate phase of Chagas' disease. Am J Trop Med Hyg 1998;59(4):526–9.

2. Rodriques Coura J, de Castro SL. A critical review on Chagas disease chemotherapy. Mem Inst Oswaldo Cruz 2002;97(1):3–24.

3. Cancado JR. Long term evaluation of etiological treatment of Chagas' disease with benznidazole. Rev Inst Med Trop Sao Paulo 2002;44(1):29–37.

4. Villar JC, Marin-Neto JA, Ebrahim S, Yusuf S. Trypanocidal drugs for chronic asymptomatic *Trypanosoma cruzi* infection. Cochrane Database Syst Rev 2002;(1):CD003463.

5. Castro JA, Diaz de Toranzo EG. Toxic effects of nifurtimox and benznidazole, two drugs used against American trypanosomiasis (Chagas' disease). Biomed Environ Sci 1988;1(1):19–33.

Benzocaine

See also Local anesthetics

General Information

Benzocaine is a poorly soluble local anesthetic, an ester of para-aminobenzoic acid. It is used in many countries as a component of some free-sale formulations for topical use, for example in skin creams, as a dry powder for skin ulcers, as throat lozenges, and as teething formulations for young children. It is also used in aerosol sprays when anesthetizing the oropharynx. Relatively high concentrations of local anesthetic are required to be effective topically, increasing tissue penetration and the risk of subsequent toxicity. Benzocaine formulations are available in concentrations of 1–20%.

Organs and Systems

Hematologic

Methemoglobinemia is a classical complication of benzocaine (SEDA-12, 256) (SEDA-21, 135) (SEDA-22, 141). The problem arises in both adults and children (1–4), and the risk has led to criticism of its free availability. It has, amongst other things, been suggested that it should be eliminated from products for use in children, that concentrations in over-the-counter products should be limited, and that there should be explicit label warnings of the hematological risk (SED-12, 256) (SEDA-17, 135) (1). Early diagnosis and treatment are crucial, as the condition is potentially fatal, particularly in neonates.

Five cases of benzocaine-induced methemoglobinemia were reported in 1998, following its use for transesophageal echocardiography (5–8). Methemoglobin concentrations over 15% can lead to cyanosis, whilst concentrations over 70% lead to circulatory collapse and death (7,8). The degree of methemoglobinemia depends on the total dose of drug and any factors that enhance systemic absorption. The elderly and neonates are particularly susceptible to methemoglobinemia, as are those with inherited methemoglobin reductase deficiency or the abnormal hemoglobin M. Adequate monitoring and observation of patients both during and after transesophageal echocardiography is essential, as this rare complication of benzocaine and other local anesthetics, such as prilocaine, is both potentially fatal and eminently treatable.

- Severe methemoglobinemia was suspected in a 1-year-old infant after topical application of 10% benzocaine ointment around an enterostomy; on postoperative day 3 the SpO_2 was 90% and arterial blood was dark red in color (9).

The authors pointed out the serious potential for toxicity in infants of a local anesthetic that is commonly used for this purpose in adults.

However, adult cases have been reported with Cetacaine (a proprietary mixture of 14% benzocaine,

2% tetracaine, and 2% butylaminobenzoate) (10–12) and with benzocaine alone (13).

Cetacaine spray used to anesthetize the oropharynx before endoscopy led to dyspnea, central cyanosis, and an oxygen saturation of 80%; methemoglobinemia was diagnosed, and the patient recovered rapidly with methylthioninium chloride 1 mg/kg over 5 minutes.

- A 77-year-old woman received two sprays of Cetacaine for an attempted emergency nasotracheal intubation. After intubation she became cyanosed. The arterial blood was chocolate-brown in color and the SaO_2 by CO oximetry was 54–58%, despite a high PaO_2. The methemoglobin concentration was 39% and she was treated with methylthioninium chloride. Three weeks later Cetacaine again caused cyanosis with a drop in SpO_2 to 76% and a methemoglobin concentration of 24%, which resolved spontaneously.
- A 74-year-old man received Cetacaine spray to his oropharynx for transesophageal echocardiography. His SpO_2 fell to 85%. He became drowsy, then unresponsive, cyanotic, and apneic, and required intubation. His PaO_2 was 37 kPa (280 mmHg), SaO_2 40%, and methemoglobin concentration 60%. Intravenous methylthioninium chloride produced an immediate improvement in the cyanosis and the methemoglobin concentration fell to 0.6%.
- A 71-year-old man received 20% benzocaine spray to the upper airway for bronchoscopy. His SpO_2 gradually fell to under 85% and he required intubation. His methemoglobin concentration was 19%, SaO_2 75%, and PaO_2 44 kPa (329 mmHg). After intravenous methylthioninium chloride the methemoglobin concentration fell to 1.8%.

Several other cases of methemoglobinemia after the administration of topical benzocaine formulations have been reported (14–19). All recovered completely without sequelae after the intravenous administration of methylthioninium chloride 1–2 mg/kg.

- A 69-year-old man developed methemoglobinemia (68%) after pharyngeal anesthesia using 20% benzocaine 15 ml (swish and swallow) for transesophageal echocardiography (20). He responded to intravenous methylthioninium chloride, but a diagnosis of non-Q wave myocardial infarction was made on the basis of raised cardiac enzymes and a normal electrocardiogram.

Whether benzocaine-induced methemoglobinemia is a hypersusceptibility or collateral reaction is controversial. There has been a retrospective review of 188 benzocaine exposures in children under 18 years of age, reported to four regional poison information centers, in 1993–96 (21). Mean and median ingested dosages were 87 and 50 mg/kg respectively and 55% patients had an exposure over 40 mg/kg. In all, 92% patients were asymptomatic. Reported symptoms included oral numbness ($n=8$), vomiting ($n=3$), and oral irritation, dizziness, and nausea ($n=1$ each). Methemoglobin concentrations were measured in eight patients, seven of whom had concentrations over 1%. A child, who had

had 5–10 applications of over-the-counter teething gel applied in 24 hours, had a methemoglobin concentration of 19% and was the only patient to have cyanosis. The authors concluded that accidental ingestion of over-the-counter benzocaine-containing products rarely causes cyanosis. The lack of dose dependence suggests that this reaction is a hypersusceptibility reaction.

Four cases of methemoglobinemia have again been described after the use of benzocaine spray for topical anesthesia of the airways.

- A 42-year-old woman had a superior laryngeal nerve block with lidocaine, topical anesthesia with benzocaine spray, and intravenous midazolam for awake fiberoptic intubation (22). Her SpO_2 fell from about 85% to about 30%, and despite high-frequency jet ventilation with 100% oxygen she had persistent SpO_2 readings in the low 80s. Her arterial blood was chocolate-brown in color, with a PaO_2 of 44 kPa (330 mmHg) and an oxyhemoglobin saturation (SaO_2) of 51%. This discrepancy between PaO_2 and SaO_2 suggested methemoglobinemia, and co-oximetry showed a concentration of 51%. Methylthioninium chloride 140 mg produced an immediate improvement in her color, and her SaO_2 improved over the next 10 minutes.
- An elderly man received benzocaine 20% spray to the throat in preparation for transesophageal echocardiography. He became unwell 1 hour later, with lethargy, central cyanosis, hypoxia, dyspnea, tachypnea, and tachycardia (23). His arterial blood was burgundy-colored and the methemoglobin concentration was 41%. He was treated with two doses of methylthioninium chloride 2 mg/kg and was weaned from oxygen within 10 hours.
- Significant methemoglobinemia occurred in a 65-year-old man on re-exposure to topical 20% benzocaine spray for anesthesia of the airways in preparation for awake fiberoptic intubation (24). This occurred despite exposure 3 days before to 14% benzocaine for the same procedure. During attempted intubation, he suddenly desaturated to 80% and had significant hypotension and bradycardia, necessitating external cardiac massage and cricothyroid puncture. His SaO_2 did not improve significantly, despite seemingly adequate resuscitation with 100% oxygen and intravenous adrenaline. His arterial methemoglobin concentration was 55%. Methylthioninium chloride 100 mg intravenously led to rapid improvement in the SaO_2, allowing surgery to continue.
- A 57-year-old man developed severe methemoglobinemia after receiving topical benzocaine spray and lidocaine jelly during awake fiberoptic intubation (25). After intubation, his oxygen saturation fell to 65% on 100% oxygen. He was cyanosed and had dark arterial blood sample with normal gas tensions. His methemoglobin concentration was 60% and treatment with methylthioninium chloride was successful.

These cases illustrate the importance of co-oximetry on grounds of clinical suspicion. Methemoglobin concentrations of 10–15% can cause dark-colored blood and cyanosis. Concentrations of 20–45% can cause lethargy,

dizziness, headache, and collapse. Higher concentrations (50–70%) can cause seizures, dysrhythmias, coma, and death.

Skin

Granuloma gluteale adultorum is a rare skin condition of unknown etiology, characterized by reddish purple granulomatous nodules on the gluteal surfaces and groin areas.

- Granuloma gluteale adultorum occurred in a 40-year-old woman who presented with a 3-year history of the condition associated with the use of topical benzocaine (26).

Immunologic

Benzocaine can cause sensitization, and being a para-aminobenzoic acid derivative it can cross-react with para-phenylenediamine, sulfonamides, aniline dyes, and related local anesthetics. However, in a recent retrospective study of 5464 patients it was concluded that benzocaine allergy is not common in the UK, confirming earlier reports that benzocaine should not be used as a single screening agent for local anesthetic allergy (27).

Allergic contact dermatitis has been attributed to local benzocaine (28).

- A 72-year-old woman was treated for thoracic *Herpes zoster* with oral aciclovir and topical benzocaine 20% ointment. She subsequently developed painful pruritic erythematous dermatitis in the area of the lesions, spreading to her arm. The dermatitis was initially misdiagnosed as aciclovir resistance, but on patch testing she had a positive reaction to benzocaine.

The authors highlighted the problem in diagnosing allergic contact dermatitis in patients who have other skin lesions in that area. They emphasized the importance of patch testing to identify the causative agent.

References

1. Gentile DA. Severe methemoglobinemia induced by a topical teething preparation. Pediatr Emerg Care 1987;3(3):176–8.
2. Cooper HA. Methemoglobinemia caused by benzocaine topical spray. South Med J 1997;90(9):946–8.
3. Gilman CS, Veser FH, Randall D. Methemoglobinemia from a topical oral anesthetic. Acad Emerg Med 1997;4(10):1011–13.
4. Guerriero SE. Methemoglobinemia caused by topical benzocaine. Pharmacotherapy 1997;17(5):1038–40.
5. McGrath PD, Moloney JF, Riker RR. Benzocaine-induced methemoglobinemia complicating transesophageal echocardiography: a case report. Echocardiography 1998;15(4):389–92.
6. Malhotra S, Kolda M, Nanda NC. Local anesthetic-induced methemoglobinemia during transesophageal echocardiography. Echocardiography 1998;15(2):165–8.
7. Ho RT, Nanevicz T, Yee R, Figueredo VM. Benzocaine-induced methemoglobinemia—two case reports related to transesophageal echocardiography premedication. Cardiovasc Drugs Ther 1998;12(3):311–12.
8. Fisher MA, Henry D, Gillam L, Chen C. Toxic methemoglobinemia: a rare but serious complication of transesophageal echocardiography Can J Cardiol 1998;14(9):1157–60.

9. Adachi T, Fukumoto M, Uetsuki N, Yasui O, Hayashi M. Suspected severe methemoglobinemia caused by topical application of an ointment containing benzocaine around the enterostomy. Anesth Analg 1999;88(5):1190–1.

10. Maher P. Methemoglobinemia: an unusual complication of topical anesthesia. Gastroenterol Nurs 1998;21(4):173–5.

11. Khan NA, Kruse JA. Methemoglobinemia induced by topical anesthesia: a case report and review. Am J Med Sci 1999;318(6):415–18.

12. Stoiber TR. Toxic Methemoglobinemia complicating transesophageal echocardiography. Echocardiography 1999;16(4):383–5.

13. Slaughter MS, Gordon PJ, Roberts JC, Pappas PS. An unusual case of hypoxia from benzocaine-induced methemoglobinemia. Ann Thorac Surg 1999;67(6):1776–8.

14. Haynes JM. Acquired methemoglobinemia following benzocaine anesthesia of the pharynx. Am J Crit Care 2000;9(3):199–201.

15. Gregory PJ, Matsuda K. Cetacaine spray-induced methemoglobinemia after transesophageal echocardiography. Ann Pharmacother 2000;34(9):1077.

16. Nguyen ST, Cabrales RE, Bashour CA, Rosenberger TE Jr, Michener JA, Yared JP, Starr NJ. Benzocaine-induced methemoglobinemia. Anesth Analg 2000;90(2):369–71.

17. Kern K, Langevin PB, Dunn BM. Methemoglobinemia after topical anesthesia with lidocaine and benzocaine for a difficult intubation. J Clin Anesth 2000;12(2):167–72.

18. Gupta PM, Lala DS, Arsura EL. Benzocaine-induced methemoglobinemia. South Med J 2000;93(1):83–6.

19. Gunaratnam NT, Vazquez-Sequeiros E, Gostout CJ, Alexander GL. Methemoglobinemia related to topical benzocaine use: is it time to reconsider the empiric use of topical anesthesia before sedated EGD? Gastrointest Endosc 2000;52(5):692–3.

20. Wurdeman RL, Mohiuddin SM, Holmberg MJ, Shalaby A. Benzocaine-induced methemoglobinemia during an outpatient procedure. Pharmacotherapy 2000;20(6):735–8.

21. Spiller HA, Revolinski DH, Winter ML, Weber JA, Gorman SE. Multi-center retrospective evaluation of oral benzocaine exposure in children. Vet Hum Toxicol 2000;42(4):228–31.

22. Singh RK, Kambe JC, Andrews LK, Russell JC. Benzocaine-induced methemoglobinemia accompanying adult respiratory distress syndrome and sepsis syndrome: case report. J Trauma 2001;50(6):1153–7.

23. Ramsakal A, Lezama JL, Adelman HM. A potentially fatal effect of topical anesthesia. Hosp Pract (Off Ed) 2001;36(6):13–14.

24. Udeh C, Bittikofer J, Sum-Ping ST. Severe methemoglobinemia on reexposure to benzocaine. J Clin Anesth 2001;13(2):128–30.

25. Keld DB, Hein L, Dalgaard M, Krogh L, Rodt SA. The incidence of transient neurologic symptoms (TNS) after spinal anaesthesia in patients undergoing surgery in the supine position. Hyperbaric lidocaine 5% versus hyperbaric bupivacaine 0.5%. Acta Anaesthesiol Scand 2000;44(3):285–90.

26. Dytoc MT, Fiorillo L, Liao J, Krol AL. Granuloma gluteale adultorum associated with use of topical benzocaine preparations: case report and literature review. J Cutan Med Surg 2002;6(3):221–5.

27. Sidhu SK, Shaw S, Wilkinson JD. A 10-year retrospective study on benzocaine allergy in the United Kingdom. Am J Contact Dermat 1999;10(2):57–61.

28. Roos TC, Merk HF. Allergic contact dermatitis from benzocaine ointment during treatment of *Herpes zoster*. Contact Dermatitis 2001;44(2):104.

Benzodiazepines

See also Individual agents

General Information

The benzodiazepines typically share hypnotic, anxiolytic, myorelaxant, and anticonvulsant activity. Because their efficacy and tolerability are generally good, especially in the short term, they have been used extensively and are likely to continue to be used for many years to come. However, their less specific use in the medically or psychiatrically ill, and in healthy individuals experiencing the stresses of life or non-specific symptoms has often been inappropriate and sometimes dangerous (SEDA-18, 43). The pharmacoepidemiology of benzodiazepine use has been carefully studied in various countries (1), including the USA (2) and France, where 7% of the adult population (17% of those over 65 years) are regular users (3). In Italy, consumption of benzodiazepines remained stable (50 defined daily doses per 1000 population) from 1995 to 2003, while expenditure increased by 43% to €565M per annum (4). The need to limit spending on pharmaceutical products, as well as the very real likelihood of inducing iatrogenic disease (for example cognitive impairment, accidents, drug dependence, withdrawal syndromes), has prompted many reviews and policy statements aimed at discouraging inappropriate use. Despite this, the available evidence suggests that there continues to be expensive and inappropriate use in several countries (5).

A comprehensive review of manufacture, distribution, and use has described the rather marked international variation in use of the drugs and the role of the International Narcotics Control Board, a United Nations agency, in the restriction of these drugs (1). Most countries are signatories to the UN Convention on Psychotropic Substances 1971, and are thus obliged to implement controls on the international trade in abusable drugs, including benzodiazepines. Some countries, such as Australia and New Zealand, have imposed further stringent controls on certain drugs, such as flunitrazepam, which are thought to have particular abuse liability (6). A wide-ranging discussion of benzodiazepine regulation has pointed out both the potential merits of the approach and the fact that some restrictions in the past have turned out to be counterproductive (7).

A comprehensive review of benzodiazepine-induced adverse effects and liability to abuse and dependence, in which it was concluded that most benzodiazepine use is both appropriate and helpful (2), has been challenged (8–10). Balanced clinical reviews of benzodiazepine use (11,12) include sets of recommendations on appropriate prescribing and avoiding adverse effects, including tolerance/dependence. Similarly, guidelines for the management of insomnia and the judicious use of hypnotics have been reviewed (13,14). Benzodiazepines are often over-prescribed in hospital (SEDA-17, 42), and their continued prescription after discharge constitutes a significant source of long-term users. Anxiety symptoms and insomnia are common in the medically ill population and can be due to specific physical causes, a reaction to illness, or a co-morbid psychiatric illness, such as depression. Moreover, caffeine, alcohol, nicotine, and a variety of medications can cause insomnia (15). Accordingly, the systematic assessment of such patients allows remediable causes to be identified and the use of hypnosedatives to be minimized. Elderly people and medically ill patients are susceptible to the adverse effects of benzodiazepines, and alternatives are worth considering (11,16), particularly given evidence that behavioral therapies can be more effective and more durable than drug therapy (17).

The important advantages of the benzodiazepines over their predecessors are that they cause relatively less psychomotor impairment, drowsiness, and respiratory inhibition, and are consequently relatively safe in overdose. However, it must be emphasized that these advantages are relative, and that the low toxicity potential does not apply when they are combined with other agents, particularly alcohol (18) and opioids (19).

As well as the added toxicity seen in co-administration with other CNS depressants, benzodiazepines facilitate self-injurious behavior by disinhibiting reckless or suicidal impulses (20). Benzodiazepines are commonly used in both attempted and completed suicide (21). A German study has suggested that hypnosedatives are the commonest drugs used in self-poisoning, that most are prescribed by physicians, and that in nearly half of those taking them chronically, adverse effects were considered to be a possible cause of self-poisoning (22). Before prescribing any drugs of this class, clinicians are exhorted to assess both suicidality and alcohol problems; there is a quick screen for the latter, the Alcohol Use Disorders Identification Test (AUDIT), which consists of a 10-item questionnaire and an 8-item clinical procedure (23).

Hypersensitivity reactions are rare. A few cases of anaphylaxis have been described, although usually these have been with the injectable forms and may have involved the stabilizing agents (24). Serious skin reactions to clobazam (SEDA-21, 38) and tetrazepam (25) have been reported. Lesser reactions have also been reported with diazepam, clorazepate (via N-methyldiazepam) (26), and midazolam (SEDA-17, 44, 45).

Tumor-inducing effects have been observed in animals (SEDA-6, 39), but human reports are essentially negative.

First-trimester exposure appears to confer a small but definite increased risk (from a baseline of 0.06% up to 0.7%) of oral cleft in infants (27). However, second-generation effects are infrequent and usually reversible (28), although some doubt remains about the extent of developmental delay in children who have been exposed in utero (27). A review has emphasized that concerns about second-generation effects are mainly theoretical, and has concluded that some agents (for example chlordiazepoxide) are probably safe during pregnancy and lactation and that others (for example alprazolam) are best avoided (29).

Pharmacokinetics

As far as is currently known, benzodiazepines and similar drugs (zopiclone, zolpidem) act by a single mechanism, interacting at the GABA receptor complex to enhance the ability of GABA to open a chloride ion channel and thereby hyperpolarize the neuronal membrane. It is usual, therefore, to classify benzodiazepines, and recommend their clinical use, on the basis of their duration of action or their half-life. While this is without doubt a useful classification, it is simplistic and does not take into account other important pharmacokinetic factors.

The first factor that is considered significant is the metabolism of benzodiazepines to pharmacologically active metabolites. Many newer benzodiazepines intended for use as long-acting anxiolytic or sedative agents were in fact intended to be so metabolized to ensure stable blood concentrations over prolonged periods. Drugs with long durations of effect, attributable at least in part to the formation of active metabolites, are listed in Table 1. Individuals vary considerably in their metabolism of benzodiazepines, and interpatient variation in concentrations of the parent compounds and of (generally active) metabolites is usual. In addition, ethnicity plays a major role in determining the frequency of poor and extensive metabolizers, with notable differences between Caucasians and East Asians (30).

Another, often neglected, aspect of the pharmacokinetics of benzodiazepines is their rate of onset of action, since their properties and therapeutic benefits depend to a considerable degree on the rapidity of onset of their perceived effects. Within a given drug class, the more rapidly the hypnotic effect occurs, the greater the abuse potential. For most drugs of abuse, it is the affective and behavioral changes associated with a rapid rise in drug blood concentration that is sought, whether the drug is abused by intravenous injection, nasal or bronchial absorption, or (as with alcohol) rapid oral absorption from an empty stomach (31). Diazepam and flunitrazepam are effective hypnotics because they are rapidly absorbed and there is a quick rise in blood concentrations, even though after tissue redistribution and loss of their immediate effects they have long half-lives. It also explains the preference, and so the increased liability for abuse, for drugs like diazepam (31) and flunitrazepam, especially when the latter is snorted (32). In general, polar molecules, such as lorazepam, oxazepam, and temazepam (all of which have a hydroxyl group), gain access to the

Table 1 Benzodiazepines with active metabolites that have long half-lives; metabolism and predominant metabolite half-lives

To desmethyldiazepam*	$t_{1/2}$ (hours)	To other metabolites	$t_{1/2}$ (hours)
Lorazepate	40–100	Chlordiazepoxide	40–100
Diazepam	36	Clobazam	30–150
Halazepam	20	Flurazepam	40–120
Medazepam	2	Quazepam	40–75
Prazepam	120+		

* Half-life about 60 hours.

Table 2 Rates of absorption and half-lives of benzodiazepines

	t_{max} (hours)	$t_{1/2}$ (hours)
Slow absorption		
Clonazepam	2–4	20–40
Loprazolam	2–5	5–15
Lorazepam	2	10–20
Oxazepam	2	5–15
Temazepam (hard capsules)	3	8–20
Intermediate absorption and elimination		
Alprazolam	1–2	12–15
Bromazepam	1–4	10–25
Chlordiazepoxide	1–2	10–25
Intermediate absorption, slow elimination (with active metabolites)		
Flurazepam	1.5	40–120
Clobazam	1–2	20–40
Chlorazepate	1	40–100
Quazepam	1.5	15–35
Rapid absorption, slow elimination, but rapid redistribution		
Diazepam	1	20–70
Flunitrazepam	1	10–40
Nitrazepam	1	20–30
Rapid absorption, rapid elimination, rapid redistribution		
Lormetazepam (soft capsules)	1	8–20
Temazepam (soft capsules)	1	8–20
Rapid absorption, rapid elimination		
Brotizolam	1	4–7
Zolpidem	1.5	2–5
Zopiclone	1.5	5–8
Rapid absorption, very rapid elimination		
Midazolam	0.3	1–4
Triazolam	1	2–5

CNS more slowly than their more lipophilic cousins. Since temazepam is much more quickly absorbed from a soft gelatin liquid-containing capsule than from a hard capsule or tablet, it is the preferred form for both hypnotic use (Table 2) and recreational use (and for this reason is restricted in some countries). Kinetic differences between drugs and between formulations partially explain why comparing equipotent doses of benzodiazepines is difficult.

The route of metabolism can also be significant, particularly in those with liver disease or who are taking concomitant hepatic enzyme inhibitors, such as erythromycin (SEDA-20, 31). The complex interaction between hepatic dysfunction and benzodiazepines has been reviewed (33); these drugs more readily affect liver function in individuals with liver disease and may also directly contribute to hepatic encephalopathy, as shown by the ability of benzodiazepine antagonists to reverse coma transiently in such patients (33). Elderly people appear to be at increased risk only if they are physically unwell, and particularly if they are taking many medications.

Rapid absorption, often followed by rapid redistribution to tissue stores with consequent falls in brain and blood drug concentrations, plays a significant role in the quick onset and cessation of perceived effects, but long-term actions, for example mild sedative and antianxiety effects, are a consequence of slow hepatic clearance, either by hydroxylation and subsequent conjugation to a glucuronide or by microsomal metabolism to other possibly pharmacologically active metabolites. Agents that are subject to microsomal metabolism and/or oxidation accumulate more rapidly in patients with reduced liver function (for example frail elderly people); only the metabolism of drugs such as oxazepam, lorazepam, and temazepam, which predominantly undergo glucuronidation, is not affected by liver function (Table 3) nor suffer from interference by drugs, such as cimetidine, estrogens, or erythromycin, which compete for the enzyme pathways (see Drug–Drug Interactions).

Pharmacodynamics

The use of techniques of molecular biology to clone the benzodiazepine receptor and the other components of the GABA receptor/chloride channel complex has shown that there are likely to be many variant forms of the receptor, owing to the multiplicity of protein subunits that constitute it. This has given rise to the hope that more selective agonist drugs, for example the "Z drugs" (zaleplon, zolpidem, and zopiclone), may produce fewer adverse effects (35,36); however, this hope appears to have been overoptimistic (10). There are also many ways in which different drugs interact with receptor sites to produce their effects, including agonism, partial agonism, antagonism, inverse agonism (contragonism), and even partial inverse agonism; this increases the complexity considerably. The

Table 3 Predominant metabolic pathways for benzodiazepines and related agonists

Via CYP3A oxidation	Via glucuronidation
Alprazolam	Lorazepam
Anidazolam	Oxazepam
Bromazepam	Temazepam
Brotizolam	
Chlordiazepoxide	
Clobazam (also CYP2C19)	
Clonazepam	
Chlorazepate	
Diazepam (also CYP2C19)	
Estazolam	
Flunitrazepam	
Flurazepam	
Halazepam	
Loprazolam	
Lormetazepam	
Medazepam	
Midazolam	
Nitrazepam	
Prazepam	
Quazepam	
Triazolam	
Zaleplon	
Zolpidem	
Zopiclone	

NB: Drugs other than diazepam and clobazam, in particular the so-called "Z drugs" (zaleplon, zolpidem, zopiclone) (34), are also likely to have multiple oxidative pathways.

suggestion that partial agonists (such as alpidem and abecarnil) have greater anxiolytic than sedative potency (37), or that they will be less likely to give rise to abuse (35) or dependence (38), is yet to be established.

Medicolegal considerations

Medicolegal problems, especially with the use of triazolam, have been discussed (SEDA-13, 33); debate continues on the interpretation of evidence that points to an increased incidence of adverse behavioral effects with triazolam (39), flunitrazepam, and other short-acting high-potency agents (12). A review has highlighted a substantial rate (0.3–0.7%) of aggressive reactions to benzodiazepines, and the fact that a majority so affected may have intended a disinhibitory effect, with clear forensic implications (40). High rates of benzodiazepine consumption, much of it illicit, continue in prison populations.

Efforts to restrict benzodiazepines in New York State (2,7) and to ban triazolam (Halcion) in the UK (7,41) and the Netherlands (42)(SEDA-4,V) have likewise been fraught with controversy. For example, the requirement to use triplicate prescription forms in New York has been effective in reducing prescription volumes, including arguably necessary and appropriate prescriptions (43). A 1979 suspension of triazolam availability in the Netherlands was overturned in 1990, while a 1993 formal ban in the UK has remained in force (44). Two extensive reports have included recommendations for resolving the special problems posed by the Halcion controversy (44,45).

General adverse effects

Benzodiazepines have a high therapeutic index of safety, with little effect on most systems (other than the CNS) in high doses. However, their toxicity increases markedly when they are combined with other CNS depressant drugs, such as alcohol or opioid analgesics. Medically ill and brain injured patients are particularly susceptible to adverse neurological or behavioral effects (SEDA-18, 43) (SEDA-20, 30) (46).

The most frequent adverse effect which occurs in at least one-third of patients is drowsiness, often accompanied by incoordination or ataxia. Problems with driving, operating machinery, or falls can result, particularly in the elderly, and can be an important source of morbidity, loss of physical function, and mortality (47,48). Memory impairment, loss of insight, and transient euphoria are common; "paradoxical" reactions of irritability or aggressive behavior have been well documented (11) and appear to occur more often in individuals with a history of impulsiveness or a personality disorder (40), and in the context of interpersonal stress and frustration (49). Tolerance to the sedative and hypnotic effects generally occurs more rapidly than to the anxiolytic or amnestic effects (1).

Physical dependence on benzodiazepines is recognized as a major problem, and occurs after relatively short periods of treatment (50,51), particularly in patients with a history of benzodiazepine or alcohol problems. Abrupt withdrawal can cause severe anxiety, perceptual changes, convulsions, or delirium. It can masquerade as a return of the original symptoms in a more severe form (rebound), or present with additional features (SEDA-17, 42) (11). Up to 90% of regular benzodiazepine users have adverse symptoms on withdrawal. The differences between rebound, withdrawal syndrome, and recurrence have been reviewed in detail (3).

Rebound insomnia or heightened daytime anxiety can occur, particularly after short-acting benzodiazepine hypnotics (12,52,53), and constitute a major reason for continuing or resuming drug use (11).

The use of intravenous benzodiazepines administered by paramedics for the treatment of out-of-hospital status epilepticus has been evaluated in a double-blind, randomized trial in 205 adults (54). The patients presented either with seizures lasting 5 minutes or more or with repetitive generalized convulsive seizures, and were randomized to receive intravenous diazepam 5 mg, lorazepam 2 mg, or placebo. Status epilepticus was controlled on arrival at the hospital in significantly more patients taking benzodiazepines than placebo (lorazepam 59%, diazepam 43%, placebo 21%). The rates of respiratory or circulatory complications related to drug treatment were 11% with lorazepam, 10% with diazepam, and 23% with placebo, but these differences were not significant.

Intranasal midazolam 0.2 mg/kg and intravenous diazepam 0.3 mg/kg have been compared in a prospective randomized study in 47 children (aged 6 months to 5 years) with prolonged (over 10 minutes) febrile seizures (55). Intranasal midazolam controlled seizures significantly earlier than intravenous diazepam. None of the children had respiratory distress, bradycardia, or other adverse effects. Electrocardiography, blood pressure, and pulse oximetry were normal in all children during seizure activity and after cessation of seizures.

Organs and Systems

Cardiovascular

Hypotension follows the intravenous injection of benzodiazepines, but is usually mild and transient (SED-11, 92) (56), except in neonates who are particularly sensitive to this effect (57). Local reactions to injected diazepam are quite common and can progress to compartment syndrome (SEDA-17, 44). In one study (58), two-thirds of the patients had some problem, and most eventually progressed to thrombophlebitis. Flunitrazepam is similar to diazepam in this regard (59). Altering the formulation by changing the solvent or using an emulsion did not greatly affect the outcome (60). Midazolam, being water-soluble, might be expected to produce fewer problems; in five separate studies there were no cases of thrombophlebitis, and in two others the incidence was 8–10%, less than with diazepam but similar to thiopental and saline (61).

Respiratory

Respiratory depression has been reported as the commonest adverse effect of intravenous diazepam (56), especially at the extremes of age. Midazolam has similar effects (62). All benzodiazepines can cause respiratory depression, particularly in bronchitic patients, through drowsiness and reduction in exercise tolerance (63). Rectal administration of, for example, diazepam can offer advantages in unconscious or uncooperative patients, and is less likely than parenteral administration to produce respiratory depression.

A previous report that rectal and intravenous diazepam can cause respiratory depression in children with seizures (SEDA-24, 84) has been challenged (64,65). The authors of the second comment stated that this complication does not occur when rectal diazepam gel is used without other benzodiazepines; they also recommended that during long-term therapy families should be instructed not to give rectal diazepam more than once every 5 days or five times in 1 month.

In a prospective study of children admitted to an accident and emergency department because of seizures, there were 122 episodes in which diazepam was administered rectally and/or intravenously; there was respiratory depression in 11 children, of whom 8 required ventilation (66). The authors questioned the use of rectal or intravenous diazepam as first-line therapy for children with acute seizures.

Nervous system

Falls

The role of different types of benzodiazepines in the risk of falls in a hospitalized geriatric population has been examined in a prospective study of 7908 patients, consecutively admitted to 58 clinical centers during 8 months (67). Over 70% of the patients were older than 65 years, 50% were women, and 24% had a benzodiazepine prescription during the hospital stay. The findings suggested that the use of benzodiazepines with short and very short half-lives is an important and independent risk factor for falls. Their prescription for older hospitalized patients should be carefully evaluated.

In a case-control study using the Systematic Assessment of Geriatric Drug Use via Epidemiology (SAGE) database, the records of 9752 patients hospitalized for fracture of the femur during the period 1992–1996 were extracted and matched by age, sex, state, and index date to the records of 38 564 control patients (68). Among older individuals, the use of benzodiazepines slightly increased the risk of fracture of the femur. Overall, non-oxidative benzodiazepines do not seem to confer a lower risk than oxidative agents. However, the latter may be more dangerous among very old individuals (85 years of age or older), especially if used in high dosages.

In a similar case-control study, 245 elderly patients were matched with 817 controls (69). Benzodiazepines as a group were not associated with a higher risk of hip fracture, but patients who used lorazepam or two or more benzodiazepines had a significantly higher risk.

Effects on performance

All benzodiazepines can cause drowsiness and sedation, and can affect motor and mental performance. Driving is one motor and mental task that is particularly likely to be impaired (SEDA-7, 46), with dangerous consequences; hypnosedatives, like alcohol, impair both actual driving performance (70) and laboratory psychomotor tests (35), and are over-represented in blood samples from delinquent drivers (71). As with alcohol, the maximal impairment occurs while the drug blood concentrations are rising (72), rather than when they have peaked, are stable, or are falling. Somewhat surprisingly, zopiclone 7.5 mg, but not triazolam 0.25 mg, produced deficits in simulated aircraft flight performance 2 and 3 hours after the dose (73). The motor and mental performance reductions induced by hypnotics, especially in elderly people (74), result in an increased incidence of falls (SEDA-21, 38) which can cause hip fractures (75). Agents with short half-lives, including the "Z drugs", were previously thought to carry a reduced risk or even none, but earlier reassuring data have been supplanted by convincing evidence of harm, particularly during the first 2 weeks of prescription (48,76).

Fit young subjects had no impairment of their exercise ability after temazepam or nitrazepam, although nitrazepam caused a subjective feeling of hangover (77).

Seizures

Benzodiazepines can provoke seizures and occasionally precipitate status epilepticus.

- A 28-year-old man with complex partial status, which lasted for 2 months, had a paradoxical worsening of seizure activity in response to diazepam and midazolam (78).

Of 63 neonates receiving lorazepam, diazepam, or both in an intensive care unit, 10 had serious adverse events, including 6 with seizures (57).

Psychological, psychiatric

Cognition

The amnestic effects of benzodiazepines are pervasive and appear to derive from disruption of the consolidation of short-term into long-term memory (79). Amnesia appears to underlie the tendency of regular hypnotic users to overestimate their time asleep, because they simply forget the wakeful intervals (80); in contrast, the same patients underestimate their time spent asleep when drug-free. This amnestic property (SEDA-17, 42) (SEDA-19, 33) has been used to advantage in minor surgery, particularly with midazolam and other short-acting compounds (although male doctors and dentists are advised to have a chaperone present when performing benzodiazepine-assisted procedures with female patients). However, unwanted amnesia can occur, particularly with triazolam, when used as a hypnotic or as an aid for travelers (81,82). The combination of a short half-life and high potency, especially when it was used in the higher doses that were recommended when the drug was initially launched, makes triazolam particularly likely to cause this problem. Studies of low-dose lorazepam (1 mg) in healthy young adults have shown specific deficits in episodic memory (SEDA-21, 38) (SEDA-19, 35). Flurazepam and temazepam have initiated relatively few reports of adverse effects on memory, although flurazepam did cause daytime sedation. Temazepam was uncommonly mentioned in adverse reaction reports, but was also reported more often as being without adequate hypnotic effect. Ironically, temazepam produces more, and oxazepam less, sedation than other benzodiazepines in overdose (83).

The role of benzodiazepines in brain damage has been reviewed (SEDA-14, 36). Cognitive impairment in long-term users can be detected in up to half of the subjects, compared with 16% of controls, but the issue of reversibility with prolonged abstinence is unresolved. Cognitive toxicity is more common with benzodiazepines than other anticonvulsants, with the possible exception of phenobarbital (84).

Patients often have memory deficits after taking benzodiazepines and alcohol. In a study of hippocampal presynaptic glutamate transmission in conjunction with memory deficits induced by benzodiazepines and ethanol, reductions in hippocampal glutamate transmission closely correlated with the extent of impairment of spatial memory performance. The results strongly suggested that presynaptic dysfunction in dorsal hippocampal glutamatergic neurons would be critical for spatial memory deficits induced by benzodiazepines and ethanol (85).

When the relation between benzodiazepine use and cognitive function was evaluated in a prospective study of 2765 elderly subjects, the authors concluded that current benzodiazepine use, especially in recommended or higher dosages, is associated with worse memory among community-dwelling elderly people (86).

In a prospective study, 1389 people aged 60–70 years were recruited from the electoral rolls of the city of Nantes, France (Epidemiology of Vascular Aging Study) (87). A range of symptoms was examined, including cognitive functioning and symptoms of depressive anxiety, and data were also collected on psychotropic and other drugs, as well as tobacco use and alcohol consumption at baseline and thereafter at 2 and 4 years. Users of benzodiazepines were divided into episodic users, recurrent users, and chronic users. Chronic users of benzodiazepines had a significantly higher risk of cognitive decline in the global cognitive test and two attention tests than non-users. Overall, episodic and recurrent users had lower cognitive scores compared with non-users, but the differences were not statistically significant. These findings suggest that long-term use of benzodiazepines is a risk factor for increased cognitive decline in elderly people.

Delirium

Excessive anxiety and tremulousness, hyperexcitability, confusion, and hallucinations were all reported more often with triazolam than with temazepam or flurazepam, when spontaneous reporting was analysed (81). Whether this is dose-related, and perhaps related to the rapid changes in blood concentration with triazolam, is not clear. Delirium is common, particularly in elderly people, who may have impaired drug clearance, and must always be regarded as possibly drug-induced. Of considerable relevance to hospital practice is the finding of a three-fold increased risk of postoperative delirium in patients given a benzodiazepine (88). Dose- and age-related increases in adverse cognitive and other central nervous effects from benzodiazepines (82) are well documented. The use of these drugs in elderly people has been reviewed, with recommendations about maximizing the benefit-to-harm balance in this group of individuals who are susceptible to cognitive and other adverse effects (89,90).

Sleep

The benzodiazepines typically suppress REM sleep, with consequent rebound dreaming and restlessness on withdrawal, leading to poorer sleep patterns (SEDA-12, 42) (91).

The use of benzodiazepines, particularly the short-acting compounds such as triazolam, for the induction of sleep has provoked much discussion (SEDA-17, 42). The debate rages over the risks and benefits of short-acting compounds, in inducing bizarre behavior or rapid withdrawal with daytime anxiety, compared with the possibility of hangover sedation and performance deficits with longer-acting compounds (92). The treatment of sleep disorders is multifaceted, because of the complex nature of sleep and the variety of factors that can give rise to sleep disorders (82). Consequently, such treatment should be selected and proffered carefully, with due regard for all the factors, not treated cavalierly with the latest flavor-of-the-month benzodiazepine receptor agonist. Non-drug treatments are effective (17) and should be considered first; pharmacological treatment should take into consideration any pre-existing factors, for example anxiety, depression, the duration and nature of medical problems (including any painful condition), concomitant medications, and other substance use (13).

Psychoses

Depression is commonly seen (93), either during benzodiazepine treatment or as a complication of withdrawal (SEDA-17, 42). Relief of anxiety symptoms can uncover pre-existing depression, rather than causing depression per se. In addition to their euphoriant effects in some individuals, benzodiazepines can directly increase irritability and depression and, less commonly, lead to full-blown manic episodes (94,95).

Review of a Canadian adverse drug reactions database showed several cases of previously unreported benzodiazepine-induced adverse effects, including hallucinations and encephalopathy (96), although whether benzodiazepines alone were responsible is difficult to confirm. Visual hallucinations have also been reported in association with zolpidem (97).

Benzodiazepine withdrawal, like alcohol withdrawal, can cause schizophreniform auditory hallucinations (98).

Behavior

While they are generally regarded as being tranquillizers, benzodiazepines and related hypnosedatives can release aggression and induce antisocial behavior (99), particularly in combination with alcohol (100) and in the presence of frustration (49). Aggression can occur during benzodiazepine intoxication and withdrawal (99). Non-medical use of flunitrazepam (101) seems particularly likely to reveal paradoxical rage and aggression, with consequent forensic problems. The combination of abnormal disinhibited behavior and amnesia produced by benzodiazepines can be singularly dangerous. Anecdotal cases suggest that hypnosedatives can also disinhibit violent behavior in individuals taking antidepressants. A literature review of behavioral adverse effects associated with benzodiazepines (clonazepam, diazepam, and lorazepam) has shown that 11–25% of patients with mental retardation have these adverse effects (102). In two controlled studies, lorazepam was more likely to provoke aggression than oxazepam (103,104).

Gastrointestinal

Nausea due to benzodiazepines has been reported as being commoner in children, but the incidence does not usually greatly exceed that found with placebo. Gastrointestinal disturbances are more common with the newer non-benzodiazepine agents, for example zopiclone and buspirone (105,106).

Liver

Jaundice has been reported after benzodiazepines, although in only a few cases have they been the only drugs involved (SED-12, 97).

Sexual function

Female orgasm is inhibited by some central depressant and psychotropic drugs, including antipsychotic drugs, antidepressants, and anxiolytic benzodiazepines (107). A survey of patients with bipolar affective disorder taking lithium showed that the co-administration of benzodiazepines was associated with a significantly increased risk (49%) of sexual dysfunction in both men and women (108). Reduced libido is uncommonly reported, as is sexual inhibition, but the actual incidences of these complications may be considerably higher. Hypnosedatives, particularly flunitrazepam and gammahydroxybutyrate, are implicated in sexual assault and "date rape" (109).

Long-Term Effects

Drug tolerance

Animal studies have suggested a possible mechanism for tolerance, in that chronic treatment of rats with triazolam reduced the mRNA coding for certain GABA receptor proteins (110).

Drug dependence

The likelihood and possible severity of dependence on benzodiazepines has been discussed (50).

Drug withdrawal

The likelihood and possible severity of withdrawal from benzodiazepines has been discussed, especially with regard to the newer short-acting compounds (50).

Withdrawal symptoms occur in at least one-third of long-term users (over 1 year), even if the dose is gradually tapered (111). Symptoms come on within 2–3 days of withdrawal of a short-acting or medium-acting benzodiazepine, or 7–10 days after a long-acting drug; short-acting benzodiazepines tend to produce a more marked withdrawal syndrome (35). Lorazepam and alprazolam are particularly difficult to quit. Symptoms usually last 1–6 weeks, but can persist for many months, leaving the patient in a vulnerable state, with likely recurrence of the original disorder and of self-medication. Withdrawal symptoms can occur within 4–6 weeks of daily long-acting benzodiazepine use (112), and possibly earlier in susceptible individuals.

Symptoms on withdrawal are variable in nature and degree. Rebound insomnia can occur one or two nights after withdrawal of short-acting drugs. Anxiety is common, with both psychological and physical manifestations, including apprehension, panic, insomnia, palpitation, sweating, tremor, and gastrointestinal disturbances. Irritability and aggression also occur, notably after triazolam. Depression has been reported after benzodiazepine withdrawal (113). There may be increased or distorted sensory perceptions, such as photophobia, altered (metallic) taste, and hypersensitivity to touch and pain. Flu-like muscle aches and spasms, unsteadiness, and clumsiness are common. Perceptual distortions include burning or creeping of the skin and apparent movement or changes in objects or self (111). General malaise with loss of appetite can occur. As with alcohol, paranoid psychosis, delirium, and epileptic fits are possible on withdrawal (SED-12, 97). With careful handling, often involving psychological and sometimes adjunctive pharmacological support, motivated patients who depend on benzodiazepines can usually be successfully withdrawn. In particular, the combination of gradual dose-tapering and cognitive behavioral therapy can be helpful (114). Guidelines on the management of such patients have been concisely presented (51).

Second-Generation Effects

Teratogenicity

Benzodiazepines readily pass from the mother to fetus through the placenta (115). There may be a risk of congenital malformations, particularly oral cleft, if a pregnant woman takes a benzodiazepine during the first trimester, but the data are inconsistent across drugs (alprazolam having the most clearly defined risk), and any overall effect is probably small (27,28). The risk of benzodiazepine-induced birth defects thus remains uncertain (116), despite two cases of fetal-alcohol syndrome reported after benzodiazepine exposure alone (117).

The occurrence of congenital abnormalities associated with the use of benzodiazepines (alprazolam, clonazepam, medazepam, nitrazepam, and tofisopam) during pregnancy has been analysed in a matched case-control study (118). The cases and controls were drawn from the Hungarian Case-Control Surveillance of Congenital Abnormalities from 1980 to 1996. Of the 38 151 pregnant women who delivered babies without congenital anomalies, 75 had taken benzodiazepines during pregnancy, compared with 57 of 22 865 who delivered offspring with anomalies. Thus, treatment with these benzodiazepines during pregnancy did not cause a detectable teratogenic risk. However, the true relevance of these findings needs to be supported by prospective case ascertainment.

Fetotoxicity

Benzodiazepines readily pass from the mother to fetus through the placenta (115). There is a further concern about cognitive development after in utero exposure to benzodiazepines. It now appears that the slowed intellectual progress seen in some children exposed in utero will "catch up" in most cases by age 4 (28). Unfortunately, the impact of sedative-hypnotic use during pregnancy is often complicated by the abuse of multiple agents and poor maternal nutrition and antenatal care, and may be further confounded by social and environmental deprivation, which the infant often faces after birth (28,119). More definite but short-lived problems occur with benzodiazepines given in late pregnancy and during labor; here floppiness, apnea, and withdrawal in the infant can pose problems (28,120) but usually resolve uneventfully (SEDA-21, 38). Pregnant women should avoid benzodiazepines if possible, especially during late pregnancy and labor; if required, chlordiazepoxide appears to have the best established record (29). On the other hand, alprazolam should be avoided, and temazepam plus diphenhydramine appears to be a particularly toxic combination in late pregnancy, based on animal research and one case report of fetal activation followed by stillbirth (121).

Lactation

Benzodiazepines are secreted into the milk in relatively small amounts (28). During lactation, longer-acting agents are relatively contraindicated, particularly with continued administration beyond 3–5 days, owing to the likelihood of infant sedation (120,122). Short-acting benzodiazepines and zopiclone are probably safe, especially if restricted to single doses or for short courses of therapy (28,123). Zopiclone and midazolam, for example, become undetectable in breast milk 4–5 hours after a dose (124).

Susceptibility Factors

Age

The safety of benzodiazepines in neonates has been assessed in a retrospective chart review of 63 infants who received benzodiazepines (lorazepam and/or midazolam) as sedatives or anticonvulsants (57). Five infants had hypotension and three had respiratory depression. In all cases of respiratory depression, ventilatory support was initiated or increased. Significant hypotension was treated with positive inotropic drugs in two cases. Thus, respiratory depression and hypotension are relatively common when benzodiazepines are prescribed in these patients. However, both depression and hypotension could also have been due to the severe underlying illnesses and concomitant medications. Matched controls were not studied.

Other features of the patient

Benzodiazepines are more likely to cause adverse effects in patients with HIV infection and other causes of organic brain syndrome (46).

Drug Administration

Drug overdose

Overdosage of benzodiazepines alone is generally thought to be safe, but deaths have occasionally been reported (125–127). In 204 consecutive suicides seen by the San Diego County Coroner during 1981–1982, drugs were detected in 68%, and anxiolytics and hypnotics in 11% and 12% respectively; although benzodiazepines were found in under 10% of the group as a whole, they were found in one-third of those who died by overdose (128). In one series of 2827 intentional cases of poisoning, in which there were ten deaths, three were associated with benzodiazepines; death was related to a delay between ingestion and medical intervention (129), and advanced age has also been described as a risk factor (130). In other cases death has been attributed to combined overdose with other drugs, such as alcohol (126), oxycodone (131,132), tramadol (133), and amitriptyline (134).

Concomitant benzodiazepine overdose has also been reported to be an independent risk factor in the development of hepatic encephalopathy (OR = 1.91; CI = 1.00, 3.65) and renal dysfunction (OR = 1.81; CI = 1.00, 3.22) in patients who take a paracetamol overdose (135).

Drug–Drug Interactions

Antibiotics

Antibiotics (erythromycin, chloramphenicol, isoniazid) compete for hepatic oxidative pathways that metabolize most benzodiazepines, as well as zolpidem, zopiclone, and buspirone (SEDA-22, 39) (SEDA-22, 41).

Macrolides cause increases in the serum concentrations, AUCs, and half-lives and reductions in the clearance of triazolam and midazolam (136–138). These changes can result in clinical effects, such as prolonged psychomotor impairment, amnesia, or loss of consciousness (139). Erythromycin can increase concentrations of midazolam and triazolam by inhibition of CYP3A4, and dosage reductions of 50% have been proposed if concomitant therapy is unavoidable (140).

Antifungal imidazoles

Antifungal imidazoles (ketoconazole, itraconazole, and analogues) compete for hepatic oxidative pathways that metabolize most benzodiazepines, as well as zolpidem, zopiclone, and buspirone (SEDA-22, 39, 41–43).

Antihistamines

The potentiation of sedative effects from benzodiazepines when combined with centrally acting drugs with antihistamine properties (for example first-generation antihistamines, tricyclic antidepressants, and neuroleptic drugs) can pose problems (141). Antihistamines that do not have central actions do not interact with benzodiazepines as in the case of mizolastine and lorazepam (142), ebastine and diazepam (143), and terfenadine and diazepam (141).

Calcium channel blockers

Diltiazem and verapamil compete for hepatic oxidative pathways that metabolize most benzodiazepines, as well as zolpidem, zopiclone, and buspirone (SEDA-22, 39) (SEDA-22, 41).

Central stimulants

Caffeine and other central stimulants can reverse daytime sedation from benzodiazepine use. There was a positive effect of caffeine (250 mg) on early-morning performance after both placebo and flurazepam (30 mg) given the night before (144,145), particularly in terms of subjective assessments of mood and sleepiness. However, one cannot assume that the alerting effect of caffeine necessarily reverses the amnestic, disinhibiting, or insight-impairing effects of benzodiazepines. Indeed, caffeine can actually worsen learning and performance already impaired by lorazepam (146). Other drugs with direct or indirect CNS stimulant activity (theophylline, ephedrine, amphetamine, and their analogues) have similar effects and can counteract the effects of benzodiazepines, at least subjectively. Another worrying feature of stimulant use, particularly in drug misusers, is that it commonly increases the perceived need for hypnosedatives.

Cimetidine

Cimetidine can impair benzodiazepine metabolism and lead to adverse effects (SEDA-18, 43). In contrast, a few benzodiazepines are metabolized exclusively by glucuronide conjugation (lorazepam, oxazepam, temazepam), and are therefore unaffected by concomitant therapy with cimetidine and other oxidation inhibitors (121).

Clozapine

Caution has been recommended when starting clozapine in patients taking benzodiazepines (SEDA-19, 55). Three cases of delirium associated with clozapine and benzodiazepines (147) have been reported. There have been several reports of synergistic reactions, resulting in increased sedation and ataxia, when lorazepam was begun in patients already taking clozapine (148).

- Syncope and electrocardiographic changes (sinus bradycardia of 40/minute with deep anteroseptal inverted T waves and minor ST changes in other leads) have been observed with the concurrent administration of clozapine (after the dosage was increased to 300 mg/day) and diazepam (30 mg/day) in a 50-year-old man (149).

CNS depressants

The interactions of benzodiazepines with other nervous system depressants, especially alcohol and other GABA-ergic drugs, have been reviewed (150). Other drugs with nervous system depressant effects (opioids, anticonvulsants, general anesthetics) also can add to, and complicate, the depressant action of benzodiazepines.

Phenothiazines and butyrophenones can counteract intoxication from lysergic acid diethylamide (LSD); benzodiazepines can inhibit this useful effect of antipsychotic drugs (151).

Disulfiram

Disulfiram competes for hepatic oxidative pathways that metabolize most benzodiazepines, as well as zolpidem, zopiclone, and buspirone (SEDA-22, 39) (SEDA-22, 41).

Enzyme inducers

Enzyme induction can be problematic with co-administration of benzodiazepines and rifampicin or certain anticonvulsants (phenobarbital, phenytoin, carbamazepine). However, despite enzyme stimulation, the net effect of adding these anticonvulsants can be augmentation of benzodiazepine-induced sedation.

Rifampicin, and presumably other enzyme inducers, reduces concentrations of zolpidem, zopiclone, and buspirone (SEDA-22, 42). Drugs that are solely glucuronidated (lorazepam, oxazepam, and temazepam) are not affected.

HIV protease inhibitors

Some protease inhibitors (saquinavir) compete for hepatic oxidative pathways that metabolize most benzodiazepines, as well as zolpidem, zopiclone, and buspirone (SEDA-22, 39) (SEDA-22, 41).

Levodopa

The question of whether starting a benzodiazepine in patients taking levodopa is followed by a faster increase in antiparkinsonian drug requirements has been studied using drug dispensing data for all the residents in six Dutch cities (152). All were 55 years old or older and had used levodopa for at least 360 days. There were 45 benzodiazepine starters and 169 controls. Antiparkinsonian drug doses increased faster in the benzodiazepine group, but the difference was not significant (RR = 1.44; 95% CI = 0.89, 2.59).

Lithium

In 18 patients treated with benzodiazepines and/or antipsychotic drugs there were increased chromosomal aberrations and increased sister chromatid exchange, but there were no significant differences between this group and another group of 18 patients taking lithium in addition to benzodiazepines and/or antipsychotic drugs (153).

Moxonidine

Moxonidine can potentiate the effect of benzodiazepines (154).

Muscle relaxants

Laboratory investigations have shown that some benzodiazepines can produce biphasic effects on the actions of neuromuscular blocking agents (155,156), higher doses potentiating the effects (155,157); however, several human investigations have failed to show a significant effect (158–160). It has been suggested that agents that are added to commercial formulations of some benzodiazepines to render them more water-soluble may mask the benzodiazepine effect (160).

Nevertheless, some interactions of benzodiazepines with muscle relaxants used in anesthesia have been described. Diazepam has been reported to potentiate the effects of tubocurare (161) and gallamine (162) and to reduce the effects of suxamethonium (162). However, in 113 patients undergoing general anesthesia, intravenous diazepam 20 mg, lorazepam 5 mg, and lormetazepam 2 mg did not potentiate the neuromuscular blocking effects of vecuronium or atracurium (160).

In 113 patients undergoing general anesthesia, intravenous midazolam 15 mg slowed recovery of the twitch height after vecuronium and atracurium compared with diazepam. The recovery index was not altered (160). However, in another study in 20 patients, midazolam 0.3 mg/kg did not affect the duration of blockade, recovery time, intensity of fasciculations, or adequacy of relaxation for tracheal intubation produced by suxamethonium 1 mg/kg, nor the duration of blockade and adequacy of relaxation for tracheal intubation produced by pancuronium 0.025 mg/kg in incremental doses until 99% depression of muscle-twitch tension was obtained (159). Furthermore, in 60 patients undergoing maintenance anesthesia randomly assigned to one of six regimens (etomidate, fentanyl, midazolam, propofol, thiopental plus nitrous oxide, or isoflurane plus nitrous oxide), midazolam did not alter rocuronium dosage requirements (163).

Neuroleptic drugs

Because of the frequency of co-administration of benzodiazepines with neuroleptic drugs, it is important to consider possible adverse effects that can result from such combinations. In a brief review, emphasis has been placed on pharmacokinetic interactions between neuroleptic drugs and benzodiazepines, as much information on their metabolic pathways is emerging (164). Thus, the enzyme CYP3A4, which plays a dominant role in the metabolism of benzodiazepines, also contributes to the metabolism of clozapine, haloperidol, and quetiapine, and neuroleptic drug plasma concentrations can rise. Intramuscular levomepromazine in combination with an intravenous benzodiazepine has been said to increase the risk of airways obstruction, on the basis of five cases of respiratory impairment; the doses of levomepromazine were higher in the five cases that had accompanying airways obstruction than in another 95 patients who did not (165).

Omeprazole

Omeprazole can impair benzodiazepine metabolism and lead to adverse effects (SEDA-18, 43).

Opioids

Fentanyl competes for hepatic oxidative pathways that metabolize most benzodiazepines, as well as zolpidem, zopiclone, and buspirone (SEDA-22, 39) (SEDA-22, 41).

Oral contraceptives

Oral contraceptives alter the metabolism of some benzodiazepines that undergo oxidation (alprazolam, chlordiazepoxide, diazepam) or nitroreduction (nitrazepam) (166). For these drugs, oral contraceptives inhibit enzyme activity and reduce clearance. There is nevertheless no evidence that this interaction is of clinical importance. It should be noted that for other benzodiazepines that undergo oxidative metabolism, such as bromazepam or clotiazepam, no change has ever been found in oral contraceptive users. Some other benzodiazepines, such as lorazepam, oxazepam, and temazepam, are metabolized by glucuronic acid conjugation. The clearance of temazepam was increased when oral contraceptives were co-administered, but the clearances of lorazepam and oxazepam were not (167). Again, it is unlikely that this is an interaction of clinical importance.

Selective serotonin reuptake inhibitors (SSRIs)

Some SSRIs (notably fluvoxamine and to a lesser extent fluoxetine) and their metabolites inhibit hepatic oxidative enzymes, particularly CYP2C19 and CYP3A, that metabolize most benzodiazepines, as well as zaleplon, zolpidem, zopiclone, and buspirone (SEDA-22, 39) (SEDA-22, 41) (168,169). Apart from fluvoxamine, SSRIs do not generally have a clinically prominent effect on hypnosedative effects; studies vary from those that have found that fluoxetine has a moderate but functionally unimportant impact on diazepam concentrations (170) to results that suggest significant aggravation of the cognitive effects of alprazolam when co-prescribed with the SSRI (171).

Tricyclic antidepressants

Four patients developed adverse effects attributable to combinations of benzodiazepines with tricyclic antidepressants, including exacerbations of delusional disorder (172).

Nefazodone competes for hepatic oxidative pathways that metabolize most benzodiazepines, as well as zolpidem, zopiclone, and buspirone (SEDA-22, 39) (SEDA-22, 41).

References

1. Fraser AD. Use and abuse of the benzodiazepines. Ther Drug Monit 1998;20(5):481–9.
2. Woods JH, Winger G. Current benzodiazepine issues. Psychopharmacology (Berl) 1995;118(2):107–15.
3. Pelissolo A, Bisserbe JC. Dependance aux benzodiazepines. Aspects clinique et biologiques. [Dependence on benzodiazepines. Clinical and biological aspects.] Encephale 1994;20(2):147–57.
4. Ciuna A, Andretta M, Corbari L, Levi D, Mirandola M, Sorio A, Barbui C. Are we going to increase the use of antidepressants up to that of benzodiazepines? Eur J Clin Pharmacol 2004;60(9):629–34.
5. Anonymous. What's wrong with prescribing hypnotics? Drug Ther Bull 2004;42(12):89–93.
6. Judd F. Flunitrazepam—schedule 8 drug. Australas Psychiatry 1998;6:265.
7. Woods JH. Problems and opportunities in regulation of benzodiazepines. J Clin Pharmacol 1998;38(9):773–82.
8. Griffiths RR. Commentary on review by Woods and Winger. Benzodiazepines: long-term use among patients is a concern and abuse among polydrug abusers is not trivial. Psychopharmacology (Berl) 1995; 118(2):116–17.
9. Lader M. Commentary on review by Woods and Winger. Psychopharmacology (Berl) 1995;118:118.
10. Holbrook AM. Treating insomnia. BMJ 2004; 329(7476):1198–9.
11. Lader M. Psychiatric disorders. Speight T, Holford N, editors. Avery's Drug Treatment 4th ed. Auckland: ADIS International Press, 1997:1437.
12. Ashton H. Guidelines for the rational use of benzodiazepines. When and what to use. Drugs 1994;48(1):25–40.
13. Pagel JF. Treatment of insomnia. Am Fam Physician 1994;49(6):1417–21, 1423–4.
14. Mendelson WB, Jain B. An assessment of short-acting hypnotics. Drug Saf 1995;13(4):257–70.
15. Mellinger GD, Balter MB, Uhlenhuth EH. Insomnia and its treatment. Prevalence and correlates. Arch Gen Psychiatry 1985;42(3):225–32.
16. Wise MG, Griffies WS. A combined treatment approach to anxiety in the medically ill. J Clin Psychiatry 1995;56(Suppl 2):14–19.
17. Morin CM, Colecchi C, Stone J, Sood R, Brink D. Behavioral and pharmacological therapies for late-life insomnia: a randomized controlled trial. JAMA 1999;281(11):991–9.
18. Gaudreault P, Guay J, Thivierge RL, Verdy I. Benzodiazepine poisoning. Clinical and pharmacological considerations and treatment. Drug Saf 1991;6(4):247–65.
19. Megarbane B, Gueye P, Baud F. Interactions entre benzodiazepines et produits opioides. [Interactions between benzodiazepines and opioids.] Ann Med Interne (Paris) 2003;154(Spec No 2):S64–72.
20. Taiminen TJ. Effect of psychopharmacotherapy on suicide risk in psychiatric inpatients. Acta Psychiatr Scand 1993;87(1):45–7.
21. Michel K, Waeber V, Valach L, Arestegui G, Spuhler T. A comparison of the drugs taken in fatal and nonfatal self-poisoning. Acta Psychiatr Scand 1994;90(3):184–9.
22. Schwarz UI, Ruder S, Krappweis J, Israel M, Kirch W. Epidemiologie medikamentöser Parasuizide. Eine Erhebung aus dem Universitätsklinikum Dresden. [Epidemiology of attempted suicide using drugs. An inquiry from the Dresden University Clinic.] Dtsch Med Wochenschr 2004;129(31–32):1669–73.
23. Bohn MJ, Babor TF, Kranzler HR. The Alcohol Use Disorders Identification Test (AUDIT): validation of a screening instrument for use in medical settings. J Stud Alcohol 1995;56(4):423–32.
24. Deardon DJ, Bird GL. Acute (type 1) hypersensitivity to i.v. Diazemuls. Br J Anaesth 1987;59(3):391.
25. Pirker C, Misic A, Brinkmeier T, Frosch PJ. Tetrazepam drug sensitivity—usefulness of the patch test. Contact Dermatitis 2002;47(3):135–8.
26. Sachs B, Erdmann S, Al-Masaoudi T, Merk HF. In vitro drug allergy detection system incorporating human liver microsomes in chlorazepate-induced skin rash: drug-specific proliferation associated with interleukin-5 secretion. Br J Dermatol 2001;144(2):316–20.
27. Altshuler LL, Cohen L, Szuba MP, Burt VK, Gitlin M, Mintz J. Pharmacologic management of psychiatric illness during pregnancy: dilemmas and guidelines. Am J Psychiatry 1996;153(5):592–606.
28. McElhatton PR. The effects of benzodiazepine use during pregnancy and lactation. Reprod Toxicol 1994;8(6):461–75.
29. Iqbal MM, Sobhan T, Ryals T. Effects of commonly used benzodiazepines on the fetus, the neonate, and the nursing infant. Psychiatr Serv 2002;53(1):39–49.
30. Kim K, Johnson JA, Derendorf H. Differences in drug pharmacokinetics between East Asians and Caucasians and the role of genetic polymorphisms. J Clin Pharmacol 2004;44(10):1083–105.
31. Griffiths RR, McLeod DR, Bigelow GE, Liebson IA, Roache JD, Nowowieski P. Comparison of diazepam and oxazepam: preference, liking and extent of abuse. J Pharmacol Exp Ther 1984;229(2):501–8.
32. Bond A, Seijas D, Dawling S, Lader M. Systemic absorption and abuse liability of snorted flunitrazepam. Addiction 1994;89(7):821–30.
33. Ananth J, Swartz R, Burgoyne K, Gadasally R. Hepatic disease and psychiatric illness: relationships and treatment. Psychother Psychosom 1994;62(3–4):146–59.
34. Hesse LM, von Moltke LL, Greenblatt DJ. Clinically important drug interactions with zopiclone, zolpidem and zaleplon. CNS Drugs 2003;17(7):513–32.
35. Lader M. Clin pharmacology of anxiolytic drugs: Past, present and future. Biggio G, Sanna E, Costa E, editors. GABA-A Receptors and Anxiety. From Neurobiology to Treatment. New York: Raven Press, 1995:135.
36. Anonymous. Zopiclone, zolpidem and zaleplon. Get your "zzz's" without affecting performance the next day. Drugs Ther Perspect 2004;20(2):16–18.
37. Haefely W, Martin JR, Schoch P. Novel anxiolytics that act as partial agonists at benzodiazepine receptors. Trends Pharmacol Sci 1990;11(11):452–6.
38. Rickels K, DeMartinis N, Aufdembrinke B. A double-blind, placebo-controlled trial of abecarnil and diazepam in the treatment of patients with generalized anxiety disorder. J Clin Psychopharmacol 2000; 20(1):12–18.
39. O'Donovan MC, McGuffin P. Short acting benzodiazepines. BMJ 1993;306(6883):945–6.
40. Michel L, Lang JP. Benzodiazepines et passage à l'acte criminel. [Benzodiazepines and forensic aspects.] Encephale 2003;29(6):479–85.
41. Dyer C. Halcion edges its way back into Britain in low doses. BMJ 1993;306:1085.
42. Te Lintelo J, Pieters T. Halcion: de lotgevallen van de "Dutch Hysteria". Pharm Wkbl 2003;138(46):1600–5.
43. Wagner AK, Soumerai SB, Zhang F, Mah C, Simoni-Wastila L, Cosler L, Fanning T, Gallagher P, Ross-Degnan D. Effects of state surveillance on new post-hospitalization benzodiazepine use. Int J Qual Health Care 2003;15(5):423–31.
44. Abraham J. Transnational industrial power, the medical profession and the regulatory state: adverse drug reactions and the crisis over the safety of Halcion in

the Netherlands and the UK. Soc Sci Med 2002;55(9): 1671–90.

45. Klein DF. The report by the Institute of Medicine and postmarketing surveillance. Arch Gen Psychiatry 1999;56(4):353–4.

46. Ayuso JL. Use of psychotropic drugs in patients with HIV infection. Drugs 1994;47(4):599–610.

47. Gray SL, LaCroix AZ, Blough D, Wagner EH, Koepsell TD, Buchner D. Is the use of benzodiazepines associated with incident disability? J Am Geriatr Soc 2002;50(6):1012–18.

48. Wagner AK, Zhang F, Soumerai SB, Walker AM, Gurwitz JH, Glynn RJ, Ross-Degnan D. Benzodiazepine use and hip fractures in the elderly: who is at greatest risk? Arch Intern Med 2004;164(14):1567–72.

49. Salzman C, Kochansky GE, Shader RI, Porrino LJ, Harmatz JS, Swett CP Jr. Chlordiazepoxide-induced hostility in a small group setting. Arch Gen Psychiatry 1974;31(3):401–5.

50. Woods JH, Katz JL, Winger G. Abuse liability of benzodiazepines. Pharmacol Rev 1987;39(4):251–413.

51. Ashton H. The treatment of benzodiazepine dependence. Addiction 1994;89(11):1535–41.

52. Adam K, Oswald I. Can a rapidly-eliminated hypnotic cause daytime anxiety? Pharmacopsychiatry 1989;22(3):115–19.

53. Kales A, Manfredi RL, Vgontzas AN, Bixler EO, Vela-Bueno A, Fee EC. Rebound insomnia after only brief and intermittent use of rapidly eliminated benzodiazepines. Clin Pharmacol Ther 1991;49(4):468–76.

54. Alldredge BK, Gelb AM, Isaacs SM, Corry MD, Allen F, Ulrich S, Gottwald MD, O'Neil N, Neuhaus JM, Segal MR, Lowenstein DH. A comparison of lorazepam, diazepam, and placebo for the treatment of out-of-hospital status epilepticus. N Engl J Med 2001;345(9):631–7.

55. Wassner E, Morris B, Fernando L, Rao M, Whitehouse WP. Intranasal midazolam for treating febrile seizures in children. Buccal midazolam for childhood seizures at home preferred to rectal diazepam. BMJ 2001;322(7278):108.

56. Donaldson D, Gibson G. Systemic complications with intravenous diazepam. Oral Surg Oral Med Oral Pathol 1980;49(2):126–30.

57. Ng E, Klinger G, Shah V, Taddio A. Safety of benzodiazepines in newborns. Ann Pharmacother 2002;36(7–8):1150–5.

58. Glaser JW, Blanton PL, Thrash WJ. Incidence and extent of venous sequelae with intravenous diazepam utilizing a standardized conscious sedation technique. J Periodontol 1982;53(11):700–3.

59. Mikkelsen H, Hoel TM, Bryne H, Krohn CD. Local reactions after i.v. injections of diazepam, flunitrazepam and isotonic saline. Br J Anaesth 1980;52(8):817–19.

60. Jensen S, Huttel MS, Schou Olesen A. Venous complications after i.v. administration of Diazemuls (diazepam) and Dormicum (midazolam). Br J Anaesth 1981;53(10):1083–5.

61. Reves JG, Fragen RJ, Vinik HR, Greenblatt DJ. Midazolam: pharmacology and uses. Anesthesiology 1985;62(3):310–24.

62. Dundee JW, Halliday NJ, Harper KW, Brogden RN. Midazolam. A review of its pharmacological properties and therapeutic use. Drugs 1984;28(6):519–43.

63. Woodcock AA, Gross ER, Geddes DM. Drug treatment of breathlessness: contrasting effects of diazepam and promethazine in pink puffers. BMJ (Clin Res Ed) 1981;283(6287):343–6.

64. Mackereth S. Use of rectal diazepam in the community. Dev Med Child Neurol 2000;42(11):785.

65. Kriel RL, Cloyd JC, Pellock JM. Respiratory depression in children receiving diazepam for acute seizures: a prospective study. Dev Med Child Neurol 2000;42(6):429–30.

66. Norris E, Marzouk O, Nunn A, McIntyre J, Choonara I. Respiratory depression in children receiving diazepam for acute seizures: a prospective study. Dev Med Child Neurol 1999;41(5):340–3.

67. Passaro A, Volpato S, Romagnoni F, Manzoli N, Zuliani G, Fellin R. Benzodiazepines with different half-life and falling in a hospitalized population. The GIFA study. Gruppo Italiano di Farmacovigilanza nell'Anziano. J Clin Epidemiol 2000;53(12):1222–9.

68. Sgadari A, Lapane KL, Mor V, Landi F, Bernabei R, Gambassi G. Oxidative and nonoxidative benzodiazepines and the risk of femur fracture. The Systematic Assessment of Geriatric Drug Use Via Epidemiology Study Group. J Clin Psychopharmacol 2000;20(2):234–9.

69. Pierfitte C, Macouillard G, Thicoipe M, Chaslerie A, Pehourcq F, Aissou M, Martinez B, Lagnaoui R, Fourrier A, Begaud B, Dangoumau J, Moore N. Benzodiazepines and hip fractures in elderly people: case-control study. BMJ 2001;322(7288):704–8.

70. O'Hanlon JF, Volkerts ER. Hypnotics and actual driving performance. Acta Psychiatr Scand 1986;332(Suppl):95–104.

71. Heinemann A, Grellner W, Preu J, Kratochwil M, Cordes O, Lignitz E, Wilske J, Puschel K. Zur Straßenverkehrsdelinquenz durch psychotrope Substanzen bei Senioren in drei Regionen Deutschlands. Teil I: Medikamente und Betäubungsmittel. Blutalkohol 2004;41:117–27.

72. Ellinwood EH Jr. Linnoila M, Easler ME, Molter DW. Onset of peak impairment after diazepam and after alcohol. Clin Pharmacol Ther 1981;30(4):534–8.

73. Jing BS, Zhan H, Li YF, Zhou YJ, Guo H. Effects of short-action hypnotics triazolam and zopiclone on simulated flight performance. Space Med Med Eng (Beijing) 2003;16(5):329–31.

74. Kruse WH. Problems and pitfalls in the use of benzodiazepines in the elderly. Drug Saf 1990;5(5):328–44.

75. Ray WA, Griffin MR, Schaffner W, Baugh DK, Melton LJ 3rd. Psychotropic drug use and the risk of hip fracture. N Engl J Med 1987;316(7):363–9.

76. Vermeeren A. Residual effects of hypnotics: epidemiology and clinical implications. CNS Drugs 2004;18(5):297–328.

77. Charles RB, Kirkham AJ, Guyatt AR, Parker SP. Psychomotor, pulmonary and exercise responses to sleep medication. Br J Clin Pharmacol 1987;24(2):191–7.

78. Al Tahan A. Paradoxic response to diazepam in complex partial status epilepticus. Arch Med Res 2000;31(1):101–4.

79. Ghoneim MM, Mewaldt SP. Benzodiazepines and human memory: a review. Anesthesiology 1990;72(5):926–38.

80. Schneider-Helmert D. Why low-dose benzodiazepine-dependent insomniacs can't escape their sleeping pills. Acta Psychiatr Scand 1988;78(6):706–11.

81. Bixler EO, Kales A, Brubaker BH, Kales JD. Adverse reactions to benzodiazepine hypnotics: spontaneous reporting system. Pharmacology 1987;35(5):286–300.

82. Gillin JC, Byerley WF. Drug therapy: the diagnosis and management of insomnia. N Engl J Med 1990;322(4):239–48.

83. Buckley NA, Dawson AH, Whyte IM, O'Connell DL. Relative toxicity of benzodiazepines in overdose. BMJ 1995;310(6974):219–21.

84. Meador KJ. Cognitive side effects of antiepileptic drugs. Can J Neurol Sci 1994;21(3):S12–16.

85. Shimizu K, Matsubara K, Uezono T, Kimura K, Shiono H. Reduced dorsal hippocampal glutamate release significantly correlates with the spatial memory deficits produced by benzodiazepines and ethanol. Neuroscience 1998;83(3):701–6.

86. Hanlon JT, Horner RD, Schmader KE, Fillenbaum GG, Lewis IK, Wall WE Jr. Landerman LR, Pieper CF, Blazer DG, Cohen HJ. Benzodiazepine use and cognitive

function among community-dwelling elderly. Clin Pharmacol Ther 1998;64(6):684–92.

87. Paterniti S, Dufouil C, Alperovitch A. Long-term benzodiazepine use and cognitive decline in the elderly: the epidemiology of vascular aging study. J Clin Psychopharmacol 2002;22(3):285–93.

88. Marcantonio ER, Juarez G, Goldman L, Mangione CM, Ludwig LE, Lind L, Katz N, Cook EF, Orav EJ, Lee TH. The relationship of postoperative delirium with psychoactive medications. JAMA 1994; 272(19):1518–22.

89. Shorr RI, Robin DW. Rational use of benzodiazepines in the elderly. Drugs Aging 1994;4(1):9–20.

90. Madhusoodanan S, Bogunovic OJ. Safety of benzodiazepines in the geriatric population. Expert Opin Drug Saf 2004;3(5):485–93.

91. Gillin JC, Spinweber CL, Johnson LC. Rebound insomnia: a critical review. J Clin Psychopharmacol 1989;9(3):161–72.

92. McClure DJ, Walsh J, Chang H, Olah A, Wilson R, Pecknold JC. Comparison of lorazepam and flurazepam as hypnotic agents in chronic insomniacs. J Clin Pharmacol 1988;28(1):52–63.

93. Patten SB, Williams JV, Love EJ. Self-reported depressive symptoms following treatment with corticosteroids and sedative-hypnotics. Int J Psychiatry Med 1996;26(1):15–24.

94. Strahan A, Rosenthal J, Kaswan M, Winston A. Three case reports of acute paroxysmal excitement associated with alprazolam treatment. Am J Psychiatry 1985;142(7):859–61.

95. Rigby J, Harvey M, Davies DR. Mania precipitated by benzodiazepine withdrawal. Acta Psychiatr Scand 1989;79(4):406–7.

96. Patten SB, Love EJ. Neuropsychiatric adverse drug reactions: passive reports to Health and Welfare Canada's adverse drug reaction database (1965–present). Int J Psychiatry Med 1994;24(1):45–62.

97. Tsai MJ, Huang YB, Wu PC. A novel clinical pattern of visual hallucination after zolpidem use. J Toxicol Clin Toxicol 2003;41(6):869–72.

98. Roberts K, Vass N. Schneiderian first-rank symptoms caused by benzodiazepine withdrawal. Br J Psychiatry 1986;148:593–4.

99. Bond AJ. Drug-induced behavioural disinhibition. CNS Drugs 1998;9:41–57.

100. Brahams D. Iatrogenic crime: criminal behaviour in patients receiving drug treatment. Lancet 1987;1(8537):874–5.

101. Dobson J. Sedatives/hypnotics for abuse. NZ Med J 1989;102(881):651.

102. Kalachnik JE, Hanzel TE, Sevenich R, Harder SR. Benzodiazepine behavioral side effects: review and implications for individuals with mental retardation. Am J Ment Retard 2002;107(5):376–410.

103. Kochansky GE, Salzman C, Shader RI, Harmatz JS, Ogeltree AM. The differential effects of chlordiazepoxide and oxazepam on hostility in a small group setting. Am J Psychiatry 1975;132(8):861–3.

104. Bond A, Lader M. Differential effects of oxazepam and lorazepam on aggressive responding. Psychopharmacology (Berl) 1988;95(3):369–73.

105. Monchesky TC, Billings BJ, Phillips R. Zopiclone: a new nonbenzodiazepine hypnotic used in general practice. Clin Ther 1986;8(3):283–91.

106. Newton RE, Marunycz JD, Alderdice MT, Napoliello MJ. Review of the side-effect profile of buspirone. Am J Med 1986;80(3B):17–21.

107. Shen WW, Sata LS. Inhibited female orgasm resulting from psychotropic drugs. A five-year, updated, clinical review. J Reprod Med 1990;35(1):11–14.

108. Ghadirian AM, Annable L, Belanger MC. Lithium, benzodiazepines, and sexual function in bipolar patients. Am J Psychiatry 1992;149(6):801–5.

109. Smith KM, Larive LL, Romanelli F. Club drugs: methylenedioxymethamphetamine, flunitrazepam, ketamine hydrochloride, and gamma-hydroxybutyrate. Am J Health Syst Pharm 2002;59(11):1067–76.

110. Ramsey-Williams VA, Carter DB. Chronic triazolam and its withdrawal alters GABA$_A$ receptor subunit mRNA levels: an in situ hybridization study. Brain Res Mol Brain Res 1996;43(1–2):132–40.

111. Lader M, Morton S. Benzodiazepine problems. Br J Addict 1991;86(7):823–8.

112. Miller NS, Gold MS. Benzodiazepines: tolerance, dependence, abuse, and addiction. J Psychoactive Drugs 1990;22(1):23–33.

113. Olajide D, Lader M. Depression following withdrawal from long-term benzodiazepine use: a report of four cases. Psychol Med 1984;14(4):937–40.

114. Baillargeon L, Landreville P, Verreault R, Beauchemin JP, Gregoire JP, Morin CM. Discontinuation of benzodiazepines among older insomniac adults treated with cognitive-behavioural therapy combined with gradual tapering: a randomized trial. CMAJ 2003;169(10):1015–20.

115. Ashton H. Disorders of the foetus and infant. Davies DM, editor. Textbook of Adverse Drug Reactions, 3rd ed. Oxford: Oxford University Press, 1985:77.

116. Rosenberg L, Mitchell AA, Parsells JL, Pashayan H, Louik C, Shapiro S. Lack of relation of oral clefts to diazepam use during pregnancy. N Engl J Med 1983;309(21):1282–5.

117. Laegreid L, Olegard R, Wahlstrom J, Conradi N. Abnormalities in children exposed to benzodiazepines in utero. Lancet 1987;1(8524):108–9.

118. Eros E, Czeizel AE, Rockenbauer M, Sorensen HT, Olsen J. A population-based case-control teratologic study of nitrazepam, medazepam, tofisopam, alprazolum and clonazepam treatment during pregnancy. Eur J Obstet Gynecol Reprod Biol 2002;101(2):147–54.

119. Thadani PV. Biological mechanisms and perinatal exposure to abused drugs. Synapse 1995;19(3):228–32.

120. Boutroy MJ. Drug-induced apnea. Biol Neonate 1994;65(3–4):252–7.

121. Anonymous. Benzodiazepines: general statement. AHFS Drug Information 1998;1934.

122. Spigset O. Anaesthetic agents and excretion in breast milk. Acta Anaesthesiol Scand 1994;38(2):94–103.

123. Pons G, Rey E, Matheson I. Excretion of psychoactive drugs into breast milk. Pharmacokinetic principles and recommendations. Clin Pharmacokinet 1994;27(4):270–89.

124. Matheson I, Lunde PK, Bredesen JE. Midazolam and nitrazepam in the maternity ward: milk concentrations and clinical effects. Br J Clin Pharmacol 1990;30(6):787–93.

125. Michalodimitrakis M, Christodoulou P, Tsatsakis AM, Askoxilakis I, Stiakakis I, Mouzas I. Death related to midazolam overdose during endoscopic retrograde cholangiopancreatography. Am J Forensic Med Pathol 1999;20(1):93–7.

126. Drummer OH, Syrjanen ML, Cordner SM. Deaths involving the benzodiazepine flunitrazepam. Am J Forensic Med Pathol 1993;14(3):238–43.

127. Aderjan R, Mattern R. Eine tödlich verlaufene Monointoxikation mit Flurazepam (Dalmadorm). Probleme bei der toxikologischen Beurteilung. [A fatal monointoxication by flurazepam (Dalmadorm). Problems of the toxicological interpretation.] Arch Toxicol 1979;43(1):69–75.

128. Mendelson WB, Rich CL. Sedatives and suicide: the San Diego study. Acta Psychiatr Scand 1993;88(5):337–41.

129. Bruyndonckx RB, Meulemans AI, Sabbe MB, Kumar AA, Delooz HH. Fatal intentional poisoning cases admitted to

the University Hospitals of Leuven, Belgium from 1993 to 1996. Eur J Emerg Med 2002;9(3):238–43.

130. Shah R, Uren Z, Baker A, Majeed A. Trends in suicide from drug overdose in the elderly in England and Wales, 1993–1999. Int J Geriatr Psychiatry 2002;17(5): 416–21.

131. Burrows DL, Hagardorn AN, Harlan GC, Wallen ED, Ferslew KE. A fatal drug interaction between oxycodone and clonazepam. J Forensic Sci 2003;48(3):683–6.

132. Drummer OH, Syrjanen ML, Phelan M, Cordner SM. A study of deaths involving oxycodone. J Forensic Sci 1994;39(4):1069–75.

133. Michaud K, Augsburger M, Romain N, Giroud C, Mangin P. Fatal overdose of tramadol and alprazolam. Forensic Sci Int 1999;105(3):185–9.

134. Kudo K, Imamura T, Jitsufuchi N, Zhang XX, Tokunaga H, Nagata T. Death attributed to the toxic interaction of triazolam, amitriptyline and other psychotropic drugs. Forensic Sci Int 1997;86(1–2):35–41.

135. Schmidt LE, Dalhoff K. Concomitant overdosing of other drugs in patients with paracetamol poisoning. Br J Clin Pharmacol 2002;53(5):535–41.

136. Warot D, Bergougnan L, Lamiable D, Berlin I, Bensimon G, Danjou P, Puech AJ. Troleandomycin–triazolam interaction in healthy volunteers: pharmacokinetic and psychometric evaluation. Eur J Clin Pharmacol 1987;32(4):389–93.

137. Phillips JP, Antal EJ, Smith RB. A pharmacokinetic drug interaction between erythromycin and triazolam. J Clin Psychopharmacol 1986;6(5):297–9.

138. Gascon MP, Dayer P, Waldvogel F. Les interactions médicamenteuses du midazolam. [Drug interactions of midazolam.] Schweiz Med Wochenschr 1989;119(50):1834–6.

139. Hiller A, Olkkola KT, Isohanni P, Saarnivaara L. Unconsciousness associated with midazolam and erythromycin. Br J Anaesth 1990;65(6):826–8.

140. Amsden GW. Macrolides versus azalides: a drug interaction update. Ann Pharmacother 1995;29(9):906–17.

141. Moser L, Huther KJ, Koch-Weser J, Lundt PV. Effects of terfenadine and diphenhydramine alone or in combination with diazepam or alcohol on psychomotor performance and subjective feelings. Eur J Clin Pharmacol 1978;14(6):417–23.

142. Patat A, Perault MC, Vandel B, Ulliac N, Zieleniuk I, Rosenzweig P. Lack of interaction between a new antihistamine, mizolastine, and lorazepam on psychomotor performance and memory in healthy volunteers. Br J Clin Pharmacol 1995;39(1):31–8.

143. Mattila MJ, Aranko K, Kuitunen T. Diazepam effects on the performance of healthy subjects are not enhanced by treatment with the antihistamine ebastine. Br J Clin Pharmacol 1993;35(3):272–7.

144. Johnson LC, Spinweber CL, Gomez SA, Matteson LT. Daytime sleepiness, performance, mood, nocturnal sleep: the effect of benzodiazepine and caffeine on their relationship. Sleep 1990;13(2):121–35.

145. Johnson LC, Spinweber CL, Gomez SA. Benzodiazepines and caffeine: effect on daytime sleepiness, performance, and mood. Psychopharmacology (Berl) 1990;101(2):160–7.

146. Rush CR, Higgins ST, Bickel WK, Hughes JR. Acute behavioral effects of lorazepam and caffeine, alone and in combination, in humans. Behav Pharmacol 1994;5(3): 245–54.

147. Jackson CW, Markowitz JS, Brewerton TD. Delirium associated with clozapine and benzodiazepine combinations. Ann Clin Psychiatry 1995;7(3):139–41.

148. Cobb CD, Anderson CB, Seidel DR. Possible interaction between clozapine and lorazepam. Am J Psychiatry 1991;148(11):1606–7.

149. Tupala E, Niskanen L, Tiihonen J. Transient syncope and ECG changes associated with the concurrent administration of clozapine and diazepam. J Clin Psychiatry 1999;60(9):619–20.

150. Hollister LE. Interactions between alcohol and benzodiazepines. Recent Dev Alcohol 1990;8:233–9.

151. Vardy MM, Kay SR. LSD psychosis or LSD-induced schizophrenia? A multimethod inquiry. Arch Gen Psychiatry 1983;40(8):877–83.

152. van de Vijver DA, Roos RA, Jansen PA, Porsius AJ, de Boer A. Influence of benzodiazepines on antiparkinsonian drug treatment in levodopa users. Acta Neurol Scand 2002;105(1):8–12.

153. Bigatti MP, Corona D, Munizza C. Increased sister chromatid exchange and chromosomal aberration frequencies in psychiatric patients receiving psychopharmacological therapy. Mutat Res 1998;413(2):169–75.

154. Wesnes K, Simpson PM, Jansson B, Grahnen A, Weimann HJ, Kuppers H. Moxonidine and cognitive function: interactions with moclobemide and lorazepam. Eur J Clin Pharmacol 1997;52(5):351–8.

155. Driessen JJ, Vree TB, van Egmond J, Booij LH, Crul JF. In vitro interaction of diazepam and oxazepam with pancuronium and suxamethonium. Br J Anaesth 1984;56(10):1131–8.

156. Wali FA. Myorelaxant effect of diazepam. Interactions with neuromuscular blocking agents and cholinergic drugs. Acta Anaesthesiol Scand 1985;29(8):785–9.

157. Driessen JJ, Vree TB, van Egmond J, Booij LH, Crul JF. Interaction of midazolam with two non-depolarizing neuromuscular blocking drugs in the rat in vivo sciatic nerve–tibialis anterior muscle preparation. Br J Anaesth 1985;57(11):1089–94.

158. Asbury AJ, Henderson PD, Brown BH, Turner DJ, Linkens DA. Effect of diazepam on pancuronium-induced neuromuscular blockade maintained by a feedback system. Br J Anaesth 1981;53(8):859–63.

159. Cronnelly R, Morris RB, Miller RD. Comparison of thiopental and midazolam on the neuromuscular responses to succinylcholine or pancuronium in humans. Anesth Analg 1983;62(1):75–7.

160. Driessen JJ, Crul JF, Vree TB, van Egmond J, Booij LH. Benzodiazepines and neuromuscular blocking drugs in patients. Acta Anaesthesiol Scand 1986;30(8):642–6.

161. Feldman SA, Crawley BE. Diazepam and muscle relaxants. BMJ 1970;1(697):691.

162. Feldman SA, Crawley BE. Interaction of diazepam with the muscle-relaxant drugs. BMJ 1970;1(5705):336–8.

163. Olkkola KT, Tammisto T. Quantifying the interaction of rocuronium (Org 9426) with etomidate, fentanyl, midazolam, propofol, thiopental, and isoflurane using closed-loop feedback control of rocuronium infusion. Anesth Analg 1994;78(4):691–6.

164. Bourin M, Baker GB. Therapeutic and adverse effect considerations when using combinations of neuroleptics and benzodiazepines. Saudi Pharm J 1998;3–4:262–5.

165. Hatta K, Takahashi T, Nakamura H, Yamashiro H, Endo H, Kito K, Saeki T, Masui K, Yonezawa Y. A risk for obstruction of the airways in the parenteral use of levomepromazine with benzodiazepine. Pharmacopsychiatry 1998;31(4):126–30.

166. Jochemsen R, van der Graaff M, Boeijinga JK, Breimer DD. Influence of sex, menstrual cycle and oral contraception on the disposition of nitrazepam. Br J Clin Pharmacol 1982;13(3):319–24.

167. Patwardhan RV, Mitchell MC, Johnson RF, Schenker S. Differential effects of oral contraceptive steroids on the metabolism of benzodiazepines. Hepatology 1983;3(2): 248–53.

168. Nemeroff CB, DeVane CL, Pollock BG. Newer anti-depressants and the cytochrome P450 system. Am J Psychiatry 1996;153(3):311–20.

169. Dresser GK, Spence JD, Bailey DG. Pharmacokinetic–pharmacodynamic consequences and clinical relevance of cytochrome P450 3A4 inhibition. Clin Pharmacokinet 2000;38(1):41–57.

170. Lemberger L, Rowe H, Bosomworth JC, Tenbarge JB, Bergstrom RF. The effect of fluoxetine on the pharmacokinetics and psychomotor responses of diazepam. Clin Pharmacol Ther 1988;43(4):412–19.

171. Lasher TA, Fleishaker JC, Steenwyk RC, Antal EJ. Pharmacokinetic pharmacodynamic evaluation of the combined administration of alprazolam and fluoxetine. Psychopharmacology (Berl) 1991;104(3):323–7.

172. Beresford TP, Feinsilver DL, Hall RC. Adverse reactions to benzodiazepine–tricyclic antidepressant compound. J Clin Psychopharmacol 1981;1(6):392–4.

Benzoxonium chloride

See also Disinfectants and antiseptics

General Information

Benzoxonium is a quaternary ammonium compound with antibacterial, antiviral, and antimycotic activity. It can be used in topical disinfection, disinfection of surgical instruments, inhibition of plaque formation, and in veterinary products.

Organs and Systems

Immunologic

Contact allergic reactions have been rarely reported, with potential cross-reactivity with benzalkonium chloride and domiphen bromide (1,2).

- A 37-year-old woman developed intense burning and pruritic eczema where she had applied a cream containing benzoxonium for seborrheic dermatitis for 5 months (3). The reaction disappeared on withdrawal of the cream. Patch tests were positive to benzoxonium chloride 0.1% aqueous on days 2 and 4. Patch tests with benzalkonium chloride and benzoxonium chloride in 20 controls were negative.

References

1. de Groot AC, Conemans J, Liem DH. Contact allergy to benzoxonium chloride (Bradophen). Contact Dermatitis 1984;11(5):324–5.

2. Bruynzeel DP, de Groot AC, Weyland JW. Contact dermatitis to lauryl pyridinium chloride and benzoxonium chloride. Contact Dermatitis 1987;17(1):41–2.

3. Diaz-Ramon L, Aguirre A, Raton-Nieto JA, de Miguel M. Contact dermatitis from benzoxonium chloride. Contact Dermatitis 1999;41(1):53–4.

Benzoyl peroxide

General Information

Benzoyl peroxide is an antimicrobial and keratolytic agent used in the treatment of acne; it is also added to some foods. It is a catalyst for cross-linking in the production of plastics and is occasionally used in acrylic resin systems (for example composite dental fillings, dental prostheses) in which it is formed during the cross-linking process.

Organs and Systems

Skin

Allergic contact dermatitis has been attributed to topical benzoyl peroxide in a variety of settings (1–4).

- An 80-year-old man developed dermatitis in his leg amputation stump. He had been using stretching tapes containing benzoyl peroxide, and a patch test showed a positive reaction to benzoyl peroxide (1% in petrolatum) on days 2 and 3 (5).

References

1. Shwereb C, Lowenstein EJ. Delayed type hypersensitivity to benzoyl peroxide. J Drugs Dermatol 2004;3(2):197–9.

2. Forschner K, Zuberbier T, Worm M. Benzoyl peroxide as a cause of airborne contact dermatitis in an orthopaedic technician. Contact Dermatitis 2002;47(4):241.

3. Hernandez-Nunez A, Sanchez-Perez J, Pascual-Lopez M, Aragues M, Garcia-Diez A. Allergic contact dermatitis from benzoyl peroxide transferred by a loving son. Contact Dermatitis 2002;46(5):302.

4. Dejobert Y, Piette F, Thomas P. Contact dermatitis from benzoyl peroxide in dental prostheses. Contact Dermatitis 2002;46(3):177–8.

5. Greiner D, Weber J, Kaufmann R, Boehncke WH. Benzoyl peroxide as a contact allergen in adhesive tape. Contact Dermatitis 1999;41(4):233.

Benzydamine

General Information

Benzydamine is 1-benzyl-3-(3-dimethylaminopropoxy)-*H*-indazole, used for medical purposes as the hydrochloride. It has analgesic, anti-inflammatory, antipyretic, and local anesthetic effects. In the past it has been especially used in the symptomatic treatment of edematous post-operative or traumatic swelling, non-specific inflammation of the upper respiratory tract, and inflammation of connective tissues and joints. Nowadays, Tantum verde is the only such formulation listed in Germany; it is used for the treatment of oral and pharyngeal inflammation from any cause, for example radiotherapy-induced mucositis, stomatitis, Vincent's angina, necrotic oropharyngeal neoplasms, after surgical operations on the mouth and pharynx, after intubation, and after endoscopic laryngeal surgery. It can be administered as a spray, a gargle solution, a rinsing solution, or lozenges.

Organs and Systems

Skin

Skin reactions, including photosensitivity and contact dermatitis (when used topically), have been reported (1–7).

- A 67-year-old woman with pharyngitis gargled with Tantum verde, and after 3 weeks, during a holiday, developed an erythematous rash on sun-exposed skin, worsening within the next few days (8). She had not used a sunscreen. There were mainly well-demarcated areas of eczema on the face, neck, neckline, forearms, and lower legs. After oral and topical corticosteroids, the skin lesions improved within a few days.

There have been two other case reports of photoallergic dermatitis after local pharyngeal treatment with formulations containing benzydamine (6). This presumably occurs because of oral or intestinal absorption.

References

1. Turner M, Laitt R. Benzydamine oral rinse and rash. BMJ (Clin Res Ed) 1988;296(6628):1071.
2. Bruynzeel DP. Contact allergy to benzydamine. Contact Dermatitis 1986;14(5):313–14.
3. Anonymous. Difflam—a topical NSAID. Drug Ther Bull 1986;24(5):19–20.
4. Goncalo S, Souso L, Greitas JD. Dermatitis de fotosensibilizacion por benzidamine. Dermatitis Contacto 1982;3:21.
5. Vincenzi C, Cameli N, Tardio M, Piraccini BM. Contact and photocontact dermatitis due to benzydamine hydrochloride. Contact Dermatitis 1990;23(2):125–6.
6. Fernandez de Corres L. Photodermatitis from benzydamine. Contact Dermatitis 1980;6(4):285.
7. Frosch PJ, Weickel R. Photokontaktallergie durch Benzydamin (Tantum). [Photocontact allergy caused by benzydamine (Tantum).] Hautarzt 1989;40(12):771–3.
8. Henschel R, Agathos M, Breit R. Photocontact dermatitis after gargling with a solution containing benzydamine. Contact Dermatitis 2002;47(1):53.

Benzyl alcohol

See also Disinfectants and antiseptics

General Information

Benzyl alcohol is commonly used as a preservative in multidose injectable pharmaceutical formulations. For this purpose, concentrations in the range of 0.5–2.0% are used and the whole amount of benzyl alcohol injected is generally very well tolerated. Concentrations of 0.9% are used in Bacteriostatic Sodium Chlorine (USP), which is often used in the management of critically ill patients to flush intravascular catheters after the addition of medications or the withdrawal of blood, and in Sterile Bacteriostatic Water for injection (USP), used to dilute or reconstitute medications for intravenous use. The content of benzyl alcohol in a lot of injectable pharmaceutical formulations needs to be considered carefully. The view still taken in many countries that the additives and excipients in medicines are trade secrets must be deplored. The duty to declare them is only realized in some countries.

The toxic effects of benzyl alcohol include respiratory vasodilatation, hypertension, convulsions, and paralysis.

Organs and Systems

Nervous system

The data on reported cases of neurological disorders after intrathecal chemotherapy with methotrexate or cytosine arabinoside that could be attributed to benzyl alcohol or to other preservatives have been reviewed in the context of a case of flaccid paraplegia after intrathecal administration of cytosine arabinoside diluted in bacteriostatic water containing 1.5% benzyl alcohol (1). Most commonly, flaccid paraparesis, with absent reflexes, developed rapidly, often with pain and anesthesia. Very often there was full recovery. The prognosis depended mainly on the concentration of the preservative and on the time of exposure. In some cases, the paralysis ascended to cause respiratory distress, cardiac arrest, and death. Only preservative-free sterile CSF substitute or saline, or preferably the patient's own CSF, should be used to dilute chemotherapeutic agents (SEDA-11, 475).

Skin

Allergic contact dermatitis, characterized by erythema, palpable edema, and raised borders, was attributed to benzyl alcohol (2). In this case, the benzyl alcohol was present as a preservative in an injectable solution of sodium tetradecyl sulfate, a sclerosing agent used for the treatment of varicose veins. The author provided a list of 151 injectable formulations (48 for subcutaneous administration) that contained benzyl alcohol as a preservative in the range 0.5–2.0%. The list included hormones and steroids, antihypertensive drugs (reserpine), vitamin formulations (vitamins B_{12} and B_6), ammonium sulfate, antihistamines, antibiotics, heparin (17 brands), tranquillizers, and sclerosing agents (sodium morrhuate and sodium tetradecyl sulfate).

- A patient with a contact allergic reaction to a topical antimycotic drug formulation that contained benzoyl alcohol had positive patch tests on day 4 and a positive repeated open application test to benzoyl alcohol 5% in petroleum jelly (3).

The authors noted that although contact allergic reactions to benzoyl alcohol are rarely reported, they can be responsible for contact allergy to topical glucocorticoid formulations.

Immunologic

Various allergic reactions have been attributed to benzyl alcohol.

- A 55-year-old man developed fatigue, nausea, and diffuse angioedema shortly after an intramuscular injection of vitamin B12 containing benzyl alcohol (4).
- In another male patient, fever developed, and a maculopapular rash occurred on his chest and arms after an injection of cytarabine, vincristine, and heparin in a dilution solution containing benzyl alcohol (5).

Susceptibility Factors

Age

A gasping syndrome in small premature infants who had been exposed to intravenous formulations containing benzyl alcohol 0.9% as a preservative has been described (SEDA-10, 421) (SEDA-11, 475) (6–8). The affected infants presented with a metabolic acidosis, seizures, neurological deterioration, hepatic and renal dysfunction, and cardiovascular collapse. Death was reported in 16 children who received a minimum of 99 mg/kg/day of benzyl alcohol. This metabolic acidosis is caused by accumulation of the metabolite benzoic acid and is mainly related to an excessive body burden relative to body weight, so that the load of the metabolite may exceed the capacity of the immature liver and kidney for detoxification. The FDA has recommended that neither intramuscular flushing solutions containing benzyl alcohol nor dilutions with this preservative should be used in newborn infants.

In a review of the hospital and autopsy records of infants admitted to a nursery during the previous 18 months, 218 patients had been given fluids containing benzyl alcohol as flush solutions and they were compared with 218 neonates admitted during the following 18 months (9). Withdrawal of benzyl alcohol as a preservative had no demonstrable effect on mortality, but the development of kernicterus was significantly associated with benzyl alcohol in 15 of 49 exposed patients, and no cases occurred after withdrawal of the preservative. However, this apparent association was not confirmed in a 5-year study of the use of benzyl alcohol as a preservative in intravenous medications in a neonatal intensive care unit (10). In 129 neonates who died between the ages of 2 and 28 days, there was no difference in the rate of kernicterus and the exposure to benzyl alcohol between neonates who developed kernicterus and the control group of unaffected infants who were born during the same period and who were of the same birth weight and gestation age. In this study, only estimates of the extent of exposure to benzyl alcohol were given, rather than exact doses and serum concentrations.

References

1. Hahn AF, Feasby TE, Gilbert JJ. Paraparesis following intrathecal chemotherapy. Neurology 1983;33(8):1032–8.
2. Shmunes E. Allergic dermatitis to benzyl alcohol in an injectable solution. Arch Dermatol 1984;120(9):1200–1.
3. Podda M, Zollner T, Grundmann-Kollmann M, Kaufmann R, Boehncke WH. Allergic contact dermatitis from benzyl alcohol during topical antimycotic treatment. Contact Dermatitis 1999;41(5):302–3.
4. Grant JA, Bilodeau PA, Guernsey BG, Gardner FH. Unsuspected benzyl alcohol hypersensitivity. N Engl J Med 1982;306(2):108.
5. Wilson JP, Solimando DA Jr, Edwards MS. Parenteral benzyl alcohol-induced hypersensitivity reaction. Drug Intell Clin Pharm 1986;20(9):689–91.
6. Gershanik J, Boecler B, George W, et al. Gasping syndrome: benzyl alcohol poisoning. Clin Res 1981;29:895a.
7. Gershanik J, Boecler B, Ensley H, McCloskey S, George W. The gasping syndrome and benzyl alcohol poisoning. N Engl J Med 1982;307(22):1384–8.
8. Gershanik J, Boecler B, George W, et al. Neonatal deaths associated with use of benzyl alcohol—United States. Munch Med Wochenschr 1982;31:290.
9. Jardine DS, Rogers K. Relationship of benzyl alcohol to kernicterus, intraventricular hemorrhage, and mortality in preterm infants. Pediatrics 1989;83(2):153–60.
10. Cronin CM, Brown DR, Ahdab-Barmada M. Risk factors associated with kernicterus in the newborn infant: importance of benzyl alcohol exposure. Am J Perinatol 1991;8(2):80–5.

Bephenium

General Information

Bephenium hydroxynaphthoate is an antihelminthic drug that has been used in the treatment of hookworm infections due to *Ancylostoma duodenale* in a single dose (1). It is well tolerated, and reactions are confined to mild gastrointestinal disturbances (unpleasant taste, nausea, abdominal pain, and sometimes also vomiting and diarrhea), headache, and dizziness. It is reputed to be safe in pregnancy but is better avoided in conditions in which purgation could be dangerous; these naturally include the last few months of pregnancy, because of the risk of miscarriage.

Reference

1. Botero D. Chemotherapy of human intestinal parasitic diseases. Annu Rev Pharmocol Toxicol 1978;18:1–15.

Bepridil

See also Antidysrhythmic drugs

General Information

Bepridil is an antidysrhythmic drug with unusual pharmacological properties in that it belongs to both class I and class IV. In other words, it blocks both the fast inward sodium current and the slow outward calcium current in excitable cardiac cells (SEDA-13, 141). It was withdrawn because of its serious prodysrhythmic effects.

Bepridil has been the subject of a brief general review (1) and its pharmacokinetics have been specifically reviewed (2). Although it is highly protein-bound, bepridil does not take part in protein-binding displacement interactions (2).

The main adverse effect of bepridil is torsade de pointes due to QT interval prolongation. After intravenous infusion bepridil can cause local reactions (3) and phlebothrombosis (4). Other minor adverse effects that have been reported include urticaria (5), gastrointestinal disturbances (especially diarrhea) (6,7), and dizziness (6–8). Hepatic enzymes can rise (9,10).

Organs and Systems

Cardiovascular

Bepridil can cause hypotension after rapid intravenous injection (6,11), but not during long-term oral therapy (12,13).

Bepridil prolongs the QT interval (3,7,8,14), an effect that is dose-related (14). It can therefore cause dysrhythmias, including polymorphous ventricular tachycardia, the risk of which is greater in patients with potassium depletion, those with pre-existing prolongation of the QT interval, those with a history of serious ventricular dysrhythmias, and those who are also taking other drugs that prolong the QT interval (15).

Of 75 elderly patients who took bepridil 200 mg/day, 23 had prolongation of the QT interval. The factors that were associated with this were hypokalemia, bradycardia, renal insufficiency, and an increased plasma bepridil concentration (16).

Drug–Drug Interactions

Antidysrhythmic drugs

Because it prolongs the QT interval, bepridil can potentiate the effects of other drugs with the same effect (for example other Class I antidysrhythmic drugs and amiodarone).

Beta-adrenoceptor antagonists

The effect of a beta-blocker (metoprolol 30–40 mg/day or bisoprolol 2.5–5.0 mg/day for 1 month) on the change in QT interval, QT dispersion, and transmural dispersion of repolarization caused by bepridil has been studied in 10 patients with paroxysmal atrial fibrillation resistant to various antidysrhythmic drugs (17). Bepridil significantly prolonged the QTc interval from 0.42 to 0.50 seconds, QT dispersion from 0.07 to 0.14 seconds, and transmural dispersion of repolarization from 0.10 to 0.16 seconds. The addition of a beta-blocker shortened the QTc interval from 0.50 to 0.47 seconds, QTc dispersion from 0.14 to 0.06 seconds, and transmural dispersion of repolarization from 0.16 to 0.11 seconds. The authors therefore suggested that combined therapy with bepridil and a beta-blocker might be useful for intractable atrial fibrillation.

Bepridil does not interact with propranolol (8).

Digoxin

Bepridil does not interact with digoxin (18).

Phenazone

Bepridil increases the rate of clearance of phenazone (antipyrine) and might therefore be expected to enhance the rate of clearance of other drugs that are metabolized (19).

References

1. Anonymous. Bepridil. Lancet 1988;1(8580):278–9.
2. Benet LZ. Pharmacokinetics and metabolism of bepridil. Am J Cardiol 1985;55(7):C8–13.
3. Ponsonnaille J, Citron B, Threil F, Heiligenstein D, Gras H. Etude des effets electrophysiologiques du bepridil utilisé par voie veineuse. [The electrophysiologic effects of intravenously administered bepridil.] Arch Mal Coeur Vaiss 1982;75(12):1415–23.
4. Rowland E, McKenna WJ, Krikler DM. Electrophysiologic and antiarrhythmic actions of bepridil. Comparison with verapamil and ajmaline for atrioventricular reentrant tachycardia. Am J Cardiol 1985;55(13 Pt 1):1513–19.
5. Brembilla-Perrot B, Aliot E, Clementy J, Cosnay P, Djiane P, Fauchier JP, Kacet S, Lellouche D, Mabo P, Richard M, Victor J. Evaluation of bepridil efficacy by electrophysiologic testing in patients with recurrent ventricular tachycardia: comparison of two regimens. Cardiovasc Drugs Ther 1992;6(2):187–93.
6. Fauchier JP, Cosnay P, Neel C, Rouesnel P, Bonnet P, Quilliet L. Traitement des tachycardies supraventriculaires et ventriculaires paroxystiques par le bépridil. [Treatment of supraventricular and paroxysmal ventricular tachycardia with bepridil.] Arch Mal Coeur Vaiss 1985;78(4):612–19.
7. Roy D, Montigny M, Klein GJ, Sharma AD, Cassidy D. Electrophysiologic effects and long-term efficacy of bepridil for recurrent supraventricular tachycardias. Am J Cardiol 1987;59(1):89–92.
8. Frishman WH, Charlap S, Farnham DJ, Sawin HS, Michelson EL, Crawford MH, DiBianco R, Kostis JB, Zellner SR, Michie DD, et al. Combination propranolol and bepridil therapy in stable angina pectoris. Am J Cardiol 1985;55(7):C43–9.
9. DiBianco R, Alpert J, Katz RJ, Spann J, Chesler E, Ferri DP, Larca LJ, Costello RB, Gore JM, Eisenman MJ. Bepridil for chronic stable angina pectoris: results of a prospective multicenter, placebo-controlled, dose-ranging study in 77 patients. Am J Cardiol 1984;53(1):35–41.
10. Hill JA, O'Brien JT, Alpert JS, Gore JM, Zusman RM, Christensen D, Boucher CA, Vetrovec G, Borer JS, Friedman C, et al. Effect of bepridil in patients with chronic stable angina: results of a multicenter trial. Circulation 1985;71(1):98–103.
11. Flammang D, Waynberger M, Jansen FH, Paillet R, Coumel P. Electrophysiological profile of bepridil, a new anti-anginal drug with calcium blocking properties. Eur Heart J 1983;4(9):647–54.
12. Canicave JC, Deu J, Jacq J, Paillet R. Un nouvel antiangoreux, le bépridil: appreciation de son efficacité par l'epreuve d'effort au cours d'un essai a double insu contre placébo. [A new antianginal drug, bepridil: efficacy estimation by exertion test during a double blind test against a placebo.] Therapie 1980;35(5):607–12.
13. Upward JW, Daly K, Campbell S, Bergman G, Jewitt DE. Electrophysiologic, hemodynamic and metabolic effects of intravenous bepridil hydrochloride. Am J Cardiol 1985;55(13 Pt 1):1589–95.
14. Perelman MS, McKenna WJ, Rowland E, Krikler DM. A comparison of bepridil with amiodarone in the treatment of established atrial fibrillation. Br Heart J 1987;58(4):339–44.
15. Singh BN. Bepridil therapy: guidelines for patient selection and monitoring of therapy. Am J Cardiol 1992;69(11):D79–85.
16. Viallon A, Laporte-Simitsidis S, Pouzet V, Venet C, Tardy B, Zeni F, Bertrand JC. Bépridil: intérêt du dosage sérique dans la surveillance du traitement. [Bepridil:

importance of serum level in treatment surveillance.] Presse Méd 2000;29(12):645–7.

17. Yoshiga Y, Shimizu A, Yamagata T, Hayano T, Ueyama T, Ohmura M, Itagaki K, Kimura M, Matsuzaki M. Betablocker decreases the increase in QT dispersion and transmural dispersion of repolarization induced by bepridil. Circ J 2002;66(11):1024–8.
18. Stern H, Aust P, Belz GG, Schneider HT. Interaction entre bépridil et digoxine. Rev Med 1983;24:1279.
19. Funck-Brentano C, Chaffin PL, Wilkinson GR, McAllister B, Woosley RL. Effect of oral administration of a new calcium channel blocking agent, bepridil on antipyrine clearance in man. Br J Clin Pharmacol 1987;24(4):559–60.

Beraprost

See also Prostaglandins

General Information

Beraprost is a stable, orally active analogue of PGI_2. It has been tested in patients with intermittent claudication in a randomized, placebo-controlled trial (1). Beraprost improved walking distance more often than placebo. It also reduced the incidence of critical cardiovascular events, but the trial was not powered for statistical validation of this effect. As with iloprost, headache and flushing were the most common adverse effects.

Reference

1. Lievre M, Morand S, Besse B, Fiessinger JN, Boissel JP. Oral Beraprost sodium, a prostaglandin I(2) analogue, for intermittent claudication: a double-blind, randomized, multicenter controlled trial. Beraprost et Claudication Intermittente (BERCI) Research Group. Circulation 2000;102(4):426–31.

Berberidaceae

See also Herbal medicines

General Information

The genera in the family of Berberidaceae (Table 1) include lychee and soapberry.

Berberis vulgaris

Barberry (pipperidge bush) is a vernacular name for *Berberis vulgaris* (the European barberry), but it can also refer to *Mahonia aquifolium* and *Mahonia nervosa*. In the USA only the *Mahonia* species have had official status as a source of barberry, but *Berberis vulgaris* is said to serve similar medicinal purposes and to contain similar principles. Its root bark yields the quaternary isoquinoline alkaloid berberine and several other tertiary and quaternary alkaloids. Berberine is also found

Table 1 The genera of Berberidaceae

Achlys (achlys)
Berberis L (barberry)
Caulophyllum (cohosh)
Diphylleia (umbrellaleaf)
Epimedium (epimedium)
Jeffersonia (jeffersonia)
Mahonia (barberry)
Nandina (nandina)
Podophyllum (may apple)
Vancouveria (insideout flower)

in *Hydrastis canadensis* (goldenseal) and *Coptis chinensis* (goldenthread).

Adverse effects

In man berberine has positive inotropic, negative chronotropic, antidysrhythmic, and vasodilator properties (1) and there is experimental evidence that it can cause arterial hypotension (2,3).

Berberine displaces bilirubin from albumin and there is therefore a risk of kernicterus in jaundiced neonates (4).

In a study of the effect of berberine in acute watery diarrhea, oral doses of 400 mg were well tolerated, except for complaints about its bitter taste and a few instances of transient nausea and abdominal discomfort. However, patients with cholera given tetracycline plus berberine were more ill, suffered longer from diarrhea, and required larger volumes of intravenous fluid than those given tetracycline alone (5).

Caulophyllum thalictroides

Caulophyllum thalictroides (blue cohosh) contains vasoactive glycosides and quinolizidine alkaloids that produce toxic effects on the myocardium in animals.

Adverse effects

Heart failure occurred in the fetus of a mother who used blue cohosh.

- A 41-week-old boy weighing 3.66 kg developed respiratory distress, acidosis, and shock shortly after a spontaneous vaginal delivery (6). His 36-year-old mother had a history of adequately controlled hypothyroidism and had taken tablets of blue cohosh for 1 month to induce uterine contractions. Subsequently she felt more contractions and less fetal activity. After delivery, the baby continued to be critically ill for several weeks and required treatment for respiratory failure and cardiogenic shock. He gradually improved and was extubated after 21 days. There were no congenital abnormalities or other reasons to explain the infant's problems. He remained in hospital for 31 days and an electrocardiogram at discharge was consistent with a resolving anterolateral myocardial infection. Two years later he had fully recovered, but cardiomegaly and impaired left ventricular function persisted.

The authors believed that the consumption of blue cohosh by the mother had caused heart failure in the child.

Dysosma pleianthum

Dysosma pleianthum (bajiaolian), a species of May apple, is a traditional Chinese herbal medicine rich in podophyllotoxin. It has been widely used in China for thousands of years as a general remedy and for the treatment of snake bite, weakness, condyloma accuminata, lymphadenopathy, and tumors.

Adverse effects

Five people developed nausea, vomiting, diarrhea, abdominal pain, thrombocytopenia, leukopenia, abnormal liver function tests, sensory ataxia, altered consciousness, and persistent peripheral tingling or numbness after drinking infusions of bajiaolian (7). These effects were consistent with podophyllum intoxication.

Mahonia species

Barberry is a vernacular name for members of the *Berberis* species, such as *Berberis vulgaris* (European barberry), but is also used to refer to members of the *Mahonia* species, such as *Mahonia aquifolium* and *Mahonia nervosa*. In the USA only the latter species have had official status as a source of barberry, but *Berberis vulgaris* is said to serve similar medicinal purposes and to contain similar principles. Its root bark yields the quaternary isoquinoline alkaloid berberine and several other tertiary and quaternary alkaloids. It has been used to treat a variety of skin conditions (8,9). The literature sometimes cautions that barberry alkaloids can cause arterial hypotension.

References

1. Lau CW, Yao XQ, Chen ZY, Ko WH, Huang Y. Cardiovascular actions of berberine. Cardiovasc Drug Rev 2001;19(3):234–44.
2. Sabir M, Bhide NK. Study of some pharmacological actions of berberine. Indian J Physiol Pharmacol 1971;15(3):111–32.
3. Chun YT, Yip TT, Lau KL, Kong YC, Sankawa U. A biochemical study on the hypotensive effect of berberine in rats. Gen Pharmacol 1979;10(3):177–82.
4. Chan E. Displacement of bilirubin from albumin by berberine. Biol Neonate 1993;63(4):201–8.
5. Khin-Maung-U, Myo-Khin, Nyunt-Nyunt-Wai, Aye-Kyaw, Tin-U. Clinical trial of berberine in acute watery diarrhoea. BMJ (Clin Res Ed) 1985;291(6509):1601–5.
6. Jones TK, Lawson BM. Profound neonatal congestive heart failure caused by maternal consumption of blue cohosh herbal medication. J Pediatr 1998;132(3 Pt 1):550–2.
7. Kao WF, Hung DZ, Tsai WJ, Lin KP, Deng JF. Podophyllotoxin intoxication: toxic effect of Bajiaolian in herbal therapeutics. Hum Exp Toxicol 1992;11(6):480–7.
8. Turner NJ, Hebda RJ. Contemporary use of bark for medicine by two Salishan native elders of southeast Vancouver Island, Canada. J Ethnopharmacol 1990;29(1):59–72.
9. Grimme H, Augustin M. Phytotherapie bei chronischen Dermatosen und Wunden: was ist gesichert? [Phytotherapy in chronic dermatoses and wounds: what is the evidence?] Forsch Komplementarmed 1999;6(Suppl 2):5–8.

Beta$_2$-adrenoceptor agonists

See also Individual agents

General Information

Beta$_2$-adrenoceptor agonists are widely used in asthma and have inevitably been associated with a number of problems. Some of these are attributable to the drugs themselves, others to the formulations in which they are given.

Organs and Systems

Cardiovascular

Eight men with mild asthma underwent measurement of forearm blood flow, a surrogate marker for peripheral vasodilatation (1). All received in sequential order the following: normoxia plus placebo, normoxia plus inhaled salbutamol 800 micrograms, hypoxia (SpO$_2$ 82%) plus placebo, and hypoxia plus inhaled salbutamol 800 micrograms. The period of mask breathing was 60 minutes and inhalation of salbutamol/placebo started after 30 minutes. While there were non-significant differences in blood pressure and potassium concentrations between the different treatments, forearm blood flow increased significantly by 45% in hypoxic patients inhaling salbutamol versus normoxic patients inhaling placebo. The authors concluded that the combination of hypoxia and inhalation of beta$_2$-agonists has serious systemic vascular adverse effects, potentially leading to pulmonary shunting and reduced venous return, which may be associated with sudden death. Furthermore, asthmatic patients in respiratory distress should be given beta$_2$-agonists and oxygen concomitantly whenever possible.

Intravenous and intracoronary salbutamol (10–30 micrograms/minute and 1–10 micrograms/minute respectively), and intravenous isoprenaline (1–5 micrograms/ minute), a mixed beta$_1$/beta$_2$-adrenoceptor agonist, were infused in 85 patients with coronary artery disease and 22 healthy controls during fixed atrial pacing (2). Both salbutamol and isoprenaline produced large increases in QT dispersion (QT$_{onset}$, QT$_{peak}$, and QT$_{end}$), more pronouncedly in patients with coronary artery disease. Dispersion of the QT interval is thought to be a surrogate marker for cardiac dysrhythmia (3). The authors concluded that beta$_2$-adrenoceptors mediate important electrophysiological effects in human ventricular myocardium and can trigger dysrhythmias in susceptible patients.

In a blind, randomized study, 29 children aged under 2 years, with moderate to severe acute exacerbations of hyper-reactive airways disease, were treated with either a standard dose of nebulized salbutamol (0.15 mg/kg) or a low dose of nebulized salbutamol (0.075 mg/kg) plus nebulized ipratropium bromide 250 micrograms (4). Standard and low-dose nebulized salbutamol was given three times at intervals of 20 minutes and nebulized ipratropium bromide was given once. Clinical improvement, measured as O$_2$ saturation and relief of respiratory distress, was similar in both groups. QT dispersion was measured at baseline and after treatment and was significantly increased only by the standard dose of nebulized salbutamol.

Respiratory

Beta-adrenoceptor agonists can produce or worsen hypoxia acutely in patients with asthma by increasing ventilation–perfusion inequality. It is not known whether this effect is clinically important in patients with asthma not severe enough to require hospital treatment (where supplementary oxygen is standard therapy).

Metabolism

In obstetrics, the classic effects of beta$_2$-adrenoceptor agonists on glucose metabolism can be absent or harmless in the non-diabetic, but dangerous in women with diabetes, in whom they can cause metabolic acidosis (5); the hyperglycemic effect can be aggravated if glucocorticoids are given (as they may be to prevent hyaline membrane disease in prematurity).

Immunologic

The possibility of a causal relation between the administration of beta$_2$-adrenoceptor agonists and reduced serum immunoglobulin concentrations has been raised in various studies. In one study, adults with asthma taking steroids were compared with patients taking beta$_2$-adrenoceptor agonists (6). The patients who were using beta$_2$-adrenoceptor agonists had significantly lower serum IgG concentrations, irrespective of any history of steroid use. However, in patients using both treatments this depressive effect was even more pronounced; its mechanism is unclear.

Beta$_2$-adrenoceptor agonists and the response to allergens

Following inhalation of an allergen by a sensitized asthmatic, an immediate or type I response is seen. This occurs rapidly and is characterized by dyspnea, wheeze, and a fall in the FEV$_1$ or peak expiratory flow. The response can be prevented or reversed by inhalation of a beta$_2$-agonist. Several hours later, however, a proportion of asthmatics develop a delayed or type III response. This response is prolonged and associated with inflammatory changes in the airways. For some time after it resolves there is an increase in non-specific reactivity of the airways. This can be quantified by measuring the PC$_{20}$ of histamine or methacholine. This is the provocative concentration necessary to cause a 20% fall in the FEV$_1$ or peak expiratory flow. The delayed response is not prevented by prior inhalation of a beta$_2$-agonist. It can be prevented by prior treatment with cromoglicate or a corticosteroid.

Treatment with a beta$_2$-agonist aerosol, before allergen inhalation, allows inhalation of significantly greater amounts of allergen before the type I response occurs. In asthmatics who only have a type I response before treatment with a beta$_2$-agonist, a late response to the increased allergen dose results. In asthmatics who already have a type III response, this response is increased (7). Treatment with an oral beta$_2$-agonist for 2 weeks

increases sensitivity to inhaled allergen. In addition, reversal of allergen-induced bronchoconstriction by an inhaled beta$_2$-agonist is significantly impaired (8). Treatment for 1 week with an inhaled beta$_2$-agonist increases the late (type III) asthmatic response to the same dose of inhaled allergen. The increase in airway reactivity to methacholine following the late response is also increased (9). Sufficient inhaled beta$_2$-agonist needs to be taken to produce this effect. The effect is seen with salbutamol 0.8 mg/day, but not with 0.2 or 0.4 mg/day (10). Pretreatment with an inhaled beta$_2$-agonist not only increases the response to allergen but also attenuates the protective effect of a beta$_2$-agonist against both allergen and methacholine, that is both specific and non-specific airway reactivity is increased (11).

Clearly, the combined use of a regular inhaled beta$_2$-agonist and allergen exposure can cause more airway inflammation than allergen exposure alone. It has been suggested that regular use of beta$_2$-agonists may induce dysfunction of beta-receptors on the mast cells making the mast cells more prone to release mediator (12). Regular treatment with beta$_2$-agonists alone will result in greater airway inflammation and persistent asthma. This emphasizes the importance of regular prophylactic medication with cromoglicate or inhaled corticosteroids.

Death

Increased mortality among asthmatic patients has been correlated with an increase in the use of beta-adrenoceptor agonist aerosols on two occasions, first in the UK in 1966, and then in New Zealand in the late 1970s and 1980s. On both occasions the rise in deaths correlated well with increasing use of beta-agonist aerosols. However, when the death rates subsequently fell, the use of beta-agonist aerosols did not fall to the same extent (SEDA-13, 427) (SEDA-21, 179), suggesting that the correlation may have been due to the way the aerosols were used rather than with the fact of their use.

The sharp rise in asthma mortality in 1977 in New Zealand provoked debate about the safety of beta$_2$-adrenoceptor agonists, especially the short-acting compound fenoterol. This led to the withdrawal of fenoterol in New Zealand and amendment of the American Asthma Guidelines, suggesting caution in the regular use of beta$_2$-agonists (13). Although there is evidence linking fenoterol to increased morbidity and mortality in asthma (14), the underlying mechanisms were not known. It was suggested that the increase in mortality might be linked to fatal cardiac dysrhythmias, developing under conditions of asthma-induced hypoxia and high doses of beta$_2$-adrenoceptor agonists (15).

One likely explanation for the events of 1966 and later can be found in the fact, discussed below, that with progressive use of beta-agonists the response tends to fall, as a result of which the patient takes increasing doses, without relief. An association between increasing use of beta-agonist aerosols and asthma deaths is therefore to be expected, unless this accumulation of dosage can be avoided by proper guidance. There is still a possibility that the association between the use of these products and fatal reactions could have been due to an as yet unrecognized adverse effect of beta-agonist aerosols that becomes prevalent only under particular conditions.

Identification of susceptible patients

An alternative explanation for the epidemic of asthma fatalities among users of beta-adrenoceptor agonist aerosols postulates the existence of a subset of asthmatic patients who are more sensitive than others to an adverse effect of beta-agonists. In this view the occurrence of a peak incidence of deaths will eliminate this subset and the overall death rate will thus fall once more without a proportionate reduction in the use of beta-agonists. A subset of asthmatic patients who develop a significant reduction in bronchodilator response to salbutamol after a short period of treatment has indeed been identified, although the number of patients studied was small. The subset developed a significant reduction in the B_{max} for beta$_2$-adrenoceptors in the lung. This was measured in vivo by PET scanning using a beta-antagonist ligand. Patients in the subset were homozygous for glycine at codon 16 on the beta$_2$-adrenoceptor gene (SEDA-21, 180).

However, another and larger study failed to identify any polymorphism or haplotype of the gene associated with fatal/near fatal asthma, and the authors concluded that the beta$_2$-adrenoceptor genotype was not a major factor in fatal or near fatal asthma (16). A third study similarly found no relation between genotype (coding for amino acids 16 and 27) and change in overall asthma control (17).

On the other hand, other workers have found that homozygotes for arginine 16 were 5.3 times (CI = 1.6, 17.7) more likely than homozygotes for glycine 16 to have a positive response to salbutamol, while heterozygotes for codon 16 on the beta$_2$-adrenoceptor gene were 2.3 times (CI = 1.3, 4.2) more likely to have a positive response to salbutamol than homozygotes for glycine 16 (18).

Finally, in a subset of patients with homozygous glycine on codon 16 of the beta$_2$-adrenoceptor gene, lymphocyte beta$_2$-adrenoceptor density was reduced after treatment for 1 week with a long-acting beta$_2$-agonist. There was also a reduction in maximal response to salbutamol (19).

The upshot of all this is that patients who are homozygous for glycine at codon 16 of the beta$_2$-adrenoceptor gene have a reduced bronchodilator response to salbutamol and this response is further reduced by repeated administration, which also causes a reduction in beta$_2$-adrenoceptor number. So far no genotype has been associated with overall asthma control or the frequency of fatal or near fatal attacks of asthma. Further documentation of the effect of the beta$_2$-adrenoceptor genotype on the response to beta$_2$-agonists may lead to the use of alternative bronchodilators in patients who are homozygous for glycine at codon 16.

Long-Term Effects

Drug tolerance

Reduced responsiveness to beta$_2$-adrenoceptor agonists

The bronchodilator effects of short-acting beta$_2$-agonists are not significantly reduced on chronic administration. However the bronchoprotective effect of beta$_2$-agonists,

as measured by prevention of the response to spasmogens and exercise, becomes significantly reduced. This has been documented by measuring the PC_{20}, the concentration of methacholine or other spasmogen that provokes a 20% fall in lung function. Bronchoprotection results in a rise in PC_{20} and as bronchoprotection is lost, the PC_{20} falls.

Inhalation of salbutamol four times a day for 1 week did not affect the bronchodilator response to salbutamol, but there was a significant reduction in PC_{20} to methacholine (10).

Co-administration of a corticosteroid may mitigate the loss of bronchoprotective effect. The methacholine PC_{20} for salbutamol was significantly greater after 3 weeks treatment with the inhaled corticosteroid budesonide. However, addition of the long-acting beta$_2$-agonist salmeterol 0.05 mg bd significantly reduced the bronchoprotective effect of salbutamol, despite concurrent treatment with inhaled glucocorticoids (20). The bronchoprotective effect of salmeterol itself fell after only two doses (21). On the other hand, despite the administration of inhaled corticosteroids, the bronchodilator effect of another long-acting beta$_2$-agonist, formoterol, was reduced after treatment for 3 weeks. Administration of prednisolone 50 mg and hydrocortisone 100 mg rapidly reversed the reduction in response (22).

However, it is difficult to extrapolate PC_{20} changes after treatment with beta$_2$-agonists to the clinical outcome. There is an assumption that if PC_{20} falls, the patient is more likely to suffer acute attacks when exposed to spasmogens, allergens, and exercise. However, the loss of bronchoprotective effect has not so far been shown to increase morbidity or mortality in asthmatic patients.

Regular salbutamol has been compared with salbutamol, taken as needed, in mild asthmatics. There was no change in asthma control nor any increase in the frequency or severity of exacerbation (23). As the bronchodilator response is maintained, patients can be advised to use short-acting beta$_2$-agonists to relieve acute bronchoconstriction and if necessary to increase the dose.

The significance of stereoisomers of beta$_2$-adrenoceptor agonists

An alternative hypothesis has been proposed to explain why beta$_2$-agonists lose their bronchoprotective effect while retaining a bronchodilator effect. The beta$_2$-agonists currently available for treating asthma consist of racemic mixtures of equal amounts of two stereoisomers, the *R*-isomer (or L-isomer), which is the beta-adrenoceptor agonist, and the *S*-isomer (D-isomer) which is inactive.

In guinea-pig airways, the constrictor response to platelet activating factor (PAF), histamine, and prostaglandin $F_{2\alpha}$ are all prevented by infusion of racemic isoprenaline. After the isoprenaline is stopped, the constrictor response is markedly potentiated. Infusion of the *S*-isomer alone does not prevent the constrictor responses in contrast to the infusion of racemic isoprenaline. After infusion of the *S*-isomer is stopped there is an increase in the response to the constrictor agents, equivalent to that seen after racemic isoprenaline. This can be compared to asthma, in which prolonged exposure to racemates of beta$_2$-agonists produces a loss of the bronchoprotective effect while maintaining the immediate bronchodilator effect (24).

Regular exposure to a racemate, especially during or after an allergic reaction, will cause hyper-reactivity to spasmogens, and this could be due to an effect of the S-isomer. This effect is not seen immediately, because of beta$_2$-adrenoceptor-mediated bronchodilatation by the R-isomer.

Most of the clinical work on this phenomenon has been undertaken with salbutamol. In one major investigation, after administration of racemic salbutamol to healthy volunteers, both the peak plasma concentration of R-salbutamol and the systemic availability (measured by the AUC) were higher than when R-salbutamol was given in an equivalent dose as the R-isomer alone. It was concluded that R-salbutamol was more efficiently metabolized in the absence of S-salbutamol. S-salbutamol is a competitive inhibitor at the active site of the phenol-sulfotransferase enzyme, and its absence allows more R-salbutamol to be metabolized, resulting in lower systemic availability of R-salbutamol when the R-isomer alone is administered. Although the plasma concentrations of R-salbutamol were lower, the rise in plasma glucose and fall in plasma potassium were greater when the pure R-isomer was given alone. There was also a greater increase in heart rate and finger tremor. The greater potency of R-salbutamol given alone suggests inhibition of the effects of the R-isomer by the S-isomer (25).

In another investigation, a single dose of 1.25 mg nebulized R-salbutamol, administered to asthmatics, produced equivalent bronchoprotection, bronchodilatation, tachycardia, and restlessness to that given by 2.5 mg of racemic salbutamol (26). In a further study, asthmatic patients were treated for 28 days with racemic or R-salbutamol administered by nebulizer three times a day. Improvement in FEV$_1$ was similar after R-salbutamol 0.63 mg and racemic salbutamol 2.5 mg and greatest with R-salbutamol 1.25 mg. Racemic salbutamol 1.25 mg had the least bronchodilator effect, especially after chronic dosing (27).

It is not known if this phenomenon is specific to salbutamol or is shared by other racemic beta$_2$-agonists.

Second-Generation Effects

Pregnancy

Use of beta$_2$-adrenoceptor agonists in threatened premature labor
The adverse effects of the beta$_2$-adrenoceptor agonists when given (as a rule by injection) to arrest premature uterine contractions are very similar to those experienced when the classic drug in the series (salbutamol) is used for other purposes. In the special circumstances of obstetrics, however, there are several particular safety problems.

Choice of drugs
Probably most or all beta$_2$-agonists could be used in obstetrics as well as in asthma, and some are used for both purposes; however, manufacturers have tended to develop their individual compounds for one purpose or the other. Surprisingly, one large survey suggested that when used in pregnancy, salbutamol may be less well tolerated by the mother (stimulation, cardiovascular

effects) than the much less selective isoxsuprine (SED-12, 321).

In one large survey, salbutamol was less well tolerated by the mother (stimulation, cardiovascular effects) than the much less selective isoxsuprine (SED-12, 321).

Cardiovascular
None of the beta$_2$-adrenoceptor agonists used to delay delivery can be given in effective doses either orally or by injection without affecting the maternal heart rate (and to a lesser extent the fetal heart rate) in a high proportion of cases. It is not possible to say whether this effect is more likely to occur with certain drugs of this type than with others (particularly because the obstetric situation itself affects the fetal heart rate) (SEDA-17, 145), but in effective doses a maternal heart rate increase of some 30 beats/minute or more is common, with a fetal heart rate increase of up to 20 beats/minute. A substantial proportion of mothers (with intravenous use up to 30%) experience such symptoms as headache, tremulousness, tightness of the chest, palpitation, and flushing. There is clear and direct evidence that tocolytics also exert toxic effects on the myocardial tissue of the infant, especially if given for long periods (28,29). The calcium channel blocker verapamil does not protect either the maternal heart or the fetal heart against the toxic effects of tocolysis (SEDA-9, 126). Pulmonary edema is a rare but potentially life-threatening complication of beta$_2$-agonists (SEDA-10, 115) (30).

Metabolism
In obstetrics the classic effects of beta$_2$-adrenoceptor agonists on glucose metabolism can be absent or harmless in those without diabetes, but dangerous in those with diabetes, in whom they can cause metabolic acidosis (5). The hyperglycemic effect can be aggravated if glucocorticoids are also given (as they may be to prevent hyaline membrane disease in prematurity).

Susceptibility Factors

Age

The use of long-acting beta$_2$-adrenoceptor agonists in the management of asthma in children has been comprehensively reviewed (31). In children, as in adults, regular long-acting beta$_2$-adrenoceptor agonists can produce bronchodilator subsensitivity to short-acting beta-agonists and tolerance to the bronchoprotective effects of long-acting beta-agonists against challenges with exercise and methacholine. The clinical significance of these findings is unclear.

References

1. Burggraaf J, Westendorp RG, in't Veen JC, Schoemaker RC, Sterk PJ, Cohen AF, Blauw GJ. Cardiovascular side effects of inhaled salbutamol in hypoxic asthmatic patients. Thorax 2001;56(7):567–9.
2. Lowe MD, Rowland E, Brown MJ, Grace AA. Beta(2) adrenergic receptors mediate important electrophysiological effects in human ventricular myocardium. Heart 2001;86(1):45–51.

3. Pye M, Quinn AC, Cobbe SM. QT interval dispersion: a non-invasive marker of susceptibility to arrhythmia in patients with sustained ventricular arrhythmias? Br Heart J 1994;71(6):511–14.

4. Yuksel H, Coskun S, Polat M, Onag A. Lower arrhythmogenic risk of low dose albuterol plus ipratropium. Indian J Pediatr 2001;68(10):945–9.

5. Thomas DJ, Gill B, Brown P, Stubbs WA. Salbutamol-induced diabetic ketoacidosis. BMJ 1977;2(6084):438.

6. Mansfield LE, Nelson HS. Effect of beta-adrenergic agents on immunoglobulin G levels of asthmatic subjects. Int Arch Allergy Appl Immunol 1982;68(1):13–16.

7. Lai CK, Twentyman OP, Holgate ST. The effect of an increase in inhaled allergen dose after rimiterol hydrobromide on the occurrence and magnitude of the late asthmatic response and the associated change in nonspecific bronchial responsiveness Am Rev Respir Dis 1989;140(4):917–23.

8. Larsson K, Martinsson A, Hjemdahl P. Influence of beta-adrenergic receptor function during terbutaline treatment on allergen sensitivity and bronchodilator response to terbutaline in asthmatic subjects. Chest 1992;101(4):953–60.

9. Cockcroft DW, O'Byrne PM, Swystun VA, Bhagat R. Regular use of inhaled albuterol and the allergen-induced late asthmatic response. J Allergy Clin Immunol 1995;96(1):44–9.

10. Bhagat R, Swystun VA, Cockcroft DW. Salbutamol-induced increased airway responsiveness to allergen and reduced protection versus methacholine: dose response. J Allergy Clin Immunol 1996;97(1 Pt 1):47–52.

11. Cockcroft DW, McParland CP, Britto SA, Swystun VA, Rutherford BC. Regular inhaled salbutamol and airway responsiveness to allergen. Lancet 1993;342(8875):833–7.

12. Cockcroft DW. Inhaled beta2-agonists and airway responses to allergen. J Allergy Clin Immunol 1998;102(5):S96–9.

13. National Asthma Education Program, National Institutes of Health. Guidelines for the Diagnosis and Management of Asthma. Publication No 91-3042. Bethesda: United States Department of Health and Human Services, 1991.

14. Sears MR, Taylor DR. The beta2-agonist controversy. Observations, explanations and relationship to asthma epidemiology. Drug Saf 1994;11:259–83.

15. Bremner P, Burgess CD, Crane J, McHaffie D, Galletly D, Pearce N, Woodman K, Beasley R. Cardiovascular effects of fenoterol under conditions of hypoxaemia. Thorax 1992;47(10):814–17.

16. Weir TD, Mallek N, Sandford AJ, Bai TR, Awadh N, Fitzgerald JM, Cockcroft D, James A, Liggett SB, Pare PD. Beta2-adrenergic receptor haplotypes in mild, moderate and fatal/near fatal asthma. Am J Respir Crit Care Med 1998;158(3):787–91.

17. Hancox RJ, Sears MR, Taylor DR. Polymorphism of the beta2-adrenoceptor and the response to long-term beta2-agonist therapy in asthma. Eur Respir J 1998;11(3):589–93.

18. Martinez FD, Graves PE, Baldini M, Solomon S, Erickson R. Association between genetic polymorphisms of the beta2-adrenoceptor and response to albuterol in children with and without a history of wheezing. J Clin Invest 1997;100(12):3184–8.

19. Aziz I, Hall IP, McFarlane LC, Lipworth BJ. Beta2-adrenoceptor regulation and bronchodilator sensitivity after regular treatment with formoterol in subjects with stable asthma. J Allergy Clin Immunol 1998;101(3):337–41.

20. Yates DH, Kharitonov SA, Barnes PJ. An inhaled glucocorticoid does not prevent tolerance to the bronchoprotective effect of a long-acting inhaled beta 2-agonist. Am J Respir Crit Care Med 1996;154(6 Pt 1):1603–7. Erratum in: Am J Respir Crit Care Med 1997;155(4):1491.

21. Drotar DE, Davis EE, Cockcroft DW. Tolerance to the bronchoprotective effect of salmeterol 12 hours after starting twice daily treatment. Ann Allergy Asthma Immunol 1998;80(1):31–4.

22. Tan KS, Grove A, McLean A, Gnosspelius Y, Hall IP, Lipworth BJ. Systemic corticosteroid rapidly reverses bronchodilator subsensitivity induced by formoterol in asthmatic patients. Am J Respir Crit Care Med 1997;156(1):28–35.

23. Drazen JM, Israel E, Boushey HA, Chinchilli VM, Fahy JV, Fish JE, Lazarus SC, Lemanske RF, Martin RJ, Peters SP, Sorkness C, Szefler SJ. Comparison of regularly scheduled with as-needed use of albuterol in mild asthma. Asthma Clinical Research Network. N Engl J Med 1996;335(12):841–7.

24. Handley DA, McCullough JR, Crowther SD, Morley J. Sympathomimetic enantiomers and asthma. Chirality 1998;10(3):262–72.

25. Boulton DW, Fawcett JP. Pharmacokinetics and pharmacodynamics of single oral doses of albuterol and its enantiomers in humans. Clin Pharmacol Ther 1997;62(2):138–44.

26. Cockcroft DW, Swystun VA. Effect of single doses of S-salbutamol, R-salbutamol, racemic salbutamol, and placebo on the airway response to methacholine. Thorax 1997;52(10):845–8.

27. Nelson HS, Bensch G, Pleskow WW, DiSantostefano R, DeGraw S, Reasner DS, Rollins TE, Rubin PD. Improved bronchodilation with levalbuterol compared with racemic albuterol in patients with asthma. J Allergy Clin Immunol 1998;102(6 Pt 1):943–52.

28. Bohm N, Adler CP. Focal necroses, fatty degeneration and subendocardial nuclear polyploidization of the myocardium in newborns after beta-sympathicomimetic suppression of premature labor. Eur J Pediatr 1981;136(2):149–57.

29. Fletcher SE, Fyfe DA, Case CL, Wiles HB, Upshur JK, Newman RB. Myocardial necrosis in a newborn after long-term maternal subcutaneous terbutaline infusion for suppression of preterm labor. Am J Obstet Gynecol 1991;165(5 Pt 1):1401–4.

30. Wagner JM, Morton MJ, Johnson KA, O'Grady JP, Speroff L. Terbutaline and maternal cardiac function. JAMA 1981;246(23):2697–701.

31. Bisgaard H. Long-acting beta(2)-agonists in management of childhood asthma: a critical review of the literature. Pediatr Pulmonol 2000;29(3):221–34.

Beta-adrenoceptor antagonists

See also Individual agents

General Information

Many beta-adrenoceptor antagonists (beta-blockers) have been developed, and their adverse effects have been comprehensively reviewed (1). The spectrum of adverse effects is broadly similar for all beta-blockers, despite differences in their pharmacological properties, notably cardioselectivity, partial agonist activity, membrane-stabilizing activity, and lipid solubility (see Table 1). The influence of these properties is mentioned in the general discussion when appropriate and is summarized at the end of the section. Individual differences in toxicity are largely unimportant but will be mentioned briefly.

Although beta-blockers have been available for many years, new members of this class with novel pharmacological profiles continue to be developed. These new drugs are claimed to have either greater cardioselectivity or vasodilatory and beta$_2$-agonist properties. The claimed

Table 1 Properties of beta-adrenoceptor antagonists (where known)

Drug	Lipid solubility[a]	Cardioselectivity	Partial agonist activity	Membrane-stabilizing activity
Acebutolol	0.7	±	+	+
Alprenolol	31	−	+	+
Amosulalol		−		
Arotinolol				
Atenolol	0.02	+	−	
Befunolol				
Betaxolol		+	−	±
Bevantolol	Low	+	−	+
Bisoprolol		++		−
Bopindolol				
Bucindolol				
Bufetolol				
Bufuralol	+	−	+	
Bunitrolol	+	−	++	±
Bupranolol				
Butofilolol				
Carazolol				
Carteolol	−	+		
Carvedilol	++	−	−	
Celiprolol		±	+[b]	−
Cetamolol				
Cicloprolol				
Cloranolol				
Dexpropranolol				
Diacetolol				
Dilevalol				
Draquinolol				
Epanolol	Minimal	+	+	
Esmolol	−	+	−	
Flestolol	−	−	−	
Indenolol				
Labetalol	+	−	−	
Levobetaxolol				
Levobunolol		−		
Levomoprolol				
Medroxalol				
Mepindolol				
Metipranolol				
Metoprolol	0.2	+	−	±
Moprolol				
Nadolol	0.03	−	−	−
Nebivolol		+	−	−
Nifenalol				
Nipradilol				
Oxprenolol	0.7	−	+	+
Penbutolol	−	−	+	+
Pindolol	0.2	−	++	±
Practolol	0.02	+	+	−
Pronethalol				
Propranolol	4.3	−	−	++
Sotalol	0.02	−	−	−
Talinolol		+		
Tertatolol				
Tilisolol				
Timolol	0.03	−	±	±
Xamoterol		+	++	

[a] Octanol:water partition coefficient
[b] Partial beta$_2$-adrenoceptor agonist

advantages of these new drugs serve to highlight the supposed disadvantages of the older members of the class (their adverse constrictor effects on the airways and peripheral blood vessels). Strong commercial emphasis is being placed on these new properties, and papers extolling these effects often appear in non-peer-reviewed supplements or even in reputable journals (2).

Although the toxicity of the beta-adrenoceptor antagonists has been fairly well documented, there has been a subtle change in perceptions of their potential benefits and drawbacks. The cardioprotective effect of beta-blockers after myocardial infarction and their efficacy in reducing "silent" myocardial ischemia have persuaded some clinicians to use them preferentially. On the other hand, they can significantly impair the quality of life (3) and are contraindicated in some patients. A few patients cannot tolerate beta-blockade at all. These include patients with bronchial asthma, patients with second- or third-degree heart block, and those with seriously compromised limb perfusion causing claudication, ischemic rest pain, and pregangrene.

General adverse effects

The adverse effects of beta-blockers are usually mild, with occurrence rates of 10–20% for the most common in most studies. Most are predictable from the pharmacological and physicochemical properties of these drugs. Examples include fatigue, cold peripheries, bradycardia, heart failure, sleep disturbances, bronchospasm, and altered glucose tolerance. Gastrointestinal upsets are also relatively common. Serious adverse cardiac effects and even sudden death can follow abrupt withdrawal of therapy in patients with ischemic heart disease. Most severe adverse reactions can be avoided by careful selection of patients and consideration of individual beta-blockers. Hypersensitivity reactions have been relatively rare since the withdrawal of practolol. Tumor-inducing effects have not been established in man.

Fatigue

Fatigue is one of the most commonly reported adverse effects of beta-adrenoceptor antagonists, with reported occurrence rates of up to 20% or more, particularly in those who exert themselves. It has to be viewed alongside the ability to produce fatigue and lethargy by a possible effect on the nervous system. The precise cause of physical fatigue is not known, but hypotheses include impaired muscle blood supply, effects on intermediary metabolism, and a direct effect on muscle contractility (4).

Theoretically, $beta_1$-selective drugs are less likely to alter these variables, and might therefore have an advantage over non-selective drugs. However, this has not always been shown in single-dose studies in volunteers (5,6), although in two such studies atenolol produced less exercise intolerance than propranolol at comparable dosages (7,8). For an unexplained reason, cardioselectivity impaired performance relatively less in subjects with a high proportion of slow-twitch muscle fibers than it did in those whose muscle biopsy specimens showed a high percentage of fast-twitch fibers (9). The muscle fibers of long-distance runners are predominantly of the slow-twitch type, and this probably explains the superiority of atenolol over propranolol when exercise performance was assessed in such subjects (7). The release of lactic acid from skeletal muscle cells is impaired to a

greater extent by non-selective beta-blockers than by cardioselective drugs, and cardioselectivity was associated with a less marked fall in blood glucose during and after maximal and submaximal exercise (10,11). Partial agonist activity might have been the reason for the superiority of oxprenolol over propranolol in terms of exercise duration (12).

Differences among beta-blockers

Although there are now many different beta-adrenoceptor antagonists, and the number is still increasing, there are only a few important characteristics that distinguish them in terms of their physicochemical and pharmacological properties: lipid solubility, cardioselectivity, partial agonist activity, and membrane-stabilizing activity. The characteristics of the currently available compounds are shown in Table 1.

Lipid solubility

Lipid solubility (13) determines the extent to which a drug partitions between an organic solvent and water. Propranolol, oxprenolol, metoprolol, and timolol are the most lipid-soluble beta-adrenoceptor antagonists, and atenolol, nadolol, and sotalol are the most water-soluble; acebutolol and pindolol are intermediate (14).

The more lipophilic drugs are extensively metabolized in the gut wall and liver (first-pass metabolism). This first-pass clearance is variable and can result in 20-fold differences in plasma drug concentrations between patients who have taken the same dose. It also produces susceptibility to drug interactions with agents that alter hepatic drug metabolism, for example cimetidine, and can result in altered kinetics and hence drug response in patients with hepatic disease, particularly cirrhosis. Lipid-soluble drugs pass the blood–brain barrier more readily (15) and should be more likely to cause adverse nervous system effects, such as disturbance of sleep, but the evidence for this is not very convincing.

In contrast, water-soluble drugs are cleared more slowly from the body by the kidneys. These drugs therefore tend to accumulate in patients with renal disease, do not interact with drugs that affect hepatic metabolism, and gain access to the brain less readily.

Cardioselectivity

Cardioselectivity (16), or more properly $beta_1$-adrenoceptor selectivity, is the term used to indicate that there are at least two types of beta-adrenoceptors, and that while some drugs are non-selective (that is they are competitive antagonists at both $beta_1$- and $beta_2$-adrenoceptors), others appear to be more selective antagonists at $beta_1$-adrenoceptors, which are predominantly found in the heart. Bronchial tissue, peripheral blood vessels, the uterus, and pancreatic beta-cells contain principally $beta_2$-adrenoceptors. Thus, cardioselective beta-adrenoceptor antagonists, such as atenolol and metoprolol, might offer theoretical benefits to patients with bronchial asthma, peripheral vascular disease, and diabetes mellitus.

Cardioselective drugs may have relatively less effect on the airways, but they are in no way cardiospecific and they should be used with great care in patients with evidence of reversible obstructive airways disease.

The benefits of cardioselective drugs in patients with Raynaud's phenomenon or intermittent claudication have been difficult to prove. Because of vascular sparing, cardioselective agents may also be preferable in stress, when adrenaline is released.

Cardioselective drugs are less likely to produce adverse effects in patients with type I diabetes than non-selective drugs. At present, hypoglycemia in patients with type I diabetes mellitus is the only clinical problem in which cardioselectivity is considered important. Even there, any potential advantages of cardioselective drugs in minimizing adverse effects apply only at low dosages, since cardioselectivity is dose-dependent.

Partial agonist activity

Partial agonist activity (17,18) is the property whereby a molecule occupying the beta-adrenoceptor exercises agonist effects of its own at the same time as it competitively inhibits the effects of other extrinsic agonists. The effects of these drugs depend on the degree on endogenous tone of the sympathetic nervous system. When there is high endogenous sympathetic tone they tend to act as beta-blockers; when endogenous sympathetic tone is low they tend to act as beta-agonists. Thus, xamoterol had a beneficial effect in patients with mild heart failure (NYHA classes I and II), through a positive inotropic effect on the heart; however, in severe heart failure (NYHA classes III and IV), in which sympathetic tone is high, it acted as a beta-blocker and worsened the heart failure, through a negative inotropic effect (19).

Partial agonists, such as acebutolol, oxprenolol, pindolol, practolol, and xamoterol, produce less resting bradycardia. It has also been claimed that such agents cause a smaller increase in airways resistance in asthmatics, less reduction in cardiac output (and consequently a lower risk of congestive heart failure), and fewer adverse effects in patients with cold hands, Raynaud's phenomenon, or intermittent claudication. However, none of these advantages has been convincingly demonstrated in practice, and patients with bronchial asthma or incipient heart failure must be considered at risk with this type of compound.

Drugs with partial agonist activity can produce tremor (20).

Drugs that combine beta$_1$-antagonism or partial agonism with beta$_2$-agonism (celiprolol, dilevalol, labetalol, pindolol) or with alpha-antagonism (carvedilol, labetalol) have been developed (21). Both classes have significant peripheral vasodilating effects. Drugs with significant agonist activity at beta$_1$-adrenoceptors have poor antihypertensive properties (22).

Membrane-stabilizing activity

Drugs with membrane-stabilizing activity reduce the rate of rise of the cardiac action potential and have other electrophysiological effects. Membrane-stabilizing activity has only been shown in human cardiac muscle in vitro in concentrations 100 times greater than those produced by therapeutic doses (23). It is therefore likely to be of clinical relevance only if large overdoses are taken.

Use in heart failure

Traditionally, beta-blockers have been contraindicated in patients with heart failure. However, there are some patients with systolic heart failure who benefit from a

beta-blocker (24). Early evidence was strongest for idiopathic dilated cardiomyopathy rather than ischemic heart disease (25). However, several randomized controlled trials of beta-blockers in patients with mild to moderate heart failure have been published. These include the CIBIS II trial with bisoprolol (26), the MERIT-HF trial with metoprolol (27), and the PRECISE trial with carvedilol (28). These have shown that cardiac mortality in these patients can be reduced by one-third, despite concurrent treatment with conventional therapies of proven benefit (that is ACE inhibitors).

Diastolic dysfunction can lead to congestive heart failure, even when systolic function is normal (29,30). Since ventricular filling occurs during diastole, failure of intraventricular pressure to fall appropriately during diastole leads to increased atrial pressure, which eventually leads to increased pulmonary and systemic venous pressures, causing a syndrome of congestive heart failure indistinguishable clinically from that caused by systolic pump failure (31). Diastolic dysfunction occurs in systemic arterial hypertension, hypertrophic obstructive cardiomyopathy, and infiltrative heart diseases, which reduce ventricular compliance or increase ventricular stiffness (32). As energy is required for active diastolic myocardial relaxation, a relative shortage of adenosine triphosphate in ischemic heart disease also often leads to co-existing diastolic and systolic dysfunction (33). Beta-blockers improve diastolic function in general, and this may be beneficial in patients with congestive heart failure associated with poor diastolic but normal systolic function.

Beta-blockade reduces mortality in patients with heart failure by at least a third when initiated carefully, with gradual dose titration, in those with stable heart failure (34,35). Similarly, beta-blocker prescribing should be encouraged in people with diabetes, since they have a worse outcome after cardiac events and beta-blockade has an independent secondary protective effect (36,37). The small risk of masking metabolic and autonomic responses to hypoglycemia, which was only a problem with non-selective agents in type I diabetes, is a very small price worth paying in diabetics with coronary heart disease.

Use in glaucoma

It has been more than a quarter of a century since the discovery that oral propranolol reduces intraocular pressure in patients with glaucoma. However, the use of propranolol for glaucoma was limited by its local anesthetic action (membrane-stabilizing activity).

Topical timolol was released for general use in 1978. That timolol is systemically absorbed was suggested by early reports of reduced intraocular pressure in the untreated eyes of patients using monocular treatment. About 80–90% of a topically administered drop drains through the nasolacrimal duct and enters the systemic circulation through the highly vascular nasal mucosa, without the benefit of first-pass metabolism in the liver; only a small fraction is swallowed. Thus, topical ophthalmic dosing is probably more akin to intravenous delivery than to oral dosing, and systemic adverse reactions are potentially serious. However, although patients may give their physicians a detailed list of current medications, they often fail to mention the use of eye-drops, about which physicians are often either unaware or do not have time to ask specific questions.

Betaxolol is a beta$_1$-selective adrenoceptor antagonist without significant membrane-stabilizing activity or intrinsic sympathomimetic activity. It may be no more effective than other drugs in reducing intraocular pressure, but it may be safer for some patients, particularly those with bronchospastic disease (but see the section on Respiratory under Drug administration route) (38).

Partial agonist activity of beta-blockers may help to prevent ocular nerve damage and subsequent visual field loss associated with glaucoma. Such damage may be related to a reduction in ocular perfusion, as might occur if an ocular beta-blocker caused local vasoconstriction. An agent with intrinsic sympathomimetic activity might preserve ocular perfusion through local vasodilatation or by minimizing local vasoconstriction. The data are sparse and inconclusive, but carteolol appears to have no effect on retinal blood flow or may even increase it, making it potentially suitable as a neuroprotective drug (38,39).

Organs and Systems

Cardiovascular

A randomized comparison of oral atenolol and bisoprolol in 334 patients with acute myocardial infarction was associated with drug withdrawal in 70 patients (21%) because of significant bradydysrhythmias, hypotension, heart failure, and abnormal atrioventricular conduction (40). Logistic regression analysis suggested that critical events were more likely to occur in patients who were pretreated with dihydropyridine calcium antagonists.

Heart failure
Beta-adrenoceptor antagonists reduce cardiac output through their negative inotropic and negative chronotropic effects. They can therefore cause worsening systolic heart failure or new heart failure in patients who depend on high sympathetic drive to maintain cardiac output. Plasma noradrenaline is increased in patients with heart failure, and the extent of this increase is directly related to the degree of ventricular impairment (41). Since the greatest effect on sympathetic activity occurs with the first (and usually the lowest) doses, heart failure associated with beta-blockade seems to be independent of dosage. Heart failure is one of the most serious adverse effects of the beta-adrenoceptor antagonists (42), but it is usually predictable and can be attenuated by pretreatment with diuretics and angiotensin-converting enzyme inhibitors in patients who are considered to be at risk.

It has been suggested that drugs with partial agonist activity (see Table 1), which have a minimal depressant effect on normal resting sympathetic tone, might cause less reduction in cardiac output (43) and thus protect against the development of cardiac decompensation (44). However, this has not been satisfactorily shown for drugs with high partial agonist activity, for example acebutolol, oxprenolol, and pindolol (45), and these drugs should therefore be given with the same caution as others

in compromised patients. Xamoterol, a beta-antagonist with substantial beta$_1$ partial agonist activity, was hoped to be of benefit in mild congestive heart failure (46), but its widespread use by non-specialists in more severe degrees of heart failure resulted in many reports of worsening heart failure (47). Heart failure has also been produced by labetalol (48) and after the use of timolol eye-drops in the treatment of glaucoma (49).

Hypotension
Beta-adrenoceptor antagonists lower blood pressure, probably by a variety of mechanisms, including reduced cardiac output. More severe reductions in blood pressure can occur and can be associated with syncope (42). It has been suggested that this is more likely to occur in old people, but comprehensive studies have stressed the safety of beta-blockers in this age group (50).

- Profound hypotension, resulting in renal insufficiency, has been reported in a single patient after the administration of atenolol 100 mg orally (51); however, large doses of furosemide and diazoxide were also given in this case, and this appears more likely to have been a consequence of a drug interaction.

Cardiac dysrhythmias and heart block
Beta-blockade can result in sinus bradycardia, because blockade of sympathetic tone allows unopposed parasympathetic activity. Drugs with partial agonist activity may prevent bradycardia (52). However, heart rates under 60/minute often worry the physician more than the patient: in a retrospective study of nearly 7000 patients taking beta-adrenoceptor antagonists, apart from dizziness in patients with heart rates under 40/minute (0.4% of the total group), slow heart rates were well tolerated (53).

All beta-blockers cause an increase in atrioventricular conduction time; this is most pronounced with drugs that have potent membrane-depressant properties and no partial agonist activity. Sotalol differs from other beta-blockers in that it increases the duration of the action potential in the cardiac Purkinje fibers and ventricular muscle at therapeutic doses. This is a class III antidysrhythmic effect, and because of this, sotalol has been used to treat ventricular (54–56) and supraventricular dysrhythmias (57). The main serious adverse effect of sotalol is that it is prodysrhythmic in certain circumstances, and can cause torsade de pointes (58,59).

Acute chest pain
Worsening of angina pectoris has been attributed to beta-blocker therapy. The reports include 35 cases in a series of 296 elderly patients admitted to hospital with suspected myocardial infarction; in these 35 the pain disappeared within 7 hours of withdrawing beta-blocker therapy (60).

Worsening of angina has been reported at very low heart rates (61). Propranolol resulted in vasotonic angina in six patients during a double-blind trial, with prolongation of the duration of pain and electrocardiographically assessed ischemia. It has been suggested that this reflects a reduction in coronary perfusion as a result of reduced cardiac output, and also coronary arterial spasm provoked by non-selective agents by inhibition of beta$_2$-mediated vasodilatation

(62). The latter explanation is controversial, and the use of beta-blockers in patients with arteriographic evidence of coronary artery spasm has not consistently caused worsening of the disorder (63).

Unstable angina has also followed treatment for hypertension with cardioselective drugs such as betaxolol (64).

Peripheral vascular effects

Cold extremities or exacerbation of Raynaud's phenomenon are amongst the commonest adverse effects reported with beta-blockers (5.8% of nearly 800 patients taking propranolol) (42); Raynaud's phenomenon occurs in 0.5–6% of patients (65). The mechanism may be potentiation of the effects of a cold environment on an already abnormal circulation, but whether symptoms can be produced de novo is more difficult to determine. However, a retrospective questionnaire study in 758 patients taking antihypertensive drugs showed that 40% of patients taking beta-blockers noted cold extremities, compared with 18% of those taking diuretics; there were no significant differences among patients taking alprenolol, atenolol, metoprolol, pindolol, and propranolol (66). Similarly, a large randomized study showed that the incidence of Raynaud's phenomenon was the same for atenolol and pindolol (67). In another study, vasospastic symptoms improved when labetalol was substituted for a variety of beta-blockers (68). On the other hand, a small, double-blind, placebo-controlled study in patients with established Raynaud's phenomenon showed that the prevalence of symptoms with both propranolol and labetalol was no greater than that with placebo (69).

Intermittent claudication has also been reported to be worsened by beta-adrenoceptor antagonists, but has been difficult to document because of the difficulty of study design in patients with advanced atherosclerosis. As early as 1975 it was reported from one small placebo-controlled study that propranolol did not exacerbate symptoms in patients with intermittent claudication (70). This has subsequently been supported by the results of several large placebo-controlled trials of beta-blockers in mild hypertension and reports of trials of the secondary prevention of myocardial infarction, in which intermittent claudication was not mentioned as an adverse effect, even though it was not a specific contraindication to inclusion (71). In addition, a comprehensive study of the effects of beta-adrenoceptor antagonists in patients with intermittent claudication did not show beta-blockade to be an independent risk factor for the disease (72). In men with chronic stable intermittent claudication, atenolol (50 mg bd) had no effect on walking distance or foot temperature (73). These findings have been confirmed in a recent meta-analysis of 11 randomized, controlled trials to determine whether beta-blockers exacerbate intermittent claudication (SEDA-17, 234).

Patchy skin necrosis has been described in hypertensive patients with small-vessel disease in the legs who were taking beta-blockers. Characteristically, pedal pulses remained palpable and the lesions occurred during cold weather and healed on withdrawal of the drugs (74–76). Three cases have been reported in which long-lasting incipient gangrene of the leg was immediately overcome when a beta-blocker was withdrawn (77,78), showing how easily these drugs are overlooked in such circumstances. In several cases of beta-blocker-induced gangrene, recovery did not follow withdrawal of therapy, and amputation was necessary (79,80). Thus, when possible, other forms of therapy should be used in patients with critical ischemia or rest pain.

It has also been suggested that beta-blockade may compromise the splanchnic vasculature. Intravenous propranolol reduces splanchnic blood flow experimentally by 29% while reducing cardiac output by only 6% (81).

Five patients developed mesenteric ischemia, four with ischemic colitis, and one with abdominal angina, while taking beta-adrenoceptor antagonists (82). Although causation was not proven, it was possible.

Respiratory

The respiratory and cardiovascular adverse effects of topical therapy with timolol or betaxolol have been studied in a randomized, controlled trial in 40 elderly patients with glaucoma (83). Five of the 20 allocated to timolol discontinued treatment for respiratory reasons, compared with three of the 20 patients allocated to betaxolol. There were no significant differences in mean values of spirometry, pulse, or blood pressure between the groups. This study confirms that beta-blockers administered as eye-drops can reach the systemic circulation and that serious adverse respiratory events can occur in elderly people, even if they are screened before treatment for cardiac and respiratory disease. These events can occur using either the selective betaxolol agent or the non-selective timolol.

Airways obstruction

Since the introduction of propranolol, it has been recognized that patients with bronchial asthma treated with beta-adrenoceptor antagonists can develop severe airways obstruction (84), which can be fatal (85) or near fatal (86,87); this has even followed the use of eye-drops containing timolol (88). Beta-blockers upset the balance of bronchial smooth muscle tone by blocking the bronchial $beta_2$-adrenoceptors responsible for bronchodilation. They also promote degranulation of mast cells and depress central responsiveness to carbon dioxide (89,90).

Although $beta_1$-selective drugs are theoretically safer, there are reports of serious reductions in ventilatory function (91,92), even when used as eye-drops (93). However, it has been concluded that if beta-blockade is necessary in the treatment of glaucoma, cardioselective beta-blocking drugs should be preferred (94). While cardioselectivity is dose-dependent (95), and higher dosages might therefore be expected to produce adverse effects, metoprolol and bevantolol, even in dosages that are lower than those usually required for a therapeutic effect, may be poorly tolerated by patients with asthma (96).

Whether drugs with partial agonist activity confer any advantage is uncertain. Some of the evidence that patients with asthma tolerate beta-blockers is probably misleading, relating to patients with chronic obstructive airways disease who have irreversible changes and who do not respond to either bronchoconstricting or bronchodilating drugs (97). In contrast, a few patients who have never had asthma or chronic bronchitis develop severe bronchospasm when given a beta-blocker. Some, but not all, of these cases (98) may have been allergic reactions to the dyestuffs (for example tartrazine) that are used to color some formulations. Other patients, who need not have a history of chest disease, only develop increased airways resistance with beta-blockers during respiratory infections.

It is against this background that claims that some asthmatic subjects will tolerate certain beta-blockers (99) must be viewed. Some asthmatic patients may indeed tolerate either cardioselective beta-blockers (such as atenolol and metoprolol) or labetalol (100,101), and in patients taking atenolol beta$_2$-adrenoceptor agonists may continue to produce bronchodilatation (102), but in most instances other therapeutic options are preferable (103). Celiprolol is a beta$_1$-adrenoceptor antagonist that has partial beta$_2$-agonist activity. Small studies have suggested that it may be useful in patients with asthma (104), but worsening airways obstruction has been reported (105); it has been concluded that celiprolol has no advantage over existing beta-blockers in the treatment of hypertension (106).

Bronchospasm, which can be life-threatening, can be precipitated by beta-blocker eye-drops. Even beta$_1$-selective antagonists, such as betaxolol, can cause a substantial reduction in forced expiratory volume. Wheezing and dyspnea have been reported among patients using betaxolol: the symptoms resolved after withdrawal. A cross-sectional study has shown that ophthalmologists were more aware than chest physicians about the use of beta-blocker eye-drops by patients with obstructive airways disease; patient awareness was also poor (38,107).

Attention has also been drawn to the increased risks of the adverse effects of beta-blockers on respiratory function in old people (108).

Central ventilatory suppression

Reduced sensitivity of the respiratory center to carbon dioxide has been reported (89,109). The clinical significance of this is unknown, but lethal synergism between morphine and propranolol in suppressing ventilation in animals has been described (110).

Pneumonitis, pulmonary fibrosis, and pleurisy

Pulmonary fibrosis (111) and pleural fibrosis (112) have both been described as infrequent complications associated with practolol. Pulmonary fibrosis has also occurred during treatment with pindolol (113) and acebutolol (114,115). Pleuritic and pneumonitic reactions to acebutolol have been reported (116).

Ear, nose, throat

Nasal polyps, rhinitis, and sinusitis resistant to long courses of antibiotics and surgical intervention have been described in five patients taking non-selective beta-adrenoceptor antagonists (propranolol and timolol) (117). The symptoms resolved when the drugs were withdrawn and did not recur when beta$_1$-selective adrenoceptor blockers (metoprolol or atenolol) were given instead.

Nervous system

Some minor neuropsychiatric adverse effects, such as light-headedness, visual and auditory hallucinations, illusions, sleep disturbances, vivid dreams, and changes in mood and affect, have been causally related to long-term treatment with beta-adrenoceptor antagonists (118,119). Other occasional nervous system effects of beta-blockers include hearing impairment (120), episodic diplopia (121), and myotonia (122).

Although some migraine sufferers use beta-adrenoceptor antagonists prophylactically, there are also reports of the development of migraine on exposure to propranolol or rebound aggravation when the drug is withdrawn (123). Stroke, a rare complication of migraine, has been reported in three patients using propranolol for prophylaxis (124–126). Seizures have been reported with the short-acting beta-blocker esmolol, usually with excessive doses (117). Myasthenia gravis has been associated with labetalol (127), oxprenolol, and propranolol (128), and carpal tunnel syndrome has been reported with long-term beta-blockade, the symptoms gradually disappearing on withdrawal of therapy (129).

Propranolol and gabapentin are both effective in essential tremor. However, pindolol, which has substantial partial agonist activity, can cause tremor (130), and gabapentin can occasionally cause reversible movement disorders. A patient who developed dystonic movements after the combined use of gabapentin and propranolol has been described (131).

- A 68-year-old man with a 10-year history of essential tremor was initially treated with propranolol (120 mg/day), which was only slightly effective. Propranolol was replaced by gabapentin (900 mg/day). The tremor did not improve and propranolol (80 mg/day) was added. Two days later he developed paroxysmal dystonic movements in both hands. Between episodes, neurological examination was normal. When propranolol was reduced to 40 mg/day the abnormal movements progressively disappeared.

This case suggests that there is a synergistic effect between propranolol and gabapentin.

In addition, tiredness, fatigue, and lethargy, probably the commonest troublesome adverse effects of beta-blockers and often the reason for withdrawal (132), may have a contributory nervous system component, although they are probably primarily due to reduced cardiac output and altered muscle metabolism (65) (see also the section on Fatigue in this monograph). In general, a definite neurological association has been difficult to prove, and studies of patients taking beta-adrenoceptor antagonists for hypertension, which incorporated control groups of patients taking either other antihypertensive drugs or a placebo, appear to have shown that the incidence of symptoms that can be specifically attributed to beta-adrenoceptor antagonists is lower than anticipated (133).

The more lipophilic drugs, such as propranolol and oxprenolol, would be expected to pass the blood–brain barrier more readily than hydrophilic drugs, such as atenolol and nadolol, and there is some evidence that they do so (15). In theory, therefore, hydrophilic drugs might be expected to produce fewer neuropsychiatric adverse effects. A double-blind, placebo-controlled evaluation of the effects of four beta-blockers (atenolol, metoprolol, pindolol, and propranolol) on central nervous function (134) showed that disruption of sleep was similar with the three lipid-soluble drugs, averaging six to seven wakenings per night, compared with an average of three wakenings per night for atenolol and placebo. Only pindolol, which has a higher CSF/plasma concentration ratio than metoprolol and propranolol, significantly altered rapid eye movement sleep and latency (135). Patients who took pindolol and propranolol also had high depression scores.

In a placebo-controlled sleep laboratory study of atenolol, metoprolol, pindolol, and propranolol, the three lipophilic drugs reduced dreaming (equated with rapid eye movement sleep) but increased the recollection of dreaming and the amount of wakening; in contrast, although atenolol also reduced sleep, it had no effect on subjective measures of sleep (136).

The published data on the effects of beta-blockers on the nervous system have been extensively reviewed (137). The overall incidence of effects was low, and lowest with the hydrophilic drugs. However, a meta-analysis of 55 studies of the cognitive effects of beta-blockade did not show any firm evidence that lipophilic drugs caused more adverse effects than hydrophilic ones (138). Recent data confirming a correlation between lipophilicity and serum concentrations on the one hand and nervous system effects on the other (139) have fuelled this controversy.

Car-driving and other specialized skills

In view of the large numbers of people who take beta-adrenoceptor antagonists regularly for hypertension or ischemic heart disease, the question arises whether these drugs impair performance in tasks that require psychomotor coordination. The occupations under scrutiny include car-driving, the operation of industrial machinery, and the piloting of aeroplanes. The current evidence is conflicting and controversial. One report suggested that propranolol and pindolol given for 5 days impaired slalom driving in a manner comparable with the coordination defects caused by alcohol (140). In contrast, other studies have shown that driving skills were not impaired during long-term beta-blocker therapy and might even be improved (141,142). There is also a suggestion that tolerance to the central effects of these drugs can develop within 3 weeks of starting therapy, provided the dosage does not change (143). Until more information is available from well-controlled studies, it is advisable to inform patients who are starting treatment with beta-blockers that they should exercise special care in the performance of skills requiring psychomotor coordination for the first 1 or 2 weeks.

Sensory systems

Eyes

Keratopathy in association with the practolol syndrome is the major serious ocular effect ascribed to beta-adrenoceptor antagonists. Conjunctivitis and visual disturbances have also been reported, and a case of ocular pemphigoid has been described in a patient taking timolol

eye-drops for glaucoma (144). Anterior uveitis has been reported in patients taking betaxolol (145) and metipranolol (146,147). Corneal anesthesia and epithelial sloughing with continuing use of topical beta-blockers have also been reported (148), as have ocular myasthenia and worsened sicca syndrome. Patients who lack CYP2D6 are more likely to have higher systemic concentrations of beta-blockers after topical application, making them susceptible to adverse effects.

- Recurrent retinal arteriolar spasm with associated visual loss has been described in a 68-year-old man with hypertension treated with atenolol (SEDA-17, 236).
- A 60-year-old man with open-angle glaucoma developed an allergic contact conjunctivitis and dermatitis from carteolol, a topical non-cardioselective beta-blocker (149). He had extensive cross-reactivity to other topical beta-blockers, such as timolol and levobunolol. Cross-reactivity among different beta-blockers is possibly due to a common lateral aliphatic chain.

Psychological, psychiatric

Disturbances of psychomotor function

Beta-adrenoceptor antagonists impair performance in psychomotor tests after single doses. These include effects of atenolol, oxprenolol, and propranolol on pursuit rotor and reaction times (150,151). However, other studies with the same drugs have failed to show significant effects (152–156), and the issue has remained controversial. A report that sotalol improved psychomotor performance in 12 healthy individuals in a dose of 320 mg/day but impaired performance at 960 mg/day (157) has been interpreted to indicate that the water-soluble beta-adrenoceptor antagonists would be less likely than the fat-soluble drugs to produce nervous system effects. Both atenolol and propranolol alter the electroencephalogram; atenolol affects body sway and alertness and propranolol impairs short-term memory and the ability to concentrate (158,159). These results suggest that both lipophilic and hydrophilic beta-adrenoceptor antagonists can affect the central nervous system, although the effects may be subtle and difficult to demonstrate.

In 27 hypertensive patients aged 65 years or more, randomized to continue atenolol treatment for 20 weeks or to discontinue atenolol and start cilazapril, there was a significant improvement in the choice reaction time in the patients randomized to cilazapril (160). This study has confirmed previous reports that chronic beta-blockade can determine adverse effects on cognition in elderly patients. Withdrawal of beta-blockers should be considered in any elderly patient who has signs of mental impairment.

In a placebo-controlled trial of propranolol in 312 patients with diastolic hypertension, 13 tests of cognitive function were assessed at baseline, 3 months, and 12 months (161). Propranolol had no significant effects on 11 of the 13 tests. Compared with placebo, patients taking propranolol had fewer correct responses at 3 months and made more errors of commission.

Psychoses
Bipolar affective disorder
Bipolar depression affects 1% of the general population, and treatment resistance is a significant problem. The addition of pindolol can lead to significant improvement in depressed patients who are resistant to antidepressant drugs, such as selective serotonin reuptake inhibitors or phenelzine. Of 17 patients with refractory bipolar depression, in whom pindolol was added to augment the effect of antidepressant drugs, eight responded favorably (162). However, two developed transient hypomania, and one of these became psychotic after the resolution of hypomanic symptoms. In both cases transient hypomanic symptoms resolved without any other intervention, while psychosis required pindolol withdrawal.

Anxiety and depression have been reported after the use of nadolol, which is hydrophilic (163). In a study of the co-prescribing of antidepressants in 3218 new users of beta-blockers (164), 6.4% had prescriptions for antidepressant drugs within 34 days, compared with 2.8% in a control population. Propranolol had the highest rate of co-prescribing (9.5%), followed by other lipophilic beta-blockers (3.9%) and hydrophilic beta-blockers (2.5%). In propranolol users, the risk of antidepressant use was 4.8 times greater than the control group, and was highest in those aged 20–39 (RR = 17; 95% CI = 14, 22).

Organic brain syndrome
The development of a severe organic brain syndrome has been reported in several patients taking beta-adrenoceptor antagonists regularly without a previous history of psychiatric illness (165–167). A similar phenomenon was seen in a young healthy woman who took propranolol 160 mg/day (168). The psychosis can follow initial therapy or dosage increases during long-term therapy (169). The symptoms, which include agitation, confusion, disorientation, anxiety, and hallucinations, may not respond to treatment with neuroleptic drugs, but subsides rapidly when the beta-blockers are withdrawn. Symptoms are also ameliorated by changing from propranolol to atenolol (170).

Schizophrenia
A schizophrenia-like illness has also been seen in close relation to the initiation of propranolol therapy (171).

Endocrine

Prolactin

- Reversible hyperprolactinemia with galactorrhea occurred in a 38-year-old woman taking atenolol for hypertension (172).

Thyroid
Propranolol inhibits the conversion of thyroxine (T4) to tri-iodothyronine (T3) by peripheral tissues (173), resulting in increased formation of inactive reverse T3. There have been several reports of hyperthyroxinemia in clinically euthyroid patients taking propranolol for non-thyroid reasons in high dosages (320–480 mg/day) (174,175). The incidence was considered to be higher than could be accounted for by the development of spontaneous hyperthyroidism, but the mechanism is unknown.

The effect of beta-adrenoceptor antagonists on thyroid hormone metabolism is unlikely to play a significant role in their use in hyperthyroidism. Since D-propranolol has similar effects on thyroxine metabolism to those seen with the racemic mixture, membrane-stabilizing activity may be involved (176).

In one case, beta-adrenoceptor blockade masked an unexpected thyroid crisis, resulting in severe cerebral dysfunction before the diagnosis was made (177).

Metabolism

Hypoglycemia
Hypoglycemia, producing loss of consciousness in some cases, can occur in non-diabetic individuals who are taking beta-adrenoceptor antagonists, particularly those who undergo prolonged fasting (178) or severe exercise (179,180). Patients on maintenance dialysis are also at risk (181). It has been suggested that non-selective drugs are most likely to produce hypoglycemia and that cardioselective drugs are to be preferred in at-risk patients (182), but the same effect has been reported with atenolol under similar circumstances (180).

Two children in whom propranolol was used to treat attention deficit disorders and anxiety became unarousable, with low heart rates and respiratory rates, due to hypoglycemia (183). Hypoglycemia can be caused by reduced glucose intake (fasting), increased utilization (hyperinsulinemia), or reduced production (enzymatic defects). One or more of these mechanisms can be responsible for hypoglycemia secondary to drugs. Children treated with propranolol may be at increased risk of hypoglycemia, particularly if they are fasting. Concomitant treatment with methylphenidate can increase the risk of this metabolic disorder.

However, contrary to popular belief, beta-adrenoceptor antagonists do not by themselves increase the risk of hypoglycemic episodes in insulin-treated diabetics, in whom their use was concluded to be generally safe (184). Indeed, in 20 such patients treated with diet or diet plus oral hypoglycemic agents, both propranolol and metoprolol produced small but significant increases in blood glucose concentrations after 4 weeks (185). The rise was considered clinically important in only a few patients.

However, in insulin-treated diabetics who become hypoglycemic, non-selective beta-adrenoceptor antagonists can mask the adrenaline-mediated symptoms, such as palpitation, tachycardia, and tremor; they can cause a rise in mean and diastolic blood pressures, due to unopposed alpha-adrenoceptor stimulation from catecholamines, because the $beta_2$-adrenoceptor-mediated vasodilator response is blocked (186); they can also impair the rate of rise of blood glucose toward normal (187). In contrast, cardioselective drugs mask hypoglycemic symptoms less (188); because of vascular sparing, they are less likely to be associated with a diastolic pressor response in the presence of catecholamines, although this has been reported with metoprolol (189); and delay in recovery from hypoglycemia is either less marked or undetectable with cardioselective drugs, such as atenolol or metoprolol. Thus, if insulin-requiring diabetics need to be treated with a beta-adrenoceptor antagonist, a cardioselective agent should always be chosen for reasons of safety, while allowing that this type of beta-blocker is associated with insulin resistance and can impair insulin sensitivity by 15–30% (SEDA-17, 235), and hence increase insulin requirements.

People with diabetes have a much worse outcome after acute myocardial infarction, with a mortality rate at least twice that in non-diabetics. However, tight control of blood glucose, with immediate intensive insulin treatment during the peri-infarct period followed by intensive subcutaneous insulin treatment, was associated with a 30% reduction in mortality at 1 year, as reported in the DIGAMI study. In addition, the use of beta-blockers in this group of patients had an independent secondary preventive effect (190). The use of beta-blockers in diabetics with ischemic heart disease should be encouraged (37).

In 686 hypertensive men treated for 15 years, beta-blockers were associated with a higher incidence of diabetes than thiazide diuretics (191). This was an uncontrolled study, but the observation deserves further study.

Blood lipids

There is increasing evidence that beta-adrenoceptor antagonists increase total triglyceride concentrations in blood and reduce high-density lipoprotein (HDL) cholesterol. Comparisons of non-selective and cardioselective drugs have shown that lipid changes are less marked but still present with beta$_1$-selective agents (192). Current information suggests that beta$_1$-selective drugs may be preferable in patients with hypertriglyceridemia (193). Topical beta-blockers can cause rises in serum triglyceride concentrations and falls in serum high-density lipoprotein concentrations; this makes them less suitable in patients with coronary heart disease (38,194).

The importance of these effects for the long-term management of patients with hypertension or ischemic heart disease is unknown, but it is recognized that a high serum total cholesterol and a low HDL cholesterol are associated with an increased risk of ischemic heart disease. However, a significant reduction in HDL cholesterol after treatment for 1 year with timolol was of no prognostic significance and did not attenuate the protective effect of the drug (195). In a 4-year randomized, placebo-controlled study of six antihypertensive monotherapies, acebutolol produced only a small and probably clinically irrelevant (0.17 mmol/l) reduction in total cholesterol (196), which was not statistically different from four of the other antihypertensive drugs.

Obesity

It has been suggested that beta-blockers may predispose to obesity by reducing basal metabolic rate via beta-adrenoceptor blockade (197). Thermogenesis in response to heat and cold, meals, stress, and anxiety is also reduced by beta-adrenoceptor blockade, promoting weight gain (SEDA-16, 193). Beta$_3$-adrenoceptors have been implicated in this mechanism (198,199). Since propranolol blocks beta$_3$-receptors in vivo (200), it would be wise on theoretical grounds to avoid propranolol in obese patients; nadolol is another non-selective beta-blocker that does not act on beta$_3$-adrenoceptors.

A systematic review of eight prospective, randomized trials in 7048 patients with hypertension (3205 of whom were taking beta-blockers) confirmed that body weight was higher in those taking beta-blockers than in controls at the end of the studies (201). The median difference in body weight was 1.2 kg (range –0.4–3.5 kg). There was no relation between demographic characteristics and changes in body weight. The weight gain was observed in the first few months of treatment and thereafter there was no further weight gain compared with controls. This observation suggests that first-line use of beta-blockers in obese patients with hypertension should be considered with caution.

Electrolyte balance

Hypokalemia

Adrenaline by infusion produces a transient increase in plasma potassium, followed by a prolonged fall; pretreatment with beta-adrenoceptor antagonists results in a rise in plasma potassium (202). These effects may be mediated via beta$_2$-adrenoceptors (203), and cardioselective drugs should have smaller effects (202). In the Treatment of Mild Hypertension Study (TOMHS), acebutolol did not change serum potassium after 4 years (196).

It has been argued that drug combinations that contain a beta-adrenoceptor antagonist in combination with a thiazide diuretic minimize the hypokalemic effect of the latter; however, marked hypokalemia in the absence of primary hyperaldosteronism has been reported in a patient taking Sotazide (a combination of hydrochlorothiazide and the non-selective drug sotalol) (204). The use of a combination formulation of chlortalidone and atenolol has also produced hypokalemia (205), in one case complicated by ventricular fibrillation after myocardial infarction (206).

In addition to a rise in serum potassium, timolol increases plasma uric acid concentrations (207). In the TOMHS study, acebutolol increased serum urate by 7 μmol/l (196).

Mineral balance

A fall in serum calcium has been reported with atenolol (208), but whether this was causal has been disputed (209).

Hematologic

Thrombocytopenia has been reported in patients taking oxprenolol (210,211) and alprenolol (212,213); it can recur on rechallenge. This effect is presumed to have an immunological basis.

In the International Agranulocytosis and Aplastic Anemia Study the relation between cardiovascular drugs and agranulocytosis was examined: there was a relative risk of 2.5 (95% CI = 1.1, 6.1) for propranolol (214). Other beta-blockers did not increase risk and propranolol had no association with aplastic anemia. There are also anecdotal reports of this association (215).

Gastrointestinal

Mild gastrointestinal adverse effects, such as nausea, dyspepsia, constipation, or diarrhea, have been reported in

5–10% of patients taking beta-adrenoceptor antagonists (42). A reduction in dosage or a change to another member of the group will usually produce amelioration. Severe reactions of this type are very infrequent, but severe diarrhea, dehydration, hypokalemia, and weight loss, recurring after rechallenge, occurred with propranolol in a single case (216).

Nausea and vomiting have been attributed to timolol eye-drops (217).

- Severe nausea and vomiting occurred in a 77-year-old woman treated with timolol eye-drops for glaucoma. Her weight had fallen by 8 kg (13%). All physical, laboratory, and instrumental examinations were negative. Gastroduodenoscopy and duodenal biopsy were unremarkable and *Helicobacter pylori* was absent. When timolol was replaced by betaxolol, her complaints disappeared and she gained 2 kg. On rechallenge 3 months later she developed severe nausea, vomiting, and anorexia after some days of treatment. She immediately stopped taking the treatment and 4 days later the symptoms disappeared.

Since timolol has been satisfactorily used by millions of patients, the incidence of serious gastrointestinal events appears to be very low. Absence of symptoms after betaxolol therapy in this patient is in agreement with its lower risk of non-cardiac adverse reactions compared with the non-selective agent timolol.

Beta-adrenoceptor antagonists can cause non-anginal chest pain because of esophagitis (218), due to adherence of the tablet mass, resulting in esophageal spasm, inflammatory change, and even perforation.

Sclerosing peritonitis and retroperitoneal fibrosis

Sclerosing peritonitis was described as part of the practolol syndrome (219–221), and it can also occur with other beta-adrenoceptor antagonists (222,223).

Retroperitoneal fibrosis has been reported in patients taking oxprenolol (224), atenolol (225), propranolol (226), metoprolol (227), sotalol (228), and timolol (including eye-drops) (229,230). However, this disorder often occurs spontaneously and has been reported very infrequently in patients taking beta-blockers (231). Thus, in the absence of any causal relation it is most likely that it reflects the spontaneous incidence in patients taking a common therapy. This conclusion has been supported by an analysis of 100 cases of retroperitoneal fibrosis (232).

Liver

Many beta-adrenoceptor antagonists undergo substantial first-pass hepatic metabolism; these include alprenolol, metoprolol, oxprenolol, and propranolol. Hepatic cirrhosis, with consequent portosystemic shunting, can therefore result in increased systemic availability and higher plasma concentrations, perhaps resulting in adverse effects. Beta-blockers may also reduce liver blood flow and cause interactions with drugs with flow-dependent hepatic clearance.

The oxidative clearance of the lipophilic drugs, metoprolol, timolol, and bufuralol, is influenced by the debrisoquine hydroxylation gene locus, resulting in polymorphic metabolism (233). This might result in an increase in the adverse effects of these beta-blockers in poor metabolizers, but to date there is no objective evidence of such an association (234).

Beta-adrenoceptor antagonists, used in the prevention of bleeding from esophageal varices in patients with hepatic cirrhosis, have reportedly caused hepatic encephalopathy in several patients (235–239). Thus, extreme caution is required, particularly because resuscitation can be difficult when beta-blockers are given to patients with gastrointestinal bleeding or encephalopathy (240).

Biliary tract

Biliary cirrhosis was reported as part of the practolol syndrome (241), but there have been no comparable reports with other beta-adrenoceptor antagonists.

Urinary tract

Propranolol reduces renal blood flow and glomerular filtration rate after acute administration, associated with, and probably partly due to, falls in cardiac output and blood pressure (242,243). There has been some argument about whether these effects persist during long-term therapy (244). Despite early suggestions that renal function might be worsened by such therapy, particularly in patients with chronic renal insufficiency (245), the clinical significance of these changes is debatable (246). Claims that nadolol increases renal blood flow and that cardioselective drugs such as atenolol reduce renal blood flow less than non-selective agents in old people (247) are thus probably relatively unimportant. The vasodilating beta-blocker carvedilol maintains renal blood flow whilst reducing glomerular filtration rate, suggesting that renal vasodilatation occurs (248), although a single case of reversible renal insufficiency has been described in a clinical trial in patients with severe heart failure (249).

Skin

Rashes were part of the practolol (oculomucocutaneous) syndrome, but are infrequent with other beta-adrenoceptor antagonists. The eruptions can be urticarial, morbilliform, eczematous, vesicular, bullous, psoriasiform, or lichenoid (250–255).

Beta-blocker eye-drops can cause skin rashes (256).

- A 70-year-old woman treated with topical timolol for glaucoma developed a papular eruption on the arms and back, consistent with prurigo. All tests were within the reference ranges. There was no improvement after 1 month of topical corticosteroids. The eruption cleared completely within 1 month of timolol withdrawal. Betaxolol eye-drops were introduced and the eruption recurred within 1 week. When beta-blocker therapy was replaced by synthetic cholinergic eye-drops (drug unspecified) the eruption cleared completely without any recurrence a year later.
- Allergic contact dermatitis due to carteolol eye drops occurred in a 61-year-old woman (257). Withdrawal of carteolol and the use of timolol instead led to improvement within 10 days, suggesting that in some cases there is no cross-reactivity between different beta-blockers.

Although cutaneous adverse effects have been previously described after oral beta-blockers, including timolol, this observation further suggests a class effect of topical beta-blockers. This case also suggests a cross-reaction between timolol and betaxolol.

In a review of 588 patients with established psoriasis it was concluded that about two-thirds of such patients are likely to have a flare-up with a beta-adrenoceptor antagonist, regardless of the agent used (258). In patients with vitiligo, beta-blockers rarely exacerbate depigmentation (7/548 patients) (259). In a separate report, topical betaxolol used for glaucoma was associated with periocular cutaneous pigmentary changes (260).

Some patients have positive patch tests and/or a positive response to oral rechallenge. There can also be cross-sensitivity to other beta-blockers in compromised patients. The mechanisms appear to include both immunological and pharmacological effects; in the latter case the drug may modify growth regulation in the epidermis (261).

Contact allergy to topical beta-blockers can occur.

- A 68-year-old woman developed contact allergy after many years of using befunolol (262). Patch-testing showed cross-sensitivity to carteolol. Evidence of such cross-sensitivity has not previously been reported.

Sweat glands

Hyperhydrosis or sweating with beta-blockers has been reported with both oral formulations (sotalol and acebutolol) (263) and topical formulations (carteolol) (264), although the patients described in these reports were not rechallenged to ascertain the link. However, it was suggested that beta-blockade increased exercise-related sweating in healthy volunteers, more so with a non-selective beta-blocker (propranolol), than a selective one (atenolol) (265). The mechanism for this was uncertain, but was thought to be due to an imbalance between beta- and alpha-adrenergic activity. In some instances, clonidine, an alpha-adrenoceptor antagonist, was effective in treating hyperhydrosis (266), whereas in other cases, propranolol was paradoxically effective (267).

Hair

There have been single case reports of alopecia in association with propranolol (268) and metoprolol (269).

Musculoskeletal

It has been suggested that arthralgia is a not an uncommon adverse effect of beta-adrenoceptor antagonists, particularly metoprolol (270), although the association was not confirmed by rechallenge in any patient. A later case-control study in 127 patients attending a hypertension clinic who had arthropathy showed no significant relation between the arthropathy and the use of beta-blockers (271). On the other hand, five cases of metoprolol-associated arthralgia, most with negative serological tests for collagenases, have been reported to the FDA (272).

Muscle cramps have been reported in patients taking beta-blockers with partial agonist activity (273); it has been suggested (274) that this might be a beta$_2$-partial agonist effect, although this has not subsequently been

supported (275). However, a crossover study in 78 hypertensive patients suggested that beta-blockers with partial agonist activity (pindolol and carteolol) caused muscle cramps in up to 40% of these patients, with an associated rise in serum CK and CK-MB, although the severity of the cramps did not correlate with the enzyme activities (276).

Sexual function

Uncontrolled studies of the effect of beta-adrenoceptor antagonists on sexual function have often shown a high incidence of absence of erections, reduced potency, and reduced libido (277). Several large controlled trials in hypertension and ischemic heart disease have provided more exact information. In a large-scale, prospective, placebo-controlled study, reduced sexual activity was an adverse effect of sufficient severity to lead to the withdrawal of some patients in the propranolol-treated group (278). In the TOMHS study, the incidence of difficulty in obtaining and maintaining an erection over 48 months was 17% with both acebutolol and placebo (196). In the TAIM study (279), a randomized, placebo-controlled study lasting 6 months, atenolol did not cause a significant increase in erectile problems in men (11%; 95% CI 2, 20%) compared with placebo (3%; 0, 9%). Loss of libido and difficulty in sustaining an erection can be induced in young healthy volunteers (134); although these effects may be more common with lipophilic drugs, such as propranolol (280) and pindolol (281), they have also been reported with atenolol (282).

Peyronie's disease

Peyronie's disease is a fibrotic condition of the penis that has been associated with beta-blockers, such as propranolol (283), metoprolol (284), and labetalol (284). However, 100 consecutive cases of Peyronie's disease included only five men who had taken a beta-blocker before the onset of the condition (285); the authors concluded that the syndrome was likely to be associated with chronic degenerative arterial disease and not with beta-adrenoceptor antagonists.

Immunologic

Leukocytoclastic vasculitis has been reported with sotalol (286).

- A progressive cutaneous vasculitis occurred in a 66-year-old man taking sotalol for prevention of a symptomatic atrial fibrillation. After 7 days he noted a petechial eruption on his wrists and ankles. This progressed during the next days to palpable purpura on the hands, wrists, ankles, and feet. A biopsy specimen showed changes consistent with leukocytoclastic vasculitis. After withdrawal of sotalol the skin rash cleared completely without any other intervention.

Other beta-blockers associated with leukocytoclastic vasculitis include acebutolol, alprenolol, practolol, and propranolol.

Antinuclear antibodies in high titers were detected in a number of patients with the practolol oculomucocutaneous syndrome. Tests in patients taking acebutolol (287,288) and celiprolol (289) have also shown a high frequency of antinuclear antibodies. Positive lupus erythematosus cell preparations have been observed in patients taking acebutolol (288).

The lupus-like syndrome was part of the practolol syndrome and has also been attributed to acebutolol (290,291), atenolol (SEDA-16, 194), labetalol (292), pindolol (293), and propranolol (294). However, apart from practolol, it seems to be very rare during treatment with beta-adrenoceptor antagonists.

Anaphylactic reactions have been attributed to beta-adrenoceptor antagonists only very infrequently (295). However, it appears that anaphylactic reactions precipitated by other agents can be particularly severe in patients taking beta-blockers, especially non-selective drugs, and may require higher-than-usual doses of adrenaline for treatment (296–299). The view that allergy skin testing or immunotherapy is inadvisable in patients taking beta-blockers (300) has been disputed, bearing in mind the low incidence of this adverse effect (301).

Long-Term Effects

Drug withdrawal

Interest in the possible effects of the sudden withdrawal of beta-adrenoceptor antagonists followed a 1975 report of two deaths and four life-threatening complications of coronary artery disease within 2 weeks of withdrawal of propranolol (302). Subsequent analyses did not always confirm these findings (303,304), and it has not been easy to distinguish between natural progression and deterioration caused by drug withdrawal under such circumstances. However, a case-control study in hypertensive patients showed a relative risk of 4.5 (95% CI = 1.1, 19) associated with recent withdrawal of beta-blockers and the development of myocardial infarction or angina (305).

The symptoms attributed to the sudden withdrawal of beta-adrenoceptor antagonists (severe exacerbation of angina pectoris, acute myocardial infarction, sudden death, malignant tachycardia, sweating, palpitation, and tremor) are consistent with transient adrenergic hypersensitivity. Unequivocal signs of rebound hypersensitivity have been observed after drug withdrawal in patients with ischemic heart disease (306), but not in hypertensive patients (307–309). The density of beta-adrenoceptors on human lymphocyte membranes increased by 40% during treatment with propranolol for 8 days (310), and hypersensitivity to isoprenaline can be shown in hypertensive patients after the withdrawal of different beta-adrenoceptor antagonists, including propranolol (311), metoprolol (312), and atenolol (313). This hypersensitivity occurs within 2 days of drug withdrawal, can persist for up to 14 days, and is presumed to reflect the up-regulation of beta-adrenoceptors that occurs with prolonged treatment. This phenomenon is said to be diminished by gradual withdrawal of therapy and by the use of drugs with partial agonist activity, such as pindolol (314). Whether this is directly relevant to the effects of the sudden withdrawal of beta-adrenoceptor antagonists in patients with ischemic heart disease is speculative.

Although there is evidence that abrupt withdrawal of long-acting beta-blockers is not associated with the development of the beta-blocker withdrawal syndrome (315),

current information suggests that withdrawal of beta-adrenoceptor antagonists, particularly in patients with ischemic heart disease, should be accomplished by gradual dosage reduction over 10–14 days. However, even gradual withdrawal may not always prevent rebound effects (316).

Second-Generation Effects

Pregnancy

Great concern at one time accompanied the use of beta-adrenoceptor antagonists in pregnancy, particularly in the management of hypertension. On theoretical grounds beta-adrenoceptor antagonists might be expected to increase uterine contractions, impair placental blood flow, cause intrauterine growth retardation, accentuate fetal and neonatal distress, and increase the risk of neonatal hypoglycemia and perinatal mortality. There are many anecdotal reports of such complications attributed to beta-adrenoceptor antagonists, often propranolol. However, many of the adverse effects listed above are also potential complications of hypertension in pregnancy, and in the absence of a properly controlled trial of therapy, definite conclusions of cause and effect have been impossible on the basis of these anecdotes alone.

Many of the fears expressed were set aside by a double-blind, randomized, placebo-controlled trial of atenolol in pregnancy-associated hypertension in 120 women (316), which showed that babies in the placebo group had a higher morbidity, that atenolol reduced the occurrence of respiratory distress syndrome and intrauterine growth retardation, and that neonatal hypoglycemia and hyperbilirubinemia were equally common in the treated and placebo groups. Although bradycardia was more common with atenolol, it had no deleterious consequences. However, the offspring of women taking atenolol had lower body weights on follow up, the significance of which is unclear (316).

It is reasonable to consider that beta-adrenoceptor antagonists can be used in pregnancy without serious risks, provided patients are kept under careful clinical observation. Since all beta-blockers cross the placenta freely, major differences in effects or toxicity among the various drugs are unlikely, and in a review of beta-blockers in pregnancy it was concluded that no single beta-blocker is superior (317). However, in a small study in 51 women with pregnancy-induced hypertension the combination of hydralazine and propranolol was associated with lower blood glucose and weight at birth compared with the combination of hydralazine and pindolol (with partial agonist activity), despite similar blood pressure control. It was suggested that beta-adrenoceptor antagonists without partial agonist activity might reduce uteroplacental blood flow (318).

Fetotoxicity

The adverse effects of beta-adrenoceptor antagonists on the fetus have been reviewed (319). Beta blockers cross the placenta, and can have adverse maternal and fetal effects. Studies of the use of beta-blockers during pregnancy have generally been small, and the gestational age at the start of the study was generally 29–33 weeks, leaving substantially unanswered the possibility that treatment of more patients and/or longer treatment durations may reveal unrecognized adverse events. These observations underline the fact that the safety of beta-blockers remains uncertain and that they are therefore better not given before the third trimester.

Non-cardioselective beta-adrenoceptor antagonists

Observations derived from uncontrolled studies have shown an association between maternal use of propranolol and intrauterine growth retardation, neonatal respiratory depression, bradycardia, hypoglycemia, and increased perinatal mortality. However, in randomized, placebo-controlled studies of metoprolol and oxprenolol, there was no evidence of effects on birth weight.

- Two infants with features of severe beta-blockade (bradycardia, persistent hypotension), persistent hypoglycemia, pericardial effusion, and myocardial hypertrophy were born before term to mothers taking long-term oral labetalol for hypertension in pregnancy.

Although labetalol is considered to be generally safe in neonates, impaired urinary excretion and lower albumin binding in preterm infants can prolong the half-life of labetalol and increase its systemic availability and toxicity (320).

Cardioselective beta-adrenoceptor antagonists

There is reluctance to use atenolol in pregnancy, especially if treatment starts early. In placebo-controlled studies, birth weight was significantly lower with atenolol groups. The same was true when atenolol was compared with non-cardioselective agents: the weight of infants born to women taking atenolol was significantly lower. When atenolol was started later there was no difference in birth weight between infants born to women treated with atenolol or other beta-blockers, suggesting the relevance of the time of initiation of atenolol. Atenolol should therefore be avoided in the early stages of pregnancy and given with caution in the later stages.

- Fetal bradycardia and pauses after each two normal beats occurred at 21 weeks gestation in a 37-year-old woman using timolol eye-drops for glaucoma; when timolol was withdrawn, the fetal heart rate recovered (321).

The authors concluded that when a woman taking glaucoma therapy becomes pregnant, it is usually possible to interrupt therapy during pregnancy. Treatment may be deferred until delivery of the infant.

Lactation

The list of beta-adrenoceptor antagonists that have been detected in breast milk includes atenolol (322), acebutolol and its active N-acetyl metabolite (323), metoprolol (324), nadolol (325), oxprenolol and timolol (326), propranolol (327), and sotalol (328). Most authors have concluded that the estimated daily infant dose derived from breast-feeding is likely to be too low to produce untoward effects in the suckling infant, and indeed such effects were not noted in the above cases. However, in the case of

acebutolol it was considered that clinically important amounts of drug could be transferred after increasing plasma concentrations were noted in two breastfed infants.

Susceptibility Factors

Genetic factors

Most beta-blockers undergo extensive oxidation (329). There have been anecdotal reports of high plasma concentrations of some beta-blockers in poor metabolizers of debrisoquine, and controlled studies have shown that debrisoquine oxidation phenotype is a major determinant of the metabolism, pharmacokinetics, and some of the pharmacological effects of metoprolol, bufuralol, timolol, and bopindolol. The poor metabolizer phenotype is associated with increased plasma drug concentrations, a prolonged half-life, and more intense and sustained beta-blockade. There are also phenotypic differences in the pharmacokinetics of the enantiomers of metoprolol and bufuralol.

Renal disease

The hydrophilic drugs atenolol and sotalol are eliminated largely unchanged in the urine; with deteriorating renal function their half-lives can be prolonged as much as 10-fold (330,331). Other beta-adrenoceptor antagonists, for example acebutolol and metoprolol, have active metabolites that can accumulate (332). Massive retention of the metabolite propranolol gluconate has also been reported in patients with renal insufficiency taking long-term oral propranolol (333); this metabolite is then deconjugated, and concentrations of propranolol can be significantly increased in these patients. Thus, in a patient with a low creatinine clearance, either dosage adjustment or a change of beta-blocker may be necessary.

Other features of the patient

Heart failure

Untreated congestive heart failure secondary to systolic pump failure is a contraindication to the use of beta-adrenoceptor antagonists. Patients in frank or incipient heart failure have reduced sympathetic drive to the heart, and acute life-threatening adverse effects can therefore follow beta-blockade. This is one of the recognized potentially serious complications of beta-blockers in the management of thyrotoxic crisis (334). However, patients with heart failure treated with ACE inhibitors and/or diuretics and digoxin may well gain long-term benefit from beta-adrenoceptor antagonists (34,35).

Heart block

Second-degree or third-degree heart block is a contraindication to beta-adrenoceptor blockade. If it is considered necessary for the control of dysrhythmias, a beta-blocker can be given after the institution of pacing.

Acute myocardial infarction

After many trials including thousands of patients, it is increasingly accepted that treatment of acute myocardial infarction with beta-adrenoceptor antagonists is beneficial. Given intravenously within 4–6 hours of the onset of the infarction these drugs can prevent ventricular dysrhythmias and cardiac rupture (335,336). When given orally during the first year after infarction, beta-adrenoceptors reduce mortality by about 25% (337) and probably more in diabetic subjects (37). Since heart failure, hypotension, and bradycardia are complications of both myocardial infarction and beta-adrenoceptor blockade, it might be assumed that these effects would be more common when the two are combined. However, reviews of the relevant studies (335,338–346) do not suggest that beta-adrenoceptor antagonists, given after acute myocardial infarction, either acutely intravenously or for secondary prophylaxis, increase the incidence of adverse effects or the risk of any particular adverse effect. Nevertheless, patients were rigorously selected for inclusion in these trials; less careful decisions to treat may carry increased risks.

Bronchial asthma

Beta-adrenoceptor antagonists should not be given to patients with bronchial asthma or obstructive airways disease, unless there are no other treatment options, because of the risk of precipitating bronchospasm resistant to bronchodilators. Celiprolol, a beta$_1$-antagonist with beta$_2$-agonist activity, has a theoretical but unproven advantage. Alternatively, cardioselective drugs should be chosen in the lowest possible dosages and in conjunction with a beta$_2$-adrenoceptor agonist, such as salbutamol or terbutaline, to minimize bronchoconstriction.

Smoking

Some common activities, such as mental effort (347), cigarette smoking, and coffee drinking (348,349), can produce stress associated with increased catecholamine secretion. In the presence of a non-selective beta-adrenoceptor antagonist, there can be a marked diastolic pressor response, due to mechanisms identical to those described above in hypoglycemia in diabetes. This effect may be smaller with cardioselective drugs.

Theoretically, frequent rises in diastolic blood pressure associated with smoking whilst taking a non-selective beta-adrenoceptor antagonist could be harmful; in a patient with ischemic heart disease or hypertension a cardioselective drug might offer advantages. There is no evidence of differences in morbidity or mortality in patients taking non-selective and cardioselective agents, but both the MRC and IPPPSH trials of mild hypertension showed increases in the incidence of coronary events in patients taking non-selective beta-adrenoceptor antagonists who were also cigarette smokers (350). The explanation that cigarette smoking increases the hepatic metabolism of beta-adrenoceptor blockers, reducing their effectiveness (351), does not extend to the use of cardioselective beta-blockers in smokers, as reported in the HAPPHY and MAPHY trials.

Insulin-treated diabetes

Beta-adrenoceptor antagonists may mask the symptoms of hypoglycemia, result in a catecholamine-mediated rise in diastolic blood pressure, and delay the return of blood glucose concentrations to normal. These effects are minimized or abolished by using a beta$_1$-selective drug, and this type of drug should always be used in preference to a non-selective drug in insulin-treated diabetes.

Anaphylaxis

Beta-blockers can make anaphylactic reactions more difficult to diagnose and treat (348). Even patients with spontaneous attacks of angioedema or urticaria can be at risk when given beta-blockers (352).

Drug Administration

Drug administration route

Beta-adrenoceptor antagonists are used as ocular tension-lowering drugs without notable effects on pupillary size or refraction. Their systemic effects are greater than one would expect, since there is no first-pass metabolism after ocular administration and the plasma concentration can therefore attain therapeutic concentrations (353).

The systemic adverse effects of ophthalmic beta-blockers have been reviewed (354). Symptomatic bradycardia from systemic or ophthalmic use of beta-blockers alone suggests underlying cardiac conduction disturbances. Beta$_2$-adrenoceptor blockade can exacerbate or trigger bronchospasm in patients with asthma or pulmonary disease associated with hyper-reactive airways. Occasionally, adverse systemic reactions can be severe enough to require drug withdrawal. Obtaining a careful medical history and checking pulse rate and rhythm and peak expiratory flow rate should identify the vast majority of patients with potential cardiac and respiratory contraindications.

Beta-blockers that are available as eye-drops include timolol, metipranolol, and levobunolol, which are non-selective beta$_1$- and beta$_2$-adrenoceptor antagonists, and betaxolol, a relatively cardioselective beta$_1$-adrenoceptor antagonist. Although selective beta$_1$-blockers are less likely to precipitate bronchospasm, this and other systemic effects can nevertheless occur (SED-12, 1200).

In 165 patients who used timolol 0.5% eye-drops, adverse effects were reported in 23%, including psychiatric effects (40%), cardiovascular effects (19%), respiratory effects (7%), and local effects (26%) (355).

Cardiovascular

Hemodynamic changes after the topical ocular use of beta-blockers sometimes include only small reductions in heart rate and resting pulse rate and an insignificant reduction in blood pressure. However, patients with cardiovascular disorders, especially those with an irregular heart rate and dysrhythmias, are certainly at risk (SEDA-4, 339). Bradycardia, cardiac arrest, heart block, hypotension, palpitations, syncope, and cerebral ischemia and stroke can occur (356). Rebound tachycardia has been reported after withdrawal of ophthalmic timolol (88,357). Continuous 24-hour monitoring of blood pressure has shown that beta-blocker eye-drops for glaucoma can increase the risk of nocturnal arterial hypotension (358).

Respiratory

Beta-blockers can aggravate or precipitate bronchospasm (SEDA-4, 339) (SEDA-5, 426) and potentially life-threatening respiratory failure can occur.

- A 58-year-old patient using topical timolol maleate for open-angle glaucoma developed cough and dyspnea due to interstitial pneumonitis. Three months after withdrawal of the eye-drops, he was asymptomatic with normal lung function, chest X-ray, and thoracic CT scan (359).

Nervous system

Light-headedness, mental depression, weakness, fatigue, acute anxiety, dissociative behaviour, disorientation, and memory loss can develop a few days to some months after the start of timolol therapy (88). Central nervous system complaints are most common in patients who have the greatest reduction in intraocular pressure (SEDA-5, 426). Patients may be unaware of the symptoms until the medication is stopped.

Sensory systems

Dry eyes have been reported after the systemic or ocular use of timolol (360). A sensation of dryness in the eyes can develop and is usually transitory. There can be a reduction in the Schirmer test and tear film break-up time. Symptomatic superficial punctate keratitis in association with complete corneal anesthesia has been observed (361).

Amaurosis fugax has been reported in association with topical timolol (362).

Endocrine

Ophthalmic beta-blockers can cause hypoglycemia in insulin-dependent diabetes (363). Conversely, in diabetic patients taking oral hypoglycemic drugs, hyperglycemia can develop because of impaired insulin secretion (SEDA-21, 487).

Electrolyte balance

Severe hyperkalemia has been reported in association with topical timolol, confirmed by rechallenge (364).

Skin

Cutaneous changes secondary to instillation of betaxolol have been described (260).

Musculoskeletal

Aggravation of myasthenia gravis has been observed during ophthalmic timolol therapy (365). Bilateral pigmentation of the fingernails and toenails, marked hyperkalemia, and arthralgia after ocular timolol have all been reported (SED-12, 1200).

Sexual function

Erectile impotence can occur after ophthalmic use of beta-blockers (88).

Susceptibility factors

All of the susceptibility factors that apply to systemically administered beta-blockers also apply to eye-drops. This particularly applies to asthma (260).

Glaucoma

Eyes with potential angle closure require a miotic drug and should not be treated with beta-blockers alone. To exclude the risk of precipitating glaucoma in a susceptible individual, gonioscopy is recommended before starting topical beta-adrenoceptor antagonist therapy.

Drug tolerance

Tachyphylaxis can develop after treatment with ophthalmic beta-blockers (366). There are two forms, short-term "escape," which occurs over a few days, and long-term "drift," which occurs over months and years.

Drug overdose

The increasing use of beta-adrenoceptor antagonists appears to have resulted in more frequent reports of severe high-dose intoxication (367,368), in which beta-adrenoceptor antagonists are often taken in combination with sedatives or alcohol. There can be a very short latency from intake of the drug until fulminant symptoms occur (369). The clinical features are well established. Cardiovascular suppression results in bradycardia, heart block, and congestive heart failure, and intraventricular conduction abnormalities are common (370). Ventricular tachycardias with sotalol intoxication may reflect its class III antidysrhythmic properties, leading to prolongation of the QT interval (371) and torsade de pointes, which may respond to lidocaine (372). Bronchospasm and occasionally hypoglycemia can also occur. Coma and epileptiform seizures are often seen (370,373) and may not be secondary to circulatory changes. The outcome is seldom fatal, but 16 fatal cases of intoxication with talinolol (which is beta$_1$-selective) have been described. Deaths have also occurred with metoprolol and acebutolol. Acebutolol has membrane-stabilizing activity, and it has been suggested that drugs with this property carry greater risk when taken in overdose (374). Lipid solubility influences the rate of nervous system penetration of a drug, and overdosage with highly lipophilic drugs, such as oxprenolol and propranolol, has been associated with rapid loss of consciousness and coma (375–377).

Treatment should include isoprenaline (although massive doses may be required), glucagon, and atropine. If a beta$_1$-selective antagonist has been taken, isoprenaline may reduce diastolic blood pressure by its unopposed vasodilator effect on beta$_2$-adrenoceptors (378). The beta$_1$-selective agonist dobutamine may be preferable in such patients (379). A temporary transvenous pacemaker should be inserted if significant heart block or bradycardia occur. Seizures in overdosage with a beta-adrenoceptor antagonist respond poorly to diazepam and barbiturates; muscle relaxants and artificial ventilation may be required. In general, the lipid-soluble drugs are highly protein-bound with a large apparent volume of distribution; forced diuresis or hemodialysis are therefore unlikely to be of use.

Propranolol intoxication can cause central nervous system depression in the absence of clinical signs of cardiac toxicity.

- A 16-year-old boy developed central nervous system depression and an acute dilated cardiomyopathy after taking 3200 mg of propranolol in a suicide attempt (380). He was treated with gastric lavage, activated charcoal, and mechanical ventilation. Echocardiography showed a poorly contracting severely dilated left ventricle. After intravenous isoprenaline hydrochloride and glucagon, echocardiography showed normal left ventricular size and function. He became fully alert 20 hours later and made a good recovery without sequelae.

Early echocardiographic evaluation is important in beta-blocker overdose and can prevent delay in the diagnosis and treatment of cardiac toxicity.

Two regional poison centers in the USA have reviewed 280 cases of beta-blocker overdose (381). All patients with symptoms developed them within 6 hours of ingestion. Four patients died as a result of overdosage. There was cardiovascular morbidity in 41 patients (15%), requiring treatment with cardioactive drugs. Propranolol, atenolol, and metoprolol were responsible for 87% of the cases and 84% of cardiovascular morbidity. Beta-blockers with membrane-stabilizing activity (acebutolol, labetalol, metoprolol, pindolol, and propranolol) accounted for 62% of beta-blocker exposures and 73% of cardiovascular morbidity. Symptomatic bradycardia (heart rate less than 60/minute) or hypotension (systolic blood pressure less than 90 mmHg) were observed in all cases classified as having cardiovascular morbidity. Beta-blocker exposure was complicated by a history of at least one co-ingestant in 73% of the cases, benzodiazepines and ethanol being the most frequent. Cardioactive co-ingestants were reported in 26% of cases: calcium channel blockers, cyclic antidepressants, neuroleptic drugs, and ACE inhibitors were the most common. Multivariate analysis showed that the only independent variable significantly associated with cardiovascular morbidity was the presence of another cardioactive drug. When patients who took another cardioactive drug were excluded, the only variable associated with cardiovascular morbidity was the ingestion of a beta-blocker with membrane-stabilizing activity.

Two fatal cases of acebutolol intoxication (6 and 4 g) have been reported (382). In both cases, the onset of symptoms was sudden (within 2 hours of ingestion), with diminished consciousness, PR, QRS, and QT prolongation, and hypotension unresponsive to inotropic drugs. In both cases there were episodes of repetitive polymorphous ventricular tachycardia.

These cases have confirmed the potential toxicity of beta-blockers with membrane stabilizing activity; they predispose the patient to changes in ventricular repolarization, which can cause QT prolongation and serious ventricular dysrhythmias. This is generally not seen in cases of propranolol intoxication.

Drug–Drug Interactions

General

Drug interactions with beta-adrenoceptor antagonists can be pharmacokinetic or pharmacodynamic (383–385).

Pharmacokinetic interactions
Absorption interactions
The absorption of some beta-adrenoceptor antagonists is altered by aluminium hydroxide, ampicillin, and food; these are interactions of doubtful clinical relevance.

Metabolism interactions
Beta-adrenoceptor antagonists that are cleared predominantly by the liver (for example metoprolol, oxprenolol, propranolol, and timolol) are more likely to participate in drug interactions involving changes in liver blood flow, hepatic drug metabolism, or both. Thus, enzyme-inducing drugs, such as phenobarbital and rifampicin, increase the clearance of drugs such as propranolol and metoprolol and reduce their systemic availability (386,387). Similarly, the histamine H_2 receptor antagonist cimetidine increases the systemic availability of labetalol, metoprolol, and propranolol by inhibiting hepatic oxidation (388–391). The disposition of drugs with high extraction ratios, such as propranolol and metoprolol, is also affected by changes in liver blood flow, and this may be the mechanism by which hydralazine reduces the first-pass clearance of oral propranolol and metoprolol (392).

Lipophilic beta-adrenoceptor antagonists are metabolized to varying degrees by oxidation by liver microsomal cytochrome P450 (for example propranolol by CYP1A2 and CYP2D6 and metoprolol by CYP2D6). These agents can therefore reduce the clearance and increase the steady-state plasma concentrations of other drugs that undergo similar metabolism, potentiating their effects. Drugs that are affected in this way include theophylline (393), thioridazine (394), chlorpromazine (395), warfarin (396), diazepam (397), isoniazid (398), and flecainide (399). These interactions are most likely to be of clinical significance when the affected drug has a low therapeutic ratio, for example theophylline or warfarin.

Beta-blockers can also affect the clearance of high clearance drugs by altering hepatic blood flow. This occurs when propranolol is co-administered with lidocaine (400), but it appears that this interaction is due more to inhibition of enzyme activity than to a reduction in hepatic blood flow (401). Atenolol inhibits the clearance of disopyramide, but the mechanism is unknown (402). Conversely, quinidine doubles propranolol plasma concentrations in extensive but not poor metabolizers (403) and oral contraceptives increase metoprolol plasma concentrations (404).

Pharmacodynamic interactions
The pharmacodynamic interactions of the beta-adrenoceptor antagonists can mostly be predicted from their pharmacology.

Blood pressure
The antihypertensive effect of beta-blockers can be impaired by the concurrent administration of some non-steroidal anti-inflammatory drugs (NSAIDs), possibly because of inhibition of the synthesis of renal vasodilator prostaglandins. This interaction is probably common to all beta-blockers, but may not occur with all NSAIDs; for example, sulindac appears to affect blood pressure less than indometacin (405–407).

The hypertensive crisis that can follow the withdrawal of clonidine can be accentuated by beta-blockers. It has also been reported that when beta-blockers are used in conjunction with drugs that cause arterial vasoconstriction they can have an additional effect on peripheral perfusion, which can be hazardous. Thus, combining beta-blockers with ergot alkaloids, as has been recommended for migraine, can cause severe peripheral ischemia and even tissue necrosis (408).

The hypotensive effects of halothane and barbiturates can be exaggerated by beta-adrenoceptor antagonists. However, they are not contraindicated in anesthesia, provided the anesthetist is aware of what the patient is taking.

The combination of caffeine with beta-blockers causes a raised blood pressure (409).

Cardiac dysrhythmias

The bradycardia produced by digoxin can be enhanced by beta-adrenoceptor antagonists. Neostigmine enhances vagal activity and can aggravate bradycardia (410). An apparent interaction between sotalol and thiazide-induced hypokalemia, resulting in torsade de pointes (411), has prompted the withdrawal of the combination formulation Sotazide.

- The co-prescription of sotalol 80 mg bd with terfenadine 60 mg bd (both drugs that can prolong the QT interval) in a 71-year-old lady with hypertension, atrial fibrillation, and nasal congestion was complicated by recurrent torsade de pointes, causing dizzy spells and confusion after 8 days (412). She was treated with temporary pacing, but her symptoms resolved 72 hours after drug withdrawal.

Cardiac contractility

The negative inotropic effects of class I antidysrhythmic agents, such as disopyramide, procainamide, quinidine, and tocainide can be accentuated by beta-blockers; this is most pronounced in patients with pre-existing myocardial disease and can result in left ventricular failure or even asystole (413). Digoxin can obviate the negative inotropic effect of beta-blockers in patients with poor left ventricular function.

References

1. Cruickshank JM, Prichard BNC. Beta-blockers in Clinical Practice. Edinburgh: Churchill Livingstone, 1988.
2. Brennan TA. Buying editorials. N Engl J Med 1994;331(10):673–5.
3. Croog SH, Levine S, Testa MA, Brown B, Bulpitt CJ, Jenkins CD, Klerman GL, Williams GH. The effects of antihypertensive therapy on the quality of life. N Engl J Med 1986;314(26):1657–64.
4. Anonymous. Fatigue as an unwanted effect of drugs. Lancet 1980;1(8181):1285–6.
5. Pearson SB, Banks DC, Patrick JM. The effect of beta-adrenoceptor blockade on factors affecting exercise tolerance in normal man. Br J Clin Pharmacol 1979;8(2):143–8.
6. Anderson SD, Bye PT, Perry CP, Hamor GP, Theobald G, Nyberg G. Limitation of work performance in normal adult males in the presence of beta-adrenergic blockade. Aust NZ J Med 1979;9(5):515–20.
7. Kaiser P. Running performance as a function of the dose–response relationship to beta-adrenoceptor blockade. Int J Sports Med 1982;3(1):29–32.
8. Kaijser L, Kaiser P, Karlsson J, Rossner S. Beta-blockers and running. Am Heart J 1980;100(6 Pt 1):943–4.
9. Bowman WC. Effect of adrenergic activators and inhibitors on the skeletal muscles. Szekeres L, editor. Adrenergic Activators and Inhibitors. Berlin: Springer Verlag; 1980.
10. Frisk-Holmberg M, Jorfeldt L, Juhlin-Dannfelt A. Metabolic effects in muscle during antihypertensive therapy with beta 1- and beta 1/beta 2-adrenoceptor blockers. Clin Pharmacol Ther 1981;30(5):611–18.
11. Koch G, Franz IW, Lohmann FW. Effects of short-term and long-term treatment with cardio-selective and non-selective beta-receptor blockade on carbohydrate and lipid metabolism and on plasma catecholamines at rest and during exercise. Clin Sci (Lond) 1981;61(Suppl 7):S433–5.
12. Franciosa JA, Johnson SM, Tobian LJ. Exercise performance in mildly hypertensive patients. Impairment by propranolol but not oxprenolol. Chest 1980;78(2):291–9.
13. McDevitt DG. Differential features of beta-adrenoceptor blocking drugs for therapy. Laragh J, Buhler F, editors. Frontiers in Hypertension Research. New York: Springer Verlag, 1981:473.
14. Woods PB, Robinson ML. An investigation of the comparative liposolubilities of beta-adrenoceptor blocking agents. J Pharm Pharmacol 1981;33(3):172–3.
15. Neil-Dwyer G, Bartlett J, McAinsh J, Cruickshank JM. Beta-adrenoceptor blockers and the blood–brain barrier. Br J Clin Pharmacol 1981;11(6):549–53.
16. McDevitt DG. Clinical significance of cardioselectivity: state of the art. Drugs 1983;25(Suppl 2):219.
17. McDevitt DG. Beta-adrenoceptor blocking drugs and partial agonist activity. Is it clinically relevant? Drugs 1983;25(4):331–8.
18. Cruickshank JM. Measurement and cardiovascular relevance of partial agonist activity (PAA) involving beta 1- and beta 2-adrenoceptors. Pharmacol Ther 1990;46(2):199–242.
19. Cruickshank JM. The xamoterol experience in the treatment of heart failure. Am J Cardiol 1993;71(9):C61–4.
20. McCaffrey PM, Riddell JG, Shanks RG. An assessment of the partial agonist activity of Ro 31–1118, flusoxolol and pindolol in man. Br J Clin Pharmacol 1987;24(5):571–80.
21. Prichard BN. Beta-blocking agents with vasodilating action. J Cardiovasc Pharmacol 1992;19(Suppl 1):S1–4.
22. Prichard BN, Owens CW. Mode of action of beta-adrenergic blocking drugs in hypertension. Clin Physiol Biochem 1990;8(Suppl 2):1–10.
23. Coltart DJ, Meldrum SJ, Hamer J. The effect of propranolol on the human and canine transmembrane action potential. Br J Pharmacol 1970;40(1):148P.
24. Barnett DB. Beta-blockers in heart failure: a therapeutic paradox. Lancet 1994;343(8897):557–8.
25. Waagstein F, Bristow MR, Swedberg K, Camerini F, Fowler MB, Silver MA, Gilbert EM, Johnson MR, Goss FG, Hjalmarson A. Beneficial effects of metoprolol in idiopathic dilated cardiomyopathy. Metoprolol in Dilated Cardiomyopathy (MDC) Trial Study Group. Lancet 1993;342(8885):1441–6.
26. The Cardiac Insufficiency Bisoprolol Study II (CIBIS-II): a randomised trial. Lancet 1999;353(9146):9–13.
27. Merit-HF Study Group. Effect of metoprolol CR/XL in chronic heart failure: Metoprolol CR/XL Randomised Intervention Trial in Congestive Heart Failure (MERIT-HF). Lancet 1999;353(9169):2001–7.

28. Packer M, Colucci WS, Sackner-Bernstein JD, Liang CS, Goldscher DA, Freeman I, Kukin ML, Kinhal V, Udelson JE, Klapholz M, Gottlieb SS, Pearle D, Cody RJ, Gregory JJ, Kantrowitz NE, LeJemtel TH, Young ST, Lukas MA, Shusterman NH. Double-blind, placebo-controlled study of the effects of carvedilol in patients with moderate to severe heart failure. The PRECISE Trial. Prospective Randomized Evaluation of Carvedilol on Symptoms and Exercise. Circulation 1996;94(11):2793–9.

29. Dougherty AH, Naccarelli GV, Gray EL, Hicks CH, Goldstein RA. Congestive heart failure with normal systolic function. Am J Cardiol 1984;54(7):778–82.

30. Wheeldon NM, MacDonald TM, Flucker CJ, McKendrick AD, McDevitt DG, Struthers AD. Echocardiography in chronic heart failure in the community. Q J Med 1993;86(1):17–23.

31. Clarkson P, Wheeldon NM, Macdonald TM. Left ventricular diastolic dysfunction. Q J Med 1994;87(3):143–8.

32. Wheeldon NM, Clarkson P, MacDonald TM. Diastolic heart failure. Eur Heart J 1994;15(12):1689–97.

33. Pouleur H. Diastolic dysfunction and myocardial energetics. Eur Heart J 1990;11(Suppl C):30–4.

34. Krumholz HM. Beta-blockers for mild to moderate heart failure. Lancet 1999;353(9146):2–3.

35. Sharpe N. Benefit of beta-blockers for heart failure: proven in 1999. Lancet 1999;353(9169):1988–9.

36. Gottlieb SS, McCarter RJ, Vogel RA. Effect of beta-blockade on mortality among high-risk and low-risk patients after myocardial infarction. N Engl J Med 1998;339(8):489–97.

37. MacDonald TM, Butler R, Newton RW, Morris AD. Which drugs benefit diabetic patients for secondary prevention of myocardial infarction? DARTS/MEMO Collaboration. Diabet Med 1998;15(4):282–9.

38. Frishman WH, Kowalski M, Nagnur S, Warshafsky S, Sica D. Cardiovascular considerations in using topical, oral, and intravenous drugs for the treatment of glaucoma and ocular hypertension: focus on beta-adrenergic blockade. Heart Dis 2001;3(6):386–97.

39. Girkin CA. Neuroprotection: does it work for any neurological diseases? Ophthalmic Pract 2001;19:298–302.

40. Van De Ven LLM, Spanjaard JN, De Jongste MJL, Hillege H, Verkenne P, Van Gilst WH, Lie KI. Safety of beta-blocker therapy with and without thrombolysis: A comparison or bisoprolol and atenolol in acute myocardial infarction. Curr Ther Res Clin Exp 1996;57:313.

41. Thomas JA, Marks BH. Plasma norepinephrine in congestive heart failure. Am J Cardiol 1978;41(2):233–43.

42. Greenblatt DJ, Koch-Weser J. Clinical toxicity of propranolol and practolol: a report from the Boston Collaborative Drug Surveillance Program. Avery GS, editor. Cardiovascular Drugs. Vol 2. Beta-Adrenoceptor Blocking Drugs, Chapter VIII. Sydney: Adis Press; 1977:179.

43. Aellig WH. Pindolol—a beta-adrenoceptor blocking drug with partial agonist activity: clinical pharmacological considerations. Br J Clin Pharmacol 1982;13(Suppl 2):S187–92.

44. Imhof P. The significance of beta1-beta2-selectivity and intrinsic sympathomimetic activity in beta-blockers, with particular reference to antihypertensive treatment. Adv Clin Pharmacol 1976;11:26–32.

45. Davies B, Bannister R, Mathias C, Sever P. Pindolol in postural hypotension: the case for caution. Lancet 1981;2(8253):982–3.

46. Anonymous. Xamoterol: stabilising the cardiac beta receptor? Lancet 1988;2(8625):1401–2.

47. Anonymous. New evidence on xamoterol. Lancet 1990;336(8706):24.

48. Frais MA, Bayley TJ. Left ventricular failure with labetalol. Postgrad Med J 1979;55(646):567–8.

49. Britman NA. Cardiac effects of topical timolol. N Engl J Med 1979;300(10):566.

50. Wikstrand J, Berglund G. Antihypertensive treatment with beta-blockers in patients aged over 65. BMJ (Clin Res Ed) 1982;285(6345):850.

51. Montoliu J, Botey A, Darnell A, Revert L. Hipotension prolongada tras la primera dosis de atenolol. [Prolonged hypotension after the first dose of atenolol.] Med Clin (Barc) 1981;76(8):365–6.

52. McNeil JJ, Louis WJ. A double-blind crossover comparison of pindolol, metoprolol, atenolol and labetalol in mild to moderate hypertension. Br J Clin Pharmacol 1979;8(Suppl 2):S163–6.

53. Cruickshank JM. Beta-blockers, bradycardia and adverse effects. Acta Ther 1981;7:309.

54. Anastasiou-Nana MI, Anderson JL, Askins JC, Gilbert EM, Nanas JN, Menlove RL. Long-term experience with sotalol in the treatment of complex ventricular arrhythmias. Am Heart J 1987;114(2):288–96.

55. Obel IW, Jardine R, Haitus B, Millar RN. Efficacy of oral sotalol in reentrant ventricular tachycardia. Cardiovasc Drugs Ther 1990;4(Suppl 3):613–18.

56. Griffith MJ, Linker NJ, Garratt CJ, Ward DE, Camm AJ. Relative efficacy and safety of intravenous drugs for termination of sustained ventricular tachycardia. Lancet 1990;336(8716):670–3.

57. Juul-Moller S, Edvardsson N, Rehnqvist-Ahlberg N. Sotalol versus quinidine for the maintenance of sinus rhythm after direct current conversion of atrial fibrillation. Circulation 1990;82(6):1932–9.

58. Desoutter P, Medioni J, Lerasle S, Haiat R. Bloc auriculo-ventriculaire et torsade de pointes après surdosage par le sotalol. [Atrioventricular block and torsade de pointes following sotalol overdose.] Nouv Presse Méd 1982;11(52):3855.

59. Belton P, Sheridan J, Mulcahy R. A case of sotalol poisoning. Ir J Med Sci 1982;151(4):126–7.

60. Pathy MS. Acute central chest pain in the elderly. A review of 296 consecutive hospital admissions during 1976 with particular reference to the possible role of beta-adrenergic blocking agents in inducing substernal pain. Am Heart J 1979;98(2):168–70.

61. Warren V, Goldberg E. Intractable angina pectoris. Combined therapy with propranolol and permanent pervenous pacemaker. JAMA 1976;235(8):841–2.

62. Robertson RM, Wood AJ, Vaughn WK, Robertson D. Exacerbation of vasotonic angina pectoris by propranolol. Circulation 1982;65(2):281–5.

63. McMahon MT, McPherson MA, Talbert RL, Greenberg B, Sheaffer SL. Diagnosis and treatment of Prinzmetal's variant angina. Clin Pharm 1982;1(1):34–42.

64. Aubran M, Trigano JA, Allard-Laour G, Ebagosti A, Torresani J. Angor accéléré sous béta-bloquants. [Angina accelerated under betablockers.] Ann Cardiol Angeiol (Paris) 1986;35(2):99–101.

65. Hall PE, Kendall MJ, Smith SR. Beta blockers and fatigue. J Clin Hosp Pharm 1984;9(4):283–91.

66. Feleke E, Lyngstam O, Rastam L, Ryden L. Complaints of cold extremities among patients on antihypertensive treatment. Acta Med Scand 1983;213(5):381–5.

67. Greminger P, Vetter H, Boerlin JH, Havelka J, Baumgart P, Walger P, Lüscher T, Siegenthaler W, Vetter W. A comparative study between 100 mg atenolol and 20 mg pindolol slow-release in essential hypertension. Drugs 1983;25 (Suppl 2):37–41.

68. Eliasson K, Danielson M, Hylander B, Lindblad LE. Raynaud's phenomenon caused by beta-receptor blocking drugs. Improvement after treatment with a combined

alpha- and beta-blocker. Acta Med Scand 1984;215(4): 333–9.

69. Steiner JA, Cooper R, Gear JS, Ledingham JG. Vascular symptoms in patients with primary Raynaud's phenomenon are not exacerbated by propranolol or labetalol. Br J Clin Pharmacol 1979;7(4):401–3.

70. Reichert N, Shibolet S, Adar R, Gafni J. Controlled trial of propranolol in intermittent claudication. Clin Pharmacol Ther 1975;17(5):612–15.

71. Breckenridge A. Which beta blocker? BMJ (Clin Res Ed) 1983;286(6371):1085–8.

72. Lepantalo M. Chronic effects of labetalol, pindolol, and propranolol on calf blood flow in intermittent claudication. Clin Pharmacol Ther 1985;37(1):7–12.

73. Solomon SA, Ramsay LE, Yeo WW, Parnell L, Morris-Jones W. Beta-blockade and intermittent claudication: placebo controlled trial of atenolol and nifedipine and their combination. BMJ 1991;303(6810):1100–4.

74. Gokal R, Dornan TL, Ledingham JGG. Peripheral skin necrosis complicating beta-blockage. BMJ 1979; 1(6165):721–2.

75. Hoffbrand BI. Peripheral skin necrosis complicating beta-blockade. BMJ 1979;1(6170):1082.

76. Rees PJ. Peripheral skin necrosis complicating beta-blockade. BMJ 1979;1(6168):955.

77. O'Rourke DA, Donohue MF, Hayes JA. Beta-blockers and peripheral gangrene. Med J Aust 1979;2(2):88.

78. Fogoros RN. Exacerbation of intermittent claudication by propranolol. N Engl J Med 1980;302(19):1089.

79. Stringer MD, Bentley PG. Peripheral gangrene associated with beta-blockade. Br J Surg 1986;73(12):1008.

80. Dompmartin A, Le Maitre M, Letessier D, Leroy D. Nécrose digitales sous béta-bloquants. [Digital necroses induced by beta-blockers.] Ann Dermatol Venereol 1988;115(5):593–6.

81. Price HL, Cooperman LH, Warden JC. Control of the splanchnic circulation in man. Role of beta-adrenergic receptors. Circ Res 1967;21(3):333–40.

82. Schneider R. Do beta-blockers cause mesenteric ischemia? J Clin Gastroenterol 1986;8(2):109–10.

83. Diggory P, Cassels-Brown A, Vail A, Hillman JS. Randomised, controlled trial of spirometric changes in elderly people receiving timolol or betaxolol as initial treatment for glaucoma. Br J Ophthalmol 1998;82(2):146–149.

84. McNeill RS. Effect of a beta-adrenergic-blocking agent, propranolol, on asthmatics. Lancet 1964;13:1101–2.

85. Harries AD. Beta-blockade in asthma. BMJ (Clin Res Ed) 1981;282(6272):1321.

86. Australian Adverse Drug Reactions Advisory Committee. Beta-blockers. Med J Aust 1980;2:130.

87. Raine JM, Palazzo MG, Kerr JH, Sleight P. Near-fatal bronchospasm after oral nadolol in a young asthmatic and response to ventilation with halothane. BMJ (Clin Res Ed) 1981;282(6263):548–9.

88. McMahon CD, Shaffer RN, Hoskins HD Jr, Hetherington J Jr. Adverse effects experienced by patients taking timolol. Am J Ophthalmol 1979;88(4):736–8.

89. Mustchin CP, Gribbin HR, Tattersfield AE, George CF. Reduced respiratory responses to carbon dioxide after propranolol: a central action. BMJ 1976;2(6046):1229–31.

90. Trembath PW, Taylor EA, Varley J, Turner P. Effect of propranolol on the ventilatory response to hypercapnia in man. Clin Sci (Lond) 1979;57(5):465–8.

91. Chang LC. Use of practolol in asthmatics: a plea for caution. Lancet 1971;2(7719):321.

92. Waal-Manning HJ, Simpson FO. Practolol treatment in asthmatics. Lancet 1971;2(7736):1264–5.

93. Harris LS, Greenstein SH, Bloom AF. Respiratory difficulties with betaxolol. Am J Ophthalmol 1986;102(2): 274–5.

94. Diggory P, Cassels-Brown A, Vail A, Abbey LM, Hillman JS. Avoiding unsuspected respiratory side-effects of topical timolol with cardioselective or sympathomimetic agents. Lancet 1995;345(8965):1604–6.

95. Formgrein H. The effect of metoprolol and practolol on lung function and blood pressure in hypertensive asthmatics. Br J Clin Pharmacol 1976;3:1007.

96. Wilcox PG, Ahmad D, Darke AC, Parsons J, Carruthers SG. Respiratory and cardiac effects of metoprolol and bevantolol in patients with asthma. Clin Pharmacol Ther 1986;39(1):29–34.

97. Nordstrom LA, MacDonald F, Gobel FL. Effect of propranolol on respiratory function and exercise tolerance in patients with chronic obstructive lung disease. Chest 1975;67(3):287–92.

98. Fraley DS, Bruns FJ, Segel DP, Adler S. Propranolol-related bronchospasm in patients without history of asthma. South Med J 1980;73(2):238–40.

99. Mue S, Sasaki T, Shibahara S, Takahashi M, Ohmi T, Yamauchi K, Suzuki S, Hida W, Takishima T. Influence of metoprolol on hemodynamics and respiratory function in asthmatic patients. Int J Clin Pharmacol Biopharm 1979;17(8):346–50.

100. Assaykeen TA, Michell G. Metoprolol in hypertension: an open evaluation. Med J Aust 1982;1(2):73–7.

101. Jackson SH, Beevers DG. Comparison of the effects of single doses of atenolol and labetalol on airways obstruction in patients with hypertension and asthma. Br J Clin Pharmacol 1983;15(5):553–6.

102. Ellis ME, Sahay JN, Chatterjee SS, Cruickshank JM, Ellis SH. Cardioselectivity of atenolol in asthmatic patients. Eur J Clin Pharmacol 1981;21(3):173–6.

103. Committee on Safety of Medicines. Fatal bronchospasm associated with beta-blockers. Curr Probl 1987;20:2.

104. van Zyl AI, Jennings AA, Bateman ED, Opie LH. Comparison of respiratory effects of two cardioselective beta-blockers, celiprolol and atenolol, in asthmatics with mild to moderate hypertension. Chest 1989;95(1):209–13.

105. Waal-Manning HJ, Simpson FO. Safety of celiprolol in hypertensives with chronic obstructive respiratory disease. NZ Med J 1990;103:222.

106. Anonymous. Celiprolol—a better beta blocker? Drug Ther Bull 1992;30(9):35–6.

107. Malik A, Memon AM. Beta blocker eye drops related airway obstruction. J Pak Med Assoc 2001;51(5):202–4.

108. Tattersfield AE. Respiratory function in the elderly and the effects of beta blockade. Cardiovasc Drugs Ther 1991;4(Suppl 6):1229–32.

109. Campbell SC, Lauver GL, Cobb RB Jr. Central ventilatory depression by oral propranolol. Clin Pharmacol Ther 1981;30(6):758–64.

110. Davis WM, Hatoum NS. Lethal synergism between morphine or other narcotic analgesics and propranolol. Toxicology 1979;14(2):141–51.

111. Erwteman TM, Braat MC, van Aken WG. Interstitial pulmonary fibrosis: a new side effect of practolol. BMJ 1977;2(6082):297–8.

112. Marshall AJ, Eltringham WK, Barritt DW, Davies JD, Griffiths DA, Jackson LK, Laszlo G, Read AE. Respiratory disease associated with practolol therapy. Lancet 1977;2(8051):1254–7.

113. Musk AW, Pollard JA. Pindolol and pulmonary fibrosis. BMJ 1979;2(6190):581–2.

114. Wood GM, Bolton RP, Muers MF, Losowsky MS. Pleurisy and pulmonary granulomas after treatment with acebutolol. BMJ (Clin Res Ed) 1982;285(6346):936.

115. Akoun GM, Herman DP, Mayaud CM, Perrot JY. Acebutolol-induced hypersensitivity pneumonitis. BMJ (Clin Res Ed) 1983;286(6361):266–7.

116. Akoun GM, Touboul JL, Mayaud CM, et al. Pneumopathie d'hypersensibilité à l'acébutolol: données en faveur d'un mécanisme immunologique et médiation cellulaire. Rev Fr Allergol 1985;75:85.

117. Das G, Ferris JC. Generalized convulsions in a patient receiving ultrashort-acting beta-blocker infusion. Drug Intell Clin Pharm 1988;22(6):484–5.

118. Fleminger R. Visual hallucinations and illusions with propranolol. BMJ 1978;1(6121):1182.

119. Greenblatt DJ, Shader RI. On the psychopharmacology of beta adrenergic blockade. Curr Ther Res Clin Exp 1972;14(9):615–25.

120. Faldt R, Liedholm H, Aursnes J. Beta blockers and loss of hearing. BMJ (Clin Res Ed) 1984;289(6457):1490–2.

121. Weber JC. Beta-adrenoreceptor antagonists and diplopia. Lancet 1982;2(8302):826–7.

122. Turkewitz LJ, Sahgal V, Spiro A. Propranolol-induced myotonia. Mt Sinai J Med 1984;51(2):207.

123. Robson RH. Recurrent migraine after propranolol. Br Heart J 1977;39(10):1157–8.

124. Prendes JL. Considerations on the use of propranolol in complicated migraine. Headache 1980;20(2):93–5.

125. Gilbert GJ. An occurrence of complicated migraine during propranolol therapy. Headache 1982;22(2):81–3.

126. Bardwell A, Trott JA. Stroke in migraine as a consequence of propranolol. Headache 1987;27(7):381–3.

127. Leys D, Pasquier F, Vermersch P, Gosset D, Michiels H, Kassiotis P, Petit H. Possible revelation of latent myasthenia gravis by labetalol chlorhydrate. Acta Clin Belg 1987;42(6):475–6.

128. Komar J, Szalay M, Szel I. Myasthenische Episode nach Einnahme grosser Mengen Beta-blocker. [A myasthenic episode following intake of large amounts of a beta blocker.] Fortschr Neurol Psychiatr 1987;55(6):201–2.

129. Emara MK, Saadah AM. The carpal tunnel syndrome in hypertensive patients treated with beta-blockers. Postgrad Med J 1988;64(749):191–2.

130. Hod H, Har-Zahav J, Kaplinsky N, Frankl O. Pindolol-induced tremor. Postgrad Med J 1980;56(655):346–7.

131. Palomeras E, Sanz P, Cano A, Fossas P. Dystonia in a patient treated with propranolol and gabapentin. Arch Neurol 2000;57(4):570–1.

132. Medical Research Council Working Party on Mild to Moderate Hypertension. Adverse reactions to bendrofluazide and propranolol for the treatment of mild hypertension. Lancet 1981;2(8246):539–43.

133. Bengtsson C, Lennartsson J, Lindquist O, Noppa H, Sigurdsson J. Sleep disturbances, nightmares and other possible central nervous disturbances in a population sample of women, with special reference to those on antihypertensive drugs. Eur J Clin Pharmacol 1980;17(3):173–7.

134. Kostis JB, Rosen RC. Central nervous system effects of beta-adrenergic-blocking drugs: the role of ancillary properties. Circulation 1987;75(1):204–12.

135. Patel L, Turner P. Central actions of beta-adrenoceptor blocking drugs in man. Med Res Rev 1981;1(4):387–410.

136. Betts TA, Alford C. Beta-blockers and sleep: a controlled trial. Eur J Clin Pharmacol 1985;28(Suppl):65–8.

137. McAinsh J, Cruickshank JM. Beta-blockers and central nervous system side effects. Pharmacol Ther 1990;46(2):163–97.

138. Dimsdale JE, Newton RP, Joist T. Neuropsychological side effects of beta-blockers. Arch Intern Med 1989;149(3):514–25.

139. Dahlof C, Dimenas E. Side effects of beta-blocker treatments as related to the central nervous system. Am J Med Sci 1990;299(4):236–44.

140. Braun P, Reker K, Friedel B, et al. Driving tests with beta-receptor blockers. Blutalkohol 1979;16:495.

141. Betts T. Effects of beta blockade on driving. Aviat Space Environ Med 1981;52(11 Pt 2):S40–5.

142. Panizza D, Lecasble M. Effect of atenolol on car drivers in a prolonged stress situation. Eur J Clin Pharmacol 1985;28(Suppl):97–9.

143. Broadhurst AD. The effect of propranolol on human psychomotor performance. Aviat Space Environ Med 1980;51(2):176–9.

144. Fiore PM, Jacobs IH, Goldberg DB. Drug-induced pemphigoid. A spectrum of diseases. Arch Ophthalmol 1987;105(12):1660–3.

145. Jain S. Betaxolol-associated anterior uveitis. Eye 1994;8(Pt 6):708–9.

146. Schultz JS, Hoenig JA, Charles H. Possible bilateral anterior uveitis secondary to metipranolol (optipranolol) therapy. Arch Ophthalmol 1993;111(12):1606–7.

147. O'Connor GR. Granulomatous uveitis and metipranolol. Br J Ophthalmol 1993;77(8):536–8.

148. Fraunfelder FT. Drug-induced ocular side effects. Folia Ophthalmol Jpn 1996;47:770.

149. Kellner U, Kraus H, Foerster MH. Multifocal ERG in chloroquine retinopathy: regional variance of retinal dysfunction. Graefes Arch Clin Exp Ophthalmol 2000;238(1):94–7.

150. Bryan PC, Efiong DO, Stewart-Jones J, Turner P. Propranolol on tests of visual function and central nervous activity. Br J Clin Pharmacol 1974;1:82.

151. Glaister DH, Harrison MH, Allnutt MF. Environmental influences on cardiac activity. Burley DM, Frier JH, Rondel RK, Taylor SH, editors. New Perspectives in Beta-blockade. Horsham, UK: Ciba Laboratories; 1973:241.

152. Landauer AA, Pocock DA, Prott FW. Effects of atenolol and propranolol on human performance and subjective feelings. Psychopharmacology (Berl) 1979;60(2):211–15.

153. Salem SA, McDevitt DG. Central effects of beta-adrenoceptor antagonists. Clin Pharmacol Ther 1983;33(1):52–7.

154. Ogle CW, Turner P, Markomihelakis H. The effects of high doses of oxprenolol and of propranolol on pursuit rotor performance, reaction time and critical flicker frequency. Psychopharmacologia 1976;46(3):295–9.

155. Turner P, Hedges A. An investigation of the central effects of oxprenolol. Burley DM, Frier JH, Rondel RK, Taylor SH, editors. New Perspectives in Beta-blockade. Horsham, UK: Ciba Laboratories; 1973:269.

156. Tyrer PJ, Lader MH. Response to propranolol and diazepam in somatic and psychic anxiety. BMJ 1974;2(909):14–16.

157. Greil W. Central nervous system effects. Curr Ther Res 1980;28:106.

158. Currie D, Lewis RV, McDevitt DG, Nicholson AN, Wright NA. Central effects of beta-adrenoceptor antagonists. I—Performance and subjective assessments of mood. Br J Clin Pharmacol 1988;26(2):121–8.

159. Nicholson AN, Wright NA, Zetlein MB, Currie D, McDevitt DG. Central effects of beta-adrenoceptor antagonists. II—Electroencephalogram and body sway. Br J Clin Pharmacol 1988;26(2):129–41.

160. Hearing SD, Wesnes KA, Bowman CE. Beta blockers and cognitive function in elderly hypertensive patients: withdrawal and consequences of ACE inhibitor substitution. Int J Geriatr Psychopharmacol 1999;2:13–17.

161. Perez-Stable EJ, Halliday R, Gardiner PS, Baron RB, Hauck WW, Acree M, Coates TJ. The effects of propranolol on cognitive function and quality of life: a randomized trial among patients with diastolic hypertension. Am J Med 2000;108(5):359–65.

162. Yatham LN, Lint D, Lam RW, Zis AP. Adverse effects of pindolol augmentation in patients with bipolar depression. J Clin Psychopharmacol 1999;19(4):383–4.

163. Russell JW, Schuckit NA. Anxiety and depression in patient on nadolol. Lancet 1982;2(8310):1286–7.

164. Thiessen BQ, Wallace SM, Blackburn JL, Wilson TW, Bergman U. Increased prescribing of antidepressants subsequent to beta-blocker therapy. Arch Intern Med 1990;150(11):2286–90.

165. Topliss D, Bond R. Acute brain syndrome after propranolol treatment. Lancet 1977;2(8048):1133–4.

166. Helson L, Duque L. Acute brain syndrome after propranolol. Lancet 1978;1(8055):98.

167. Kurland ML. Organic brain syndrome with propranolol. N Engl J Med 1979;300(7):366.

168. Gershon ES, Goldstein RE, Moss AJ, van Kammen DP. Psychosis with ordinary doses of propranolol. Ann Intern Med 1979;90(6):938–9.

169. Kuhr BM. Prolonged delirium with propanolol. J Clin Psychiatry 1979;40(4):198–9.

170. McGahan DJ, Wojslaw A, Prasad V, Blankenship S. Propranolol-induced psychosis. Drug Intell Clin Pharm 1984;18(7–8):601–3.

171. Steinhert J, Pugh CR. Two patients with schizophrenic-like psychosis after treatment with beta-adrenergic blockers. BMJ 1979;1(6166):790.

172. Lee ST. Hyperprolactinemia, galactorrhea, and atenolol. Ann Intern Med 1992;116(6):522.

173. Harrower AD, Fyffe JA, Horn DB, Strong JA. Thyroxine and triiodothyronine levels in hyperthyroid patients during treatment with propranolol. Clin Endocrinol (Oxf) 1977;7(1):41–4.

174. Cooper DS, Daniels GH, Ladenson PW, Ridgway EC. Hyperthyroxinemia in patients treated with high-dose propranolol. Am J Med 1982;73(6):867–71.

175. Mooradian A, Morley JE, Simon G, Shafer RB. Propranolol-induced hyperthyroxinemia. Arch Intern Med 1983;143(11):2193–5.

176. Heyma P, Larkins RG, Higginbotham L, Ng KW. D-propranolol and DL-propranolol both decrease conversion of L-thyroxine to L-triiodothyronine. BMJ 1980;281(6232):24–5.

177. Jones DK, Solomon S. Thyrotoxic crisis masked by treatment with beta-blockers. BMJ (Clin Res Ed) 1981;283(6292):659.

178. Gold LA, Merimee TJ, Misbin RI. Propranolol and hypoglycemia: the effects of beta-adrenergic blockade on glucose and alanine levels during fasting. J Clin Pharmacol 1980;20(1):50–8.

179. Uusitupa M, Aro A, Pietikainen M. Severe hypoglycaemia caused by physical strain and pindolol therapy. A case report. Ann Clin Res 1980;12(1):25–7.

180. Holm G, Herlitz J, Smith U. Severe hypoglycaemia during physical exercise and treatment with beta-blockers. BMJ (Clin Res Ed) 1981;282(6273):1360.

181. Zarate A, Gelfand M, Novello A, Knepshield J, Preuss HG. Propranolol-associated hypoglycemia in patients on maintenance hemodialysis. Int J Artif Organs 1981;4(3):130–4.

182. Belton P, O'Dwyer WF, Carmody M, Donohoe J. Propranolol associated hypoglycaemia in non-diabetics. Ir Med J 1980;73(4):173.

183. Chavez H, Ozolins D, Losek JD. Hypoglycemia and propranolol in pediatric behavioral disorders. Pediatrics 1999;103(6 Pt 1):1290–2.

184. Barnett AH, Leslie D, Watkins PJ. Can insulin-treated diabetics be given beta-adrenergic blocking drugs? BMJ 1980;280(6219):976–8.

185. Wright AD, Barber SG, Kendall MJ, Poole PH. Beta-adrenoceptor-blocking drugs and blood sugar control in diabetes mellitus. BMJ 1979;1(6157):159–61.

186. Davidson NM, Corrall RJ, Shaw TR, French EB. Observations in man of hypoglycaemia during selective and non-selective beta-blockade. Scott Med J 1977;22(1):69–72.

187. Deacon SP, Barnett D. Comparison of atenolol and propranolol during insulin-induced hypoglycaemia. BMJ 1976;2(6030):272–3.

188. Blohme G, Lager I, Lonnroth P, Smith U. Hypoglycemic symptoms in insulin-dependent diabetics. A prospective study of the influence of beta-blockade. Diabete Metab 1981;7(4):235–8.

189. Shepherd AM, Lin MS, Keeton TK. Hypoglycemia-induced hypertension in a diabetic patient on metoprolol. Ann Intern Med 1981;94(3):357–8.

190. Malmberg K, Ryden L, Hamsten A, Herlitz J, Waldenstrom A, Wedel H. Mortality prediction in diabetic patients with myocardial infarction: experiences from the DIGAMI study. Cardiovasc Res 1997;34(1):248–53.

191. Samuelsson O, Hedner T, Berglund G, Persson B, Andersson OK, Wilhelmsen L. Diabetes mellitus in treated hypertension: incidence, predictive factors and the impact of non-selective beta-blockers and thiazide diuretics during 15 years treatment of middle-aged hypertensive men in the Primary Prevention Trial Goteborg, Sweden. J Hum Hypertens 1994;8(4):257–63.

192. Van Brammelen P. Lipid changes induced by beta-blockers. Curr Opin Cardiol 1988;3:513.

193. Bielmann P, Leduc G, Jequier JC, et al. Changes in the lipoprotein composition after chronic administration of metoprolol and propranolol in hypertriglyceridemic-hypertensive subjects. Curr Ther Res 1981;30:956.

194. Gavalas C, Costantino O, Zuppardi E, Scaramucci S, Doronzo E, Aharrh-Gnama A, Nubile M, Di Nuzzo S, De Nicola GC. Variazioni della colesterolemia in pazienti sottoposti a terapia topica con il timololo. Ann Ottalmol Clin Ocul 2001;127:9–14.

195. Northcote RJ. Beta blockers, lipids, and coronary atherosclerosis: fact or fiction? BMJ (Clin Res Ed) 1988;296(6624):731–2.

196. Neaton JD, Grimm RH Jr, Prineas RJ, Stamler J, Grandits GA, Elmer PJ, Cutler JA, Flack JM, Schoenberger JA, McDonald R, et al. Treatment of Mild Hypertension Study. Final results. Treatment of Mild Hypertension Study Research Group. JAMA 1993;270(6):713–24.

197. Astrup AV. Fedme og diabetes som bivirkninger til beta-blokkere. [Obesity and diabetes as side-effects of beta-blockers.] Ugeskr Laeger 1990;152(40):2905–8.

198. Connacher AA, Jung RT, Mitchell PE. Weight loss in obese subjects on a restricted diet given BRL 26830A, a new atypical beta adrenoceptor agonist. BMJ (Clin Res Ed) 1988;296(6631):1217–20.

199. Wheeldon NM, McDevitt DG, McFarlane LC, Lipworth BJ. Do beta 3-adrenoceptors mediate metabolic responses to isoprenaline. Q J Med 1993;86(9):595–600.

200. Emorine LJ, Marullo S, Briend-Sutren MM, Patey G, Tate K, Delavier-Klutchko C, Strosberg AD. Molecular characterization of the human beta 3-adrenergic receptor. Science 1989;245(4922):1118–21.

201. Sharma AM, Pischon T, Hardt S, Kunz I, Luft FC. Hypothesis: Beta-adrenergic receptor blockers and weight gain: a systematic analysis. Hypertension 2001;37(2):250–4.

202. Saunders J, Prestwich SA, Avery AJ, Kilborn JR, Morselli PL, Sonksen PH. The effect of non-selective and selective beta-1-blockade on the plasma potassium response to hypoglycaemia. Diabete Metab 1981;7(4):239–42.

203. Arnold JMO, Shanks RG, McDevitt DG. Beta-adrenoceptor antagonism of isoprenaline induced metabolic changes in man. Br J Clin Pharmacol 1983;16:621P.

204. Skehan JD, Barnes JN, Drew PJ, Wright P. Hypokalaemia induced by a combination of a beta-blocker and a thiazide. BMJ (Clin Res Ed) 1982;284(6309):83.

205. Walters EG, Horswill CE, Shelton JR, Ali Akbar F. Hazards of beta-blocker/diuretic tablets. Lancet 1985; 2(8448):220–1.

206. Odugbesan O, Chesner IM, Bailey G, Barnett AH. Hazards of combined beta-blocker/diuretic tablets. Lancet 1985;1(8439):1221–2.

207. Pedersen OL, Mikkelsen E. Serum potassium and uric acid changes during treatment with timolol alone and in combination with a diuretic. Clin Pharmacol Ther 1979;26(3):339–43.

208. Bushe CJ. Does atenolol have an effect on calcium metabolism? BMJ (Clin Res Ed) 1987;294(6583):1324–5.

209. Freestone S, MacDonald TM. Does atenolol have an effect on calcium metabolism? BMJ (Clin Res Ed) 1987; 295(6589):53.

210. Dodds WN, Davidson RJ. Thrombocytopenia due to slow-release oxprenolol. Lancet 1978;2(8091):683.

211. Hare DL, Hicks BH. Thrombocytopenia due to oxprenolol. Med J Aust 1979;2(5):259.

212. Caviet NL, Klaassen CH. Trombocuytopenie veroorzaakt door alprenolol. [Thrombocytopenia caused by alprenolol.] Ned Tijdschr Geneeskd 1979;123(1):18–20.

213. Magnusson B, Rodjer S. Alprenolol-induced thrombocytopenia. Acta Med Scand 1980;207(3):231–3.

214. Kelly JP, Kaufman DW, Shapiro S. Risks of agranulocytosis and aplastic anemia in relation to the use of cardiovascular drugs: The International Agranulocytosis and Aplastic Anemia Study. Clin Pharmacol Ther 1991;49(3):330–41.

215. Nawabi IU, Ritz ND. Agranulocytosis due to propranolol. JAMA 1973;223(12):1376–7.

216. Robinson JD, Burtner DE. Severe diarrhea secondary to propranolol. Drug Intell Clin Pharm 1981;15(1):49–50.

217. Wolfhagen FH, van Neerven JA, Groen FC, Ouwendijk RJ. Severe nausea and vomiting with timolol eye drops. Lancet 1998;352(9125):373.

218. Carlborg B, Kumlien A, Olsson H. Medikamentella esofagusstrikturen. [Drug-induced esophageal strictures.] Lakartidningen 1978;75(49):4609–11.

219. Windsor WO, Durrein F, Dyer NH. Fibrinous peritonitis: a complication of practolol therapy. BMJ 1975;2(5962):68.

220. Eltringham WK, Espiner HJ, Windsor CW, Griffiths DA, Davies JD, Baddeley H, Read AE, Blunt RJ. Sclerosing peritonitis due to practolol: a report on 9 cases and their surgical management. Br J Surg 1977;64(4):229–35.

221. Marshall AJ, Baddeley H, Barritt DW, Davies JD, Lee RE, Low-Beer TS, Read AE. Practolol peritonitis. A study of 16 cases and a survey of small bowel function in patients taking beta adrenergic blockers. Q J Med 1977;46(181):135–49.

222. Ahmad S. Sclerosing peritonitis and propranolol. Chest 1981;79(3):361–2.

223. Nillson BV, Pederson KG. Sclerosing peritonitis associated with atenolol. BMJ (Clin Res Ed) 1985;290:518.

224. McClusky DR, Donaldson RA, McGeown MG. Oxprenolol and retroperitoneal fibrosis. BMJ 1980;281(6253):1459–60.

225. Johnson JN, McFarland J. Retroperitoneal fibrosis associated with atenolol. BMJ 1980;280(6217):864.

226. Pierce JR Jr, Trostle DC, Warner JJ. Propranolol and retroperitoneal fibrosis. Ann Intern Med 1981;95(2):244.

227. Thompson J, Julian DG. Retroperitoneal fibrosis associated with metoprolol. BMJ (Clin Res Ed) 1982;284(6309):83–4.

228. Laakso M, Arvala I, Tervonen S, Sotarauta M. Retroperitoneal fibrosis associated with sotalol. BMJ (Clin Res Ed) 1982;285(6348):1085–6.

229. Rimmer E, Richens A, Forster ME, Rees RW. Retroperitoneal fibrosis associated with timolol. Lancet 1983;1(8319):300.

230. Benitah E, Chatelain C, Cohen F, Herman D. Fibrose retropéritonéale: effet systémique d'un collyre bétabloquant? [Retroperitoneal fibrosis: a systemic effect of beta-blocker eyedrops?] Presse Méd 1987;16(8):400–1.

231. Bullimore DW. Retroperitoneal fibrosis associated with atenolol. BMJ 1980;281(6239):564.

232. Pryor JP, Castle WM, Dukes DC, Smith JC, Watson ME, Williams JL. Do beta-adrenoceptor blocking drugs cause retroperitoneal fibrosis? BMJ (Clin Res Ed) 1983;287(6393):639–41.

233. Mahgoub A, Idle JR, Dring LG, Lancaster R, Smith RL. Polymorphic hydroxylation of debrisoquine in man. Lancet 1977;2(8038):584–6.

234. Smith RL. Polymorphic metabolism of the beta-adrenoreceptor blocking drugs and its clinical relevance. Eur J Clin Pharmacol 1985;28(Suppl):77–84.

235. Sherlock S. Diseases of the Liver and Biliary System6th edn. Oxford: Blackwell Scientific Publications; 1981:163.

236. Conn HO. Propranolol in the treatment of portal hypertension: a caution. Hepatology 1982;2(5):641–4.

237. Hayes PC, Shepherd AN, Bouchier IA. Medical treatment of portal hypertension and oesophageal varices. BMJ (Clin Res Ed) 1983;287(6394):733–6.

238. Tarver D, Walt RP, Dunk AA, Jenkins WJ, Sherlock S. Precipitation of hepatic encephalopathy by propranolol in cirrhosis. BMJ (Clin Res Ed) 1983;287(6392):585.

239. Watson P, Hayes JR. Cirrhosis, hepatic encephalopathy, and propranolol. BMJ (Clin Res Ed) 1983;287(6398):1067.

240. Anonymous. Beta-adrenergic blockers in cirrhosis. Lancet 1985;1(8442):1372–3.

241. Brown PJ, Lesna M, Hamlyn AN, Record CO. Primary biliary cirrhosis after long-term practolol administration. BMJ 1978;1(6127):1591.

242. Falch DK, Odegaard AE, Norman N. Decreased renal plasma flow during propranolol treatment in essential hypertension. Acta Med Scand 1979;205(1–2):91–5.

243. Bauer JH, Brooks CS. The long-term effect of propranolol therapy on renal function. Am J Med 1979;66(3):405–10.

244. Kincaid-Smith P, Fang P, Laver MC. A new look at the treatment of severe hypertension. Clin Sci Mol Med 1973;45(Suppl 1):s75–87.

245. Warren DJ, Swainson CP, Wright N. Deterioration in renal function after beta-blockade in patients with chronic renal failure and hypertension. BMJ 1974;2(912):193–4.

246. Wilkinson R. Beta-blockers and renal function. Drugs 1982;23(3):195–206.

247. Britton KE, Gruenwald SM, Nimmon CC. Nadolol and renal haemodynamics. International Experience With Nadolol, No. 37, International Congress and Symposium Series. London: Royal Society of Medicine; 1981:77.

248. Dupont AG. Effects of carvedilol on renal function. Eur J Clin Pharmacol 1990;38(Suppl 2):S96–100.

249. Krum H, Sackner-Bernstein JD, Goldsmith RL, Kukin ML, Schwartz B, Penn J, Medina N, Yushak M, Horn E, Katz SD, et al. Double-blind, placebo-controlled study of the long-term efficacy of carvedilol in patients with severe chronic heart failure. Circulation 1995;92(6):1499–506.

250. Hawk JL. Lichenoid drug eruption induced by propanolol. Clin Exp Dermatol 1980;5(1):93–6.

251. Guillet G, Chouvet V, Perrot H. Un accident des bétabloquants: lichen induit par le pindolol avec anticorps pemphigus-like. Bordeaux Med 1981;14:95.

252. Faure M, Hermier C, Perrot H. Accidents cutanés provoqués par le propranolol. [Cutaneous reactions to propranolol.] Ann Dermatol Venereol 1979;106(2):161–5.

253. Newman BR, Schultz LK. Epinephrine-resistant anaphylaxis in a patient taking propranolol hydrochloride. Ann Allergy 1981;47(1):35–7.

254. Kauppinen K, Idanpaan-Heikkila J. Cutaneous reactions to beta-blocking agents. Proceedings. XV International Congress of Dermatology, Mexico, 1977. 1979:702.

255. Halevy S, Feuerman EJ. Psoriasiform eruption induced by propranolol. Cutis 1979;24(1):95–8.

256. Girardin P, Derancourt C, Laurent R. A new cutaneous side-effect of ocular beta-blockers. Clin Exp Dermatol 1998;23(2):95.

257. Sanchez-Perez J, Cordoba S, Bartolome B, Garcia-Diez A. Allergic contact dermatitis due to the beta-blocker carteolol in eyedrops. Contact Dermatitis 1999;41(5):298.

258. Gold MH, Holy AK, Roenigk HH Jr. Beta-blocking drugs and psoriasis. A review of cutaneous side effects and retrospective analysis of their effects on psoriasis. J Am Acad Dermatol 1988;19(5 Pt 1):837–41.

259. Schallreuter KU. Beta-adrenergic blocking drugs may exacerbate vitiligo. Br J Dermatol 1995;132(1):168–9.

260. Arnoult L, Bowman ZL, Kimbrough RL, Stewart RH. Periocular cutaneous pigmentary changes associated with topical betaxolol. J Glaucoma 1995;4:263–7.

261. Neumann HAM, Van Joost TH. Dermatitis as a side-effect of long-term treatment with beta-adrenoceptor blocking agents. Br J Dermatol 1980;103:566.

262. Nino M, Suppa F, Ayala F, Balato N. Allergic contact dermatitis due to the beta-blocker befunolol in eyedrops, with cross-sensitivity to carteolol. Contact Dermatitis 2001;44(6):369.

263. Schmutz JL, Houet C, Trechot P, Barbaud A, Gillet-Terver MN. Sweating and beta-adrenoceptor antagonists. Dermatology 1995;190(1):86.

264. Schmutz JL, Barbaud A, Reichert S, Vasse JP, Trechot P. First report of sweating associated with topical beta-blocker therapy. Dermatology 1997;194(2):197–8.

265. Gordon NF. Effect of selective and nonselective beta-adrenoceptor blockade on thermoregulation during prolonged exercise in heat. Am J Cardiol 1985;55(10):D74–8.

266. Feder R. Clonidine treatment of excessive sweating. J Clin Psychiatry 1995;56(1):35.

267. Tanner CM, Goetz CG, Klawans HL. Paroxysmal drenching sweats in idiopathic parkinsonism: response to propanolol. Neurology 1982;32(Suppl A):162.

268. Hilder RJ. Propranolol and alopecia. Cutis 1979;24(1):63–4.

269. Graeber CW, Lapkin RA. Metoprolol and alopecia. Cutis 1981;28(6):633–4.

270. Savola J. Arthropathy induced by beta blockade. BMJ (Clin Res Ed) 1983;287(6401):1256–7.

271. Waller PC, Ramsay LE. Do beta blockers cause arthropathy? A case control study. BMJ (Clin Res Ed) 1985;291(6510):1684.

272. Sills JM, Bosco L. Arthralgia associated with beta-adrenergic blockade. JAMA 1986;255(2):198–9.

273. Zimlichman R, Krauss S, Paran E. Muscle cramps induced by beta-blockers with intrinsic sympathomimetic activity properties: a hint of a possible mechanism. Arch Intern Med 1991;151(5):1021.

274. Tomlinson B, Cruickshank JM, Hayes Y, Renondin JC, Lui JB, Graham BR, Jones A, Lewis AD, Prichard BN. Selective beta-adrenoceptor partial agonist effects of pindolol and xamoterol on skeletal muscle assessed by plasma creatine kinase changes in healthy subjects. Br J Clin Pharmacol 1990;30(5):665–72.

275. Wheeldon NM, Newnham DM, Fraser GC, McDevitt DG, Lipworth BJ. The effect of pindolol on creatine kinase is not due to beta 2-adrenoceptor partial agonist activity. Br J Clin Pharmacol 1991;31(6):723–4.

276. Imai Y, Watanabe N, Hashimoto J, Nishiyama A, Sakuma H, Sekino H, Omata K, Abe K. Muscle cramps and elevated serum creatine phosphokinase levels induced by beta-adrenoceptor blockers. Eur J Clin Pharmacol 1995;48(1):29–34.

277. Burnett WC, Chahine RA. Sexual dysfunction as a complication of propranolol therapy in man. Cardiovasc Med 1979;4:811.

278. Beta-blocker Heart Attack Trial Research Group. A randomized trial of propranolol in patients with acute myocardial infarction. I. Mortality results. JAMA 1982;247(12):1707–14.

279. Wassertheil-Smoller S, Blaufox MD, Oberman A, Davis BR, Swencionis C, Knerr MO, Hawkins CM, Langford HG. Effect of antihypertensives on sexual function and quality of life: the TAIM Study. Ann Intern Med 1991;114(8):613–20.

280. Croog SH, Levine S, Sudilovsky A, Baume RM, Clive J. Sexual symptoms in hypertensive patients. A clinical trial of antihypertensive medications. Arch Intern Med 1988;148(4):788–94.

281. Kostis JB, Rosen RC, Holzer BC, Randolph C, Taska LS, Miller MH. CNS side effects of centrally-active antihypertensive agents: a prospective, placebo-controlled study of sleep, mood state, and cognitive and sexual function in hypertensive males. Psychopharmacology (Berl) 1990;102(2):163–70.

282. Suzuki H, Tominaga T, Kumagai H, Saruta T. Effects of first-line antihypertensive agents on sexual function and sex hormones. J Hypertens Suppl 1988;6(4):S649–51.

283. Osborne DR. Propranolol and Peyronie's disease. Lancet 1977;1(8021):1111.

284. Kristensen BO. Labetalol-induced Peyronie's disease? A case report. Acta Med Scand 1979;206(6):511–12.

285. Pryor JP, Castle WM. Peyronie's disease associated with chronic degenerative arterial disease and not with beta-adrenoceptor blocking agents. Lancet 1982;1(8277):917.

286. Rustmann WC, Carpenter MT, Harmon C, Botti CF. Leukocytoclastic vasculitis associated with sotalol therapy. J Am Acad Dermatol 1998;38(1):111–12.

287. Booth RJ, Bullock JY, Wilson JD. Antinuclear antibodies in patients on acebutolol. Br J Clin Pharmacol 1980;9(5):515–17.

288. Cody RJ Jr, Calabrese LH, Clough JD, Tarazi RC, Bravo EL. Development of antinuclear antibodies during acebutolol therapy. Clin Pharmacol Ther 1979;25(6):800–5.

289. Huggins MM, Menzies CW, Quail D, Rumfitt IW. An open multicenter study of the effect of celiprolol on serum lipids and antinuclear antibodies in patient with mild to moderate hypertension. J Drug Dev 1991;4:125–33.

290. Bigot MC, Trenque T, Moulin M, Beguin J, Loyau G. Acebutolol-induced lupus syndrome. Therapie 1984;39:571–5.

291. Hourdebaigt-Larrusse P, Grivaux M. Une nouvelle obscuration de lupus induit par un béta-bloquant. Sem Hop 1984;60:1515.

292. Griffiths ID, Richardson J. Lupus-type illness associated with labetalol. BMJ 1979;2(6188):496–7.

293. Clerens A, Guilmot-Bruneau MM, Defresne C, Bourlond A. Beta-blocking agents: side effects. Biomedicine 1979;31(8):219.

294. Harrison T, Sisca TS, Wood WH. Case report. Propranolol-induced lupus syndrome? Postgrad Med 1976;59(1):241–4.

295. Holzbach E. Ein Beta-blocker als Zusatztherapie beim Delirium tremens. [Beta-Blockers as adjuvant therapy in delirium tremens.] MMW Munch Med Wochenschr 1980;122(22):837–40.

296. Jacobs RL, Rake GW Jr, Fournier DC, Chilton RJ, Culver WG, Beckmann CH. Potentiated anaphylaxis in patients with drug-induced beta-adrenergic blockade. J Allergy Clin Immunol 1981;68(2):125–7.

297. Hannaway PJ, Hopper GD. Severe anaphylaxis and drug-induced beta-blockade. N Engl J Med 1983;308(25):1536.

298. Cornaille G, Leynadier F, Modiano, Dry J. Gravité du choc anaphylactic chez les malades traités par béta-bloqueurs. [Severity of anaphylactic shock in patients treated with beta-blockers.] Presse Méd 1985;14(14):790–1.

299. Raebel MA. Potentiated anaphylaxis during chronic beta-blocker therapy. DICP Ann Pharmacother 1988;22:720.

300. Toogood JH. Beta-blocker therapy and the risk of anaphylaxis. CMAJ 1987;136(9):929–33.

301. Arkinstall WW, Toogood JH. Beta-blocker therapy and the risk of anaphylaxis. CMAJ 1987;137(5):370–1.

302. Miller RR, Olson HG, Amsterdam EA, Mason DT. Propranolol-withdrawal rebound phenomenon. Exacerbation of coronary events after abrupt cessation of antianginal therapy. N Engl J Med 1975;293(9):416–18.

303. Myers MG, Wisenberg G. Sudden withdrawal of propranolol in patients with angina pectoris. Chest 1977;71(1):24–6.

304. Shiroff RA, Mathis J, Zelis R, Schneck DW, Babb JD, Leaman DM, Hayes AH Jr. Propranolol rebound—a retrospective study. Am J Cardiol 1978;41(4):778–80.

305. Psaty BM, Koepsell TD, Wagner EH, LoGerfo JP, Inui TS. The relative risk of incident coronary heart disease associated with recently stopping the use of beta-blockers. JAMA 1990;263(12):1653–7.

306. Olsson G, Hjemdahl P, Rehnqvist N. Rebound phenomena following gradual withdrawal of chronic metoprolol treatment in patients with ischemic heart disease. Am Heart J 1984;108(3 Pt 1):454–62.

307. Maling TJ, Dollery CT. Changes in blood pressure, heart rate, and plasma noradrenaline concentration after sudden withdrawal of propranolol. BMJ 1979;2(6186):366–7.

308. Lederballe Pedersen O, Mikkelsen E, Lanng Nielsen J, Christensen NJ. Abrupt withdrawal of beta-blocking agents in patients with arterial hypertension. Effect on blood pressure, heart rate and plasma catecholamines and prolactin. Eur J Clin Pharmacol 1979;15(3):215–17.

309. Webster J, Hawksworth GM, Barber HE, Jeffers TA, Petrie JC. Withdrawal of long-term therapy with atenolol in hypertensive patients. Br J Clin Pharmacol 1981;12(2):211–14.

310. Aarons RD, Nies AS, Gal J, Hegstrand LR, Molinoff PB. Elevation of beta-adrenergic receptor density in human lymphocytes after propranolol administration. J Clin Invest 1980;65(5):949–57.

311. Nattel S, Rangno RE, Van Loon G. Mechanism of propranolol withdrawal phenomena. Circulation 1979;59(6):1158–64.

312. Rangno RE, Langlois S, Lutterodt A. Metoprolol withdrawal phenomena: mechanism and prevention. Clin Pharmacol Ther 1982;31(1):8–15.

313. Walden RJ, Bhattacharjee P, Tomlinson B, Cashin J, Graham BR, Prichard BN. The effect of intrinsic sympathomimetic activity on beta-receptor responsiveness after beta-adrenoceptor blockade withdrawal. Br J Clin Pharmacol 1982;13(Suppl 2):S359–64.

314. Rangno RE, Langlois S. Comparison of withdrawal phenomena after propranolol, metoprolol and pindolol. Br J Clin Pharmacol 1982;13(Suppl 2):S345–51.

315. Krukemyer JJ, Boudoulas H, Binkley PF, Lima JJ. Comparison of hypersensitivity to adrenergic stimulation after abrupt withdrawal of propranolol and nadolol: influence of half-life differences. Am Heart J 1990;120(3):572–9.

316. Rubin PC, Butters L, Clark DM, Reynolds B, Sumner DJ, Steedman D, Low RA, Reid JL. Placebo-controlled trial of atenolol in treatment of pregnancy-associated hypertension. Lancet 1983;1(8322):431–4.

317. Lowe SA, Rubin PC. The pharmacological management of hypertension in pregnancy. J Hypertens 1992;10(3):201–7.

318. Paran E, Holzberg G, Mazor M, Zmora E, Insler V. Beta-adrenergic blocking agents in the treatment of pregnancy-induced hypertension. Int J Clin Pharmacol Ther 1995;33(2):119–23.

319. Khedun SM, Maharaj B, Moodley J. Effects of antihypertensive drugs on the unborn child: what is known, and how should this influence prescribing? Paediatr Drugs 2000;2(6):419–36.

320. Crooks BN, Deshpande SA, Hall C, Platt MP, Milligan DW. Adverse neonatal effects of maternal labetalol treatment. Arch Dis Child Fetal Neonatal Ed 1998;79(2):F150–1.

321. Wagenvoort AM, van Vugt JM, Sobotka M, van Geijn HP. Topical timolol therapy in pregnancy: is it safe for the fetus? Teratology 1998;58(6):258–62.

322. White WB, Andreoli JW, Wong SH, Cohn RD. Atenolol in human plasma and breast milk. Obstet Gynecol 1984;63(Suppl 3):S42–4.

323. Boutroy MJ, Bianchetti G, Dubruc C, Vert P, Morselli PL. To nurse when receiving acebutolol: is it dangerous for the neonate? Eur J Clin Pharmacol 1986;30(6):737–9.

324. Sandstrom B, Regardh CG. Metoprolol excretion into breast milk. Br J Clin Pharmacol 1980;9(5):518–19.

325. Devlin RG, Duchin KL, Fleiss PM. Nadolol in human serum and breast milk. Br J Clin Pharmacol 1981;12(3):393–6.

326. Fidler J, Smith V, De Swiet M. Excretion of oxprenolol and timolol in breast milk. Br J Obstet Gynaecol 1983;90(10):961–5.

327. Smith MT, Livingstone I, Hooper WD, Eadie MJ, Triggs EJ. Propranolol, propranolol glucuronide, and naphthoxylactic acid in breast milk and plasma. Ther Drug Monit 1983;5(1):87–93.

328. O'Hare MF, Murnaghan GA, Russell CJ, Leahey WJ, Varma MP, McDevitt DG. Sotalol as a hypotensive agent in pregnancy. Br J Obstet Gynaecol 1980;87(9):814–20.

329. Lennard MS, Tucker GT, Woods HF. The polymorphic oxidation of beta-adrenoceptor antagonists. Clinical pharmacokinetic considerations. Clin Pharmacokinet 1986;11(1):1–17.

330. McAinsh J, Holmes BF, Smith S, Hood D, Warren D. Atenolol kinetics in renal failure. Clin Pharmacol Ther 1980;28(3):302–9.

331. Berglund G, Descamps R, Thomis JA. Pharmacokinetics of sotalol after chronic administration to patients with renal insufficiency. Eur J Clin Pharmacol 1980;18(4):321–6.

332. Verbeeck RK, Branch RA, Wilkinson GR. Drug metabolites in renal failure: pharmacokinetic and clinical implications. Clin Pharmacokinet 1981;6(5):329–45.

333. Stone WJ, Walle T. Massive retention of propranolol metabolites in maintenance hemodialysis patients. Clin Pharmacol Ther 1980;27:288.

334. McDevitt DG. Beta-adrenoceptor blockade in hyperthyroidism. Shanks RG, editor. Advanced Medicine: Topics in Therapeutics 3. London: Pitman Medical; 1977:100.

335. Rossi PR, Yusuf S, Ramsdale D, Furze L, Sleight P. Reduction of ventricular arrhythmias by early intravenous atenolol in suspected acute myocardial infarction. BMJ (Clin Res Ed) 1983;286(6364):506–10.

336. Ryden L, Ariniego R, Arnman K, Herlitz J, Hjalmarson A, Holmberg S, Reyes C, Smedgard P, Svedberg K, Vedin A, Waagstein F, Waldenstrom A, Wilhelmsson C, Wedel H, Yamamoto M. A double-blind trial of metoprolol in acute myocardial infarction. Effects on ventricular tachyarrhythmias. N Engl J Med 1983;308(11):614–18.

337. Anonymous. Long-term and short-term beta-blockade after myocardial infarction. Lancet 1982;1(8282):1159–61.

338. Baber NS, Evans DW, Howitt G, Thomas M, Wilson T, Lewis JA, Dawes PM, Handler K, Tuson R. Multicentre

post-infarction trial of propranolol in 49 hospitals in the United Kingdom, Italy, and Yugoslavia. Br Heart J 1980;44(1):96–100.

339. Beta-Blocker Heart Attack Study Group. The Beta-blocker Heart Attack Trial. JAMA 1981;246(18):2073–4.

340. Wilhelmsson C, Vedin JA, Wilhelmsen L, Tibblin G, Werko L. Reduction of sudden deaths after myocardial infarction by treatment with alprenolol. Preliminary results. Lancet 1974;2(7890):1157–60.

341. Andersen MP, Bechsgaard P, Frederiksen J, Hansen DA, Jurgensen HJ, Nielsen B, Pedersen F, Pedersen-Bjergaard O, Rasmussen SL. Effect of alprenolol on mortality among patients with definite or suspected acute myocardial infarction. Preliminary results. Lancet 1979;2(8148):865–8.

342. Ahlmark G, Saetre H, Korsgren M. Reduction of sudden deaths after myocardial infarction. Lancet 1974; 2(7896):1563.

343. Hjalmarson A, Elmfeldt D, Herlitz J, Holmberg S, Malek I, Nyberg G, Ryden L, Swedberg K, Vedin A, Waagstein F, Waldenstrom A, Waldenstrom J, Wedel H, Wilhelmsen L, Wilhelmsson C. Effect on mortality of metoprolol in acute myocardial infarction. A double-blind randomised trial. Lancet 1981;2(8251):823–7.

344. Norwegian Multicentre Study Group. Timolol-induced reduction in mortality and reinfarction in patients surviving acute myocardial infarction. N Engl J Med 1981;304(14):801–7.

345. Julian DG, Prescott RJ, Jackson FS, Szekely P. Controlled trial of sotalol for one year after myocardial infarction. Lancet 1982;1(8282):1142–7.

346. Hansteen V, Moinichen E, Lorentsen E, Andersen A, Strom O, Soiland K, Dyrbekk D, Refsum AM, Tromsdal A, Knudsen K, Eika C, Bakken J Jr, Smith P, Hoff PI. One year's treatment with propranolol after myocardial infarction: preliminary report of Norwegian multicentre trial. BMJ (Clin Res Ed) 1982;284(6310):155–60.

347. Heidbreder E, Pagel G, Rockel A, Heidland A. Beta-adrenergic blockade in stress protection. Limited effect of metoprolol in psychological stress reaction. Eur J Clin Pharmacol 1978;14(6):391–8.

348. Trap-Jensen J, Carlsen JE, Svendsen TL, Christensen NJ. Cardiovascular and adrenergic effects of cigarette smoking during immediate non-selective and selective beta adrenoceptor blockade in humans. Eur J Clin Invest 1979;9(3):181–3.

349. Freestone S, Ramsay LE. Effect of coffee and cigarette smoking in untreated and diuretic-treated hypertensive patients. Br J Clin Pharmacol 1981;11:428.

350. Ramsay LE. Antihypertensive drugs. Curr Opin Cardiol 1987;1:524.

351. Deanfield J, Wright C, Krikler S, Ribeiro P, Fox K. Cigarette smoking and the treatment of angina with propranolol, atenolol, and nifedipine. N Engl J Med 1984;310(15):951–4.

352. Howard PJ, Lee MR. Beware beta-adrenergic blockers in patients with severe urticaria! Scott Med J 1988;33(5):344–5.

353. Korte JM, Kaila T, Saari KM. Systemic bioavailability and cardiopulmonary effects of 0.5% timolol eyedrops. Graefes Arch Clin Exp Ophthalmol 2002;240(6):430–5.

354. Caballero F, Lopez-Navidad A, Cotorruelo J, Txoperena G. Ecstasy-induced brain death and acute hepatocellular failure: multiorgan donor and liver transplantation. Transplantation 2002;74(4):532–7.

355. Fraunfelder FT. Ocular beta-blockers and systemic effects. Arch Intern Med 1986;146(6):1073–4.

356. Stewart WC, Castelli WP. Systemic side effects of topical beta-adrenergic blockers. Clin Cardiol 1996;19(9):691–7.

357. Nelson WL, Fraunfelder FT, Sills JM, Arrowsmith JB, Kuritsky JN. Adverse respiratory and cardiovascular events attributed to timolol ophthalmic solution, 1978–1985. Am J Ophthalmol 1986;102(5):606–11.

358. Hayreh SS, Podhajsky P, Zimmerman MB. Beta-blocker eyedrops and nocturnal arterial hypotension. Am J Ophthalmol 1999;128(3):301–9.

359. Vandezande LM, Gallouj K, Lamblin C, Fourquet B, Maillot E, Wallaert B. Pneumopathie interstitielle induite par un collyre de timolol. [Interstitial lung disease induced by timolol eye solution.] Rev Mal Respir 1999;16(1):91–3.

360. Heel RC, Brogden RN, Speight TM, Avery GS. Timolol: a review of its therapeutic efficacy in the topical treatment of glaucoma. Drugs 1979;17(1):38–55.

361. Van Buskirk EM. Corneal anesthesia after timolol maleate therapy. Am J Ophthalmol 1979;88(4):739–43.

362. Coppeto JR. Transient ischemic attacks and amaurosis fugax from timolol. Ann Ophthalmol 1985;17(1):64–5.

363. Silverstone BZ, Marcus T. [Hypoglycemia due to ophthalmic timolol in a diabetic.] Harefuah 1990;118(12):693–4.

364. Swenson ER. Severe hyperkalemia as a complication of timolol, a topically applied beta-adrenergic antagonist. Arch Intern Med 1986;146(6):1220–1.

365. Shaivitz SA. Timolol and myasthenia gravis. JAMA 1979;242(15):1611–12.

366. Boger WP 3rd. Shortterm "escape" and longterm "drift." The dissipation effects of the beta adrenergic blocking agents. Surv Ophthalmol 1983;28(Suppl):235–42.

367. Anonymous. Self-poisoning with beta-blockers. BMJ 1978;1(6119):1010–11.

368. Anonymous. Beta-blocker poisoning. Lancet 1980;1(8172):803–4.

369. Tynan RF, Fisher MM, Ibels LS. Self-poisoning with propranolol. Med J Aust 1981;1(2):82–3.

370. Buiumsohn A, Eisenberg ES, Jacob H, Rosen N, Bock J, Frishman WH. Seizures and intraventricular conduction defect in propranolol poisoning. A report of two cases. Ann Intern Med 1979;91(6):860–2.

371. Neuvonen PJ, Elonen E, Vuorenmaa T, Laakso M. Prolonged Q-T interval and severe tachyarrhythmias, common features of sotalol intoxication. Eur J Clin Pharmacol 1981;20(2):85–9.

372. Assimes TL, Malcolm I. Torsade de pointes with sotalol overdose treated successfully with lidocaine. Can J Cardiol 1998;14(5):753–6.

373. Lagerfelt J, Matell G. Attempted suicide with 5.1 g of propranolol. A case report. Acta Med Scand 1976;199(6):517–18.

374. Henry JA, Cassidy SL. Membrane stabilising activity: a major cause of fatal poisoning. Lancet 1986;1(8495):1414–17.

375. Aura ED, Wexler LF, Wirtzburg RA. Massive propranolol overdose: successful treatment with high dose isoproterenol and glucagon. Am J Med 1986;80:755.

376. Weinstein RS. Recognition and management of poisoning with beta-adrenergic blocking agents. Ann Emerg Med 1984;13(12):1123–31.

377. Nicolas F, Villers D, Rozo L, Haloun A, Bigot A. Severe self-poisoning with acebutolol in association with alcohol. Crit Care Med 1987;15(2):173–4.

378. Richards DA, Prichard BN. Self-poisoning with beta-blockers. BMJ 1978;1(6127):1623–4.

379. Freestone S, Thomas HM, Bhamra RK, Dyson EH. Severe atenolol poisoning: treatment with prenalterol. Hum Toxicol 1986;5(5):343–5.

380. Lifshitz M, Zucker N, Zalzstein E. Acute dilated cardiomyopathy and central nervous system toxicity following propranolol intoxication. Pediatr Emerg Care 1999;15(4):262–3.

381. Love JN, Howell JM, Litovitz TL, Klein-Schwartz W. Acute beta blocker overdose: factors associated with the development of cardiovascular morbidity. J Toxicol Clin Toxicol 2000;38(3):275–81.

382. Love JN. Acebutolol overdose resulting in fatalities. J Emerg Med 2000;18(3):341–4.

383. McDevitt DG. Clinically important adverse drug interactions. Petrie JC, editor. Cardiovascular and Respiratory Disease Therapy. Amsterdam: Elsevier/North Holland, Biomedical Press; 1980;1:21.

384. Lewis RV, McDevitt DG. Adverse reactions and interactions with beta-adrenoceptor blocking drugs. Med Toxicol 1986;1(5):343–61.

385. Kendall MJ, Beeley L. Beta-adrenoceptor blocking drugs: adverse reactions and drug interactions. Pharmacol Ther 1983;21(3):351–69.

386. Alvan G, Piafsky K, Lind M, von Bahr C. Effect of pentobarbital on the disposition of alprenolol. Clin Pharmacol Ther 1977;22(3):316–21.

387. Bennett PN, John VA, Whitmarsh VB. Effect of rifampicin on metoprolol and antipyrine kinetics. Br J Clin Pharmacol 1982;13(3):387–91.

388. Feely J, Wilkinson GR, Wood AJ. Reduction of liver blood flow and propranolol metabolism by cimetidine. N Engl J Med 1981;304(12):692–5.

389. Daneshmend TK, Roberts CJ. Cimetidine and bioavailability of labetalol. Lancet 1981;1(8219):565.

390. Kirch W, Kohler H, Spahn H, Mutschler E. Interaction of cimetidine with metoprolol, propranolol, or atenolol. Lancet 1981;2(8245):531–2.

391. Sax MJ. Analysis of possible drug interactions between cimetidine (and ranitidine) and beta-blockers. Adv Ther 1988;5:210.

392. McLean AJ, Skews H, Bobik A, Dudley FJ. Interaction between oral propranolol and hydralazine. Clin Pharmacol Ther 1980;27(6):726–32.

393. Conrad KA, Nyman DW. Effects of metoprolol and propranolol on theophylline elimination. Clin Pharmacol Ther 1980;28(4):463–7.

394. Greendyke RM, Kanter DR. Plasma propranolol levels and their effect on plasma thioridazine and haloperidol concentrations. J Clin Psychopharmacol 1987;7(3):178–82.

395. Peet M, Middlemiss DN, Yates RA. Pharmacokinetic interaction between propranolol and chlorpromazine in schizophrenic patients. Lancet 1980;2(8201):978.

396. Bax ND, Lennard MS, Tucker GT, Woods HF, Porter NR, Malia RG, Preston FE. The effect of beta-adrenoceptor antagonists on the pharmacokinetics and pharmacodynamics of warfarin after a single dose. Br J Clin Pharmacol 1984;17(5):553–7.

397. Ochs HR, Greenblatt DJ, Verburg-Ochs B. Propranolol interactions with diazepam, lorazepam, and alprazolam. Clin Pharmacol Ther 1984;36(4):451–5.

398. Santoso B. Impairment of isoniazid clearance by propranolol. Int J Clin Pharmacol Ther Toxicol 1985;23(3):134–6.

399. Lewis GP, Holtzman JL. Interaction of flecainide with digoxin and propranolol. Am J Cardiol 1984;53(5):B52–7.

400. Ochs HR, Carstens G, Greenblatt DJ. Reduction in lidocaine clearance during continuous infusion and by coadministration of propranolol. N Engl J Med 1980;303(7):373–7.

401. Bax ND, Tucker GT, Lennard MS, Woods HF. The impairment of lignocaine clearance by propranolol—major contribution from enzyme inhibition. Br J Clin Pharmacol 1985;19(5):597–603.

402. Bonde J, Bodtker S, Angelo HR, Svendsen TL, Kampmann JP. Atenolol inhibits the elimination of disopyramide. Eur J Clin Pharmacol 1985;28(1):41–3.

403. Leemann T, Dayer P, Meyer UA. Single-dose quinidine treatment inhibits metoprolol oxidation in extensive metabolizers. Eur J Clin Pharmacol 1986;29(6):739–41.

404. Kendall MJ, Jack DB, Quarterman CP, Smith SR, Zaman R. Beta-adrenoceptor blocker pharmacokinetics and the oral contraceptive pill. Br J Clin Pharmacol 1984;17(Suppl 1):S87–9.

405. Watkins J, Abbott EC, Hensby CN, Webster J, Dollery CT. Attenuation of hypotensive effect of propranolol and thiazide diuretics by indomethacin. BMJ 1980;281(6242):702–5.

406. Wong DG, Spence JD, Lamki L, Freeman D, McDonald JW. Effect of non-steroidal anti-inflammatory drugs on control of hypertension by beta-blockers and diuretics. Lancet 1986;1(8488):997–1001.

407. Lewis RV, Toner JM, Jackson PR, Ramsay LE. Effects of indomethacin and sulindac on blood pressure of hypertensive patients. BMJ (Clin Res Ed) 1986;292(6525):934–5.

408. Venter CP, Joubert PH, Buys AC. Severe peripheral ischaemia during concomitant use of beta blockers and ergot alkaloids. BMJ (Clin Res Ed) 1984;289(6440):288–9.

409. Smits P, Hoffmann H, Thien T, Houben H, van't Laar A. Hemodynamic and humoral effects of coffee after beta 1-selective and nonselective beta-blockade. Clin Pharmacol Ther 1983;34(2):153–8.

410. Eldor J, Hoffman B, Davidson JT. Prolonged bradycardia and hypotension after neostigmine administration in a patient receiving atenolol. Anaesthesia 1987;42(12):1294–7.

411. McKibbin JK, Pocock WA, Barlow JB, Millar RN, Obel IW. Sotalol, hypokalaemia, syncope, and torsade de pointes. Br Heart J 1984;51(2):157–62.

412. Feroze H, Suri R, Silverman DI. Torsades de pointes from terfenadine and sotalol given in combination. Pacing Clin Electrophysiol 1996;19(10):1519–21.

413. Ikram H. Hemodynamic and electrophysiologic interactions between antiarrhythmic drugs and beta blockers, with special reference to tocainide. Am Heart J 1980;100(6 Pt 2):1076–80.

Beta-lactam antibiotics

See also Individual agents

General Information

The beta-lactam antibiotics still comprise roughly half of the antibiotic market worldwide. The common structure that defines the whole family of beta-lactam antibiotics is the four-membered, highly reactive beta-lactam ring, which is essential for antimicrobial activity (1). The following simplifying classification is practical:

1. penicillins
2. cephalosporins
3. monobactams (containing no second ring system besides the beta-lactam ring)
4. carbapenems

In addition, beta-lactamase inhibitors also contain the beta-lactam structure.

The crucial event that initiates the antimicrobial effects of beta-lactam antibiotics is binding to and inhibition of bacterial enzymes located in the cell membrane, the so-called penicillin-binding proteins (2). This happens by covalent binding, through opening of the beta-lactam ring. Enzyme activities of penicillin-binding proteins are involved in the last steps of bacterial cell wall (peptidoglycan) synthesis, and their inhibition halts cell growth, causing cell death and lysis (3). Beta-lactamases are genetically and structurally closely related to penicillin-binding proteins.

Despite their chemical diversity, their adverse effects profiles share various common aspects. There are several reasons why beta-lactam antibiotics belonging to different classes can cause comparable reactions. Besides the beta-lactam ring, other structural similarities (for example side chains) or antimicrobial activity can be relevant. However, the incidence of a given reaction, and in particular instances also the severity, varies among beta-lactam classes.

Incidence and cause–effect relations

It is difficult to establish clearly the incidence and cause–effect relations of many reactions and hence to identify patients at risk. The following factors are important:

1. The range of recommended daily doses varies by more than an order of magnitude, according to clinical need. Hence, the incidence of some collateral and toxic reactions varies greatly among different populations.
2. Combinations of beta-lactam antibiotics with antimicrobial drugs from other molecular classes are often used, especially in severe infection.
3. The spectrum of potential beta-lactam-antibiotic-induced reactions is especially broad, and in most cases no test procedure is available to distinguish beta-lactam antibiotics from other causes of a reaction, in particular from the consequences of the treated infection.

Relation to dose

Many reactions to beta-lactam antibiotics are clearly not immune mediated. These include bleeding disorders, neurotoxicity, and most cases of diarrhea. In addition, many reactions, the pathogenesis of which is still being discussed, clearly depend on the daily and the cumulative dose of beta-lactam antibiotics and hence the duration of treatment. Although the rare, but well-understood, immune hemolysis after penicillin is seen mostly with high-dose and long-term treatment, dose dependency and time dependency point to direct toxicity rather than to immunological mechanisms. Indeed, direct toxic effects of beta-lactam antibiotics on eukaryotic cells and specific interactions with receptor proteins and enzymes have been shown (4) and may underlie particular reactions.

There are three lines of evidence that beta-lactam antibiotics cause a variety of reactions by toxic mechanisms:

1. Certain reactions are overwhelmingly reported to be dose-dependent and time-dependent.
2. Particular compounds cause adverse effects with unexpectedly high frequencies in certain circumstances (for example cystic fibrosis, bacterial endocarditis, and osteomyelitis) that require particularly high doses and prolonged treatment.
3. Beta-lactam antibiotics affect a variety of cultured eukaryotic cells.

For other reactions, the underlying mechanisms are less clear. The body of individual reports and some published series suggest that their incidence increases disproportionately with prolonged, high-dosage treatment, that is, with accumulation. This is particularly the case in the following reactions:

- severe neutropenia up to total agranulocytosis, as observed with virtually all beta-lactam antibiotics.
- acute interstitial nephritis, seen with methicillin but more rarely also with other beta-lactams, for example penicillin G.
- one type of hepatitis induced by isoxazolyl penicillins;
- varying combinations of symptoms positively referred to or not as "serum sickness-like syndromes."

There have been reports of high overall frequencies of adverse effects after the use of very high cumulative doses of beta-lactam antibiotics in healthy volunteers and in patients with, for example, chronic osteomyelitis, pulmonary exacerbations in cystic fibrosis, and infective endocarditis (5–9). In one series, 23% of patients treated with an average cumulative dose of carbenicillin of 925 g and 68% of those treated with ureidopenicillins 329 g developed adverse effects, including rash, fever, leukopenia, eosinophilia, thrombocytopenia, and hepatic damage, requiring change of therapy in 52% of cases in the latter group (10). Another study included a total of 292 treatment courses with five different beta-lactams for infective endocarditis (6). With a treatment duration of 9 days or less, drug was withdrawn in only 3% because of adverse reactions. However, treatment courses ranging from 10 days to 6 weeks were associated with adverse reactions in 33%, one-quarter of which consisted of neutropenia. Fourteen of 44 patients receiving piperacillin up to 900 mg/kg/day for acute pulmonary exacerbations in cystic fibrosis developed a syndrome that resembled serum sickness; the symptoms were mainly fever, malaise, anorexia, eosinophilia, and rashes (8). The reaction occurred after a minimum of 9 days and the frequency of symptoms was dose-related. All patients who developed the reaction were re-admitted at 4–28 months after the initial episode and in every case re-exposure to piperacillin did not evoke the reaction.

The dose-relation of reactions to piperacillin in patients with cystic fibrosis has created a debate about its usefulness in this condition (11–15). However, comparable dose-related patterns and frequencies of adverse effects were found in other patients treated with piperacillin (15) and with other beta-lactam antibiotics (16), as well as in patients with both cystic fibrosis and other conditions (6,10,16). Three later studies showed that piperacillin more often caused fever, rash, and other reactions per treatment course in patients with cystic fibrosis compared with a large variety of other beta-lactam or non-beta-lactam antibiotics (17–19). Of particular interest is a study in which volunteers who took high doses of cefalotin or cefapirin for up to 4 weeks developed comparable syndromes, with an overall incidence of adverse effects of 100% (9). Despite these astonishingly high frequencies, these reactions were predominantly regarded as being allergic, although their pathogenesis was mostly unclear.

Thus, a disproportionately high frequency of apparently unrelated adverse effects occurs in a relatively small group of patients, those needing high-dose prolonged treatment, who are at particular risk.

Mechanisms

Degradation products spontaneously formed in aqueous solutions, for example culture media, rather than the parent molecules themselves, may be responsible for the observed effects (4). Antiproliferative activities were generally more pronounced with cephalosporins than with penicillins, while monobactams appear to be practically free from such effects. Carbapenems have not been thoroughly studied in this respect, and some data on clavulanic acid and two other beta-lactamase inhibitors do not clearly reflect the same kind of toxicity as observed with penicillins and cephalosporins (20).

The selectivity of beta-lactam antibiotics for bacterial target proteins is not absolute. A specific interaction of modified cephalosporins with mammalian serine proteases has been shown (21) and the affinity of various penicillins for the benzodiazepine receptor may be part of the chain of events leading to neurotoxicity (22) However, most intriguing are observations made in proliferating cultured cells. Biological effects associated with proliferation were dose-dependently inhibited by a large array of beta-lactam antibiotics in a variety of cells from both man and animals (4,23). Resting cells, on the other hand, were not susceptible, even to very high concentrations.

The clinical impact of the inhibitory effects of beta-lactam antibiotics on proliferating eukaryotic cells is as yet unknown, and formal proof of a correlation with toxicity in patients is lacking. However, there are reasons for considering this type of toxicity as the cause of neutropenia and thrombocytopenia (SEDA-13, 230). In dogs, high-dose cefonicid and cefazedone for up to several months caused bone marrow damage, resembling the findings in clinical cases of neutropenia, which could explain peripheral cytopenias (24,25). In addition, mild thrombocytopenia and reticulocytopenia, which have been concomitantly found respectively in 30 and 17% of cases of neutropenia (26), are also paralleled by results in dogs. On the other hand, in the same dogs, IgG associated with erythrocytes, neutrophils, and platelets was found after high-dose treatment with cefazedone (27) Antigranulocyte IgG antibodies in beta-lactam-induced neutropenia have also been described in man (28–30). However, the relevance of these findings is unclear, since high cumulative doses of beta-lactams often induce beta-lactam-specific IgG antibodies in patients with and without adverse effects (6,31). Newer data from human and animal cell culture investigations suggest that ceftazidime-induced myelosuppression could be the consequence of multiple effects on various myeloid and nonmyeloid cells in the bone marrow (32–34). They also give hints of a more rational basis for using G-CSF or other cytokines in beta-lactam-antibiotic-induced neutropenia (32,34). Hence, there is still controversy about whether beta-lactam antibiotics can cause neutropenia by both toxic and immunological mechanisms and how both mechanisms could act in concert with each other.

For evaluation of local tolerability, human peritoneal cells (35), human osteoblasts (36), and human as well as animal endothelial cells (37) have been studied in culture. The type of toxicity and rank efficacy among various compounds were congruent with the results from earlier studies on other cells (4,23). The clinical relevance of these data remains to be established.

The Jarisch–Herxheimer reaction

The Jarisch–Herxheimer reaction is a systemic reaction that occurs hours after initial treatment of spirochete infections, such as syphilis, leptospirosis, Lyme disease, and relapsing fever, and presents with fever, rigors, hypotension, and flushing (38,39). In patients with syphilis the reaction is more frequent in secondary syphilis and can cause additional manifestations, such as flare-up of cutaneous lesions, sudden aneurysmal dilatation of the aortic arch (40), and angina pectoris or acute coronary occlusion (SED-8, 559). It can easily be mistaken for a drug-induced hypersensitivity reaction. The underlying mechanism is initiated by antibiotic-induced release of spirochete-derived pyrogens. Transient rises in TNF, IL-6, and IL-8 have been detected (41). The role of TNF-alpha in the pathogenesis of the Jarisch–Herxheimer reaction is further underscored by the observation that in patients undergoing penicillin treatment for louse-borne relapsing fever, pretreatment with anti-TNF antibody Fab fragments partially protected against the reaction (42). The reaction lasts 12–24 hours and can be alleviated by aspirin. Alternatively, prednisone can be used and is recommended as adjunctive treatment of symptomatic cardiovascular syphilis or neurosyphilis.

Organs and Systems

Respiratory

Allergic bronchospasm can principally be a consequence of IgE antibody-mediated allergy to all beta-lactam antibiotics.

Nervous system

Since the first observation of convulsions after intraventricular administration of penicillin more than 50 years ago (43), neurotoxicity has been attributed to most beta-lactam antibiotics. Its manifestations are considered to be the consequence of GABAergic inhibition (44,45)and include clear epileptic manifestations as well as more atypical reactions, such as asterixis, drowsiness, and hallucinations. Epileptogenic activity of beta-lactam antibiotics has also been documented in animals and in brain slices in vitro (46). With penicillins and cephalosporins, integrity of the beta-lactam ring is a prerequisite, and epileptogenic activity is extinguished by beta-lactamase (47,48). However, this may not be true of the carbapenems, the neurotoxicity of which is differently related to their structure (49). However, clinical manifestations are always clearly dose-dependent, and brain tissue concentrations appear to be more relevant than CSF or blood concentrations (46). Accordingly, the major risk factor is impaired renal function, particularly when it is not recognized. Other risk factors are age (very young or very old), meningitis, intraventricular therapy, and a history of epilepsy (50).

The neurotoxic potential differs considerably among the various beta-lactam antibiotics, and experimental models have been developed for investigating this (51,52). Currently, imipenem + cilastatin appears to cause the highest frequency of neurotoxic effects (53,54) and the above-mentioned risk factors have been particularly confirmed with this compound (SEDA-18, 261) (55). Quinolone antibiotics, which themselves are proconvulsant, can potentiate excitation of the central nervous system by beta-lactam antibiotics, at least in animals (56,57).

Sensory systems

In vitro, methicillin and ceftazidime in high concentrations produced toxic effects on corneal and endothelial cells of the eye (58,59).

Metabolism

Pivaloyl-containing compounds (baccefuconam, cefetamet pivoxil, cefteram pivoxil, pivampicillin, pivmecillinam) can significantly increase urinary carnitine excretion (60,61). These compounds are esterified prodrugs, which become effective only after the release of pivalic acid, which in turn is esterified with carnitine. Carnitine loss induced by pivaloyl-containing beta-lactams was first described in children and can produce symptoms similar to other types of carnitine deficiency, for example secondary to organic acidurias (60). Carnitine is essential for the transport of fatty acids through the mitochondrial membrane for beta-oxidation. Consequences of its deficiency include skeletal damage, cardiomyopathy, hypoglycemia and reduced ketogenesis, encephalopathy, hepatomegaly, and Reye-like syndromes (62).

The administration of pivaloyl-conjugated beta-lactam antibiotics to healthy volunteers for 54 days reduced mean serum carnitine 10-fold and muscle carnitine, as measured per non-collagen protein, more than 2-fold (62). Long-term treatment of children for 12–37 months to prevent urinary tract infection resulted in serum carnitine concentrations of 0.9–3.6 µmol/l (reference range 23–60 µmol/l). In four cases, muscle carnitine was 0.6–1.4 µmol/g non-collagen protein (reference range 7.1–19) (63).

Although oral carnitine aided the elimination of the pivaloyl moiety, its simultaneous use did not fully compensate for the adverse metabolic effects of pivaloyl-containing beta-lactams (64,65). The consequences of pivaloyl-induced carnitine loss seem to be generally reversible. But as long as the risk of pivaloyl-induced urinary loss of carnitine and particular risk factors are not better defined, it is prudent to use pivaloyl-containing prodrugs only in short-term treatment.

Electrolyte balance

Since beta-lactam antibiotics contain sodium or potassium, they can cause or at least aggravate electrolyte disturbances when given in sufficiently high doses. The most frequent manifestations are hypernatremia and hypokalemia. The sodium content of injectable beta-lactam antibiotics per gram of active compound varies by up to a factor of three (66).

Hematologic

Neutropenia

While in large series of several thousands of patients, neutropenia has generally been reported as an adverse effect in under 0.1–1.0% (SEDA-13, 212), an overview in 1985 estimated that neutropenia (neutrophil count below 1.0×10^9/l) occurs in up to 15% of all patients treated with high-dose intravenous beta-lactam antibiotics for more than 10 days (26). In subsequent series of patients treated for several weeks with various beta-lactam antibiotics, up to 25% developed neutropenia (5,21,67–69).

In one series, 22 of 128 patients receiving cloxacillin for staphylococcal infections became neutropenic (67). Neutropenia appeared, on average, 23 days after the start of therapy. The same authors, in a somewhat bigger population, found neutropenia in 1.1% of patients who received cumulative doses of oxacillin below 150 g, but in 43% (22 of 51) who received more than 150 g (5). Similarly, in 132 patients, cefapirin in a cumulative dose of less than 90 g did not cause neutropenia, but did in 26% (five of 19) of those who used higher total doses (21).

In addition, for a given compound, higher daily doses increase the risk of neutropenia. In one study, seven of 14 patients became neutropenic with a mean dose of penicillin G of 17 g/day after 9–23 days (68), while in another study only 12 of 193 patients developed neutropenia with a mean dose of 11 g/day for an average duration of 20 days (69). A considerable extension of the aforementioned study (68) corroborated this: neutropenia occurred in 35% of those treated with a mean daily dose of 17 g of penicillin G for an average of 23 days, while it was found in only 8% of those who received 12 g for 22 days (6).

Epidemiological studies (7,70) as well as single cases of severe neutropenia observed with newer compounds have invariably confirmed the dose- and time-dependent pattern described above. For example, cefepime, a fourth-generation cephalosporin, possibly or probably caused neutropenia in only 0.2% of 3314 treatment courses, while 7.1% of those who received cefepime for several weeks developed neutropenia (71). Accordingly, high-dose cefepime (150 mg/kg/day) was given for 7–10 days to 43 children for bacterial meningitis without causing neutropenia (72), while there were two cases in adults after total doses of 112 g (over 28 days) and 120 g (30 days) respectively (73).

It is therefore not surprising that after consecutive or simultaneous treatment with more than one beta-lactam antibiotic, neutropenia is similarly observed, suggesting additive toxicity (6,74,75).

There is so far no clear evidence about the different risks of different compounds. The data best fit the assumption that the risk of neutropenia correlates with the cumulative dose, or probably more precisely with the area under the serum concentration versus time curve (AUC). Hence, renal insufficiency is a potential risk factor. In addition, beta-lactam-antibiotic-induced leukopenia has been associated with hepatic dysfunction (76).

Recovery in most cases is rapid and uneventful. In patients who were re-exposed to the same or other beta-lactam antibiotics, there was similar dependence of neutropenia on the duration of treatment and the cumulative dose (26). Whether the use of hemopoietic growth factors, and in particular G-CSF, is useful is unclear. There are case reports of positive clinical effects (77–79). However, the recovery time in these reports did not differ from that observed in a large population of untreated patients (26). Theoretically, early use of growth factors could even be counterproductive, since some toxic effects of beta-lactam antibiotics on bone marrow cells appear to be related to the S-phase of the cell cycle (4). On the other hand, G-CSF maintained the proliferative activity of bone marrow cells exposed to ceftazidime in vitro, if it was added at the beginning of the culture process (32).

Neutropenia is accompanied by fever, eosinophilia, and/or a rash in more than 80% of cases.

Hemolytic anemia

Immune hemolytic anemia was originally described with penicillin G, but subsequently also with other penicillins and cephalosporins. It is usually seen during treatment with very high doses after the so-called "drug absorption" mechanism. The beta-lactam antibiotic binds covalently to the erythrocyte surface, forming complete antigens, which can in turn bind drug-specific circulating IgG antibody. Typically, direct and indirect Coombs' tests are positive, but complement is not activated (80–82). Rarely, other immunological mechanisms have been observed, for example the so-called "innocent bystander" type of hemolysis (82), in which complement can be detected on the erythrocyte surface. Some cephalosporins, clavulanic acid, and imipenem + cilastatin can cause positive direct antiglobulin tests (83). The phenomenon is due to non-specific serum protein absorption on to the erythrocyte membrane and is not related to immune hemolytic processes. Detection of non-immunologically bound serum proteins is improved if the reagents used include additional anti-albumin activity (84). The phenomenon is a known source of difficulties in evaluating suspected immune hemolysis or routine cross-matching of blood products (85). The true frequency of the phenomenon is unclear, since it has not been positively sought.

Thrombocytosis

Thrombocytosis is frequently mentioned as an adverse effect of beta-lactam antibiotics. However, it has been suggested that this reflects healing from infection rather than toxicity (86).

Eosinophilia

Virtually all beta-lactam antibiotics can cause eosinophilia, either isolated or in the context of very different reactions.

Bleeding disorders

Treatment with beta-lactam antibiotics can result in impaired hemostasis and bleeding. The true incidence of bleeding is difficult to assess, since many non-antibiotic

factors can be involved, such as malnutrition with vitamin K depletion (87), renal insufficiency (88), and serious infection (89). Cancer, the use of cytotoxic drugs, and surgery have made conclusive interpretation of coagulation disorders difficult (90). Between the different beta-lactam antibiotics, the reported incidence of clinical relevant bleeding varies widely, and was highest with moxalactam (22% of patients), now withdrawn (SED-12, 625). With other cephalosporins, bleeding was observed with frequencies ranging from 2.7% (cefazolin/cefalotin) to 8.2% (cefoxitime) (91). Two basic mechanisms have been proposed.

Altered coagulation

Both direct inhibition of the hepatic production of vitamin K-dependent clotting factors and alterations in the intestinal flora, with subsequent reduction of microbial supply of vitamin K, have been implicated (92,93). The relative role of either mechanism is difficult to assess, but experimental support for the flora theory is weak (94,95).

Several of the cephalosporins that contain either a non-substituted N-methylthiotetrazole (NMTT) side chain, such as cefamandole, cefamazole, cefmenoxime, cefmetazole, cefoperazone, cefotetan, and moxalactam, as well as a substituted NMTT side chain (ceforanide, ceforicid, or cefotiam), or the structurally similar N-methylthiotriazine ring in ceftriaxone and the 2-methyl-1,2,4-thiadiazole-5-thiol (MTD) ring of cefazolin interfere with vitamin K-dependent clotting factor synthesis in the liver (factors II, VII, IX, and X). The molecular mechanism involves dose-dependent inhibition of microsomal carboxylase function, as shown in animals (96), and inhibition of the epoxide reductase system in both animals and man (97–100). Cefoxitin, a non-NMTT compound, was implicated significantly more often than the NMTT-containing compounds cefamandole and cefoperazone (101).

The NMTT must leave the parent antibiotic to inhibit the carboxylation reaction (102). The NMTT molecule leaves the parent cephalosporin either during spontaneous hydrolysis in the blood or during nucleophilic cleavage of the beta-lactam ring by intestinal bacteria, and is reabsorbed from the gut into the portal circulation (103). Studies in healthy volunteers show compound-related differences in the ability of NMTT antibiotics to generate free NMTT, reflecting drug-specific differences in susceptibility to in vitro hydrolysis or differences in gut NMTT production, which may be a function of biliary excretion of the drug (104).

Altered platelet numbers and function

Platelet dysfunction occurs dose-dependently with carbenicillin, ticarcillin, and, infrequently, other broad-spectrum penicillins (105), but the NMTT cephalosporin moxalactam has also been associated with altered platelet function in both healthy subjects and in patients treated with standard regimens (106–110). In contrast, clinical studies including cefotaxime, ceftizoxime, cefoperazone, and ceftracone did not show platelet dysfunction attributable to these compounds (109–111). There is evidence that beta-lactam-antibiotic-induced platelet dysfunction is at least partially irreversible (112).

From a practical point of view it can be concluded that:

1. the use of cephalosporins containing an NMTT side chain is associated with a risk of dose-dependent inhibition of vitamin K-dependent clotting factor synthesis.
2. platelet dysfunction occurs primarily with the broad-spectrum penicillins, but the NMTT cephalosporins, notably moxalactam, have also been implicated; monitoring of bleeding time should be considered in patients at risk (bleeding history, clinical bleeding, concomitant thrombocytopenia, or the use of other drugs known to interfere with platelet function.
3. the presence of non-antibiotic factors, such as therapy with vitamin K antagonists or NSAIDs, renal insufficiency, hepatic dysfunction, impaired gastrointestinal function, and malnutrition, can increase the risk of bleeding in cephalosporin-treated patients; close monitoring of homeostasis (prothrombin time, bleeding time), as well as prophylactic supplementation with vitamin K or, if necessary, therapeutic administration of fresh-frozen plasma and/or platelets is warranted according to the clinical context.

Gastrointestinal

Gastrointestinal upsets, nausea, and vomiting have been observed with virtually all beta-lactam antibiotics, both oral and parenteral. Even when comparing analogous applications and doses, no particular risk can be clearly ascribed to a given compound. Acute hemorrhagic colitis without pseudomembrane formation has been described after treatment with various penicillins and cephalosporins (SEDA-21, 261).

Antibiotic-induced diarrhea

There are three types of antibiotic-induced diarrhea:

- simple diarrhea due to altered bowel flora; this is quite common, for example it occurs in about 8% of patients who take ampicillin (113).
- diarrhea due to loss of bowel flora and overgrowth of *Clostridium difficile*, with toxin production; this is much less common.
- a rare form of diarrhea that is due to allergy.

Almost all antibacterial agents have been observed to cause diarrhea in a variable proportion of patients (114,115). The proportion depends not only on the antibiotic, but also on the clinical setting (in-patient/out-patient), age, race, and the definition of diarrhea. Severe colonic inflammation develops in a variable proportion of cases, and in some cases pseudomembranous colitis occurs (116–121). Since 1977, much evidence has accumulated that the most important causative agent in antibiotic-associated diarrhea is an anaerobic, Gram-positive, toxin-producing bacterium, *C. difficile* (122–124).

Pseudomembranous colitis was known before the introduction of antimicrobial agents and can still occur without previous antibiotic use, for example after antineoplastic chemotherapy (125) or even spontaneously. However, the number of cases has increased dramatically since antibiotics began to be used (126). Patients treated with lincomycin or clindamycin, cephalosporins, penicillinase-resistant penicillins, or combinations of several antibiotics

are at especially high risk (127–130). A low risk is usually associated with sulfonamides, co-trimoxazole, chloramphenicol, and tetracyclines (116). Although few data have yet been published on this subject for the quinolones, they seldom seem to cause diarrhea and pseudomembranous colitis (131).

Presentation

In pseudomembranous colitis the stools are generally watery, with occult blood loss, which is seldom gross. Common findings include abdominal pain, cramps, fever, and leukocytosis. Especially severe forms can run such a rapid course that diarrhea does not occur; they present with symptoms of severe toxicity and shock (132). As a rare complication, marked dilatation of the colon and paralytic ileus can develop, that is, toxic megacolon.

Pseudomembranes are described as initially punctuate creamy to yellow plaques, 0.2–2.0 cm in size, which may be confluent, with "skip areas" of edematous mucosa. Histologically they are composed of fibrin, mucous, necrotic epithelial cells, and leukocytes.

An acute colitis, different from pseudomembranous colitis, was observed in five patients taking penicillin and penicillin derivatives (133). There was considerable rectal bleeding. The radiographic findings were those of ischemic colitis (spasm, transverse ridging, "thumbprinting," and punctuate ulceration). On sigmoidoscopy and biopsy, the mucosa was normal, except for an inflammatory cell infiltration in one case. Conservative treatment resulted in rapid remission.

Occurrence and frequency

Clostridium difficile has been isolated in 11–33% of patients with antibiotic-associated diarrhea, 60–75% of patients with antibiotic-associated colitis, and 96–100% of patients with pseudomembranous colitis (117,134,135). However, about 2% of the adult population are asymptomatic carriers (127). Primary symptomless colonization with *C. difficile* reduces the risk of antibiotic-associated diarrhea (136). Infants up to 2 years seem to be refractory to pseudomembranous colitis, although a high percentage may be carriers of *C. difficile* (135,137). The reasons for this are unknown. It has been speculated that infants lack receptors for the toxin.

There have been several reports of frequent diarrhea in patients treated with combinations of ampicillin or amoxicillin with beta-lactamase inhibitors, such as sulbactam or clavulanic acid (138–141). A double-blind crossover study in healthy volunteers showed disturbances of small bowel motility after oral co-amoxiclav (142).

The appearance of pseudomembranous colitis in clusters of patients (143–146) may explain the wide variation in occurrence, and suggests that the disease may result from cross-contamination among patients rendered susceptible by antibiotic treatment. This is especially true for epidemic outbreaks in hospitals, where the disease may be considered a nosocomial infection favored by serious illness, frequent and prolonged use of broad-spectrum antibiotics (especially cephalosporins), and poor compliance with the rules of hospital hygiene (147). In such an epidemic, a variable proportion of patients will harbor the organism as asymptomatic carriers. An additional possible explanation for the large differences in reported frequencies may be the use of different methods of detection and differences in the definition of the disease. If colonoscopy was routinely performed in all patients with diarrhea taking clindamycin, pseudomembranous colitis was found in as many as 10% (148).

Although the first antibiotics reported to cause pseudomembranous colitis were lincomycin and clindamycin, the disease was later described with all other antimicrobial drugs, even topically applied (149). Vancomycin (150) and metronidazole (151), which may be used as specific treatments, have also been implicated.

Susceptibility factors
Besides the type of antibiotic therapy, other factors such as the age of the patient, the severity of the underlying disease, colonic stasis, cytostatic therapy, surgical interventions, and gastrointestinal manipulations are predisposing factors for antibiotic-associated colitis (152–156).

It is still not established if there is a correlation between toxin production or genotype of the *C. difficile* and the clinical manifestations of the infection (157,158). Although hospital-acquired antibiotic-associated colitis is by far the major problem, community-acquired diarrhea associated with *C. difficile* has also been described (159).

Mechanism
Clostridium difficile produces two well-characterized toxins (124,160)—toxin A, an enterotoxin, and toxin B, an extremely potent cytotoxin—which are thought to be responsible for the disease. The toxigenicity of toxins A and B varies between different strains of *C. difficile* and seems to correlate with symptomatic disease (161). Pseudomembranes were found in a higher percentage of patients with stools positive for cytotoxin than in patients whose stools were positive for *C. difficile*, but toxin-negative (153) Although there is also a high association with *C. difficile* (about 20% are toxin-positive) in antibiotic-associated diarrhea without pseudomembranes, it is possible that this microorganism plays no pathogenic role in some of these usually milder forms of the disease. In these cases the diarrhea may be due to impaired metabolism of carbohydrates, altered fatty acid profiles, or the composition and deconjugation of bile acids by quantitatively and qualitatively altered fecal flora (114,115,135).

Diagnosis
The diagnosis of antibiotic-related colitis should be considered in any patient with severe diarrhea during or within 4–6 weeks after antibiotic therapy. The single best diagnostic procedure is sigmoidoscopy, although in a number of cases the typical pseudomembranous lesions may be seen only above the rectosigmoid area (162). Radiographic investigations (barium enema and air contrast) may show typical findings, but are dangerous in advanced cases and should be avoided. Computerized tomography showed typical but not pathognomonic patterns in two patients (163).

Clostridium difficile can be cultured from the stool, and toxins A and B can be assessed by different techniques (116). The most accurate method is still a cytotoxin tissue culture assay. This detects the cytopathic effect of cytotoxin B, which can be neutralized by *Clostridium sordellii* antitoxin, but it takes 24–48 hours to show a result. Alternative tests that produce faster results have been developed. A latex agglutination test lacks sensitivity and specificity, and does not distinguish toxigenic from non-toxigenic strains. An enzyme immunoassay for toxin A may be an acceptable alternative to the cell cytotoxin assay and the results are rapidly available. A dot immunobinding assay has not yet been extensively studied (164).

Management
Therapy consists of withdrawal of the antibiotic when diarrhea occurs and replacement of fluid and electrolyte losses. In less severe cases of antibiotic-associated diarrhea, no further treatment is needed. However, in patients with pseudomembranous colitis, a more intensive approach is usually required. When a toxic syndrome develops, fluid losses within the bowel can be very large. In these cases, a central venous line offers the chance to measure central venous pressure. Usually there is also loss of serum proteins and in some cases blood, which need appropriate replacement. In the rare cases with fulminant colitis and toxic megacolon, surgical intervention may be necessary (165,166).

In pseudomembranous colitis (typical endoscopic findings, positive test for *C. difficile* or its toxin), the preferred treatment is oral metronidazole, 250 mg qds or 500 mg tds (120,167). Metronidazole is as effective as vancomycin 125–250 mg qds, which is significantly more expensive (168). Oral bacitracin 25 000 U qds (169) and oral teicoplanin (170) are acceptable alternatives.

Relapses are similarly frequent after treatment with metronidazole and vancomycin (116). In 189 adult patients, a first relapse occurred in up to 24% and a second relapse in 46% (169). Relapse may be due to sporulation of *C. difficile* and not to the development of resistance. Relapses usually respond to further courses of the initial treatment. Some alternative treatments have been proposed for repeatedly relapsing cases, including the combination of vancomycin with rifampicin for 10 days (171).

The role of anion exchange resins (colestyramine and colestipol), which bind *C. difficile* toxin, is still controversial (172). If ion exchange resins are given at all, they should not be given together with vancomycin, because they also bind the antibiotic (173). Attempts to restore the intestinal flora with *Lactobacillus GG* (174), or with fecal enemas (175) from healthy volunteers have shown some favorable results in less severe cases. However, esthetic and infectious concerns may be an obstacle. It also has been suggested that treatment with *Saccharomyces boulardii* may help prevent the development of antibiotic-associated diarrhea (176). Its value in the prevention and treatment of relapses has still to be demonstrated. Antimotility agents have been associated with an increased incidence of antibiotic-related diarrhea and can worsen symptoms when the disease is already established (177). They should therefore be avoided.

There is little evidence that re-exposure to the same antibiotic that caused pseudomembranous colitis confers a further risk for relapse. Still, it would be wise to avoid the antibiotics that are most often related to pseudo-membranous colitis in a patient who has had this complication.

Liver

Increases in serum transaminases and alkaline phosphatase, largely without additional symptoms, have been reported with the majority of beta-lactam antibiotics. With different compounds the estimated frequencies vary by up to a factor of 10. However, the frequency also depends on patient-related factors; in one study only a minority of transaminase increases could not be explained by factors other than antibiotic treatment (86).

More severe liver disease, presenting as hepatitis and/or intrahepatic cholestasis, has been seen with beta-lactam antibiotics of various classes, the isoxazolyl penicillins being most frequently involved. Co-amoxiclav has repeatedly been associated with cholestatic hepatitis.

Hepatitis is accompanied by fever, eosinophilia, and/or a rash in more than 80% of cases. This hints at the possibility of overlapping pathogenetic steps and sheds some doubt on the reliability of these accompanying symptoms as indicators of immune-mediated reactions, for example serum sickness-like syndromes.

One type of hepatitis is mainly associated with oxacillin (178,179). Eight of 54 patients developed this reaction after a mean cumulative dose of oxacillin 157 g (180).

Prolonged duration of treatment and increasing age were risk factors for flucloxacillin-induced jaundice (181), and cholestatic liver injury has been described most often with flucloxacillin (182,183) and other isoxazolylpenicillins (184). Whether cholestatic hepatitis after the combination of amoxicillin with clavulanic acid (co-amoxiclav) is related to one of these categories is not yet clear.

Urinary tract

Methicillin-induced acute interstitial nephritis follows a similar pattern of dose-dependence and time-dependence to that of neutropenia (185,186). This reaction occurred in 16% of all children treated with high-dose methicillin (187). Nephritis occurred after a mean of 17 days and a mean cumulative dose of 120 g.

With other beta-lactams, mainly penicillin G, acute interstitial nephritis is rare, but it can follow the same pattern (188).

Nephritis is accompanied by fever, eosinophilia, and/or a rash in more than 80% of cases. This hints at the possibility of overlapping pathogenetic steps and sheds some doubt on the reliability of these accompanying symptoms as indicators of immune-mediated reactions, for example serum sickness-like syndromes.

Acute renal insufficiency, with or without skin rash and eosinophilia, has been reported with various beta-lactam antibiotics, most often with methicillin. Hence, the designation "methicillin-nephritis" is still sometimes used. The pathogenesis is largely unknown and is different from the nephrotoxicity of older cephalosporins (cefaloridine and cefalotin).

Skin

Rashes are among the most common adverse reactions to drugs in general and occur in 2–3% of hospitalized patients (189). Most distinct mucocutaneous reactions that can be induced by drugs have been associated with the use of individual beta-lactam antibiotics. These reactions include urticaria, angioedema, maculopapular rash, fixed drug eruption, erythema multiforme, Stevens–Johnson syndrome, toxic epidermal necrolysis, allergic vasculitis, serum sickness-like syndrome, eczematous lesions, pruritus, and stomatitis (190–193). The maculopapular rash, starting on the trunk or areas of pressure or trauma, is more frequent than all other skin manifestations together (189,194). Involvement of mucous membranes, palms, and soles is variable; the eruption can be associated with moderate to severe pruritus and fever. In addition, an indistinguishable rash often accompanies various reactions in other organs.

Pustular drug eruptions due to penicillin (195), amoxicillin (196), ampicillin (197), bacampicillin (198), cefazolin (199,200), cefradine (201), cefalexin (202), cefaclor (203), or imipenem + cilastin (204) seem to form a distinct clinical entity that has to be differentiated from pustular psoriasis, which can be drug-induced as well (204). A history of drug exposure, rapid disappearance of the eruption after the drug is stopped, and eosinophils in the inflammatory infiltrate argue in favor of pustular drug eruptions.

In patients with mononucleosis, aminopenicillins, and, less so, cephalosporins evoke rashes in a much higher percentage than usual (205). The incidence of rashes in infectious mononucleosis without antibiotics is 3–15%, compared with 40–100% with ampicillin. The underlying mechanism is speculative.

Immunologic

The adverse effects of early penicillin use consisted almost exclusively of anaphylaxis. This stimulated extensive research into the immune responses associated with penicillin and made penicillin the most prominent model for immune reactions to drugs.

The pathogenesis of many presumably immunologically mediated reactions to beta-lactam antibiotics is still unknown. Reliable and standardized tests to predict hypersensitivity only exist for a minority of allergic reactions, that is, IgE-mediated reactions. The matter is further complicated by the fact that beta-lactams can readily induce immune responses that by themselves do not necessarily result in disease. This is the case, for example, when antierythrocyte antibodies directed against beta-lactam bound to the erythrocyte surface are formed. This biological property (immunogenicity) has to be distinguished from allergenicity, that is, immune responses causing disease.

Cross-reactivity, that is, hypersensitivity reactions initially induced by one compound but triggered by another, is an important and as yet unresolved problem, complicated by the fact that beta-lactams undergo structural modifications after administration, and that different parts of the molecule (such as the nucleus or side chains) can be involved. Data from cross-exposed patients (skin tests or drug challenge) suggest a high degree of cross-reactivity between compounds belonging to the same class and between the penicillins and carbapenems, but a low degree of cross-reactivity between penicillins and cephalosporins and between monobactams and the other beta-lactams.

Mechanisms

Drug allergy or hypersensitivity represents an acquired capacity of the organism to mount an immunologically mediated reaction to a compound. This ultimately involves covalent or exceptionally non-covalent binding to and modification of host molecules (presumably proteins) by the drug, to which the host becomes sensitized (induction phase). Re-exposure to the sensitizing drug can trigger a series of immunological effector mechanisms (effector phase). These can be defined as pathways of inflammation or tissue injury, but they also represent mechanisms of immune protection from infectious agents.

Traditionally, the classification scheme defined by Gell and Coombs (206) distinguishes four types of reactions:

- type I reactions, which are IgE-mediated immediate hypersensitivity reactions.
- type II reactions, which are mediated by cytotoxic IgM and/or IgG.
- type III reactions, which are mediated by immune complexes.
- type IV reactions, which are cell-mediated hypersensitivity responses.

However, this classification fails to account for the complex and sequential involvement of several cell types and mediators in the immune response, as recognized today (207).

IgE-antibody-mediated adverse reactions

IgE-antibody-mediated hypersensitivity can serve as a paradigm to demonstrate some important features of beta-lactam hypersensitivity. Beta-lactams are small molecules that have to combine with a host macromolecule to be recognized by the immune system. In the case of penicillin, this reaction involves coupling of reactive degradation products to a protein-containing carrier (208). There are several degradation pathways, which result in the formation of reactive compounds, most importantly penicilloyl (209), also called the major determinant. Other less abundant degradation products include penilloate, benzylpenicilloate, and benzylpenilloate, the so-called minor determinants.

The complex contains haptens, often multiple, coupled to a protein-containing carrier molecule, and can induce T cell-dependent B cell activation, leading to the formation of antihapten antibodies. The mechanisms that govern the selection of the different immunoglobulin isotypes are reviewed elsewhere (207).

The time required for sensitization is called "latency" and is variable, depending on factors such as route of exposure, hapten dose, and chemical reactivity of the drug, as well as on genetic and acquired host factors.

The period between the last exposure to the drug and the first appearance of symptoms has been termed the "reaction time." It is part of the clinical description of an adverse event and may help to attribute it to a specific drug (SED-12, 594).

Once sensitivity has been established, that is, once hapten-specific IgE-producing B cells have been formed, exposure to even small amounts of hapten can induce a cascade of events that lead to immediate reactions, such as anaphylaxis (210). Briefly, preformed IgE antibodies to drug determinants recognize the hapten-carrier complex and fix to the surface of mast cells or basophils, triggering the release of a series of mediators, such as histamine, neutral proteases, biologically active arachidonic acid products, and cytokines. This ultimately leads to a clinical spectrum that ranges from a mild local reaction to anaphylactic shock.

Non-IgE-antibody-mediated immunological reactions

Modification of erythrocyte surface components due to binding of beta-lactams or their metabolic products is thought to be the cause of the formation of antierythrocyte antibodies and the development of a positive Coombs' test implicated in the development of immune hemolytic anemia (211). About 3% of patients receiving large doses of intravenous penicillin (10–20 million units/day) will develop a positive direct Coombs' test (212). However, only a small fraction of Coombs' positive patients will develop frank hemolytic anemia (213). Antibody-coated erythrocytes are probably eliminated by the reticuloendothelial system (extravascular hemolysis) (214), or less often by complement-mediated intravascular erythrocyte destruction (215). Another mechanism implicates circulating immune complexes (anti-beta-lactam antibody/beta-lactam complexes), resulting in erythrocyte elimination by an "innocent bystander" mechanism (82). Similar mechanisms have been implicated in thrombocytopenia associated with beta-lactam antibiotics (216,217).

Contact dermatitis was often observed when penicillin was used in topical formulations and still continues to be described in cases of occupational exposure to beta-lactams (218,219). The underlying mechanism is thought to involve chemical modification of antigen-presenting cells in the epidermis, leading to sensitization of drug-specific T cells (220,221).

The underlying mechanism of a series of clinical entities associated with beta-lactams, such as maculopapular rash, drug fever, eosinophilia, serum sickness-like disease, vesicular and bullous skin reactions, erythema nodosum, and acute interstitial nephritis, is suspected to be immunological but is still largely unknown.

Reactions specific to side chains

Side chain–specific allergic reactions to beta-lactams are a steadily increasing problem (SEDA-21, 260) (222–224). Apart from epitopes generated by the beta-lactam nucleus, side chains attached to it can serve as additional epitopes recognized by the host immune response. Side chain–specific antibodies can be detected in patients who are allergic to beta-lactam antibiotics, even in the absence of reactivity to the mother compound. The clinical importance of this is debated. Serious anaphylactic reactions to amoxicillin occurred in three patients who tolerated benzylpenicillin (225). The phenomenon is mostly relevant for patients given semisynthetic penicillins, cephalosporins, carbapenems, and monobactams: compounds derived from each of these classes of drugs share certain side chains that may be cross-recognized by preformed antibody. Diagnosis of side chain–specific allergy requires a panel of diagnostic tools available only at selected research centers.

Pseudoallergy

The term "hypersensitivity" includes both immunoallergic and pseudoallergic reactions. Immunoallergic reactions occur when highly specific mechanisms involving immunological memory and recognition are involved. Pseudoallergic reactions are reactions that mimic immunoallergic reactions, but in which a specific immune-mediated mechanism is not involved. The so-called ampicillin rash is an example of a pseudoallergic reaction. Some major mediators of pseudoallergic reactions have been reviewed (226). The roles of newer putative mechanisms, involving cytokines, kinins, and other host-derived substances, remain to be ascertained. Most important is the fact that currently there are no standardized and validated animal models for predicting pseudoallergic reactions (227).

Animal models

Guinea pigs have been used for years in studies of systemic anaphylaxis. However, variations in predictability and sensitivity limit their value (228,229). Passive cutaneous anaphylaxis is another guinea pig model, but it is no more sensitive than systemic anaphylaxis (228). Respiratory sensitization, resulting in IgE-mediated immediate hypersensitivity has been investigated in mice and guinea pigs (230,231). Most often highly reactive chemicals have been used, and the models are of limited value in testing antimicrobial drugs.

Contact sensitizers have been studied in guinea pigs and mice, and it has been stated that "these models can reasonably identify the majority of human contact sensitizers" (227).

The best approach to induce a specific immune response against substances of low molecular weights is to use hapten-carrier conjugates. This method is of value in assessing the potential for cross-reactivity between closely related compounds, such as beta-lactam antibiotics (232).

It is obvious that the development of new animal models, for example transgenic and knock-out mice, should create new possibilities for predicting the sensitizing potential of new antimicrobials. The sad fact that hypersensitivity reactions are among the most commonly occurring adverse effects when antibiotics are used underlines the urgent need for research efforts in academia and industry (227).

Incidence

The true incidence of immunologically mediated reactions to beta-lactam antibiotics is hard to evaluate. This is mainly because of problems associated with the case definition of hypersensitivity reactions. The pathogenetic mechanism for a significant number of reactions presumed to be immunological in nature has not yet been conclusively determined. Furthermore, studies that address the incidences of adverse reactions face the problem of dealing with heterogeneous patient populations, treated with different types of beta-lactams, and administered by diverse routes in various dosages. The issue can be illustrated by reviewing data derived from four pharmacoepidemiological studies.

1. The International Rheumatic Fever Study, a prospective multicenter study that recorded allergic reactions, defined as hypotension, dyspnea, pruritus, urticaria, angioedema, arthralgia, and maculopapular rash in 1790 patients treated with monthly intramuscular benzathine penicillin for prophylaxis of rheumatic fever (32 430 injections during 2736 patient years). There was a 3.2% case incidence of allergic reactions and a 0.2% case incidence of anaphylaxis (12/100 000 injections), including one death (0.05%, equivalent to 3.1/100 000 injections) (233).
2. A large national study by venereal disease clinics in the USA, including four cooperative surveys conducted at 5-year intervals (1954, 1959, 1964, and 1969). The study included data from 94 655 patients unselected with regard to a history of penicillin allergy. The frequency of anaphylaxis was 0.055%, including one death (234).
3. A retrospective analysis of allergic reactions (drug-induced fever and rash) in 90 adults with cystic fibrosis, of whom 26 developed probable allergic reactions to parenteral beta-lactams. There was drug-induced fever in 54 and skin reactions in 28 of 897 treatment courses (6 and 3.1% respectively). There was one case of non-fatal anaphylaxis. The numbers of allergic reactions per number of patients receiving specific antibiotics were: carbenicillin 4/56, mezlocillin 7/42, piperacillin 11/31, ticarcillin 1/20, cefazolin 0/24, ceftazidime 1/35, imipenem + cilastatin 4/16, and nafcillin 3/36 (17).
4. The Boston Collaborative Drug Surveillance Program. In this classic study in in-patients during 1966–82, beta-lactams headed the list of drugs causing skin reactions, presumably allergic. The overall reaction rate (the number of drug-related skin reactions per 1000 treated patients) was 51 for amoxicillin, 42 for ampicillin, 29 for semisynthetic penicillins, 16 for penicillin G, and 13 for cephalosporins (18,193).

These four sets of data illustrate a spectrum of diverse settings of beta-lactam administration: single-dose parenteral use (in venereal disease clinics), intermittent parenteral use (in rheumatic fever), and continuous high-dose parenteral use (in cystic fibrosis). Factors other than route of administration and dosing, such as drug history, underlying disease, co-administered drugs, and the risk profile of a particular compound, will be important in assessing the risk of giving a beta-lactam to a particular patient, as discussed in more detail below.

Table 1 contains a list of presumably immunologically mediated effects of beta-lactams, according to their estimated frequencies. The mechanisms of most of these reactions are not completely understood, which implies that some of the entities listed may be due to non-immunological mechanisms. The frequencies of the various adverse effects vary among different beta-lactams and depend on additional factors, discussed below. A compilation of reported frequencies of occurrence related to different compounds has been published and was used and extended to prepare Table 1 (194).

Presentation

The requirement for sensitization explains why a drug may be administered for a variable length of time without adverse effects. Once the organism is sensitized, the manifestation of hypersensitivity will depend on the route and dose of the allergen as well as the type of effector mechanism involved, preformed IgE being the most rapid, others evolving more slowly, typically over days. Generally much less drug is required to trigger a hypersensitivity reaction in a sensitized subject than for induction. Anaphylactic reactions have been described after ingestion of meat from penicillin-fed animals or after sexual intercourse in a penicillin-sensitive patient (269,270).

The time for sensitization to occur is often difficult to establish in a patient who develops symptoms during continuous therapy. A classification scheme that distinguishes between immediate, accelerated, and late reactions is of limited clinical use, since it will only allow distinction between IgE-mediated reactions (that is, rapid reactions) and non-IgE-mediated reactions (that is, more slowly evolving reactions) in the setting of re-exposure of a sensitized subject (80).

In contrast to hypersensitivity, other adverse reactions do not require sensitization and require similar doses of drug for recurrence. A special case is a syndrome (Hoigné's syndrome) that resembles an immediate allergic reaction combined with hallucinations, aggressive behavior, anxiety, and auditory and visual disturbances, which has been described after intramuscular procaine penicillin and benzathine penicillin. It is probably due to accidental intravascular injection and results from microembolism of the penicillin depot formulation (271–275).

Susceptibility factors

Several factors that influence hypersensitivity have been recognized and reviewed (276).

Patient-related factors

Patient-related factors include an increased incidence of allergic reactions to beta-lactams in patients with systemic lupus erythematosus (277) but not with atopic diseases (278). Genetic factors that influence drug metabolism and excretion, as well as the underlying disease of the patient and host immune reactivity, are likely to modulate the risk and severity of hypersensitivity reactions.

Table 1 Presumably immunologically mediated adverse reactions to beta-lactams

Adverse reaction	References
Expected in one or more of 100 treatment courses	
Maculopapular rash[a]	(193,194,235)
Expected once in 100–1000 treatment courses	
Urticaria, angioedema	(80,194,235,236)
Drug fever [b]	(17,237)
Eosinophilia[c]	(238–240)
Expected once in 1000–10 000 treatment courses	
Anaphylactic shock	(210,241,242)
Bronchospasm and acute severe dyspnea	(243,244)
Thrombocytopenia	(91,245)
Serum sickness-like disease	(246–249)
Vasculitis	
Expected less than once in 10 000 treatment courses	
Hemolytic anemia	(81,82,250–253)
Vesicular and bullous skin reactions (including Stevens–Johnson syndrome and toxic epidermal necrolysis)	(254,260)
Erythema multiforme[d]	(257,261)
Erythema nodosum[e]	(257,261)
Interstitial nephritis[f]	(262)
Observed after occupational exposure	
Contact sensitivity	(219,263)
Anaphylaxis	(210)
Asthma, pneumonitis	(264–268)

[a] Occurs with all beta-lactams; more often with aminopenicillins, penicillinase-resistant penicillins, and anti-*Pseudomonas* penicillins
[b] Occurs with all beta-lactams; probably more often with piperacillin + tazobactam and aztreonam
[c] Occurs with all beta-lactams; probably more often with meticillin, nafcillin, oxacillin, second- and third-generation cephalosporins, aztreonam, and imipenem
[d] Occurs with all beta-lactams; probably more often with penicillins G and V, antipseudomonal penicillins, cefaclor, cefadroxil, cefalexin, loracarbef, aztreonam, and imipenem
[e] Occurs probably with all beta-lactams, but more often with penicillins G and V, cefuroxime, cefoperazone, cefaclor, and imipenem
[f] Occurs probably with all beta-lactams; well documented for methicillin

A history of a prior penicillin reaction increases the risk of a subsequent exposure. A classic study showed a frequency of allergic reactions to penicillin of 0.62% (155 of 24 906 treatment courses) in patients without a history of penicillin allergy compared with 13% (10 of 78 treatment courses) in patients with a history of penicillin allergy (234). Reaction rates are higher in patients with a history that suggests IgE-mediated reactions (279).

Patients with chronic lymphatic leukemia or with concurrent infection with Epstein–Barr virus or HIV have an increased frequency of ampicillin- and amoxicillin-associated rashes (280).

Drug-related factors
Drug dosage, mode of administration, and duration of treatment probably influence the frequency of allergic reactions. Topical administration has been associated with a high incidence of sensitization, in contrast to a low incidence with the oral route. For IgE-mediated reactions, a frequent and intermittent course of treatment is more likely to cause allergy than a prolonged course without a drug-free interval (208). High doses of parenteral beta-lactams are usually required for the induction of penicillin-induced hemolytic anemia (212). Similarly, it is likely that the high dosages of beta-lactams used in patients with cystic fibrosis result in a high incidence of drug fever (17).

Co-administration of beta-blockers has been associated with an increased risk of severe allergic drug reactions and reduces the effect of adrenaline in the immediate treatment of anaphylactic shock. The mechanism involves changes in the regulation of anaphylactic mediators (281).

Evidence that allopurinol potentiates skin reactions to ampicillin is controversial (192,282).

Long-Term Effects

Drug resistance

The introduction of penicillin G more than 50 years ago was one of the milestones in the treatment of infectious diseases, leading to a drastic reduction in mortality from severe infections (283–285). Two years later the emergence of the first penicillin-resistant *Staphylococcus aureus* rapidly cooled clinicians' enthusiasm. Since then microorganisms have developed various mechanisms to survive antibiotic pressure, including the following:

1. Modification of the targets of beta-lactam antibiotics, that is, the penicillin-binding proteins (286,287), resulting in a reduced affinity of the antibiotic.
2. The synthesis of new penicillin-binding proteins with very low affinity for the antibiotic, providing a high degree of resistance.
3. The production and secretion into the periplasmic space of beta-lactamases, that is, enzymes sharing structural analogies with the penicillin-binding proteins without fulfilling any function in the cell wall synthesis but hydrolysing and inactivating the beta-lactam ring. The genes encoding for these beta-lactamases are usually located on a plasmid but can also be anchored in the bacterial genome (288,289).
4. Structural modification of porines, proteins that form channels in the outer membrane of Gram-negative bacteria, preventing the antibiotics from reaching the penicillin-binding proteins by impairing their penetration through channels of the outer membrane (290,291).

All of these mechanisms are mainly based on interbacterial exchange of DNA or on point mutations (292), the predominant mechanisms for genetic exchange being transformation, transduction, and conjugation (293). Transformation is the simplest way to transfer DNA to another bacterium, provided that this is ready to accept foreign DNA (= competent bacteria). This mechanism of genetic transfer is mostly used by several human pathogens: *Streptococcus pneumoniae, Hemophilus influenzae, Neisseria meningitidis, Neisseria gonorrhoeae,* and *Bacillus subtilis.* The transduction needs a bacteriophage (a virus) as a vector to inject DNA into a bacterium. This elaborate system is limited by the restricted specificity of the vectors for few microorganisms. The most sophisticated system is conjugation. This mechanism was first observed in *E. coli* in 1952 by Hayes, who described the first transfer of genetic material (F-Factor, or fertility factor) by conjugation (294). Microorganisms use conjugation to transfer several types of genetic material, either extrachromosomal (that is, plasmids) or intrachromosomal (that is, transposons).

In summary, microorganisms can exchange and acquire genetic material in order to adapt to a changing environment, the antibiotic pressure. Furthermore, DNA exchange between prokaryotes and eukaryotic cells (yeasts) and some plants has been observed (295). A review has addressed in detail the problem of emergence and spread of resistance among clinical isolates (296). Here we shall only briefly discuss as examples the development of resistance by two major pathogens, *S. pneumoniae* and *S. aureus.*

One of the most striking features in microbiology is the rapid emergence and worldwide spread of penicillin-resistant *S. pneumoniae* (pneumococci), mainly due to the uncontrolled use of penicillin in certain countries (297). The first cases of penicillin-resistant pneumococci were reported in the 1960s in New Guinea and Australia. Penicillin-resistant pneumococci have now been registered in all continents. The highest rate was reported in 1989 in Hungary, amounting to 57% of all clinical isolates (298). Until now, pneumococci have not acquired the genes encoding for beta-lactamases. Accordingly, the underlying mechanism of penicillin resistance is structural modification of penicillin-binding proteins, leading to reduced affinity to the penicillin molecule (see above). These modifications of the penicillin-binding protein usually require several genetic steps. Moreover, horizontal transfer of pieces of penicillin-binding protein genes has been described between *Streptococcus mitis* and *Streptococcus pneumoniae* (299). Such modifications of penicillin-binding proteins lead to reduced affinity of these enzymes for their natural substrates (disaccharide-pentapeptides) (300) and eventually to the synthesis of a structurally different cell wall harboring more branched peptides. This is the biological price that pneumococci pay to survive antibiotic pressure (301). Usually in an epidemic area a few clones of penicillin-resistant pneumococci are responsible for the majority of the registered cases (302). Furthermore, DNA polymorphism analysis has shown that isolates have been imported from one continent to another, causing new epidemics (303–306).

Another major pathogen *S. aureus* has developed two different mechanisms of resistance:

- synthesis of beta-lactamase (nowadays more than 80% of *S. aureus* secrete beta-lactamase).
- the emergence of so-called methicillin-resistant *S. aureus* (MRSA), which can grow even in the presence of high concentrations of methicillin (up to 800 μg/ml).

The unique feature of MRSA is based on the acquisition of a low-affinity penicillin-binding protein for beta-lactam antibiotic molecules (the penicillin-binding protein 2A), which allows the bacteria to carry on synthesis of its cell wall, whereas the other penicillin-binding proteins are already inactivated by the high concentration of methicillin or other beta-lactamase-resistant beta-lactam antibiotics.

The origin of the penicillin-binding protein 2A is a matter of debate. Until now the only antibiotics that inhibit MRSA are the glycopeptides, such as vancomycin. A nightmare scenario would be the transfer of vancomycin resistance from enterococci to MRSA, which would cause a major epidemiological and therapeutic problem in the treatment of staphylococcal infections. There have been a few cases of vancomycin-resistant coagulase-negative *S. aureus* (307,308), but none of vancomycin-resistant MRSA, although transfer of vancomycin resistance to staphylococci has been achieved experimentally (309).

The continuous spread of resistance among clinical isolates, especially of multiresistant microorganisms represents a unique challenge in the treatment of infectious diseases. The detection of asymptomatic carriers of pneumococci, especially young children in day care centers, makes early detection even more difficult (310). Uncontrolled use of antibiotics in agriculture selects multiresistant fecal flora in animals, and meat can be contaminated by imperfect processing.

The problem of increasing resistance of micro-organisms is a major worldwide issue that necessitates close collaboration of clinicians, epidemiologists, and basic research laboratories. Newer and fast diagnostic tools (such as the polymerase chain reaction), routinely introduced into clinical laboratories, and better understanding at the molecular level of mechanisms of resistance of microorganisms are key prerequisites for the prevention of further spread of resistant microorganisms. Additional measures, for example broad use of vaccines and restrictions on antibiotic use imposed by health authorities, will require global cooperation and will have to be addressed by international organizations such as the WHO.

Second-Generation Effects

Teratogenicity

Since the days of the thalidomide disaster about 40 years ago, resulting in the birth of some thousands of malformed babies, it has been well recognized that drugs taken by pregnant mothers can have severe adverse effects on their unborn children. A consequence of the thalidomide disaster was worldwide awareness that drugs can cause congenital malformations and the necessity to investigate this possibility in animals. Since thalidomide, around 30 drugs have been proven to be teratogenic, not all of which are currently in clinical use (311). For most drugs, however, safety in pregnancy has still to be established. With the risk of teratogenicity and dysmorphogenesis ever present, clinicians are in general very cautious in prescribing drugs for pregnant women. Despite this, over 60% of pregnant women consume therapeutic agents not directly related to their pregnancy, and it has been estimated that about 5% of birth defects are caused by maternal drug therapy (312).

Even if a drug is generally recognized as being safe after animal experiments, it is wise to be suspicious when giving it to a pregnant woman. One major obstacle in evaluating safety in humans is the sample size required to reach sound conclusions. For example, in Europe, neural tube defects and cleft lips both occur with a prevalence of around seven per 10 000 live births (313). It has been calculated that for an uncommon drug exposure (that is, a frequency of under one per 1000 pregnant women and a background malformation prevalence of 0.001), one would have to monitor more than 1 000 000 births in order to detect a teratogenic effect, even though the relative risk associated with the drug might be as high as 20 (that is, a 20-fold increased risk of a particular malformation). In contrast, for formulations that are commonly used in pregnancy (for example by 2% of women, as was the case with thalidomide) and that are associated with an extremely high relative risk (such as 175), 1000 births would be sufficient to detect the teratogenic potential, even when the background prevalence of the malformation was as low as 0.0024 (314).

Another issue that has to be taken into consideration is the temporal relation between drug exposure and the effect on the embryo or fetus (315). Exposure to harmful drugs in the 2 weeks after conception usually leads to abortion, which may not be noticed. In the next 6–7 weeks the embryo is assumed to be extremely sensitive to teratogens (316). However, different organs and systems may be susceptible to teratogens at different times during this period. Therefore, in order to link drug use during pregnancy to a congenital malformation, drug intake must have taken place when the organ or organ system was sensitive to its harmful effects (315). It goes without saying that exact information on the timing of exposure is crucial.

In an ideal world, no drug would become available before it had been thoroughly tested for safety and effectiveness in a randomized, double-blind, placebo-controlled trial in pregnant women (317). However, because of ethical concerns about the welfare of the mother and fetus, pregnant women are traditionally excluded from drug trials. Therefore, usage is most often based on indirect measures of safety, such as in vitro studies and animal models. However, the thalidomide affair reminds us of the potential inadequacy of animal models.

In reality, most information about the safety of antimicrobial drugs in pregnancy comes from a history of long-term use with no reported adverse outcomes. As has been emphasized (317) most practitioners are happy to prescribe penicillin and its derivatives although there are no data from formal trials. However, there are data that show that penicillin V is safe during pregnancy (318). The study took place in Hungary between 1980 and 1996. The case group consisted of 22 865 malformed infants or fetuses, of whom 173 (0.8%) had mothers who had taken penicillin V during pregnancy. Two control neonates without malformations were matched with every case according to sex, week of birth, and the district of the parent's residence. Of the 38 151 infants in the control group, 218 had been treated with penicillin V. This difference was explained mainly by recall bias and confounders, because there was no difference in the adjusted odds ratio for medically documented phenoxymethylpenicillin treatment during the second and third months of gestation, that is, during the critical period for most major congenital abnormalities in case-matched control pairs. Thus, treatment with oral phenoxymethylpenicillin during pregnancy presents very little, if any, teratogenic risk.

There have also been two studies of the teratogenic potential of other penicillins. In the first study, in 791 women who had redeemed a prescription for pivampicillin during their first pregnancy, birth outcomes (malformations, pre-term delivery, and low birth weight) were matched with similar outcomes in 7472 reference pregnancies in which the mother had not redeemed any prescription for pivampicillin during pregnancy (319). There were no significant effects of pivampicillin. In the second study, in 78 women who took cefuroxime axetil during pregnancy, none of the 13 women who were treated in the first trimester gave birth to a malformed child, but one baby with hip dysplasia was found among 20 babies from mothers treated in their second trimester, and there was one case of hypospadias and one of imperforate anus in 47 children of mothers treated in the third trimester (320). The authors correctly concluded that the number of patients who had taken cefuroxime in the first trimester of pregnancy was small, and that cefuroxime should be used with caution in the early months of pregnancy.

Susceptibility Factors

Renal disease

Renal insufficiency is a risk factor for the toxic effects of the beta-lactams (321,322), including neurotoxic reactions (323), inhibition of platelet aggregation (324), and to some extent interaction with vitamin K-dependent synthesis of coagulation factors (325).

Drug–Drug Interactions

Antacids

Antacids increase gastric pH and can result in impaired dissolution of some cephalosporins (326–328).

Anticoagulants

Some beta-lactam antibiotics impair coagulation by inhibiting hepatic and intestinal vitamin K production and impairing platelet function.

- A patient suffered significant postoperative bleeding 4 days after dental surgery in a patient taking amoxicillin, despite the use of a tranexamic acid (4.8%) mouth rinse to control hemostasis (329).

Interactions with drugs that affect coagulation and platelet function must therefore be borne in mind.

- A 58-year-old woman developed a raised INR and microscopic hematuria while taking warfarin and co-amoxiclav (330). This was attributed to an interaction of the two drugs.

In contrast, some penicillinase-resistant penicillins (dicloxacillin, nafcillin) provoke resistance to warfarin, lasting for up to 3 weeks after withdrawal of the antibiotic (331,332).

- A patient experienced the effects of interactions of warfarin with nafcillin and dicloxacillin (333). During co-administration of nafcillin, warfarin doses were increased to as much as 4.5 times the previous amounts needed to provide adequate anticoagulation. During co-administration of dicloxacillin, warfarin doses gradually fell, but still stabilized at a higher maintenance dose than before.
- A 41-year-old man taking warfarin 22 mg/week with a prothrombin time of 20.7 seconds was given dicloxacillin 500 mg qds for 10 days (331). The prothrombin time and S- and R-warfarin concentrations fell by 17, 25, and 20% respectively after 5 days. In a retrospective review of seven other patients, the mean prothrombin time fell by 17% (range 11–26%) within 4 days of starting dicloxacillin.

This type of interaction may be due to induction of warfarin metabolism.

Digoxin

In 10% of patients taking digoxin, there is inactivation of up to 40% of the drug before absorption, by intestinal *Eubacterium lentum*. This can be reversed by antibiotics (334,335). The lack of effects of some beta-lactam antibiotics on serum digoxin concentrations in one study (336) might have been due to the small sample size or resistance of the bacteria.

Nifedipine

An active dipeptide transport system that depends on hydrogen ions takes up non-ester amino-beta-lactams (penicillin, amoxicillin, and oral first-generation cephalosporins) (337–339) and specific cephalosporins that lack the alpha-amino group (cefixime, ceftibuten, cefdinir, cefprozil) (340,341). Nifedipine increases amoxicillin and cefixime absorption, probably by stimulating the dipeptide transport system, since the serum concentrations of passively absorbed drugs and intestinal blood flow did not change (342–344).

Oral contraceptive steroids

There have been anecdotal reports that oral antibiotics reduced the efficacy of oral contraceptives. The proposed mechanism is that the antibiotics reduce the amount of gut bacteria that normally deconjugate excreted estrogens prior to reabsorption. However, in small formal studies this effect has not been confirmed (345–347). It is nevertheless possible that this is the mechanism, but that it occurs in too few women to be detected in small formal studies.

As early as 1971, it was observed that there was an increased incidence of intermenstrual bleeding in women who were reliably taking oral contraceptives and rifampicin for tuberculosis (348). Subsequent studies showed that pregnancy was a possible adverse effect of the combined use of antibiotics and oral contraceptives, the most commonly involved antimicrobial drugs being ampicillin, co-trimoxazole, and tetracyclines (349). In an analysis based on reports to the Committee on Safety of Medicines in the UK between 1968 and 1984, 63 pregnancies were identified in women taking this combination of drugs (345). Tetracyclines and penicillin were the drugs most often involved. However, the question of under-reporting was underlined. Over the years, there have been a few reports of the possibility of ineffectiveness of oral contraceptives during the use of antimicrobial drugs.

- A healthy 21-year-old woman, using an oral contraceptive, became pregnant while taking minocycline 100 mg/day for acne (350).

At least three different mechanisms have been proposed.

1. Antibiotics, for example rifampicin (SEDA-8, 256), interfere with the hepatic metabolism of the compounds in oral contraceptives.
2. Antibiotics increase gastric emptying and small intestinal motility. This in turn alters gastrointestinal absorption (and reabsorption) of oral contraceptives (probably both estrogens and progestogens). Increased gastrointestinal motility has been best studied in relation to macrolide antibiotics (SEDA-18, 269). However, there is no evidence of reduced efficacy of oral contraceptives through an effect of macrolides on gastrointestinal motility, which is in any case an unlikely mechanism.
3. Antibiotics interfere with the normal flora in the gastrointestinal tract, thereby also interfering with the normal enterohepatic circulation of the compounds that are included in oral contraceptives. This is a complex story. Oral contraceptives contain estrogens and progestogens. There are several different derivatives in each group and the amounts of each compound vary from formulation to formulation. However, most (if not all) of the compounds have an enterohepatic circulation—they are excreted into the bile, usually as conjugates, and are reabsorbed from the intestinal tract. The efficacy of their absorption and reabsorption depends on physicochemical factors in the gut (such as pH, conjugated versus unconjugated compounds, and adsorption to microbes and dietary constituents). In addition to this basic physiological circulation, intestinal microbes interact with the compounds, most often by splitting conjugates, but also by acting on double bonds, hydroxyl groups, and keto groups, present in the original compounds. These derivatives may have different absorption rates from the original ones. Partly because of their complexity, these microbial interactions have been very little studied. However, it is well known that microbes

interfere with the enterohepatic circulation of other molecules with similar structures, such as androgens (SEDA-13, 215) (SEDA-16, 262) and bile acids (351). A similar effect can take place in patients with gastrointestinal bacterial infections. In addition, and at least from a theoretical point of view, an effect on this enterohepatic circulation may also occur in individuals with a high load of living microbes, as is the case when ingesting probiotics (products that contain live bacteria such as Bifidobacterium and Lactobacillus). This possibility has not been adequately addressed by any of the companies that sell tons of probiotics to fertile women taking oral contraceptives.

Given the problems of under-reporting, the lack of proper investigations, and the possibility of an unwanted pregnancy, the concern can be reduced to a practical one: what should women be told? An excellent recommendation has been published in the UK (352): "Your doctor has prescribed antibiotics, which are necessary to treat [your] infection. However, the antibiotics can interfere with the pill and make it less effective. This means that you may not be protected from pregnancy if you have sex, even though you are taking the pill. You are advised that you should take precautions, that is use of a condom, during the time you are taking the antibiotics, and for 7 days after completing the course of antibiotics ···." For the time being, this is the best advice. However, more investigations in this important field are needed.

Phenobarbital

There was an unexpectedly high frequency of adverse effects in a pediatric intensive care unit with the combination of high-dose phenobarbital and beta-lactam antibiotics, mainly cefotaxime (353). The reactions, which mostly affected the skin and blood, were only rarely reproduced by a single component, suggesting an interaction. However, these findings have not been confirmed, and their impact is unclear.

Probenecid

Probenecid inhibits the tubular resorption of anions and inhibits the renal excretion of most beta-lactam antibiotics (354,355).

Vecuronium

There are various conflicting reports about acute interactions of beta-lactam antibiotics, especially acylaminopenicillins (apalcillin, azlocillin, mezlocillin, piperacillin), with vecuronium, leading to prolongation of muscle blockade. Reports of clinically relevant effects (356–358) conflict with reports of no effect (359).

Food–Drug Interactions

Co-administration of acid-labile beta-lactams, such as penicillin and ampicillin, with food reduces their systemic availability by lowering gastric pH and delaying gastric emptying (360).

Food increases the systemic availability of some cephalosporin prodrug esters, possibly by improving dissolution or blocking premature hydrolysis (361,362).

Interference with Diagnostic Tests

Aminoglycosides

Plasma aminoglycoside concentrations can be falsely low because they are inactivated by penicillins and cephalosporins. This effect occurred in plasma stored for 24 hours or longer before measurement (363–365).

Coombs' test

There are often false-positive antiglobulin tests by non-immunologically bound serum proteins, especially with cephalosporins, clavulanic acid, and imipenem + cilastin. This is a source of difficulty in cross-matching blood products.

Glycosuria

Urine samples containing beta-lactams should be tested for glucose by the glucose oxidase method, since falsely high values are observed with the copper reduction method (366,367).

Ciclosporin measurement

A retrospective study found an increased risk of ciclosporin-associated early nephrotoxicity in nafcillin-treated patients, despite the fact that ciclosporin concentrations were not different from controls (368). Possible interference of nafcillin with ciclosporin measurement, giving rise to falsely low concentrations, was considered as a possible explanation.

References

1. Morin RB, Gorman M, editors. The Chemistry and Biology of the Beta-lactam Antibiotics. New York: Academic Press, 1982;1–3.
2. Waxman DJ, Strominger JL. Penicillin-binding proteins and the mechanism of action of beta-lactam antibiotics. Annu Rev Biochem 1983;52:825–69.
3. Frere JM, Joris B. Penicillin-sensitive enzymes in peptidoglycan biosynthesis. Crit Rev Microbiol 1985;11(4):299–396.
4. Neftel KA, Hafkemeyer P, Cottagnoud P, Eich G, Hübscher U. Did evolutionary forerunners of betalactam antibiotics bind to nucleid acid replication enzymes? In: 50 Years of Penicillin Application. Berlin, Prague: Technische Universität Berlin, 1993:394.
5. Rello J, Gatell JM, Miro JM, Martinez JA, Soriano E, Garcia San Miguel J. Effectos secundarios asociados a la cloxacillina. [Secondary effects associated with cloxacillin.] Med Clin (Barc) 1987;89(15):631–3.
6. Olaison L, Belin L, Hogevik H, Alestig K. Incidence of beta-lactam-induced delayed hypersensitivity and neutropenia during treatment of infective endocarditis. Arch Intern Med 1999;159(6):607–15.
7. Himelright IM, Keerasuntonpong A, McReynolds JA, Smith EA, Abell E, Smith RJ, Baddour LM. Gender predilection of antibiotic-induced granulocytopenia in outpatients with septic arthritis or osteomyelitis. Infect Dis Clin Pract 1997;6:183.
8. Reed MD, Stern RC, Myers CM, Klinger JD, Yamashita TS, Blumer JL. Therapeutic evaluation of piperacillin for acute pulmonary exacerbations in cystic fibrosis. Pediatr Pulmonol 1987;3(2):101–9.
9. Sanders WE Jr, Johnson JE 3rd, Taggart JG. Adverse reactions to cephalothin and cephapirin. Uniform occurrence on prolonged intravenous administration of high doses. N Engl J Med 1974;290(8):424–9.
10. Lang R, Lishner M, Ravid M. Adverse reactions to prolonged treatment with high doses of carbenicillin and ureidopenicillins. Rev Infect Dis 1991;13(1):68–72.
11. Stead RJ, Kennedy HG, Hodson ME, Batten JC. Adverse reactions to piperacillin in cystic fibrosis. Lancet 1984;1(8381):857–8.
12. Strandvik B. Adverse reactions to piperacillin in patients with cystic fibrosis. Lancet 1984;1(8390):1362.
13. Brock PG, Roach M. Adverse reactions to piperacillin in cystic fibrosis. Lancet 1984;1(8385):1070–1.
14. McDonnell TJ, FitzGerald MX. Cystic fibrosis and penicillin hypersensitivity. Lancet 1984;1(8389):1301–2.
15. Stead RJ, Kennedy HG, Hodson ME, Batten JC. Adverse reactions to piperacillin in adults with cystic fibrosis. Thorax 1985;40(3):184–6.
16. Koch C, Hjelt K, Pedersen SS, Jensen ET, Jensen T, Lanng S, Valerius NH, Pedersen M, Hoiby N. Retrospective clinical study of hypersensitivity reactions to aztreonam and six other beta-lactam antibiotics in cystic fibrosis patients receiving multiple treatment courses. Rev Infect Dis 1991;13(Suppl 7):S608–11.
17. Pleasants RA, Walker TR, Samuelson WM. Allergic reactions to parenteral beta-lactam antibiotics in patients with cystic fibrosis. Chest 1994;106(4):1124–8.
18. Wills R, Henry RL, Francis JL. Antibiotic hypersensitivity reactions in cystic fibrosis. J Paediatr Child Health 1998;34(4):325–9.
19. Mallon P, Murphy P, Elborn S. Fever associated with intravenous antibiotics in adults with cystic fibrosis. Lancet 1997;350(9092):1676–7.
20. Yamabe S, Adachi K, Watanabe M, Ueda S. The effects of three beta-lactamase inhibitors: YTR830H, sulbactam and clavulanic acid on the growth of human cells in culture. Chemioterapia 1987;6(5):337–40.
21. Vidal Pan C, Gonzalez Quintela A, Roman Garcia J, Millan I, Martin Martin F, Moya Mir M. Cephapirin-induced neutropenia. Chemotherapy 1989;35(6):449–53.
22. Antoniadis A, Muller WE, Wollert U. Benzodiazepine receptor interactions may be involved in the neurotoxicity of various penicillin derivatives. Ann Neurol 1980;8(1):71–3.
23. Neftel KA, Hubscher U. Effects of beta-lactam antibiotics on proliferating eucaryotic cells. Antimicrob Agents Chemother 1987;31(11):1657–61.
24. Bloom JC, Lewis HB, Sellers TS, Deldar A. The hematologic effects of cefonicid and cefazedone in the dog: a potential model of cephalosporin hematotoxicity in man. Toxicol Appl Pharmacol 1987;90(1):135–42.
25. Deldar A, Lewis H, Bloom J, Weiss L. Cephalosporin-induced changes in the ultrastructure of canine bone marrow. Vet Pathol 1988;25(3):211–18.
26. Neftel KA, Hauser SP, Muller MR. Inhibition of granulopoiesis in vivo and in vitro by beta-lactam antibiotics. J Infect Dis 1985;152(1):90–8.
27. Bloom JC, Thiem PA, Sellers TS, Deldar A, Lewis HB. Cephalosporin-induced immune cytopenia in the dog: demonstration of erythrocyte-, neutrophil-, and platelet-associated IgG following treatment with cefazedone. Am J Hematol 1988;28(2):71–8.
28. Rouveix B, Lassoued K, Regnier B. Neutropénies induites par les bétalactamines: mécanisme toxique ou immun? [Beta lactam-induced neutropenia: toxic or immune mechanism?] Therapie 1988;43(6):489–92.
29. Murphy MF, Riordan T, Minchinton RM, Chapman JF Amess JA, Shaw EJ, Waters AH. Demonstration of an immune-mediated mechanism of penicillin-induced

neutropenia and thrombocytopenia. Br J Haematol 1983;55(1):155–60.

30. Murphy MF, Metcalfe P, Grint PC, Green AR, Knowles S, Amess JA, Waters AH. Cephalosporin-induced immune neutropenia. Br J Haematol 1985;59(1):9–14.

31. Lee D, Dewdney JM, Edwards RG, Neftel KA, Walti M. Measurement of specific IgG antibody levels in serum of patients on regimes comprising high total dose beta-lactam therapy. Int Arch Allergy Appl Immunol 1986;79(4):344–8.

32. Charak BS, Brown EG, Mazumder A. Role of granulocyte colony-stimulating factor in preventing ceftazidime-induced myelosuppression in vitro. Bone Marrow Transplant 1995;15(5):749–55.

33. Hauser SP, Udupa KB, Lipschitz DA. Murine marrow stromal response to myelotoxic agents in vitro. Br J Haematol 1996;95(4):596–604.

34. Hauser SP, Allewelt MC, Lipschitz DA. Effects of myelotoxic agents on cytokine production in murine long-term bone marrow cultures. Stem Cells 1998;16(4):261–70.

35. Yen CJ, Tsai TJ, Chen HS, Fang CC, Yang CC, Lee PH, Lin RH, Tsai KS, Hung KY, Yen TS. Effects of intraperitoneal antibiotics on human peritoneal mesothelial cell growth. Nephron 1996;74(4):694–700.

36. Edin ML, Miclau T, Lester GE, Lindsey RW, Dahners LE. Effect of cefazolin and vancomycin on osteoblasts in vitro. Clin Orthop Relat Res 1996;(333):245–51.

37. Lanbeck P, Paulsen O. Cytotoxic effects of four antibiotics on endothelial cells. Pharmacol Toxicol 1995;77(6):365–70.

38. Friedland JS, Warrell DA. The Jarisch–Herxheimer reaction in leptospirosis: possible pathogenesis and review. Rev Infect Dis 1991;13(2):207–10.

39. Maloy AL, Black RD, Segurola RJ Jr. Lyme disease complicated by the Jarisch–Herxheimer reaction. J Emerg Med 1998;16(3):437–8.

40. Young EJ, Weingarten NM, Baughn RE, Duncan WC. Studies on the pathogenesis of the Jarisch–Herxheimer reaction: development of an animal model and evidence against a role for classical endotoxin. J Infect Dis 1982;146(5):606–15.

41. Negussie Y, Remick DG, DeForge LE, Kunkel SL, Eynon A, Griffin GE. Detection of plasma tumor necrosis factor, interleukins 6, and 8 during the Jarisch–Herxheimer reaction of relapsing fever. J Exp Med 1992;175(5):1207–12.

42. Fekade D, Knox K, Hussein K, Melka A, Lalloo DG, Coxon RE, Warrell DA. Prevention of Jarisch–Herxheimer reactions by treatment with antibodies against tumor necrosis factor alpha. N Engl J Med 1996;335(5):311–15.

43. Johnson HC, Walker A. Convulsive factor in commercial penicillin. Arch Surg 1945;50:69.

44. Macdonald RL, Barker JL. Pentylenetetrazol and penicillin are selective antagonists of GABA-mediated postsynaptic inhibition in cultured mammalian neurones. Nature 1977;267(5613):720–1.

45. Chow P, Mathers D. Convulsant doses of penicillin shorten the lifetime of GABA-induced channels in cultured central neurones. Br J Pharmacol 1986;88(3):541–7.

46. Schliamser SE, Cars O, Norrby SR. Neurotoxicity of beta-lactam antibiotics: predisposing factors and pathogenesis. J Antimicrob Chemother 1991;27(4):405–25.

47. Gutnick MJ, Prince DA. Penicillinase and the convulsant action of penicillin. Neurology 1971;21(7):759–64.

48. Sobotka P, Safanda J. The epileptogenic action of penicillins: structure–activity relationship. J Mol Med 1976;1:151.

49. Sunagawa M, Nouda H. [Neurotoxicity of carbapenem compounds and other beta-lactam antibiotics.] Jpn J Antibiot 1996;49(1):1–16.

50. Barrons RW, Murray KM, Richey RM. Populations at risk for penicillin-induced seizures. Ann Pharmacother 1992;26(1):26–9.

51. Grondahl TO, Langmoen IA. Epileptogenic effect of antibiotic drugs. J Neurosurg 1993;78(6):938–43.

52. De Sarro A, Ammendola D, Zappala M, Grasso S, De Sarro GB. Relationship between structure and convulsant properties of some beta-lactam antibiotics following intracerebroventricular microinjection in rats. Antimicrob Agents Chemother 1995;39(1):232–7.

53. Winston DJ, Ho WG, Bruckner DA, Champlin RE. Beta-lactam antibiotic therapy in febrile granulocytopenic patients. A randomized trial comparing cefoperazone plus piperacillin, ceftazidime plus piperacillin, and imipenem alone. Ann Intern Med 1991;115(11):849–59.

54. Rolston KV, Berkey P, Bodey GP, Anaissie EJ, Khardori NM, Joshi JH, Keating MJ, Holmes FA, Cabanillas FF, Elting L. A comparison of imipenem to ceftazidime with or without amikacin as empiric therapy in febrile neutropenic patients. Arch Intern Med 1992;152(2):283–91.

55. Pestotnik SL, Classen DC, Evans RS, Stevens LE, Burke JP. Prospective surveillance of imipenem/cilastatin use and associated seizures using a hospital information system. Ann Pharmacother 1993;27(4):497–501.

56. De Sarro A, Zappala M, Chimirri A, Grasso S, De Sarro GB. Quinolones potentiate cefazolin-induced seizures in DBA/2 mice. Antimicrob Agents Chemother 1993;37(7):1497–503.

57. De Sarro A, Ammendola D, De Sarro G. Effects of some quinolones on imipenem-induced seizures in DBA/2 mice. Gen Pharmacol 1994;25(2):369–79.

58. Berry M, Gurung A, Easty DL. Toxicity of antibiotics and antifungals on cultured human corneal cells: effect of mixing, exposure and concentration. Eye 1995;9(Pt 1):110–15.

59. Duch-Samper AM, Capdevila C, Menezo JL, Hurtado-Sarrio M. Endothelial toxicity of ceftazidime in anterior chamber irrigation solution Exp Eye Res 1996;63(6):739–45.

60. Holme E, Greter J, Jacobson CE, Lindstedt S, Nordin I, Kristiansson B, Jodal U. Carnitine deficiency induced by pivampicillin and pivmecillinam therapy. Lancet 1989;2(8661):469–73.

61. Melegh B, Kerner J, Bieber LL. Pivampicillin-promoted excretion of pivaloylcarnitine in humans. Biochem Pharmacol 1987;36(20):3405–9.

62. Abrahamsson K, Eriksson BO, Holme E, Jodal U, Jonsson A, Lindstedt S. Pivalic acid-induced carnitine deficiency and physical exercise in humans. Metabolism 1996;45(12):1501–7.

63. Holme E, Jodal U, Linstedt S, Nordin I. Effects of pivalic acid-containing prodrugs on carnitine homeostasis and on response to fasting in children. Scand J Clin Lab Invest 1992;52(5):361–72.

64. Nakashima M, Kosuge K, Ishii I, Ohtsubo M. [Influence of multiple-dose administration of cefetamet pivoxil on blood and urinary concentrations of carnitine and effects of simultaneous administration of carnitine with cefetamet pivoxil.] Jpn J Antibiot 1996;49(10):966–79.

65. Melegh B, Pap M, Molnar D, Masszi G, Kopcsanyi G. Carnitine administration ameliorates the changes in energy metabolism caused by short-term pivampicillin medication. Eur J Pediatr 1997;156(10):795–9.

66. Baron DN, Hamilton-Miller JM, Brumfitt W. Sodium content of injectable beta-lactam antibiotics. Lancet 1984;1(8386):1113–14.

67. Gatell JM, Rello J, Miro JM, Martinez JA, Soriano E, SanMiguel Garcia J. Cloxacillin-induced neutropenia. J Infect Dis 1986;154(2):372.

68. Olaison L, Alestig K. A prospective study of neutropenia induced by high doses of beta-lactam antibiotics. J Antimicrob Chemother 1990;25(3):449–53.

69. Neftel KA, Walti M, Schulthess HK, Gubler J. Adverse reactions following intravenous penicillin-G relate to degradation of the drug in vitro. Klin Wochenschr 1984;62(1):25–9.

70. Vial T, Pofilet C, Pham E, Payen C, Evreux JC. Agranulocytoses aiguës médicamenteuses: expérience du Centre Régional de Pharmacovigilance de Lyon sur 7 ans. [Acute drug-induced agranulocytosis: experience of the Regional Center of Pharmacovigilance of Lyon over 7 years.] Therapie 1996;51(5):508–15.

71. Neu HC. Safety of cefepime: a new extended-spectrum parenteral cephalosporin. Am J Med 1996;100(6A):S68–75.

72. Saez-Llorens X, Castano E, Garcia R, Baez C, Perez M, Tejeira F, McCracken GH Jr. Prospective randomized comparison of cefepime and cefotaxime for treatment of bacterial meningitis in infants and children. Antimicrob Agents Chemother 1995;39(4):937–40.

73. Dahlgren AF. Two cases of possible cefepime-induced neutropenia. Am J Health Syst Pharm 1997;54(22):2621–2.

74. Gerber L, Wing EJ. Life-threatening neutropenia secondary to piperacillin/tazobactam therapy. Clin Infect Dis 1995;21(4):1047–8.

75. Wilson C, Greenhood G, Remington JS, Vosti KL. Neutropenia after consecutive treatment courses with nafcillin and piperacillin. Lancet 1979;1(8126):1150.

76. Oldfield EC 3rd. Leukopenia associated with the use of beta-lactam antibiotics in patients with hepatic dysfunction. Am J Gastroenterol 1994;89(8):1263–4.

77. Ramos Fernandez de Soria R, Martin Nunez G, Sanchez Gil F. Agranulocitosis inducida por drogas. Rapida recuperacion con el uso precoz de G-CSF. [Agranulocytosis induced by drugs. Rapid recovery with the early use of G-CSF.] Sangre (Barc) 1994;39(2):145–6.

78. Bradford CR, Ong EL, Hendrick DJ, Saunders PW. Use of colony stimulating factors for the treatment of drug-induced agranulocytosis. Br J Haematol 1993;84(1):182–3.

79. Borgbjerg BM, Hovgaard D, Laursen JB, Aldershvile J. Granulocyte colony stimulating factor in neutropenic patients with infective endocarditis. Heart 1998;79(1):93–5.

80. Levine BB, Redmond AP, Fellner MJ, Voss HE, Levytska V. Penicillin allergy and the heterogenous immune responses of man to benzylpenicillin. J Clin Invest 1966;45(12):1895–906.

81. Petz LD, Fudenberg HH. Coombs-positive hemolytic anemia caused by penicillin administration. N Engl J Med 1966;274(4):171–8.

82. Funicella T, Weinger RS, Moake JL, Spruell M, Rossen RD. Penicillin-induced immunohemolytic anemia associated with circulating immune complexes. Am J Hematol 1977;3:219–23.

83. Garratty G. Review: Immune hemolytic anemia and/or positive direct antiglobulin tests caused by drugs. Immunohematol 1994;10(2):41–50.

84. Petz LD, Garratty G. Acquired Immune Hemolytic Anemias. New York: Churchill Livingstone, 1980.

85. Williams ME, Thomas D, Harman CP, Mintz PD, Donowitz GR. Positive direct antiglobulin tests due to clavulanic acid. Antimicrob Agents Chemother 1985;27(1):125–7.

86. Norrby SR. Side effects of cephalosporins. Drugs 1987;34(Suppl 2):105–20.

87. Barza M, Furie B, Brown AE, Furie BC. Defects in vitamin K-dependent carboxylation associated with moxalactam treatment. J Infect Dis 1986;153(6):1166–9.

88. Andrassy K, Koderisch J. An open study on hemostasis in 20 patients with normal and impaired renal function treated with cefotetan alone or combined with tobramycin. In: Abstracts, 15th International Congress of Chemotherapy. Istanbul, 1987.

89. Conly JM, Ramotar K, Chubb H, Bow EJ, Louie TJ. Hypoprothrombinemia in febrile, neutropenic patients with cancer: association with antimicrobial suppression of intestinal microflora. J Infect Dis 1984;150(2):202–12.

90. Holt J. Hypoprothrombinemia and bleeding diathesis associated with cefotetan therapy in surgical patients. Arch Surg 1988;123(4):523.

91. Hicks MJ, Flaitz CM. The role of antibiotics in platelet dysfunction and coagulopathy. Int J Antimicrob Agents 1993;2:129.

92. Shirakawa H, Komai M, Kimura S. Antibiotic-induced vitamin K deficiency and the role of the presence of intestinal flora. Int J Vitam Nutr Res 1990;60(3):245–51.

93. Williams KJ, Bax RP, Brown H, Machin SJ. Antibiotic treatment and associated prolonged prothrombin time. J Clin Pathol 1991;44(9):738–41.

94. Lipsky JJ. Antibiotic-associated hypoprothrombinaemia. J Antimicrob Chemother 1988;21(3):281–300.

95. Sattler FR, Weitekamp MR, Sayegh A, Ballard JO. Impaired hemostasis caused by beta-lactam antibiotics. Am J Surg 1988;155(5A):30–9.

96. Lipsky JJ. Mechanism of the inhibition of the gamma-carboxylation of glutamic acid by N-methylthiotetrazole-containing antibiotics. Proc Natl Acad Sci USA 1984; 81(9):2893–7.

97. Suttie JW, Engelke JA, McTigue J. Effect of N-methyl-thiotetrazole on rat liver microsomal vitamin K-dependent carboxylation. Biochem Pharmacol 1986;35(14): 2429–33.

98. Uchida K, Yoshida T, Komeno T. Mechanism for hypoprothrombinemia caused by N-methyltetrazolethiol (NNTT)-containing antibiotics. Abstracts, 15th International Congress of Chemotherapy. Istanbul, 1987:1153.

99. Shearer MJ, Bechtold H, Andrassy K, Koderisch J, McCarthy PT, Trenk D, Jahnchen E, Ritz E. Mechanism of cephalosporin-induced hypoprothrombinemia: relation to cephalosporin side chain, vitamin K metabolism, and vitamin K status. J Clin Pharmacol 1988;28(1):88–95.

100. Jones P, Bodey GP, Rolston K, Fainstein V, Riccardi S. Cefoperazone plus mezlocillin for empiric therapy of febrile cancer patients. Am J Med 1988;85(1A):3–8.

101. Brown RB, Klar J, Lemeshow S, Teres D, Pastides H, Sands M. Enhanced bleeding with cefoxitin or moxalactam. Statistical analysis within a defined population of 1493 patients. Arch Intern Med 1986;146(11):2159–64.

102. Boyd DB, Lunn WH. Electronic structures of cephalosporins and penicillins. 9. Departure of a leaving group in cephalosporins. J Med Chem 1979;22(7):778–84.

103. Mizojiri K, Norikura R, Takashima A, Tanaka H, Yoshimori T, Inazawa K, Yukawa T, Okabe H, Sugeno K. Disposition of moxalactam and N-methyl-tetrazolethiol in rats and monkeys. Antimicrob Agents Chemother 1987;31(8):1169–76.

104. Schentag JJ, Welage LS, Williams JS, Wilton JH, Adelman MH, Rigan D, Grasela TH. Kinetics and action of N-methylthiotetrazole in volunteers and patients. Population-based clinical comparisons of antibiotics with and without this moiety. Am J Surg 1988;155(5A):40–4.

105. Fletcher C, Pearson C, Choi SC, Duma RJ, Evans HJ, Qureshi GD. In vitro comparison of antiplatelet effects of beta-lactam penicillins. J Lab Clin Med 1986;108(3): 217–23.

106. Bang NU, Tessler SS, Heidenreich RO, Marks CA, Mattler LE. Effects of moxalactam on blood coagulation and platelet function. Rev Infect Dis 1982; 4(Suppl): S546–54.

107. Weitekamp MR, Aber RC. Prolonged bleeding times and bleeding diathesis associated with moxalactam administration. JAMA 1983;249(1):69–71.

108. Weitekamp MR, Caputo GM, Al-Mondhiry HA, Aber RC. The effects of latamoxef, cefotaxime, and cefoperazone on platelet function and coagulation in normal volunteers. J Antimicrob Chemother 1985;16(1):95–101.

109. Weitekamp MR, Holmes P, Walker ME. A double blind study on the effects of cefoperazone (CPZ), ceftizoxime (CTZ), moxalactam (MOX) on platelet function and prothrombin time in normal volunteers. In: Abstracts, 25th Interscience Conference on Antimicrobial Agents and Chemotherapy. Minneapolis, Minnesota, 1985:959.

110. Fass RJ, Copelan EA, Brandt JT, Moeschberger ML, Ashton JJ. Platelet-mediated bleeding caused by broadspectrum penicillins. J Infect Dis 1987;155(6):1242–8.

111. Norrby R, Foord RD, Hedlund P. Clinical and pharmacokinetic studies on cefuroxime. J Antimicrob Chemother 1977;3(4):355–62.

112. Burroughs SF, Johnson GJ. Beta-lactam antibiotic-induced platelet dysfunction: evidence for irreversible inhibition of platelet activation in vitro and in vivo after prolonged exposure to penicillin. Blood 1990;75(7):1473–80.

113. Knudsen ET, Harding JW. A multicentre comparative trial of talampicillin and ampicillin in general practice. Br J Clin Pract 1975;29(10):255–64.

114. Ewe K. Diarrhoea and constipation. Baillieres Clin Gastroenterol 1988;2(2):353–84.

115. Hooker KD, DiPiro JT. Effect of antimicrobial therapy on bowel flora. Clin Pharm 1988;7(12):878–88.

116. Bartlett JG. Antibiotic-associated diarrhea. Clin Infect Dis 1992;15(4):573–81.

117. Kelly CP, Pothoulakis C, LaMont JT. Clostridium difficile colitis. N Engl J Med 1994;330(4):257–62.

118. George WL. Antimicrobial agent-associated colitis and diarrhea: historical background and clinical aspects. Rev Infect Dis 1984;6(Suppl 1):S208–13.

119. Talbot RW, Walker RC, Beart RW Jr. Changing epidemiology, diagnosis, and treatment of Clostridium difficile toxin-associated colitis. Br J Surg 1986;73(6):457–60.

120. Hogenauer C, Hammer HF, Krejs GJ, Reisinger EC. Mechanisms and management of antibiotic-associated diarrhea. Clin Infect Dis 1998;27(4):702–10.

121. Johnson S, Gerding DN. Clostridium difficile-associated diarrhea. Clin Infect Dis 1998;26(5):1027–34.

122. Larson HE, Price AB. Pseudomembranous colitis: Presence of clostridial toxin. Lancet 1977;2(8052–8053):1312–14.

123. Borriello SP. 12th C. L. Oakley lecture. Pathogenesis of Clostridium difficile infection of the gut. J Med Microbiol 1990;33(4):207–15.

124. Bartlett JG. Clostridium difficile: history of its role as an enteric pathogen and the current state of knowledge about the organism. Clin Infect Dis 1994;18(Suppl 4):S265–72.

125. Anand A, Glatt AE. Clostridium difficile infection associated with antineoplastic chemotherapy: a review. Clin Infect Dis 1993;17(1):109–13.

126. Bartlett JG. Antibiotic-associated pseudomembranous colitis. Rev Infect Dis 1979;1(3):530–9.

127. Aronsson B, Mollby R, Nord CE. Antimicrobial agents and Clostridium difficile in acute enteric disease: epidemiological data from Sweden, 1980–1982. J Infect Dis 1985;151(3):476–81.

128. Aronsson B, Mollby R, Nord CE. Clostridium difficile and antibiotic associated diarrhoea in Sweden. Scand J Infect Dis Suppl 1982;35:53–8.

129. Fekety R, Shah AB. Diagnosis and treatment of Clostridium difficile colitis. JAMA 1993;269(1):71–5.

130. Barbut F, Corthier G, Charpak Y, Cerf M, Monteil H, Fosse T, Trevoux A, De Barbeyrac B, Boussougant Y, Tigaud S, Tytgat F, Sedallian A, Duborgel S, Collignon A, Le Guern ME, Bernasconi P, Petit JC. Prevalence and pathogenicity of Clostridium difficile in hospitalized patients. A French multicenter study. Arch Intern Med 1996;156(13):1449–54.

131. Zehnder D, Kunzi UP, Maibach R, Zoppi M, Halter F, Neftel KA, Muller U, Galeazzi RL, Hess T, Hoigne R. Die Häufigkeit der Antibiotika-assoziierten Kolitis bei hospitalisierten Patienten der Jahre 1974–1991 im 'Comprehensive Hospital Drug Monitoring' Bern/St. Gallen. [Frequency of antibiotics-associated colitis in hospitalized patients in 1974–1991 in "Comprehensive Hospital Drug Monitoring," Bern/St. Gallen.] Schweiz Med Wochenschr 1995;125(14):676–83.

132. Burke GW, Wilson ME, Mehrez IO. Absence of diarrhea in toxic megacolon complicating Clostridium difficile pseudomembranous colitis. Am J Gastroenterol 1988;83(3):304–7.

133. Toffler RB, Pingoud EG, Burrell MI. Acute colitis related to penicillin and penicillin derivatives. Lancet 1978;2(8092 Pt 1):707–9.

134. Finegold SM. Clinical considerations in the diagnosis of antimicrobial agent-associated gastroenteritis. Diagn Microbiol Infect Dis 1986;4(Suppl 3):S87–91.

135. Viscidi R, Willey S, Bartlett JG. Isolation rates and toxigenic potential of Clostridium difficile isolates from various patient populations. Gastroenterology 1981;81(1):5–9.

136. Shim JK, Johnson S, Samore MH, Bliss DZ, Gerding DN. Primary symptomless colonisation by Clostridium difficile and decreased risk of subsequent diarrhoea. Lancet 1998;351(9103):633–6.

137. Mardh PA, Helin I, Colleen I, Oberg M, Holst E. Clostridium difficile toxin in faecal specimens of healthy children and children with diarrhoea. Acta Paediatr Scand 1982;71(2):275–8.

138. Pitts NE, Gilbert GS, Knirsch AK, Noguchi Y. Worldwide clinical experience with sultamicillin. APMIS Suppl 1989;5:23–34.

139. McLinn SE, Moskal M, Goldfarb J, Bodor F, Aronovitz G, Schwartz R, Self P, Ossi MJ. Comparison of cefuroxime axetil and amoxicillin–clavulanate suspensions in treatment of acute otitis media with effusion in children. Antimicrob Agents Chemother 1994;38(2):315–18.

140. Todd PA, Benfield P. Amoxicillin/clavulanic acid. An update of its antibacterial activity, pharmacokinetic properties and therapeutic use. Drugs 1990;39(2):264–307.

141. Friedel HA, Campoli-Richards DM, Goa KL. Sultamicillin. A review of its antibacterial activity, pharmacokinetic properties and therapeutic use. Drugs 1989;37(4):491–522.

142. Caron F, Ducrotte P, Lerebours E, Colin R, Humbert G, Denis P. Effects of amoxicillin–clavulanate combination on the motility of the small intestine in human beings. Antimicrob Agents Chemother 1991;35(6):1085–8.

143. Cerquetti M, Pantosti A, Gentile G, D'Ambrosio F, Mastrantonio P. Epidemie ospedaliere di diarrea da Clostridium difficile: dimostrazione di infezione crociata mediante tecniche di tipizzazione. [Hospital epidemic of Clostridium difficile diarrhea: demonstration of cross-infection using a typing technic.] Ann Ist Super Sanita 1989;25(2):327–32.

144. McFarland LV, Surawicz CM, Stamm WE. Risk factors for Clostridium difficile carriage and C. difficile-associated diarrhea in a cohort of hospitalized patients. J Infect Dis 1990;162(3):678–84.

145. Nolan NP, Kelly CP, Humphreys JF, Cooney C, O'Connor R, Walsh TN, Weir DG, O'Briain DS. An epidemic of pseudomembranous colitis: importance of person to person spread. Gut 1987;28(11):1467–73.

146. Impallomeni M, Galletly NP, Wort SJ, Starr JM, Rogers TR. Increased risk of diarrhoea caused by Clostridium difficile in elderly patients receiving cefotaxime. BMJ 1995;311(7016):1345–6.

147. Starr JM, Rogers TR, Impallomeni M. Hospital-acquired *Clostridium difficile* diarrhoea and herd immunity. Lancet 1997;349(9049):426–8.

148. Tedesco FJ. Clindamycin and colitis: a review. J Infect Dis 1977;135(Suppl):S95–8.

149. Milstone EB, McDonald AJ, Scholhamer CF Jr. Pseudomembranous colitis after topical application of clindamycin. Arch Dermatol 1981;117(3):154–5.

150. Hecht JR, Olinger EJ. *Clostridium difficile* colitis secondary to intravenous vancomycin. Dig Dis Sci 1989;34(1):148–9.

151. Saginur R, Hawley CR, Bartlett JG. Colitis associated with metronidazole therapy. J Infect Dis 1980;141(6):772–4.

152. Brown E, Talbot GH, Axelrod P, Provencher M, Hoegg C. Risk factors for *Clostridium difficile* toxin-associated diarrhea. Infect Control Hosp Epidemiol 1990;11(6):283–90.

153. Gerding DN, Olson MM, Peterson LR, Teasley DG, Gebhard RL, Schwartz ML, Lee JT Jr. *Clostridium difficile*-associated diarrhea and colitis in adults. A prospective case-controlled epidemiologic study. Arch Intern Med 1986;146(1):95–100.

154. Church JM, Fazio VW. A role for colonic statis in the pathogenesis of disease related to *Clostridium difficile*. Dis Colon Rectum 1986;146:95.

155. Pierce PF Jr, Wilson R, Silva J Jr, Garagusi VF, Rifkin GD, Fekety R, Nunez-Montiel O, Dowell VR Jr, Hughes JM. Antibiotic-associated pseudomembranous colitis: an epidemiologic investigation of a cluster of cases. J Infect Dis 1982;145(2):269–74.

156. de Lalla F, Privitera G, Ortisi G, Rizzardini G, Santoro D, Pagano A, Rinaldi E, Scarpellini P. Third generation cephalosporins as a risk factor for *Clostridium difficile*-associated disease: a four-year survey in a general hospital. J Antimicrob Chemother 1989;23(4):623–31.

157. Cheng SH, Lu JJ, Young TG, Perng CL, Chi WM. *Clostridium difficile*-associated diseases: comparison of symptomatic infection versus carriage on the basis of risk factors, toxin production, and genotyping results. Clin Infect Dis 1997;25(1):157–8.

158. Samore M, Killgore G, Johnson S, Goodman R, Shim J, Venkataraman L, Sambol S, DeGirolami P, Tenover F, Arbeit R, Gerding D. Multicenter typing comparison of sporadic and outbreak *Clostridium difficile* isolates from geographically diverse hospitals. J Infect Dis 1997;176(5):1233–8.

159. Hirschhorn LR, Trnka Y, Onderdonk A, Lee ML, Platt R. Epidemiology of community-acquired *Clostridium difficile*-associated diarrhea. J Infect Dis 1994;169(1):127–33.

160. Lyerly DM, Krivan HC, Wilkins TD. *Clostridium difficile*: its disease and toxins. Clin Microbiol Rev 1988;1(1):1–18.

161. Wren B, Heard SR, Tabaqchali S. Association between production of toxins A and B and types of *Clostridium difficile*. J Clin Pathol 1987;40(12):1397–401.

162. Seppala K, Hjelt L, Sipponen P. Colonoscopy in the diagnosis of antibiotic-associated colitis. A prospective study. Scand J Gastroenterol 1981;16(4):465–8.

163. Mukai JK, Janower ML. Diagnosis of pseudomembranous colitis by computed tomography: a report of two patients. Can Assoc Radiol J 1987;38(1):62–3.

164. Woods GL, Iwwen PC. Comparison of a dot immunobinding assay, latex agglutination, and cytotoxin assay for laboratory diagnosis of *Clostridium difficile*-associated diarrhea. J Clin Microbiol 1990;28(5):855–7.

165. Morris JB, Zollinger RM Jr, Stellato TA. Role of surgery in antibiotic-induced pseudomembranous enterocolitis. Am J Surg 1990;160(5):535–9.

166. Van Ness MM, Cattau EL Jr. Fulminant colitis complicating antibiotic-associated pseudomembranous colitis: case report and review of the clinical manifestations and treatment. Am J Gastroenterol 1987;82(4):374–7.

167. Wenisch C, Parschalk B, Hasenhundl M, Hirschl AM, Graninger W. Comparison of vancomycin, teicoplanin, metronidazole, and fusidic acid for the treatment of *Clostridium difficile*-associated diarrhea. Clin Infect Dis 1996;22(5):813–18.

168. Teasley DG, Gerding DN, Olson MM, Peterson LR, Gebhard RL, Schwartz MJ, Lee JT Jr. Prospective randomised trial of metronidazole versus vancomycin for *Clostridium-difficile*-associated diarrhoea and colitis. Lancet 1983;2(8358):1043–6.

169. Bartlett JG. Treatment of antibiotic-associated pseudomembranous colitis. Rev Infect Dis 1984;6(Suppl 1):S235–41.

170. de Lalla F, Santoro D, Rinaldi E, Suter F, Cruciani M, Guaglianone MH, Rizzardini G, Pellegata G. Teicoplanin in the treatment of infections by staphylococci, *Clostridium difficile* and other Gram-positive bacteria. J Antimicrob Chemother 1989;23(1):131–42.

171. Buggy BP, Fekety R, Silva J Jr. Therapy of relapsing *Clostridium difficile*-associated diarrhea and colitis with the combination of vancomycin and rifampin. J Clin Gastroenterol 1987;9(2):155–9.

172. Ariano RE, Zhanel GG, Harding GK. The role of anion-exchange resins in the treatment of antibiotic-associated pseudomembranous colitis. CMAJ 1990;142(10):1049–51.

173. Taylor NS, Bartlett JG. Binding of *Clostridium difficile* cytotoxin and vancomycin by anion-exchange resins. J Infect Dis 1980;141(1):92–7.

174. Gorbach SL, Chang TW, Goldin B. Successful treatment of relapsing *Clostridium difficile* colitis with *Lactobacillus* GG. Lancet 1987;2(8574):1519.

175. Bowden TA Jr, Mansberger AR Jr, Lykins LE. Pseudomembraneous enterocolitis: mechanism for restoring floral homeostasis. Am Surg 1981;47(4):178–83.

176. McFarland LV, Surawicz CM, Greenberg RN, Elmer GW, Moyer KA, Melcher SA, Bowen KE, Cox JL. Prevention of beta-lactam-associated diarrhea by *Saccharomyces boulardii* compared with placebo. Am J Gastroenterol 1995;90(3):439–48.

177. Novak E, Lee JG, Seckman CE, Phillips JP, DiSanto AR. Unfavorable effect of atropine-diphenoxylate (Lomotil) therapy in lincomycin-caused diarrhea. JAMA 1976;235(14):1451–4.

178. Olans RN, Weiner LB. Reversible oxacillin hepatotoxicity. J Pediatr 1976;89(5):835–8.

179. Michelson PA. Reversible high dose oxacillin-associated liver injury. Can J Hosp Pharm 1981;34:83.

180. Onorato IM, Axelrod JL. Hepatitis from intravenous high-dose oxacillin therapy: findings in an adult inpatient population. Ann Intern Med 1978;89(4):497–500.

181. Fairley CK, McNeil JJ, Desmond P, Smallwood R, Young H, Forbes A, Purcell P, Boyd I. Risk factors for development of flucloxacillin associated jaundice. BMJ 1993;306(6872):233–5.

182. Turner IB, Eckstein RP, Riley JW, Lunzer MR. Prolonged hepatic cholestasis after flucloxacillin therapy. Med J Aust 1989;151(11–12):701–5.

183. Devereaux BM, Crawford DH, Purcell P, Powell LW, Roeser HP. Flucloxacillin associated cholestatic hepatitis. An Australian and Swedish epidemic? Eur J Clin Pharmacol 1995;49(1–2):81–5.

184. Kleinman MS, Presberg JE. Cholestatic hepatitis after dicloxacillin-sodium therapy. J Clin Gastroenterol 1986;8(1):77–8.

185. Ditlove J, Weidmann P, Bernstein M, Massry SG. Methicillin nephritis. Medicine (Baltimore) 1977;56(6):483–91.

186. Galpin JE, Shinaberger JH, Stanley TM, Blumenkrantz MJ, Bayer AS, Friedman GS, Montgomerie JZ, Guze LB, Coburn JW, Glassock RJ. Acute interstitial nephritis due to methicillin. Am J Med 1978;65(5):756–65.

187. Sanjad SA, Haddad GG, Nassar VH. Nephropathy, an underestimated complication of methicillin therapy. J Pediatr 1974;84(6):873–7.

188. Neftel KA. Verträglichkeit der hochdosierten Therapie mit Betalactam-Antibiotika-Pathogenese der Nebenwirkungen insbesondere der Neutropenie. Fortschr Antimikr Antineoplast Chemother 1984;3–1:71.

189. Bigby M, Jick S, Jick H, Arndt K. Drug-induced cutaneous reactions. A report from the Boston Collaborative Drug Surveillance Program on 15,438 consecutive inpatients, 1975 to 1982. JAMA 1986;256(24):3358–63.

190. Zurcher K, Krebs A. Cutaneous Drug Reactions. Basel: Karger-Verlag, 1991.

191. Stubb S, Heikkila H, Kauppinen K. Cutaneous reactions to drugs: a series of in-patients during a five-year period. Acta Derm Venereol 1994;74(4):289–91.

192. Hoigne R, Sonntag MR, Zoppi M, Hess T, Maibach R, Fritschy D. Occurrence of exanthema in relation to aminopenicillin preparations and allopurinol. N Engl J Med 1987;316(19):1217.

193. Arndt KA, Jick H. Rates of cutaneous reactions to drugs. A report from the Boston Collaborative Drug Surveillance Program. JAMA 1976;235(9):918–23.

194. Hunziker T, Hoigné RV, Kuenzi UP, et al. Comprehensive hospital drug monitoring (CHDM), the adverse skin reactions, a 20-years survey. Pharmacoepidemiology 1995;4(Suppl 1):S13.

195. Katz M, Seidenbaum M, Weinrauch L. Penicillin-induced generalized pustular psoriasis. J Am Acad Dermatol 1987;17(5 Pt 2):918–20.

196. Prieto A, de Barrio M, Lopez-Saez P, Baeza ML, de Benito V, Olalde S. Recurrent localized pustular eruption induced by amoxicillin. Allergy 1997;52(7):777–8.

197. Beylot C, Bioulac P, Doutre MS. Pustuloses exanthéma-tiques aiguës généralisées. [Acute generalized exanthematic pustuloses (four cases).] Ann Dermatol Venereol 1980;107(1–2):37–48.

198. Isogai Z, Sunohara A, Tsuji T. Pustular drug eruption due to bacampicilin hydrochloride in a patient with psoriasis. J Dermatol 1998;25(9):612–15.

199. Stough D, Guin JD, Baker GF, Haynie L. Pustular eruptions following administration of cefazolin: a possible interaction with methyldopa. J Am Acad Dermatol 1987;16(5 Pt 1):1051–2.

200. Fayol J, Bernard P, Bonnetblanc JM. Pustular eruption following administration of cefazolin: a second case report. J Am Acad Dermatol 1988;19(3):571.

201. Kalb RE, Grossman ME. Pustular eruption following administration of cephradine. Cutis 1986; 38(1):58–60.

202. Jackson H, Vion B, Levy PM. Generalized eruptive pustular drug rash due to cephalexin. Dermatologica 1988;177(5):292–4.

203. Ogoshi M, Yamada Y, Tani M. Acute generalized exanthematic pustulosis induced by cefaclor and acetazolamide. Dermatology 1992;184(2):142–4.

204. Spencer JM, Silvers DN, Grossman ME. Pustular eruption after drug exposure: is it pustular psoriasis or a pustular drug eruption? Br J Dermatol 1994;130(4):514–19.

205. McCloskey GL, Massa MC. Cephalexin rash in infectious mononucleosis. Cutis 1997;59(5):251–4.

206. Gell PGH, Coombs RRA. Classification of allergic reactions responsible for clinical hypersensitivity and disease. In: Gell PGH, Coombs RRA, Lachmann PJ, editors. Clinical Aspects of Immunology. Oxford: Blackwell Scientific Publications, 1975:251–4.

207. Plaut M, Zimmerman EM. Allergy and mechanisms of hypersensitivity. In: Paul WE, editor. Fundamental Immunology. 3rd ed. New York: Raven Press, 1993:1399.

208. De Weck AL. Pharmacologic and immunochemical mechanisms of drug hypersensitivity. Immunol Allergy Clin North Am 1991;11:461.

209. Lafaye P, Lapresle C. Fixation of penicilloyl groups to albumin and appearance of anti-penicilloyl antibodies in penicillin-treated patients. J Clin Invest 1988;82(1):7–12.

210. Bochner BS, Lichtenstein LM. Anaphylaxis. N Engl J Med 1991;324(25):1785–90.

211. Levine B, Redmond A. Immunochemical mechanisms of penicillin induced Coombs positivity and hemolytic anemia in man. Int Arch Allergy Appl Immunol 1967;31(6):594–606.

212. Abraham GN, Petz LD, Fudenberg HH. Immunohaematological cross-allergenicity between penicillin and cephalothin in humans. Clin Exp Immunol 1968;3(4):343–57.

213. Garratty G, Petz LD. Drug-induced immune hemolytic anemia. Am J Med 1975;58(3):398–407.

214. Worlledge SM. Immune drug-induced hemolytic anemias. Semin Hematol 1973;10(4):327–44.

215. Kerr RO, Cardamone J, Dalmasso AP, Kaplan ME. Two mechanisms of erythrocyte destruction in penicillin-induced hemolytic anemia. N Engl J Med 1972;287(26):1322–5.

216. Christie DJ, Lennon SS, Drew RL, Swinehart CD. Cefotetan-induced immunologic thrombocytopenia. Br J Haematol 1988;70(4):423–6.

217. Gharpure V, O'Connell B, Schiffer CA. Mezlocillin-induced thrombocytopenia. Ann Intern Med 1993;119(8):862.

218. Moller NE, Nielsen B, von Wurden K. Contact dermatitis to semisynthetic penicillins in factory workers. Contact Dermatitis 1986;14(5):307–11.

219. Tadokoro K, Niimi N, Ohtoshi T, Nakajima K, Takafuji S, Onodera K, Suzuki S, Muranaka M. Cefotiam-induced IgE-mediated occupational contact anaphylaxis of nurses; case reports, RAST analysis, and a review of the literature. Clin Exp Allergy 1994;24(2):127–33.

220. Hertl M, Geisel J, Boecker C, Merk HF. Selective generation of CD8+ T cell clones from the peripheral blood of patients with cutaneous reactions to beta-lactam antibiotics. Br J Dermatol 1993;128(6):619–26.

221. Scheper RJ, von Blomberg BM. Immunoregulation of T cell-mediated skin hypersensitivity. Arch Toxicol Suppl 1994;16:63–70.

222. Adkinson NF Jr. Beta-lactam crossreactivity. Clin Exp Allergy 1998;28(Suppl 4):37–40.

223. Bolzacchini E, Meinardi S, Orlandi M, Rindone B. 'In vivo' models of hapten generation. Clin Exp Allergy 1998;28(Suppl 4):83–6.

224. Perez Pimiento A, Gomez Martinez M, Minguez Mena A, Trampal Gonzalez A, de Paz Arranz S, Rodriguez Mosquera M. Aztreonam and ceftazidime: evidence of in vivo cross allergenicity. Allergy 1998;53(6):624–5.

225. Blanca M, Perez E, Garcia J, Miranda A, Fernandez J, Vega JM, Terrados S, Avila M, Martin A, Suau R. Anaphylaxis to amoxycillin but good tolerance for benzyl penicillin. In vivo and in vitro studies of specific IgE antibodies. Allergy 1988;43(7):508–10.

226. Dejarnatt AC, Grant JA. Basic mechanisms of anaphylaxis and anaphylactoid reactions. Immunol Allergy Clin North Am 1992;12:33–46.

227. Choquet-Kastylevsky G, Descotes J. Value of animal models for predicting hypersensitivity reactions to medicinal products. Toxicology 1998;129(1):27–35.

228. Chazal I, Verdier F, Virat M, Descotes J. Prediction of drug induced immediate hypersensitivity in guinea-pigs. Toxicol In Vitro 1994;8:1045–9.

229. Nagami K, Matsumoto H, Maki E, Motegi K, Aoyagi K, Naruse S, Samura K, Losos GJ, Ikemoto F. Experimental methods for immunization and challenge in antigenicity studies in guinea pigs. J Toxicol Sci 1995;20(5):579–94.

230. Sarlo K, Karol MH. Guinea pig predictive tests for allergy. In: Dean JH, Luster MI, Munson AE, Kiber I, editors. Immunotoxicology and Immunopharmacology, 2nd ed. New York: Raven Press; 1994:703–20.

231. Hilton J, Dearman RJ, Boylett MS, Fielding I, Basketter DA, Kimber I. The mouse IgE test for the identification of potential chemical respiratory allergens: considerations of stability and controls. J Appl Toxicol 1996;16(2):165–70.

232. Saxon A, Swabb EA, Adkinson NF Jr. Investigation into the immunologic cross-reactivity of aztreonam with other beta-lactam antibiotics. Am J Med 1985;78(2A):19–26.

233. International Rheumatic Fever Study Group. Allergic reactions to long-term benzathine penicillin prophylaxis for rheumatic fever. Lancet 1991;337(8753):1308–10.

234. Rudolph AH, Price EV. Penicillin reactions among patients in venereal disease clinics. A national survey. JAMA 1973;223(5):499–501.

235. Shepherd GM. Allergy to beta-lactam antibiotics. Immunol Allergy Clin North Am 1991;11:611.

236. Hantson P, de Coninck B, Horn JL, Mahieu P. Immediate hypersensitivity to aztreonam and imipenem. BMJ 1991;302(6771):294–5.

237. Mackowiak PA, LeMaistre CF. Drug fever: a critical appraisal of conventional concepts. An analysis of 51 episodes in two Dallas hospitals and 97 episodes reported in the English literature. Ann Intern Med 1987;106(5):728–33.

238. Calandra GB, Wang C, Aziz M, Brown KR. The safety profile of imipenem/cilastatin: worldwide clinical experience based on 3470 patients. J Antimicrob Chemother 1986;18(Suppl E):193–202.

239. Sanders CV, Greenberg RN, Marier RL. Cefamandole and cefoxitin. Ann Intern Med 1985;103(1):70–8.

240. Swabb EA. Review of the clinical pharmacology of the monobactam antibiotic aztreonam. Am J Med 1985;78(2A):11–18.

241. Delage C, Irey NS. Anaphylactic deaths: a clinicopathologic study of 43 cases. J Forensic Sci 1972;17(4):525–40.

242. Weiss ME, Adkinson NF. Immediate hypersensitivity reactions to penicillin and related antibiotics. Clin Allergy 1988;18(6):515–40.

243. Hoigné RV, Braunschweig S, Zehnder D, et al. Pharmacoepidemiology 1994;4(Suppl 1):S90.

244. Hoigné R, Jaeger MD, Hess T, Wymann R, Muller U, Galeazzi R, Maibach R, Kunzi UP. Akute schwere Dyspnoea als Medikamentennebenwirkung. [Acute severe dyspnea as a side effect of drugs. Report from the CHDM (Comprehensive Hospital Drug Monitoring).] Schweiz Med Wochenschr 1990;120(34):1211–16.

245. Adkinson NF Jr. Immunogenicity and cross-allergenicity of aztreonam. Am J Med 1990;88(3C):S12–15.

246. Platt R, Dreis MW, Kennedy DL, Kuritsky JN. Serum sickness-like reactions to amoxicillin, cefaclor, cephalexin, and trimethoprim–sulfamethoxazole. J Infect Dis 1988;158(2):474–7.

247. Levine LR. Quantitative comparison of adverse reactions to cefaclor vs. amoxicillin in a surveillance study. Pediatr Infect Dis 1985;4(4):358–61.

248. Moskovitz BL. Clinical adverse effects during ceftriaxone therapy. Am J Med 1984;77(4C):84–8.

249. Stricker BH, Tijssen JG. Serum sickness-like reactions to cefaclor. J Clin Epidemiol 1992;45(10):1177–84.

250. White JM, Brown DL, Hepner GW, Worlledge SM. Penicillin-induced haemolytic anaemia. BMJ 1968;3(609):26–9.

251. Tuffs L, Manoharan A. Flucloxacillin-induced haemolytic anaemia. Med J Aust 1986;144(10):559–60.

252. Garratty G, Postoway N, Schwellenbach J, McMahill PC. A fatal case of ceftriaxone (Rocephin)-induced hemolytic anemia associated with intravascular immune hemolysis. Transfusion 1991;31(2):176–9.

253. Chambers LA, Donovan LM, Kruskall MS. Ceftazidime-induced hemolysis in a patient with drug-dependent antibodies reactive by immune complex and drug adsorption mechanisms. Am J Clin Pathol 1991;95(3):393–6.

254. Fellner MJ. Adverse reactions to penicillin and related drugs. Clin Dermatol 1986;4(1):133–41.

255. Schopf E, Stuhmer A, Rzany B, Victor N, Zentgraf R, Kapp JF. Toxic epidermal necrolysis and Stevens–Johnson syndrome. An epidemiologic study from West Germany. Arch Dermatol 1991;127(6):839–42.

256. Wakelin SH, Allen J, Zhou S, Wojnarowska F. Drug-induced linear IgA disease with antibodies to collagen VII. Br J Dermatol 1998;138(2):310–14.

257. Fellner MJ, Mark AS. Penicillin- and ampicillin-induced pemphigus vulgaris. Int J Dermatol 1980;19(7):392–3.

258. Manders SM, Heymann WR. Acute generalized exanthemic pustulosis. Cutis 1994;54(3):194–6.

259. McDonald BJ, Singer JW, Bianco JA. Toxic epidermal necrolysis possibly linked to aztreonam in bone marrow transplant patients. Ann Pharmacother 1992;26(1):34–5.

260. Brenner S, Wolf R, Ruocco V. Drug-induced pemphigus. I. A survey Clin Dermatol 1993;11(4):501–5.

261. Blacker KL, Stern RS, Wintroub BU. Cutaneous reactions to drugs. In: Fitzpatrick TB, editor. Dermatology in General Medicine. 4th ed. New York: McGraw-Hill, 1993:1783.

262. Murray KM, Keane WR. Review of drug-induced acute interstitial nephritis. Pharmacotherapy 1992;12(6):462–7.

263. Schulz KH, Schopf E, Wex O. Allergische Berufsekzeme durch Ampicillin. [Allergic occupational eczemas caused by ampicillin.] Berufsdermatosen 1970;18(3):132–43.

264. Davies RJ, Hendrick DJ, Pepys J. Asthma due to inhaled chemical agents: ampicillin, benzyl penicillin, 6 amino penicillanic acid and related substances. Clin Allergy 1974;4(3):227–47.

265. Wengrower D, Tzfoni EE, Drenger B, Leitersdorf E. Erythroderma and pneumonitis induced by penicillin? Respiration 1986;50(4):301–3.

266. de Hoyos A, Holness DL, Tarlo SM. Hypersensitivity pneumonitis and airways hyperreactivity induced by occupational exposure to penicillin. Chest 1993;103(1):303–4.

267. Stenton SC, Dennis JH, Hendrick DJ. Occupational asthma due to ceftazidime. Eur Respir J 1995;8(8):1421–3.

268. Moscato G, Galdi E, Scibilia J, Dellabianca A, Omodeo P, Vittadini G, Biscaldi GP. Occupational asthma, rhinitis and urticaria due to piperacillin sodium in a pharmaceutical worker. Eur Respir J 1995;8(3):467–9.

269. Kanny G, Puygrenier J, Beaudoin E, Moneret-Vautrin DA. Choc anaphylactique alimentaire: implication des residues de pénicilline. [Alimentary anaphylactic shock: implication of penicillin residues.] Allerg Immunol (Paris) 1994;26(5):181–3.

270. Green RL, Green MA. Postcoital urticaria in a penicillin-sensitive patient. Possible seminal transfer of penicillin. JAMA 1985;254(4):531.

271. Hoigne R. Akute Nebenreaktionen auf Penicillinpräparate. [Acute side-reactions to penicillin preparations.] Acta Med Scand 1962;171:201–8.

272. Silber TJ, D'Angelo L. Psychosis and seizures following the injection of penicillin G procaine. Hoigné's syndrome. Am J Dis Child 1985;139(4):335–7.

273. Kraus SJ, Green RL. Pseudoanaphylactic reactions with procaine penicillin. Cutis 1976;17(4):765–7.

274. Kryst L, Wanyura H. Hoigné's syndrome—its course and symptomatology. J Maxillofac Surg 1979;7(4):320–6.

275. Tompsett R. Pseudoanaphylactic reactions to procaine penicillin G. Arch Intern Med 1967;120(5):565–7.

276. Van Arsdel PP Jr. Classification of risk factors for drug allergy. Immunol Allergy Clin North Am 1991;11:475.

277. Petri M, Albritton J. Antibiotic allergy in systemic lupus erythematosus: a case control study. J Rheumatol 1992;20:399.

278. Capaul R, Maibach R, Kuenzi UP, et al. Atopy, bronchial asthma and previous adverse drug reactions (ADRs): risk factors for ADRs? Post Marketing Surveillance 1993;7:331.

279. Green GR, Rosenblum AH, Sweet LC. Evaluation of penicillin hypersensitivity: value of clinical history and skin testing with penicilloyl-polylysine and penicillin G. A cooperative prospective study of the penicillin study group of the American Academy of Allergy. J Allergy Clin Immunol 1977;60(6):339–45.

280. Battegay M, Opravil M, Wuthrich B, Luthy R. Rash with amoxycillin–clavulanate therapy in HIV-infected patients. Lancet 1989;2(8671):1100.

281. Toogood JH. Risk of anaphylaxis in patients receiving beta-blocker drugs. J Allergy Clin Immunol 1988;81(1):1–5.

282. Jick H, Porter JB. Potentiation of ampicillin skin reactions by allopurinol or hyperuricemia. J Clin Pharmacol 1981;21(10):456–8.

283. Fleming A. On the bactericidal action of cultures of a Penicillium with a special reference to their use in the isolation of B. influenzae. Br J Exp Pathol 1929;10:226.

284. Abraham EP. Further observation on penicillin. Lancet 1941;1:177.

285. Florey HW. Penicillins in war wounds. A report from the Mediterranean. Lancet 1943;2:742.

286. Tomasz A. Penicillin-binding proteins and the antibacterial effectiveness of beta-lactam antibiotics. Rev Infect Dis 1986;8(Suppl 3):S260–78.

287. Georgopapadakou NH. Penicillin-binding proteins and bacterial resistance to beta-lactams. Antimicrob Agents Chemother 1993;37(10):2045–53.

288. Ghuysen JM. Serine beta-lactamases and penicillin-binding proteins. Annu Rev Microbiol 1991;45:37–67.

289. Philippon A, Labia R, Jacoby G. Extended-spectrum beta-lactamases. Antimicrob Agents Chemother 1989;33(8):1131–6.

290. Nikaido H. Prevention of drug access to bacterial targets: permeability barriers and active efflux. Science 1994;264(5157):382–8.

291. Livermore DM. Interplay of impermeability and chromosomal beta-lactamase activity in imipenem-resistant Pseudomonas aeruginosa. Antimicrob Agents Chemother 1992;36(9):2046–8.

292. Moreillon P. La résistance bactérienne aux antibiotiques. [Bacterial resistance to antibiotics.] Schweiz Med Wochenschr 1995;125(23):1151–61.

293. Watson JD, Hopkins NH, Roberts JW, et al. The genetic systems provided by E. coli and its viruses. In: Gillen JR, editor. Molecular Biology of the Gene. Menlo Park: Benjamin/Cummings, 1987:176.

294. Hayes W. Recombination in Bact. coli K 12; unidirectional transfer of genetic material Nature 1952;169(4290):118–19.

295. Amabile-Cuevas CF, Chicurel ME. Bacterial plasmids and gene flux. Cell 1992;70(2):189–99.

296. Neu HC. The crisis in antibiotic resistance. Science 1992;257(5073):1064–73.

297. Friedland IR, McCracken GH Jr. Management of infections caused by antibiotic-resistant Streptococcus pneumoniae. N Engl J Med 1994;331(6):377–82.

298. Marton A, Gulyas M, Munoz R, Tomasz A. Extremely high incidence of antibiotic resistance in clinical isolates of Streptococcus pneumoniae in Hungary. J Infect Dis 1991;163(3):542–8.

299. Coffey TJ, Dowson CG, Daniels M, Spratt BG. Genetics and molecular biology of beta-lactam-resistant pneumococci. Microb Drug Resist 1995;1(1):29–34.

300. Tomasz A. Multiple-antibiotic-resistant pathogenic bacteria. A report on the Rockefeller University Workshop. N Engl J Med 1994;330(17):1247–51.

301. Garcia-Bustos J, Tomasz A. A biological price of antibiotic resistance: major changes in the peptidoglycan structure of penicillin-resistant pneumococci. Proc Natl Acad Sci USA 1990;87(14):5415–19.

302. Appelbaum PC. Antimicrobial resistance in Streptococcus pneumoniae: an overview. Clin Infect Dis 1992;15(1):77–83.

303. Barnes DM, Whittier S, Gilligan PH, Soares S, Tomasz A, Henderson FW. Transmission of multidrug-resistant serotype 23F Streptococcus pneumoniae in group day care: evidence suggesting capsular transformation of the resistant strain in vivo. J Infect Dis 1995;171(4):890–6.

304. Munoz R, Coffey TJ, Daniels M, Dowson CG, Laible G, Casal J, Hakenbeck R, Jacobs M, Musser JM, Spratt BG, et al. Intercontinental spread of a multiresistant clone of serotype 23F Streptococcus pneumoniae. J Infect Dis 1991;164(2):302–6.

305. Soares S, Kristinsson KG, Musser JM, Tomasz A. Evidence for the introduction of a multiresistant clone of serotype 6B Streptococcus pneumoniae from Spain to Iceland in the late 1980s. J Infect Dis 1993;168(1):158–63.

306. Tomasz A. The pneumococcus at the gates. N Engl J Med 1995;333(8):514–15.

307. Cherubin CE, Corrado ML, Sierra MF, Gombert ME, Shulman M. Susceptibility of Gram-positive cocci to various antibiotics, including cefotaxime, moxalactam, and N-formimidoyl thienamycin. Antimicrob Agents Chemother 1981;20(4):553–5.

308. Schwalbe RS, Stapleton JT, Gilligan PH. Emergence of vancomycin resistance in coagulase-negative staphylococci. N Engl J Med 1987;316(15):927–31.

309. Noble WC, Virani Z, Cree RG. Co-transfer of vancomycin and other resistance genes from Enterococcus faecalis NCTC 12201 to Staphylococcus aureus. FEMS Microbiol Lett 1992;72(2):195–8.

310. Reichler MR, Allphin AA, Breiman RF, Schreiber JR, Arnold JE, McDougal LK, Facklam RR, Boxerbaum B, May D, Walton RO, et al. The spread of multiply resistant Streptococcus pneumoniae at a day care center in Ohio. J Infect Dis 1992;166(6):1346–53.

311. Koren G, Pastuszak A, Ito S. Drugs in pregnancy. N Engl J Med 1998;338(16):1128–37.

312. Rao JM, Arulappu R. Drug use in pregnancy: how to avoid problems. Drugs 1981;22(5):409–14.

313. EUROCAT Working Group. EUROCAT Report 7:15 years of surveillance of congenital anomalies in Europe 1980–1994. Brussels: Scientific Institute of Public Health—Louis Pasteur, 1997.

314. Khoury MJ, Holtzman NA. On the ability of birth defects monitoring to detect new teratogens. Am J Epidemiol 1987;126(1):136–43.

315. Irl C, Hasford J. Assessing the safety of drugs in pregnancy: the role of prospective cohort studies. Drug Saf 2000;22(3):169–77.

316. Lenz W. Kindliche Missbildungen nach Medikamenten wärhend der Gravidität. Dtsch Med Wochenschr 1961;86:2555–6.

317. Weller TM, Rees EN. Antibacterial use in pregnancy. Drug Saf 2000;22(5):335–8.

318. Czeizel AE, Rockenbauer M, Olsen J, Sorensen HT. Oral phenoxymethylpenicillin treatment during pregnancy. Results of a population-based Hungarian case-control study. Arch Gynecol Obstet 2000;263(4):178–81.

319. Larsen H, Nielsen GL, Sorensen HT, Moller M, Olsen J, Schonheyder HC. A follow-up study of birth outcome in users of pivampicillin during pregnancy. Acta Obstet Gynecol Scand 2000;79(5):379–83.

320. Manka W, Solowiow R, Okrzeja D. Assessment of infant development during an 18-month follow-up after treatment of infections in pregnant women with cefuroxime axetil. Drug Saf 2000;22(1):83–8.

321. Fossieck B Jr, Parker RH. Neurotoxicity during intravenous infusion of penicillin. A review. J Clin Pharmacol 1974;14(10):504–12.

322. Andrassy K, Weischedel E, Ritz E, Andrassy T. Bleeding in uremic patients after carbenicillin. Thromb Haemost 1976;36(1):115–26.

323. Schliamser SE, Bolander H, Kourtopoulos H, Norrby SR. Neurotoxicity of benzylpenicillin: correlation to concentrations in serum, cerebrospinal fluid and brain tissue fluid in rabbits. J Antimicrob Chemother 1988;21(3):365–72.

324. Bang NU, Kammer RB. Hematologic complications associated with betalactam antibiotics. Rev Infect Dis 1983;5(Suppl):380.

325. Sattler FR, Weitekamp MR, Ballard JO. Potential for bleeding with the new beta-lactam antibiotics. Ann Intern Med 1986;105(6):924–31.

326. Hughes GS, Heald DL, Barker KB, Patel RK, Spillers CR, Watts KC, Batts DH, Euler AR. The effects of gastric pH and food on the pharmacokinetics of a new oral cephalosporin, cefpodoxime proxetil. Clin Pharmacol Ther 1989;46(6):674–85.

327. Saathoff N, Lode H, Neider K, Depperman KM, Borner K, Koeppe P. Pharmacokinetics of cefpodoxime proxetil and interactions with an antacid and an H2 receptor antagonist. Antimicrob Agents Chemother 1992;36(4):796–800.

328. Blouin RA, Kneer J, Ambros RJ, Stoeckel K. Influence of antacid and ranitidine on the pharmacokinetics of oral cefetamet pivoxil. Antimicrob Agents Chemother 1990;34(9):1744–8.

329. Bandrowsky T, Vorono AA, Borris TJ, Marcantoni HW. Amoxicillin-related postextraction bleeding in an anticoagulated patient with tranexamic acid rinses. Oral Surg Oral Med Oral Pathol Oral Radiol Endod 1996;82(6):610–12.

330. Davydov L, Yermolnik M, Cuni LJ. Warfarin and amoxicillin/clavulanate drug interaction. Ann Pharmacother 2003;37(3):367–70.

331. Mailloux AT, Gidal BE, Sorkness CA. Potential interaction between warfarin and dicloxacillin. Ann Pharmacother 1996;30(12):1402–7.

332. Heilker GM, Fowler JW Jr, Self TH. Possible nafcillin–warfarin interaction. Arch Intern Med 1994;154(7):822–4.

333. Taylor AT, Pritchard DC, Goldstein AO, Fletcher JL Jr. Continuation of warfarin–nafcillin interaction during dicloxacillin therapy. J Fam Pract 1994;39(2):182–5.

334. Lindenbaum J, Rund DG, Butler VP Jr, Tse-Eng D, Saha JR. Inactivation of digoxin by the gut flora: reversal by antibiotic therapy. N Engl J Med 1981;305(14):789–94.

335. Saha JR, Butler VP Jr, Neu HC, Lindenbaum J. Digoxin-inactivating bacteria: identification in human gut flora. Science 1983;220(4594):325–7.

336. Rhodes KM, Brown SN. Do the penicillin antibiotics interact with digoxin? Eur J Clin Pharmacol 1994;46(5):479–80.

337. Ganapathy ME, Prasad PD, Mackenzie B, Ganapathy V, Leibach FH. Interaction of anionic cephalosporins with the intestinal and renal peptide transporters PEPT 1 and PEPT 2. Biochim Biophys Acta 1997;1324(2):296–308.

338. Matsumoto S, Saito H, Inui K. Transcellular transport of oral cephalosporins in human intestinal epithelial cells, Caco-2: interaction with dipeptide transport systems in apical and basolateral membranes. J Pharmacol Exp Ther 1994;270(2):498–504.

339. Sugawara M, Iseki K, Miyazaki K, Shiroto H, Kondo Y, Uchino J. Transport characteristics of ceftibuten, cefixime and cephalexin across human jejunal brush-border membrane. J Pharm Pharmacol 1991;43(12):882–4.

340. Dantzig AH, Duckworth DC, Tabas LB. Transport mechanisms responsible for the absorption of loracarbef, cefixime, and cefuroxime axetil into human intestinal Caco-2 cells. Biochim Biophys Acta 1994;1191(1):7–13.

341. Winstanley PA, Orme ML. The effects of food on drug bioavailability. Br J Clin Pharmacol 1989;28(6):621–8.

342. Westphal JF, Trouvin JH, Deslandes A, Carbon C. Nifedipine enhances amoxicillin absorption kinetics and bioavailability in humans. J Pharmacol Exp Ther 1990;255(1):312–17.

343. Duverne C, Bouten A, Deslandes A, Westphal JF, Trouvin JH, Farinotti R, Carbon C. Modification of cefixime bioavailability by nifedipine in humans: involvement of the dipeptide carrier system. Antimicrob Agents Chemother 1992;36(11):2462–7.

344. Deslandes A, Camus F, Lacroix C, Carbon C, Farinotti R. Effects of nifedipine and diltiazem on pharmacokinetics of cefpodoxime following its oral administration. Antimicrob Agents Chemother 1996;40(12):2879–81.

345. Back DJ, Grimmer SF, Orme ML, Proudlove C, Mann RD, Breckenridge AM. Evaluation of Committee on Safety of Medicines yellow card reports on oral contraceptive-drug interactions with anticonvulsants and antibiotics. Br J Clin Pharmacol 1988;25(5):527–32.

346. Orme ML, Back DJ. Factors affecting the enterohepatic circulation of oral contraceptive steroids. Am J Obstet Gynecol 1990;163(6 Pt 2):2146–52.

347. Hanker JP. Gastrointestinal disease and oral contraception. Am J Obstet Gynecol 1990;163(6 Pt 2):2204–7.

348. Reimers D, Jezek A. Rifampicin und andere Antituberkulotika bei gleichzeitiger oraler Kontrazeption. [The simultaneous use of rifampicin and other antitubercular agents with oral contraceptives.] Prax Pneumol 1971;25(5):255–62.

349. Szoka PR, Edgren RA. Drug interactions with oral contraceptives: compilation and analysis of an adverse experience report database. Fertil Steril 1988;49(5 Suppl 2):S31–8.

350. de Groot AC, Eshuis H, Stricker BH. Ineffectiviteit van orale anticonceptie tijdens gebruik van minocycline. [Inefficacy of oral contraception during use of minocycline.] Ned Tijdschr Geneeskd 1990;134(25):1227–9.

351. Midtvedt T. Microbial functional activities. In: Hanson LA, Yolken RH, editors. Probiotics, Other Nutritional Factors, and Intestinal Microflora. Philadelphia: Lippincott-Raven, 1999:79–96.

352. Mastrantonio M, Minhas H, Gammon A. Antibiotics, the pill, and pregnancy. J Accid Emerg Med 1999;16(4):268–70.

353. Harder S, Schneider W, Bae ZU, Bock U, Zielen S. Unerwünschte Arzneimittel-reaktionen bei gleichzeitiger Gabe von hochdosiertem Phenobarbital und Betalaktam-Antibiotika. [Undesirable drug reactions in simultaneous administration of high-dosage phenobarbital and beta-lactam antibiotics.] Klin Padiatr 1990;202(6):404–7.

354. Young DS. Effects of Drugs on Clinical Laboratory Tests. 3rd ed. Washington: AACC Press, 1990.

355. Garton AM, Rennie RP, Gilpin J, Marrelli M, Shafran SD. Comparison of dose doubling with probenecid for sustaining serum cefuroxime levels. J Antimicrob Chemother 1997;40(6):903–6.

356. Singh YN, Harvey AL, Marshall IG. Antibiotic-induced paralysis of the mouse phrenic nerve-hemidiaphragm preparation, and reversibility by calcium and by neostigmine. Anesthesiology 1978;48(6):418–24.

357. Segredo V, Caldwell JE, Matthay MA, Sharma ML, Gruenke LD, Miller RD. Persistent paralysis in critically

ill patients after long-term administration of vecuronium. N Engl J Med 1992;327(8):524–8.

358. Tryba M. Wirkungsverstarkung nicht-depolarisierender Muskelrelakantien durch Acylaminopencilline. Untersuchungen am Beispiel von Vecuronium. [Potentiation of the effect of non-depolarizing muscle relaxants by acylami-nopenicillins. Studies on the example of vecuronium.] Anaesthesist 1985;34(12):651–5.

359. Condon RE, Munshi CA, Arfman RC. Interaction of vecuronium with piperacillin or cefoxitin evaluated in a prospective, randomized, double-blind clinical trial. Am Surg 1995;61(5):403–6.

360. Welling PG. Interactions affecting drug absorption. Clin Pharmacokinet 1984;9(5):404–34.

361. Finn A, Straughn A, Meyer M, Chubb J. Effect of dose and food on the bioavailability of cefuroxime axetil. Biopharm Drug Dispos 1987;8(6):519–26.

362. Sommers DK, van Wyk M, Moncrieff J, Schoeman HS. Influence of food and reduced gastric acidity on the bio-availability of bacampicillin and cefuroxime axetil. Br J Clin Pharmacol 1984;18(4):535–9.

363. Tindula RJ, Ambrose PJ, Harralson AF. Aminoglycoside inactivation by penicillins and cephalosporins and its impact on drug-level monitoring. Drug Intell Clin Pharm 1983;17(12):906–8.

364. Pickering LK, Rutherford I. Effect of concentration and time upon inactivation of tobramycin, gentamicin, netilmicin and amikacin by azlocillin, carbenicillin, mecillinam, mezlocillin and piperacillin. J Pharmacol Exp Ther 1981;217(2):345–9.

365. Blair DC, Duggan DO, Schroeder ET. Inactivation of amikacin and gentamicin by carbenicillin in patients with end-stage renal failure. Antimicrob Agents Chemother 1982;22(3):376–9.

366. LeBel M, Paone RP, Lewis GP. Effect of ten new beta-lactam antibiotics on urine glucose test methods. Drug Intell Clin Pharm 1984;18(7–8):617–20.

367. Kowalsky SF, Wishnoff FG. Evaluation of potential inter-action of new cephalosporins with Clinitest. Am J Hosp Pharm 1982;39(9):1499–501.

368. Jahansouz F, Kriett JM, Smith CM, Jamieson SW. Potentiation of cyclosporine nephrotoxicity by nafcillin in lung transplant recipients. Transplantation 1993;55(5):1045–8.

Beta-lactamase inhibitors

General Information

Beta-lactamases are genetically and structurally closely related to penicillin-binding proteins. Their production by bacteria is a major mechanism of resistance to the action of beta-lactam antibiotics. Drugs have therefore been developed that inhibit beta-lactamase, as a way of overcoming this resistance (SEDA-20, 229). They are beta-lactam compounds with particularly high affinities for beta-lactamases (1,2), which therefore act as competitive inhibitors of beta-lactamases. Beta-lactamase inhibitors have no important antimicrobial activity and are only given in combination with an antimicrobial beta-lactam.

The following beta-lactamase inhibitors are in use:

- clavulanic acid (rINN), produced naturally by *Streptomyces clavuligerus*, used in combination with amoxicillin or ticarcillin; the combination clavulanic acid + amoxicillin is also called co-amoxiclav (BAN);
- sulbactam (rINN), a halogenated derivative of penicillanic acid, used in combination with ampicillin or cefoperazone;
- tazobactam (rINN), a halogenated derivative of peni-cillanic acid, used in combination with piperacillin.

In order to improve absorption, sulbactam has also been bound to ampicillin in the single molecule sultamicillin, which is hydrolysed to the active components after absorption.

An inherent obstacle in evaluating the adverse effects of beta-lactamase inhibitors is that they are only co-administered with antimicrobial beta-lactams, the doses of which are usually several times higher. For the most part, combinations of beta-lactam antibiotics with beta-lactamase inhibitors produce the adverse effects of the individual drugs. However, it is not always possible to say whether an adverse effect is due to one drug alone or to the combina-tion. For example, cholestatic hepatitis occurs more often with co-amoxiclav than with ampicillin alone; however, this could be because it is primarily due to clavulanic acid or because the combination somehow increases the risk.

Organs and Systems

Respiratory

Interstitial pneumonitis has been attributed to ampicill-in + sulbactam in two Japanese patients (3).

Psychological, psychiatric

Behavioral changes occurred in four children aged 1.5–10.5 years, taking co-amoxiclav (4).

Hematologic

Parallel to a well-known phenomenon seen with cephalo-sporins, clavulanic acid can be associated with a positive direct antiglobulin test. In three patients antibiotic courses, including intravenous ticarcillin + clavulanic acid, were associated with positive direct antiglobulin tests in over 50% of cases (5–7). Corresponding observa-tions were made in patients taking ampicillin + sulbactam (8). In vitro studies showed that clavulanic acid and sul-bactam caused non-immunological absorption of plasma proteins on to the erythrocyte surface (5,9). There seems to be no clinical impact of this phenomenon, but it can interfere with cross-matching of blood products or with the investigation of true hemolysis.

Reversible bone marrow suppression after high-dose piperacillin + tazobactam was seen in an underweight woman and was thought to be a dose-dependent and piperacillin-related effect (10).

Gastrointestinal

Two cases of hemorrhagic colitis, apparently not related to *Clostridium difficile*, have been reported after co-amoxi-clav (11,12). However, the same type of colitis has repeat-edly been observed with aminopenicillins alone (12).

Co-amoxiclav often causes diarrhea and other gastro-intestinal problems. Oral administration was associated with motor disturbances of the small intestine (13).

Liver

Cholestatic hepatitis
DoTS classification

Dose-relation: hypersusceptibility effect

Time-course: immediate

Susceptibility factors: genetic (DRB1*1501*DRB5-DRB5*0101-DQB1*0602 haplotypes); age over 55 years; male sex; duration of treatment

Co-amoxiclav can cause cholestatic hepatitis. The first report appeared in 1988 (14), since when several hundreds of cases have been reported, for example to health authorities (15), and over 100 cases have been described in detail (16–31). Clavulanic acid is instrumental, either alone or in combination with amoxicillin, since the risk of acute liver injury is much smaller with amoxicillin alone (32).

The relative contributions of amoxicillin and clavulanate to co-amoxiclav-induced hepatotoxicity are incompletely understood. In patients with co-amoxiclav hepatotoxicity, previous use of amoxicillin and rechallenge with amoxicillin were both uneventful, pointing to clavulanic acid as the more likely culprit (16). In a report from the UK, the incidence of liver injury with amoxicillin alone was 0.3 per 10 000 prescriptions versus 1.7 with co-amoxiclav (32). The risk increased after multiple use and with increasing age to 1 per 1000 prescriptions of co-amoxiclav. The main message is that the combination should be used with caution in elderly patients. A patient who has had documented hepatotoxicity related to co-amoxiclav should be well informed about this adverse drug reaction and any future use should be prohibited.

Ticarcillin + clavulanic acid, which is only used intravenously, has also been reported to induce a similar syndrome (33,34) and can also aggravate pre-existing hepatitis (35). One cholestatic reaction has been reported with intravenous sulbactam + ampicillin (36).

The importance of taking a careful history in patients in whom drug-related hepatitis is suspected has been underlined (37).

Incidence
Considering the large number of patients who take this very widely used combination, the risk of hepatitis was initially estimated to be very low, probably below 1/100 000 (23). Newer data, however, have suggested a risk of 1/10 000 or higher (32). In a retrospective cohort study of family practitioners' records, with a high proportion of mild cases, there was a rate of 1 per 4449 prescriptions (32). If this is the case, it is wise to reserve co-amoxiclav (and maybe also ticarcillin + clavulanate) for use in infections caused by strains producing beta-lactamases that can destroy amoxicillin (or ticarcillin).

The syndrome is practically unknown in children; only one pediatric case has been reported so far, in a 4-year-old boy with spherocytosis (16) and causality was disputed (17).

Presentation
The hepatitis usually develops acutely, although an interval of up to 4 weeks between the end of treatment and the first signs of hepatitis is frequent and can prevent rapid diagnosis. Although the clinical effects can be impressive, the condition is usually reversible within 4–6 weeks.

- A 40-year-old woman with a history of chronic sinusitis and asthma developed nausea, vomiting, abdominal pain, and diarrhea (38). Six weeks before, she had taken a 10-day course of co-amoxiclav for acute sinusitis. Her transaminase activities were markedly increased, as was total bilirubin. All drugs were withdrawn, her symptoms progressively improved, and she was discharged without a clearly identified cause of her illness. Liver function tests normalized completely within a few weeks. Two months later she had another episode of acute sinusitis and was again given co-amoxiclav. A few days later she developed nausea, vomiting, a skin rash, abdominal pain, and reduced appetite. Her alanine transaminase activity was 199 U/l (0–65), aspartate transaminase 99 U/l (0–60), and alkaline phosphatase 362 U/l (50–180). The antibiotic was withdrawn, and she completely recovered in 2 weeks and had normal liver function tests over the next several months.

- A 33-month-old boy took co-amoxiclav (dose not stated) for 10 days for otitis media (39). He had taken it twice before. One day after completing the course he developed a rash over his entire body, followed 3 days later by lethargy, jaundice, pale stools, and pruritus. The jaundice persisted, the liver was markedly enlarged, and all liver function tests were abnormal. Tests for known viral and metabolic causes of cholestasis were negative. A percutaneous liver biopsy showed centrilobular cholestasis "consistent with a drug reaction." He was given ursodeoxycholic acid (30 mg/kg/day) and vitamins A, D, and K; later prednisolone was added. However, his jaundice persisted, as did severe pruritus. He also developed extensive xanthomatosis and failure to grow. A liver transplantation was successfully performed 8 months after the onset of symptoms. His explanted liver had features of biliary cirrhosis, with ductular proliferation and ductopenia.

One fatal outcome was described in a patient who was also taking ethinylestradiol, which can itself cause cholestasis (40).

In isolated cases, Stevens–Johnson syndrome together with cholestasis and bone marrow aplasia have been associated with either amoxicillin alone (41) or with co-amoxiclav (42).

Histological features
Liver biopsy shows predominantly centrilobular or panlobular cholestasis, and occasionally granulomatous hepatitis (43).

Mechanism
The mechanism of the syndrome and its possible relation to the liver injury that other beta-lactams, particularly isoxazolylpenicillins, can cause are unclear. A slight eosinophilia has been seen in many cases (26,43,44) and some of the sporadic cases of rechallenge were positive (16). However, there is no other evidence supporting an

immunoallergic basis. Hepatic accumulation or biliary secretion of clavulanic acid or its metabolites have not been demonstrated (45).

Two other theories have been proposed (46). One is based on the metabolic formation of neo-antigens, and subsequent recognition of these antigens as foreign by the immune system. This "immune allergic hypothesis" is supported by the strong association with an HLA class II haplotype. The authors argued that "HLA class II molecules are required for antigen presentation to CD4-positive T cells. HLA alleles may differ by a little as a single codon, and one amino acid residue difference at a critical site in the resulting polypeptide may be functionally significant, determining not only the affinity with which a given antigen is presented but also the interaction of the HLA peptide complex with the T cell receptor." Their other theory was that the liver disease may arise through linkage with another gene on chromosome 6p. This "linked-gene" hypothesis, they proposed, may explain why jaundice is rare after treatment with co-amoxiclav, although this particular HLA haplotype is common in Northern Europe, where co-amoxiclav is commonly prescribed.

Whatever the mechanisms might be, at present it is reasonable to look on clavulanate as the main contributor to the development of hepatotoxicity with co-amoxiclav. Hepatotoxicity has also been reported with clavulanate plus ticarcillin (34). So far, however, there has been no genetic evaluation of patients with hepatotoxic reactions after therapy with clavulanate and ticarcillin.

Susceptibility factors
Increasing age (over 55 years), male sex, and duration of treatment are risk factors (26,32,47), while drug dose and route of administration, other medications, previous drug allergies, or prior use of co-amoxiclav were not significantly associated with the reaction.

The importance of HLA antigens in the pathogenesis of some liver diseases (autoimmune hepatitis, primary biliary cirrhosis, primary cholangitis) is also reasonably well established (48), and there is a significant association between co-amoxiclav-induced liver damage and an HLA haplotype (49,50). HLA-class antigens have been investigated in 35 patients with biopsy-documented liver damage due to co-amoxiclav and 300 controls (volunteer bone marrow donors) (46). HLA-A and HLA-B were typed using alloantisera and HLA-DBR and HLA-DWB were typed by PCR. The patients with hepatitis were characterized by a higher frequency of the DRB1*1501*DRB5-DRB5*0101-DQB1*0602 haplotype (57 versus 12% in controls). Patients with that haplotype tended to have a cholestatic rather than a hepatocellular type of hepatitis. However, these data also suggest that other factors must act concurrently. These factors may involve heterogeneity of the formed antigens and/or polymorphism of the T cell receptor. A reaction to (unknown) metabolites of clavulanic acid also has to be kept in mind. The authors suggested that "metabolic factors may play a greater role in the pathogenesis of hepatocellular cases, whereas immunological factors may be more involved in the pathogenesis of cholestatic ones." This HLA association has been confirmed in a study in which there was an increased frequency of homozygous status for this haplotype (51). This might reflect population differences and the small sample size in both studies (46). It is reasonable to assume that HLA characterization will be implemented in a future diagnostic armamentarium.

Urinary tract

The combination of piperacillin + tazobactam was thought to have caused acute interstitial nephritis in a 51-year-old woman (52). It remains open whether the combination or one of the components was the culprit.

Immunologic

Clavulanic acid has a very low immunogenic and allergenic potential in animals. The possible impact of its co-administration with other beta-lactam antibiotics is unknown (53). Two patients with IgE-mediated hypersensitivity to oral co-amoxiclav and positive skin tests for clavulanic acid, but not for penicillins, both tolerated oral amoxicillin. One patient was also challenged with clavulanic acid and developed urticaria, conjunctivitis, and bronchial obstruction (54). Since co-amoxiclav has been widely used since its introduction in 1981, the frequency of hypersensitivity reactions is low. The clinical data available on sulbactam and tazobactam are still limited and do not allow an assessment of the frequency and pattern of associated hypersensitivity reactions (55).

Body temperature

A woman immediately developed hyperpyrexia up to 40°C after a first dose of intravenous ampicillin + sulbactam, having previously tolerated ampicillin alone for 10 days. Hyperpyrexia was repeatedly observed after six more doses of sulbactam (56).

Interference with Diagnostic Tests

Leukocyte dipstick test

Clavulanic acid caused false-positive dipstick tests for leukocytes; sulbactam and tazobactam did not (57).

References

1. Rolinson GN. Evolution of beta-lactamase inhibitors. Rev Infect Dis 1991;13(Suppl 9):S727–32.
2. Hoover JRE. Betalactam antibiotics: structure-activity relationships. Demain AL, Solomon NA, editors. Antibiotics Containing the Betalactam-Structure, Part II. Berlin: Springer-Verlag, 1983:119.
3. Miyashita N, Nakajima M, Kuroki M, Kawabata S, Hashiguchi K, Niki Y, Kawane H, Matsushima T. [Sulbactam/ampicillin-induced pneumonitis.] Nihon Kokyuki Gakkai Zasshi 1998;36(8):684–9.
4. Macknin ML. Behavioral changes after amoxicillin–clavulanate Pediatr Infect Dis J 1987;6(9):873–4.
5. Williams ME, Thomas D, Harman CP, Mintz PD, Donowitz GR. Positive direct antiglobulin tests due to clavulanic acid. Antimicrob Agents Chemother 1985;27(1):125–7.
6. Finegold SM, Johnson CC. Lower respiratory tract infection. Am J Med 1985;79(5B):73–7.
7. Blanchard M, Oppliger R, Bucher U. Positiver direkter Coombs-Test bei akuten Leukämien und anderen Hämoblastosen: Zusammenhang mit clavulansäurehaltigen Antibiotika? [Positive direct Coombs' test in acute leukemias

and other hemoblastoses: relation to clavulanic acid-containing antibiotics?] Schweiz Med Wochenschr 1989;119(2):39–45.

8. Lutz P, Dzik W. Very high incidence of a positive direct antiglobulin test (+DAT) in patients receiving Unasyn. Transfusion 1992;32:23.

9. Garratty G, Arndt PA. Positive direct antiglobulin tests and haemolytic anaemia following therapy with beta-lactamase inhibitor containing drugs may be associated with non-immunologic adsorption of protein onto red blood cells. Br J Haematol 1998;100(4):777–83.

10. Ruiz-Irastorza G, Barreiro G, Aguirre C. Reversible bone marrow depression by high-dose piperacillin/tazobactam. Br J Haematol 1996;95(4):611–12.

11. Klotz F, Barthet M, Perreard M. A propos d'un cas de colite aiguë hémorragique après la prise orale d'Augmentin. [A case of acute hemorrhagic colitis after oral ingestion of Augmentin.] Ann Med Interne (Paris) 1990;141(3):276.

12. Heer M, Sulser H, Hany A. Segmentale, hämorrhagische Kolitis nach Amoxicillin-Therapie. [Segmental hämorrhagic colitis following amoxicillin therapy.] Schweiz Med Wochenschr 1989;119(21):733–5.

13. Caron F, Ducrotte P, Lerebours E, Colin R, Humbert G, Denis P. Effects of amoxicillin–clavulanate combination on the motility of the small intestine in human beings. Antimicrob Agents Chemother 1991;35(6):1085–8.

14. van den Broek JW, Buennemeyer BL, Stricker BH. Cholestatische hepatitis door de combinatic amoxicilline en clavulaanzuur (Augmentin). [Cholestatic hepatitis caused by a combination of amoxicillin and clavulanic acid (Augmentin).] Ned Tijdschr Geneeskd 1988;132(32):1495–7.

15. Thomson JA, Fairley CK, McNeil JJ, Purcell P. Augmentin-associated jaundice. Med J Aust 1994;160(11):733–4.

16. Stricker BH, Van den Broek JW, Keuning J, Eberhardt W, Houben HG, Johnson M, Blok AP. Cholestatic hepatitis due to antibacterial combination of amoxicillin and clavulanic acid (Augmentin) Dig Dis Sci 1989;34(10):1576–80.

17. Reddy KR, Brillant P, Schiff ER. Amoxicillin–clavulanate potassium-associated cholestasis. Gastroenterology 1989; 96(4):1135–41.

18. Reddy KR, Schiff ER. Hepatitis and Augmentin. Dig Dis Sci 1990;35(8):1045–6.

19. Verhamme M, Ramboer C, Van de Bruaene P, Inderadjaja N. Cholestatic hepatitis due to an amoxycillin/clavulanic acid preparation. J Hepatol 1989;9(2):260–4.

20. Dowsett JF, Gillow T, Heagerty A, Radcliffe M, Toadi R, Isle I, Russell RC. Amoxycillin/clavulanic acid (Augmentin)-induced intrahepatic cholestasis. Dig Dis Sci 1989;34(8):1290–3.

21. Schneider JE, Kleinman MS, Kupiec JW. Cholestatic hepatitis after therapy with amoxicillin/clavulanate potassium. NY State J Med 1989;89(6):355–6.

22. Pelletier G, Ink O, Fabre M, Hagege H. Hépatite cholestatique probablement due à l'association d'amoxilline et d'acide clavulanique. [Hepatic cholestasis probably due to the combination of amoxicillin and clavulanic acid.] Gastroenterol Clin Biol 1990;14(6–7):601.

23. Larrey D, Vial T, Micaleff A, Babany G, Morichau-Beauchant M, Michel H, Benhamou JP. Hepatitis associated with amoxycillin–clavulanic acid combination report of 15 cases. Gut 1992;33(3):368–71.

24. Hanssens M, Mast A, Van Maele V, Pauwels W. Cholestatische icterus door amoxicilline–clavulaanzuur bij 4 patienten. [Cholestatic jaundice caused by amoxicillin–clavulanic acid in 4 patients.] Ned Tijdschr Geneeskd 1994;138(29):1481–3.

25. Wong FS, Ryan J, Dabkowski P, Dudley FJ, Sewell RB, Smallwood RA. Augmentin-induced jaundice. Med J Aust 1991;154(10):698–701.

26. Alexander P, Roskams T, Van Steenbergen W, Peetermans W, Desmet V, Yap SH. Intrahepatic cholestasis

induced by amoxicillin/clavulanic acid (Augmentin): a report on two cases. Acta Clin Belg 1991;46(5):327–32.

27. Maggini M, Raschetti R, Agostinis L, Cattaruzzi C, Troncon MG, Simon G. Use of amoxicillin and amoxicillin-clavulanic acid and hospitalization for acute liver injury Ann Ist Super Sanita 1999;35(3):429–33.

28. Soza A, Riquelme F, Alvarez M, Duarte I, Glasinovic JC, Arrese M. Hepatotoxicidad por amoxicilina/acido clavulanico: caso clinico. [Hepatotoxicity by amoxicillin/clavulanic acid: case report.] Rev Med Chil 1999;127(12):1487–91.

29. Ma C, Bayliff CD, Ponich T. Amoxicillin–clavuanic acid-induced hepatotoxicity. Can J Hosp Pharm 1999;52:30–2.

30. Richardet JP, Mallat A, Zafrani ES, Blazquez M, Bognel JC, Campillo B. Prolonged cholestasis with ductopenia after administration of amoxicillin/clavulanic acid. Dig Dis Sci 1999;44(10):1997–2000.

31. Limauro DL, Chan-Tompkins NH, Carter RW, Brodmerkel GJ Jr, Agrawal RM. Amoxicillin/clavulanate-associated hepatic failure with progression to Stevens–Johnson syndrome. Ann Pharmacother 1999;33(5):560–4.

32. Garcia Rodriguez LA, Stricker BH, Zimmerman HJ. Risk of acute liver injury associated with the combination of amoxicillin and clavulanic acid. Arch Intern Med 1996;156(12):1327–32.

33. Ryan J, Dudley FJ. Cholestasis with ticarcillin–potassium clavulanate (Timentin). Med J Aust 1992;156(4):291.

34. Sweet JM, Jones MP. Intrahepatic cholestasis due to ticarcillin–clavulanate. Am J Gastroenterol 1995;90(4):675–6.

35. Van der Auwera P, Legrand JC. Ticarcillin–clavulanic acid therapy in severe infections. Drugs Exp Clin Res 1985;11(11):805–13.

36. Lode H, Springsklee M. Klinische Ergebnisse mit Sulbactam/Ampicillin in einer multizentrischen Studie an 425 Patienten. [Clinical results with sulbactam/ampicillin in a multicenter study of 425 patients.] Med Klin (Munich) 1989;84(5):236–41.

37. Aithal PG, Day CP. The natural history of histologically proved drug induced liver disease. Gut 1999;44(5):731–5.

38. Nathani MG, Mutchnick MG, Tynes DJ, Ehrinpreis MN. An unusual case of amoxicillin/clavulanic acid-related hepatotoxicity. Am J Gastroenterol 1998;93(8):1363–5.

39. Chawla A, Kahn E, Yunis EJ, Daum F. Rapidly progressive cholestasis: an unusual reaction to amoxicillin/clavulanic acid therapy in a child. J Pediatr 2000;136(1):121–3.

40. Hebbard GS, Smith KG, Gibson PR, Bhathal PS. Augmentin-induced jaundice with a fatal outcome. Med J Aust 1992;156(4):285–6.

41. Cavanzo FJ, Garcia CF, Botero RC. Chronic cholestasis, paucity of bile ducts, red cell aplasia, and the Stevens–Johnson syndrome. An ampicillin-associated case. Gastroenterology 1990;99(3):854–6.

42. Escallier F, Dalac S, Caillot D, Boulitrop C, Collet E, Lambert D. Erythème polymorphe, aplasie, hépatite cholestatique au cours d'un traitement par Augmentin (amoxicilline acide clavulanique). [Erythema multiforme, aplasia, cholestatic hepatitis during treatment with Augmentin (amoxicillin + clavulanic acid).] Rev Med Interne 1990;11(1):73–5.

43. Silvain C, Fort E, Levillain P, Labat-Labourdette J, Beauchant M. Granulomatous hepatitis due to combination of amoxicillin and clavulanic acid. Dig Dis Sci 1992;37(1):150–2.

44. Belknap MK, McClelland KJ. Cholestatic hepatitis associated with amoxicillin–clavulanate. Wis Med J 1993;92(5):241–2.

45. Reading C, Slocombe B. Augmentin: clavulanate-potentiated amoxicillin. In: Queener SF, Webber JA, Queener SW, editors. Betalactam Antibiotics for Clinical Use. New York: Marcel Dekker, 1986;527.

46. Hautekeete ML, Horsmans Y, Van Waeyenberge C, Demanet C, Henrion J, Verbist L, Brenard R, Sempoux C,

Michielsen PP, Yap PS, Rahier J, Geubel AP. HLA association of amoxicillin–clavulanate-induced hepatitis. Gastroenterology 1999;117(5):1181–6.

47. Thomson JA, Fairley CK, Ugoni AM, Forbes AB, Purcell PM, Desmond PV, Smallwood RA, McNeil JJ. Risk factors for the development of amoxycillin–clavulanic acid associated jaundice. Med J Aust 1995;162(12):638–40.

48. Berson A, Freneaux E, Larrey D, Lepage V, Douay C, Mallet C, Fromenty B, Benhamou JP, Pessayre D. Possible role of HLA in hepatotoxicity. An exploratory study in 71 patients with drug-induced idiosyncratic hepatitis. J Hepatol 1994;20(3):336–42.

49. Van Waeryenberge C, Hautekeete ML, Horsmans Y. Demanet C, et al. Amoxycillin–clavulanate-induced hepatitis is linked to the DRB11501-DRB50101-DQB10602 haplotype but not to DPB antigens. Europ J Immunogen 1998;25(Suppl 1):66.

50. Donaldson PT, Underhill JA, Clare M, O'Donohue J, et al. Is there a genetic basis for Augmentin associated jaundice? A link with HLA DRB11501-DQA10102-DQB10602 haplotype. Hepatology 1998;28:256A.

51. O'Donohue J, Oien KA, Donaldson P, Underhill J, Clare M, MacSween RN, Mills PR. Co-amoxiclav jaundice: clinical and histological features and HLA class II association. Gut 2000;47(5):717–20.

52. Pill MW, O'Neill CV, Chapman MM, Singh AK. Suspected acute interstitial nephritis induced by piperacillin-tazobactam Pharmacotherapy 1997;17(1):166–9.

53. Edwards RG, Dewdney JM, Dobrzanski RJ, Lee D. Immunogenicity and allergenicity studies on two beta-lactam structures, a clavam, clavulanic acid, and a carbapenem: structure-activity relationships. Int Arch Allergy Appl Immunol 1988;85(2):184–9.

54. Fernandez-Rivas M, Perez Carral C, Cuevas M, Marti C, Moral A, Senent CJ. Selective allergic reactions to clavulanic acid. J Allergy Clin Immunol 1995;95(3):748–50.

55. Wilson SE, Nord CE. Clinical trials of extended spectrum penicillin/beta-lactamase inhibitors in the treatment of intra-abdominal infections. European and North American experience. Am J Surg 1995;169(Suppl 5A):S21–6.

56. Olivencia-Yurvati AH, Sanders SP. Sulbactam-induced hyperpyrexia. Arch Intern Med 1990;150(9):1961.

57. Beer JH, Vogt A, Neftel K, Cottagnoud P. False positive results for leucocytes in urine dipstick test with common antibiotics. BMJ 1996;313(7048):25.

Bethanechol

General Information

Bethanechol is a quaternary ammonium compound that shares both the muscarinic and nicotinic actions of acetylcholine but it is much more slowly deactivated. It has been used to treat clomipramine-induced orgasmic dysfunction (1).

Organs and Systems

Nervous system

An acute dystonic reaction to bethanecol has been reported in a 10-month-old boy (SEDA-12, 124). This reaction was unexpected since bethanecol does not normally penetrate the blood–brain barrier; the authors assumed that the barrier may not be impenetrable to the drug in young infants.

During a controlled clinical trial of intraventricular bethanecol in patients with Alzheimer's disease, reversible drug-induced parkinsonism was observed in one patient (SEDA-15, 5). The frequent co-existence of Alzheimer's disease and Parkinson's disease presents potential problems for therapy and adverse effects when the cholinergic system is manipulated.

Reference

1. Bernik M, Kieira AH, Nunes PV. Bethanecol chloride for treatment of clomipramine-induced orgasmic dysfunction in males. Rev Hosp Clin Fac Med Sao Paulo 2004;59(6):357–60.

Bevantolol

See also Beta-adrenoceptor antagonists

General Information

Bevantolol, a hydrophilic cardioselective beta-blocker with membrane-stabilizing activity, may have a higher incidence of fatigue, headache, and dizziness than atenolol or propranolol (1,2).

References

1. Maclean D. Bevantolol vs propranolol: a double-blind controlled trial in essential hypertension. Angiology 1988;39(6):487–96.

2. Rodrigues EA, Lawrence JD, Dasgupta P, Hains AD, Lahiri A, Wilkinson PR, Raftery EB. Comparison of bevantolol and atenolol in chronic stable angina. Am J Cardiol 1988;61(15):1204–9.

Biguanides

General Information

Biguanides (1) and metformin (2–4) have been reviewed. Metformin (rINN) is the only biguanide commonly used; buformin (rINN) and phenformin (rINN) have been withdrawn in many countries (SEDA-4, 306) because of dangerous adverse effects. However, they are still available in a few countries, and with increasing travel, adverse effects of drugs no longer available in one country can occur if the drug is obtained elsewhere.

The biguanides have a special affinity for the mitochondrial membrane, which causes an alteration in electron transport and results in reduced oxygen consumption. Inhibition of the active transport of glucose in the intestinal mucosa, absent activation of glucose transporters, inhibition of gluconeogenesis, and inhibition of fatty acid oxidation and of lipid synthesis are the effects that are considered to cause lowering of the blood glucose and improving blood lipids in diabetes mellitus. The blood glucose lowering effect of metformin was comparable to that of sulfonylureas, according to a meta-analysis, but body weight increases with sulfonylureas and falls with metformin, leading to a mean weight change difference of 2.9 kg (5).

Most (70–90%) of a dose of metformin is eliminated via the kidneys with a half-life of 9 hours (6). In contrast, phenformin is mostly eliminated by metabolism; its half-life is about 11 hours (7).

Observational studies

In a large American study in 3234 non-diabetic people with a raised fasting blood glucose and a raised blood glucose 2 hours after a glucose load, diabetes occurred in 7.8 cases per 100 participants per year after a mean treatment period of 2.8 years with metformin 850 mg bd; there were 11 cases per 100 participants per year after placebo and 4.8 cases per 100 participants per year after a life-style intervention program (8). Gastrointestinal symptoms were most frequent in those who took metformin. In a later study, glucose tolerance tests were performed after a 14-day washout period of metformin and placebo in the patients who had not developed diabetes (9). Diabetes was more frequently diagnosed in the metformin group, but when the diabetes conversions during treatment and washout were combined, diabetes was still significantly less common in the metformin group.

Comparative studies

Metformin and troglitazone have been compared in 21 patients with type 2 diabetes unresponsive to glibenclamide 10 mg bd (10). Metformin stabilized weight and reduced adipocyte size, leptin concentrations, and glucose transport. GLUT1 and GLUT4 in isolated adipocytes were not changed. Insulin-stimulated whole-body glucose disposal rate increased by 20%. Troglitazone caused increases in body weight, adipocyte size, leptin concentrations, and basal and insulin-stimulated glucose transport. GLUT4 protein expression was increased two-fold and insulin-stimulated whole-body glucose disposal rate increased by 44%.

Placebo-controlled studies

In a placebo-controlled study in 40 patients with impaired glucose tolerance metformin 500 mg bd for 6 months increased insulin-stimulated glucose metabolism by 20% with minimal improvement in glucose tolerance; this effect was maintained after 12 months (11).

In 82 children aged 10–16 years with type 2 diabetes, metformin lowered HbA_{1c} and fasting blood glucose compared with placebo (12). More patients who took placebo had to drop out because more medication was necessary. Most of the adverse events (abdominal pain, diarrhea, nausea, vomiting) occurred during metformin treatment.

Combinations of oral hypoglycemic drugs

The different mechanisms of action of the various classes of hypoglycemic drugs makes combined therapy feasible: the sulfonylureas and meglitinides stimulate insulin production by different mechanisms, the biguanides reduce glucose production by the liver and excretion from the liver, acarbose reduces the absorption of glucose from the gut, and the thiazolidinediones reduce insulin resistance in fat. It is not necessary to wait until the maximal dose of one drug has been reached before starting another. However, sulfonylureas and meglitinides should no longer be used when endogenous insulin production is minimal. Combinations of insulin with sulfonylureas or meglitinides should only be used while the patient is changing to insulin, except when long-acting insulin is given at night in order to give the islets a rest and to stimulate daytime insulin secretion.

This subject has been reviewed in relation to combined oral therapy. In a systematic review of 63 studies with a duration of at least 3 months and involving at least 10 patients at the end of the study, and in which HbA_{1c} was reported, five different classes of oral drugs were almost equally effective in lowering blood glucose concentrations (13). HbA_{1c} was reduced by about 1–2% in all cases. Combination therapy gave additive effects. However, long-term vascular risk reduction was demonstrated only with sulfonylureas and metformin.

In a placebo-controlled study in 116 patients who responded insufficiently to metformin 2.5 g/day, rosiglitazone 2 or 4 mg bd was added for 26 weeks (14). HbA_{1c} and fasting plasma glucose improved and hemoglobin fell. Edema was reported in 5.2% of the patients who took rosiglitazone and two patients withdrew because of headache.

Biguanides + meglitinides

Patients with type 2 diabetes with unsatisfactory control after taking metformin for 6 months were randomized to metformin alone, repaglinide alone, or metformin + repaglinide (each 27 patients) (15). Combined therapy reduced HbA_{1c} after 3 months by 1.4% and fasting glucose by 2.2 mmol/l. Repaglinide alone or in combination with metformin increased insulin concentrations. The most common adverse effects were hypoglycemia, diarrhea, and headache. Gastrointestinal adverse effects were common in those taking metformin alone, and body weight increased in both groups taking repaglinide.

In 12 patients with type 2 diabetes, a combination of nateglinide 120 mg or placebo with metformin 500 mg before each meal on two separate days was well tolerated (16). One patient taking nateglinide had a headache. One patient was withdrawn because of a myocardial infarction and had multivessel coronary artery disease on catheterization.

In a prospective, randomized, double-blind, placebo-controlled study for 24 weeks, 701 patients took nateglinide 120 mg before the three main meals, or metformin 500 mg tds, or the combination of the two, or placebo (17). The most frequent adverse effect was hypoglycemia, and it was most common in the combination group. There were no differences between those who took nateglinide only or metformin only and there were no episodes of serious hypoglycemia. Diarrhea was more frequent in those taking metformin or the combination, but infection, nausea, headache, and abdominal pain were comparable in the two groups.

Of 82 patients insufficiently controlled by metformin, 27 continued to take metformin with placebo, 28 took titrated repaglinide with placebo, and 27 took metformin with titrated repaglinide for 4–5 months (18). There were no serious adverse effects. Nine patients taking metformin + repaglinide reported 30 hypoglycemic events and three patients taking repaglinide reported 9 events.

Insulin + biguanides

Metformin was given as an adjunct to insulin in a double-blind, placebo-controlled study in 28 adolescents needing more than 1 U/kg/day (19). The dose of metformin was 1000 mg/day when body weight was under 50 kg, 1500 mg/day when it was 50–75 kg, and 2000 mg/day when it was over 75 kg. Metformin lowered insulin requirements. The number of episodes of hypoglycemia increased compared with placebo. There was gastrointestinal discomfort in six patients taking metformin and five taking placebo.

A comparable placebo-controlled study was reported in 353 patients with type 2 diabetes for 48 weeks. All were taking insulin, and HbA$_{1c}$ fell in those who also took metformin. Body weight was reduced by 0.4 kg by metformin and increased by 1.2 kg by placebo. Symptomatic episodes of hypoglycemia were more common with metformin. There were mild transient gastrointestinal complaints in 56 and 13% respectively (20).

Insulin plus metformin (27 patients, 2000 mg/day) or troglitazone (30 patients, 600 mg/day) in patients with type 2 diabetes using at least 30 U/day was compared with insulin alone (30 patients) for 4 months (21). Body weight increased in the insulin and the insulin plus troglitazone groups. In the insulin plus metformin group there were significantly more gastrointestinal adverse effects but less hypoglycemia than the other groups.

In 80 patients taking metformin 850 or 1000 mg tds plus NPH insulin at bedtime, metformin was withdrawn and repaglinide 4 mg tds added in half of the patients for 16 weeks (22). In the repaglinide group the dose of insulin increased slightly and weight gain was 1.8 kg more. Mild hypoglycemia occurred more often in the metformin group; nightly episodes of hypoglycemia occurred only with repaglinide. One patient taking repaglinide had a myocardial infarction, and one had three separate hospitalizations for chest pain (myocardial infarction was excluded). No specific data were presented about gastrointestinal adverse effects or infections.

Contraindications

Contraindications to treatment with biguanides are:

1. impaired renal function (serum creatinine may not be a sufficient indicator; creatinine clearance must be estimated)
2. an increased risk of impaired renal function in intercurrent diseases with fever, congestive heart failure, or infections of the urinary tract, during treatment with diuretics, intravenous pyelography, or severe dieting
3. states associated with tissue hypoxia (respiratory insufficiency, heart insufficiency, anemia, and peripheral vascular disease)
4. hepatitis and hepatic cirrhosis
5. excessive use of alcohol
6. wasting diseases
7. preoperatively and postoperatively.

In general, biguanides should not be used in people aged over 75 years (23).

Of 308 patients 73% had contraindications, risk factors, or intercurrent illnesses necessitating withdrawal of metformin (24): 19% had renal impairment, 25% heart failure, 6.5% respiratory insufficiency, and 1.3% hepatic impairment; 51% had advanced coronary heart disease, 9.8% atrial fibrillation, 3.3% chronic alcohol abuse, 2% advanced peripheral arterial disease, and 0.7% were pregnant.

Four fatal cases in 18 months in a community hospital were reported; three had clear contraindications (25): a 45-year-old woman with liver cirrhosis, a 64-year-old man with coronary artery disease, and a 65-year-old man with peripheral arterial disease and asthma; a 74-year-old man had renal insufficiency.

In a retrospective study of 1874 patients with type 2 diabetes taking metformin, 25% had contraindications, including acute myocardial infarction, cardiac failure, renal impairment, and chronic liver disease (26). However, contraindications often did not lead to withdrawal of metformin: in 621 episodes, only 10% stopped taking it. Only 25 and 18% stopped taking metformin when they developed renal impairment or myocardial infarction, respectively. One patient developed lactic acidosis, but this may have been a consequence of myocardial infarction.

Organs and Systems

Cardiovascular

The cardiovascular effects of metformin have been reviewed (27). Metformin reduces blood pressure and has a beneficial effect on blood lipid concentrations.

In a retrospective study, cardiovascular deaths in patients using a sulfonylurea only ($n = 741$) were compared with deaths in patients taking a sulfonylurea + metformin ($n = 169$) (28). In patients taking the combination the adjusted odds ratios (95% CI) were:

- overall mortality 1.63 (1.27, 2.09);
- mortality from ischemic heart disease 1.73 (1.17, 2.55);
- stroke 2.33 (1.17, 4.63).

The patients taking the combination were younger, had had diabetes for longer, were more obese, and had higher blood glucose concentrations.

Metabolism

Biguanides cause hypoglycemia in 0.24 cases per 100 patient-years and it is more common when they are used in combination with a sulfonylurea (29). In 102 consecutive patients with drug-induced hospital-related hypoglycemic coma, 13 were taking metformin + glibenclamide and 3 were taking metformin + insulin (30).

Lactic acidosis

DoTS classification

Adverse effect: Lactic acidosis due to biguanides
Dose-relation: toxic effect
Time-course: time-independent
Susceptibility factors: genetic (slow phenformin metabolizers); age; disease (impaired liver, kidney, or cardiac function, alcoholism)

Biguanides can cause lactic acidosis, which is fatal in 50% of cases (31).

- A 65-year-old man with a creatinine clearance of 67 ml/minute taking metformin 850 mg bd developed lactic acidosis (lactate 25 mmol/l, pH 7.13, bicarbonate 5 mmol/l) (32). Despite the relatively small dosage of metformin, he had unexplained very high metformin concentrations (61 µg/ml).

A possible explanation for the high metformin concentration in this case was that an unknown substance related to intestinal inclusion inhibited its tubular excretion. Other cases involving metformin have included the following:

- a 62-year-old woman: pH 6.60, blood lactate 45 mmol/l, creatinine 133 µmol/l (33);
- a 72-year-old woman: pH 6.84, creatinine 125 µmol/l (34);
- a 75-year-old woman: pH 6.73, lactate 18 mmol/l (34);
- a patient with creatinine 91 µmol/l, creatinine clearance 52 ml/minute, metformin concentration 61 µg/ml (target under 5 µg/ml) (35);
- a 52-year-old woman, a chronic alcohol user: pH 6.74, lactate over 30 mmol/l, creatinine 710 µmol/l (36);
- an 83-year-old woman with mild renal insufficiency (37).

All survived, but all needed hemodialysis. In all cases there were contraindications to metformin.

Five patients with metformin-associated severe lactic acidosis, seen between 1 September 1998 and 31 May 2001, have been reported (38). Two had attempted suicide. All had severe metabolic acidosis with a high anion gap and raised blood lactate concentrations. Four developed profound hypotension and three had acute respiratory failure. Three had normal preceding renal function. Three required conventional hemodialysis and two continuous renal replacement therapy.

Cases also continue to be reported with buformin and phenformin (39).

- A 67-year-old man who had taken phenformin and glibenclamide for 2 years became lethargic and confused (40). His pH was 6.91, serum lactate 25 mmol/l and later 30 mmol/l, and blood glucose very low (0.5 mmol/l), possibly because of vomiting, anorexia, and glibenclamide. Hemodialysis was advised but not performed, since he recovered spontaneously.

Incidence

In patients taking metformin, lactic acidosis is rare (3 per 100 000 patient-years) and is most often seen when contraindications to metformin (impaired kidney or liver function, alcoholism, circulatory problems, old age) are neglected or not detected (41). Although the relative risk of lactic acidosis with metformin is significantly lower than with phenformin or buformin (42), it has been repeatedly reported (SEDA-6, 371) (43), even in the absence of known contraindications (44).

Experience with metformin in a large American health organization in 9875 patients has been presented (45). There was one probable case of lactic acidosis in an 82-year-old woman who developed renal impairment while taking metformin 500 mg/day.

In 11 797 patients (22 296 person-years) in Saskatchewan who took metformin from 1980–95 there were 9 cases of lactic acidosis per 100 000 patient-years (46), a much lower incidence than the estimated rate of 40–64 cases for phenformin.

The lower frequency of lactic acidosis during treatment with metformin compared with other biguanides may be caused by its short non-polar hydrophobic side chains substituted with two CH_3 groups. This has a lower affinity for hydrophobic structures, such as phospholipids in mitochondrial and cellular membranes, than the longer monosubstituted side-chains of the other biguanides (41).

Mechanism and susceptibility factors

Biguanides in high doses inhibit the oxidation of carbohydrate substrates by affecting mitochondrial function. Anoxidative carbohydrate metabolism stimulates the production of lactate. High lactate production leads to lactic acidosis (type B) with a low pH (<6.95). Hyperlactatemia was common in patients taking buformin, even without alcoholism or impaired liver, kidney, or cardiac function (47).

In reaction to a report of lactic acidosis at a therapeutic metformin concentration (SEDA-22, 476), in which a mitochondrial defect was supposed to have increased susceptibility to metformin, it has been observed that diabetes itself may dispose to hyperlactatemia (48). Others (49) have taken issue with the opinion (SEDA-22, 476) that the association of lactic acidosis with metformin may be coincidental, as lactic acidosis can also emerge during critical illnesses (type A lactic acidosis, caused by circulatory insufficiency). However, patients with type B lactic acidosis, with high biguanide concentrations, will also develop circulatory insufficiency after some hours.

The main susceptibility factor for lactic acidosis due to metformin is renal insufficiency (33). In patients taking phenformin, poor oxidative metabolism may contribute (50).

All patients admitted to a hospital during 6 months who had taken at least one dose of metformin were retrospectively evaluated for susceptibility factors for metformin-associated lactic acidosis (8). There were 263 hospitalizations in 204 patients. In 71 admissions there was at least one contraindication, such as renal or liver disease, renal dysfunction, congestive cardiac failure, metabolic acidosis, or an intravenous iodinated contrast medium given within 48 hours of metformin. In 29 (41%) metformin was continued despite the contraindication. The most frequent contraindication was a raised serum creatinine, but in only eight of the 32 admissions was metformin withdrawn. Of nine patients using metformin who died (not necessarily directly related to metformin), six had an absolute contraindication. In two patients who died and in one who survived, blood lactate was increased and this was temporally related to the use of metformin.

Whether metformin in therapeutic doses can cause lactic acidosis in the absence of renal insufficiency has been investigated by studying case histories of metformin-associated lactic acidosis in various databases published from May 1995 to January 2000 (51). Overdoses and lactic acidosis caused by contrast media were excluded. There were 21 reports of 26 cases, of which five did not comply with the criteria (lactate over 5 mmol/l, pH 7.35 or less). Plasma metformin concentration was measured in only four cases. The authors distinguished between lactic acidosis precipitated by metformin, which was defined as occurring without accumulation of metformin, and lactic acidosis that occurred during primary acute or chronic renal insufficiency, with accumulation of metformin. In the first group, six of the eight patients died. In the second group, notwithstanding a mean lactate concentration of nearly 15 mmol/l, only one of the 12 patients died, having refused dialysis. They concluded that there is no relation between the use of metformin and lactic acidosis, except when metformin accumulates. This has been illustrated by the case of a 76-year-old woman taking 850 mg metformin bd who developed lactic acidosis due to metformin accumulation during deteriorating kidney function (52).

Drugs that can precipitate lactic acidosis in patients taking metformin include ACE inhibitors, thiazide diuretics, NSAIDs, and drugs such as furosemide, nifedipine, cimetidine, amiloride, triamterene, trimethoprim, and digoxin, which are all secreted in the renal tubules, compete with metformin, and can contribute to increased plasma metformin concentrations (53).

The need to follow recommended guidelines strictly in order to avoid lactic acidosis in patients taking metformin has been emphasized (54).

Presentation

The early symptoms of lactic acidosis are nausea, vomiting, and diarrhea; since these are common adverse effects of biguanides, a careful watch should be kept for their sudden onset or aggravation, which might point to lactic acidosis (55).

In retrospective studies, neither the degree of hyperlactatemia nor accumulation of metformin had prognostic significance, but mortality was linked to the underlying disease (56,57).

Management

The best therapy of metformin-induced lactic acidosis is immediate hemodialysis, but metformin in the tissues continues to produce lactate while the drug is being removed during dialysis. Sodium bicarbonate is not very effective and can paradoxically lower the pH and cause hypernatremia and fluid overload. Tracheal intubation and mechanical ventilation may be necessary (53). Theophylline and dichloroacetate have also been used. Theophylline stimulates oxygen exchange in the lungs. Dichloroacetate activates pyruvate dehydrogenase, inhibiting lactate formation, but it is neurotoxic, can cause cataract, and is mutagenic (SEDA-7, 410).

The results of hemodialysis in biguanide-induced lactic acidosis are variable. Metformin and buformin are dialysable, but phenformin is poorly eliminated.

Successful continuous venovenous hemofiltration has been reported (58).

- A 68-year-old woman with type 2 diabetes and hypertension took phenformin 90 mg/day and glibenclamide 6 mg/day. She developed a urinary tract infection and oliguria followed by respiratory distress and mental confusion without neurological defects. Her pH was 6.84, serum lactate 28 mmol/l, creatinine 186 µmol/l, and glucose 10.4 mmol/l, and there were no ketone bodies. She received assisted ventilation, bicarbonate, dopamine + obutamine, glucose + insulin, and antibiotics. Her serum lactate increased to 44 mmol/l and continuous venovenous hemofiltration was started. After 5 days her lactate concentration was in the reference range (0.5–2.2 mmol/l). The serum phenformin concentration was almost 600 ng/ml (10 times the therapeutic value).

Nutrition

Vitamin B_{12} deficiency can be caused by metformin.

- A 63-year-old man with type 2 diabetes, who had taken metformin for at least 5 years, had a low serum vitamin B_{12} concentration (110 pg/ml; reference range 200–230) and a normal serum folate (59). There were no autoantibodies. A Schilling test showed malabsorption of vitamin B_{12}. Metformin was withdrawn and 2 months later a Schilling test showed no malabsorption.
- This case prompted a report of 10 metformin-associated patients with cobalamin deficiency among 162 patients with vitamin B_{12} concentrations below 200 pg/ml (60). They had taken a mean dose of metformin of 2015 mg/day for an average of 8.9 years. The mean vitamin B_{12} concentration was 140 pg/ml. All had normal serum folate and creatinine concentrations and no antibodies to intrinsic factor. In one patient there was malabsorption.

Hematologic

Megaloblastic anemia is rare with metformin, but vitamin B_{12} concentrations can be reduced by metformin and phenformin (61) because of reduced absorption, and pre-existing deficiency can be exacerbated (41).

Metformin can occasionally cause a hemolytic anemia.

- A 68-year-old woman of North African Jewish descent with a raised HbA_{1c} was given metformin 850 mg tds and repaglinide 1 mg tds, and 14 days later developed extreme weakness and anemia, her hemoglobin having fallen from 12 to 8 g/dl within 1 week (62). Her reticulocyte count was 11%, with polychromasia. The bilirubin rose to 35 µmol/l (27 µmol/l direct). The haptoglobin concentration was low and a direct Coombs' test was negative. Metformin was withdrawn. Two units of erythrocytes were transfused and the hemoglobin rose to 11 g/dl and remained stable. Glucose-6-phosphate dehydrogenase (G6PD) activity was significantly reduced. There were no other precipitating factors for hemolysis due to G6PD deficiency.

It is unclear whether metformin caused hemolysis directly in this case or via G6PD deficiency. Two other patients have been reported with normal G6PD activity (63,64); one had a positive Coombs' test (64).

Gastrointestinal

Abdominal discomfort is frequent with metformin (15–25%), and nausea, vomiting, and diarrhea occur even in the absence of lactic acidosis. Other effects include flatulence, abdominal bloating, anorexia, and a metallic taste. Anorexia and weight loss are often seen at the beginning of treatment. Phenformin can cause hemorrhagic gastritis (65).

The gastrointestinal adverse effects of metformin can be reduced by giving the metformin during or immediately after meals, starting with a low dose and increasing it gradually (41).

In 43 patients with poorly controlled type 2 diabetes using insulin, the addition of metformin improved HbA_{1c} and reduced the dose of insulin (66). Seven patients in the metformin group and four in the placebo group had nausea; nine versus four had diarrhea.

- Three patients who had taken metformin for more than 2 years developed diarrhea (67). After withdrawal of metformin the diarrhea resolved within 1 month. A fourth patient developed diarrhea after taking metformin for 4 months, which stopped after withdrawal; rechallenge with metformin 8 months later led to recurrence. Three of these patients had bowel disease (diverticulosis, irritable bowel syndrome, and diabetic neuropathy).
- A 49-year-old woman developed chronic diarrhea after using metformin 850 mg tds and insulin for 5 years (68). After 5 months, metformin was withdrawn and the diarrhea resolved within 3 days. On rechallenge the diarrhea returned.
- A 44-year-old non-diabetic man took metformin 1700 mg/day for some weeks for obesity (69). He developed severe gastrointestinal hemorrhage needing blood transfusion. A bleeding Meckel's diverticulum was removed and he had no further hemorrhage. Coagulation studies, to investigate whether reduced platelet aggregation or altered coagulation factors (increased tissue plasminogen activator (tPA) or reduced tPA-Ag, or PAI-1) could have contributed, were not done.

Liver

Metformin can cause hepatitis (70).

- A 52-year-old woman took glipizide and enalapril and then, because of persistent hyperglycemia, metformin 1000 mg/day (71). Her liver enzymes were normal, and after 2 weeks the dosage of metformin was increased to 2000 mg/day. Two weeks later she became icteric and her bilirubin and liver enzymes were increased. Serological studies were negative. All drugs were withdrawn. A liver biopsy was consistent with toxic hepatitis. She had normal liver enzymes after a month.

Hepatitis after sulfonylureas is known, and this patient had taken glipizide for several years. The combination of glipizide and metformin may have been to blame.

- A 75-year-old man taking insulin about 40 U/day was given metformin 500 mg bd (72). He also used enteric-coated aspirin, diltiazem XR, ibuprofen, and lovastatin. Two months later his liver enzymes were raised, but he felt well. Hepatitis antibodies were negative. After withdrawal of metformin his liver enzymes became normal. He agreed to restart metformin. His liver enzymes remained normal, but he finally preferred insulin monotherapy.

It is not clear what caused the hepatitis in this case, although it seems that metformin was not to blame.

- A 64-year-old man developed cholestatic jaundice 2 weeks after starting to take metformin 500 mg bd (73). It resolved slowly over several months after withdrawal.

Pancreas

Phenformin can cause pancreatitis (74).

Skin

Urticaria and rashes are seen occasionally with metformin. Lichen ruber planus has been reported (75).

Immunologic

Leukocytoclastic vasculitis and pneumonitis have been attributed to metformin (76,77).

Death

In 2275 diabetic patients aged 45–74 years compared with 9047 non-diabetics with proven coronary artery disease, 32% of those taking metformin and 44% of those taking combined metformin and glibenclamide died during 7.7 years (78). After 4 years the risks of death with metformin alone and combined therapy were equal, but after 7 years combined therapy had a worse prognosis.

Second-Generation Effects

Lactation

Metformin is increasingly being used in the polycystic ovarian syndrome and therefore in lactating women. In seven breastfeeding mothers taking a median dose of 1500 mg/day, the mean relative infant dose transferred in the milk was 0.28% (79). Serum metformin concentrations were very low or undetectable in infants and they appeared to be healthy. A specific warning was given for children with impaired renal function (prematurity, renal insufficiency).

Susceptibility Factors

Age

The effect of age on the response to metformin has been studied in 174 patients aged over 70 years, not well-controlled on glibenclamide 7.5 mg/day or gliclazide 120 mg/day (80). They were given either maximal doses of a sulfonylurea (glibenclamide 15 mg/day or gliclazide 240 mg/day) or a sulfonylurea + metformin (1700 mg/day). Renal function and liver function were normal. There were nine cases of non-severe hypoglycemia in the first group. In the second group there were two cases of hypoglycemia after delayed meals and 35% had transient mild gastrointestinal discomfort. There were no increases in lactic acid. Lipid concentrations were a little lower in the second group. The authors concluded that age as such is not a contraindication to metformin, provided that contraindications, such as renal impairment, are absent and that blood glucose is measured regularly.

Drug Administration

Drug overdose

The regional poison centers certified by the American Association of Poison Control have reported 55 cases of metformin ingestion by children (81). Unintentional ingestion of 1700 mg of metformin did not pose health risks. In 21 children tested for blood glucose, lactate, or electrolytes, there was no evidence of lactic acidosis. Plasma metformin concentrations were not determined.

- A 37-year-old woman purposely took metformin 10 g (82). She did not develop hypoglycemia, but the serum lactate increased to 3.2 mmol/l (reference range under 2.1 mmol/l) and she became nauseated. She recovered.
- A healthy 21-year-old woman took metformin 45 g (53×850 mg) in a suicide attempt and developed acute pancreatitis with metabolic acidosis (pH 6.96), hypoglycemia (1.3 mmol/l), and an anion gap of 37 mmol/l (83). She was given 290 g of dextrose, and her blood glucose rose to 25 mmol/l. Other laboratory tests were normal. When later measured, serum amylase was 121 U/l, urinary amylase 97 U/l (both twice the upper limit of the reference range), and serum lipase 724 U/l (5–6 times raised). A CT scan with contrast showed stage B acute pancreatitis. Serum amylase and serum lipase rose to 368 and 1900 U/l respectively. She recovered after 8 days. A CT scan 1 month later was normal. Lactic acid and metformin were not determined. The use of alcohol or other drugs that can cause pancreatitis could not be established. Gallstones and hyperlipidemia were not present. The initial hypoglycemia could have been a direct effect of metformin; hyperglycemia is more often seen during lactic acidosis.
- A non-diabetic 25-year-old woman died after 2 days of lactic acidosis and multiple organ failure, having taken an unknown amount of her father's metformin (38,84).
- A 58-year-old woman with type 2 diabetes took an overdose of metform in 55 g plus 100 mg of glibenclamide and 3.1 g of acarbose (38,84). She developed lactic acidosis and survived with hemodialysis.

When a patient in coma has an unexplained anion gap, a suicide attempt with metformin should be considered.

Drug–Drug Interactions

Alpha-glucosidase inhibitors

Metformin can be effectively combined with miglitol (SEDA-25, 514) but metformin may accumulate in the gastrointestinal wall, and the combination of metformin with acarbose or miglitol may reduce the absorption of metformin (85,86).

Cephalexin

In a double-blind, randomized, crossover study in 12 healthy volunteers, cefalexin 500 mg increased the C_{max} and AUC of a single dose of metformin 500 mg by 34 and 24% respectively and reduced its renal clearance to 14% (87). The authors suggested that cefalexin inhibits the renal tubular secretion of metformin.

Contrast media for radiological investigations

Radiocontrast media can induce acute renal insufficiency in patients taking metformin (88,89). Metformin should be withdrawn 2 days before an iodinated contrast medium is given (SEDA-21, 445) and the following protocol has been suggested (90):

- take a blood sample for creatinine baseline estimation before giving a contrast medium;
- withdraw metformin 48 hours before the investigation;
- if the urine output is normal for 48 hours after the radiological procedure the patient can resume metformin;
- when it is discovered after a procedure that the preinvestigation creatinine was raised (since the procedure may be carried out before the creatinine is known), the patient's physician should be contacted and the creatinine must be measured again within 48 hours.

Since January 1998 the package insert approved by the FDA has stated: "Glucophage (metformin) should be discontinued at the time of or prior to the procedure and withheld for 48 hours subsequent to the procedure and reinstituted only after renal function has been re-evaluated and found to be normal" (91).

Multiple drugs

The combination of metformin with other drugs that can lower the blood glucose concentration can result in severe hypoglycemia.

- A 79-year-old woman was admitted to hospital stuporose and unresponsive (92). She had taken metformin 850 mg bd for 14 days, during which time she complained of loss of appetite and consumed little starch. On that morning she had had nausea and dizziness. Her blood glucose was 2.0 mmol/l and her serum potassium 3.3 mmol/l. A CT scan of the head was normal.

The combination of metformin, which itself does not cause hypoglycemia, with an ACE inhibitor, nitrofurantoin, and an NSAID, which all have glucose-lowering effects, and poor food intake may have led to hypoglycemia in this case.

NSAIDs

Drug interactions can precipitate metformin-induced lactic acidosis, as has been reported after the addition of indometacin (93).

- A 57-year-old woman, who had taken metformin 500 mg bd for 15 years, took indometacin 50 mg qds for 2 months. She developed oliguria and acidosis (pH 6.82, serum lactate 21 mmol/l, creatinine 480 µmol/l). After stopping metformin and indometacin she improved and left hospital with stable impaired kidney function.

The authors reported that two other cases of metformin-associated lactic acidosis with concurrent NSAID therapy have been reported to the Committee on Safety of Medicines in the UK. Indometacin can impair kidney function and may have done so in this case. Phenformin can cause tubular damage and oliguria in animals (94) and so it is conceivable that metformin-induced renal damage may also have contributed.

Phenprocoumon

The clearance of phenprocoumon was increased by metformin, perhaps because of increased liver blood flow (95).

Rosiglitazone

In 16 male volunteers aged 22–55 years, rosiglitazone 2 mg bd had no effect on the steady-state pharmacokinetics of oral metformin 500 mg bd; there were no clinically significant episodes of hypoglycemia and blood lactic acid concentrations did not increase (96).

Warfarin

Potentiation of the anticoagulant action of warfarin by phenformin has been reported (97).

References

1. Bailey CJ. Biguanides and NIDDM. Diabetes Care 1992;15(6):755–72.
2. Bailey CJ, Turner RC. Metformin. N Engl J Med 1996;334(9):574–9.
3. Pugh J. Metformin monotherapy for type II diabetes. Adv Ther 1997;14:338–47.
4. Scheen AJ. Clinical pharmacokinetics of metformin. Clin Pharmacokinet 1996;30(5):359–71.
5. Johansen K. Efficacy of metformin in the treatment of NIDDM. Meta-analysis. Diabetes Care 1999;22(1):33–7.
6. Pentikainen PJ, Neuvonen PJ, Penttila A. Pharmacokinetics of metformin after intravenous and oral administration to man. Eur J Clin Pharmacol 1979;16(3):195–202.
7. Alkalay D, Khemani L, Wagner WE, Bartlett MF. Pharmacokinetics of phenformin in man. J Clin Pharmacol 1975;15(5-6):446–8.
8. Knowler WC, Barrett-Connor E, Fowler SE, Hamman RF, Lachin JM, Walker EA, Nathan DM; Diabetes Prevention Program Research Group. Reduction in the incidence of type 2 diabetes with lifestyle intervention or metformin. N Engl J Med 2002;346(6):393–403.
9. Diabetes Prevention Program Research Group. Effects of withdrawal from metformin on the development of diabetes in the diabetes prevention program. Diabetes Care 2003;26(4):977–80.
10. Ciaraldi TP, Kong AP, Chu NV, Kim DD, Baxi S, Loviscach M, Plodkowski R, Reitz R, Caulfield M, Mudaliar S, Henry RR. Regulation of glucose transport and insulin signaling by troglitazone or metformin in adipose tissue of type 2 diabetic subjects. Diabetes 2002;51(1):30–6.
11. Lehtovirta M, Forsen B, Gullstrom M, Haggblom M, Eriksson JG, Taskinen MR, Groop L. Metabolic effects of metformin in patients with impaired glucose tolerance. Diabet Med 2001;18(7):578–83.
12. Jones KL, Arslanian S, Peterokova VA, Park JS, Tomlinson MJ. Effect of metformin in pediatric patients with type 2 diabetes: a randomized controlled trial. Diabetes Care 2002;25(1):89–94.
13. Van Gaal LF, De Leeuw IH. Rationale and options for combination therapy in the treatment of Type 2 diabetes. Diabetologia 2003;46(Suppl 1):M44–50.
14. Gomez-Perez FJ, Fanghanel-Salmon G, Antonio Barbosa J, Montes-Villarreal J, Berry RA, Warsi G, Gould EM. Efficacy and safety of rosiglitazone plus metformin in Mexicans with type 2 diabetes. Diabetes Metab Res Rev 2002;18(2):127–34.
15. Moses R, Slobodniuk R, Boyages S, Colagiuri S, Kidson W, Carter J, Donnelly T, Moffitt P, Hopkins H. Effect of repaglinide addition to metformin monotherapy on glycemic control in patients with type 2 diabetes. Diabetes Care 1999;22(1):119–24.
16. Hirschberg Y, Karara AH, Pietri AO, McLeod JF. Improved control of mealtime glucose excursions with co-administration of nateglinide and metformin. Diabetes Care 2000;23(3):349–53.
17. Horton ES, Clinkingbeard C, Gatlin M, Foley J, Mallows S, Shen S. Nateglinide alone and in combination with metformin improves glycemic control by reducing mealtime glucose levels in type 2 diabetes. Diabetes Care 2000;23(11):1660–5.
18. Moses R. Repaglinide in combination therapy with metformin in Type 2 diabetes. Exp Clin Endocrinol Diabetes 1999;107(Suppl 4):S136–9.
19. Hamilton J, Cummings E, Zdravkovic V, Finegood D, Daneman D. Metformin as an adjunct therapy in adolescents with type 1 diabetes and insulin resistance: a randomized controlled trial. Diabetes Care 2003;26(1):138–43.
20. Wulffele MG, Kooy A, Lehert P, Bets D, Ogterop JC, Borger van der Burg B, Donker AJ, Stehouwer CD. Combination of insulin and metformin in the treatment of type 2 diabetes. Diabetes Care 2002;25(12):2133–40.
21. Strowig SM, Aviles-Santa ML, Raskin P. Comparison of insulin monotherapy and combination therapy with insulin and metformin or insulin and troglitazone in type 2 diabetes. Diabetes Care 2002;25(10):1691–8.
22. Furlong NJ, Hulme SA, O'Brien SV, Hardy KJ. Repaglinide versus metformin in combination with bedtime NPH insulin in patients with type 2 diabetes established on insulin/metformin combination therapy. Diabetes Care 2002;25(10):1685–90.
23. Sulkin TV, Bosman D, Krentz AJ. Contraindications to metformin therapy in patients with NIDDM. Diabetes Care 1997;20(6):925–8.
24. Holstein A, Nahrwold D, Hinze S, Egberts EH. Contraindications to metformin therapy are largely disregarded. Diabet Med 1999;16(8):692–6.
25. Beis SJ, Goshman LM, Newkirk GL. Risk factors for metformin-associated lactic acidosis. WMJ 1999;98(4):56–7.
26. Emslie-Smith AM, Boyle DI, Evans JM, Sullivan F, Morris AD; DARTS/MEMO Collaboration. Contraindications to metformin therapy in patients with Type 2 diabetes—a population-based study of adherence to prescribing guidelines. Diabet Med 2001;18(6):483–8.
27. Howes LG, Sundaresan P, Lykos D. Cardiovascular effects of oral hypoglycaemic drugs. Clin Exp Pharmacol Physiol 1996;23(3):201–6.
28. Olsson J, Lindberg G, Gottsater M, Lindwall K, Sjostrand A, Tisell A, Melander A. Increased mortality in Type II diabetic patients using sulphonylurea and metformin in combination: a population-based observational study. Diabetologia 2000;43(5):558–60.
29. Guariglia A, Gonzi GL, Regolisti G, Vinci S. Treatment of biguanide-induced lactic acidosis: reproposal of the

"physiological" approach and review of the literature. Ann Ital Med Int 1994;9(1):35–9.

30. Ben-Ami H, Nagachandran P, Mendelson A, Edoute Y. Drug-induced hypoglycemic coma in 102 diabetic patients. Arch Intern Med 1999;159(3):281–4.

31. Cohen RD, Woods HF. Lactic acidosis revisited. Diabetes 1983;32(2):181–91.

32. Lalau JD, Race JM, Brinquin L. Lactic acidosis in metformin therapy. Relationship between plasma metformin concentration and renal function. Diabetes Care 1998;21(8):1366–7.

33. Reeker W, Schneider G, Felgenhauer N, Tempel G, Kochs E. Metformin-induzierte Laktatazidose. [Metformin-induced lactic acidosis.] Dtsch Med Wochenschr 2000;125(9):249–51.

34. Lovas K, Fadnes DJ, Dale A. Metforminassosiert laktacidose–pasienteksempel og litteraturgjennomgang. [Metformin associated lactic acidosis—case reports and literature review.] Tidsskr Nor Laegeforen 2000;120(13):1539–41.

35. Soomers AJ, Tack CJ. Ernstige lactaatacidose bij metforminegebruik bij een patient met contra-indicaties voor metformine. [Severe lactic acidosis due to metformin ingestion in a patient with contra-indication for metformin.] Ned Tijdschr Geneeskd 2001;145(2):104–5.

36. Houwerzijl EJ, Snoek WJ, van Haastert M, Holman ND. Ernstige lactaatacidose bij metforminegebruik bij een patient met contra-indicates voor metformine. [Severe lactic acidosis due to metformin therapy in a patient with contra-indications for metformin.] Ned Tijdschr Geneeskd 2000;144(40):1923–6.

37. Berner B, Hummel KM, Strutz F, Ritzel U, Ramadori G, Hagenlocher S, Kleine P, Muller GA. Metformin-assoziierte Lactatazidose mit akutem Nierenversagen bei Diabetes mellitus Typ 2. [Metformin-associated lactic acidosis with acute renal failure in type 2 diabetes mellitus.] Med Klin (Munich) 2002;97(2):99–103.

38. Chang CT, Chen YC, Fang JT, Huang CC. Metformin-associated lactic acidosis: case reports and literature review. J Nephrol 2002;15(4):398–402.

39. Irsigler K, Kritz H, Kaspar L, Lageder H, Regal H. Vier todliche Laktazidosen unter Biguanidtherapie. [Four cases of fatal lactic acidosis during biguanide therapy (author's transl).] Wien Klin Wochenschr 1978;90(6):201–6.

40. Kwong SC, Brubacher J. Phenformin and lactic acidosis: a case report and review. J Emerg Med 1998;16(6):881–6.

41. Cusi K, DeFronzo RA. Metformin: a review of its metabolic effects. Diabetes Rev 1998;6:89–131.

42. Berger W. Zur Problematik der Biguanidbehandlung. Pharma-Kritik (Bern) 1979;1:9.

43. Hermann LS. Metformin: a review of its pharmacological properties and therapeutic use. Diabete Metab 1979;5(3):233–45.

44. Tymms DJ, Leatherdale BA. Lactic acidosis due to metformin therapy in a low risk patient. Postgrad Med J 1988;64(749):230–1.

45. Selby JV, Ettinger B, Swain BE, Brown JB. First 20 months' experience with use of metformin for type 2 diabetes in a large health maintenance organization. Diabetes Care 1999;22(1):38–44.

46. Stang M, Wysowski DK, Butler-Jones D. Incidence of lactic acidosis in metformin users. Diabetes Care 1999;22(6):925–7.

47. Perusicova J, Skrha J, Hodinar A, Bernovska A, Cacakova V, Richtrova A. Hladiny kyseliny mlecne u diabetiku II. Typu lecenych buforminem. [Levels of lactic acid in type II diabetics treated with buformin.] Vnitr Lek 1996;42(1):7–11.

48. Chan NN, Darko D, O'Shea D. Lactic acidosis with therapeutic metformin blood level in a low-risk diabetic patient. Diabetes Care 1999;22(1):178.

49. Cohen RD, Woods HF. Metformin and lactic acidosis. Diabetes Care 1999;22(6):1010–11.

50. Oates NS, Shah RR, Idle JR, Smith RL. Influence of oxidation polymorphism on phenformin kinetics and dynamics. Clin Pharmacol Ther 1983;34(6):827–34.

51. Lalau JD, Race JM. Lactic acidosis in metformin therapy: searching for a link with metformin in reports of "metformin-associated lactic acidosis". Diabetes Obes Metab 2001;3(3):195–201.

52. Kruse JA. Metformin-associated lactic acidosis. J Emerg Med 2001;20(3):267–72.

53. Lothholz H, Rahn A, Thurman P. Metformin-assoziierte Lactatazidose mit akutem Nierenversagen bei Diabetes mellitus Typ 2. [Metformin-associated lactic acidosis with acute renal failure in type 2 diabetes mellitus.] Med Klin (Munich) 2002;97(7):434–5.

54. Chan NN, Brain HP, Feher MD. Metformin-associated lactic acidosis: a rare or very rare clinical entity? Diabet Med 1999;16(4):273–81.

55. Vigneri R, Goldfine ID. Role of metformin in treatment of diabetes mellitus. Diabetes Care 1987;10(1):118–22.

56. Lalau JD, Race JM. Lactic acidosis in metformin therapy. Drugs 1999;58(Suppl 1):55–60.

57. Lalau JD, Race JM. Lactic acidosis in metformin-treated patients. Prognostic value of arterial lactate levels and plasma metformin concentrations. Drug Saf 1999;20(4):377–84.

58. Mariano F, Benzi L, Cecchetti P, Rosatello A, Merante D, Goia F, Capra L, Lanza G, Curto V, Cavalli PL. Efficacy of continuous venovenous haemofiltration (CVVH) in the treatment of severe phenformin-induced lactic acidosis. Nephrol Dial Transplant 1998;13(4):1012–15.

59. Gilligan MA. Metformin and vitamin B12 deficiency. Arch Intern Med 2002;162(4):484–5.

60. Andres E, Noel E, Goichot B. Metformin-associated vitamin B12 deficiency. Arch Intern Med 2002; 162(19):2251–2.

61. Adams JF, Clark JS, Ireland JT, Kesson CM, Watson WS. Malabsorption of vitamin B12 and intrinsic factor secretion during biguanide therapy. Diabetologia 1983;24(1):16–18.

62. Meir A, Kleinman Y, Rund D, Da'as N. Metformin-induced hemolytic anemia in a patient with glucose-6-phosphate dehydrogenase deficiency. Diabetes Care 2003;26(3):956–7.

63. Lin KD, Lin JD, Juang JH. Metformin-induced hemolysis with jaundice. N Engl J Med 1998;339(25):1860–1.

64. Kashyap AS, Kashyap S. Haemolytic anaemia due to metformin. Postgrad Med J 2000;76(892):125–6.

65. Florianello F, Gatti C, Marinoni M, Bagni CM. Gastrite emorragica da antidiabetici. Acta Chir Ital 1978;34:597.

66. Aviles-Santa L, Sinding J, Raskin P. Effects of metformin in patients with poorly controlled, insulin-treated type 2 diabetes mellitus. A randomized, double-blind, placebo-controlled trial. Ann Intern Med 1999;131(3):182–8.

67. Raju B, Resta C, Tibaldi JT. Metformin and late gastrointestinal complications. Am J Med 2000;109(3):260–1.

68. Foss MT, Clement KD. Metformin as a cause of late-onset chronic diarrhea. Pharmacotherapy 2001;21(11):1422–4.

69. Burrull-Madero MA, Del-Villar-Ruiz A, Grau-Cerrato S, Andreu-Garcia M, Goday-Arno A. Digestive hemorrhage caused by a Meckel's diverticulum in a metformin-treated patient: is there any connection? Pharm World Sci 2001;23(3):120–1.

70. Cubukcu A, Yilmaz MT, Satman I, Buyukdevrim AS. Metformin kullanimina bag_li bir akut hepatit vakasi. [Metformin-induced hepatitis.] Istanb Tip Fak Mecm 1991;54:447–52.

71. Babich MM, Pike I, Shiffman ML. Metformin-induced acute hepatitis. Am J Med 1998;104(5):490–2.

72. Swislocki AL, Noth R. Pseudohepatotoxicity of metformin. Diabetes Care 1998;21(4):677–8.

73. Desilets DJ, Shorr AF, Moran KA, Holtzmuller KC. Cholestatic jaundice associated with the use of metformin. Am J Gastroenterol 2001;96(7):2257–8.

74. Graeber GM, Marmor BM, Hendel RC, Gregg RO. Pancreatitis and severe metabolic abnormalities due to phenformin therapy. Arch Surg 1976;111(9):1014–16.

75. Azzam H, Bergman R, Friedman-Birnbaum R. Lichen planus associated with metformin therapy. Dermatology 1997;194(4):376.

76. Klapholz L, Leitersdorf E, Weinrauch L. Leucocytoclastic vasculitis and pneumonitis induced by metformin. BMJ (Clin Res Ed) 1986;293(6545):483.

77. Dore P, Perault MC, Recart D, Dejean C, Meurice JC, Fougere MC, Vandel B, Patte F. Pneumopathie medicamenteuse a la metformine? [Pulmonary diseases induced by metformin?] Therapie 1994;49(5):472–3.

78. Fisman EZ, Tenenbaum A, Boyko V, Benderly M, Adler Y, Friedensohn A, Kohanovski M, Rotzak R, Schneider H, Behar S, Motro M. Oral antidiabetic treatment in patients with coronary disease: time-related increased mortality on combined glyburide/metformin therapy over a 7.7-year follow-up Clin Cardiol 2001;24(2):151–8.

79. Hale TW, Kristensen JH, Hackett LP, Kohan R, Ilett KF. Transfer of metformin into human milk. Diabetologia 2002;45(11):1509–14.

80. Gregorio F, Ambrosi F, Manfrini S, Velussi M, Carle F, Testa R, Merante D, Filipponi P. Poorly controlled elderly Type 2 diabetic patients: the effects of increasing sulphonylurea dosages or adding metformin. Diabet Med 1999;16(12):1016–24.

81. Spiller HA, Weber JA, Winter ML, Klein-Schwartz W, Hofman M, Gorman SE, Stork CM, Krenzelok EP. Multicenter case series of pediatric metformin ingestion. Ann Pharmacother 2000;34(12):1385–8.

82. Bates D, Caton B. Metformin overdose. Can J Hosp Pharm 1999;52:173–5.

83. Ben MH, Thabet H, Zaghdoudi I, Amamou M. Metformin associated acute pancreatitis. Vet Hum Toxicol 2002;44(1):47–8.

84. Chang CT, Chen YC, Fang JT, Huang CC. High anion gap metabolic acidosis in suicide: don't forget metformin intoxication—two patients' experiences. Ren Fail 2002;24(5):671–5.

85. Dachman AH. New contraindication to intravascular iodinated contrast material. Radiology 1995;197(2):545.

86. Scheen AJ, Lefebvre PJ. Potential pharmacokinetics interference between alpha-glucosidase inhibitors and other oral antidiabetic agents. Diabetes Care 2002; 25(1):247–8.

87. Jayasagar G, Krishna Kumar M, Chandrasekhar K, Madhusudan Rao C, Madhusudan Rao Y. Effect of cephalexin on the pharmacokinetics of metformin in healthy human volunteers. Drug Metabol Drug Interact 2002;19(1):41–8.

88. Zandijk E, Demey HE, Bossaert LL. Lactic acidosis due to metformin. Tijdschr Geneeskd 1997;53:543–6.

89. Safadi R, Dranitzki-Elhalel M, Popovtzer M, Ben-Yehuda A. Metformin-induced lactic acidosis associated with acute renal failure. Am J Nephrol 1996;16(6):520–2.

90. Rasuli P, Hammond DI. Metformin and contrast media: where is the conflict? Can Assoc Radiol J 1998;49(3):161–6.

91. Hammond DI, Rasuli P. Metformin and contrast media. Clin Radiol 1998;53(12):933–4.

92. Zitzmann S, Reimann IR, Schmechel H. Severe hypoglycemia in an elderly patient treated with metformin. Int J Clin Pharmacol Ther 2002;40(3):108–1089.

93. Chan NN, Fauvel NJ, Feher MD. Non-steroidal anti-inflammatory drugs and metformin: a cause for concern? Lancet 1998;352(9123):201.

94. Schwarzbeck A. Non-steroidal anti-inflammatory drugs and metformin. Lancet 1998;352(9130):818.

95. Ohnhaus EE, Berger W, Duckert F, Oesch F. The influence of dimethylbiguanide on phenprocoumon elimination and its mode of action. A drug interaction study. Klin Wochenschr 1983;61(17):851–8.

96. Di Cicco RA, Allen A, Carr A, Fowles S, Jorkasky DK, Freed MI. Rosiglitazone does not alter the pharmacokinetics of metformin. J Clin Pharmacol 2000;40(11):1280–5.

97. Hamblin TJ. Interaction between warfarin and phenformin. Lancet 1971;2(7737):1323.

Bile acids

General Information

The bile acids are used in the long-term treatment of cholesterol gallstones. Ursodeoxycholic acid is the 7-epimer of chenodeoxycholic acid. Tauroursodeoxycholic acid is a derivative of ursodeoxycholic acid.

Observational studies

In a retrospective review of medical records over 12 months, ursodeoxycholic acid (20 mg/kg/day) reduced serum bilirubin concentrations in four of five children with cholestasis and hyperbilirubinemia (1). No adverse effects were reported.

Placebo-controlled studies

In a randomized placebo-controlled study in 219 patients with histology-proven chronic hepatitis (44 HbsAg-positive and 149 anti-HCV antibody-positive) and persistently raised transaminases, oral ursodeoxycholic acid 300 mg bd for 6 months produced significant improvement in clinical and biochemical markers (2). Apart from diarrhea, which was reported by a few patients, it was well tolerated.

The combinations of oral ursodeoxycholic acid 13–15 mg/kg/day plus interferon (3 MU three times a week) and interferon plus placebo for 6 months have been compared in a randomized, placebo-controlled study in 91 patients with chronic hepatitis C resistant to interferon (3). Combined interferon plus ursodeoxycholic acid was more effective than interferon alone in terms of normalizing alanine transaminase at 6 months (but not at 12 months), but not in terms of virological response. The frequency of adverse effects was similar in the two groups. Diarrhea, which was reported by a few patients, was the only adverse effect attributable to ursodeoxycholic acid.

The long-term effects of ursodeoxycholic acid 14–16 mg/kg/day has been investigated in a double-blind, placebo-controlled, multicenter trial in 192 patients with primary biliary cirrhosis (4). Ursodeoxycholic acid was associated with significant improvement in liver function tests and liver histology, but it did not affect the time to death or liver transplantation. Adverse effects were mild: abdominal pain, flatulence, and diarrhea were reported in nine patients taking ursodeoxycholic acid and six taking placebo.

High-dose ursodeoxycholic acid (20 mg/kg/day) has been compared with placebo in the treatment of primary sclerosing cholangitis in a 2-year double-blind preliminary study in 26 patients (5). High-dose ursodeoxycholic acid did not influence symptoms, but resulted in significant improvement in liver biochemistry and a significant reduction in the progression of cholangiographic appearances and liver fibrosis, as assessed by disease staging. No significant adverse effects were reported.

Ursodeoxycholic acid 250 mg tds plus ofloxacin 200 mg bd has been compared with ursodeoxycholic acid alone in the prevention of occlusion of biliary stents in a randomized trial in 52 patients with inoperable obstructive jaundice (6). Combination treatment was not superior to ursodeoxycholic acid alone. There was no significant difference in the frequency of adverse events between the two groups.

General adverse effects

Mild diarrhea and slightly raised serum transaminases are very common with chenodeoxycholic acid, while ursodeoxycholic acid seldom causes significant diarrhea or hypertransaminasemia. This difference is puzzling, since ursodeoxycholic acid, like chenodeoxycholate, is metabolized to lithocholate, and some if not all animal studies have shown evidence of hepatotoxicity. One undesirable property of ursodeoxycholic acid is that occasionally treatment is followed by the development of resistant (and radio opaque) coatings to gallstones, thus retarding or preventing further dissolution. Neither hypersensitivity nor tumor-inducing effects reactions have been reported.

Experience with tauroursodeoxycholic acid is limited. It is less effective than ursodeoxycholic acid and causes more adverse effects. Two patients who took tauroursodeoxycholic acid for primary biliary cirrhosis developed severe right upper quadrant pain, and rechallenge with tauroursodeoxycholic acid was positive (7).

Organs and Systems

Metabolism

Although most studies have shown no consistent effects of chenodeoxycholic acid on serum cholesterol concentrations, in the National Cooperative Gallstone Study there was a 10% increase over a 2-year period in treated people compared with a 5% rise in controls (8). Low-density lipoprotein concentrations rose in association; other varieties were unaffected.

Gastrointestinal

About half of all patients given the usual dose of chenodeoxycholic acid, 15 mg/kg/day, develop diarrhea, because the unabsorbed bile acid causes water to be secreted into the large bowel (9). The symptoms remit with dosage reduction and may not recur if the dose is then slowly increased again. It is best avoided in inflammatory bowel disease.

Liver

Serum transaminases tend to double or triple in the early weeks of treatment with chenodeoxycholic acid in about one-third of patients (10). There is a hypothesis that this is due to impaired lithocholate sulfation. Lithocholic acid is

formed by the 7-dehydroxylation of chenodeoxycholic acid and is ordinarily inactivated by sulfation. However, hypertransaminasemia has been detected in nearly 75% of people with a low sulfation capacity (this capacity being bimodally distributed) and in less than one in 10 of those with a high capacity. All the same, chenodeoxycholic acid is substantially, if not totally, devoid of serious hepatotoxic actions. Liver biopsy has shown no significant changes; minor changes can include fatty change and lipofuscin accumulation.

Skin

- Lichenoid skin eruptions have been reported in a 1-month-old infant with neonatal hepatitis 3 weeks after the administration of ursodeoxycholic acid (11). There was complete resolution after withdrawal of ursodeoxycholic acid and treatment with glucocorticoids.
- Lichenoid eruptions have been reported in a 61-year-old man with gallstones who took ursodeoxycholic acid 600 mg/day for a few weeks (12). The eruption improved on withdrawal, but recurred when ursodeoxycholic acid was reintroduced 3 months later.

Lichen planus developed in one patient taking a combination of chenodeoxycholic and ursodeoxycholic acid (SEDA-17, 428).

Second-Generation Effects

Teratogenicity

The clinical and biological effects and safety of ursodeoxycholic acid in intrahepatic cholestasis of pregnancy have been reported in 19 patients, 14 of whom had clinical improvement, with reduction or disappearance of pruritus, and 11 of whom had an improvement in biochemical liver function tests (13). The only birth defect reported was pyloric stenosis in a boy whose mother had taken ursodeoxycholic acid for 10 days at 34 weeks gestation.

References

1. George R, Stevens A, Berkenbosch JW, Turpin J, Tobias J. Ursodeoxycholic acid in the treatment of cholestasis and hyperbilirubinemia in pediatric intensive care unit patients. South Med J 2002;95(11):1276–9.
2. Berlotti M, Morselli-Labate AM, Rusticali AG, Loria P, Carulli N, the Investigators of the Italian Multicenter Study on UDCA in Chronic Hepatitis N. Ursodeoxycholic acid improves liver tests in chronic hepatitis. Clin Drug Invest 1999;17:425–34.
3. Poupon RE, Bonnand AM, Queneau PE, Trepo C, Zarski JPi, Vetter D, Raabe JJ, Thieffin G, Larrey D, Grange JD, Capron JP, Serfaty L, Chretien Y, St Marc Girardin MF, Mathiex-Fortunet H, Zafrani ES, Guechot J, Beuers U, Paumgartner G, Poupon R. Randomized trial of interferon-alpha plus ursodeoxycholic acid versus interferon plus placebo in patients with chronic hepatitis C resistant to interferon. Scand J Gastroenterol 2000;35(6):642–9.
4. Pares A, Caballeria L, Rodes J, Bruguera M, Rodrigo L, Garcia-Plaza A, Berenguer J, Rodriguez-Martinez D, Mercader J, Velicia R, Gines A, Linares-Rodriguez A, Cano-Ruiz A, Martin-Scapa A, Berenguer M, Fernandez-Rodriguez C, Obrador A, Vaquer P, Clemente G, Arenas-

Mirave JI, Castiella A, Vargas V, Martin-Vivaldi R, Vidan JM, Zozaya JM, Planas R, Viver JM, De la Mata M, Pons F, Diaz F. Long-term effects of ursodeoxycholic acid in primary biliary cirrhosis: results of a double-blind controlled multicentric trial. UDCA-Cooperative Group from the Spanish Association for the Study of the Liver. J Hepatol 2000;32(4):561–6.

5. Mitchell SA, Bansi DS, Hunt N, Von Bergmann K, Fleming KA, Chapman RW. A preliminary trial of high-dose ursodeoxycholic acid in primary sclerosing cholangitis. Gastroenterology 2001;121(4):900–7.

6. Halm U, Schiefke, Fleig WE, Mossner J, Keim V. Ofloxacin and ursodeoxycholic acid versus ursodeoxycholic acid alone to prevent occlusion of biliary stents: a prospective, randomized trial. Endoscopy 2001;33(6):491–4.

7. Pratt DS, Kaplan MM. Abdominal pain after taking ursodiol. N Engl J Med 1993;328(20):1502.

8. Albers JJ, Grundy SM, Cleary PA, Small DM, Lachin JM, Schoenfield LJ. National Cooperative Gallstone Study: the effect of chenodeoxycholic acid on lipoproteins and apolipoproteins. Gastroenterology 1982;82(4):638–46.

9. Schoenfiled J, Coyne MJ, Conley BR, Chung A, Bonorris GG. In: Quantitative Aspects of Structure and Function. Aulendorf: Edite Cantor, 1976:413–18.

10. Dowling RH. Chenodeoxycholic acid therapy of gallstones. Philadelphia: WB Saunders Company, 1977.

11. Buyukgebiz B, Arslan N, Ozturk Y, Soyal C, Lebe B. Drug reaction to ursodeoxycholic acid: lichenoid drug eruption in an infant using ursodeoxycholic acid for neonatal hepatitis. J Pediatr Gastroenterol Nutr 2002;35(3):384–6.

12. Horiuchi Y. Lichenoid eruptions due to ursodeoxycholic acid administration. Gastroenterology 2001;121(2):501–2.

13. Berkane N, Cocheton JJ, Brehier D, Merviel P, Wolf C, Lefevre G, Uzan S. Ursodeoxycholic acid in intrahepatic cholestasis of pregnancy. A retrospective study of 19 cases. Acta Obstet Gynecol Scand 2000;79(11):941–6.

Bimatoprost

See also Prostaglandins

General Information

Bimatoprost is an analogue of $PGF_{2\alpha}$, used to treat glaucoma. It is believed to lower intraocular pressure by increasing the outflow of aqueous humor through both the trabecular meshwork and uveoscleral routes.

Organs and Systems

Sensory systems

Bimatoprost can cause gradual darkening of the color of the eyes and the eyelid skin, increased thickness, numbers and darkness of eyelashes, conjunctival hyperemia, and ocular pruritus [1]. Darkening of the iris occurs in 1.1% of patients [2].

Hair

Eyelash growth was reported in 36–48% of patients after 6 months of using bimatoprost [2].

References

1. Cantor LB. Bimatoprost: a member of a new class of agents, the prostamides, for glaucoma management. Expert Opin Investig Drugs 2001;10(4):721–31.

2. Sherwood M, Brandt J; Bimatoprost Study Groups 1 and 2. Six-month comparison of bimatoprost once-daily and twice-daily with timolol twice-daily in patients with elevated intra-ocular pressure. Surv Ophthalmol 2001;45(Suppl 4):S361–8.

Biotin

See also Vitamins

General Information

Biotin is a water-soluble vitamin of the B complex (vitamin B_{10}, also called vitamin H), and is found in many foods, especially eggs and liver. Biotin is involved in the action of four carboxylases:

- acetyl-CoA carboxylase, which catalyses the binding of bicarbonate to acetyl-CoA to form malonyl-CoA in the synthesis of fatty acids
- pyruvate carboxylase, which is involved in gluconeogenesis
- methylcrotonyl-CoA carboxylase, which catalyses an essential step in the metabolism of leucine
- propionyl-CoA carboxylase, which catalyses essential steps in the metabolism of amino acids, cholesterol, and fatty acids.

Although biotin has been proposed as a treatment for diabetes mellitus, brittle nails, and hair loss, there is little good evidence of its efficacy in these conditions. It has also been used as a skin-conditioning agent in many cosmetic products in concentrations of 0.0001–0.6% [1].

Organs and Systems

Cardiovascular

Eosinophilic pleural effusion with eosinophilic pericardial tamponade has been attributed to concomitant use of pantothenic acid and biotin [2].

- A 76-year-old woman developed chest pain and difficulty in breathing. She had no history of allergy and had been taking biotin 10 mg/day and pantothenic acid 300 mg/day for 2 months for alopecia. Chest X-rays showed pleural effusions and cardiac enlargement. Blood tests showed an inflammatory syndrome, with an erythrocyte sedimentation rate of 51 mm/hour and an eosinophil count of $1.2–1.5 \times 10^9/l$. Pericardiotomy showed an eosinophilic infiltrate. There was no evidence of vasculitis. Serological studies were negative for antinuclear antibodies, rheumatoid factor, viruses, bacteria, and Lyme disease. Stool examination and parasitological serologies were negative. A malignant tumor was excluded by mammography, thoracoscopy, and a CT scan. Myelography, a biopsy specimen of the iliac crest bone, and the concentrations of IgE, lysozyme, and vitamin B_{12} were also normal. A week after withdrawal of pantothenic acid and biotin she improved dramatically and her eosinophilia resolved.

References

1. Fiume MZ; Cosmetic Ingredient Review Expert Panel. Final report on the safety assessment of biotin. Int J Toxicol 2001;20(Suppl 4):1–12.
2. Debourdeau PM, Djezzar S, Estival JL, Zammit CM, Richard RC, Castot AC. Life-threatening eosinophilic pleuropericardial effusion related to vitamins B5 and H. Ann Pharmacother 2001;35(4):424–6.

Biperiden

See also Anticholinergic drugs

General Information

Biperiden is given orally in doses rising from 2 to 6 mg/day, more being given in individual cases. Of the anticholinergic effects that biperiden can cause, drowsiness seems to be one of the most prominent, and it should not be given to patients who have to drive motor vehicles. A dose of 12 mg has been reported to precipitate involuntary movements in some cases of parkinsonism (SEDA-1, 120).

Organs and Systems

Skin

Contact dermatitis has been attributed to biperiden (1).

Long-Term Effects

Drug withdrawal

Insomnia occurred after biperiden withdrawal in two patients with schizophrenia (2).

Drug-Drug Interactions

Haloperidol

In eight healthy men volunteers biperiden 2 mg reduced the serum haloperidol concentrations increased by carteolol 10 mg (3).

References

1. Torinuki W. Contact dermatitis to biperiden and photocontact dermatitis to phenothiazines in a pharmacist. Tohoku J Exp Med 1995;176(4):249–52.
2. Hirose S. Insomnia related to biperiden withdrawal in two schizophrenic patients. Int Clin Psychopharmacol 2000;15(6):357–9.
3. Isawa S, Murasaki M, Miura S, Yoshioka M, Uchiumi M, Kumagai Y, Aoki S, Hisazumi H, Kudo S. Pharmacokinetic and pharmacodynamic interactions among haloperidol, carteolol hydrochloride and biperiden hydrochloride. Nihon Shinkei Seishin Yakurigaku Zasshi 1999;19(3):111–18.

Bismuth

General Information

Bismuth is a brittle reddish-white metallic element (symbol Bi; atomic no. 83). It enjoyed great popularity up to the early 20th century, and thereafter continued to be used in the form of insoluble bismuth compounds, used for their supposed effects on the gastric wall as antacids, protective coatings, or inhibitors of proteolytic activity. The use of bismuth was particularly heavy in Australia, where bismuth subgallate was commonly used in postcolectomy or postileostomy patients, and in France, where bismuth subnitrate and other salts were widely self-administered for both gastric and intestinal conditions.

Bismuth salts are still in use. Tripotassium dicitratobismuthate and bicitropeptide (a bismuth-peptide complex) are used in the eradication of *Helicobacter pylori* in combination with antibiotics (SEDA-21, 233) (1–4), and ranitidine bismuth citrate is used to treat peptic ulcer (5). Bismuth salicylates are used in other intestinal diseases, such as microscopic colitis (6,7) and collagenous colitis (8). Bismuth subnitrate plus iodoform is used to pack surgical cavities. Bismuth oxide and bismuth subgallate are found in some topical formulations that are used for treating hemorrhoids. Bismuth is also used topically as a bacteriostatic.

Bismuth compounds are also used as hemostatic compounds (9). A uniform technique of tonsillectomy, including the use of bismuth subgallate and re-assessment of the tonsillar fossae after a 3-minute observation period, reduced the incidence of primary tonsillar hemorrhage in a retrospective study of 705 children (10). However, in a randomized study of 204 patients the evidence for the use of bismuth subgallate as a hemostatic agent in tonsillectomy was weak (11). Bismuth iodoform paraffin paste is commonly used in ear, nose, and throat surgery and in oral and maxillofacial surgery. A new area for the use of bismuth compounds may be in oncology as anticancer agents (12).

Due to the formation of an insoluble bismuth chloride complex in the gastric juice after oral administration of bismuth salts, the diffusion of the bismuth ion into the circulation is delayed. During treatment with tripotassium dicitratobismuthate, plasma concentrations of bismuth rise to 10–20 µmol/l which are not regarded as toxic. From experience over somewhat more than 20 years it would seem that the inherent risks of bismuth intoxication are relatively small if these compounds are used within the recommended ranges of dosage and length of treatment. However, they too can be abused, resulting in renal tubular damage (SEDA-18, 241) and attention has been drawn to the possible risks resulting from the ready absorption of citrate (13).

Placebo-controlled studies

Data from 20 clinical studies in 5000 patients who had taken ranitidine bismuth citrate (200, 400, or 800 mg bd) have been reported (14). The incidence of adverse events was not different from that associated with placebo and was independent of dose. The most common events (>1% of patients) were upper respiratory tract infections, constipation, diarrhea, nausea, vomiting, dizziness, and headache, the last being the only event reported by over 2% of the patients. Adverse events considered by the clinical investigator to be adverse reactions occurred with a similar frequency amongst patients given ranitidine bismuth citrate (8%), ranitidine hydrochloride (6%), and placebo (6%). The incidence of adverse reactions was greater when amoxicillin (11%) or clarithromycin (20%) were co-prescribed.

Organs and Systems

Respiratory

There has been a single report of a lung disorder with cough, which was traced to intravenous injection of a so-called "health tonic" containing bismuth, which had resulted in bismuth-containing subpleural opacities in the lungs (15).

Two cases of respiratory complications following the use of bismuth gallate have been reported (9).

- A 19-month-old boy with reactive airways disease had a tonsillectomy and adenoidectomy and bismuth-coated sponges were used for hemostasis. Excessive bleeding was not reported. In the recovery room he developed difficulty in breathing, and required oxygen followed by bronchodilators and deep suctioning. A chest X-ray showed speckled opacities throughout the lung fields and in the oropharynx and nasopharynx, probably due to aspiration of bismuth particles. He went on to develop a pneumonitis.
- An 8-year-old girl with asthma underwent tonsillectomy and adenoidectomy; hemostasis was performed with bismuth–adrenaline paste. A small amount of bismuth was noted in the endotracheal tube before extubation, and in the recovery room she developed respiratory difficulty associated with nasal flaring and sternal retraction. A chest X-ray showed aspirated radio-opaque material outlining the tracheobronchial tree and early pulmonary infiltrates.

Both patients had a history of refractory airway disease that put them at risk of respiratory complications after bismuth aspiration. Fortunately neither developed any serious respiratory compromise immediately after aspiration or required intubation.

Nervous system

From 1973 onward many cases of an encephalopathy were reported among bismuth users. By 1979, 945 cases had been recorded in France alone, 72 of them fatal; the world-wide total exceeded 1000 cases. Bismuth encephalopathy is characterized by ataxia, confusion, speech disorder, and myoclonus. The subgallate and oxychloride have been implicated, as has the subcitrate when used in a patient with impaired bismuth clearance. The chelate tripotassium dicitratobismuthate, which contains very small amounts of bismuth, appears to be safe in this respect for normal use, as does the occasional use of more traditional bismuth products for conditions such as travelers' diarrhea. Use of bismuth subnitrate ("Roter" tablets) does not seem to lead to metal absorption (16), but such absorption does occur from bismuth salicylate (17).

- A 49-year-old woman with chronic gastric ulcers and 5 years of bismuth abuse developed bismuth encephalopathy, with progressive dementia, dysarthria, and myoclonic jerks 1 week after increasing the dosage of bismuth (18). Electroencephalography showed generalized spike-wave complexes, suggesting that the myoclonus was epileptic in nature. Bismuth was withdrawn and she was given valproate, which reduced the frequency of the myoclonic jerks. Administration of the chelator dimercaptopropane sulfonic acid (DMPS) enhanced bismuth elimination but aggravated the clinical symptoms and it was therefore withdrawn. She slowly recovered.
- An 86-year-old woman underwent partial maxillectomy for squamous cell carcinoma of the right alveolus and hard palate, and the maxillary antrum was packed with a length of bismuth iodoform paraffin paste (19). Postoperatively she developed delirium and by day 5 was exhausted, light-headed, and unsteady. She became increasingly aggressive and by day 11 was eating very little and having fainting episodes. Worsening confusion and some paranoid ideation was apparent and tremor was pronounced, but there were no focal neurological signs. The bismuth iodoform paraffin pack was removed on day 14 and 7 days later she had improved and was very cooperative and alert when she was discharged 5 days later. The bismuth serum concentration on day 14 was 146 nmol/l (reference range 0–4 nmol/l) and on day 22 was 81 nmol/l. The original peak bismuth concentration was extrapolated to over 300 nmol/l.

Three phases of the encephalopathy that bismuth can cause can be distinguished (SEDA-4 167) (20):

1. *Prodromal phase* This is characterized by such vague complaints as weakness, mental slowness, short memory, reduced working capacity, insomnia, headache, and anxiety. These symptoms can easily be dismissed as non-specific, and can persist for more than 2 years before further signs develop. In general, however, the course is gradually progressive toward the symptoms of the next phase.
2. *Acute phase* Sudden deterioration to an acute encephalopathy occurs over a period ranging from several hours to 1–2 days. Patients develop dysarthria, severe locomotor disturbances such as ataxia, difficulty in walking, intention tremor, myoclonic jerks (especially of the upper limbs, face, and trunk), incontinence due to loss of sphincter control, hyper-reflexia, and sometimes generalized convulsions. The patient may be confused, disoriented, and agitated. Excitation, hallucinations, delirium, and fluctuations of mental alertness, ranging from dizziness to loss of consciousness and coma, can occur. In about 7–9% of cases the outcome is fatal,

owing to bronchopulmonary, cardiovascular, thromboembolic, or infectious complications.

3. *Recovery phase* After withdrawal of bismuth, the toxic symptoms usually abate rapidly, although physical and psychological weakness, depressive mood, memory impairment, intellectual deterioration, sleep disturbances, headache, and other symptoms occasionally persist for several months, and in isolated cases for more than a year. Exceptionally, psychic and intellectual capacity remain permanently impaired.

The reason for the suddenness of the outbreak of bismuth encephalopathy in the 1970s after the drug had been used for so many years is uncertain. A major French epidemiological study undertaken at the time (SEDA-6, 217) failed to detect any clear link to particular dosage habits, topographical factors, or drug interactions. Unknown environmental factors may have altered either the effects of bismuth itself or the sensitivity of the brain. It was later suggested that a change in intestinal flora converted bismuth salts into more soluble neurotoxic compounds (21), although it is not clear why this should have happened during the 1970s. Since measures were taken to counter the traditional use of bismuth, only very occasional new cases of encephalopathy have been reported since then. It is currently unresolved whether the lower doses of bismuth in gastric powders, antacids, astringents, demulcents, purgatives, and antidiarrheal formulations that are still in use are in the long run innocuous; if an unknown environmental factor did indeed lead to toxic manifestations with the older products, it might similarly modify the effects of others; watchfulness is therefore essential. In fact, one suspects something of a renaissance of bismuth encephalopathy in the 1990s; in 1993 cases were reported from several countries, associated inter alia with abuse of bismuth subsalicylate (Pepto-Bismol) (22) and the use of bismuth subgallate (23).

As late as 1994 a toxic encephalopathy, relapsing but reversible, was reported in a woman who had received a large dose of bismuth when bismuth iodoform paraffin paste was inserted extradurally (24). Elsewhere neurotoxicity has been reported (SEDA-19, 446).

Mouth and teeth

A black tongue was reportedly caused by exogenous pigment in chewable bismuth subsalicylate tablets.

- A 51-year-old white woman developed black discoloration of her tongue (25). The black substance was easily removed by scraping the surface of the tongue. She denied using tobacco products or alcohol. Her medications included alprazolam, montelukast, amitriptyline, hydroxychloroquine, triamcinolone acetonide, omeprazole, cisapride, and calcium carbonate. She had recently started to chew three to six bismuth subsalicylate tablets daily. She was advised to stop using bismuth subsalicylate and to brush her tongue with a soft-bristled toothbrush. The discoloration improved within a couple of hours and eventually disappeared completely. She continued to take hydroxychloroquine, a known cause of oral mucosal pigmentation.

Gastrointestinal

The results of a comparative trial suggested that the adverse reactions most commonly encountered during courses of treatment including bismuth and designed to eliminate *H. pylori* are vomiting, diarrhea, abdominal pain, headache, and a metallic taste in the mouth (SEDA-22, 393) (26).

Constipation is an occasional adverse effect of bismuth therapy. The feces are grey or black, and can be mistaken for melena (27).

Biliary tract

- Acute cholecystitis caused by non-O1 *Vibrio cholerae* has been described in a 55-year-old healthy traveler immediately after a vacation in Cancun, Mexico (28). During his vacation he had taken the Pepto-Bismol brand of bismuth subsalicylate 30 ml tds as prophylaxis against traveler's diarrhea. At surgery his gall bladder was acalculous, inflamed, distended, and nearly ruptured. Pathogenetic factors may have included the use of bismuth subsalicylate, distension of the gall bladder from illness-induced fasting, and bacterial toxins in the gall bladder.

The authors implied that bismuth subsalicylate could have prevented the secretory diarrhea that is seen in many infections with non-O1 *V. cholerae*. Diarrhea would result in evacuation of many organisms from the small bowel. Bismuth subsalicylate might have impaired this mechanism and increased the number of organisms with access to the common bile duct at the ampulla of Vater.

Urinary tract

Some reviewers have claimed that bismuth can cause reversible acute renal insufficiency, but if this indeed occurs it must be excessively rare; it might be part of a nephrotic syndrome.

Skin

- A man who had taken bismuth subsalicylate after heavy meals once or twice a month for the previous 4 years developed crops of small, black, carbon-like particles (size range 0.2–0.5 mm) on the skin (29). The palms and soles were not involved. These particles appeared at intervals of 15–30 days and persisted for 2 or 3 days if not removed by soap and water. They were located in follicular orifices and caused no symptoms; they tested positive for bismuth. The condition receded completely after bismuth was withdrawn (30).

Musculoskeletal

Osteoarthropathy was an associated feature in some 3% of patients with bismuth encephalopathy. However, at least one case is on record in which a bismuth osteoarthropathy developed without any manifestation of encephalopathy (31). The symptoms mainly involve one or both shoulders, of which painful restriction of movement is usually the first sign in the postacute phase of bismuth encephalopathy. This can persist for several months after bismuth has been withdrawn. X-ray examination shows an osteolytic deforming glenohumeral osteoarthropathy with necrosis of the humeral head. Unilateral or bilateral fractures can occur. The lesions described can regress without sequelae over several months and osteonecrosis can also proceed to complete lysis of the humeral head.

The fact that much bismuth is ordinarily stored in the skeleton may be relevant in the etiology of bismuth osteoarthropathy. In two reported cases a differing type of osteopathy occurred, associated with different localization of the pathological lesions and with unusually high bismuth concentrations in the bone: both patients had received bismuth injections for syphilis many months or even years before (SEDA-4, 169).

Immunologic

Sensitization to bismuth derivatives has been reported but is rare.

- A 33-year-old woman with atopic hand eczema and allergic rhinitis was given Noviform, an eye ointment containing bibrocathol (bismuth oxide and tetrabromo-cathechol), for periorbital dermatitis and noticed an exacerbation of her dermatitis (32). A patch test was positive for bismuth oxide.

Anaphylaxis to bismuth subsalicylate (Pepto-Bismol) has been observed (33).

- A 25-year-old man with symptoms of acute gastroenteritis took Pepto-Bismol, a total of eight caplets over 6 hours. About 30 minutes after the last dose, he developed generalized acute urticaria. He had previously tolerated Pepto-Bismol well, but had presumably become sensitized. He was successfully treated with intravenous fluids and histamine H_1 receptor antagonists.

Second-Generation Effects

Teratogenicity

Very little is known about the use of bismuth in pregnancy, but in documented cases mothers affected with bismuth encephalopathy during pregnancy gave birth to healthy infants.

Susceptibility Factors

Renal disease

Bismuth is predominantly excreted via the kidney and would be expected to accumulate in patients with renal insufficiency. It is not impossible that combined exposure to bismuth and other metals could render the patient more susceptible to bismuth toxicity; the parallels between the complications seen here and with other light metals (zinc, aluminium) are striking.

Drug Administration

Drug administration route

Severe systemic intoxication in the past has been observed after incautious use of bismuth salts on extensive wound areas.

Drug overdose

Renal damage has been reported in cases of bismuth overdose.

- A 17-year-old girl took 25 tablets of bismuth subcitrate 300 mg (total 7.5 g) in a suicide attempt and developed severe renal insufficiency (34). Renal biopsy showed evidence of acute tubular necrosis, with epithelial flattening, lumen widening, and atrophic changes in the convoluted tubules and mononuclear cell infiltration and edema in the interstitium. She was managed with hemodialysis and recovered.
- A 22-year-old woman took 5.4 g of colloidal bismuth subcitrate in a suicide attempt and developed Fanconi's syndrome and acute renal insufficiency (35). She received hemodialysis and intravenous sodium 2,3-mercapto-1-propanesulfonate 60 hours after intoxication. Her serum bismuth concentrations fell from 640 to 15 µg/l within 6 days, her renal function improved, and her tonsillar ulceration healed. Hemodialysis was discontinued on day 14. She had normal renal function 6 weeks later.
- Reversible bismuth nephrotoxicity was reported in a 16-year-old girl who had nausea, vomiting, and dizziness for 4–5 days and oliguria for 2 days (36). She had taken an overdose of tripotassium dicitratobismuthate tablets containing a total amount of 3.0–4.5 g of bismuth. Blood urea and serum creatinine were increased and there was proteinuria and erythrocytes in the urine. Acute tubular necrosis was observed on biopsy.

References

1. Wermeille J, Zelger G, Cunningham M. The eradication treatments of *Helicobacter pylori*. Pharm World Sci 1998;20(1):1–17.
2. van der Hulst RW, van't Hoff BW, van der Ende A, Tytgat GN. Behandeling van *Helicobacter pylori*-infectie. [Treatment of *Helicobacter pylori* infections.] Ned Tijdschr Geneeskd 1999;143(8):395–400.
3. Houben MH, van de Beek D, Hensen EF, Craen AJ, Rauws EA, Tytgat GN. A systematic review of *Helicobacter pylori* eradication therapy—the impact of antimicrobial resistance on eradication rates. Aliment Pharmacol Ther 1999;13(8):1047–55.
4. Trust TJ, Alm RA, Pappo J. *Helicobacter pylori*: today's treatment, and possible future treatment. Eur J Surg Suppl 2001;(586):82–8.
5. Van Oijen AH, Verbeek AL, Jansen JB, De Boer WA. Review article: treatment of *Helicobacter pylori* infection with ranitidine bismuth citrate- or proton pump inhibitor-based triple therapies. Aliment Pharmacol Ther 2000;14(8):991–9.
6. Fine KD, Lee EL. Efficacy of open-label bismuth subsalicylate for the treatment of microscopic colitis. Gastroenterology 1998;114(1):29–36.
7. Schiller LR. Microscopic colitis syndrome: lymphocytic colitis and collagenous colitis. Semin Gastrointest Dis 1999;10(4):145–55.
8. Amaro R, Poniecka A, Rogers AI. Collagenous colitis treated successfully with bismuth subsalicylate. Dig Dis Sci 2000;45(7):1447–50.

9. Murray AD, Gibbs SR, Billings KR, Biavati MJ. Respiratory difficulty following bismuth subgallate aspiration. Arch Otolaryngol Head Neck Surg 2000;126(1):79–81.

10. Conley SF, Ellison MD. Avoidance of primary post-tonsillectomy hemorrhage in a teaching program. Arch Otolaryngol Head Neck Surg 1999;125(3):330–3.

11. Sorensen WT, Henrichsen J, Bonding P. Does bismuth subgallate have haemostatic effects in tonsillectomy? Clin Otolaryngol Allied Sci 1999;24(1):72–4.

12. Tiekink ER. Antimony and bismuth compounds in oncology. Crit Rev Oncol Hematol 2002;42(3):217–24.

13. Slikkerveer A, De Wolff FA. Bismuth: Biokinetics and neurotoxicity. Vinken PJ, Bruyn GW, editors. Handbook of Clinical Neurology. Vol. 64. Intoxication of the Nervous System. Part I. Amsterdam: Elsevier, 1994;331–51.

14. Pipkin GA, Mills JG, Kler L, Dixon JS, Wood JR. The safety of ranitidine bismuth citrate in controlled clinical studies. Pharmacoepidemiol Drug Saf 1996;5(6):399–407.

15. Addrizzo-Harris DJ, Churg A, Rom WN. Radio-opaque punctate opacities on the chest radiograph following intravenous injection of a bismuth compound. Thorax 1997;52(3):303–4.

16. Nwokolo CU, Prewett EJ, Sawyer AA, et al. Lack of bismuth absorption from bismuth subnitrate (Roter) tablets. Eur J Gastroenterol Hepatol 1989;5:433.

17. Nwokolo CU, Mistry P, Pounder RE. The absorption of bismuth and salicylate from oral doses of Pepto-Bismol (bismuth salicylate). Aliment Pharmacol Ther 1990;4(2):163–9.

18. Teepker M, Hamer HM, Knake S, Bandmann O, Oertel WH, Rosenow F. Myoclonic encephalopathy caused by chronic bismuth abuse. Epileptic Disord 2002;4(4):229–33.

19. Harris RA, Poole A. Beware of bismuth: post maxillectomy delirium. ANZ J Surg 2002;72(11):846–7.

20. Martin-Bouyer G. Intoxications par les sels de bismuth administrés par voie orale. [Poisoning by orally administered bismuth salts.] Gastroenterol Clin Biol 1978;2(4):349–56.

21. Menge H, Gregor M, Brosius B, Hopert R, Lang A. Pharmacology of bismuth. Eur J Gastroenterol Hepatol 1992;4(Suppl 2):41–7.

22. Jungreis AC, Schaumburg HH. Encephalopathy from abuse of bismuth subsalicylate (Pepto-Bismol). Neurology 1993;43(6):1265.

23. Friedland RP, Lerner AJ, Hedera P, Brass EP. Encephalopathy associated with bismuth subgallate therapy. Clin Neuropharmacol 1993;16(2):173–6.

24. Sharma RR, Cast IP, Redfern RM, O'Brien C. Extradural application of bismuth iodoform paraffin paste causing relapsing bismuth encephalopathy: a case report with CT and MRI studies. J Neurol Neurosurg Psychiatry 1994;57(8):990–3.

25. Ioffreda MD, Gordon CA, Adams DR, Naides SJ, Miller JJ. Black tongue. Arch Dermatol 2001;137(7):968–9.

26. Lerang F, Moum B, Ragnhildstveit E, Haug JB, Hauge T, Tolas P, Aubert E, Henriksen M, Efskind PS, Nicolaysen K, Soberg T, Odegaard A, Berge T. A comparison between omeprazole-based triple therapy and bismuth-based triple therapy for the treatment of *Helicobacter pylori* infection: a prospective randomized 1-yr follow-up study. Am J Gastroenterol 1997;92(4):653–8.

27. Sainz MI, Redin MD, San Miguel R, Baleztena J, Santos MA, Petri M, Notivol MP. Problemas de utilizacion de medicamentos en pacientes enterostomizados. [Problems in the use of medicines in enterostomized patients.] An Sist Sanit Navar 2003;26(3):383–403.

28. West BC, Silberman R, Otterson WN. Acalculous cholecystitis and septicemia caused by non-O1 Vibrio cholerae: first reported case and review of biliary infections with *Vibrio cholerae*. Diagn Microbiol Infect Dis 1998;30(3):187–91.

29. Ellenberg R, King AL, Sica DA, Posner M, Savory J. Cerebrospinal fluid aluminum levels following deferoxamine. Am J Kidney Dis 1990;16(2):157–9.

30. Ruiz-Maldonado R, Contreras-Ruiz J, Sierra-Santoyo A, Lopez-Corella E, Guevara-Flores A. Black granules on the skin after bismuth subsalicylate ingestion. J Am Acad Dermatol 1997;37(3 Pt 1):489–90.

31. Gaucher A, Netter P, Faure G, Hutin MF, Burnel D. Bismuth-induced osteoarthropathies. Med J Aust 1979;1(4):129–30.

32. Wictorin A, Hansson C. Allergic contact dermatitis from a bismuth compound in an eye ointment. Contact Dermatitis 2001;45(5):318.

33. More D, Whisman B, Johns J, Hagan L. Anaphylaxis to Pepto-Bismol. Allergy 2002;57(6):558.

34. Sarikaya M, Sevinc A, Ulu R, Ates F, Ari F. Bismuth subcitrate nephrotoxicity. A reversible cause of acute oliguric renal failure. Nephron 2002;90(4):501–2.

35. Hruz P, Mayr M, Low R, Drewe J, Huber G. Fanconi's syndrome, acute renal failure, and tonsil ulcerations after colloidal bismuth subcitrate intoxication. Am J Kidney Dis 2002;39(3):E18.

36. Akpolat I, Kahraman H, Arik N, Akpolat T, Kandemir B, Cengiz K. Acute renal failure due to overdose of colloidal bismuth. Nephrol Dial Transplant 1996;11(9):1890–1.

Bisoprolol

See also Beta-adrenoceptor antagonists

General Information

Bisoprolol is a highly selective beta$_1$-adrenoceptor antagonist. Its adverse effects profile is similar to that of atenolol (1), and despite theoretical benefits there is no convincing clinical evidence that bisoprolol has an advantage (2).

Organs and Systems

Metabolism

Bisoprolol can increase serum triglycerides and reduce HDL cholesterol (3).

References

1. Neutel JM, Smith DH, Ram CV, Kaplan NM, Papademetriou V, Fagan TC, Lefkowitz MP, Kazempour MK, Weber MA. Application of ambulatory blood pressure monitoring in differentiating between antihypertensive agents. Am J Med 1993;94(2):181–7.

2. Wheeldon NM, MacDonald TM, Prasad N, Maclean D, Peebles L, McDevitt DG. A double-blind comparison of bisoprolol and atenolol in patients with essential hypertension. QJM 1995;88(8):565–70.

3. Lancaster SG, Sorkin EM. Bisoprolol. A preliminary review of its pharmacodynamic and pharmacokinetic properties, and therapeutic efficacy in hypertension and angina pectoris. Drugs 1988;36(3):256–85.

Bisphosphonates

General Information

The development of bisphosphonates for clinical purposes began with the discovery that inorganic pyrophosphate is present in blood and urine and inhibits the precipitation of calcium and phosphate (1). Derivatives of pyrophosphate had been widely used for industrial purposes, because they inhibit the precipitation of calcium carbonate. Their principal use was as antiscaling additives in washing powders, water, and oil brines, to prevent deposition of calcium carbonate scale. It was then found that pyrophosphate binds strongly to calcium phosphate, prevents both the formation and dissolution of calcium phosphate crystals, and inhibits calcification in vitro. The bisphosphonates are used to treat bone diseases characterized by increased osteoclastic bone resorption (2). Long-term administration of low doses of oral bisphosphonates is considered to be valuable in patients with postmenopausal osteoporosis (3,4).

Adverse effects of the bisphosphonates include low-grade transient fever and headache; other effects are asymptomatic hypocalcemia, hypophosphatemia, and hypomagnesemia (5–7).

Alendronate

Alendronate is an aminobisphosphonate with general properties similar to those of the other bisphosphonates. It inhibits bone resorption and is used in osteoporosis and Paget's disease of bone. It has also been used in the treatment of bone metastases and hypercalcemia of malignancy.

Clodronate

Clodronate is a bisphosphonate that has demonstrated efficacy in patients with a variety of disorders of enhanced bone resorption, including Paget's disease, osteolytic bone metastases, and hypercalcemia of malignancy (8,9). In preclinical studies, clodronate prevented bone loss during immobilization (10).

Etidronate

Etidronate, an alkylbisphosphonate, was the first to be introduced for the management of bone resorption disorders. Subsequently, a cyclic regimen of etidronate followed by calcium supplementation was established in the treatment of osteoporosis.

Pamidronate

Pamidronate in the disodium form, a second-generation bisphosphonate, has an intermediate antiresorptive activity; its continuous administration produces rapid suppression of bone resorption. Unlike etidronate, it does not impair bone mineralization at therapeutic dosages in patients with Paget's disease. Pamidronate inhibits osteoclast activity primarily by binding with hydroxyapatite crystals in the bone matrix, preventing the attachment of osteoclast precursor cells. Other mechanisms of action of matrix-bound pamidronate may include direct inhibition of mature osteoclast function, promotion of osteoclast apoptosis, and interference with osteoblast-mediated osteoclast activation. In patients with osteoporosis, pamidronate increased bone mineral density by 6.8% over 2.2 years (11). The frequently observed adverse effects with pamidronate therapy were gastrointestinal: gastritis due to either a local reaction when a high concentration of the drug stays in the mucus or by chelation with calcium ions (12).

Residronate

Residronate is a pyridinylbisphosphonate with potent antiresorptive properties. In animal studies it was about 1000 times more potent than etidronate and 3-5 times more potent than alendronate (13), which enables the use of a lower dose and a shorter treatment regimen, with consequent potential minimization of adverse effects. In a randomized, double-blind, multicenter study of the efficacy, safety, and tolerability of residronate in 62 patients taking oral residronate for Paget's disease of bone, adverse effects were recorded in 29 patients (14). Twelve had upper gastrointestinal adverse events, of which three were moderate to severe. Four other patients withdrew because of adverse events, but one only was considered to be possibly drug-related (mild colitis). There was a transient reduction in serum calcium and phosphorus concentrations, greatest at 1 month after the start of treatment, and followed by a gradual return toward baseline concentrations.

Comparative studies

In 72 postmenopausal women (mean age 65 years) with established osteoporosis who took elemental calcium 1.0 g/day and vitamin D 400 U/day, etidronate and hormones were compared (15). The Hormone Replacement Therapy (HRT) group ($n = 18$) took cyclical estrogen and progesterone; the etidronate group ($n = 17$) took intermittent cyclical etidronate; and the combined therapy group ($n = 19$) took both HRT and etidronate. Three patients in the HRT group and two patients in the combined therapy group withdrew owing to estrogen-related adverse effects. One patient each from the control group and the etidronate group withdrew because of inability to tolerate the medications. Two patients each from the control and combined therapy groups, and one from the etidronate group withdrew owing to other medical problems. There was one death due to myocardial infarction in the etidronate group, and one patient in the control group was lost to follow-up. Six patients complained of nausea after etidronate, but symptoms improved with time.

In 32 women treated for postmenopausal osteoporosis for 2 years with either pamidronate or with oral fluoride, adverse effects were a transient fever with influenza-like symptoms in five patients after the first infusion of pamidronate, and rigors and mild phlebitis in one patient (16).

Placebo-controlled studies

Of 300 patients, 221 (111 pamidronate, 110 placebo) withdrew prematurely (17). The majority of withdrawals

($n = 115$) were due to disease progression or death due to multiple myeloma. The number of patients who withdrew because of adverse experiences ($n = 30$) was small in both groups, and no deaths occurred due to the treatment. Adverse gastrointestinal events were reported in patients who received both pamidronate and placebo, but although the rates were not significantly different in the two groups, there were more cases of nausea, dysphagia/dyspepsia, and gastrointestinal ulceration in the pamidronate group.

In a long-term follow-up of two randomized, placebo-controlled trials of pamidronate in women with breast carcinoma and osteolytic bone metastases, adverse events caused premature withdrawal of therapy in 22% of 367 patients taking pamidronate 90 mg/day and 20% of 38 patients taking placebo (18).

- A 75-year-old woman was withdrawn after developing an allergic reaction in her left eye possibly related to pamidronate.
- Another patient discontinued pamidronate after an episode of symptomatic hypocalcemia.
- Two other serious and unexpected adverse events occurred in patients taking pamidronate.
- A 45-year-old woman who had been taking placebo developed an interstitial pulmonary infiltrate and dyspnea 4 days after taking pamidronate on a compassionate basis after completing the study.
- An 83-year-old woman developed increased weakness, fatigue, and dyspnea 3 weeks after her last dose of pamidronate.

These adverse events were both assessed by the treating physician as being possibly related to pamidronate. Fatigue related to the study drug was reported slightly more often by patients taking pamidronate (40%) than those taking placebo (29%). Fever related to the study drug was reported in 14% of pamidronate patients and in 5% of placebo patients.

The effect of oral pamidronate on bone mineral density and its adverse effect profile has been investigated in a double-blind, placebo-controlled study in 122 patients aged 55–75 years with established vertebral osteoporosis (19). The patients took disodium pamidronate 300 mg/day for 4 weeks every 16 weeks (group A), 150 mg/day for 4 weeks every 8 weeks (group B), or placebo (group C). All also took calcium 500 mg/day and vitamin D 400 IU/day. In groups A and B there were significant reductions in serum osteocalcin and urinary deoxypuridinoline and an excess of gastrointestinal adverse effects, particularly in group A. The authors concluded that intermittent pamidronate therapy can prevent bone loss in both the lumbar spine and femoral neck in patients with established vertebral osteoporosis, although the 300 mg dose did not appear suitable for clinical use because of gastrointestinal adverse effects.

Organs and Systems

Neuromuscular function

The efficacy and safety of amidronate in recalcitrant reflex sympathetic dystrophy have been assessed in 10 women and 13 men, mean age 44 years (20). Amidronate was given intravenously in a dose of 1 mg/kg/day for 1–3 days. There were adverse events in 14 patients: transient fever ($n = 6$), venous inflammation ($n = 2$), transient symptomless hypocalcemia ($n = 3$), nausea ($n = 1$), lymphopenia ($n = 1$), transient hypertension ($n = 1$).

Sensory systems

Eyes

Adverse effects with various forms of pamidronate included 23 cases of suspected ocular adverse drug reactions associated with the use of intravenous pamidronate disodium (21). Bilateral anterior uveitis occurred 24–48 hours after administration in six cases; three reports involved unilateral episcleritis, occurring 1–6 days after administration; and 13 patients complained of non-specific transient conjunctivitis 6–8 hours after administration.

The first case of uveitis due to pamidronate was reported in 1993 (22). A review of reports published as of 1994 (21) found 23 cases, including 7 cases of anterior uveitis, 3 of episcleritis or scleritis, and 13 of non-specific transient conjunctivitis. Since then, other cases of anterior uveitis have been reported (23,24).

Of 16 cases of pamidronate-induced anterior uveitis (23,24), 11 were bilateral and 5 unilateral. In most cases, the onset was within 24–48 hours of initiation of the pamidronate infusion, although in one patient the interval was 17 days. The severity, when specified, ranged from mild to severe. Treatment was by watchful waiting in two patients, oral glucocorticoid therapy or hospital admission in four, and topical glucocorticoids with or without cycloplegic agents in nine. The time to recovery, when specified, ranged from a few days to a month. The cumulative pamidronate dose was 30–240 mg.

Ears

Serious adverse effects of aminobisphosphonates were reported in otospongiosis. Of two patients with stapedial otosclerosis and sensorineural hearing loss one developed total bilateral deafness and the other retained minimal auditory function in the low frequencies (25). It was recommended that sensorineural deafness in selected patients with otosclerosis should be treated with sodium fluoride, and that patients with Paget's disease treated with aminobisphosphonates should be closely monitored and the drug discontinued immediately if hearing deteriorates. Elsewhere, ototoxicity has been reported (SEDA-20, 440).

Psychological, psychiatric

Olfactory hallucinations have been attributed to etidronate (26).

Endocrine

A patient who was receiving disodium pamidronate developed gynecomastia, and of another 13 patients, two more men had gynecomastia and one woman had tender swollen breasts (27).

Mineral balance

Pamidronate can cause asymptomatic hypocalcemia (SEDA-20, 440). In a study of the use of pamidronate to treat immobilization hypercalcemia after acute spinal cord injury in nine patients, one patient had transient drug-related fever and four had asymptomatic hypocalcemia (28).

- A 39-year-old normocalcemic patient with subclinical hypoparathyroidism and bone metastases from breast carcinoma was given pamidronate 60 mg parenterally and developed hypocalcemia (1.42 mmol/l) and carpopedal spasm (29). Hypocalcemia due to latent hypoparathyroidism had been compensated by extensive osteolysis due to bone metastases.

Gastrointestinal

The aminobisphosphonates cause severe gastrointestinal adverse effects: of greatest concern is their capacity to cause esophageal lesions. A report identified three patients with severe esophagitis from alendronate (30). Four episodes of esophagitis occurred in 49 patients in a study of a new timed-release formulation of pamidronate (31). Severe esophagitis or esophageal ulceration have been reported in seven patients taking bisphosphonates (six alendronate and one etidronate); the lesions healed on withdrawal (32).

In 57 patients with advanced prostate cancer resistant to first-line hormonal therapy treated with estramustine and clodronate, the main adverse effect was nausea (33). Therapeutic efficacy was small. Reasons for premature withdrawal of clodronate in one study included refusal to continue treatment (five patients) and progressive disease of the bone (four patients) (34). One patient refused to take clodronate from the start; seven discontinued clodronate after a median of 13 (range 0.2–23) months because of adverse events. In five patients the cause was nausea, combined with vomiting in four and diarrhea in one. After 0.9, 1.0, and 1.3 months the dosage of clodronate was reduced to 800 mg/day in three patients (one had nausea, another dyspepsia, and a third had uncharacteristic sensations in the skeleton).

The safety of cyclic etidronate has been evaluated in 550 general practices in the UK in 7977 patients taking cyclic etidronate (7244 women) (35). The findings were consistent with the conclusions of several reviews of the safety and tolerability of cyclic etidronate (36,37). The most common adverse effects reported in these reviews were minor gastrointestinal events, such as diarrhea, nausea, and flatulence. Etidronate has not been associated with an increased incidence of serious gastrointestinal adverse events.

Liver

Although adverse events associated with bisphosphonates are usually gastrointestinal, raised transaminases (aspartate transaminase and alanine transaminase) have also been described in many cases. However, the frequency of such changes has been poorly investigated. The Probone study was a phase II trial in 610 osteopenic women randomized for 3 years to receive placebo or clodronate 65, 400, 800 mg/day, or 400 mg/day for 15 days out of 90 (intermittent group) (38). During the first study year, gastrointestinal adverse events were reported by 20–26% of the patients in the five study groups, but there were no differences between groups. The high-dose clodronate groups (400 and 800 mg/day) had no more hepatic adverse effects than the low-dose groups, and there were no serious adverse effects on the liver. However, these higher doses of clodronate caused a significant mean increase in alanine transaminase of 5.4–5.8 IU compared with placebo. In volunteers with initially normal transaminase activity, the risk ratio for an increase to above normal was 1.8 with clodronate 400 mg/day and 2.5 with clodronate 800 mg/day. In these groups, aspartate transaminase and alanine transaminase, respectively, rose above the top of the reference ranges in 12 and 18% of the volunteers. The respective percentages in the placebo group were 6.2 and 7.2%. All bilirubin concentrations were normal. The authors concluded that oral clodronate may increase the activity of serum transaminases, and that these enzymes most likely come from the liver.

Skin

Necrobiotic palisading granuloma has been attributed to intravenous disodium clodronate (39).

Musculoskeletal

Of 12 patients given pamidronate (seven men, mean age 25 years) with either corticosteroid-induced or postmenopausal osteoporosis, none of whom had undergone transplantation, nine reported severe bone pain, starting at about 12 hours after the infusion and lasting for up to 3 days (40). The bone pain typically started in the spine then migrated to the ribs and finally to the lower limbs. The pain was excruciating in seven patients, rendering them bed-bound and making sputum expectoration and physiotherapy difficult. Paracetamol and diclofenac were unsuccessful in preventing or relieving pain. Two of the nine patients also had febrile reactions and one developed phlebitis around the infusion site. None of the controls developed bone pain. The high incidence of bone pain after intravenous pamidronate may be a novel drug reaction specific to cystic fibrosis. The pain may be related to the abrupt reduction in bone turnover anticipated after intravenous pamidronate.

Body temperature

In a study of the use of pamidronate to treat immobilization hypercalcemia after acute spinal cord injury in nine patients, one patient had transient drug-related fever and four had asymptomatic hypocalcemia (29).

Susceptibility Factors

Age

Caution should be exercised when using pamidronate in children, since there may be an immediate calcium-lowering effect and persistence of hypocalcemia, hypomagnesemia, and hypophosphatemia, particularly when high doses (for example 30 mg) are given intravenously (41). The authors recommended that children be given doses of 15–20 mg.

Drug Administration

Drug administration route

Intermittent intravenous clodronate is effective in preventing and treating postmenopausal bone loss (42). In Italy, it is also available for intramuscular administration, which might be an acceptable alternative for some patients. However, intramuscular injection caused substantial pain at the site of injection, which led to withdrawal in almost 50% of the patients who received a weekly dose (43). These results suggest that intermittent intramuscular clodronate can improve skeletal bone density in osteoporotic postmenopausal women, but in situ pain may limit its extensive use.

References

1. Vitte C, Fleisch H, Guenther HL. Bisphosphonates induce osteoblasts to secrete an inhibitor of osteoclast-mediated resorption. Endocrinology 1996;137(6):2324–33.
2. Adami S, Zamberlan N. Adverse effects of bisphosphonates. A comparative review. Drug Saf 1996;14(3):158–70.
3. Storm T, Thamsborg G, Steiniche T, Genant HK, Sorensen OH. Effect of intermittent cyclical etidronate therapy on bone mass and fracture rate in women with postmenopausal osteoporosis. N Engl J Med 1990;322(18):1265–71.
4. Valkema R, Vismans FJ, Papapoulos SE, Pauwels EK, Bijvoet OL. Maintained improvement in calcium balance and bone mineral content in patients with osteoporosis treated with the bisphosphonate APD. Bone Miner 1989;5(2):183–92.
5. Nussbaum SR, Younger J, Vandepol CJ, Gagel RF, Zubler MA, Chapman R, Henderson IC, Mallette LE. Single-dose intravenous therapy with pamidronate for the treatment of hypercalcemia of malignancy: comparison of 30-, 60-, and 90-mg dosages. Am J Med 1993;95(3):297–304.
6. Redalieu E, Coleman JM, Chan K, Seaman J, Degen PH, Flesch G, Brox A, Batiste G. Urinary excretion of aminohydroxypropylidene bisphosphonate in cancer patients after single intravenous infusions. J Pharm Sci 1993;82(6):665–7.
7. Daragon A, Peyron R, Serrurier D, Deshayes P. Treatment of hypercalcemia of malignancy with intravenous APD. Curr Ther Res 1991;50:10–21.
8. Kanis JA. Clodronate—a new perspective in the treatment of neoplastic bone disease. Proceedings of a meeting. Helsinki. Bone 1987;8(Suppl 1):S1–86.
9. Kanis JA, McCloskey EV, Paterson AH. Use of diphosphonates in hypercalcaemia due to malignancy. Lancet 1990;335(8682):170–1.
10. Minaire P, Berard E, Meunier PJ, Edouard C, Goedert G, Pilonchery G. Effects of disodium dichloromethylene diphosphonate on bone loss in paraplegic patients. J Clin Invest 1981;68(4):1086–92.
11. Papapoulos SE. The role of bisphosphonates in the prevention and treatment of osteoporosis. Am J Med 1993;95(5A):S48–52.
12. Herrera JA, Sarabia MO, Gonzalez MM. Effects of treatment with biphosphonates on gastrointestinal and esophageal mucosa in patients with osteoporosis: pamidronate versus alendronate. Curr Ther Res 1996;60:307–13.
13. Geddes AD, D'Souza SM, Ebetino FH, Ibbotson KJ. Bisphosphonates: structure-activity relationship and therapeutic implications. Heersche JNM, Kanis JA, editors. Bone and Mineral Research. Amsterdam: Elsevier, 1994:265–74.
14. Miller PD, Brown JP, Siris ES, Hoseyni MS, Axelrod DW, Bekker PJ. A randomized, double-blind comparison of risedronate and etidronate in the treatment of Paget's disease of bone. Paget's Risedronate/Etidronate Study Group. Am J Med 1999;106(5):513–20.
15. Wimalawansa SJ. A four-year randomized controlled trial of hormone replacement and bisphosphonate, alone or in combination, in women with postmenopausal osteoporosis. Am J Med 1998;104(3):219–26.
16. Thiebaud D, Burckhardt P, Melchior J, Eckert P, Jacquet AF, Schnyder P, Gobelet C. Two years' effectiveness of intravenous pamidronate (APD) versus oral fluoride for osteoporosis occurring in the postmenopause. Osteoporos Int 1994;4(2):76–83.
17. Brincker H, Westin J, Abildgaard N, Gimsing P, Turesson I, Hedenus M, Ford J, Kandra A. Failure of oral pamidronate to reduce skeletal morbidity in multiple myeloma: a double-blind placebo-controlled trial. Danish-Swedish Co-operative study group. Br J Haematol 1998;101(2):280–6.
18. Lipton A, Theriault RL, Hortobagyi GN, Simeone J, Knight RD, Mellars K, Reitsma DJ, Heffernan M, Seaman JJ. Pamidronate prevents skeletal complications and is effective palliative treatment in women with breast carcinoma and osteolytic bone metastases: long term follow-up of two randomized, placebo-controlled trials. Cancer 2000;88(5):1082–90.
19. Ryan PJ, Blake GM, Davie M, Haddaway M, Gibson T, Fogelman I. Intermittent oral disodium pamidronate in established osteoporosis: a 2 year double-masked placebo-controlled study of efficacy and safety. Osteoporos Int 2000;11(2):171–6.
20. Cortet B, Flipo RM, Coquerelle P, Duquesnoy B, Delcambre B. Treatment of severe, recalcitrant reflex sympathetic dystrophy: assessment of efficacy and safety of the second generation bisphosphonate pamidronate. Clin Rheumatol 1997;16(1):51–6.
21. Macarol V, Fraunfelder FT. Pamidronate disodium and possible ocular adverse drug reactions. Am J Ophthalmol 1994;118(2):220–4.
22. Siris ES. Bisphosphonates and iritis. Lancet 1993;341(8842):436–7.
23. Ghose K, Waterworth R, Trolove P, Highton J. Uveitis associated with pamidronate. Aust NZ J Med 1994;24(3):320.
24. O'Donnell NP, Rao GP, Aguis-Fernandez A. Paget's disease: ocular complications of disodium pamidronate treatment. Br J Clin Pract 1995;49(5):272–3.
25. Boumans LJ, Poublon RM. The detrimental effect of aminohydroxypropylidene bisphosphonate (APD) in otospongiosis. Eur Arch Otorhinolaryngol 1991;248(4):218–21.
26. Burnet SP, Petrie JP. "Wake up and smell the roses"—a drug reaction to etidronate. Aust NZ J Med 1999;29(1):93.
27. Russell L. Disodium pamidronate. Aust Prescr 1999;22:30.
28. Massagli TL, Cardenas DD. Immobilization hypercalcemia treatment with pamidronate disodium after spinal cord injury. Arch Phys Med Rehabil 1999;80(9):998–1000.
29. Comlekci A, Biberoglu S, Hekimsoy Z, Okan I, Piskin O, Sekeroglu B, Alakavuklar M. Symptomatic hypocalcemia in a patient with latent hypoparathyroidism and breast

carcinoma with bone metastasis following administration of pamidronate. Intern Med 1998;37(4):396–7.

30. Dreyfuss BJ, Rai DS. Bisphosphonates in the treatment of osteoporosis. West J Med 1997;167(3):177–8.
31. Lufkin EG, Argueta R, Whitaker MD, Cameron AL, Wong VH, Egan KS, O'Fallon WM, Riggs BL. Pamidronate: an unrecognized problem in gastrointestinal tolerability. Osteoporos Int 1994;4(6):320–2.
32. Larsen KO, Stray N, Engh V, Sandnes D. Oesophagusskader relatert til bisfosfonater. [Esophageal lesions associated with diphosphonates.] Tidsskr Nor Laegeforen 2000;120(20):2397–9.
33. Kylmala T, Taube T, Tammela TL, Risteli L, Risteli J, Elomaa I. Concomitant i.v. and oral clodronate in the relief of bone pain—a double-blind placebo-controlled study in patients with prostate cancer. Br J Cancer 1997;76(7):939–42.
34. Kristensen B, Ejlertsen B, Groenvold M, Hein S, Loft H, Mouridsen HT. Oral clodronate in breast cancer patients with bone metastases: a randomized study. J Intern Med 1999;246(1):67–74.
35. van Staa TP, Leufkens H, Abenhaim L, Cooper C. Postmarketing surveillance of the safety of cyclic etidronate. Pharmacotherapy 1998;18(5):1121–8.
36. Fleisch H. Bisphosphonates in bone disease 1993. Berne: Stampflit Graphic Enterprise, 1993.
37. Papapoulos SE. Bisphosphonates: pharmacology and use in the treatment of osteoporosis. In: Marcus R, Feldman D, Kelsen J, editors. Osteoporosis. San Diego: Academic Press, 1996:1209–34.
38. Laitinen K, Taube T. Clodronate as a cause of aminotransferase elevation. Osteoporos Int 1999;10(2):120–2.
39. Lalinga AV, Pellegrino M, Laurini L, Miracco C. Necrobiotic palisading granuloma at injection site of disodium clodronate: a case report. Dermatology 1999;198(4):394–5.
40. Haworth CS, Selby PL, Webb AK, Mawer EB, Adams JE, Freemont TJ. Severe bone pain after intravenous pamidronate in adult patients with cystic fibrosis. Lancet 1998;352(9142):1753–4.
41. De Schepper J, de Pont S, Smitz J, De Coster D, Schots R, Otten J. Metabolic disturbances after a single dose of 30 mg pamidronate for leukaemia-associated hypercalcaemia in a 11-year-old boy. Eur J Pediatr 1999;158(9):765–6.
42. Kaastad TS, Reikeras O, Madsen JE, Narum S, Stromme JH, Obrant KJ, Nordsletten L. Effects of clodronate on cortical and trabecular bone in ovariectomized rats on a low calcium diet. Calcif Tissue Int 1997;61(2):158–64.
43. Rossini M, Braga V, Gatti D, Gerardi D, Zamberlan N, Adami S. Intramuscular clodronate therapy in postmenopausal osteoporosis. Bone 1999;24(2):125–9.

Bithionol

General Information

Bithionol is a chlorinated bisphenol with antihelminthic properties. It is active against most trematodes and has been recommended as preferable to praziquantel in fascioliasis and paragonimiasis, proving both effective and well tolerated. Bithionol also has antibacterial properties and was for this reason included for a time in cosmetic formulations. However, when given topically it caused photosensitivity reactions, and this form of application has been abandoned.

Organs and Systems

Gastrointestinal

An Egyptian report in 1991 on the use of bithionol in fascioliasis in doses of 30 mg/kg every other day for five doses noted that unpleasant symptoms were common, but some or most of them were certainly due to the underlying disease and actually abated with treatment (1). The only symptom the incidence of which actually increased as a result of treatment was diarrhea, which occurred in 12 of 14 users; one patient also developed urticaria with pruritus.

Liver

The effects of bithionol on the liver have been examined in an Egyptian study in 1990 (2). The pathology of human fascioliasis was studied before and after bithionol treatment using light and transmission electron microscopy. Fine needle biopsies were taken from five patients with established fascioliasis, before and after drug administration. By light microscopy the pathology of human fascioliasis was similar to that reported in experimental fascioliasis. The ultrastructural picture showed bile ductule hyperplasia, fibrosis of portal tracts, widening of the interhepatic spaces by many microvilli, and dilated Disse spaces with collagen fibers. Bile ductule hyperplasia may be the initial factor in fibrinogenesis, which subsequently enhances the development of microvilli on the surfaces of hepatocytes. Both light and electron microscopy showed regression of the picture of fascioliasis to normal after bithionol treatment, with no sign of adverse effects on the liver.

References

1. Bassiouny HK, Soliman NK, el-Daly SM, Badr NM. Human fascioliasis in Egypt: effect of infection and efficacy of bithionol treatment. J Trop Med Hyg 1991;94(5):333–7.
2. Abou Basha LM, Salem AI, Fadali GA. Human fascioliasis: ultrastructural study on the liver before and after bithionol treatment. J Egypt Soc Parasitol 1990;20(2):541–8.

Bitoscanate

General Information

Bitoscanate (phenylene 1,4-diisothiocyanate) enjoyed some clinical interest in the treatment of hookworm infection in around 1975 (1), but it proved highly dangerous, and deaths have occurred with as little as 300 mg. Most of the publicity that it has had in recent years relates to its listing as an "extremely hazardous substance," and the US Office of Homeland Security has actually regarded it as a possible tool for bioterrorism.

Reference

1. Samuel MR. Clinical experience with bitoscanate. Prog Drug Res 1975;19:96–107.

Bleomycin

See also Cytostatic and immunosuppressant drugs

General Information

Bleomycin is a cytostatic drug that causes double-strand breaks in DNA. It has been used to treat Hodgkin's disease and a variety of solid cancers. It is often used in combination with other anticancer drugs, for example in the regimens known as ABVD (doxorubicin + bleomycin + vinblastine + dacarbazine) and BEP (bleomycin + etoposide + cisplatin). It has also been injected intrapleurally in the management of malignant effusions.

Organs and Systems

Respiratory

Bleomycin can cause diffuse interstitial pneumonitis, with significant mortality. Bleomycin is more slowly degraded in the lungs than in other tissues, such as the bone marrow or liver, because of lower bleomycin hydrolase activity. The mechanisms of lung damage include the formation of highly reactive oxygen species; lipid peroxidation of cell membranes has been suggested, but not confirmed (1). Others have suggested a role for angiotensin-converting enzyme in production of the lung damage (2), but the data are unconvincing.

Because this is a severe adverse effect it is generally recommended that a total dose of more than 400 mg of bleomycin should be avoided in patients with normal renal function. In those over 70 years of age reduced creatinine clearance makes dosage reduction necessary.

Estimates of the incidence of bleomycin pulmonary toxicity range from 11 to 23% (3). Of 99 patients previously treated with bleomycin together with other cytostatic drugs for testicular tumors, 16 developed abnormal lung function tests; amongst those who received more than 500 mg of bleomycin cumulatively, 75% had abnormal lung function tests, Raynaud's phenomenon, or both (4). Rapid progression to fatal pulmonary fibrosis has been documented previously and, in all but one instance, there had been previous or concurrent chest radiotherapy. Two cases have been reported of rapidly progressive fatal pulmonary fibrosis in patients receiving bleomycin who had had no previous lung disease, and who had not undergone radiotherapy to the chest (5). Lung toxicity can occur at low cumulative doses of bleomycin during concurrent treatment with cyclophosphamide (which independently causes pulmonary toxicity). In 19 patients (6) there was a high (26%) incidence of fatal pulmonary toxicity in patients receiving the combination of these two drugs, which warrants special caution.

Transient but significant reductions in pulmonary function tests have been reported within 8–12 months in 35 children treated with polychemotherapy who had received a cumulative dose of 120 mg/m^2 up to 12 years after diagnosis (7). However, there were no long-term abnormalities.

In 194 patients there was a fatality rate of 2.8% from pulmonary toxicity. The incidence of fatal pulmonary toxicity increased with each decade of life above 30 and the lower the glomerular filtration rate at the time of administration the greater the death rate; the death rate may exceed 10% in those over 40 years of age (8).

Bleomycin is also associated with a hypersensitivity pneumonitis. This should be considered when interpreting cytological swabs in patients treated with the drug, since the acute cytological changes can be misinterpreted (9).

A syndrome of acute chest pain occurring during bleomycin infusion has been described in 10 patients with features that could not be ascribed to pulmonary fibrosis, hypersensitivity pneumonitis, or cardiovascular toxicity (10). The pain was sudden in onset and occurred during the first or second course, usually on the second or third day. There was retrosternal pressure or pleuritic pain, in some cases severe enough to require narcotic analgesics. Stopping or slowing the infusion produced marked improvement. In two of seven patients who received a subsequent course of treatment, the pain recurred. One patient had dyspnea and two developed an erythematous rash. One had a pleural friction rub and one a pericardial friction rub. There was fever during five episodes. There were no other physical abnormalities. There were electrocardiographic changes suggestive of pericarditis in two patients; one patient developed transient blunting of a costophrenic angle on a chest X-ray, and another a transient and small retrocardiac pulmonary infiltrate. The pain resolved spontaneously with analgesics, and there were no long-term pulmonary or cardiac sequelae. Possible underlying mechanisms include pleuropericarditis due to serosal inflammation or vascular pathology.

Severe morbidity has been reported after the use of regimens containing bleomycin: 10% of patients developed adult respiratory distress syndrome and a further 9% needed prolonged ventilation (11). The authors thought that these rates were higher than expected and attributed this to a combination of the toxic effects of bleomycin on the lung and a large retroperitoneal and/or pulmonary tumor burden.

Skin

Bleomycin can occasionally cause scleroderma-like changes in the skin (12,13), an effect that may be enhanced by radiotherapy (14).

Body temperature

When bleomycin is used as a sclerosing agent in adults, a dose of up to 1 mg/kg is generally instilled into the chest through a thoracostomy tube. Bleomycin 60 mg intrapleurally caused a fever over 39°C in two of 21 patients with malignant pleural effusions; it settled without treatment and was not associated with local discomfort (15).

Drug Administration

Drug administration route

Several antineoplastic agents have been introduced into the pleural space to achieve pleurodesis, but the largest reported experience is with bleomycin. Intrapleural bleomycin has an efficacy similar to that of tetracycline and doxycycline (16). About 45% of a dose of bleomycin is absorbed systemically, but significant adverse events are uncommon (17). Chest pain is reported in about 28% of patients, fever in 24%, and nausea in about 11% (18). A randomized comparison of bleomycin with tetracycline in 85 patients with malignant pleural effusions showed that toxicity, predominantly in the form of chest pain and fever, was similar with the two drugs (7–17%) (19). Nearly half the patients (34) died within 90 days owing to disease progression. However, one patient died within 2 days of intrapleural bleomycin, and the investigators could not exclude a contribution from the bleomycin. In another comparison of bleomycin with doxycycline there was fever in 13%, chest pain in 11%, and chills in 4% of patients treated with bleomycin (20).

References

1. Jenkinson S, Duncan C, Lawrence R, Collins J. Lack of enhancement of bleomycin lung injury in vitamin E-deficient rats. J Crit Care 1987;2:264.
2. Nussinovitch N, Peleg E, Yaron A, Ratt P, Rosenthal T. Angiotensin converting enzyme in bleomycin-treated patients. Int J Clin Pharmacol Ther Toxicol 1988;26(6):310–13.
3. Potash RJ. Acute dyspnoea in a chemotherapy recipient. Respir Care 1987;32:279.
4. Creutzig A, Polking W, Schmoll HJ, Fabel H, Alexander K. Raynaud-Syndrom und Veranderungen der Lungenfunktion als Folgen einer zytostatischen Therapie von Hodentumoren. [Raynaud syndrome and changes in lung function as sequelae of cytostatic therapy of testicular tumors.] Med Klin (Munich) 1987;82(4):131–4.
5. Dee GJ, Austin JH, Mutter GL. Bleomycin-associated pulmonary fibrosis: rapidly fatal progression without chest radiotherapy. J Surg Oncol 1987;35(2):135–8.
6. Quigley M, Brada M, Heron C, Horwich A. Severe lung toxicity with a weekly low dose chemotherapy regimen in patients with non-Hodgkin's lymphoma. Hematol Oncol 1988;6(4):319–24.
7. Kharasch VS, Lipsitz S, Santis W, Hallowell JA, Goorin A. Long-term pulmonary toxicity of multiagent chemotherapy including bleomycin and cyclophosphamide in osteosarcoma survivors. Med Pediatr Oncol 1996;27(2):85–91.
8. Simpson AB, Paul J, Graham J, Kaye SB. Fatal bleomycin pulmonary toxicity in the west of Scotland 1991–95: a review of patients with germ cell tumours. Br J Cancer 1998;78(8):1061–6.
9. Hartmann CA, Weise I, Voigt D, Reichle G. Gefahr zytologischer Fehlinterpretation bei Zytostatikapneumopathie. [Danger of false cytologic interpretation in cytostatic pneumopathy.] Prax Klin Pneumol 1987;41(6):223–6.
10. White DA, Schwartzberg LS, Kris MG, Bosl GJ. Acute chest pain syndrome during bleomycin infusions. Cancer 1987;59(9):1582–5.
11. Baniel J, Foster RS, Rowland RG, Bihrle R, Donohue JP. Complications of post-chemotherapy retroperitoneal lymph node dissection. J Urol 1995;153(3 Pt 2):976–80.
12. Kerr LD, Spiera H. Scleroderma in association with the use of bleomycin: a report of 3 cases. J Rheumatol 1992;19(2):294–6.
13. Kim KH, Yoon TJ, Oh CW, Ko GH, Kim TH. A case of bleomycin-induced scleroderma. J Korean Med Sci 1996;11(5):454–6.
14. Marck Y, Meunier L, Barneon G, Meynadier J. Sclerose cutanée en pèlerine au decours d'un traitement par l'association bleomycine et radiothérapie. [Scleroderma of the shoulders after treatment with combined bleomycin and radiotherapy.] Ann Dermatol Venereol 1994;121(10):712–14.
15. Hsu NY, Chen C. Intrapleural bleomycin in the management of malignant pleural effusion. J Surg Assoc ROC 1988;21:302.
16. Martinez-Moragon E, Aparicio J, Rogado MC, Sanchis J, Sanchis F, Gil-Suay V. Pleurodesis in malignant pleural effusions: a randomized study of tetracycline versus bleomycin. Eur Respir J 1997;10(10):2380–3.
17. Alberts DS, Chen HS, Mayersohn M, Perrier D, Moon TE, Gross JF. Bleomycin pharmacokinetics in man. II. Intracavitary administration. Cancer Chemother Pharmacol 1979;2(2):127–32.
18. Walker-Renard PB, Vaughan LM, Sahn SA. Chemical pleurodesis for malignant pleural effusions. Ann Intern Med 1994;120(1):56–64.
19. Ruckdeschel JC, Moores D, Lee JY, Einhorn LH, Mandelbaum I, Koeller J, Weiss GR, Losada M, Keller JH. Intrapleural therapy for malignant pleural effusions. A randomized comparison of bleomycin and tetracycline. Chest 1991;100(6):1528–35.
20. Patz EF Jr, McAdams HP, Erasmus JJ, Goodman PC, Culhane DK, Gilkeson RC, Herndon J. Sclerotherapy for malignant pleural effusions: a prospective randomized trial of bleomycin vs doxycycline with small-bore catheter drainage. Chest 1998;113(5):1305–11.

Blood cell transfusion and bone marrow transplantation

General Information

The most common adverse effect of routine blood transfusion is an incompatibility reaction. Massive blood transfusions can cause other adverse effects (1). Human error resulting in blood group mismatching is the leading cause of transfusion-related fatalities (2,3). Although there have been major achievements in transfusion medicine to improve the safety of blood and blood products, the risks of transfusion reactions and of the transmission of infectious agents have not been eliminated. Treatment of patients with blood or blood-derived components has therefore been the subject of great public concern, mostly because of the tragic consequences of transfusion-transmitted human immunodeficiency virus (HIV).

Most patients do not react adversely to blood products. However, some have mild to severe effects immediately or delayed for 48 hours. Information on adverse reactions to blood products collected by the New Zealand Centre for Adverse Reactions Monitoring enables the identification of unusual or unpredictable adverse reactions; risk factors such as concomitant medications, underlying diseases, rate of administration; and batch problems (4).

Minimizing the risks of blood transfusion

Because of the possible complications of blood transfusion, it is constantly emphasized that unnecessary transfusions should be avoided. In most cases therapy with blood or blood components is solely a replacement therapy and should therefore be used only when a distinct deficiency of some blood component has been demonstrated; "component blood therapy" is usually preferable to whole blood therapy, providing more specific treatment. Also, the use of autologous transfusions, although not always feasible, seems to be a strategy that might reduce complication rates (5).

In order to reduce risks to a minimum and at the same time ensure that blood products are of high quality, three measures must be enforced.

1. Proper selection of blood donors (6).
2. Screening of individual donations (7).
3. The use of production methods specifically aimed at minimizing the risks of transmitting infectious diseases (8).

Blood donor selection
Blood donors should be non-remunerated and voluntary, and their health should be checked at regular intervals. A scheme for donor selection may include permanent exclusion criteria, such as previous episodes of jaundice (including laboratory evidence of current or previous infectious hepatitis, especially hepatitis B or C), syphilis or malaria, the presence of anti-HIV antibodies, so-called risk conduct, such as homosexual or bisexual behavior, or treatment with non-recombinant growth hormone. Time-limited exclusion criteria relating to current health status should also be used; these may also include such temporary risk factors as the taking of certain kinds of medicine, a recent blood transfusion, vaccination with live vaccines, a recent pregnancy, and travel to certain geographical areas, for example regions with malaria or a high prevalence of HIV.

In most countries, people with a history of jaundice are excluded from the donor population. However, there is a substantial geographic variation in the prevalence and detection rate of hepatitis B surface antigen (HBsAg) and antibodies to hepatitis C virus (HCV) in donors (9,10). In addition, the type of donor involved influences the risk: commercial (paid) donors carry a much higher hepatitis risk than non-remunerated voluntary donors (11,12).

With respect to the risk of transmission of variant Creutzfeldt–Jakob disease by blood, some countries exclude from donation donors who lived in the UK for more than 6 months between 1980 and 1996 (13).

Laboratory screening of individual donations
Individual portions of donated blood should be tested for infectious risk whenever possible. The series of assays currently performed in most countries comprises tests for antibodies against HIV-I/-II, HCV, and HTLV-I/II, HBsAg, and a test for syphilis. However, screening for syphilis is no longer mandatory in all countries, as cost-benefit analysis has shown it to be of little value, at least with voluntary non-remunerated donors.

Now that hepatitis C can be tested for, the so-called surrogate tests such as alanine transaminase and antibodies to hepatitis B core antigen (HBcAb) are no longer carried out in all countries, and their relevance has been questioned (14).

Serological screening of every blood or plasma donation must be performed using the most sensitive techniques available. Screening may be unreliable in cases of HBsAg at low titers, as evidence has accumulated that blood that is HBsAg negative but strongly positive for HBcAg antibody may be infectious (15,16). However, routine screening for HBcAg antibodies is at present impracticable. There may also be a delay of 1–10 months before antibodies appear in patients infected with HIV or HCV.

In order to increase the sensitivity of screening, so as to minimize the so-called window period during which serological markers will not detect the infectivity marker, methods of detecting nucleic acids from, for example, the virus particle have been developed. Hepatitis C virus nucleic acid testing is obligatory in Europe, the USA, and Japan, and in many countries nucleic acid testing for other viruses has also been implemented. There is nevertheless no doubt that in future PCR-based methods will further increase the safety of blood and blood products.

Preparation of safe plasma-derived products
Infectivity can be reduced by introducing good manufacturing practice (GMP), both in blood banks and in plasma fractionation units. The sterility of the final products is checked and virus inactivation measures (for example heat treatment and/or chemical inactivation) are taken whenever appropriate. At present, virus inactivation procedures are most relevant to non-cellular products, although leukodepletion procedures using filtration have been used for infectious agents that are almost exclusively intracellular.

The virucidal methods currently in use (17) are based on different rationales. Heat treatment can involve heating solutions, heating lyophilized products, or heating in vapor under pressure, where the actual temperature, duration, and addition of stabilizers vary for the individual products (18,19). Chemical treatment of products with a mixture of an organic solvent and a detergent (S/D treatment) is highly effective against lipid-enveloped viruses (20,21). Other methods of removing or inactivating viruses use nanofiltration (22) or treatment with a combination of a colored photosensitizer and light (23).

Use of autologous blood transfusion
In some countries there has been a marked increase in the use of autologous blood transfusion, since it is known that blood-borne viruses, such as HIV, can be transmitted by allogeneic blood transfusion (24).

In 1997, 66 185 units of autologous blood (200 ml) were collected in Japan, 81% using preoperative collection and storage and 19% by perioperative hemodilution or blood salvage (24). The total volume of autologous blood collected accounted for 1.1% of the total number of units of whole blood donated in the same year. Of the autologous blood donated before surgery, 78% was used, while more than 70% of the blood that was collected by hemodilution, intraoperative salvage, and postoperative salvage was used. During whole blood donations adverse reactions were reported in 1.6% of cases, and ranged from mild reactions (for example dizziness) to severe reactions, such as angina and asthma. With respect to storage and transfusion, 288 errors or problems were reported, with a frequency of 1 per 455 units during production/storage, 1 per 213 transfusion problems/errors, 1 per 23 hemodilution procedures, and 1 per 54 salvage procedures. In 3.7% of the patients hypotension occurred during hemodilution. Clotting in blood units (0.9%) and bacterial contamination (0.4%) were the most frequent problems associated with blood salvage.

Adverse effects of massive blood transfusions

Patients who receive massive transfusions are either extremely ill and suffering from prolonged shock or are undergoing major surgery (for example organ transplantation). Patients who receive massive transfusions are exposed to several risks resulting from the addition of anticoagulant, from transfusion of cold blood, and from biochemical, hematological, and other changes in the blood during storage. The complications lead in turn to metabolic disturbances and impaired hemostasis in proportion to the transfused volume.

Acidosis
Since stored blood has a relatively low pH, transfusion can cause acidosis. Prompt and appropriate restoration of the patient's blood volume is most important, to maintain sufficient tissue and organ perfusion and to correct or avoid acidosis.

Ammonia and phosphate
Concentrations of ammonia and inorganic phosphates rise significantly during blood storage, but caution is needed only when old blood is given to patients with liver failure.

Circulatory overload
Circulatory overload with symptoms of congestive heart failure and pulmonary edema can complicate transfusion in patients with poor cardiac reserve.

Citrate toxicity
The citrate in preserved blood can cause a dangerous fall in the ionized calcium concentration in the recipient's plasma in cases of rapid and massive transfusion. The most significant warning sign of citrate intoxication is an increase in the peripheral or central venous pressure, which should be monitored during massive transfusions. An adequate intravenous dose of calcium gluconate or chloride is a reliable means of correcting dangerous hypocalcemia (25).

Coagulation factors
To correct coagulation factor deficiencies, 1–2 units of fresh frozen plasma are recommended after every 10 units of stored blood. As far as the storage lability of coagulation factors is concerned, mild falls in factors V and VIII, and occasionally fibrinogen, occur in the recipient. It must be emphasized, however, that significant coagulation disorders including disseminated intravascular coagulation (DIC) appear almost routinely during prolonged hypovolemia (26).

Hemoglobin oxygen-carrying capacity
The progressive increase in oxygen affinity of stored erythrocytes caused by a fall in the 2,3-diphosphoglycerate concentration is clinically relevant only under extreme conditions. The abnormally increased oxygen affinity of the hemoglobin is reversible in vivo within 24 hours. It is possible to restore the oxygen transport function of hemoglobin by addition of purine nucleotides to old blood (27).

Hemosiderosis
Patients who have received about 100 units of erythrocytes inevitably develop siderosis of the organs and tissues as a consequence of transfusion-induced iron overload (28). Deposition of iron results in functional damage to the heart, liver, spleen, endocrine glands, and other organs, and is often fatal. The clinical signs of iron toxicity in children are retarded growth, splenomegaly, cardiomyopathy, and endocrinopathies. Examination of the serum ferritin concentration and transferrin saturation is useful for the diagnosis of iron overload. Subcutaneous infusion of deferoxamine provides effective and relatively safe treatment by increasing iron excretion. Furthermore, ascorbic acid significantly enhances urinary iron excretion (29). Iron accumulation can be significantly reduced by transfusing young erythrocytes, since the intervals between transfusions can be extended (30,31).

Hypothermia
Transfusion of refrigerated blood, especially during massive transfusions or during exchange transfusions, can induce hypothermia, with a danger of cardiac arrest. If several units of blood are to be rapidly administered, they should be warmed, but not overheated, before transfusion (32).

Platelets
Thrombocytopenia is a well-known consequence of hemodilution. It also occurs in blood transfusions, in which thrombocytopenia constitutes a more frequent clinical problem than abnormalities of coagulation (33). If the platelet count falls below $40 \times 10^9/l$, platelet concentrates should be transfused.

In one study changes in hemostasis in surgical patients undergoing massive transfusion occurred in 93% of patients (34). The platelet count was most frequently abnormal. Well-defined hemostatic disorders, for example DIC, were detected in 48% of patients. It was suggested that the laboratory abnormalities were induced by massive transfusion. Laboratory monitoring and therapeutic measures directed at any underlying disease have been recommended.

Potassium
Hyperkalemia is an infrequent problem associated with the massive transfusion of old blood. Potassium intoxication threatens only patients with raised potassium concentrations before transfusion, for example in the crush syndrome, renal insufficiency, and extensive burns.

Cord blood

Umbilical cord blood is an alternative source of hemopoietic stem cells rather than bone marrow, especially for patients who lack an HLA-matched donor (35). Umbilical cord blood contains significantly more early and committed progenitor cells and has been used in patients with malignant and non-malignant hematological diseases. One of the advantages of cord blood is that it can be collected and stored in large scale in liquid nitro-gen below −190°C. As the number of hemopoietic cells in umbilical cord blood is limited, current experience with this type of transplantation is predominantly restricted to children, although adults have been successfully treated with umbilical cord blood transplantation (35).

In almost all patients who receive a hemopoietic stem cell transplant, fever and neutropenia will develop (36). The median duration of fever in those given cord blood is substantially longer (27 days) than in those given allo-geneic bone marrow (15 days), allogeneic peripheral blood stem cells (10 days), or autologous peripheral blood stem cells (6 days). In patients with a long period of fever, the time to engraftment and the period of neu-tropenia are longer. Therefore, aggressive prevention of infection will be necessary in these patients.

Exchange transfusion

Favorable results of exchange transfusion in a variety of diseases in adults, for example sickle cell disease, severe clotting disorders, hepatic failure, and acute hemolytic transfusion reactions, have been published (1). Today, however, machine apheresis procedures are more effec-tive and safer for patients requiring exchange of cellular elements or plasma. Exchange transfusion is the most effective therapeutic procedure in the treatment of hemo-lytic disease of the newborn. Bilirubin removal prevents damage to the central nervous system caused by hyperbi-lirubinemia. In addition, sensitized erythrocytes are replaced by normally surviving cells and anemia is cor-rected.

The risks of exchange transfusion are essentially the same as those described above for massive transfusions, and their magnitude depends on the health of the new-born infant and its gestational age and weight. The trans-fused blood should be as fresh as possible and should not have been stored for more than 4–5 days. It must be free from antigens that react with antibodies in the maternal plasma. Technical errors involving perforation of the umbilical vein, wrong placement of the cannula, or air embolism are fortunately only rare complications.

Platelet transfusion

Severe thrombocytopenia is most often observed in con-nection with cancer chemotherapy. The availability of platelet concentrates has improved the therapeutic possi-bilities. Platelet concentrates are obtained by the differ-ential centrifugation of several units of fresh blood or by apheresis from single donors using a blood cell separator. The quality of platelet concentrates obtained by apheresis deteriorates rapidly after storage for more than 24 hours. Of all blood components, platelet concentrates are the most vulnerable to bacterial contamination.

PlPlA1-negative platelets are used to treat neonatal alloimmune thrombocytopenic purpura, a rare, transient, but severe thrombocytopenia in the newborn due to pla-telet destruction by maternal antibody (1). The mother is usually a PlPlA1-negative person who has produced anti-PlPlA1 as a result of previous blood transfusions or preg-nancy. The antibody crosses the placenta and destroys the PlPlA1-positive platelets of the neonate.

Leukocyte transfusion

Centrifugal blood cell separators and techniques for fil-tration leukapheresis or reversible leukoadhesion can provide a therapeutically adequate dose of granulocytes from a single donor (37), and cells separated in this way are clinically effective. Granulocyte transfusions are indi-cated in severely granulocytopenic febrile patients with septicemia who are not responding to antibiotics. At least 2×10^{10} granulocytes per day are considered to constitute an adequate granulocyte transfusion, but larger numbers are probably required in some cases.

Complications after granulocyte transfusions occur in about 15–20% of the recipients (38), most frequently in patients given granulocytes prepared by filtration leuka-pheresis. The complications are predominantly severe febrile reactions, the transmission of cytomegalovirus infection, and graft-versus-host disease. Of particular importance are respiratory reactions with pulmonary edema, which mostly occur in allo-immunized recipients. Leukocyte aggregation may be the cause, with sequestra-tion microemboli and fluid overflow, but other causes have also been suspected. Reactions appear to be more common in patients with sepsis.

Since granulocytes prepared by centrifugation are markedly contaminated with erythrocytes, the ABO com-patibility between donor and recipient will be important unless the erythrocytes can be removed before use. Some reactions, particularly allergic and febrile complications, are associated with the presence of macromolecular agents (hydroxyethyl starch, modified gelatin, dextran), used to increase the yield of centrifugal techniques. ABO incompatibility does not alter the in vivo fate of granulo-cytes (39).

Antibodies to "passenger B lymphocytes" can pose problems after transplantation. When kidneys from a rhesus-negative cadaveric donor, whose serum contained anti-Rho (D), were transplanted into two rhesus-positive patients, anti-Rho (D) was detected in their serum and on their erythrocytes 3.5 weeks after transplantation (40). One patient had hemolysis. The antibodies persisted for nearly 6 months, despite graft rejection and nephrectomy in one case. These antibodies presumably arose from passenger B lymphocytes in the grafts from the rhesus-immunized donor.

Leukodepleted blood products

As in several other countries, the Health Council of the Netherlands has prepared recommendations on the need for routine leukodepletion by filtration of blood. The presence of leukocytes in blood products has no beneficial effect for the recipient, except in special cases, such as patients undergoing organ transplantation (41). Apart from preventing the adverse effects associated with leu-kocyte transfusion, it has been postulated that the risk of transmission of new variant Creutzfeldt–Jakob disease can be prevented by using leukodepleted blood products.

The disadvantages of leukodepletion are hypotension and adult respiratory distress syndrome (42).

Red eye syndrome, which is characterized by conjunc-tivitis, headache, and muscle aches, with spontaneous resolution, was caused by a specific filter that is not being used any more (41).

Organs and Systems

Cardiovascular

Bone marrow for transplantation is usually kept cryopreserved in dimethylsulfoxide (DMSO), and residual DMSO may be responsible for toxic reactions: in one report, all of a series of 10 patients had falls in heart rate and blood pressure (43). However, other factors, such as cell lysis or rapid intravenous infusion of large volumes, may be responsible.

Respiratory

Transfusion-related acute lung injury is an infrequent but life-threatening complication, clinically indistinguishable from adult respiratory distress syndrome (ARDS). It can occur after the administration of whole blood, erythrocytes, fresh frozen plasma, or cryoprecipitate, all of which contain variable amounts of plasma. In transfusion-related acute lung injury the symptoms of ARDS (dyspnea, pulmonary edema, severe hypoxia, fever, and hypotension) occur within 1–6 hours from the start of transfusion and usually subside within 1–4 days (44). These symptoms can vary from mild to severe and they lead to death in 5–10% of cases. The reaction may be more frequent than reported because confounding factors can mask the symptoms (45).

Transfusion-related acute lung injury has been associated with the presence of granulocyte antibodies, HLA antibodies, or biologically active lipids in the plasma. These agents activate granulocytes and endothelial cells and cause release of inflammatory mediators, which cause increased vascular permeability, fever, and hypotension (44). HLA class II antibodies can provoke transfusion-related acute lung injury, as observed in a 19-year-old woman, who developed transfusion-related acute lung injury after treatment with fresh-frozen plasma (46). Probably, monocytes are then involved in the pathogenesis of the acute lung injury (47).

Most of the fatal cases of transfusion-related acute lung injury have involved transfusions of fresh frozen plasma; whole blood, packed erythrocytes, cryoprecipitate, platelet concentrates, apheresis platelets, and occasionally intravenous immunoglobulin have also been implicated. The donors most often involved in fatal injury have been multiparous women who were antihuman lymphocyte antigen-positive or antigranulocyte antibody-positive; one or both of these antibody types have been found in 89% of reported cases. The factors that predispose to transfusion-related acute lung injury include surgery, active infection, massive transfusion, and cytokine therapy, which activate pulmonary endothelium and primes the patient's leukocytes. It has been hypothesized that transfusion-related acute lung injury results from a combination of two independent insults, the patient's clinical state and the presence of antileukocyte antibodies.

The FDA has issued a Dear Colleague letter, outlining the risk of transfusion-related acute lung injury with the use of blood products, particularly those that contain plasma (48). The agency has noted that since the first report of fatal transfusion-related acute lung injury in 1992, 45 more reports have been received by the Center for Biologics Evaluation and Research. Transfusion-related acute lung injury is now believed to be the third commonest cause of infusion-related deaths. The number of non-fatal cases of transfusion-related acute lung injury associated with blood products is also on the increase, but this may be due to better recognition and reporting.

A patient with acute myeloid leukemia developed pulmonary alveolar proteinosis during the period of leukopenia following an unrelated umbilical cord blood transplantation (49).

Hematologic

Hemolytic post-transfusion reactions (50) are most often caused by clerical and administrative errors involving misidentification (incorrect labeling of blood samples, erroneous identification of patients) rather than by mistakes in the laboratory (2,51). However, scrupulous care is demanded at all stages; in a review of hemolytic and other transfusion reactions, the importance of competent handling of whole blood and red cell suspensions (including the avoidance of freezing or osmotic damage) has been stressed (52).

Hemolysis mediated by immune reactions is usually avoided by routine antibody screening and cross-matching methods. Improved pre-transfusion testing has resulted in a significant decrease in the incidence of hemolytic transfusion reactions, although there are examples of transfusion reactions having occurred where no antibody was detectable either before or after transfusion (53).

Acute post-transfusion hemolytic reactions
Acute hemolytic post-transfusion reaction with measurable destruction of the donor's or recipient's erythrocytes due to incompatibility of antigens and antibodies is followed by hemoglobinemia. Hemoglobinemia occurs when the combined hemoglobin-binding capacity of the haptoglobins and hemopexin in plasma is saturated. The severity of the reaction depends on the nature of the antigen and antibody, on the binding strength of the antibody, and on the volume of transfused incompatible blood.

A severe acute hemolytic reaction immediately or soon after the transfusion of incompatible blood is characterized by classical symptoms: a feeling of heat along the vein into which the blood is being transfused, a sensation of severe pain in the lumbar region, substernal tightness, dyspnea, nausea, a fall in blood pressure, tachycardia, circulatory collapse, hemoglobinemia, hemoglobinuria, and jaundice. It is fatal in about 50% of cases, either because of hemolytic shock or hemorrhage due to intravascular coagulation, or because of acute renal insufficiency. Sometimes the clinical symptoms are poorly manifested, so that only fever with or without chills may be noted, or they are masked by signs of the primary disease, so that the reaction is not recognized. Especially in an anesthetized patient the only symptom of intravascular destruction of erythrocytes may be unexpected profuse bleeding from the operation wound and hypotension (54).

The overwhelming majority of such reactions (about 80%) are due to ABO incompatibility. Acute post-transfusion reactions can also occur in the presence of an irregular antibody in the recipient's plasma, usually directed against antigens of the Rh system, which can sometimes be difficult to detect; such antibodies cause hemolytic reactions only exceptionally, although several cases have been extensively described (55–59).

Delayed post-transfusion hemolytic reactions

When the signs and symptoms of a hemolytic transfusion reaction occur more than 24 hours after transfusion, the reaction is classified as a delayed reaction (60–62). It is estimated that up to 0.025% of recipients may well be at risk of delayed transfusion reactions (1); however, in one study only 1 in 10 668 transfused units cause delayed hemolysis. The severity of this type of reaction varies widely. Many of these reactions are so mild that they remain unnoticed; only a few are severe or fatal. Almost all patients with this type of complication have a history of previous transfusion and/or pregnancy, which has made sensitization possible. The symptoms comprise fever, chills, anemia, hemoglobinemia, hemoglobinuria, and reticulocytosis. Renal insufficiency can occur and the direct antiglobulin test is positive.

Delayed reactions are difficult to prevent. Incompatibility may not be demonstrable before transfusion, and at the time of the reaction the relevant antibodies may not be detectable. Post-transfusion blood samples must therefore be subjected to repeated serological testing. Delayed reactions usually occur as a result of a secondary anamnestic response within 3–21 days after the transfusion of apparently compatible blood, at a time when the antibody concentration has risen sufficiently to bring about hemolysis of the donor's erythrocytes. A primary immune response can also evoke this kind of reaction (61).

Reports of delayed transfusion reactions continue to appear and confirm the difficulty of diagnosis. Many allo-antibodies responsible for delayed reactions of various severity have been demonstrated (61,63–69). The specificities include the usual Kidd and Rh antigens/antibodies and anti-S. Delayed reactions to the Kell antigens, for example Js(a,b), have been reported (68,69), and anti-FF(b) has also been found to cause a delayed reaction (63). A delayed reaction may occur because of anti-A1 production from the group O graft and the reduction of suppressor cell activity by immunosuppressive agents (70). In sickle cell patients a more severe delayed transfusion reaction can be misdiagnosed as sickle cell crisis (71,72). This occurs particularly in patients with U variants (73).

A method for predicting the safety of transfusion is based on the use of cells labeled with radioactive chromium (74). After the administration of several milliliters of the labeled blood, the survival of erythrocytes in the recipient's circulation is examined: poor survival in vivo indicates that transfusion with these erythrocytes will be hazardous (75,76). There are two types of survival curve for incompatible erythrocytes. A curve described by a single exponential function is seen with most potent IgG antibodies that do not bind complement, including anti-D, anti-C, and anti-K, antibodies. Clearance described by more than one exponential is observed with complement-binding antibodies (77). In the latter there is a slowing of erythrocyte destruction 5–20 minutes after injection

into the circulation, probably due to acquired resistance to complement activation.

The interpretation of delayed transfusion reactions can be difficult, as the occurrence of low-grade warm acquired hemolytic anemia can resemble this form of transfusion reaction (78). Careful elution of antibody, its identification, and elucidation of its relation to the transfused erythrocytes are required to establish the nature of the reaction. If the indirect antiglobulin test is negative, autoimmune hemolysis is the likely pathogenic mechanism (79).

Hemolytic reactions after transplantation

Acquired hemolytic reactions due to anti-A or anti-B can be caused by group O allografts in renal transplantation (80–83) and can be prevented by prophylactic irradiation of the kidney (84). Cases of immune hemolytic anemia have also been attributed to donor-derived red cell antibodies after allogeneic bone marrow transplantation (85,86).

Prevention of microaggregate formation

In preserved blood, microaggregates are formed during storage. Such microaggregates are identified as cellular (platelet conglomerates, leukocyte ghosts, and platelet ghosts with fibrin co-aggregates) or proteinaceous material. Blood filters with small pore sizes seem to be effective in preventing such adverse effects as febrile non-hemolytic transfusion reactions, in preventing or delaying the development of leukocyte antibodies, and in reducing the risk of respiratory distress syndrome by removing intact or disintegrating cells, debris, and microaggregates (87).

Immunologic

Sensitization to HLA antigens

Sensitization to HLA antigens (88) is undesirable in patients awaiting organ transplantation and in patients who need long-term platelet transfusion. The success of protocols based on the use of leukocyte-depleted and frozen erythrocytes may be limited, since HLA antigens may be expressed on erythrocytes. In one study the erythrocytes of 50% of blood donors contained HLA-A, HLA-B, and HLA-C antibodies (but not antibodies to class II antigens or to leukocyte-specific antigens) (89). Neither storage at 4°C for 21 days nor cryopreservation affected the expression of these antigens. The immunogenicity of HLA antigens on red cells is unknown.

Reactions due to passive transfer of allo-antibodies

Passive transfer of allo-antibodies present in donor plasma can also cause hemolytic transfusion reactions. Low-titer erythrocyte antibodies in donor blood are considered to be relatively harmless, especially when plasma-reduced or concentrated erythrocytes are transfused in a recipient whose cells carry the relevant antigen. A complication of this type provoked by high-titer anti-E antibody has been described (90). Likewise, a hemolytic transfusion reaction occurred in a Kell-negative adult when anti-Kell contained in the plasma of a unit of whole blood reacted with Kell-positive cells transfused 4 weeks before (91).

Graft-versus-host disease

Graft-versus-host disease is a serious, potentially fatal complication of allogeneic bone marrow transplantation (92–94). It is caused by engrafted allogeneic immunocompetent T lymphocytes (passenger lymphocytes), which proliferate and react against the recipient. Graft-versus-host disease has been reported after the administration of various types of blood preparations (95), whole blood used for exchange transfusion (96), packed erythrocytes, granulocytes (97–99), and platelets (94).

Graft-versus-host disease is characterized by activated T helper cells (TH) and cytotoxic T lymphocytes (TTC) (100). Skin lesions show a reduction in antigen-presenting Langerhans cells and TTH cells and an increase in TTH/T suppressor (TTS) cells (101); these changes parallel others elsewhere in the body. Following the transfusion of blood components containing lymphocytes, graft-versus-host disease may also develop in severely immunocompromised patients, for example in patients with immunodeficiency syndrome or patients undergoing massive chemotherapy. The smallest number of lymphocytes capable of inducing graft-versus-host disease is not known, but it is known that 1 unit of blood contains a sufficient number of lymphocytes to produce graft-versus-host disease in severely immunocompromised adult patients. The finding that graft-versus-host disease is encountered more often in neonates than in adults may be explained by the immaturity of the immune defence system of neonates.

The common features of graft-versus-host disease are severe itching and persistent diarrhea. Treatment with prednisolone and, if necessary, antilymphocyte antibodies, and/or ciclosporin can help. Hepatic involvement can be mild but can progress to liver failure in spite of optimal treatment (102). Oral complications may be related to graft-versus-host disease but can also result from intensive chemotherapy/irradiation or intensive antibiotic treatment (103).

To minimize the risk of graft-versus-host disease, one can inhibit the proliferative capacity of the donor's immunocompetent lymphocytes by irradiating lymphocyte-containing blood products. A dose of 1500–3000 rads is used. A newer strategy, which seems promising, uses murine monoclonal antibodies to a pan-T cell antigen (for example CD3) to remove mature T lymphocytes from bone marrow grafts, and transplant recipients have greatly benefited from prophylactic ciclosporin (104). T cell depletion does not seem to impair (and may actually enhance) functional recovery of B cells after bone marrow transplantation (105).

The post-marrow transplantation period is followed by a period of profound immunosuppression, often complicated by life-threatening infections, for example caused by CMV (106,107).

Reactions to platelets

The major risks associated with platelet transfusion are allo-immunization and infection. Platelets rarely cause graft-versus-host disease (108,109). Allo-antibodies, especially anti-HLA antibodies, appear to be the major source of complications in patients given repeated platelet transfusions. These antibodies cause febrile reactions, but they can also be responsible for partial or complete refractoriness to platelet transfusions. It has been estimated that more than 50% of recipients become alloimmunized within 4–6 weeks after repeated platelet transfusions prepared from random donors (110,111), although there is some evidence that this problem may have been overestimated (112).

Platelet concentrates contain a considerable number of leukocytes and it is not clear whether allo-antibody formation is caused by the platelets themselves or by these contaminating leukocytes (112). There is in fact evidence that leukocyte-free platelets could prevent refractoriness to platelet transfusion (113), and also that induction of anti-HLA antibodies is reduced (114). It has also been found that that the use of HLA-matched platelets almost entirely avoids allo-immunization (114). There was severe but transient thrombocytopenia after the infusion of whole blood from a donor who was subsequently found to have a high-titer platelet-specific antibody (anti-PlA1) (115); this, however, is very rare.

Post-transfusion thrombocytopenic purpura is a rare immunological complication that develops about a week after transfusion of blood containing platelets (116–118). Most patients have been women aged 40–80 with a history of transfusions or pregnancy. The incriminated antibody in the patient's sera reacts with the recipient's own platelets. The thrombocytopenia and purpura usually last for up to 3 weeks, as the antibody disappears and the platelet count progressively rises. The responsible antibody is usually PlA1, and the patient's platelets are PlA1-negative. The precise mechanism causing this platelet destruction is uncertain, but the transient presence of an autoantibody (119) or adsorption of PlPlA1 antigen on to PlPlA1-negative platelets (120) has been suggested. There seems to be a linkage to HLA-DR3 and DRw52 (121). Anti-PlPlA2 is only seldom implicated in post-transfusion thrombocytopenia (122,123). This complication can be treated with plasma exchange, high doses of glucocorticoids, or intravenous gammaglobulin (124).

Reactions to leukocytes

Multitransfused patients often develop non-hemolytic febrile transfusion reactions. They are caused by antibodies to allo-antigens on leukocytes. The minimum number of leukocytes required to stimulate antibody production is unknown, but it is believed that these reactions occur when more than 0.5×10^9 leukocytes are transfused (125). The allo-antigens responsible for the reactions usually belong either to the HLA system, or to the granulocyte-specific antigens (126).

Allo-antibodies to these antigens can give rise to neonatal neutropenia, febrile transfusion reactions, or a poor response to granulocyte transfusions (127). The febrile reactions are usually mild, but pulmonary manifestations may be more severe. Respiratory distress may develop soon after starting the transfusion or within 24 hours. The radiologically evident pulmonary infiltrates may be associated with leukocyte aggregates and leukocyte antigen-antibody complexes. Recovery is usual.

Immune reactions to leukocytes after blood transfusion in sensitized recipients can be prevented by removing leukocytes from blood and packed erythrocytes (128–131). Numerous procedures for removing leukocytes have been described (132,133), including filtration through cotton wool and other more sophisticated filtering media. A reduction in leukocyte content of at least 80% must be achieved.

Reactions to cord blood

Compared with stem cells purified from bone marrow, there is no risk to donors in giving cord blood. The risk of graft-versus-host disease in recipients is lower, and the ability to reconstitute hemopoiesis and immunity after transplant is improved (35,134).

- In a 23-year-old man with severe aplastic anemia, graft-versus-host disease, characterized by localized erythematous plaques and papules, developed 10 months after transplantation of unrelated cord blood stem cells, but required no therapy (35). Microsatellite DNA fingerprinting indicated a stable and persistent donor–recipient mixed chimerism, whilst the circulating erythrocytes remained of host origin.

It has been suggested that the increased degree of tolerance of cord blood stem cells will yield a lower graft-versus-tumor effect (35), which might be associated with an increased risk of relapse of the malignancy (134). Unlike sibling marrow transplants, in which additional infusions of donor lymphocytes may be successful in inciting a graft-versus-tumor effect and salvaging relapses, there are no additional cellular therapy options for patients receiving unrelated cord units (135). However, interleukin-2 has antitumor activity and can augment cytotoxic effects after cord blood transplantation (134,135).

Susceptibility Factors

Oncology patients treated with intensive chemotherapy are usually immunosuppressed and in one study the overall incidence of reactions to blood transfusion was 0.3% of all transfused units, which is significantly lower than expected (136). Febrile non-hemolytic reactions and allergic urticarial reactions were the most frequent, and the number of delayed hemolytic post-transfusion reactions was much lower than in non-oncology patients. This probably reflects a relative inability of oncology patients to produce allo-antibodies against blood group antigens.

Drug Administration

Drug contamination

Immunological reactions due to contaminants

Allergic reactions to potentially allergenic drugs may explain some transfusion reactions that cannot be explained by the results of routine tests. In many countries donors are asked to volunteer their history of drug intake during the previous 24 hours, so that donation can if necessary be delayed. Nevertheless, in Canadian donors who had not admitted to drug intake 6–7% of the blood samples taken were found to have detectable

concentrations of acetylsalicylic acid and paracetamol (137). Such drugs would be potentially capable of causing untoward reactions in the recipients. The presence of drugs in donor blood can also damage some blood components, especially platelets.

Infection risk

Transmission of infectious disease by blood and blood products has remained a serious issue, especially after the unfortunate occurrence in some countries of large-scale transmission of HIV infection by blood or blood products.

It is, however, important to consider two circumstances separately: on the one hand the risk of transmitting disease with whole blood or cellular blood components under conditions where virus inactivation or virus removal methods are scarcely available, and on the other hand the far lesser risk of transmitting disease with plasma or plasma-derived products prepared in those centers where effective virus inactivation procedures can be applied to the product.

Bacteria

Transmission of bacterial infection by transfusion to recipients of blood or blood components is a dreaded complication, but is rare when modern methods (that is closed systems) are used for the collection and preparation of blood components. Since the introduction of closed systems for blood collection and of stringent regulations regarding the storage of blood at 4°C, contamination of erythrocyte products has become very uncommon. However, platelets stored at room temperature are a potential source of bacterial infection, and there have been many reports of septic episodes associated with both erythrocyte and platelet concentrate transfusions (138). These reports suggest that such reactions may occur as often as 1 per 4000 platelet transfusions or even more often (139,140). In one study, bacterial isolates from contaminated platelets included *Staphylococcus epidermidis*, *Staphylococcus aureus*, and *Bacillus cereus* (141).

Bacterial infections transmitted by contaminated erythrocyte concentrates have been caused mainly by *Yersinia enterocolitica*. This enteric organism is capable of efficient proliferation and even selective growth at refrigeration temperatures. Of the 182 reports of transfusion-related fatalities which the US FDA received between 1986 and 1991, 29 (16%) were due to bacterial contamination, and 8 of these were caused by contamination with *Yersinia enterocolitica* (142).

Spirochetes

Syphilis is one of the oldest recognized infectious risks of blood transfusion, and blood donors have been routinely screened for syphilis by serological tests for more than 50 years. In recent times, transfusion-transmitted syphilis has become extraordinarily rare, with only very few cases reported. The general use of refrigerated blood reduces the risk of transmission as *Treponema pallidum* loses its viability within a few days in whole blood stored at 4°C.

Viruses

The occurrence of viral hepatitis (143) and acquired immune deficiency syndrome (AIDS) after treatment with blood or blood products (6,144) underlines the importance of being aware of the risk of transmission of infections through blood products. More recently, human T cell lymphotropic viruses HTLV-I and HTLV-II and the parvoviruses have been recognized as blood-borne viruses that may compromise the safety of blood products. Cytomegalovirus may also be infective, especially in immunocompromised recipients.

Cytomegalovirus (CMV)

Up to about 70% of donors in Western countries are cytomegalovirus antibody positive (145) and about 10% have cytomegalovirus-infected leukocytes. In developing countries the percentage may be greater than 95%. Transfusion from such donors, especially leukocyte transfusions and massive transfusions of fresh blood, can result in a mild illness, with fever, splenomegaly, moderate rises in transaminases, atypical lymphoid cells in peripheral blood, and sometimes other symptoms. The syndrome usually appears about 4 weeks after transfusion and persists for 1–6 weeks. In immunocompetent individuals, infection with cytomegalovirus is transient and without serious consequences. Immunocompromised patients are at risk of serious, even fatal infections (146). Those at highest risk are premature low birth-weight neonates and bone marrow transplant recipients. Blood and platelets that have been screened for CMV-Ab are indicated in premature neonates and in CMV-Ab-negative recipients of seronegative bone marrow transplants. The use of seronegative donors has significantly reduced the risk of transfusion-induced cytomegalovirus infection in neonates (147–149). Emerging evidence suggests that leukodepletion may be effective in preventing transmission of cytomegalovirus by transfusion (150–152). The effect of leukodepletion suggests that the infective form of cytomegalovirus is intracellular.

Hepatitis viruses

Hepatitis transmitted by blood or blood products can be caused by several viruses. Hepatitis B virus (HBV) and hepatitis C virus (HCV), together with serologically unidentified hepatitis viruses that cause non-A, non-B, non-C hepatitis are leading pathological agents. Less important are hepatitis A virus (153,154), cytomegalovirus, Epstein–Barr virus, *Herpes simplex* virus, and other viruses that may cause liver damage.

Transmission of viral hepatitis continues to be a serious problem related to the transfusion of whole blood, cellular blood components, and to a lesser degree plasma-derived products (8,155). It is difficult and probably impossible to obtain complete data on the true incidence of hepatitis transmitted by blood or blood products: the incubation time is long, mild anicteric cases are not recognized, and systematic follow-up studies of transfused patients are difficult and expensive (156). In addition, the epidemiology of viral hepatitis is different in different regions.

Hepatitis A virus (HAV)   Only a few reports on hepatitis A virus transmission have appeared (153,154). In 1992 an outbreak of icteric hepatitis A involving at least 83 patients with hemophilia A in Italy, Belgium, Ireland, and Germany was documented; all had been treated with a high purity factor VIII concentrate produced by one manufacturer (157,158); there was icterus in 93% and a diagnosis of hepatitis A was based on the presence of IgM anti-HA. The original source of contamination was not definitively established, but it is possible that the virus did not originate from the plasma donors.

Hepatitis B virus (HBV)   Since the detection of HBsAg by Blumberg and the introduction of HBsAg screening for donors of blood and plasma in all developed countries, hepatitis B virus transmission through the use of blood and blood products has been effectively prevented. Estimates of the risk of infection, based on the sensitivities of current tests for HBsAg and for anti-HBcAg, are in the order of 1 in 200 000 per unit (159).

Passive immunization of the recipient at the time of potential exposure to hepatitis B virus is available. Prophylactic or post-exposure administration of hepatitis B immunoglobulin (HBIG) is of value in the prevention of hepatitis B. Addition of anti-hepatitis-B immunoglobulin to factor concentrates appears to abolish hepatitis B virus infectivity (160,161). Hepatitis B immunization has been used effectively in controlled trials (162,163). The prophylactic effectiveness of the vaccine administered immediately after exposure to hepatitis B virus has not been established (164).

Hepatitis C virus (HCV)   Hepatitis caused by hepatitis C virus was one form of non-A, non-B hepatitis until 1989, when a test became available that identified 50–70% of acute, self-limiting cases and more than 80% of chronic cases of transfusion-related non-A, non-B hepatitis (165). In the USA 80–90% of post-transfusion hepatitis were of the non-A, non-B type (166). Post-transfusional non-A, non-B hepatitis is in general less severe than hepatitis B, and is asymptomatic and anicteric in about 60–80% of cases. However, there is evidence that non-A, non-B hepatitis tends to progress to chronic liver disease (167,168).

The test for hepatitis C was originally based on a recombinant antigen (selected from a cDNA expression library prepared from DNA) and RNA (from plasma taken from a chimpanzee infected with non-A, non-B hepatitis originating from a patient with transfusion-mediated, non-A, non-B hepatitis) (169). Although the infectious virus particle has not yet been isolated, isolation of the genome of hepatitis C virus, expression of viral proteins and synthesis of antigenic peptides of hepatitis C virus have now permitted highly sensitive tests, based on multiple antigens from the virus.

The incidence of hepatitis C among donors varies considerably (from 0.2 to 3%); among US blood donors the prevalence was 0.36% in unpaid voluntary donors, whereas it was 10% in commercial plasma donors (11). In another study, the per unit risk of hepatitis C virus infection was 0.45% before testing had been introduced, 0.19% after the introduction of so-called surrogate tests (alanine transaminase, anti-HBcAg), and only 0.03% after the additional implementation of anti-hepatitis C virus tests (170). Now that second- or third-generation tests are available, the risk of transmitting hepatitis C virus infection is probably as low as 1 in 6000 (171).

The availability of the hepatitis C antibody test has also emphasized the relation between chronic hepatitis C, liver cirrhosis, and hepatocellular carcinoma: in Japan, 58 patients with chronic hepatitis C were followed for 7 years; 10 of them developed hepatocellular carcinoma, 14 developed cirrhosis, 30 continued with chronic hepatitis, and in 4 there was improvement of their hepatitis (172).

Hepatitis delta   When they occur with any frequency, hepatitis delta infections pose a problem, since the hepatitis tends to be more severe than hepatitis B infection alone and is more likely to progress to chronic hepatitis. Hepatitis delta virus is a defective RNA virus that can replicate only in the presence of hepatitis B virus. It has a unique hybrid structure consisting of a delta inner core encapsulated by the surface antigen of hepatitis B virus. Delta superinfection can transform asymptomatic or mild chronic hepatitis B infection to severe progressive active hepatitis and cirrhosis, and contributes substantially to fulminant hepatitis B (173,174).

Parvoviruses

Parvovirus B19 is transmissible by blood and blood products. In most cases B19 infection is of little consequence to the recipient. However, maternal infection can have serious effects on the fetus, and patients with hemolytic anemia or HIV infection may suffer an aplastic crisis as a result of B19 infection. B19 is an essentially epidemic infection and is transmitted only during the preacute phase. The virus is not lipid enveloped and is therefore not inactivated by solvent detergent treatment. Furthermore, it is highly heat-resistant. The risk of infection is generally thought to be low, perhaps in the order of 1 in 10000 to 1 in 50000, although a much higher frequency has been suggested by studies based on PCR (175,176).

Retroviruses

HIV-1   In the late 1970s, the human immunodeficiency virus (HIV) was spreading silently and was still undetected. By 1981, when AIDS was first recognized, cases had already occurred in several countries, but the worldwide spread of HIV infection was only fully realized in the mid-1980s. A still pertinent review dating from that period discussed transfusion-associated AIDS in great depth and also highlighted the fact that the scope of the problem widened with the recognition of other pathogenic retroviruses, such as HIV-2, HTLV-I, and HTLV-II (144). HIV can be transmitted by blood and blood products, and in most countries donated blood and plasma have been screened for the presence of HIV-1 antibodies since 1985, and subsequently for HIV-2 antibodies as well; HIV-positive units have been discarded. The overall level of HIV prevalence in blood donors fell from 0.035% in mid-1985 to 0.012% by mid-1987, primarily as a result of donor education and self-exclusion, and by

eliminating seropositive donors from the donor pool (177). The prevalence of HIV positivity among donors now seems to be around 1–2 per 400000 in countries with blood donation systems based on non-remunerated voluntary donors.

Before the screening of blood and plasma and before virus inactivation procedures were applied to coagulation factor products (for example factor VIII and factor IX), many hemophiliacs who were treated with substitution therapy were exposed to infection with HIV. In the USA about 70% of tested persons with hemophilia A (factor VIII deficiency) and 35% with hemophilia B (factor IX deficiency) were HIV-seropositive (177).

Up to 1987, 4% of all reported patients with AIDS in 28 European countries were likely to have been infected by blood transfusion. In these countries the percentages of patients with hemophilia or other coagulation disorders that develop AIDS were similar up to 1987 (178).

Transfusion of HIV-infected blood is likely to remain a public health problem, especially in parts of Africa (Central, Eastern, and Southern), Asia, and parts of the Caribbean. Non-sterile needles, syringes, and other skin-piercing instruments also play a role in HIV transmission.

People who have been infected do not develop antibodies for some weeks or months, and HIV infection of a minute number of transfusion recipients must therefore still be expected. Several recipients are reported to have seroconverted after transfusion of blood from donors who were anti-HIV negative at the time of donation (179). This window period has been estimated to last for an average of 45 days and it is probably less than 150 days in 90% of cases (180). The HIV antibody tests in current use are more sensitive and can detect seroconversion 5–15 days earlier than the tests used in the late 1980s (181). Since the frequency of positive tests among donors continues to fall, the actual risk of HIV infection should now be significantly less than the 1990 estimate.

HIV-2   HIV-2, which is closely related to HIV-1, was first reported to be associated with AIDS in 1986 in West Africa, where it is believed to be endemic. Several cases of HIV-2 infection have been reported among Europeans and West Africans residing in Europe and in the USA. The spectrum of disease and modes of transmission of HIV-2 seem to be similar to those of HIV-1 (182). However, there have been only relatively few reports of HIV-2 transmission in blood. The anti-HIV-1 EIA tests currently used for screening blood donors are estimated to detect from 42 to 92% of HIV-2 infections (183). Anti-HIV-2 assays are available and are used routinely in blood donor screening.

HTLV-1 and HTLV-2   The human T cell lymphotropic virus type I (HTLV-I) is endemic in some areas of Japan, the Caribbean, and Africa, and has been associated with adult T cell leukemia. In Japan, seroconversion has been observed when anti-HTLV-I-negative patients were transfused with seropositive blood or blood components; in one study the conversion rate was 62% (177). However, no case of transfusion-associated adult T cell leukemia has been reported to date (184,185). HTLV-II was originally isolated from a patient with hairy cell leukemia, but the association has not been confirmed. For both HTLV-I and HTLV-II, their natural history, their prevalence rates in blood donors, and their possible clinical consequences need to be studied further (186). In the USA the current risk of post-transfusion HTLV infection appears to be approximately 1 in 70 000 per unit (187). The risk factors for HTLV-I infection in donors are largely geographic, whereas HTLV-II infection is primarily associated with drug abuse (177). Some 97% of individuals with anti-HTLV-I show virus within their lymphocytes (179), but seroconversion has not been observed after transfusion of fresh frozen plasma or plasma-derived products from seropositive donors (177,178).

West Nile virus
A Georgia woman who died after an automobile crash was given multiple blood transfusions before she died (188). Blood samples taken at arrival in the emergency department were negative for West Nile virus, while blood samples that were taken after she had received several transfusions were positive. This finding raised concerns about transmission of West Nile virus via blood. One out of five people infected with West Nile virus will develop a mild febrile illness, lasting 3–6 days; one out of 150 people will develop meningitis or encephalitis. The West Nile virus circulates in the blood of an infected person for only a few days or weeks. Therefore, the risk of transmission of West Nile virus from transfusion of blood components is low (189).

Protozoa
Chagas' disease
In endemic areas (Central and South America), infection caused by *Trypanosoma cruzi* can be transmitted by blood. The total number of infected immigrants living in the USA has been estimated at about 50 000, and these carriers pose a risk as evidenced by reported transfusion-associated cases.

Malaria
Transfusion-induced malaria may be a life-threatening complication, especially in patients who have been repeatedly transfused, treated with immunosuppressive drugs, or splenectomized (190). The disease is readily transmitted from asymptomatic donors with latent infection. Means of preventing and treating transfusion-transmitted malaria are well defined in current literature (191,192). To prevent malaria transmission, donors from malaria-endemic areas are now only accepted after spending 3 years in a malaria-free area; this interval may well be too short.

Prion diseases
Creutzfeldt–Jakob disease (CJD), Gerstmann–Sträussler–Scheinker syndrome, fatal familial insomnia, and kuru are fatal diseases of the central nervous system, known as transmissible subacute spongiform encephalopathies (193). Creutzfeldt–Jakob disease is the most common of these and has an incidence of 1:1 000 000 in most countries. About 10% of those involved have a familial disposition, but most cases occur sporadically. There are similar diseases in sheep (scrapie), cattle (bovine spongiform encephalopathy), and other animal species. The cause of the disease was first believed to be a "slow virus," but more and more evidence points to a protein (prion) as the causative agent (194). It appears that a normally occurring protein, located primarily in neuronal cells, changes its conformation and thereby becomes diseased. This diseased protein induces the same conformational change in otherwise healthy proteins. The diseased protein is highly resistant to proteases and accumulates intracellularly and extracellularly, thereby causing the disease.

A few cases of Creutzfeldt–Jakob disease have been transmitted by corneal transplantation, dural transplantation, surgical equipment, and human growth hormone extracted from human pituitary glands (195). This has of course raised concern that Creutzfeldt–Jakob disease might prove to be transmissible by blood and blood products (196). The concern has been further accentuated by recent fears of transmission bovine spongiform encephalopathy through food consumption by humans. Some manufacturers of plasma products have reacted by recalling products from the market (197).

To date studies have shown that patients who develop Creutzfeldt–Jakob disease do not have a history of a higher rate of transfusion or treatment with blood products. Likewise, those who have received blood from donors who subsequently prove to have Creutzfeldt–Jakob disease do not acquire an increased risk. Furthermore, animal experiments have shown that blood and blood products are very low risk materials in transfer experiments from diseased to healthy animals. All the same, certain authorities are now considering the exclusion of donors from families with known cases of classic Creutzfeldt–Jakob disease.

However, the emergence of variant Creutzfeldt–Jakob disease (vCJD) in the UK and France has raised concern about a new "theoretical" risk of infection in patients treated with blood and blood products (198). Animal experiments in which blood from sheep infected with bovine spongiform encephalopathy and natural scrapie-infected sheep into scrapie-free recipient animals have suggested disease transmission by the blood transfusion route in 2 of 24 sheep with bovine spongiform encephalopathy and in 4 of 21 sheep with scrapie (199). Many European countries have incorporated leukodepletion of all blood products, as leukocytes are believed to play a key role in the pathogenesis of variant Creutzfeldt–Jakob disease (198). In some countries, people who have lived in the UK for a period longer than 6 months between 1980 and 1996 are excluded from blood donation (13). Furthermore, it has been shown that various steps used in the manufacture of plasma-derived products also contribute to reduced infectivity by bovine spongiform encephalopathy (198).

Other Environmental Interactions

Interactions of transfusion with transplantation can occur (200). Blood transfusions, and especially donor-specific transfusions, given before kidney transplantation have beneficial effects on graft survival; the mechanism for this is not known (201–203). By contrast, pre-transplant transfusions in bone marrow recipients with aplastic anemia cause major complications, and can be responsible for graft rejection and marrow transplantation failure (204).

Immunosuppressed patients with, for example, hematological malignancies are less likely to become sensitized to the histocompatibility antigens to which they are exposed by transfusion; restriction of transfusion in the pre-transplant period is therefore not necessary.

References

1. Barton JC. Nonhemolytic, noninfectious transfusion reactions. Semin Hematol 1981;18(2):95–121.
2. Linden JV, Paul B, Dressler KP. A report of 104 transfusion errors in New York State. Transfusion 1992;32(7):601–6.
3. Glover JJ, Morrill GB. Conservative treatment of over-anticoagulated patients. Chest 1995;108(4):987–90.
4. Anonymous. Blood products (manufactured)-reporting adverse reactions. WHO Pharm Newslett 1998;5/6:6–7.
5. Qutaishat S. Autologous blood transfusion: evaluation of an alternative strategy in reducing exposure to allogeneic blood transfusion. Immunol Invest 1995;24(1–2):435–41.
6. Petricciani JC, Gust ID, Hoppe PA, Krijnen HW, editors. AIDS—The Safety of Blood and Blood Products. Chichester, New York, Brisbane, Toronto, Singapore: J Wiley and Sons 1987.
7. Bray GL, Gomperts ED, Courter S, Gruppo R, Gorden EM, Manco-Johnson M, Shapiro A, Scheibel E, White G, 3rd, Lee M. A multicenter study of recombinant factor VIII (Recombinate): safety, efficacy and inhibitor risk in previously untreated patients with hemophilia A. The Recombinate Study Group. Blood 1994;83(9):2428–35.
8. Aach RD, Kahn RA. Post-transfusion hepatitis: current perspectives. Ann Intern Med 1980;92(4):539–46.
9. Alter HJ. Transfusion-associated non-A, non-B hepatitis: the first decade. In: Zuckerman AJ, editor. Viral Hepatitis and Liver Disease. New York: Alan R Liss, 1988:537.
10. Holland P, Golosova T, Szmuness W, Ketiladze E, Purcell R, Budnitskaya P, Gerety R, Vorozhbieva T, Harley E, Burlev V, Alter H, Margolina A, Lubashevskaya E. Viral hepatitis markers in Soviet and American blood donors. Transfusion 1980;20(5):504–10.
11. Dawson GJ, Lesniewski RR, Stewart JL, Boardway KM, Gutierrez RA, Pendy L, Johnson RG, Alcalde X, Rote KV, Devare SG, et al. Detection of antibodies to hepatitis C virus in U.S. blood donors. J Clin Microbiol 1991;29(3):551–6.
12. Tabor E, Goldfield M, Black HC, Gerety RJ. Hepatitis B e antigen in volunteer and paid blood donors. Transfusion 1980;20(2):192–8.
13. Regan F, Taylor C. Blood transfusion medicine. BMJ 2002;325(7356):143–7.
14. NIH Consensus. Infectious disease testing for blood transfusions. J Am Blood Resources Ass 1995;4:78–87.
15. Cossart YE, Kirsch S, Ismy SL. Post-transfusion hepatitis in Australia: report of the Australian Red Cross study. Lancet 1980;2:192.
16. Vyas GN, Perkins HA. Non-B post-transfusion hepatitis associated with hepatitis B core antibodies in donor blood. N Engl J Med 1982;306(12):749–50.
17. Suomela H. Global Blood Safety Initiative. Viral inactivation of blood and blood products. Geneva: World Health Organization, 1992.
18. Gillon J, Galea G, Wolf HM, Eibl MM, Nonnast Daniel B. Virus inactivation by heat teatment of lyophilised coagulation factor concentrates. Curr Stud Hematol Blood Transf 1989;56:44–54.
19. Heimburger N, Karges HE. Strategies to produce virus-free blood derivatives. In: Morgenthaler JJ, editor. Virus Inactivation in Plasma Products. Heidelberg: Karger, 1989:23–33.
20. Horowitz MS, Rooks C, Horowitz B, Hilgartner MW. Virus safety of solvent/detergent-treated antihaemophilic factor concentrate. Lancet 1988;2(8604):186–9.
21. Prince AM, Horowitz B, Brotman B. Sterilisation of hepatitis and HTLV-III viruses by exposure to tri(n-butyl) phosphate and sodium cholate. Lancet 1986;1(8483):706–10.
22. DiLeo AJ, Allegrezza AE Jr. Validatable virus removal from protein solutions. Nature 1991;351(6325):420–1.
23. Lambrecht B, Mohr H, Knuver-Hopf J, Schmitt H. Photoinactivation of viruses in human fresh plasma by phenothiazine dyes in combination with visible light. Vox Sang 1991;60(4):207–13.
24. Ohto H, Fuji T, Wakimoto N, Anan M, Maeda H. A survey of autologous blood collection and transfusion in Japan in 1997. Transfus Sci 2000;22(1–2):13–18.
25. Dzik WH, Kirkley SA. Citrate toxicity during massive blood transfusion. Transfus Med Rev 1988;2(2):76–94.
26. Harke H, Rahman S. Haemostatic disorders in massive transfusion. Bibl Haematol 1980;(46):179–88.
27. Valeri CR, Zaroulis CG, Vecchione JJ, Valeri DA, Anastasi J, Pivacek LE, Emerson CP. Therapeutic effectiveness and safety of outdated human red blood cells rejuvenated to improve oxygen transport function, frozen for about 1.5 years at 80 °C, washed, and stored at 4 °C for 24 hours prior to rapid infusion. Transfusion 1980; 20(3):263–76.
28. Halliday JW, Powell LW. Iron overload. Semin Hematol 1982;19(1):42–53.
29. Pippard MJ, Callender ST, Finch CA. Ferrioxamine excretion in iron-loaded man. Blood 1982;60(2):288–94.
30. Graziano JH, Piomelli S, Seaman C, Wang T, Cohen AR, Kelleher JF Jr, Schwartz E. A simple technique for preparation of young red cells for transfusion from ordinary blood units. Blood 1982;59(4):865–8.
31. Parry ES, Thomas MJG, Marcus RE, et al. Characterization and transfusion of young erythrocytes. Br J Haematol 1982;50:701.
32. Hey E, Scopes JW. Thermoregulation in the newborn. In: Avery CB, editor. Neonatology, 3rd ed. Philadelphia: JP Lippincott, 1987:201.
33. Heinrichs C. Hämostasedefekte nach Transfusionen. Anaesthesiol Reanim 1982;7:245.
34. Mannucci PM, Federici AB, Sirchia G. Hemostasis testing during massive blood replacement. A study of 172 cases. Vox Sang 1982;42(3):113–23.
35. Mao P, Liao C, Zhu Z, Wang H, Wang S, Xu Y, Mo W, Ying Y, Li Q, Liu B. Umbilical cord blood transplantation from unrelated HLA-matched donor in an adult with severe aplastic anemia. Bone Marrow Transplant 2000;26(10): 1121–3.
36. Mullen CA, Nair J, Sandesh S, Chan KW. Fever and neutropenia in pediatric hematopoietic stem cell transplant patients. Bone Marrow Transplant 2000;25(1):59–65.
37. Arnold R, Pflieger H, Wiesneth M, Bhaduri S, Bultmann B, Heimpel H. In vitro and in vivo studies on filter collected granulocytes. Scand J Haematol 1981;26(1):31–6.
38. Karp DD, Ervin TJ, Tuttle S, Gorgone BC, Lavin P, Yunis EJ. Pulmonary complications during granulocyte transfusions: incidence and clinical features. Vox Sang 1982;42(2):57–61.
39. McCullough J, Clay M, Loken M, Hurd D. Effect of ABO incompatibility on the fate in vivo of [111]indium granulocytes. Transfusion 1988;28(4):358–61.
40. Ramsey G, Israel L, Lindsay GD, Mayer TK, Nusbacher J. Anti-Rho(D) in two Rh-positive patients receiving kidney grafts from an Rh-immunized donor. Transplantation 1986;41(1):67–9.
41. van Aken WG, Brand A, van der Poel CL. Leukodepletie van bloedproducten: een maatregel ten behoeve van kwaliteit en veiligheid. [Leukodepletion of blood products: a

requirement for improvement of quality and safety.] Ned Tijdschr Geneeskd 2000;144(22):1033–6.

42. Hitzler W. Der gegenwartige Stand der Blutfiltration—Grundlagen und klinische Bedeutung von Leukozytendepletions- und Mikroaggregatfiltern bei der Bluttransfusion. [The present status of blood filtration—fundamentals and the clinical significance of leukocyte depletion and microaggregate filters in blood transfusion.] Anasthesiol Intensivmed Notfallmed Schmerzther 1993;28(6):341–51.

43. Davis JM, Rowley SD, Braine HG, Piantadosi S, Santos GW. Clinical toxicity of cryopreserved bone marrow graft infusion. Blood 1990;75(3):781–6.

44. Kopko PM, Marshall CS, MacKenzie MR, Holland PV, Popovsky MA. Transfusion-related acute lung injury: report of a clinical look-back investigation. JAMA 2002;287(15):1968–71.

45. Popovsky MA, Chaplin HC Jr, Moore SB. Transfusion-related acute lung injury: a neglected, serious complication of hemotherapy. Transfusion 1992;32(6):589–92.

46. Varela M, Mas A, Nogues N, Escorsell A, Mazzara R, Lozano M. TRALI associated with HLA class II antibodies. Transfusion 2002;42(8):1102.

47. Flesch BK, Neppert J. Transfusion-related acute lung injury caused by human leucocyte antigen class II antibody. Br J Haematol 2002;116(3):673–6.

48. Anonymous. Blood product infusions. Risk of fatal acute lung injury. WHO Pharmaceuticals Newslett 2002;1:5.

49. Tomonari A, Shirafuji N, Iseki T, Ooi J, Nagayama H, Masunaga A, Tojo A, Tani K, Asano S. Acquired pulmonary alveolar proteinosis after umbilical cord blood transplantation for acute myeloid leukemia. Am J Hematol 2002;70(2):154–7.

50. Greenwalt TJ. Pathogenesis and management of hemolytic transfusion reactions. Semin Hematol 1981;18(2):84–94.

51. Seyfried H, Walewska I. Immune hemolytic transfusion reactions. World J Surg 1987;11(1):25–9.

52. Glicher RO. Immune hemolytic transfusion reactions and pseudohemolytic transfusion reactions. Plasma Ther Transfus Technol 1985;6:7.

53. Harrison CR, Hayes TC, Trow LL, Benedetto AR. Intravascular hemolytic transfusion reaction without detectable antibodies: A case report and review of literature. Vox Sang 1986;51(2):96–101.

54. Isbister JP. Blood transfusion and blood component therapy. Clin Anaesthesiol 1984;2:643.

55. Baldwin ML, Barrasso C, Gavin J. The first example of a Raddon-like antibody as a cause of a transfusion reaction. Transfusion 1981;21(1):86–9.

56. Gorman MI, Glidden HM, Behzad O. Another example of anti-Tca. Transfusion 1981;21(5):579.

57. Kurtz SR, Kuszaj T, Ouellet R, Valeri CR. Survival of homozygous Coa (Colton) red cells in a patient with anti-Coa. Vox Sang 1982;43(1):28–30.

58. Lee EL, Bennett C. Anti-Cob causing acute hemolytic transfusion reaction. Transfusion 1982;22(2):159–60.

59. Molthan L. Intravascular hemolytic transfusion reaction due to anti-Vw+Mia with fatal outcome. Vox Sang 1981;40(2):105–8.

60. Moore SB, Taswell HF, Pineda AA, Sonnenberg CL. Delayed hemolytic transfusion reactions. Evidence of the need for an improved pretransfusion compatibility test. Am J Clin Pathol 1980;74(1):94–7.

61. Patten E, Reddi CR, Riglin H, Edwards J. Delayed hemolytic transfusion reaction caused by a primary immune response. Transfusion 1982;22(3):248–50.

62. Pineda AA, Taswell HF, Brzica SM Jr. Transfusion reaction. An immunologic hazard of blood transfusion. Transfusion 1978;18(1):1–7.

63. Boyland IP, Mufti GJ, Hamblin TJ. Delayed hemolytic transfusion reaction caused by anti-Fyb in a splenectomized patient. Transfusion 1982;22(5):402.

64. Chandeysson PL, Flye MW, Simpkins SM, Holland PV. Delayed hemolytic transfusion reaction caused by anti-P1 antibody. Transfusion 1981;21(1):77–82.

65. Furlong MB Jr, Monaghan WP. Delayed hemolytic episodes due to anti-M. Transfusion 1981;21(1):45–9.

66. Molthan L, Wick RW Jr, Gross BM. Extravascular hemolytic transfusion reactions due to anti-Yk(a)+Cs(a). Rev Fr Transfus Immunohematol 1981;24(3):263–71.

67. Pohl B, Nicodemus P, Cronin-Ladd C. Delayed hemolytic transfusion reaction caused by anti-P1. Transfusion 1981;21(6):758–9.

68. Taddie SJ, Barrasso C, Ness PM. A delayed transfusion reaction caused by anti-K6. Transfusion 1982;22(1):68–9.

69. Waheed A, Kennedy MS. Delayed hemolytic transfusion reaction caused by anti-Jsb in a Js(a+b+) patient. Transfusion 1982;22(2):161–2.

70. Contreras M, Hazlehurst GR, Armitage SE. Development of "auto-anti-A1 antibodies" following alloimmunization in an A2 recipient. Br J Haematol 1983;55(4):657–63.

71. Coles SM, Klein HG, Holland PV. Alloimmunization in two multitransfused patient populations. Transfusion 1981;21(4):462–6.

72. Diamond WJ, Brown FL Jr, Bitterman P, Klein HG, Davey RJ, Winslow RM. Delayed hemolytic transfusion reaction presenting as sickle-cell crisis. Ann Intern Med 1980;93(2):231–4.

73. Beattie KM, Sigmund KE, McGraw J, Shurafa M. U-variant blood in sickle cell patients. Transfusion 1982;22(3):257.

74. Davey RJ, Simpkins SS. ^{51}Chromium survival of Yt(a+) red cells as a determinant of the in vivo significance of anti-Yta. Transfusion 1981;21(6):702–5.

75. Davey RJ, Gustafson M, Holland PV. Accelerated immune red cell destruction in the absence of serologically detectable alloantibodies. Transfusion 1980;20(3):348–53.

76. Whitsett CF, Pierce JA. Red cell destruction in the absence of detectable antibody. Transfusion 1981;21(4):474–5.

77. Mollison PL. Survival curves of incompatible red cells. An analytical review. Transfusion 1986;26(1):43–50.

78. Rosenfield RE. Two types of delayed hemolytic transfusion reactions. Transfusion 1985;25(2):182–3.

79. Salama A, Bhakdi S, Mueller-Eckhardt C. Binding of fluid phase C3b to nonsensitized bystander human red cells. A model for in vivo effects of complement activation on blood cells. Transfusion 1985;25(6):528–34.

80. Bracey AW. Anti-A of donor lymphocyte origin in three recipients of organs from the same donor. Vox Sang 1987;53(3):181–3.

81. Bracey AW, Van Buren C. Immune anti-A1 in A2 recipients of kidneys from group O donors. Transfusion 1986;26(3):282–4.

82. Herron R, Clark M, Tate D, Kruger A, Smith DS. Immune haemolysis in a renal transplant recipient due to antibodies with anti-c specificity. Vox Sang 1986;51(3):226–7.

83. Mangal AK, Growe GH, Sinclair M, Stillwell GF, Reeve CE, Naiman SC. Acquired hemolytic anemia due to "auto"-anti-A or "auto"-anti-B induced by group O homograft in renal transplant recipients. Transfusion 1984;24(3):201–5.

84. Mangal AK, Sinclair M. Development of "auto anti-A1 antibodies" following allo immunization in an A2 recipient. Br J Haematol 1984;57(4):714–16.

85. Heim MU, Schleuning M, Eckstein R, Huhn D, Siegert W, Clemm C, Ledderose G, Kolb HJ, Wilmanns W, Mempel W. Rh antibodies against the pretransplant red cells following Rh-incompatible bone marrow transplantation. Transfusion 1988;28(3):272–5.

86. Hows J, Beddow K, Gordon-Smith E, Branch DR, Spruce W, Sniecinski I, Krance RA, Petz LD. Donor-derived red blood cell antibodies and immune hemolysis after allogeneic bone marrow transplantation. Blood 1986;67(1):177–81.

87. US Department of Health and Human Services FaDA. The Code of Federal Regulations. Title 21, Part 606. Notes: Pages: 35. Chapter Num: 122. FDA, 1987.

88. Rivera R, Scornik JC. HLA antigens on red cells. Implications for achieving low HLA antigen content in blood transfusions. Transfusion 1986;26(4):375–81.

89. Gebhardt B, Barz D, Wagner D. Zur klinischen Effektivität von kryokonservierten Blutzellen. [Clinical effectiveness of cryopreserved blood cells.] Beitr Infusionsther Transfusionsmed 1994;32:431–3.

90. Ballas SK, Bosch J, Miguel O. Passive transfer of anti-E antibody. Transfusion 1981;21(5):577–8.

91. West NC, Jenkins JA, Johnston BR, Modi N. Interdonor incompatibility due to anti-Kell antibody undetectable by automated antibody screening. Vox Sang 1986;50(3):174–6.

92. Pflieger H. Graft-versus-host disease following blood transfusions. Blut 1983;46(2):61–6.

93. Slichter SJ. Transfusion and bone marrow transplantation. Transfus Med Rev 1988;2(1):1–17.

94. von Fliedner V, Higby DJ, Kim U. Graft-versus-host reaction following blood product transfusion. Am J Med 1982;72(6):951–61.

95. Schmitz N, Kayser W, Gassmann W, Huhn A, Kruger G, Sachs V, Loffler H. Two cases of graft-versus-host disease following transfusion of nonirradiated blood products. Blut 1982;44(2):83–8.

96. Lauer BA, Githens JH, Hayward AR, Conrad PD, Yanagihara RT, Tubergen DG. Probable graft-vs-graft reaction in an infant after exchange transfusion and marrow transplantation. Pediatrics 1982;70(1):43–7.

97. Denman AM. Graft versus host diseases: new versions of old problems? BMJ (Clin Res Ed) 1985;290(6469):658–60.

98. Ritchey AK, Andiman W, McIntosh S, Berman B, Luce D. Mononucleosis syndrome following granulocyte transfusion in patients with leukemia. J Pediatr 1980;97(2):267–9.

99. Weiden PL, Zuckerman N, Hansen JA, Sale GE, Remlinger K, Beck TM, Buckner CD. Fatal graft-versus-host disease in a patient with lymphoblastic leukemia following normal granulocyte transfusion. Blood 1981;57(2):328–32.

100. Schmidmeier W, Feil W, Gebhart W, Grisold W, Gschnait F, Hinterberger W, Hocker P, Jellinger K, Krepler R, Machacek E. Fatal graft-versus-host reaction following granulocyte transfusions. Blut 1982;45(2):115–19.

101. Sloane JP, Thomas JA, Imrie SF, Easton DF, Powles RL. Morphological and immunohistological changes in the skin in allogeneic bone marrow recipients. J Clin Pathol 1984;37(8):919–30.

102. McDonald GB, Shulman HM, Sullivan KM, Spencer GD. Intestinal and hepatic complications of human bone marrow transplantation. Part I. Gastroenterology 1986;90(2):460–77.

103. Carl W, Higby DJ. Oral manifestations of bone marrow transplantation. Am J Clin Oncol 1985;8(1):81–7.

104. Filipovich AH, Krawczak CL, Kersey JH, McGlave P, Ramsay NK, Goldman A, Goldstein G. Graft-versus-host disease prophylaxis with anti-T cell monoclonal antibody OKT3, prednisone and methotrexate in allogeneic bone-marrow transplantation. Br J Haematol 1985;60(1):143–52.

105. Brenner MK, Wimperis JZ, Reittie JE, Patterson J, Asherson GL, Hoffbrand AV, Prentice HG. Recovery of immunoglobulin isotypes following T cell depleted allogeneic bone marrow transplantation. Br J Haematol 1986;64(1):125–32.

106. Grob JP, Grundy JE, Prentice HG, Griffiths PD, Hoffbrand AV, Hughes MD, Tate T, Wimperis JZ, Brenner MK. Immune donors can protect marrow-transplant recipients from severe cytomegalovirus infections. Lancet 1987;1(8536):774–6.

107. Winston DJ, Huang ES, Miller MJ, Lin CH, Ho WG, Gale RP, Champlin RE. Molecular epidemiology of cytomegalovirus infections associated with bone marrow transplantation. Ann Intern Med 1985;102(1):16–20.

108. Anonymous. Platelet transfusion therapy. Lancet 1987;2(8557):490–1.

109. National Institutes of Health Consensus Conference. Platelet transfusion therapy. Transfus Med Rev 1987;1(3):195–200.

110. Kutti J, Zaroulis CG, Dinsmore RE, Reich L, Clarkson BD, Good RA. A prospective study of platelet-transfusion therapy administered to patients with acute leukemia. Transfusion 1982;22(1):44–7.

111. Seidl S, Kilp M. The current status of platelet and granulocyte transfusions. Haematologia (Budap) 1980;13(1–4):145–54.

112. Eernisse JG, Brand A. Prevention of platelet refractoriness due to HLA antibodies by administration of leukocyte-poor blood components. Exp Hematol 1981;9(1):77–83.

113. Sirchia G, Parravicini A, Rebulla P, Bertolini F, Morelati F, Marconi M. Preparation of leukocyte-free platelets for transfusion by filtration through cotton wool. Vox Sang 1983;44(2):115–20.

114. Murphy MF, Waters AH. Immunological aspects of platelet transfusions. Br J Haematol 1985;60(3):409–14.

115. Scott EP, Moilan-Bergeland J, Dalmasso AP. Posttransfusion thrombocytopenia associated with passive transfusion of a platelet-specific antibody. Transfusion 1988;28(1):73–6.

116. Mueller-Eckhardt C. Post-transfusion purpura. Br J Haematol 1986;64(3):419–24.

117. Mueller-Eckhardt C, Lechner K, Heinrich D, Marks HJ, Mueller-Eckhardt G, Bettelheim P, Breithaupt H. Post-transfusion thrombocytopenic purpura: immunological and clinical studies in two cases and review of the literature. Blut 1980;40(4):249–57.

118. Vogelsang G, Kickler TS, Bell WR. Post-transfusion purpura: a report of five patients and a review of the pathogenesis and management. Am J Hematol 1986;21(3):259–67.

119. Stricker RB, Lewis BH, Corash L, Shuman MA. Posttransfusion purpura associated with an autoantibody directed against a previously undefined platelet antigen. Blood 1987;69(5):1458–63.

120. Kickler TS, Ness PM, Herman JH, Bell WR. Studies on the pathophysiology of posttransfusion purpura. Blood 1986;68(2):347–50.

121. de Waal LP, van Dalen CM, Engelfriet CP, von dem Borne AE. Alloimmunization against the platelet-specific Zwa antigen, resulting in neonatal alloimmune thrombocytopenia or posttransfusion purpura, is associated with the supertypic DRw52 antigen including DR3 and DRw6. Hum Immunol 1986;17(1):45–53.

122. Chapman JF, Murphy MF, Berney SI, Ord J, Metcalfe P, Amess JA, Waters AH. Post-transfusion purpura associated with anti-Baka and anti-PIA2 platelet antibodies and delayed haemolytic transfusion reaction. Vox Sang 1987;52(4):313–17.

123. Ovesen H, Taaning E, Christensen BA. [Posttransfusion purpura caused by ant-Zw b (P1(A2)).] Ugeskr Laeger 1986;148(43):2769–70.

124. Slichter SJ. Post-transfusion purpura: response to steroids and association with red blood cell and lymphocytotoxic antibodies. Br J Haematol 1982;50(4):599–605.

125. Koerner K, Kubanek B. Comparison of three different methods used in the preparation of leukocyte-poor platelet concentrates. Vox Sang 1987;53(1):26–30.

126. McCullough J, Clay M, Kline W. Granulocyte antigens and antibodies. Transfus Med Rev 1987;1(3):150–60.

127. McCullogh J. The clinical significance of granulocyte antibodies and in vivo studies of the fate of granulocytes. In: Garratty G, editor. Current Concepts in Transfusion Therapy. Arlington, VA: American Association of Blood Banks, 1985:125.

128. Hughes AS, Brozovic B. Leucocyte depleted blood: an appraisal of available techniques. Br J Haematol 1982;50(3):381–6.

129. Lieden G, Hilden JO. Febrile transfusion reactions reduced by use of buffy-coat-poor erythrocyte concentrates. Vox Sang 1982;43(5):263–5.

130. Menitove JE, McElligott MC, Aster RH. Febrile transfusion reaction: what blood component should be given next? Vox Sang 1982;42(6):318–21.

131. Ness PM, Frey E, Perkins HA. Improved blood utilization with leukocyte-poor cell masses (LPCM) prepared by cell washing. Transfusion 1981;21(1):124–6.

132. Goldfinger D, Lowe C. Prevention of adverse reactions to blood transfusion by the administration of saline-washed red blood cells. Transfusion 1981;21(3):277–80.

133. Sirchia G, Parravicini A, Rebulla P, Greppi N, Scalamogna M, Morelati F. Effectiveness of red blood cells filtered through cotton wool to prevent antileukocyte antibody production in multitransfused patients. Vox Sang 1982;42(4):190–7.

134. Laws HJ, Nurnberger W, Korholz D, Kogler G, Fischer J, Niehues T, Wernet P, Gobel U. Successful treatment of relapsed CML after cord blood transplantation with donor leukocyte infusion IL-2 and IFNalpha. Bone Marrow Transplant 2000;25(2):219–22.

135. Goldberg SL, Pecora AL, Rosenbluth RJ, Jennis AA, Preti RA. Treatment of leukemic relapse following unrelated umbilical cord blood transplantation with interleukin-2: potential for augmenting graft-versus-leukemia and graft-versus-host effects with cytokines. Bone Marrow Transplant 2000;26(3):353–5.

136. Huh YO, Lichtiger B. Transfusion reactions in patients with cancer. Am J Clin Pathol 1987;87(2):253–7.

137. MacIntyre A, Gray JD, Gorelick M, Renton K. Salicylate and acetaminophen in donated blood. CMAJ 1986;135(3):215–16.

138. Blajchman MA, Ali AM. In: Nance SJ, editor. Blood Safety: Current Challenges. Bethesda, MD: AABB, 1992:213–28.

139. Blajchman MA. Bacterial contamination of blood products and the value of pre-transfusion testing. Immunol Invest 1995;24(1–2):163–70.

140. Morrow JF, Braine HG, Kickler TS, Ness PM, Dick JD, Fuller AK. Septic reactions to platelet transfusions. A persistent problem. JAMA 1991;266(4):555–8.

141. Hogman CF, Fritz H, Sandberg L. Posttransfusion Serratia marcescens septicemia. Transfusion 1993;33(3):189–91.

142. Hoppe PA. Interim measures for detection of bacterially contaminated red cell components. Transfusion 1992;32(3):199–201.

143. Conrad ME. Diseases transmissible by blood transfusion: viral hepatitis and other infectious disorders. Semin Hematol 1981;18(2):122–46.

144. Berkman SA, Groopman JE. Transfusion associated AIDS. Transfus Med Rev 1988;2(1):18–28.

145. Silvergleid AJ, Kott TJ. Impact of cytomegalovirus testing on blood collection facilities. Vox Sang 1983;44(2):102–5.

146. Barbara JA, Tegtmeier GE. Cytomegalovirus and blood transfusion. Blood Rev 1987;1(3):207–11.

147. Kumar A, Nankervis GA, Cooper AR, Gold E, Kumar ML. Acquisition of cytomegalovirus infection in infants following exchange transfusion: a prospective study. Transfusion 1980;20(3):327–31.

148. Tegtmeier GE. The use of cytomegalovirus-screened blood in neonates. Transfusion 1988;28(3):201–3.

149. Yeager AS, Grumet FC, Hafleigh EB, Arvin AM, Bradley JS, Prober CG. Prevention of transfusion-acquired cytomegalovirus infections in newborn infants. J Pediatr 1981;98(2):281–7.

150. Bowden RA, Slichter SJ, Sayers MH, Mori M, Cays MJ, Meyers JD. Use of leukocyte-depleted platelets and cytomegalovirus-seronegative red blood cells for prevention of primary cytomegalovirus infection after marrow transplant. Blood 1991;78(1):246–50.

151. Eisenfeld L, Silver H, McLaughlin J, Klevjer-Anderson P, Mayo D, Anderson J, Herson V, Krause P, Savidakis J, Lazar A, et al. Prevention of transfusion-associated cytomegalovirus infection in neonatal patients by the removal of white cells from blood. Transfusion 1992;32(3):205–9.

152. Smith KL, Cobain T, Dunstan RA. Removal of cytomegalovirus DNA from donor blood by filtration. Br J Haematol 1993;83(4):640–2.

153. Barbara JA, Howell DR, Briggs M, Parry JV. Posttransfusion hepatitis A. Lancet 1982;1(8274):738.

154. Seeberg S, Brandberg A, Hermodsson S, Larsson P, Lundgren S. Hospital outbreak of hepatitis A secondary to blood exchange in a baby. Lancet 1981;1(8230):1155–6.

155. Blum HE, Vyas GN. Non-A, non-B hepatitis: a contemporary assessment. Haematologia (Budap) 1982;15(2):153–73.

156. Wenk RE, Brewer MK, Bass G, Bishop K. Surveillance for posttransfusion hepatitis by a community hospital. Another view. Transfusion 1981;21(5):557–9.

157. Mannucci PM. Outbreak of hepatitis A among Italian patients with haemophilia. Lancet 1992;339(8796):819.

158. Robinson SM, Schwinn H, Smith A. Clotting factors and hepatitis A. Lancet 1992;340(8833):1465.

159. Dodd RY. The risk of transfusion-transmitted infection. N Engl J Med 1992;327(6):419–21.

160. Brummelhuis HG, Over J, Duivis-Vorst CC, Wilson-de Sturler LA, Ates G, Hoek PJ, Reerink-Brongers EE. Contributions to the optimal use of human blood. IX. Elimination of hepatitis B transmission by (potentially) infectious plasma derivatives. Vox Sang 1983;45(3):205–16.

161. Tabor E, Aronson DL, Gerety RJ. Removal of hepatitis-B-virus infectivity from factor-IX complex by hepatitis-B immune-globulin. Experiments in chimpanzees. Lancet 1980;2(8185):68–70.

162. Alter HJ. The evolution, implications, and applications of the hepatitis B vaccine. JAMA 1982;247(16):2272–5.

163. Szmuness W, Stevens CE, Harley EJ, Zang EA, Oleszko WR, William DC, Sadovsky R, Morrison JM, Kellner A. Hepatitis B vaccine: demonstration of efficacy in a controlled clinical trial in a high-risk population in the United States. N Engl J Med 1980;303(15):833–41.

164. Szmuness W, Stevens CE, Oleszko WR, Goodman A. Passive-active immunisation against hepatitis B: immunogenicity studies in adult Americans. Lancet 1981;1(8220 Pt 1):575–7.

165. Alter HJ, Purcell RH, Shih JW, Melpolder JC, Houghton M, Choo QL, Kuo G. Detection of antibody to hepatitis C virus in prospectively followed transfusion recipients with acute and chronic non-A, non-B hepatitis. N Engl J Med 1989;321(22):1494–500.

166. Tremolada F, Chiappetta F, Noventa F, Valfre C, Ongaro G, Realdi G. Prospective study of posttransfusion hepatitis in cardiac surgery patients receiving only blood or also blood products. Vox Sang 1983;44(1):25–30.

167. Kiyosawa K, Akahane Y, Nagata A, Koike Y, Furuta S. The significance of blood transfusion in non-A, non-B chronic liver disease in Japan. Vox Sang 1982;43(1):45–52.

168. Realdi G, Alberti A, Rugge M, Rigoli AM, Tremolada F, Schivazappa L, Ruol A. Long-term

follow-up of acute and chronic non-A, non-B post-transfusion hepatitis: evidence of progression to liver cirrhosis. Gut 1982;23(4):270–5.

169. Choo QL, Kuo G, Weiner AJ, Overby LR, Bradley DW, Houghton M. Isolation of a cDNA clone derived from a blood-borne non-A, non-B viral hepatitis genome. Science 1989;244(4902):359–62.

170. Donahue JG, Munoz A, Ness PM, Brown DE Jr, Yawn DH, McAllister HA Jr, Reitz BA, Nelson KE. The declining risk of post-transfusion hepatitis C virus infection. N Engl J Med 1992;327(6):369–73.

171. Kleinman S, Alter H, Busch M, Holland P, Tegtmeier G, Nelles M, Lee S, Page E, Wilber J, Polito A. Increased detection of hepatitis C virus (HCV)-infected blood donors by a multiple-antigen HCV enzyme immunoassay. Transfusion 1992;32(9):805–13.

172. Kiyosawa K, Tanaka E, Sodeyama T, Furuta K, Usuda S, Yousuf M, Furuta S. Transition of antibody to hepatitis C virus from chronic hepatitis to hepatocellular carcinoma. Jpn J Cancer Res 1990;81(11):1089–91.

173. Hatzakis A, Hadziyannis S, Maclure M, Yannitsiotis A, Maudalaki T. Infection with hepatitis delta virus. N Engl J Med 1986;314(8):516–17.

174. Nishioka NS, Dienstag JL. Delta hepatitis: a new scourge? N Engl J Med 1985;312(23):1515–16.

175. Cohen BJ, Field AM, Gudnadottir S, Beard S, Barbara JA. Blood donor screening for parvovirus B19. J Virol Methods 1990;30(3):233–8.

176. McOmish F, Yap PL, Jordan A, Hart H, Cohen BJ, Simmonds P. Detection of parvovirus B19 in donated blood: a model system for screening by polymerase chain reaction. J Clin Microbiol 1993;31(2):323–8.

177. Sullivan MT, Williams AE, Fang CT, Notari EP, Poiesz BJ, Ehrlich GD. Human T-lymphotropic virus (HTLV) types I and II infection in sexual contacts and family members of blood donors who are seropositive for HTLV type I or II. American Red Cross HTLV-I/II Collaborative Study Group. Transfusion 1993;33(7):585–90.

178. Bove JR, Sandler SG. HTLV-1 and blood transfusion. Transfusion 1988;28(2):93–4.

179. Morishima Y, Ohya K, Ueda R, Fukuda T. Detection of adult T cell leukemia virus (ATLV) bearing lymphocytes in concentrated red blood cells derived from ATL associated antibody (ATLA-Ab) positive donors. Vox Sang 1986;50(4):212–15.

180. Petersen LR, Satten GA, Dodd R, Busch M, Kleinman S, Grindon A, Lenes B. Duration of time from onset of human immunodeficiency virus type 1 infectiousness to development of detectable antibody. The HIV Seroconversion Study Group. Transfusion 1994;34(4):283–9.

181. Busch MP. Retroviruses and blood transfusion: The lessons learned and the challenge yet ahead. In: Nance ST, editor. Blood Safety: Current Challenges. Bethesda: American Association of Blood Banks, 1992:1–44.

182. Broder S. Pathogenic human retroviruses. N Engl J Med 1988;318(4):243–5.

183. Centers for Disease Control (CDC). AIDS due to HIV-2 infection—New Jersey. MMWR Morb Mortal Wkly Rep 1988;37(3):33–5.

184. Editorial. HTLV-1 comes of age. Lancet 1988;1(8579):217–19.

185. Minamoto GY, Gold JW, Scheinberg DA, Hardy WD, Chein N, Zuckerman E, Reich L, Dietz K, Gee T, Hoffer J, et al. Infection with human T cell leukemia virus type I in patients with leukemia. N Engl J Med 1988;318(3):219–22.

186. Sandler SG. HTLV-I and -II. New risks for recipients of blood transfusions? JAMA 1986;256(16):2245–6.

187. Nelson KE, Donahue JG, Munoz A, Cohen ND, Ness PM, Teague A, Stambolis VA, Yawn DH, Callicott B, McAllister H, et al. Transmission of retroviruses from seronegative donors by transfusion during cardiac surgery. A multicenter study of HIV-1 and HTLV-I/II infections. Ann Intern Med 1992;117(7):554–9.

188. Stephenson J. Investigation probes risk of contracting West Nile virus via blood transfusions. JAMA 2002;288(13):1573–4.

189. Biggerstaff BJ, Petersen LR. Estimated risk of West Nile virus transmission through blood transfusion during an epidemic in Queens, New York City. Transfusion 2002;42(8):1019–26.

190. De Virgiliis S, Galanello R, Cao A. *Plasmodium malariae* transfusion malaria in splenectomized patients with thalassemia major. J Pediatr 1981;98(4):584–5.

191. Cook GC. Prevention and treatment of malaria. Lancet 1988;1(8575–6):32–7.

192. Gilcher RO, Belcher L. Posttransfusion malaria—a new look. Transfusion 1981;21:611.

193. Brown P. Transmissible human spongiform encephalopathy (infectious cerebral amyloidosis): Creutzfeldt–Jakob disease, Gerstman–Sträussler–Scheinker syndrome and Kuru. Calne DB, editor. Neurodegenerative Diseases. Philadelphia: W.B. Saunders, 1994:839–76.

194. Prusiner SB. The prion diseases. Sci Am 1995;272(1):48–51, 54–7.

195. deSilva R, Esmonde T. Transmission of Creutzfeldt–Jakob Disease. CNS Drugs 1994;2:96–101.

196. Budka H, Aguzzi A, Brown P, Brucher JM, Bugiani O, Collinge J, Diringer H, Gullotta F, Haltia M, Hauw JJ. Tissue handling in suspected Creutzfeldt–Jakob disease (CJD) and other human spongiform encephalopathies (prion diseases). Brain Pathol 1995;5(3):319–22.

197. CPMP report. Risk of transmission of Creutzfeldt–Jakob disease via medicinal products derived from human blood or plasma. CPMP report 1995;846/95.

198. Cervenakova L, Brown P, Hammond DJ, Lee CA, Saenko EL. Factor VIII and transmissible spongiform encephalopathy: the case for safety. Haemophilia 2002;8(2):63–75.

199. Hunter N, Foster J, Chong A, McCutcheon S, Parnham D, Eaton S, MacKenzie C, Houston F. Transmission of prion diseases by blood transfusion. J Gen Virol 2002;83(Pt 11):2897–905.

200. Storb R, Weiden PL. Transfusion problems associated with transplantation. Semin Hematol 1981;18(2):163–76.

201. Light JA, Metz S, Oddenino K, Strong DM, Simonis T, Biggers JA, Fernandez-Bueno C. Donor-specific transfusion with diminished sensitization. Transplantation 1982;34(6):352–5.

202. Singal DP, Ludwin D, Blajchman MA. Blood transfusion and renal transplantation. Br J Haematol 1985;61(4):595–602.

203. Whelchel JD, Shaw JF, Curtis JJ, Luke RG, Diethelm AG. Effect of pretransplant stored donor-specific blood transfusions on early renal allograft survival in one-haplotype living related transplants. Transplantation 1982;34(6):326–9.

204. Kaminski ER, Hows JM, Goldman JM, Batchelor JR. Pretransfused patients with severe aplastic anaemia exhibit high numbers of cytotoxic T lymphocyte precursors probably directed at non-HLA antigens. Br J Haematol 1990;76(3):401–5.

Blood donation

General Information

Among the various adverse effects of blood donation, vasovagal syncope and convulsive reactions are of concern to collection centers, as they may alarm potential first-time donors. First-time donors have a higher frequency of these reactions (1.7%) than repeat donors (0.2%), and donors who have such reactions donate fewer times than those without reactions (1). Donors who react are generally of lower weight and have slightly lower blood pressure than those who do not. Of the relevant social and psychological factors that have been studied, the ingestion of caffeinated beverages and shortening the duration between registration and time of phlebotomy are associated with a reduced risk of reactions (1).

Apheresis procedures are considered to be relatively safe when performed by experienced personnel. However, they are not without dangers, and there are some health risks to both patients and donors. Not unexpectedly, the risks are greater with therapeutic plasmapheresis on account of the underlying disease, with an estimated 3 deaths per 10 000 procedures (2).

Organs and Systems

Cardiovascular

Bruising in the antecubital fossa is one of the commonest adverse effects of blood donation. The common practice of flexing the arm over a cotton wool ball or swab can aggravate bleeding, and direct compression over the puncture site and elevation of the extended arm is recommended (3).

Hematologic

The only significant drawback to repeated whole blood donation is the risk of iron deficiency. In a study in 948 menstruating and 141 non-menstruating female blood donors, menstruating donors had lower mean serum ferritin concentrations than non-menstruating donors. First-time donors had a mean ferritin concentration of 24 μg/ml and regular donors 19 μg/ml. The frequency of donations was more predictive of ferritin concentrations than the number of donations (4). The authors concluded that female donors, especially those who donate three or more times a year, should have their iron status checked at appropriate intervals and should receive iron supplements.

Immunologic

Although no important adverse effects are associated specifically with multiple blood donations, depressed cell-mediated immunity and reduced lymphocyte proliferation responses have been reported in the past (5). This fear has been allayed, for example, by a 1992 study in 27 donors who had regularly given whole blood for at least 4 years; there were no abnormalities in lymphocyte subsets, neutrophil and monocyte receptors, or molecules important for host defences (6). In 25 volunteer donors undergoing regular platelet apheresis by a discontinuous process a large number of T4 and T8 lymphocytes, a moderate number of B lymphocytes, and a smaller number of monocytes were removed (7).

Frequent donations involving apheresis procedures have been reported to cause allergic reactions (urticaria, flushing, wheezing, chest pain, and in a few cases hypotension), probably due to exposure to ethylene oxide (8). Ethylene oxide is often used for sterilizing the polyvinyl chloride tubing, and similar allergic reactions in patients undergoing chronic hemodialysis have been attributed to sensitization to the ethylene oxide used for sterilizing the dialyser. One study has shown significant concentrations of IgE antibodies to ethylene dioxide in the sera of 78% of donors with allergic reactions but in only 12% of control sera.

Susceptibility Factors

Age

It has commonly been thought that donation of blood by older people might involve health risks for themselves, and in many countries healthy potential blood donors are therefore ineligible after the age of 60. However, in a study of the growing demographic group above this age, the adverse effects were no greater than in a control group of donors aged 50–65 years when the standard volume of blood (450 ml) was taken (9).

References

1. Kasprisin DO, Glynn SH, Taylor F, Miller KA. Moderate and severe reactions in blood donors. Transfusion 1992;32(1):23–6.
2. Boogaerts MA. Side effects of hemapheresis. Transfus Med Rev 1987;1(3):186–94.
3. Blackmore M. Minimising bruising in the antecubital fossa after venepuncture. BMJ (Clin Res Ed) 1987;295:332.
4. Milman N, Sondergaard M, Sorensen CM. Iron stores in female blood donors evaluated by serum ferritin. Blut 1985;51(5):337–45.
5. Strauss RG. Apheresis donor safety—changes in humoral and cellular immunity. J Clin Apher 1984;2(1):68–80.
6. Lewis SL, Kutvirt SG, Simon TL. Investigation of the effect of long-term whole blood donation on immunologic parameters. Transfusion 1992;32(1):51–6.
7. Matsui Y, Martin-Alosco S, Doenges E, Christenson L, Shapiro HM, Yunis EJ, Page PL. Effects of frequent and sustained plateletapheresis on peripheral blood mononuclear cell populations and lymphocyte functions of normal volunteer donors. Transfusion 1986;26(5):446–52.
8. Dolovich J, Sagona M, Pearson F, Buccholz D, Hiner E, Marshall C. Sensitization of repeat plasmapheresis donors to ethylene oxide gas. Transfusion 1987;27(1):90–3.
9. Pindyck J, Avorn J, Kuriyan M, Reed M, Iqbal MJ, Levine SJ. Blood donation by the elderly. Clinical and policy considerations. JAMA 1987;257(9):1186–8.

Blood glucose meters

General Information

There are various makes of meters used for measuring the blood glucose concentration. On occasion, some have been found to give false readings.

In early June 1998, the manufacturers of SureStep blood glucose meters (LifeScan) announced that they were going to replace some of the meters used by diabetics to test their blood sugar concentration because they were giving confusing error readings. SureStep home blood glucose meters manufactured before August 1997 may have been giving an error message ("Er-1") instead of "HI" (high) when a blood sugar concentration was very high—500 mg/dl (28 mmol/l) or greater. Such a concentration is potentially dangerous if not recognized and treated, and could result in hospitalization or death. The FDA had received reports of two deaths in people whose glucose was very high but who repeatedly got error message readings from the SureStep blood glucose meters and delayed seeking medical care. The FDA was concerned that some diabetics, wholesalers, and distributors who purchase these meters might not realize that this product replacement procedure concerns a potentially serious malfunction (1). The FDA classified LifeScan's recall as a Class I recall, that is a situation in which there is a reasonable probability that the use of the product will cause serious adverse health consequences or death.

People using the affected SureStep meters needed to know that an "Er-1" message might actually mean a very high concentration of blood glucose instead of an error. If users got an "Er-1" message, they needed to use the visual color change indicator to see if their blood glucose was too high. They had to compare the blue dot on the test strip to the color chart on the test strip bottle. If the dot on the strip was as dark as or darker than the color chart, it indicated a very high blood glucose, and they were advised to contact a health professional immediately.

People with diabetes who use the SureStep brand glucose meters were advised not to stop testing their blood glucose concentrations. They could continue to test with these meters as long as they knew that an "Er-1" message could actually mean a very high concentration. It was considered far more dangerous not to check blood glucose than to use a blood glucose meter that might give an unclear error message at high glucose concentrations.

Factors that alter measurements

High altitude

Sports like hiking and skiing at moderate high altitude make glucose estimation mandatory for people with diabetes. Changes in temperature, PaO_2, and humidity can result in errors in blood glucose determination. When tested at 3000 m (10 000 feet) the glucose meter Elite (Bayer Diagnostics) had a tendency to overestimate glucose concentrations, while the Life Scan One Touch II had a tendency to underestimate them (2). The bias was not clinically meaningful, although some

care may be necessary when low or intermediate blood glucose concentrations are measured with the Glucometer Elite.

Icodextrin

Icodextrin in the dialysis fluid in continuous ambulatory peritoneal dialysis can contribute to overestimation of blood glucose (SEDA-26, 461). In a comparison of a meter using the glucose oxidation method and a meter using the glucose dehydrogenase method, only the former gave results that were comparable with the laboratory method (3). The authors concluded that meters must be cross-checked with the laboratory before they can be used to measure blood glucose in patients in contact with icodextrin.

Site of blood withdrawal

The site of blood withdrawal can give different values during acute monitoring of glucose (SEDA-26, 461). Blood was tested before and 60, 90, 120, 150, and 180 minutes after a meal from the finger tips, the arms, and the thighs with the One-Touch Ultra Blood Glucose Monitoring System (LifeScan) and an extra finger prick using a blood monitoring system. When the blood glucose concentration was rising, only the finger prick gave accurate results; the readings from the other sites were lower (even after extensive rubbing) (4).

In patients with diabetes given a 75 g oral glucose load followed by a rapid-acting insulin, producing a wide range of blood glucose concentrations, of three different devices for blood glucose estimation, only finger-prick estimations followed the changes in blood glucose (5), although patients preferred other sites for testing (6).

A subcutaneous continuous glucose monitoring system was used for 24 hours in seven strictly regulated adolescents and young adults. For comparison, blood was drawn from an intravenous cannula and determined in the laboratory, and capillary samples were measured on a glucose meter. During the night-time the readings on the continuous glucose monitoring system were on average 38% lower than the other measurements, indicating a high number of false (asymptomatic) attacks of hypoglycemia (7).

Organs and Systems

Immunologic

Finger sepsis aggressive enough to cause osteomyelitis has been reported in two women, one aged 61 years with *Staphylococcus aureus*, *Staphylococcus agalactiae*, and *Enterococcus faecalis*, and another aged 57 years with a beta-hemolytic staphylococcus, *Candida non-albicans*, and unidentified anaerobic bacteria. Antibiotic treatment and local drainage were unsuccessful and the third phalanx had to be amputated. Both patients had poorly controlled diabetes (HbA_{1c} 14% and 12% respectively); they had estimated their blood glucose six times a week using an automatic lancet without changing their disposable needle (8).

References

1. Anonymous. Blood glucose meters-recalled because of error reading. WHO Newsletter 1998;9/10:16.
2. Pecchio O, Maule S, Migliardi M, Trento M, Veglio M. Effects of exposure at an altitude of 3000 m on performance of glucose meters. Diabetes Care 2000;23(1):129–31.
3. Oyibo SO, Pritchard GM, McLay L, James E, Laing I, Gokal R, Boulton AJ. Blood glucose overestimation in diabetic patients on continuous ambulatory peritoneal dialysis for end-stage renal disease. Diabet Med 2002;19(8):693–6.
4. Ellison JM, Stegmann JM, Colner SL, Michael RH, Sharma MK, Ervin KR, Horwitz DL. Rapid changes in postprandial blood glucose produce concentration differences at finger, forearm, and thigh sampling sites. Diabetes Care 2002;25(6):961–4.
5. Jungheim K, Koschinsky T. Glucose monitoring at the arm: risky delays of hypoglycemia and hyperglycemia detection. Diabetes Care 2002;25(6):956–60.
6. Tieszen KL, New JP. Alternate site blood glucose testing: do patients prefer it? Diabet Med 2003;20(4):325–8.
7. McGowan K, Thomas W, Moran A. Spurious reporting of nocturnal hypoglycemia by CGMS in patients with tightly controlled type 1 diabetes. Diabetes Care 2002;25(9):1499–503.
8. Monami M, Mannucci E, Masotti G. Finger sepsis in two poorly controlled diabetic patients with reuse of lancets. Diabetes Care 2002;25(6):1103.

Boraginaceae

See also Herbal medicines

General Information

The genera in the family of Boraginaceae (Table 1) include bluebells, borage, comfrey, and forget-me-nots.

Cynoglossum officinale

Cynoglossum officinale (hound's tongue) contains alkaloids with curare-like activity as well as hepatotoxic and carcinogenic pyrrolizidine alkaloids, which are covered in a separate monograph.

Symphytum officinale

Symphytum officinale (black wort, boneset, bruise wort, comfrey, knitback, knitbone, slippery root) contains pyrrolizidine alkaloids, such as lasiocarpine and symphytine, and their N-oxides, and has repeatedly been associated with hepatotoxicity.

Comfrey products have been withdrawn from the market in several countries, including the USA and the UK. The German Federal Health Office has restricted the availability of botanical medicines containing unsaturated pyrrolizidine alkaloids (1,2). Herbal medicines that provide more than 1 mg internally or more than 100 mg externally per day, when used as directed, are not permitted; herbal medicines that provide 0.1–1 mg internally or 10–100 mg externally per day, when used as directed, may be applied only for a maximum of 6 weeks per year, and they should not be used during pregnancy or lactation.

Adverse effects

Symphytum officinale contains pyrrolizidine alkaloids, which are the subject of a separate monograph. Certain representatives of this class and the plants in which they occur are hepatotoxic, as well as mutagenic and carcinogenic. They can produce veno-occlusive disease of the liver with clinical features like abdominal pain with ascites, hepatomegaly, splenomegaly, anorexia, nausea, vomiting, and diarrhea. Sometimes there is also damage to the lungs.

Liver

The main type of liver damage caused by *S. officinale* is veno-occlusive disease, a non-thrombotic obliteration of small hepatic veins leading to cirrhosis and eventually liver failure (3). Patients can present with acute or chronic signs; portal hypertension, hepatomegaly, and abdominal pain are the main features.

Table 1 The genera of Boraginaceae

Alkanna (alkanna)
Amsinckia (fiddleneck)
Anchusa (bugloss)
Antiphytum (saucerflower)
Argusia (sea rosemary)
Asperugo (German-madwort)
Borago (borage)
Bothriospermum (bothriospermum)
Bourreria (strongbark)
Brunnera (brunnera)
Buglossoides (buglossoides)
Carmona (scorpionbush)
Cordia (cordia)
Cryptantha (cryptantha)
Cynoglossum (hound's tongue)
Dasynotus (whitethroat)
Echium (vipersbugloss)
Ehretia (ehretia)
Eritrichium (alpine forget-me-not)
Hackelia (stickseed)
Harpagonella (grapplinghook)
Heliotropium (heliotrope)
Lappula (stickseed)
Lithospermum (stoneseed)
Macromeria (giant-trumpets)
Mertensia (bluebells)
Myosotis (forget-me-not)
Myosotidium (giant forget-me-not)
Nonea (monkswort)
Omphalodes (navelwort)
Onosmodium (marbleseed)
Onosma (onosma)
Pectocarya (combseed)
Pentaglottis (pentaglottis)
Plagiobothrys (popcorn flower)
Pulmonaria (lungwort)
Rochefortia (rochefortia)
Symphytum (comfrey)
Tiquilia (crinklemat)
Tournefortia (soldierbush)

- A 23-year-old man who had taken comfrey leaves presented with hepatic veno-occlusive disease and severe portal hypertension and subsequently died from liver failure (4). Light microscopy and hepatic angiography showed occlusion of sublobular veins and small venous radicles of the liver, associated with widespread hemorrhagic necrosis of hepatocytes.

Other reports of hepatotoxicity due to *S. officinale* have appeared (5–7).

However, the author of a review of the toxicity of *S. officinale* pointed out that since 1990 no cases of adverse events have been reported and stated that comfrey has a history of effective therapeutic use in humans and that it "might not be as dangerous to humans as current restrictions indicate" (8).

Fetotoxicity

It is prudent to avoid exposing unborn or suckling children to herbal remedies containing pyrrolizidine alkaloids. Animal studies have shown that transplacental passage and transfer to breast milk are possible, and there is a human case on record of fatal neonatal liver injury, in which the mother had used a herbal cough tea containing pyrrolizidine alkaloids throughout her pregnancy.

Heliotropium species

Heliotropium species contain various pyrrolizidine alkaloids (which are covered in a separate monograph).

Adverse effects

It is prudent to avoid exposure of unborn or suckling children to herbal remedies containing pyrrolizidine alkaloids. Animal studies have shown that transplacental passage and transfer to breast milk can occur, and fatal neonatal liver damage has been reported, when the mother used an herbal cough tea containing pyrrolizidine alkaloids throughout her pregnancy.

The German Federal Health Office has restricted the availability of botanical medicines containing unsaturated pyrrolizidine alkaloids (1,2). Herbal medicines that provide over 1 mg/day internally or over 100 mg/day externally are not permitted; herbal medicines that provide 0.1–1 mg/day internally or 10–100 mg/day may be applied only for a maximum of 6 weeks per year, and they should not be used during pregnancy or lactation.

References

1. Anonymous. Vorinformation Pyrrolizidinalkaloidhaltige Human Arzneimittel. Pharm Ztg 1990;135:2532–3; 1990;135:2623–4.
2. Anonymous. Aufbereitungsmonographien Kommission E. Pharm Ztg 1990;135:2081–2.
3. Stickel F, Seitz HK. The efficacy and safety of comfrey. Public Health Nutr 2000;3(4A):501–8.
4. Yeong ML, Swinburn B, Kennedy M, Nicholson G. Hepatic veno-occlusive disease associated with comfrey ingestion. J Gastrointest Hepatol 1990;5(2):211–14.
5. Ridker PN, McDermott WV. Hepatotoxicity due to comfrey herb tea. Am J Med 1989;87(6):701.
6. Bach N, Thung SN, Schaffner F. Comfrey herb tea-induced hepatic veno-occlusive disease. Am J Med 1989;87(1):97–9.
7. Weston CF, Cooper BT, Davies JD, Levine DF. Veno-occlusive disease of the liver secondary to ingestion of comfrey. BMJ (Clin Res Ed) 1987;295(6591):183.
8. Rode D. Comfrey toxicity revisited. Trends Pharmacol Sci 2002;23(11):497–9.

Boric acid

See also Disinfectants and antiseptics

General Information

In the past, boric acid was falsely considered to be relatively non-toxic, and had an unwarranted reputation as a germicide. However, it is only bacteriostatic, even in a saturated aqueous solution, and can cause adverse reactions. Boric acid has often proved poisonous, either by ingestion or after local use. Cases from the world literature have been reviewed (1,2). In 172 cases of boric acid intoxication, including 83 deaths, 37 deaths occurred after external use, including 23 children with nappy rash. From 1974 to 1984, the Poison Centre in Paris recorded 134 cases of intoxication with boric acid or borates, 88 of which were accidental and 31 iatrogenic.

Boric acid penetrates even intact skin, but it is readily absorbed through inflamed or otherwise damaged skin and through mucous membranes. After the application of wet compresses of boric acid to intact and eczematous skin in 21 patients over several days, blood concentrations of boric acid were generally not raised (3). One patient, however, did have a significant rise in blood boric acid concentration, which the authors ascribed to pre-existing kidney insufficiency.

Prolonged absorption of boric acid causes anorexia, weight loss, vomiting, mild diarrhea, skin rash, diffuse alopecia, convulsions, and anemia.

On account of the high toxicity and limited therapeutic value of boric acid, the borates have been abandoned as obsolete in many countries.

Organs and Systems

Skin

The skin, which is unlikely to react unfavorably to topical boric acid, can react strongly if it is absorbed systemically; resultant redness can mimic scarlet fever, and psoriasiform lesions, bullae, and alopecia can occur.

Drug Administration

Drug overdose

In acute intoxication, symptoms develop progressively, typically beginning with persistent vomiting and diarrhea (mucous and blood, with a bluish-green color). Shortly after the onset of the gastrointestinal symptoms, in some cases even earlier, a rash appears (with macules and/or papules), beginning on the abdomen, genitalia, and head, and rapidly spreading, followed by excoriation and intensive desquamation after 1–2 days. Mucous membranes are often involved, especially in young infants, in whom the mouth, pharynx, and conjunctivae are often inflamed. Later, there are central nervous system symptoms, with headache and mental confusion followed by convulsions. In children there is meningism and twitching of the facial muscles and limbs followed by convulsions. Acute tubular necrosis can occur, with oliguria or anuria, hypernatremia, hyperchloremia and hyperkalemia, proteinuria, erythrocyturia, and cylindruria. Finally, hyperthermia, a fall in blood pressure, tachycardia, and shock occur.

Fourteen cases of acute boric acid ingestion were reported in New York City over 30 months. In these patients excretion of urinary riboflavin (vitamin B_2) was determined, and in about two-thirds it was significantly increased. This is not surprising, since riboflavin and boric acid are known to form a water-soluble complex. The range of lethal doses is 1–3 g for babies, 5 g for infants, and 15–20 g for adults.

- Severe acute boric acid poisoning occurred in a 3-year-old boy after the application of a boric acid-containing talcum powder (4).
- A similar case occurred in a 27-day-old baby girl (5).
- Generalized erythema and skin desquamation, fever convulsions, and diarrhea followed repeated boric acid application to a denuded umbilical stump (6).
- Fatal intoxication has followed prostatectomy and subsequent bladder irrigation with 3% boric acid (7).

Of 172 published cases of boric acid intoxication, 83 proved fatal; the series included 37 deaths after external use of boric acid, 23 of these being children who had developed diaper rashes. The actual number of cases, mostly unpublished, must have been much greater: from 1974 to March 1984, 134 cases of intoxication by boric acid or borates were recorded in France alone, 88 being accidental and 31 associated with medicinal use.

References

1. Goldbloom RB, Goldbloom A. Boric acid poisoning; report of four cases and a review of 109 cases from the world literature. J Pediatr 1953;43(6):631–43.
2. Valdes-Dapena MA, Arey JB. Boric acid poisoning: three fatal cases with pancreatic inclusions and a review of the literature. J Pediatr 1962;61:531.
3. Schuppli R, Seiler H, Schneeberger R, Niggli H, Hoffmann K. Über die Toxizität der Borsäure. [Toxicity of boric acid.] Dermatologica 1971;143(4):227–34.
4. Skipworth GB, Goldstein N, McBride WP. Boric acid intoxication from "medicated talcum powder". Arch Dermatol 1967;95(1):83–6.
5. Baliah T, MacLeish H, Drummond KN. Acute boric acid poisoning: report of an infant successfully treated by peritoneal dialysis. Can Med Assoc J 1969;101(3):166–8.
6. Hillman DA, Hillman ES, Hall J. Boric acid poisoning. East Afr Med J 1970;47(11):572–5.
7. Schmid F, Zbinden J, Schlatter C. Zwei Fälle von letaler Borsäurevergiftung nach Blasenspülung. [Two cases of fatal boric acid poisoning after bladder irrigation.] Schweiz Med Wochenschr 1972;102(3):83–8.

Bornaprine

See also Adrenoceptor agonists

General Information

Bornaprine, a synthetic quaternary ammonium compound, has been used as an anticholinergic drug in treating Parkinson's disease (1). Its adverse effects are those characteristic of the anticholinergic drugs.

Reference

1. Cantello R, Riccio A, Gilli M, Delsedime M, Scarzella L, Aguggia M, Bergamasco B. Bornaprine vs placebo in Parkinson disease: double-blind controlled cross-over trial in 30 patients. Ital J Neurol Sci 1986;7(1):139–43.

Bosentan

See also Endothelin receptor antagonists

General Information

Bosentan is an endothelin-A and endothelin-B receptor antagonist. It is effective in pulmonary arterial hypertension (1,2) and has been marketed for this indication. The studies showed an improvement in exercise capacity and dyspnea and an increased time to clinical worsening. Efficacy in pulmonary hypertension has also been reported in an open study with a selective endothelin-A receptor antagonist (3).

The effects of bosentan (62.5 mg bd for 4 weeks followed by either 125 or 250 mg bd for a minimum of 12 weeks) have been studied in a double-blind, placebo-controlled trial in 213 patients with pulmonary arterial hypertension (2). The patients who took bosentan had improved exercise capacity, less dyspnea, and delayed worsening. There were similar results in 32 patients who took bosentan for a minimum of 12 weeks (62.5 mg bd for 4 weeks then 125 mg bd) (4). Bosentan significantly reduced pulmonary vascular resistance. The number and nature of adverse events were similar with bosentan and placebo.

Organs and Systems

Cardiovascular

In a dose-finding study with bosentan (100, 500, 1000, and 2000 mg/day) in 293 hypertensive patients (5) there were statistically significant falls in diastolic blood pressure with the 500 and 2000 mg/day doses. The effects were similar to that of enalapril 20 mg/day. The lowering of blood pressure was not associated with any changes in heart rate, plasma noradrenaline concentrations, plasma renin activity, or angiotensin II concentrations.

In the ENABLE (Endothelin Antagonist Bosentan for Lowering Cardiac Events in Heart Failure) placebo-controlled study the effects of low-dose bosentan (125 mg bd) were evaluated in 1613 patients with severe heart failure (left ventricular ejection fraction < 35%, New York Heart Association classes IIIb-IV) (6). The primary endpoint of all-cause mortality or hospitalization for heart failure was reached in 321 of 808 patients who took placebo and 312 of 805 who took bosentan. Treatment with bosentan conferred an early risk of worsening heart failure necessitating hospitalization, because of fluid retention. These results throw doubt on the potential benefits of non-specific endothelin receptor blockade in heart failure. Preliminary data suggest that in heart failure selective endothelin-A receptor antagonists (BQ-123, sitaxsentan) may be more beneficial than non-selective antagonists, especially when there is associated pulmonary hypertension (7).

Liver

The major safety issue that has emerged with bosentan, the endothelin receptor antagonist that has been most extensively studied in man, has been dose-dependent reversible impairment of hepatic function (3% with 125 mg, 7% with 250 mg), manifesting as raised transaminases (2). The effect of bosentan on hepatocanalicular bile-salt transport has been studied in rats in conjunction with a re-examination of the safety database from two clinical trials (in hypertension and congestive cardiac failure) and measurement of bile-salt concentrations in stored blood samples from these trials (8). Hepatic injury was defined as a three-fold increase in alanine transaminase activity. In the hypertension trial there were no cases of hepatic injury with placebo or enalapril. With bosentan, the frequencies were 2, 4, 11, and 8% at dosages of 100, 500, 1000, and 2000 mg/day respectively. There was a dose-dependent increase in bile-salt concentrations. In the study in patients with heart failure (New York Heart Association classes III/IV), liver injury occurred in 4% of 126 patients taking placebo and 18% of 244 patients taking bosentan 500 mg bd. A subgroup analysis showed a higher incidence of hepatic injury in patients taking concomitant bosentan and glibenclamide. Patients with hepatic injury had raised bile-salt concentrations.

In rats, intravenous bosentan produced a dose-dependent increase in plasma bile salts. The effect was potentiated when glibenclamide was co-administered. In vitro studies in rat canalicular liver plasma membranes confirmed inhibition of bile-salt transport. Three bosentan metabolites were also investigated. The M2 metabolite was more potent than bosentan, whereas the M1 and M3 metabolites produced less inhibition of bile acid transport than bosentan. The effects of bosentan and its main metabolites, both of which are eliminated in the bile, on biliary secretion have been studied in rats with biliary fistulae and with or without a genetic defect in mrp2 (9). Intravenous bosentan 0.1–10 mg/kg caused a dose-dependent increase in biliary bilirubin excretion, and doses of 10 mg/kg or over caused a sustained increase in canalicular salt-independent bile flow, combined with significant increases in the concentrations and output of glutathione and of bicarbonate in the bile. Phospholipid and cholesterol secretion were profoundly inhibited and uncoupled from bile-salt secretion. In mrp2-deficient rats, the choleretic effect of bosentan was markedly reduced. Thus, bosentan alters canalicular bile formation mostly via mrp2-mediated mechanisms. Intermittent uncoupling of

lipid from bile-salt secretion may contribute to its hepatic adverse effects.

These data suggest that bosentan causes cholestatic liver injury due to inhibition of bile-salt efflux and damage due to intracellular accumulation of bile salts.

Long-Term Effects

Drug tolerance

Despite short-term benefits of bosentan in systemic hypertension and congestive heart failure, it increases plasma concentrations of endothelin-1, probably by inhibiting its clearance via endothelin-B receptors. This may mean that its effectiveness is reduced during long-term therapy (7).

Susceptibility Factors

Renal disease

The effects of severe renal insufficiency on the pharmacokinetics and metabolism of bosentan 125 mg have been studied in an open, parallel-group study in eight patients with creatinine clearances 17–27 ml/minute and in eight healthy subjects (creatinine clearances 99–135 ml/minute) (10). The pharmacokinetics of bosentan did not differ significantly, although the concentrations of the three CYP2C9- and CYP3A4-derived metabolites increased about two-fold in the patients with renal insufficiency. It is not necessary to adjust the dosage of bosentan in patients with any grade of renal insufficiency.

References

1. Channick RN, Simonneau G, Sitbon O, Robbins IM, Frost A, Tapson VF, Badesch DB, Roux S, Rainisio M, Bodin F, Rubin LJ. Effects of the dual endothelin-receptor antagonist bosentan in patients with pulmonary hypertension: a randomised placebo-controlled study. Lancet 2001;358(9288):1119–23.
2. Rubin LJ, Badesch DB, Barst RJ, Galie N, Black CM, Keogh A, Pulido T, Frost A, Roux S, Leconte I, Landzberg M, Simonneau G. Bosentan therapy for pulmonary arterial hypertension. N Engl J Med 2002;346(12):896–903.
3. Barst RJ, Rich S, Widlitz A, Horn EM, McLaughlin V, McFarlin J. Clinical efficacy of sitaxsentan, an endothelin-A receptor antagonist, in patients with pulmonary arterial hypertension: open-label pilot study. Chest 2002;121(6):1860–8.
4. Badesch DB, Bodin F, Channick RN, Frost A, Rainisio M, Robbins IM, Roux S, Rubin LJ, Simonneau G, Sitbon O, Tapson VF. Complete results of the first randomized, placebo-controlled study of bosentan, a dual endothelin receptor antagonist, in pulmonary arterial hypertension. Curr Ther Res Clin Exp 2002;63:227–46.
5. Krum H, Viskoper RJ, Lacourciere Y, Budde M, Charlon V. The effect of an endothelin-receptor antagonist, bosentan, on blood pressure in patients with essential hypertension. Bosentan Hypertension Investigators. N Engl J Med 1998;338(12):784–90.
6. Kalra PR, Moon JC, Coats AJ. Do results of the ENABLE (Endothelin Antagonist Bosentan for Lowering Cardiac Events in Heart Failure) study spell the end for non-selective endothelin antagonism in heart failure? Int J Cardiol 2002;85(2–3):195–7.

7. Doggrell SA. The therapeutic potential of endothelin-1 receptor antagonists and endothelin-converting enzyme inhibitors on the cardiovascular system. Expert Opin Investig Drugs 2002;11(11):1537–52.

8. Fattinger K, Funk C, Pantze M, Weber C, Reichen J, Stieger B, Meier PJ. The endothelin antagonist bosentan inhibits the canalicular bile salt export pump: a potential mechanism for hepatic adverse reactions. Clin Pharmacol Ther 2001;69(4):223–31.

9. Fouassier L, Kinnman N, Lefevre G, Lasnier E, Rey C, Poupon R, Elferink RP, Housset C. Contribution of mrp2 in alterations of canalicular bile formation by the endothelin antagonist bosentan. J Hepatol 2002;37(2):184–91.

10. Dingemanse J, van Giersbergen PL. Influence of severe renal dysfunction on the pharmacokinetics and metabolism of bosentan, a dual endothelin receptor antagonist. Int J Clin Pharmacol Ther 2002;40(7):310–16.

Botulinum toxin

General Information

Botulinum toxin is one of several toxins produced by the bacterium *Clostridium botulinum*. The toxin binds with high affinity to peripheral cholinergic nerve endings, such as those at the neuromuscular junction and in the autonomic nervous system, preventing the release of the neurotransmitter acetylcholine (1). This action at the neuromuscular junction can cause weakness and even paralysis of the muscles supplied by the affected nerves. Sprouting of the terminal nerves eventually results in re-innervation of the muscles and return of function. Doses are measured in mouse units (MU), 1 MU being the LD_{50} in Swiss–Webster mice.

Botulinum toxin is used in the treatment of excessive muscle contraction disorders (dystonias), such as strabismus, blepharospasm, focal dystonias, and spasticity. One of its uses is in the removal of facial wrinkles by paralysing mimic muscles. It can reduce sweat production by blocking cholinergic innervation of eccrine sweat glands.

Therapeutic studies

For blepharospasm, injections of about 12.5–25 MU are made into the periocular muscles of each eye. When so used, adverse effects are seen in 20–50% of treatments. They consist of mild ptosis, increased or reduced tear function, diplopia, and ectropion. These effects are transient, most lasting about 2 weeks, and generally well tolerated. Occasionally ptosis is so severe as to be inconvenient for the patient. The blepharospasm is relieved for 2–4 months. Systemic effects have not been reported (2).

In the treatment of spastic torticollis there is a tendency to use larger doses (up to 1000 MU) injected into the neck muscles, and weakness of the pharyngeal muscles, resulting in dysphagia and paralysis of the vocal cords, has been reported. Difficulty in swallowing and deepening of the voice were found in up to 30% of cases in one series, resolving after 2–3 weeks (3). In one case there was severe dysphagia 2 days after an injection, with unilateral vocal cord paralysis a week later; swallowing was normal again

after 6 weeks (4). The possibility of appreciable effects from this neurotoxin at more distant neuromuscular junctions and the development of antibodies are potential dangers here.

Treatment of spasmodic torticollis with botulinum toxin has been reviewed retrospectively in 107 patients (SEDA-17, 45). It was efficacious in 93% but adverse effects occurred in 84%. Initially, 500 MU were injected into each muscle, but the incidence of adverse effects led to a reduction in dosage, 200–500 MU being injected depending on the muscle used and on neck thickness. The median dose per treatment was 1000 (range 200–1600) MU on the first visit and 800 MU subsequently. Dysphagia occurred after 44% of the treatments. This was severe in 2% of treatments, allowing only sips of fluid and necessitating hospitalization for two patients because of dehydration. Two patients developed stridor, two had substantial weight loss, and one developed pneumonia as a result of aspiration. According to the authors, the risk of dysphagia is 40% if a sternomastoid is injected and 25% if it is not. The risks of moderate or severe dysphagia are 7% and under 1% respectively. The authors estimated that there is a 3% chance of antibody production with reduced responsiveness during the first 15 months of treatment. They recommended antibody testing for patients who have initial but not subsequent improvement after repeated injections of botulinum toxin. The problem of immunological resistance to the effects of botulinum toxin associated with repeat injections has been reviewed elsewhere (5).

In a multicenter, randomized, placebo-controlled trial in 145 patients with axillary hyperhidrosis, refractory to treatment with topical aluminium chloride, both 100 and 200 MU of botulinum toxin reduced sweat production by about 80% (6). After 24 weeks, sweat production in the treated axillae was about 45% of baseline. Temporary adverse events during the first 14 weeks included headache, soreness of the muscles of the shoulder girdle, axillary itching, and increased facial sweating.

A multicenter, double-blind, randomized, placebo-controlled study in 320 patients with untreated hyperhidrosis showed a more than 50% reduction in sweat production at 4 and 16 weeks after treatment respectively in 94 and 82% of patients treated with botulinum toxin (50 MU per axilla) and in 36 and 21% of placebo-treated patients (7). The major treatment-related adverse effect was an increase in sweating in non-axillary sites after treatment. Open treatment with botulinum toxin A was offered to patients in whom sweat production was at least 50% of baseline values (8). Of 207 study subjects, 39% had one treatment, 45% had two treatments and 15% had three treatments. Response rates 4 weeks after treatment were 96, 91, and 83% after the first, second, and third treatments respectively. In one of 207 patients there was possible transient seroconversion from negative to positive for neutralizing antibodies to botulinum toxin, and subsequent treatment with botulinum toxin resulted in complete disappearance of axillary sweating 7 days after injection.

The long-term effectiveness of high-dose botulinum toxin (200 MU per axilla) has been evaluated in an open study in patients with axillary hyperhidrosis unresponsive to previous therapies (9). In 34 patients follow-up was for at least 12 months. Four relapsed within 12 months and two relapsed after 16 and 19 months. Mild pain and a burning sensation, sometimes lasting up to 1 hour after injection, were the most frequent adverse effects. No compensatory hyperhidrosis at other body sites was reported.

Organs and Systems

Nervous system

Five cases of severe headache refractory to oral analgesics have been reported in patients treated with 10–38 MU of botulinum toxin for glabella frown lines ($n = 4$) and in a patient treated with 120 MU for palmar hyperhidrosis (10). The headache lasted for 8 days to 4 weeks, did not respond to oral prednisolone, and in some patients was accompanied by photophobia, ear tenderness, or nasal congestion. Two patients had had a similar headache after a previous treatment with botulinum toxin and in another patient a similar headache occurred after the next treatment. None of the patients had a history of severe headaches.

Neuromuscular function

Muscle weakness after botulinum toxin injection is usually due to local spread of the agent. Asymptomatic systemic effects have been detected in patients with cervical dystonia after repeated botulinum toxin injections, when muscle biopsies from the vastus lateralis muscle were examined (11). However, generalized neuromuscular symptoms are rare. Patients with a reduced margin of safety with regard to neuromuscular transmission might be considered prone to systemic effects, but even in patients with myasthenia gravis symptoms distal from the injection site have been reported only occasionally (12). However, generalized muscle weakness can occur if higher doses of botulinum toxin are used, and a recent report has illustrated that this may happen in patients after many uneventful treatment sessions (13). Electrophysiological findings in these patients were suggestive of mild botulism, with doses of botulinum toxin of 600–900 units. Two similar cases had been reported previously (12). Therefore, constant long-term monitoring of patients is recommended, even if they have been receiving injections for many years without adverse effects.

Generalized muscular weakness associated with signs of systemic cholinergic autonomic impairment has been reported.

- A 25-year-old woman was treated with botulinum toxin for hyperhidrosis of the axillae and hands in one session with a total amount of 1400 MU. Six days later she complained of diffuse weakness, diplopia, mild bilateral ptosis, severe weakness in the fingers, and reduced lacrimation, salivary production, and sweating (14). She recovered completely within 2 months.

Permanent extraocular muscle damage has been reported (15).

- A 70-year-old man had increasing difficulty in maintaining binocular vision while reading. There was imbalance of his extraocular muscle activity. Botulinum toxin 2.5 MU was therefore injected into the left inferior rectus muscle under electromyography control using a 27-gauge needle. At the next visit 1 month later he complained of diplopia in all directions of gaze, in keeping with a left inferior rectus muscle palsy. Over the next 10 months there was no improvement. Magnetic resonance imaging then showed atrophy of the left inferior rectus muscle. Inferior transposition of the medial and lateral recti muscles was performed, which produced satisfactory alignment.

Botulinum-induced atrophy of extraocular muscles of the eye cannot be excluded in this case. This mechanism is supported by the observation that botulinum toxin can cause histological changes in the extraocular muscles in adult monkeys (16). The authors of the present report also suggested that intramuscular hematoma or direct damage to the nerve to the muscle may have been responsible. So far, permanent extraocular muscle damage after botulinum toxin injection seems to be rare. If additional cases are reported, patients should be informed about this possible complication before treatment.

Susceptibility Factors

In the presence of neuromuscular disorders, such as myasthenia gravis or Lambert–Eaton syndrome, botulinum toxin-induced inhibition of acetylcholine release can cause generalized weakness (17). Therefore, botulinum toxin should, if at all, be used with extreme caution in patients with neuromuscular disease, who have a reduced margin of safety with regard to neuromuscular transmission.

- An 80-year-old woman had severe difficulty in swallowing and flaccid paralysis of her cervical muscles starting 4 days after the periocular injection of botulinum toxin 120 MU for blepharospasm (12). She also developed bilateral facial nerve paralysis and slurred speech and could not fully close her eyes. Barium swallow and fluoroscopy showed signs of aspiration. The serum concentration of antiacetylcholine receptor antibodies was 6.9 units (reference range 0–0.7 units). Mestinone and prednisone improved her symptoms. She had been treated with botulinum toxin on 18 occasions over the previous 13 years without any untoward effects.

While the exact cause of muscle weakness was unclear, this case argues against the use of botulinum toxin in patients with myasthenic syndromes. When the margin of safety is reduced with regard to neuromuscular transmission, botulinum toxin can result in increased morbidity or even mortality. Generalized muscle weakness after botulinum toxin has also been reported in patients with other neuromuscular disorders (18). In addition, it should be remembered that both dysphagia and muscle weakness can occur after botulinum toxin injection, even in patients who do not suffer from generalized neuromuscular disorders (19).

Generalized weakness has been reported after botulinum toxin treatment in a patient with amyotrophic lateral sclerosis (18).

Drug Administration

Drug formulations

Pain due to injection of botulinum toxin has been reported to be less severe with botulinum toxin reconstituted in preservative-containing saline 0.9% (benzyl alcohol 0.9% w/v) than with botulinum toxin reconstituted in preservative-free saline 0.9% in patients with glabella-frown lines (20).

Drug–Drug Interactions

Neuromuscular blocking drugs

As botulinum toxin inhibits acetylcholine release it can interfere with neuromuscular blocking agents (21). It has been suggested that each dose of botulinum toxin may have two effects: first, a direct increase in sensitivity to neuromuscular blocking agents; second, compensatory synaptic remodeling resulting in reduced sensitivity (21). Thus, the effects of neuromuscular blocking agents on neuromuscular transmission cannot be predicted in patients receiving botulinum toxin.

References

1. Hambleton P. Clostridium botulinum toxins: a general review of involvement in disease, structure, mode of action and preparation for clinical use. J Neurol 1992;239(1):16–20.
2. Cohen DA, Savino PJ, Stern MB, Hurtig HI. Botulinum injection therapy for blepharospasm: a review and report of 75 patients. Clin Neuropharmacol 1986;9(5):415–29.
3. Stell R, Coleman R, Thompson P, Marsden CD. Botulinum toxin treatment of spasmodic torticollis. BMJ 1988;297(6648):616.
4. Koay CE, Alun-Jones T. Pharyngeal paralysis due to botulinum toxin injection. J Laryngol Otol 1989;103(7):698–9.
5. Borodic G, Johnson E, Goodnough M, Schantz E. Botulinum toxin therapy, immunologic resistance, and problems with available materials. Neurology 1996;46(1):26–9.
6. Heckmann M, Ceballos-Baumann AO, Plewig G; Hyperhidrosis Study Group. Botulinum toxin A for axillary hyperhidrosis (excessive sweating). N Engl J Med 2001;344(7):488–93.
7. Naumann M, Lowe NJ. Botulinum toxin type A in treatment of bilateral primary axillary hyperhidrosis: randomised, parallel group, double blind, placebo controlled trial. BMJ 2001;323(7313):596–9.
8. Naumann M, Lowe NJ, Kumar CR, Hamm H; Hyperhidrosis Clinical Investigators Group. Botulinum toxin type a is a safe and effective treatment for axillary hyperhidrosis over 16 months: a prospective study. Arch Dermatol 2003;139(6):731–6.
9. Wollina U, Karamfilov T, Konrad H. High-dose botulinum toxin type A therapy for axillary hyperhidrosis markedly prolongs the relapse-free interval. J Am Acad Dermatol 2002;46(4):536–40.
10. Alam M, Arndt KA, Dover JS. Severe, intractable headache after injection with botulinum A exotoxin: report of 5 cases. J Am Acad Dermatol 2002;46(1):62–5.
11. Ansved T, Odergren T, Borg K. Muscle fiber atrophy in leg muscles after botulinum toxin type A treatment of cervical dystonia. Neurology 1997;48(5):1440–2.
12. Borodic G. Myasthenic crisis after botulinum toxin. Lancet 1998;352(9143):1832.
13. Bhatia KP, Munchau A, Thompson PD, Houser M, Chauhan VS, Hutchinson M, Shapira AH, Marsden CD. Generalised muscular weakness after botulinum toxin injections for dystonia: a report of three cases. J Neurol Neurosurg Psychiatry 1999;67(1):90–3.
14. Tugnoli V, Eleopra R, Quatrale R, Capone JG, Sensi M, Gastaldo E. Botulism-like syndrome after botulinum toxin type A injections for focal hyperhidrosis. Br J Dermatol 2002;147(4):808–9.
15. Mohan M, Tow S, Fleck BW, Lee JP. Permanent extraocular muscle damage following botulinum toxin injection. Br J Ophthalmol 1999;83(11):1309–10.
16. Spencer RF, McNeer KW. Botulinum toxin paralysis of adult monkey extraocular muscle. Structural alterations in orbital, singly innervated muscle fibers. Arch Ophthalmol 1987;105(12):1703–11.
17. Barohn RJ, Jackson CE, Rogers SJ, Ridings LW, McVey AL. Prolonged paralysis due to nondepolarizing neuromuscular blocking agents and corticosteroids. Muscle Nerve 1994;17(6):647–54.
18. Mezaki T, Kaji R, Kohara N, Kimura J. Development of general weakness in a patient with amyotrophic lateral sclerosis after focal botulinum toxin injection. Neurology 1996;46(3):845–6.
19. Bakheit AM, Ward CD, McLellan DL. Generalised botulism-like syndrome after intramuscular injections of botulinum toxin type A: a report of two cases. J Neurol Neurosurg Psychiatry 1997;62(2):198.
20. Alam M, Dover JS, Arndt KA. Pain associated with injection of botulinum A exotoxin reconstituted using isotonic sodium chloride with and without preservative: a double-blind, randomized controlled trial. Arch Dermatol 2002;138(4):510–14.
21. Fiacchino F, Grandi L, Soliveri P, Carella F, Bricchi M. Sensitivity to vecuronium after botulinum toxin administration. J Neurosurg Anesthesiol 1997;9(2):149–53.

Bovine serum albumin (BSA)

General Information

Bovine serum albumin is often used as protein supplement in cell culture media, and residual bovine serum albumin in some formulations has occasionally caused adverse effects. Symptoms are usually mild, such as itching and urticaria. An anaphylactic reaction has been described in a patient undergoing bone marrow transplantation after the bone marrow cells had been kept in bovine serum albumin. As a component of sperm processing media, bovine serum albumin has caused adverse effects after intrauterine insemination (1). The risk of transmission of nvCJD by recombinant proteins is unknown, as cell cultures used for manufacturing them often contain bovine serum albumin (2).

References

1. Sonenthal KR, McKnight T, Shaughnessy MA, Grammer LC, Jeyendran RS. Anaphylaxis during intrauterine insemination secondary to bovine serum albumin. Fertil Steril 1991;56(6):1188–91.
2. Mauser-Bunschoten EP, Roosendaal G, van den Berg HM. Product choice and haemophilia treatment in the Netherlands. Haemophilia 2001;7(1):96–8.

Brassicaceae

See also Herbal medicines

General Information

The genera in the family of Brassicaceae (Table 1) include various types of brassica (cabbage, broccoli, brussels sprouts, kale, kohlrabi, pak choi, rape, turnip), mustard, and cress.

Table 1 The genera of Brassicaceae

Alliaria (alliaria)
Alyssum (madwort)
Anelsonia (anelsonia)
Aphragmus (aphragmus)
Arabidopsis (rock cress)
Arabis (rock cress)
Armoracia (armoracia)
Athysanus (sandweed)
Aubrieta (lilac bush)
Aurinia (aurinia)
Barbarea (yellow rocket)
Berteroa (false madwort)
Brassica (broccoli, cabbage, mustard, rape)
Braya (northern-rock cress)
Bunias (warty cabbage)
Cakile (searocket)
Calepina (ballmustard)
Camelina (false flax)
Capsella (capsella)
Cardamine (bittercress)
Cardaria (whitetop)
Caulanthus (wild cabbage)
Caulostramina (caulostramina)
Chlorocrambe (chlorocrambe)
Chorispora (chorispora)
Cochlearia (scurvy grass)
Coincya (star mustard)
Conringia (hare's ear mustard)
Coronopus (swine cress)
Crambe (crambe)
Cusickiella (cusickiella)
Descurainia (tansy mustard)
Dimorphocarpa (spectacle pod)
Diplotaxis (wallrocket)
Dithyrea (shield pod)
Draba (draba)
Dryopetalon (dryopetalon)
Eruca (rocket salad)
Erucastrum (dog mustard)
Erysimum (wallflower)
Euclidium (mustard)
Eutrema (eutrema)
Glaucocarpum (waxfruit mustard)
Guillenia (mustard)
Halimolobos (fissurewort)
Hesperis (rocket)
Heterodraba (heterodraba)
Hirschfeldia (hirschfeldia)
Hutchinsia (hutchinsia)
Iberis (candytuft)
Idahoa (idahoa)
Iodanthus (iodanthus)
Ionopsidium (ionopsidium)

Isatis (woad)
Leavenworthia (gladecress)
Lepidium (pepperweed)
Lesquerella (bladderpod)
Lobularia (lobularia)
Lunaria (lunaria)
Lyrocarpa (lyrepod)
Malcolmia (malcolmia)
Mancoa (mancoa)
Matthiola (stock)
Microthlaspi (penny cress)
Moricandia (moricandia)
Myagrum (myagrum)
Neobeckia (lake cress)
Nerisyrenia (fan mustard)
Neslia (neslia)
Parrya (parrya)
Pennellia (mock thelypody)
Phoenicaulis (phoenicaulis)
Physaria (twinpod)
Polyctenium (combleaf)
Raphanus (radish)
Rapistrum (bastard cabbage)
Rorippa (yellowcress)
Schoenocrambe (plains mustard)
Selenia (selenia)
Sibara (winged rock cress)
Sibaropsis (sibaropsis)
Sinapis (mustard)
Sisymbrium (hedge mustard)
Smelowskia (candytuft)
Stanfordia (stanfordia)
Stanleya (prince's plume)
Streptanthella (streptanthella)
Streptanthus (twist flower)
Stroganowia (stroganowia)
Subularia (awlwort)
Synthlipsis (synthlipsis)
Teesdalia (shepard's cress)
Thelypodium (thelypody)
Thelypodiopsis (tumble mustard)
Thlaspi (penny cress)
Thysanocarpus (fringepod)
Tropidocarpum (tropidocarpum)
Warea (pineland cress)

Several of the Brassicaceae contain allyl isothiocyanate, which is a potent irritant and has mutagenic activity in bacteria and fetotoxic and carcinogenic effects in rats. However, as allyl isothiocyanate also occurs in ordinary mustard, it would not be realistic to ban all botanical drugs that contain it, since they commonly provide no more than a normal daily dose of mustard (for example 5 mg of allyl isothiocyanate per 5 g of mustard).

Armoracia rusticana

Armoracia rusticana (horseradish) contains 0.05–0.2% of essential oils of which 85% is allyl isothiocyanate.

Adverse effects

Abdominal discomfort and convulsive syncope occurred after the ingestion of raw horseradish that had not been properly aired before use (1).

Brassica nigra

Brassica nigra (black mustard) contains allyl isothiocyanate. External application of preparations from black mustard has declined because of skin irritation (see *Sinapis* species).

Raphanus sativus

The root of *Raphanus sativus* var. niger (black radish) contains 0.0025% of essential oil with glycosides yielding allyl isothiocyanate and butyl isothiocyanate.

Adverse effects

The consumption of several roots of *Raphanus sativus* can produce miosis, pain, vomiting, slowed respiration, stupor, and albuminuria.

Allergic contact dermatitis has been attributed to radish (2).

Sinapis species

The *Sinapis* genus contains several different types of mustard species, including *Sinapis alba* (white mustard) and *Sinapis arvensis* (charlock mustard). Mustard has traditionally been used in heated compresses (sinapisms) to draw blood away from underlying infections and to act as a counterirritant. This can cause direct skin damage.

- A 50-year-old woman experienced a second-degree burn after applying a heated mustard compress to her chest to relieve pulmonary congestion associated with a recent episode of pneumonia (3). The injury resulted in permanent hyperpigmentation and hypertrophic scarring.

References

1. Rubin HR, Wu AW. The bitter herbs of Seder: more on horseradish horrors. JAMA 1988;259(13):1943.
2. Mitchell JC, Jordan WP. Allergic contact dermatitis from the radish, *Raphanus sativus*. Br J Dermatol 1974;91(2):183–9.
3. Linder SA, Mele JA 3rd, Harries T. Chronic hyperpigmentation from a heated mustard compress burn: a case report. J Burn Care Rehabil 1996;17(4):351–2.

Brequinar

General Information

Brequinar (DUP 785, NSC 368390) is a quinoline carboxylic acid derivative that inhibits pyrimidine synthesis by inhibiting dihydro-orotate dehydrogenase. It was originally developed as an anticancer drug, but has also been investigated for its immunosuppressant activity after transplantation. Some data suggest that that the immunosuppressant activity of brequinar may be partly due to inhibition of tyrosine phosphorylation in lymphocytes (1).

Significant adverse effects of brequinar include thrombocytopenia, maculopapular dermatitis, mucositis, and gastrointestinal disorders (2).

Susceptibility Factors

In patients with renal, hepatic, and cardiac transplants the clearance of a single oral dose of brequinar was lower than expected from previous studies (3), perhaps due to an interaction with ciclosporin, as has been shown in rats (4). Overall safety results suggest that brequinar is well tolerated in stable transplant recipients (3).

Drug–Drug Interactions

Cisplatin

Brequinar was synergistic with cisplatin in preclinical models. However, co-administration of brequinar with cisplatin does not affect the pharmacokinetics of either drug (5).

References

1. Xu X, Williams JW, Shen J, Gong H, Yin DP, Blinder L, Elder RT, Sankary H, Finnegan A, Chong AS. In vitro and in vivo mechanisms of action of the antiproliferative and immunosuppressive agent, brequinar sodium. J Immunol 1998;160(2):846–53.
2. Philip AT, Gerson B. Toxicology and adverse effects of drugs used for immunosuppression in organ transplantation. Clin Lab Med 1998;18(4):755–65.
3. Joshi AS, King SY, Zajac BA, Makowka L, Sher LS, Kahan BD, Menkis AH, Stiller CR, Schaefle B, Kornhauser DM. Phase I safety and pharmacokinetic studies of brequinar sodium after single ascending oral doses in stable renal, hepatic, and cardiac allograft recipients. J Clin Pharmacol 1997;37(12):1121–8.
4. Pally C, Smith D, Jaffee B, Magolda R, Zehender H, Dorobek B, Donatsch P, Papageorgiou C, Schuurman HJ. Side effects of brequinar and brequinar analogues, in combination with cyclosporine, in the rat. Toxicology 1998;127(1–3):207–22.
5. Burris HA 3rd, Raymond E, Awada A, Kuhn JG, O'Rourke TJ, Brentzel J, Lynch W, King SY, Brown TD, Von Hoff DD. Pharmacokinetic and phase I studies of brequinar (DUP 785; NSC 368390) in combination with cisplatin in patients with advanced malignancies. Invest New Drugs 1998;16(1):19–27.

Bretylium

See also Antidysrhythmic drugs

General Information

Bretylium, originally introduced as a hypotensive agent but no longer used as such, has not been extensively used as an antidysrhythmic drug. Its clinical pharmacology, uses, efficacy, and adverse effects have been reviewed (1–4). Adverse effects have reportedly caused the need for withdrawal in about 7% of patients (3).

Organs and Systems

Cardiovascular

Postural hypotension is common, and a significant fall in arterial pressure can occur, even in patients who are supine (5).

Occasionally bretylium causes a transient rise in blood pressure after intravenous administration, due to release of noradrenaline from sympathetic nerve endings.

Ventricular tachydysrhythmias have been reported occasionally (6).

Mouth and teeth

Long-term treatment with bretylium can cause parotid pain and swelling and pain in the tongue (7).

Body temperature

Intravenous bretylium can cause severe hyperthermia (8,9).

Drug Administration

Drug administration route

Bretylium is poorly absorbed and is therefore given parenterally. Despite its poor systemic availability, bretylium was available for some years and was often combined with a tricyclic antidepressant. After intravenous administration bretylium can cause hypotension, nausea, vomiting, and diarrhea. Bretylium should be infused over 30–60 minutes to minimize these effects.

References

1. Schwartz JB, Keefe D, Harrison DC. Adverse effects of antiarrhythmic drugs. Drugs 1981;21(1):23–45.
2. Cooper JA, Frieden J. Bretylium tosylate. Am Heart J 1971;82(5):703–6.
3. Koch-Weser J. Drug therapy: bretylium. N Engl J Med 1979;300(9):473–7.
4. Rapeport WG. Clinical pharmacokinetics of bretylium. Clin Pharmacokinet 1985;10(3):248–56.
5. Taylor SH, Saxton C, Davies PS, Stoker JB. Bretylium tosylate in prevention of cardiac dysrhythmias after myocardial infarction. Br Heart J 1970;32(3):326–9.
6. Anderson JL, Popat KD, Pitt B. Paradoxical ventricular tachycardia and fibrillation after intravenous bretylium

therapy. Report of two cases. Arch Intern Med 1981;141(6):801–2.
7. Heinrich KW, Effert S. Bretylium-Tosylat zur Behandlung maligner Arrhythmien: erste Resultate. [Bretylium tosylate in the therapy of malignant arrhythmia. First results.] Med Welt 1973;24(24):1000–2.
8. Thibault J. Hyperthermia associated with bretylium tosylate injection. Clin Pharm 1989;8(2):145–6.
9. Perlman PE, Adams WG Jr, Ridgeway NA. Extreme pyrexia during bretylium administration. Postgrad Med 1989; 85(1):111–14.

Brimonidine

General Information

Brimonidine is a highly selective potent alpha$_2$-adrenoceptor agonist, which is distinguished from clonidine by a chemical modification that reduces its ability to cross the blood–brain barrier. Like apraclonidine, brimonidine has been used to treat glaucoma. However, unlike apraclonidine, it both reduces aqueous humor production and increases aqueous outflow through the uveoscleral pathway.

The most common adverse effects of brimonidine are dry mouth, fatigue/drowsiness, and blurring of vision, which occurred significantly more often with brimonidine 0.5% than 0.2% (1,2). It can also cause allergic conjunctivitis and ocular pruritus (3). Brimonidine causes fewer adverse effects than apraclonidine, and, because it is a highly selective alpha$_2$-adrenoceptor agonist, does not cause mydriasis, lid retraction, or conjunctival blanching/rebound hyperemia (4). It is less polar than apraclonidine and is therefore more likely to cross the blood–brain barrier. However, symptoms of fatigue can occur.

Organs and Systems

Sensory systems

In a comparison with timolol, brimonidine had similar efficacy but produced more ocular allergic reactions, oral dryness, and conjunctival follicles (5). In a comparison with betaxolol 0.25% suspension, brimonidine 0.2% solution was more effective, but with a similar overall incidence of adverse effects (6).

Susceptibility Factors

Age

Brimonidine should be avoided in children, because apnea and hypotension occur.

- A 1-month-old infant with Peters anomaly had recurrent episodes of unresponsiveness, hypotension, hypotonia, and bradycardia (7). Extensive medical evaluation showed that these episodes were caused by the ophthalmic use of brimonidine.

References

1. Wilensky JT. The role of brimonidine in the treatment of open-angle glaucoma. Surv Ophthalmol 1996;41(Suppl 1): S3–7.
2. Walters TR. Development and use of brimonidine in treating acute and chronic elevations of intraocular pressure: a review of safety, efficacy, dose response, and dosing studies. Surv Ophthalmol 1996;41(Suppl 1):S19–26.
3. Chernin T. The eyes have it. FDA clears several ophthalmic drops for glaucoma in a row. Drug Topics 2001;145:20.
4. Doyle JW, Smith MF. New aqueous inflow inhibitors. Semin Ophthalmol 1999;14(3):159–63.
5. Schuman JS. Clinical experience with brimonidine 0.2% and timolol 0.5% in glaucoma and ocular hypertension. Surv Ophthalmol 1996;41(Suppl 1):S27–37.
6. Serle JB. A comparison of the safety and efficacy of twice daily brimonidine 0.2% versus betaxolol 0.25% in subjects with elevated intraocular pressure. The Brimonidine Study Group III. Surv Ophthalmol 1996;41(Suppl 1):S39–47.
7. Berlin RJ, Lee UT, Samples JR, Rich LF, Tang-Liu DD, Sing KA, Steiner RD. Ophthalmic drops causing coma in an infant. J Pediatr 2001;138(3):441–3.

Brofaromine

See also Monoamine oxidase inhibitors

General Information

Brofaromine is a selective inhibitor of monoamine oxidase (MAO) type A. In an open study in endogenous depression, adverse effects were reported in nine of 51 patients; these included dry mouth, dizziness, tremor, hypomania, anxiety, and memory problems (SEDA-17, 16).

A randomized comparison of brofaromine with imipramine in inpatients with major depression showed that brofaromine was as effective as imipramine in the treatment of major depression but had a different adverse effects profile (1). Brofaromine was more likely to cause sleep disturbances but lacked the anticholinergic and certain cardiovascular adverse effects of imipramine.

Reference

1 Volz HP, Gleiter CH, Moller HJ. Brofaromine versus imipramine in in-patients with major depression—a controlled trial. J Affect Disord 1997;44(2–3):91–9.

Bromazepam

See also Benzodiazepines

General Information

Bromazepam, a moderately short-acting benzodiazepine (half-life about 12 hours), has been used in the treatment of anxiety states and has the usual effects of benzodiazepines, for example amnesia and depressed psychomotor performance, although it causes less depression than lorazepam (SED-12, 98).

Organs and Systems

Nervous system

The mechanism of rare extrapyramidal effects with bromazepam is unexplained (SEDA-18, 44).

Long-Term Effects

Drug withdrawal

Catatonia has been described as an effect of bromazepam withdrawal (1).

- A 51-year-old man who had been taking bromazepam for 9 years in a dosage that he had gradually increased to 18 mg/day abruptly stopped taking it. He initially developed psychotic symptoms and on day 5 after withdrawal became mute and was posturing. A provisional diagnosis of a catatonic syndrome was made, and he was given oral lorazepam 3 mg and risperidone 4 mg. It was later concluded that the catatonia had most probably been due to benzodiazepine withdrawal; the risperidone was withdrawn, and diazepam was substituted for lorazepam and slowly tapered. He had no recurrence of catatonic or psychotic symptoms and his fatigue improved.

Withdrawal-induced seizures have been described in a woman taking various benzodiazepines (2).

- A 43-year-old woman had had insomnia since she was a child. At the age of 15, benzodiazepine therapy improved her sleeping, but when she gradually stopped taking benzodiazepines the insomnia returned after a few days. At the age of 26 she was abusing several benzodiazepines, including diazepam and flunitrazepam. At the age of 30 she was taking high doses of bromazepam every evening before going to sleep. After 1 month, she abruptly stopped taking bromazepam and during withdrawal had an epileptic seizure. During the next few years, she had periods of relative well-being, but also two further periods of benzodiazepine abuse, both resulting in seizures after withdrawal. She later had withdrawal seizures with zolpidem.

Drug Administration

Drug overdose

A fatal overdose of bromazepam has been reported (3).

- A 42-year-old woman with a history of depression was found unconscious, lying near her car. The lower part of her body was undressed and there were multiple purple spots and excoriations on her body, suggesting a sexual assault. She was hypothermic (core temperature 28.4°C). Her plasma bromazepam concentration was 7.7 mg/l, the highest concentration reported in a case of fatal intoxication.

Drug–Drug Interactions

Fluconazole

The interaction of bromazepam with fluconazole has been studied in 12 healthy men in a randomized, double-blind, four-way crossover study (4). The subjects took a single oral or rectal dose of bromazepam (3 mg) after pretreatment for 4 days with oral fluconazole 100 mg/day or placebo. Pharmacodynamic effects of bromazepam were assessed using self-rated drowsiness, the continuous number addition test, and electroencephalography. After rectal administration there was a higher AUC (1.7-fold) and a higher C_{max} (1.6-fold) than after oral administration; there were electroencephalographic effects and subjective drowsiness after rectal bromazepam, and the electroencephalographic effects correlated closely with mean plasma bromazepam concentrations. However, fluconazole caused no significant changes in the pharmacokinetics or pharmacodynamics of oral or rectal bromazepam.

References

1. Deuschle M, Lederbogen F. Benzodiazepine withdrawal-induced catatonia. Pharmacopsychiatry 2001;34(1):41–2.
2. Aragona M. Abuse, dependence, and epileptic seizures after zolpidem withdrawal. Review and case report. Clin Neuropharmacol 2000;23(5):281–3.
3. Michaud K, Romain N, Giroud C, Brandt C, Mangin P. Hypothermia and undressing associated with non-fatal bromazepam intoxication. Forensic Sci Int 2001;124(2–3):112–14.
4. Ohtani Y, Kotegawa T, Tsutsumi K, Morimoto T, Hirose Y, Nakano S. Effect of fluconazole on the pharmacokinetics and pharmacodynamics of oral and rectal bromazepam: an application of electroencephalography as the pharmacodynamic method. J Clin Pharmacol 2002;42(2):183–91.

Bromfenac sodium

See also Non-steroidal anti-inflammatory drugs

General Information

Bromfenac sodium (2-amino-3-(4-bromo-benzoyl)-benzeneacetic acid sodium salt sesquihydrate) has a safety profile apparently similar to that of other NSAIDs (SEDA-17, 109) (SEDA-21, 104). It was approved by the FDA in 1997 for short-term management of acute pain, but was withdrawn by the manufacturers in 1998.

Organs and Systems

Liver

In June 1998 bromfenac was withdrawn from the market because of postmarketing reports of severe hepatic failure, resulting in four deaths and eight liver transplants (SEDA-22, 115). Descriptions of some cases have appeared (1–4).

References

1. Moses PL, Schroeder B, Alkhatib O, Ferrentino N, Suppan T, Lidofsky SD. Severe hepatotoxicity associated with bromfenac sodium. Am J Gastroenterol 1999;94(5):1393–6.
2. Rabkin JM, Smith MJ, Orloff SL, Corless CL, Stenzel P, Olyaei AJ. Fatal fulminant hepatitis associated with bromfenac use. Ann Pharmacother 1999;33(9):945–7.
3. Hunter EB, Johnston PE, Tanner G, Pinson CW, Awad JA. Bromfenac (Duract)-associated hepatic failure requiring liver transplantation. Am J Gastroenterol 1999;94(8):2299–301.
4. Fontana RJ, McCashland TM, Benner KG, Appelman HD, Gunartanam NT, Wisecarver JL, Rabkin JM, Lee WM. Acute liver failure associated with prolonged use of bromfenac leading to liver transplantation. The Acute Liver Failure Study Group. Liver Transpl Surg 1999;5(6):480–4.

Bromhexine

General Information

Bromhexine is taken orally or by aerosol and reduces sputum viscosity as measured ex vivo. Although it is still used empirically by some physicians, there have been no controlled studies showing a significant improvement in clinical status or lung function. Administration by inhalation aerosol or nasal spray produces a local expectorant/mucolytic effect (1). Inhaled bromhexine (Paxirasol) reduces the amount of sputum, but does not reduce symptoms (SEDA-17, 208).

Organs and Systems

Gastrointestinal

Bromhexine can cause gastrointestinal intolerance and impair the mucous barrier in the stomach; it has been suggested it should not be given to patients with gastric ulceration. Reactivation of ulcers has been reported in a few patients, but hematemesis, melena, or other complications have not been described (2).

Drug–Drug Interactions

Antibiotics

Bromhexine increases the concentration of amoxicillin in the sputum (SEDA-17, 208) and promotes the diffusion of antibiotics into lung tissue (1).

References

1. Nagy G. The use of Paxirasol in clinical practice. Ther Hung 1993;41(3):100–6.
2. Jorgensen PH. Bromhexin. En genvurdering ud fra litteraturen. [Bromhexine. An evaluation of the literature.] Ugeskr Laeger 1982;144(18):1327–9.

Bromocriptine

General Information

Bromocriptine is an ergot derivative. High doses (for example 30–75 mg/day orally) are used in Parkinson's disease; low doses (2.5–5.0 mg/day) are used for prostatic tumors and to suppress lactation. The adverse reactions are dose-dependent and, so far as is known, reversible, but they are frequent, being experienced in up to 50% of cases. At any dose, nausea, vomiting, and postural hypotension are problematic in some patients, especially those who take high doses from the start. The gastrointestinal symptoms tend to abate as treatment is continued, but other symptoms, for example peripheral circulatory disturbances, can occur later. Psychic and psychiatric changes can be troublesome in a proportion of patients on high doses. Constipation tends to be a frequent and persistent complication.

Organs and Systems

Cardiovascular

Occasionally, patients taking low doses have postural hypotension, leading to dizziness or syncope. Raynaud's syndrome, with blanching of the extremities in response to cold, is rare. At high doses some 30% suffer a peripheral cold reaction of this type, which may not become manifest for a time, while leg cramps occur in some 10% of cases. Under 10% of patients have flushing or erythromelalgia, and hypotension occurs in some 5%. Occasional cases of bradycardia or acute left ventricular failure have been described. Patients with angina pectoris can experience aggravation of their symptoms (SED-12, 317). Even acute myocardial infarction after coronary spasm has been reported (SEDA-12, 123) (SED-12, 317).

Bromocriptine has been associated with myocardial infarction, presumably because of coronary artery spasm.

- A 29-year-old woman took bromocriptine 5 mg/day postpartum to suppress lactation (1). Four days later she developed an acute anterior myocardial infarction. Angiography showed dissection of the left main and anterior descending arteries, with occlusion of the latter. She recovered after emergency arterial grafting.
- A 21-year-old woman had an inferior myocardial infarction, in the absence of cardiovascular risks and with normal coronary arteries on angiography (2). She made a good recovery, but with some persistent posterior-wall akinesia.

In another similar case the myocardial infarction proved fatal (3).

- A 30-year-old woman collapsed and died after a first dose of bromocriptine 2.5 mg. She had severe atheroma narrowing the right coronary artery proximal to the site of thrombosis. The only obvious risk factor was heavy smoking, 30 cigarettes per day.
- A 38-year-old woman had an acute occlusion of the right popliteal artery, which gradually resolved without surgical intervention after treatment with

vasodilators, anticoagulants, and antiplatelet drugs (none of which were specified) (2). Her serum cholesterol concentration was 8 mmol/l, but she had no other risk factors.

Myocardial infarction occurred postpartum in two women taking bromocriptine (4).

- A 33-year-old woman taking bromocriptine 5 mg/day for suppression of lactation was given ergotamine 2.25 mg for acute migraine, having taken ergotamine intermittently for over 20 years. She had a myocardial infarction involving the left anterior descending coronary artery, without apparent pre-existing atherosclerosis. She made a good recovery following thrombolysis.
- A 29-year-old woman taking bromocriptine 5 mg/day postpartum had a dissection of the left anterior descending coronary artery and needed emergency bypass grafting. She made a good recovery.

These cases emphasize the potential danger of these drugs, even in young and apparently healthy individuals, although in the first case the use of two ergot derivatives simultaneously may have been ill-advised.

Edema can occur with this and other dopamine receptor agonists, the association easily being overlooked (SEDA-18, 159).

Fibrotic complications can extend to the heart, resulting in constrictive pericarditis.

Respiratory

Pulmonary reactions are rare. Pleural thickening and effusions and pleuropulmonary fibrosis have been observed in a few cases (SEDA-11, 130).

Ear, nose, throat

Nasal congestion can uncommonly occur with bromocriptine (5).

Nervous system

The high doses used in Parkinson's disease are perhaps slightly less well tolerated than equieffective doses of levodopa.

Dyskinesias can occur with bromocriptine but less often than with equieffective doses of levodopa (6).

Bromocriptine has been used successfully in patients with unilateral motor neglect, usually after a stroke.

- A 58-year-old man had a right middle cerebral artery infarction leading to, among many other neurological deficits, left-sided neglect (7). When he took bromocriptine 20 mg/day this abnormality worsened and then improved again on withdrawal.

The authors suggested that this may have been due to damage to the right putamen, while bromocriptine could still activate the striatum on the left, aggravating the hemispheric bias.

In the USA, bromocriptine has not been licensed for the suppression of lactation since 1994. Up to that time there had been no reports of intracranial hemorrhage associated with bromocriptine, but since the withdrawal of the license for this indication there have been 15 case reports of this disastrous adverse effect.

- Three women aged 22, 24, and 40 years took bromocriptine 2.5 mg bd for 2–5 days postpartum and complained of headache; two lost consciousness (8). One subsequently died and another had a residual neurological deficit. In all three cases intracerebral hemorrhage, confirmed by CT or MRI scans, occurred on the sixth day of administration. Maximal recorded blood pressures were 200/100, 173/120, and 180/118 mmHg.

Three cases of contractures of the extremities were possibly caused by bromocriptine (SEDA-14, 119).

Occasionally, paresthesia and bad dreams have been described.

When the manufacturers examined reports from physicians on adverse effects from bromocriptine in inhibition of lactation, there were 38 cases of seizures (9).

A cerebral angiopathy postpartum was also described (10).

Cerebrospinal fluid rhinorrhea has been described as an interesting but highly unusual sequel of bromocriptine administration (SEDA-8, 143). The reverse effect, air aspiration through a sellar-pharyngeal leak, has also been encountered (SEDA-9, 126).

Sensory systems

In one series, three of 18 patients developed blurred vision during high-dose treatment of Parkinson's disease (SEDA-3, 124). Diplopia has been incidentally reported. In three patients with chronic hepatic encephalopathy, reversible ototoxicity developed after the administration of bromocriptine (11).

Psychological, psychiatric

Up to 10% of patients have to be withdrawn from treatment because of psychiatric symptoms. Bromocriptine-induced psychosis is well known and particular caution is warranted in patients with a family history of mental disorders (12). Even very low doses of bromocriptine can cause psychotic reactions (SEDA-9, 126) (SEDA-10, 117), and well-recognized problems include confusion, hallucinations, delusions, and paranoia.

Endocrine

Inappropriate secretion of ADH has been described in a single patient (13).

Hematologic

One case of leukopenia and thrombocytopenia has been described (14).

Gastrointestinal

Nausea and vomiting are common with bromocriptine (15).

Liver

In one series, six of 18 patients taking high doses for Parkinson's disease developed isolated and asymptomatic increases in serum transaminases (SED-12, 317). Other

patients have also had this reaction, which is reversible (SEDA-17, 168).

Skin

- A 28-year-old woman taking bromocriptine 5 mg/day for a microprolactinoma developed numerous nodular skin lesions (16). Skin biopsy showed a polyclonal proliferation of both B and T lymphocytes in a follicular pattern, and a diagnosis of cutaneous pseudolymphoma was made. The lesions disappeared within 8 weeks of withdrawal.

Alopecia, reversible after drug withdrawal, has been reported as a rare effect of bromocriptine (SEDA-18, 159).

Hair

Treatment with bromocriptine has very rarely been associated with reversible alopecia (17).

Serosae

Retroperitoneal fibrosis (SEDA-12, 123) (18) and pulmonary fibrosis (SEDA-11, 130) during treatment with high doses of bromocriptine have been observed. The drug's structural relation to methysergide clearly has to be kept in mind. Pleural thickening and effusions can be present in up to 6% of patients treated with bromocriptine for Parkinson's disease, and this is related to duration of exposure and cumulative dose (19). The author recommended drug withdrawal in these patients. However, withdrawal does not always lead to complete resolution of the lesions (20).

- A 63-year-old woman with Parkinson's disease developed bilateral pleural thickening and effusions with interstitial shadowing in the lungs 4 years after starting treatment with bromocriptine. After replacement of the drug by levodopa there was gradual improvement, but some pleural thickening remained nearly 3 years later.

Constrictive pericarditis has also been reported.

- Constrictive pericarditis occurred in two men aged 63 and 69 years treated respectively with bromocriptine 40 mg/day for 4 years and 30 mg/day for 2 years (21). Pericardiectomy was performed in both cases, but bromocriptine was not suspected at that time. In one case the drug was continued until a pleural effusion occurred 7 months later; in the other withdrawal of bromocriptine was prompted by an episode of confusion just before pericardiectomy.

Sexual function

Increased sexual drive in patients with Parkinson's disease is common, but bromocriptine can also cause impotence, which can respond to dosage reduction (SEDA-13, 111).

Immunologic

- An allergic reaction was attributed to bromocriptine in a 26-year-old woman with a prolactin-secreting microadenoma (22).

Long-Term Effects

Mutagenicity

No chromosomal changes were found in 19 children born after bromocriptine-induced ovulation (23).

Tumorigenicity

In rats (but not in mice) high doses of bromocriptine induced malignant uterine tumors within 2 years (SEDA-3, 122). Tumor induction has not been seen in man, but enlargement of a non-invasive pituitary tumor has been observed on more than one occasion.

Second-Generation Effects

Fertility

Sudden induction of fertility in sterile women can occasionally be an embarrassing adverse reaction if the drug is being used for other purposes, for example Parkinson's disease.

Fetotoxicity

Because of its use in the treatment of female infertility, which inevitably involves early exposure of some embryos, the safety of bromocriptine in early pregnancy has been systematically evaluated in a large multicenter study with prolonged follow-up (SEDA-13, 112). There was no evidence that this use of bromocriptine was associated with an increased risk of spontaneous abortion, multiple pregnancy, or the occurrence of congenital malformations; nor did exposure in utero seem to have any adverse effects on postnatal development. Cervical incompetence may be a problem at the time of delivery, but this may well be due to a long history of infertility rather than to the drug itself.

Lactation

Bromocriptine suppresses lactation and the infant should not be breast-fed from the moment treatment is begun. If bromocriptine is deliberately (and successfully) used to suppress lactation, breast tenderness and milk leakage can ensue. It has been suggested that the use of bromocriptine for this purpose raises the risk of postpartum seizures, but the evidence is equivocal (SEDA-17, 146).

Susceptibility Factors

If bromocriptine is to be used to treat infertility, the presence of a pituitary adenoma must be excluded, since this can otherwise undergo suprasellar extension during pregnancy. Because of its adverse reactions profile, bromocriptine is better avoided in patients with cardiac disease or peripheral vascular disease. Acromegaly in patients with a history of gastrointestinal ulceration or bleeding should not be treated with bromocriptine; generally, however, it seems to be rather better tolerated by patients with acromegaly, as well as by postmenopausal women and patients with a raised serum prolactin concentration than by other patients.

It is thought that bromocriptine may aggravate hypertension of pregnancy (SEDA-15, 2); this has led to

hesitation over the continued use of bromocriptine for suppression of lactation, especially in patients with a history of pregnancy-induced hypertension.

Cocaine abusers, it is thought, may develop cerebrovascular and cardiovascular disorders if they take bromocriptine (24,25).

Drug Administration

Drug administration route

Intravaginal administration, sometimes used to reduce gastric adverse effects, has caused a vaginal burning sensation in a few patients (26).

Drug–Drug Interactions

Griseofulvin

The response to bromocriptine, at least in acromegaly, can be blocked by griseofulvin (27).

Pseudoephedrine

Psychosis has been described in a 19-year-old postpartum woman who took bromocriptine and pseudoephedrine (28).

Sympathicomimetic drugs

Dangerous hypertensive reactions can result from interactions with the sympathicomimetic drugs isometheptene and phenylpropanolamine (SEDA-17, 168).

Tamoxifen

Tamoxifen can resolve some of bromocriptine's adverse effects, offering the possibility of bromocriptine treatment to patients who cannot otherwise tolerate it (SEDA-8, 144).

References

1. Hoppe UC, Beuckelmann DJ, Bohm M, Erdmann E. A young mother with severe chest pain. Heart 1998;79(2):205.
2. Matas O, Coppere B, Dupin AC, Richalet F, Ninet J. Accidents ischémiques artériels associés à la bromocriptine. [Ischemic arterial accidents associated with bromocriptine.] JEUR 1999;1:32.
3. Dutt S, Wong F, Spurway JH. Fatal myocardial infarction associated with bromocriptine for postpartum lactation suppression. Aust NZ J Obstet Gynaecol 1998;38(1):116–17.
4. Lindner M, Rosenkranz S, Deutsch HJ, Erdmann E. Ergotamininduzierter postpartaler Myokardinfarct. [Ergotamin-induced post partum myocardial infarction.] Herz Kreisl 2000;32:65–8.
5. Jenkins PJ, Jain A, Jones SL, Besser GM, Grossman AB. Oral prednisolone supplement abolishes the acute adverse effects following initiation of depot bromocriptine therapy. Clin Endocrinol (Oxf) 1996;45(4):447–51.
6. Kondo T. Initial therapy for Parkinson's disease: levodopa vs. dopamine receptor agonists. J Neurol 2002;249(Suppl 2):II25–9.
7. Barrett AM, Crucian GP, Schwartz RL, Heilman KM. Adverse effect of dopamine agonist therapy in a patient with motor-intentional neglect. Arch Phys Med Rehabil 1999;80(5):600–3.

8. Kirsch C, Iffy L, Zito GE, McArdle JJ. The role of hypertension in bromocriptine-related puerperal intracranial hemorrhage. Neuroradiology 2001;43(4):302–4.

9. Anonymous. Postpartum hypertension, seizures, strokes reported with bromocriptine. FDA Drug Bull 1984;14(1):3–4.

10. Chartier JP, Bousigue JY, Teisseyre A, Morel C, Delpuech-Formosa F. [Postpartum cerebral angiopathy of iatrogenic origin.] Rev Neurol (Paris) 1997;153(3):212–14.

11. Lanthier PL, Morgan MY, Ballantyne J. Bromocriptine-associated ototoxicity. J Laryngol Otol 1984;98(4):399–404.

12. Le Feuvre CM, Isaacs AJ, Frank OS. Bromocriptine-induced psychosis in acromegaly. BMJ (Clin Res Ed) 1982;285(6351):1315.

13. Damase-Michel C, Sarrail E, Laens J, et al. Hyponatraemia in a patient treated with bromocriptine. Drug Invest 1993;5:285–7.

14. Giampietro O, Ferdeghini M, Petrini M. Severe leukopenia and mild thrombocytopenia after chronic bromocriptine (CB-154) administration. Am J Med Sci 1981;281(3):169–72.

15. Wilson JD, Montgomery DA, Buchanan KD. Gastrointestinal side-effects of bromocriptine. Ir J Med Sci 1980;149(12):475–8.

16. Wiesli P, Joos L, Galeazzi RL, Dummer R. Cutaneous pseudolymphoma associated with bromocriptine therapy. Clin Endocrinol (Oxf) 2000;53(5):656–7.

17. Fabre N, Montastruc JL, Rascol O. Alopecia: an adverse effect of bromocriptine. Clin Neuropharmacol 1993;16(3):266–8.

18. Hardy JC, Chevalier C, Kains JP. Fibrose rétropéritonéale. A propos de troi cas dont deux induits par la bromocriptine. [Retroperitoneal fibrosis. Apropos of 3 cases 2 of which were induced by bromocriptine.] Acta Urol Belg 1991;59(3):95–103.

19. Yaksh TL. A drug has to do what a drug has to do. Anesth Analg 1999;89(5):1075–7.

20. Faigle JW, Keberle H, Degen PH. Chemistry and pharmacokinetics of baclofen. In: Feldman RG, Young RR, Koella WP, editors. Spasticity: Disordered Motor Control. Chicago: Year Book, 1980:461–75.

21. Champagne S, Coste E, Peyriere H, Nigond J, Mania E, Pons M, Hillaire-Buys D, Balmes P, Blayac JP, Davy JM. Chronic constrictive pericarditis induced by long-term bromocriptine therapy: report of two cases. Ann Pharmacother 1999;33(10):1050–4.

22. Merola B, Sarnacchiaro F, Colao A, Di Sarno A, Di Somma C, Schettini G, Lombardi G. Allergy to ergot-derived dopamine agonists. Lancet 1992;339(8793):620.

23. Schellekens LA, Snuiverink H, Van den Berghe H. Chromosomal patterns of children born after induction of ovulation with bromocriptine. Arzneimittelforschung 1977;27(11):2151–3.

24. Bakht FR, Kirshon B, Baker T, Cotton DB. Postpartum cardiovascular complications after bromocriptine and cocaine use. Am J Obstet Gynecol 1990;162(4):1065–6.

25. Miller LG, Bakht FR, Baker T, Kirshon B. Possible cocaine predisposition to adverse cerebrovascular and cardiovascular sequelae of bromocriptine administered postpartum. J Clin Pharmacol 1989;29(9):781–5.

26. Jasonni VM, Raffelli R, de March A, Frank G, Flamigni C. Vaginal bromocriptine in hyperprolactinemic patients and puerperal women. Acta Obstet Gynecol Scand 1991;70(6):493–5.

27. Schwinn G, Dirks H, McIntosh C, Kobberling J. Metabolic and clinical studies on patients with acromegaly treated with bromocriptine over 22 months. Eur J Clin Invest 1977;7(2):101–7.

28. Reeves RR, Pinkofsky HB. Postpartum psychosis induced by bromocriptine and pseudoephedrine. J Fam Pract 1997;45(2):164–6.

Brompheniramine

See also Antihistamines

General Information

Brompheniramine is a first-generation antihistamine, an alkylamine derivative, with antimuscarinic and moderate sedative actions.

Long-Term Effects

Drug withdrawal

Withdrawal symptoms resembling cholinergic rebound (nausea, tremor, and sweating) have been described after long-term brompheniramine treatment (1).

Reference

1. Kavanagh GM, Charlwood MR, Peachey RD. Withdrawal symptoms after discontinuation of long-acting brompheniramine maleate. Br J Dermatol 1994;131(6):913–14.

Bropirimine

General Information

Oral bropirimine is an immunostimulant that has been used in the management of transitional cell carcinoma of the bladder and upper urinary tract. It is supposedly an interferon inducer. In clinical trials, bropirimine produced mild adverse effects in about 30% of patients. Nausea or vomiting were the most common (21% of patients), and headache, transient liver enzyme rises, skin rash, and arthralgia were observed in 5–14% (1). Tachycardia or chest pain occurred in 5%. Adverse effects required drug withdrawal in 15% of patients (2).

Oral bropirimine (3 g/day thrice weekly for 1 year) has been compared with weekly intravesical Bacillus Calmette-Guérin (2 cycles of 6 weeks) in 55 patients with newly diagnosed bladder carcinoma (3). Whereas the response to treatment was not significantly different between the two groups, adverse effects resulted in more withdrawals with BCG than bropirimine (14 versus 4%). Bropirimine produced more frequent systemic reactions (in particular diarrhea, fever, flu-like syndrome, headache, nausea/vomiting) but less frequent and less severe local complications.

References

1. Sarosdy MF, Lowe BA, Schellhammer PF, Lamm DL, Graham SD Jr, Grossman HB, See WA, Peabody JO, Moon TD, Flanigan RC, Crawford ED, Morganroth J. Oral bropirimine immunotherapy of carcinoma in situ of the bladder: results of a phase II trial. Urology 1996;48(1):21–7.

2. Sarosdy MF, Manyak MJ, Sagalowsky AI, Belldegrun A, Benson MC, Bihrle W, Carroll PR, Ellis WJ, Hudson MA,

Sharkey FE. Oral bropirimine immunotherapy of bladder carcinoma in situ after prior intravesical bacille Calmette-Guerin. Urology 1998;51(2):226–31.

3. Witjes WP, Konig M, Boeminghaus FP, Hall RR, Schulman CC, Zurlo M, Fittipaldo A, Riggi M, Debruyne FM. Results of a European comparative randomized study comparing oral bropirimine versus intravesical BCG treatment in BCG-naive patients with carcinoma in situ of the urinary bladder. European Bropirimine Study Group. Eur Urol 1999;36(6):576–81.

Bryostatins

General Information

Bryostatins are naturally occurring antineoplastic macrocyclic lactones derived from the marine invertebrate *Bugula neritina*, different varieties being isolated from different populations of the same species. More than 13 structurally related compounds have been isolated (1,2), and there is a variety of synthetic analogues (3). The bryostatins modulate the activity of protein kinase C.

Bryostatin 1 binds to the regulatory domain of protein kinase C; short-term exposure promotes activation of protein kinase C, whereas prolonged exposure promotes significant down-regulation (4). In preclinical and phase I clinical studies it had promising antitumor and immunomodulating effects. It amplifies expansion of myeloid and erythroid progenitor cells stimulated by the cytokines GM-CSF, M-CSF, and IL-3. Similarly, it induces the production of peripheral blood mononuclear cells with enhanced lymphokine-activated killer cell activity and proliferation in the presence of IL-2 (5).

In a phase II study, 17 patients with progressive indolent non-Hodgkin's lymphoma, previously treated with chemotherapy, received bryostatin 1 (5). Phlebitis was initially due to the 60% ethanol formulation used for administration, and the subsequent use of another formulation (60% polyethylene glycol, 30% ethanol, 10% Tween 80) reduced the incidence. In one patient, bryostatin 1 was withdrawn because of grade 2 thrombocytopenia. The dose-limiting adverse effect was myalgia, which occurred in eight patients.

Other adverse effects include fatigue, nausea, headache, vomiting, dyspnea, ataxia, anorexia, anemia, and lymphopenia (6–8).

In a phase-II study, 14 patients with metastatic cervical cancer or recurrent disease not eligible for surgery or radiation received bryostatin 1 $50–65 \, \mu g/m^2$ + cisplatin $50 \, mg/m^2$. The most common adverse effects were myalgia, anemia, and nausea or vomiting; one patient had a hypersensitivity reaction and one developed grade 3 nephrotoxicity (9).

Organs and Systems

Skin

Adverse effects of bryostatin 1 on the skin reported during phase I and II studies were alopecia, mucositis, non-specific rashes, bronzing, and hyperpigmentation in sun-exposed areas; a morbilliform eruption has also been reported (10).

Musculoskeletal

In a phase-I trial of bryostatin 1 as a 24-hour continuous infusion followed by bolus vincristine in 24 patients with refractory B cell malignancies other than acute leukemias, the dose-limiting adverse effect was myalgia (11).

References

1. Davidson SK, Haygood MG. Identification of sibling species of the bryozoan *Bugula neritina* that produce different anticancer bryostatins and harbor distinct strains of the bacterial symbiont "*Candidatus endobugula sertula*." Biol Bull 1999;196(3):273–80

2. Mutter R, Wills M. Chemistry and clinical biology of the bryostatins. Bioorg Med Chem 2000;8(8):1841–60.

3. Wender PA, Hinkle KW, Koehler MF, Lippa B. The rational design of potential chemotherapeutic agents: synthesis of bryostatin analogues. Med Res Rev 1999;19(5):388–407.

4. Kortmansky J, Schwartz GK. Bryostatin-1: a novel PKC inhibitor in clinical development. Cancer Invest 2003;21(6):924–36.

5. Blackhall FH, Ranson M, Radford JA, Hancock BW, Soukop M, McGown AT, Robbins A, Halbert G, Jayson GC; Cancer Research Campaign Phase I/II Committee. A phase II trial of bryostatin 1 in patients with non-Hodgkin's lymphoma. Br J Cancer 2001;84(4):465–9.

6. Madhusudan S, Protheroe A, Propper D, Han C, Corrie P, Earl H, Hancock B, Vasey P, Turner A, Balkwill F, Hoare S, Harris AL. A multicentre phase II trial of bryostatin-1 in patients with advanced renal cancer. Br J Cancer 2003;89(8):1418–22.

7. Armstrong DK, Blessing JA, Rader J, Sorosky JI; Gynecologic Oncology Group Study. A randomized phase II evaluation of bryostatin-1 (NSC #339555) in persistent or recurrent squamous cell carcinoma of the cervix: a Gynecologic Oncology Group Study. Invest New Drugs 2003;21(4):453–7.

8. Haas NB, Smith M, Lewis N, Littman L, Yeslow G, Joshi ID, Murgo A, Bradley J, Gordon R, Wang H, Rogatko A, Hudes GR. Weekly bryostatin-1 in metastatic renal cell carcinoma: a phase II study. Clin Cancer Res 2003;9(1):109–14.

9. Nezhat F, Wadler S, Muggia F, Mandeli J, Goldberg G, Rahaman J, Runowicz C, Murgo AJ, Gardner GJ. Phase II trial of the combination of bryostatin-1 and cisplatin in advanced or recurrent carcinoma of the cervix: a New York Gynecologic Oncology Group study. Gynecol Oncol 2004;93(1):144–8.

10. Krejci-Manwaring JM, Bogle MA, Diwan HA, Duvic MA. Morbilliform drug reaction with histologic features of pustular dermatosis associated with bryostatin-1. J Drugs Dermatol 2003;2(5):557–61.

11. Dowlati A, Lazarus HM, Hartman P, Jacobberger JW, Whitacre C, Gerson SL, Ksenich P, Cooper BW, Frisa PS, Gottlieb M, Murgo AJ, Remick SC. Phase I and correlative study of combination bryostatin 1 and vincristine in relapsed B cell malignancies. Clin Cancer Res 2003;9(16 Pt 1):5929–35.

Bucillamine

General Information

Bucillamine (mercaptomethylpropanoylcysteine) is chemically related to penicillamine and is also used in rheumatoid arthritis. Most of the information on bucillamine comes from Japan, its country of origin (1).

The patterns of adverse reactions to sulfhydryl compounds that are used in rheumatoid arthritis (bucillamine, pyritinol, and tiopronin) show remarkable similarities to those of penicillamine (SED-12, 548) (2).

Organs and Systems

Respiratory

In 10 patients with bucillamine-associated interstitial pneumonitis, the HLA antigen DR4 was present in all 10 and a positive lymphocyte stimulation test was found in three of the six patients tested (3).

Nervous system

Myasthenia gravis has been reported during the use of bucillamine (4). However, since the disease persisted after withdrawal, the role of the drug was uncertain.

Sensory systems

A change in taste has been attributed to bucillamine in a single case, without further specification (1).

Hematologic

Among 36 Korean patients with rheumatoid arthritis agranulocytosis with high fever developed in one after 3-week use of bucillamine (dose not specified) (5).

Gastrointestinal

Stomatitis, nausea, anorexia, and epigastric discomfort are common during the use of bucillamine (5).

Hemorrhagic gastritis has been reported in a single case, without further specification (1).

Liver

Increased aminotransferase activities were found in about 5% of patients using bucillamine for rheumatoid arthritis (1,5).

Urinary tract

Proteinuria occurs in about 7% of patients using bucillamine (1). Less often, nephrotic syndrome can develop (5–9). Microscopically there is membranous glomerulonephritis, with diffuse fine granular precipitation of IgG and C3 around the capillary walls, electron-dense deposits at the subepithelial side of the basement membrane and effacement of foot processes.

Skin

Bucillamine causes skin reactions in about 5% of patients (10). Rashes and pruritus are frequent and eosinophilia can occur (1,5).

Bullous pemphigoid has been attributed to bucillamine 200 mg/day (10). The mouth, pharynx, larynx, and conjunctiva were involved, as well as the skin on the chest, abdomen, and axilla. Indirect immunofluorescence showed circulating antibodies against the basement membrane.

There have been reports of bucillamine-associated pemphigus.

- A 57-year-old woman developed a generalized itchy rash 9 months after she started to take bucillamine (11). A skin biopsy showed spongiosis, lymphocytic infiltration in the epidermis, and intercellular deposition of IgG.
- Another patient had a pemphigus foliaceus-like eruption on three different occasions, in association with penicillamine, auranofin, and bucillamine (12).

A patient taking bucillamine developed an eruption that had features of both pemphigus foliaceus and pemphigus vulgaris and was associated with glomerulonephritis (13).

- A 62-year-old man with rheumatoid arthritis developed a rash on the neck, chest, and legs after taking oral bucillamine (dose not specified) for 6 months. The lesions were of two different types: small pigmented, vesicular, erythematous macules, similar to those of pemphigus foliaceus, and skin erosions, as seen in pemphigus vulgaris. There was no mucosal involvement. Serology was positive for antinuclear antibodies (1:320, nucleolar type). A biopsy showed acantholysis in the granular, spinous, and suprabasal layers. Direct immunofluorescence showed intercellular deposits of IgG and C3 throughout the epidermis, but not in the basement membrane. Indirect immunofluorescence of donor skin showed IgG reactivity in the nuclei of keratinocytes. An enzyme-linked immunoadsorbent assay (ELISA), using baculovirus-expressed recombinant desmogleins as antigen, was positive and indifferent to circulating anti-Dsg1 and anti-Dsg3 antibodies. This patient also had the nephrotic syndrome (proteinuria 8.7 g/day, total serum protein 59 g/l, serum total cholesterol 10.2 mmol/l), probably also due to bucillamine. A renal biopsy was consistent with membranous glomerulonephritis. The skin lesions improved within 1 month of bucillamine withdrawal, but full recovery of both cutaneous and renal injury was achieved only after the use of prednisone, 40 mg/day for 2 weeks.

In 13 patients with the peculiar yellow nail syndrome, bucillamine was the suspected cause in 7 (14).

Reproductive system

Gigantism of the breasts, probably induced by bucillamine, has been reported (15).

- After attempts with chrysotherapy and lobenzarit, a 24-year-old woman was given bucillamine 300 mg/day and a glucocorticoid, predonine, for rheumatoid arthritis. After 10 months she noticed bilateral breast enlargement, which over 6 months progressed to extreme proportions, the left breast ultimately reaching as far as her pubis. The skin of the breasts was thin and erythematous, with marked dilatation of the superficial veins. The nipple areola complexes were elongated and poorly defined from the surrounding skin. There were no abnormalities of prolactin, sex hormones, growth hormone, or TSH (but the values were not stated). Bilateral total mastectomy was performed and the nipple-areola complexes were removed from the resected tissue and grafted on to the breasts after insertion of a tissue expander. The breast tissue removed from the right side weighed 5 kg and that from the left side 7 kg. Histologically there was increased fibrosis and duct dilatation and no malignancy.

This effect, attributed here to bucillamine, is a rare but well-established adverse effect of penicillamine. Although the patient had also taken isoniazid for pulmonary tuberculosis, that was unlikely to have played a part, since the breast enlargement started earlier and progressed after the isoniazid had been withdrawn.

References

1. Takahashi C, Murasawi A, Nakazono K, Yoshida K, Sekiguchi H, Kikuchi M. An open clinical study of bucillamine in uncontrollable rheumatoid arthritis. Int J Immunother 1991;7:95–8.
2. Jaffe IA. Adverse effects profile of sulfhydryl compounds in man. Am J Med 1986;80(3):471–6.
3. Negishi M, Kaga S, Kasama T, Hashimoto M, Fukushima T, Yamagata N, Tabata M, Kobayashi K, Ide H, Takahashi T. [Lung injury associated with bucillamine therapy.] Ryumachi 1992;32(2):135–9.
4. Fujiyama J, Tokimura Y, Ijichi S, Arimura K, Matsuda T, Osame M. Bucillamine may induce myasthenia gravis. Jpn J Med 1991;30(1):101–2.
5. Kim SY, Lee IH, Bae SC, Yoo DH. Preliminary trial of the efficacy of bucillamine in Korean patients with rheumatoid arthritis. Clin Drug Invest 1995;9:284–90.
6. Yoshida A, Morozumi K, Suganuma T, Aoki J, Sugito K, Koyama K, Oikawa T, Fujinimi T, Matsumoto Y. [Clinicopathological study of nephropathy in patients with rheumatoid arthritis.] Ryumachi 1991;31(1):14–21.
7. Kawano M, Nomura H, Iwainaka Y, Nakashima A, Koni I, Tofuku Y, Takeda R. [Bucillamine-associated membranous nephropathy in a patient with rheumatoid arthritis.] Nippon Jinzo Gakkai Shi 1990;32(7):817–21.
8. Yoshida A, Morozumi K, Suganuma T, Sugito K, Ikeda M, Oikawa T, Fujinami T, Takeda A, Koyama K. Clinicopathological findings of bucillamine-induced nephrotic syndrome in patients with rheumatoid arthritis. Am J Nephrol 1991;11(4):284–8.
9. Baba N, Nomura T, Sakemi T, Uchida M, Watanabe T. [Membranous glomerulonephritis probably related to bucillamine therapy in two patients with rheumatoid arthritis.] Nippon Jinzo Gakkai Shi 1991;33(6):629–34.
10. Yamaguchi R, Oryu F, Hidano A. A case of bullous pemphigoid induced by tiobutarit (D-penicillamine analogue). J Dermatol 1989;16(4):308–11.
11. Amasaki Y, Sagawa A, Atsumi T, Jodo S, Nakabayashi T, Watanabe I, Mukai M, Fujisaku A, Nakagawa S, Kobayashi H. [A case of rheumatoid arthritis developing pemphigus-like skin lesion during treatment with bucillamine.] Ryumachi 1991;31(5):528–34.
12. Takashima T, Tani M. Antirheumatics-induced pemphigus foliaceus-like lesions. Hihu 1990;32:205–8.
13. Moreland LW, Russell AS, Paulus HE. Management of rheumatoid arthritis: the historical context. J Rheumatol 2001;28(6):1431–52.
14. Ichikawa Y, Shimizu H, Arimori S. "Yellow nail syndrome" and rheumatoid arthritis. Tokai J Exp Clin Med 1991;16(5–6):203–9.
15. Sakai Y, Wakamatsu S, Ono K, Kumagai N. Gigantomastia induced by bucillamine. Ann Plast Surg 2002;49(2):193–5.

Bucloxic acid

See also Non-steroidal anti-inflammatory drugs

General Information

Bucloxic acid is an NSAID that is not widely used. The usual symptoms of gastrotoxicity, nephrotoxicity, and increased blood pressure have been reported, but the major adverse effects involve skin and allergic reactions. Quincke's edema has been observed (SED-9, 152) (1) (SEDA-1, 93).

Reference

1. Penard M, Guillou M. Notre expérience de l'Esfar en cardiologie hospitalière. Ouest Med 1975;28:967.

Bucricaine

See also Local anesthetics

General Information

Bucricaine (centbucridine) is a quinolone derivative with local anesthetic activity.

Nausea, vomiting, bradycardia, backache, shivering, and hypotension can occur with a similar incidence to that of lidocaine (SED-12, 256) (1). It has been suggested that bucricaine is more potent than lidocaine and has few cardiovascular and nervous system adverse effects in animals, at high doses. One study in humans suggested that bucricaine may be associated with fewer cardiovascular adverse effects than lidocaine, but there are insufficient data to confirm this impression (2).

References

1. Dasgupta D, Garasia M, Gupta KC, Satoskar RS. Randomised double-blind study of centbucridine and lignocaine for subarachnoid block. Indian J Med Res 1983;77:512–16.
2. Samsi AB, Bhalerao RA, Shah SC, Mody BB, Paul T, Satoskar RS. Evaluation of centbucridine as a local anesthetic. Anesth Analg 1983;62(1):109–11.

Bufexamac

See also Non-steroidal anti-inflammatory drugs

General Information

Bufexamac is intended for topical use as a cream (using iontophoresis, ultrasound, and massage). Local intolerance causes burning and irritation, attributable to components of the cream. Urticaria, folliculitis, and pyoderma can occur when occlusive dressings are used. The course of contact allergy by bufexamac was particularly protracted and refractory in most of the 24 patients observed in one hospital in 1983–1987 (1). An erythema multiforme-like rash associated with contact dermatitis has been reported (SEDA-18, 103). In children, long-term topical use of bufexamac was well tolerated with few mild local adverse effects (SEDA-20, 91).

Reference

1. Geier J, Fuchs T. Kontaktallergien durch Bufexamac. [Contact allergies caused by bufexamac.] Med Klin (Munich) 1989;84(7):333–8.

Buflomedil

General Information

Buflomedil hydrochloride is a vasoactive drug with a variety of actions. It is an alpha-adrenoceptor antagonist and a weak calcium channel blocker. It inhibits platelet aggregation and improves erythrocyte deformability. However, its mechanism of action in peripheral vascular disease is not known.

Buflomedil has generally been well tolerated by most patients in clinical trials (1). The most frequently reported adverse effects include flushing, headache, vertigo, gastrointestinal discomfort, and dizziness. These rarely require drug withdrawal. In controlled trials, adverse effects have occurred in 20% of patients assigned to buflomedil and 18% of those assigned to placebo; only gastrointestinal discomfort occurred more frequently in buflomedil-treated patients (3.4 versus 2%) (2).

Organs and Systems

Nervous system

Extrapyramidal symptoms have been reported in a few frail elderly women (SEDA-13, 169). A few cases of myoclonic encephalopathy have been observed at therapeutic dosages; old people, patients of low body weight, and patients with renal insufficiency due to dehydration appear to be especially vulnerable (SEDA-9, 189) (SEDA-10, 172) (SEDA-11, 179).

Psychological, psychiatric

Depression has been reported in a few frail elderly women taking buflomedil (SEDA-13, 169).

Immunologic

An anaphylactic reaction to buflomedil has been reported (3).

- A 53-year-old woman with Raynaud's phenomenon developed an urticarial rash, pruritus, and hypotension 10 minutes after the parenteral administration of buflomedil. She received corticosteroids and recovered within 6 hours. When she later underwent skin tests with buflomedil, there was an immediate positive reaction, suggesting a type I hypersensitivity mechanism.

Drug Administration

Drug overdose

Buflomedil is generally considered to be innocuous at therapeutic dosages. Acute toxicity is due to accidental or intentional overdosage. Overdosage causes generalized seizures and cardiac conduction abnormalities, eventually leading to cardiac arrest (SEDA-21, 215).

Three cases of self-poisoning with buflomedil have been reported (4–6); two were fatal.

- A 15-year-old girl took 24 tablets of buflomedil (300 mg) and had a plasma concentration of 93.7 µg/ml. She was deeply comatose and in a convulsive state. Shortly after, she developed cardiac arrest from which she did not recover despite initially successful resuscitation.
- A young girl took a single dose of buflomedil 7.5 g and a young man 18 g. Coma with convulsions occurred in both, soon followed by rhythm and conduction disturbances. Intensive resuscitation attempts could not prevent a fatal outcome in the girl.

Chronic overdose can also lead to convulsions (7).

- A 75-year-old woman had fever and convulsions. She had diabetes mellitus and angina pectoris and took buflomedil for peripheral arterial disease. No cause for her symptoms was found, but she had a high plasma concentration of buflomedil (6.3 µg/ml, usual target range 4–4.5 µg/ml). The drug was withdrawn and the symptoms did not recur. On questioning, it appeared that she had mistakenly forgotten to abandon her old commercial formulation when her pharmacist proposed a cheaper, new, generic brand, but took both at the correctly prescribed dose.

References

1. Clissold SP, Lynch S, Sorkin EM. Buflomedil. A review of its pharmacodynamic and pharmacokinetic properties, and therapeutic efficacy in peripheral and cerebral vascular diseases. Drugs 1987;33(5):430–60.
2. Bachand RT, Dubourg AY. A review of long-term safety data with buflomedil. J Int Med Res 1990;18(3):245–52.
3. Scala E, Guerra EC, Pirrotta L, Giani M, De Pita O, Puddu P. Anaphylactic reactions to buflomedil. Allergy 1999;54(3):288–9.

4. Tomassini E, Poussel JF, Guiot P. Intoxication mortelle au buflomédil. [Fatal poisoning caused by buflomedil.] Ann Fr Anesth Reanim 1999;18(10):1091–2.
5. Perrot C, Rifler JP, Freysz M. Intoxication volontaire fatale au buflomedil: à propos d'un cas. JEUR 2000;13:135–8.
6. Vandemergel X, Biston P, Lenearts L, Marecaux G, Daune M. Buflomedil poisoning: a potentially life-threatening intoxication. Intensive Care Med 2000;26(11):1713.
7. Chiffoleau A, Yatim D, Garrec F, Veyrac G, Raoult P, Larousse C, Bourin M. Warning! One buflomedil may hide another one! Therapie 2000;55(1):221–3.

Bumadizone

See also Non-steroidal anti-inflammatory drugs

General Information

Bumadizone is an NSAID that is metabolized to phenylbutazone and oxyphenbutazone.

In a study in 647 patients, about 15% had adverse effects (gastrointestinal, fluid retention, and hypersensitivity); treatment was stopped in 7% (1).

Reference

1. Du Lac Y. Banc d'essai therapeutique d'un anti-inflammatoire Eumotol. Reumatologie 1979;8:405.

Bumetanide

See also Diuretics

General Information

Bumetanide is very similar in most respects to furosemide, although it is more potent mole for mole. An oral dose of 1–4 mg often suffices for ordinary use compared with 40–160 mg of furosemide.

Most of the adverse effects of bumetanide are the same as those of furosemide. However, it is less ototoxic and can cause muscle cramps, which furosemide does not.

Organs and Systems

Respiratory

Bumetanide has been implicated in the development of pulmonary fibrosis (SEDA-16, 223), but causality could not be determined with certainty.

Sensory systems

One advantage of bumetanide is that it is less ototoxic than furosemide (1–3). It is sensible to prefer bumetanide to furosemide in patients with hearing problems or who concurrently need ototoxic drugs, such as an aminoglycoside antibiotic.

Metabolism

It has been suggested that bumetanide has a smaller effect on blood glucose than furosemide does, but that is not at all clear.

Gastrointestinal

Very high doses of bumetanide used for renal insufficiency have sometimes produced colic (SED-10, 376).

Pancreas

A patient in whom pancreatitis was induced by both furosemide and bumetanide has been documented (SEDA-14, 184).

Skin

Bullous pemphigoid induced by bumetanide has been reported (4).

- A 67-year-old man presented with an acute bullous eruption 6 weeks after starting bumetanide. He had numerous large tense bullae on erythematous skin, with superficial ulceration on the thighs, arms, and anterior trunk. Pruritus was severe. Routine laboratory tests were normal, except for blood eosinophilia. Biopsy of a blister showed subepidermal bullae associated with dermal infiltrates of neutrophils and eosinophils. Direct immunofluorescence showed continuous linear deposits of C3 and IgG at the basement membrane zone, confirmed by immunoelectron microscopy. Circulating IgG antibasement membrane antibodies were localized in the roof of the blister. Compete clinical healing and normalization of immunology occurred within 2 months of withdrawal of bumetanide.

Pseudoporphyria (SEDA-16, 222) and Stevens–Johnson syndrome have also been reported (SED-10, 376).

Musculoskeletal

Various musculoskeletal symptoms have been reported with bumetanide, including pain, cramping, and weakness (SEDA-22, 236). The symptoms are usually mild and self-limiting, with an incidence of less than 2%, but disabling reactions have occurred after oral administration and intravenous injection, and severity correlates with dose. The onset is usually 2–4 hours after dosing; the onset may be slower during infusion.

References

1. Tuzel IH. Comparison of adverse reactions to bumetanide and furosemide. J Clin Pharmacol 1981;21(11–12 Pt 2):615–19.
2. Halstenson CE, Matzke GR. Bumetanide: a new loop diuretic (Bumex, Roche Laboratories). Drug Intell Clin Pharm 1983;17(11):786–97.
3. Ward A, Heel RC. Bumetanide. A review of its pharmacodynamic and pharmacokinetic properties and therapeutic use. Drugs 1984;28(5):426–64.
4. Boulinguez S, Bernard P, Bedane C, le Brun V, Bonnetblanc JM. Bullous pemphigoid induced by bumetanide. Br J Dermatol 1998;138(3):548–9.

Bupivacaine

See also Local anesthetics

General Information

Bupivacaine is a long-acting aminoamide local anesthetic with significantly more systemic toxicity than lidocaine.

Organs and Systems

Cardiovascular

Bupivacaine-induced cardiotoxicity, notably after epidural use, is a matter of concern and controversy (1–3). The risk can be greatly reduced or eliminated by careful dosage and/or the use of lower concentrations (SEDA-12, 108) (1).

All studies of the cardiotoxic effects of local anesthetics on the isolated heart published from 1981 to 2001 have been reviewed (4). Thirteen studies were identified, all of which studied bupivacaine, either alone or compared with other local anesthetics. The general conclusions were:

- Highly lipid-soluble, extensively protein-bound, highly potent local anesthetics, such as tetracaine, bupivacaine, and etidocaine, are much more cardiotoxic than less lipid-soluble, protein-bound, and potent local anesthetics, such as lidocaine and prilocaine.
- Bupivacaine has a potent depressant effect on electrical conduction in the heart, primarily via an action on voltage-gated sodium channels that govern the initial rapid depolarization of the cardiac action potential.
- The $S(-)$ isomer of bupivacaine is less cardiotoxic than the $R(+)$ form.
- Bupivacaine predisposes the heart to re-entrant dysrhythmias.
- The actions of bupivacaine on channels other than voltage-gated sodium channels probably contribute to the dose-dependent cardiotoxic effects of bupivacaine.

The recommended safe upper dose limit for bupivacaine is commonly 2–2.5 mg/kg. However, some authors recommend a lower dose of 1.25 mg/kg as the safe upper limit in dental practice (SEDA-20, 128) (5).

Hyperkalemia, acidosis, severe hypoxia, and myocardial ischemia increase the cardiovascular depressive effects of bupivacaine.

There has been a report of T wave changes on the electrocardiogram during caudal administration of local anesthetics (6).

- A 4.2 kg 2-month-old baby was given a caudal injection under general anesthesia for an inguinal hernia repair. A mixture of 1% lidocaine 2 ml and 0.25% bupivacaine 2 ml was injected. Every 1 ml was preceded by an aspiration test and followed by observation for 20 seconds for electrocardiographic changes. On administration of the third 1 ml dose, there was a significant increase in T wave amplitude. The aspiration test was repeated and was positive for blood. The caudal injection was stopped and the electrocardiogram returned to normal after 35 seconds. The patient remained cardiovascularly stable with no postoperative sequelae.

Previous reports have suggested that an increase in T wave amplitude could result from inadvertent intravascular administration of adrenaline-containing local anesthetics. This is the first case report of local anesthetics alone causing significant T wave changes.

Bradycardia has been reported very occasionally (7).

Bupivacaine can cause ventricular extra beats (8). Ventricular dysrhythmias and seizures were reported in a patient who received 0.5% bupivacaine 30 ml with adrenaline 5 micrograms/ml for lumbar plexus block, after a negative aspiration test (9). The patient developed ventricular fibrillation and required advanced cardiac life support for 1 hour, including 15 defibrillations, and adrenaline 40 mg before sinus rhythm could be restored. There were no neurological sequelae.

Infusions of 0.25% bupivacaine into pig coronary arteries caused ventricular fibrillation at lower rates of infusion than 0.25% bupivacaine with 1% lidocaine (10). The lidocaine/bupivacaine mixture did not have a greater myocardial depressant effect than bupivacaine alone. The authors suggested that when regional anesthesia requires high doses of local anesthetics, bupivacaine should not be used alone but in a mixture with lidocaine, and that lidocaine should be useful in the management of bupivacaine-induced ventricular fibrillation.

An animal study of the mechanism of bupivacaine-induced dysrhythmias has shown that bupivacaine facilitates early after-depolarization in rabbit sinoatrial nodal cells by blocking the delayed rectifier potassium current (11).

Inadvertent administration of bupivacaine can lead to fatal cardiovascular collapse that may be refractory to conventional resuscitation. A study in rats has suggested that in addition to its direct cardiotoxic effect, bupivacaine may have a toxic action on the brainstem, and that cardiovascular collapse may result from dysfunction of vital cardiorespiratory control systems (12).

Nervous system

Neurological symptoms subsequent to unrecognized intravascular injection are the major complications of bupivacaine: tinnitus, muscle twitching, nystagmus, and convulsions can occur. The use of vasoconstrictors is probably not advisable, as they prolong the duration of action of local anesthetics. Whether the addition of hyperbaric glucose to 0.5% bupivacaine for spinal anesthesia alters the incidence of pain from an orthopedic tourniquet is disputed; some findings suggest that it aggravates the problem (SED-12, 256) (13).

- A 13-year-old girl developed tonic-clonic seizures followed by ventricular fibrillation after subcutaneous infiltration of extensive skin abrasions with 30 mg (0.5 mg/kg) of bupivacaine over about 1 hour. She was successfully resuscitated with cardiopulmonary resuscitation and intubation, intravenous diazepam, adrenaline, and sodium bicarbonate (14).

The authors noted that although the anticonvulsant effect of diazepam is significant, some animal studies have shown that diazepam can prolong the half-life of bupivacaine. They stressed the difficulty in treating bupivacaine-induced dysrhythmias and suggested the use of phenytoin as a first-line agent in their management. However, this advice is based on only two case reports.

In seven children (aged 36–52 weeks) given caudal anesthesia with bupivacaine 3.1 mg/kg + adrenaline 5 micrograms/ml, there were significant electroencephalographic signs of central nervous system toxicity in six, and two had clinical signs of possible epileptic activity. The authors stopped the study early because of the high incidence of adverse effects. They felt that these were due to the fact that no sedative or anesthetic drugs that could have masked or alleviated local anesthetic toxicity were given, and also that infants have low concentrations of alpha$_1$ acid glycoprotein, leading to increased unbound plasma concentrations (15). However, it should be noted that 2 mg/kg is the usual upper dose limit recommended for bupivacaine. It is hardly surprising that such a high proportion of those studied showed evidence of systemic toxicity after the administration of a much higher dose of bupivacaine to such small children by a route that is known to result in rapid absorption of local anesthetic into the systemic circulation.

Reactions to local anesthetics often occur as a result of inadvertent overdose or accidental intravenous injection.

- A 53-year-old woman received postoperative epidural analgesia by nurse-administered bolus doses after a total knee replacement (16). She received her first epidural bolus of 0.25% bupivacaine 6 ml with morphine 2 mg 2 hours after the operation, with good effect. Six hours later she was accidentally given a second top-up dose intravenously. She became distressed and complained of tinnitus, palpitation, and dizziness. She was able to cooperate and was in sinus rhythm with a tachycardia of 120/minute. She was observed overnight on ICU and made a full recovery.

Despite correct epidural placement, this complication arose as a result of human error, and the authors believed that the low concentration and volume of the top-up had protected the patient from more serious sequelae.

Musculoskeletal

Muscular atrophy after intramuscular injection has been documented (17).

Immunologic

A non-IgE-mediated allergic reaction to bupivacaine has been reported (SEDA-21, 136).

- A 69-year-old woman with a history of bronchospasm after NSAID administration had heavy feelings in her arms and itchy eyes, without any change in hemodynamics, 30 minutes after an intradermal injection of bupivacaine. The same symptoms occurred during subsequent retesting 1 month later, with the addition of coughing and sneezing.

Second-Generation Effects

Pregnancy

Cardiotoxicity due to bupivacaine is more likely in pregnancy (18).

When epidural anesthesia was used for cesarean section, bupivacaine (with oxytocin) produced a higher frequency of neonatal jaundice than similar treatment using lidocaine (SEDA-14, 111).

Fetotoxicity

Adverse effects of bupivacaine on the fetus are uncommon (19), but fetal bradycardia has very occasionally been reported (20).

Susceptibility Factors

Genetic factors

Isovaleric acidemia (an autosomal recessive disorder of leucine metabolism causing episodes of acidosis during catabolic stress) and carnitine deficiency have been associated with a lowered threshold for bupivacaine-induced dysrhythmias (SEDA-22, 142).

Age

In the elderly, some local anesthetics (including lidocaine and bupivacaine) have longer durations of action (18).

Drug Administration

Drug formulations

A formulation of bupivacaine called Regibloc (bupivacaine HCl; Intramed, South Africa) was the only common factor in a series of serious complications after regional anesthesia (21).

- Three consecutive patients had prolonged blockade after retrobulbar block. One had not resolved after 3 months and three others had prolonged mydriasis for 2 weeks.
- Severe neuralgia developed in eight patients after interscalene blocks lasting 6–12 weeks.
- A 36-year-old woman developed supraclavicular skin necrosis, followed by sloughing of subcutaneous tissue down to the first rib, including the dorsal roots of the brachial plexus, after receiving an interscalene block followed by an infusion; 5 months later she still had complete sensory and motor paralysis of the C5 nerve root requiring nerve grafting.
- Skin sloughing after a penile ring-block required plastic reconstruction.
- A 16-year-old girl had a median nerve block followed by an area of skin and fat necrosis at the site of injection and a middle-aged patient received an interscalene block resulting in subsequent fat necrosis at the injection site.

No further complications were encountered after the authors changed to another formulation of bupivacaine and stopped using Regibloc.

Drug–Drug Interactions

Calcium channel blockers

Calcium channel blockers in combination with bupivacaine produce significant negative inotropic effects on the heart in animals, possibly due to reduced protein binding of the local anesthetic, as well as a generalized myocardial depressant effect (22,23).

However, bupivacaine cardiotoxicity was reduced in rats by pretreatment with low doses of calcium channel blockers (24). In vivo, the LD_{50} for bupivacaine was increased from 3.08 to 3.58 mg/kg after pretreatment with verapamil 150 micrograms/kg, and to 3.50 mg/kg after nimodipine 200 micrograms/kg. Of the rats that died, only one developed cardiac arrest first, whilst the majority developed respiratory arrest. In vitro, bupivacaine alone dose-dependently reduced heart rate, contractile force, and coronary perfusion pressure. Dysrhythmias were also noted: bradycardias, ventricular extra beats, and ventricular tachycardia were the most common. Verapamil made no difference to these adverse effects, but nimodipine significantly reduced the negative chronotropic and dysrhythmogenic effects of bupivacaine. These results, although interesting, cannot be used to reach any clinical conclusions, particularly as the mechanism of interaction between bupivacaine and calcium channel blockers has yet to be elucidated.

Clonidine

The analgesic efficacy of the addition of clonidine to an epidural solution of bupivacaine plus fentanyl has been subjected to a randomized, double-blind study in 61 parturients who received bupivacaine plus fentanyl with or without clonidine (median dose 28 micrograms/hour). There was no difference between the groups in pruritus or nausea score, but those given clonidine had less shivering and better analgesia (25).

In another randomized, double-blind study, a combination of clonidine and neostigmine was added to intrathecal bupivacaine plus fentanyl in 45 parturients (26). The combination increased the duration of labor analgesia by 83%, but was associated with significantly more nausea. However, the results were equivocal, and larger studies are needed.

Clonidine inhibits the hepatic metabolism of bupivacaine in mice (27).

Desipramine

Desipramine displaces bupivacaine from plasma proteins (28).

Mepivacaine

Bupivacaine displaces mepivacaine from protein binding sites on alpha$_1$ acid glycoprotein in vitro (29).

Pethidine

Pethidine displaces bupivacaine from plasma proteins (28). However, this interaction is probably not of clinical importance (30).

Phenytoin

Phenytoin displaces bupivacaine from plasma proteins (28).

Quinidine

Quinidine displaces bupivacaine from plasma proteins (28).

References

1. Nolte H. Zur Problematik der Cardiotoxizität von Bupivacain 0.75%. [The problem of the cardiotoxicity of bupivacaine 0.75%.] Reg Anaesth 1986;9(3):57–9.
2. Marx GF. Bupivacaine cardiotoxicity–concentration or dose? Anesthesiology 1986;65(1):116.
3. Hurley R, Feldman H. Toxicity of local anesthetics in obstetrics. I. Bupivacaine. Clin Anaesthesiol 1986;4:93.
4. Heavner JE. Cardiac toxicity of local anesthetics in the intact isolated heart model: a review. Reg Anesth Pain Med 2002;27(6):545–55.
5. Bacsik CJ, Swift JQ, Hargreaves KM. Toxic systemic reactions of bupivacaine and etidocaine. Oral Surg Oral Med Oral Pathol Oral Radiol Endod 1995;79(1):18–23.
6. Tanaka M, Nitta R, Nishikawa T. Increased T-wave amplitude after accidental intravascular injection of lidocaine plus bupivacaine without epinephrine in sevoflurane-anesthetized child. Anesth Analg 2001;92(4):915–17.
7. Exler U, Nolte H, Milatz W. Die Überwachung der Herzleitung bei Anwendung von Bupivacain 0.75% mit Hilfe der Ventrikulographie (^{99m}Tc). [Monitoring of cardiac output during use of bupivacaine 0.75% by ventriculography (^{99m}Tc).] Reg Anaesth 1986;9(3):68–73.
8. Pape R, Ammer W. Holter-EKG-Überwachung bei Periduralanaesthesie mit Bupivacain 0.75%. [Holter ECG monitoring during peridural anesthesia with bupivacaine 0.75%.] Reg Anaesth 1986;9(3):74–8.
9. Pham-Dang C, Beaumont S, Floch H, Bodin J, Winer A, Pinaud M. Accident aign toxique après bloc du plexus lombaire à la bupivacaine. [Acute toxic accident following lumbar plexus block with bupivacaine.] Ann Fr Anesth Reanim 2000;19(5):356–9.
10. Fujita Y, Endoh S, Yasukawa T, Sari A. Lidocaine increases the ventricular fibrillation threshold during bupivacaine-induced cardiotoxicity in pigs. Br J Anaesth 1998;80(2):218–22.
11. Matsuda T, Kurata Y. Effects of nicardipine and bupivacaine on early after depolarization in rabbit sinoatrial node cells: a possible mechanism of bupivacaine-induced arrhythmias. Gen Pharmacol 1999;33(2):115–25.
12. Pickering AE, Waki H, Headley PM, Paton JF. Investigation of systemic bupivacaine toxicity using the in situ perfused working heart-brainstem preparation of the rat. Anesthesiology 2002;97(6):1550–6.
13. Bridenbaugh PO, Hagenouw RR, Gielen MJ, Edstrom HH. Addition of glucose to bupivacaine in spinal anesthesia increases incidence of tourniquet pain. Anesth Analg 1986;65(11):1181–5.
14. Yan AC, Newman RD. Bupivacaine-induced seizures and ventricular fibrillation in a 13-year-old girl undergoing wound debridement. Pediatr Emerg Care 1998;14(5):354–5.
15. Breschan C, Hellstrand E, Likar R, Lonnquist PA. Toxizität und "subtoxische" Fruhzeich in Wachzustand bei Sauglingen. Bupivacain plasspiegel nach Kaudalanästhesist. [Early signs of toxicity and "subtoxic" conditions in infant monitoring. Bupivacaine plasma levels following caudal anesthesia.] Anaesthesist 1998;47(4):290–4.
16. Karaca S, Unlusoy EO. Accidental injection of intravenous bupivacaine. Eur J Anaesthesiol 2002;19(8):616–17.
17. Parris WCV, Dettbarn WD. Muscle atrophy following bupivacaine trigger point injection. Anesthesiol Rev 1989;16:50–4.

18. Chauvin M. Toxicité aiguë des anesthésiques locaux en fonction du terrain. [Acute toxicity of local anesthetics as a function of the patient's condition.] Ann Fr Anesth Reanim 1988;7(3):216–23

19. Seebacher J, Chareire F, Galli-Douant P, Viars P. L'utilisation de la Marcaine en analgésie obstétricale. [The use of Marcaine in obstetrical analgesia.] Ann Anesthesiol Fr 1978;19(4):247–53

20. Kuczkowski KM. Severe persistent fetal bradycardia following subarachnoid administration of fentanyl and bupivacaine for induction of a combined spinal-epidural analgesia for labor pain. J Clin Anesth 2004;16(1):78–9.

21. Boezaart AP, du Toit JC, van Lill G, Donald R, van der Spuy G, Bolus M. Urgent local anaesthetic drug alarm. S Afr Med J 1999;89(6):570–2.

22. Wulf H, Godicke J, Herzig S. Functional interaction between local anaesthetics and calcium antagonists in guineapig myocardium: 2. Electrophysiological studies with bupivacaine and nifedipine. Br J Anaesth 1994;73(3):364–70.

23. Herzig S, Ruhnke L, Wulf H. Functional interaction between local anaesthetics and calcium antagonists in guineapig myocardium: 1. Cardiodepressant effects in isolated organs. Br J Anaesth 1994;73(3):357–63.

24. Adsan H, Tulunay M, Onaran O. The effects of verapamil and nimodipine on bupivacaine-induced cardiotoxicity in rats: an in vivo and in vitro study. Anesth Analg 1998;86(4):818–24.

25. Paech MJ, Pavy TJ, Orlikowski CE, Evans SF. Patient-controlled epidural analgesia in labor: the addition of clonidine to bupivacaine–fentanyl. Reg Anesth Pain Med 2000;25(1):34–40.

26. Owen MD, Ozsarac O, Sahin S, Uckunkaya N, Kaplan N, Magunaci I. Low-dose clonidine and neostigmine prolong the duration of intrathecal bupivacaine-fentanyl for labor analgesia. Anesthesiology 2000;92(2):361–6.

27. Naguib M, Magboul MM, Samarkandi AH, Attia M. Adverse effects and drug interactions associated with local and regional anaesthesia. Drug Saf 1998;18(4):221–50.

28. Ghoneim MM, Pandya H. Plasma protein binding of bupivacaine and its interaction with other drugs in man. Br J Anaesth 1974;46(6):435–8.

29. Hartrick CT, Dirkes WE, Coyle DE, Raj PP, Denson DD. Influence of bupivacaine on mepivacaine protein binding. Clin Pharmacol Ther 1984;36(4):546–50.

30. Denson DD, Myers JA, Coyle DE. The clinical relevance of the drug displacement interaction between meperidine and bupivacaine. Res Commun Chem Pathol Pharmacol 1984;45(3):323–30.

Buprenorphine

See also Opioid analgesics

General Information

Buprenorphine is a partial agonist at OP_3 (μ) opioid receptors and an antagonist at OP_2 (κ) receptors.

In a double-blind, randomized study of three groups of 18 patients having abdominal surgery who received single doses of either intramuscular pethidine 75 mg, with sublingual buprenorphine 400 µg, or buprenorphine 300 µg alone, sedation and nausea were the most common adverse effects in all three groups. Patients who received sublingual buprenorphine were significantly less sedated in the immediate postoperative period (1).

In a 3-day randomized, placebo-controlled study, 40 patients with acute pancreatitis or acute-on-chronic pancreatitis were given either buprenorphine 2.4 mg/day or procaine hydrochloride 2 g/day by constant intravenous infusion (2). The patients who received buprenorphine had significantly lower pain scores than those given procaine and were significantly less likely to demand additional analgesia. The adverse effect profiles were similar in the two groups, with the exception of a significantly higher rate of sedation in those who were given buprenorphine. The authors suggested that intravenous buprenorphine is more effective and safer than procaine in acute pancreatitis.

Buprenorphine has been suggested to be useful for the treatment of cocaine and opiate dependence. In a study designed to assess its safety for this purpose (SEDA-18, 85) there were no adverse effects or serious interactions with a single dose of intravenous morphine or cocaine during daily maintenance on buprenorphine.

Organs and Systems

Cardiovascular

- A 27-year-old man injected a 2 mg suspension of crushed oral buprenorphine into his left ulnar artery, leading to acute ischemia of the hand; he was successfully treated with iloprost and dextran-40 (3).
- A 22-year-old man snorted an 8 mg crushed tablet of buprenorphine and 2 hours later had crushing chest pain, which resolved within a few minutes (4). The symptom recurred 3 weeks later after another inhalation of buprenorphine. An electrocardiogram suggested an acute anterior myocardial infarction caused by buprenorphine-induced coronary artery spasm.

Respiratory

Respiratory depression can occur with buprenorphine. It is not often a clinical problem, except in older and weaker subjects, in whom it can be fatal (5). When it occurs it is often prolonged and can be particularly difficult to reverse (SEDA-16, 87). Norbuprenorphine, a metabolite of buprenorphine via CYP3A4 causes dose-dependent respiratory depression, perhaps mediated by opioid receptors in the lung rather than the brain, and is 10 times more potent than buprenorphine (SEDA-22, 103).

Non-cardiogenic pulmonary edema has been reported after a single dose of buprenorphine (SEDA-19, 89).

Nervous system

Sedation and nausea are relatively frequent. When buprenorphine is used for patient-controlled analgesia, minor dysphoria or euphoria has been reported (SEDA-16, 88).

In one of three patients receiving epidural buprenorphine for the relief of pain from head and neck cancers, it was discontinued because of severe dizziness (SEDA-17, 87).

Mouth and teeth

There have been reports of facial and lingual ulcers, the ulceration following repeated injection of buprenorphine into the left superior cervical ganglion for trigeminal neuralgia (6) and the use of sublingual buprenorphine (7).

Gastrointestinal

Impaired gastric emptying and delayed absorption after sublingual buprenorphine have also been reported (SEDA-17, 87).

Liver

- A 33-year-old man developed severe hepatitis after an oral overdose of buprenorphine tablets 112 mg over 48 hours (8). He presented with an acute confusional state, including disorientation in time and space. The condition led to anuria and hepatorenal insufficiency. He was successfully treated with hemodialysis.

With increasing use of buprenorphine in the treatment of opioid dependence, it has been confirmed that the use of buprenorphine in opioid-dependent individuals with a history of hepatitis causes significant increases in aspartate transaminase and alanine transaminase activities (9). Liver enzymes should be monitored before giving buprenorphine to patients with hepatitis.

Four former opiate-dependent individuals with confirmed hepatitis C virus were given substitution therapy with sublingual buprenorphine. After injecting buprenorphine together with their sublingual doses, they had a marked increase in serum aspartate transaminase activity (13–50 times the upper limit of the reference range), resulting in jaundice (10). Another patient who was positive for hepatitis C and HIV developed jaundice, with panlobular liver necrosis and microvesicular steatosis, after using sublingual buprenorphine and small doses of paracetamol and aspirin (10).

Intravenous buprenorphine abuse precipitated acute-on-chronic hepatitis in a 25-year-old woman who was hepatitis C positive with a history of chronic diamorphine dependence (11).

Skin

There have been reports of severe pruritus with buprenorphine (12).

Immunologic

There have been reports of anaphylactic reactions with buprenorphine (13).

Death

Two series of 39 and 78 deaths attributed to buprenorphine have respectively been reported in Strasbourg and 13 other French forensic centers between 1996 and 2000 (14). The risks incurred by the misuse of buprenorphine seem to arise through a combination of (a) the concomitant use of other psychotropic drugs (especially benzodiazepines and neuroleptic drugs) and (b) the improper use of tablets for intravenous administration and/or massive oral doses. The total recorded number of buprenorphine-related deaths is largely underestimated, because the very low concentrations require sensitive immunoassay techniques, making them difficult to detect; furthermore different cut-off points are used by different forensic pathology laboratories in diagnosing drug-related deaths.

Long-Term Effects

Drug abuse

Abuse of buprenorphine has been reported in many countries and it is now widely dealt with under psychotropic drug legislation.

Although sublingual buprenorphine has been used in the management of heroin addiction (SEDA-16, 88), widespread abuse of buprenorphine by addicts is known (SEDA-16, 88), including the snorting of crushed sublingual tablets (SEDA-16, 88).

Buprenorphine is increasingly being used as a substitute for other opioids in the treatment of opioid abuse and is generally considered to be safe because of the ceiling effect. One report from Vienna described 50 opioid-dependent subjects who received gradual (10-day) detoxification with buprenorphine, contacting the outpatient clinic daily, so that buprenorphine could be administered according to their clinical need in a free dosage scheme (15). The mean daily dosage was 2.3 mg on day 1 and the highest mean daily dose was administered on day 2, followed by daily reduction over the study period. There was 70% compliance with the regimen and withdrawal symptoms during the study period were described as moderate.

Less satisfactory outcomes have been reported from France (16–18), where acute poisoning during buprenorphine substitution has been described in three series of patients. The first included 29 opiate addicts taking high-dosage sublingual buprenorphine with non-fatal poisoning and the second included 20 addicts who died (16). Blood concentrations of buprenorphine in the first group were low (1.0–2.3 ng/ml, mean 1.4 ng/ml), but there was concomitant intake of psychotropic medication, especially benzodiazepines, in 18 cases. Blood concentrations of buprenorphine in the fatal cases were 1.1–29 (mean 8.4) ng/ml, while concentrations of its primary metabolite, norbuprenorphine, were 0.2–13 (mean 2.6) ng/ml, within or slightly over the target range. Extensive tissue distribution buprenorphine was reported (myocardium, kidney, brain, and liver) but the highest concentrations of buprenorphine and norbuprenorphine were found in the bile, and the authors suggested that this may be the sample of choice for postmortem screening. Buprenorphine was also identified in eight of 11 hair samples assayed. Intravenous injection of crushed tablets and the concomitant use of benzodiazepines were identified as the major risk factors in the fatal cases (17).

Drug dependence

Sublingual buprenorphine is an alternative to methadone in treating opiate dependence, but its opioid agonist effects pose the risk of intravenous abuse and subsequent dependence. This abuse potential may be limited by using a combination of buprenorphine with naloxone, which will precipitate opiate withdrawal when given intravenously but not sublingually. The effects of three combinations of intravenous buprenorphine and naloxone on agonist effects and withdrawal signs and symptoms in 12 opiate-dependent patients have been described (19). After stabilization with morphine 60 mg intramuscularly the patients were challenged with intravenous doses of buprenorphine 2 mg, either alone or in combination with naloxone in ratios of 2:1, 4:1, and 8:1, with morphine alone (15 mg), or with placebo. In those given the combination there was a naloxone dose-dependent increase in opiate withdrawal signs and a reduction in the pleasurable effects that might induce abuse liability. The authors suggested that the combination of buprenorphine with naloxone in a ratio of 2:1 or 4:1 can be useful in the treatment of opiate dependence.

There have been three studies of the use of buprenorphine to treat opiate dependence.

The authors of a randomized, multicenter, placebo-controlled, double-blind study of 72 opioid-dependent individuals, who were given either buprenorphine 8 mg/day or methadone 60 mg/day for 6 months, claimed that there were no significant differences in adverse effects during induction or maintenance (20). Buprenorphine provided an alternative to methadone, with equal improvement in quality of life, psychopathology, and compliance. The results of this study should be interpreted with care, because of the unusual experimental design, which did not reflect practices in ordinary methadone maintenance programs. However, similar observations were observed during an open, flexible-dose study involving inpatient induction and outpatient maintenance in 15 opioid-dependent pregnant women (21). Sublingual buprenorphine (1–10 mg/day) was well accepted by the women, and there was a low incidence of neonatal abstinence syndrome. Further controlled and larger studies need to be done to substantiate these observations.

In a double-blind, randomized comparison of sublingual buprenorphine tablets with oral methadone in a 6-week trial in 58 patients using a flexible dosing procedure the retention rate was significantly better in those using methadone (90 versus 50%) (22). Those who completed the study had a similar number of opioid-positive urine samples, with a mean stabilization dose of 11 mg/day of buprenorphine and 70 mg/day of methadone. This study had several limitations: 6 weeks is too short a period to determine any intermediate or long-term treatment outcomes, the sample size was too small, and the comparison of non-equivalent doses makes interpretation difficult.

Drug withdrawal

The effects of buprenorphine (sublingually or by injection) in an opioid-dependent population have been studied (23,24). There was benefit in using buprenorphine to counteract opioid withdrawal effects in patients with chronic heroin use and subsequent dependence. However, the results are limited and the benefits short-term if psychosocial support is not in place as part of an overall treatment package before buprenorphine is prescribed (25).

- A 35-year-old man with a 10-year history of heroin use was given sublingual buprenorphine 24 mg/day (26). Although it was dispensed daily by a pharmacist, he

was not adequately supervised: he saved the buprenorphine tablets and continued to use heroin. He then took buprenorphine 40 mg and stopped using heroin; he immediately developed opioid withdrawal symptoms. In an attempt to relieve these symptoms, he took a further 40 or 45 mg buprenorphine in 24 hours. He subsequently came to a drug treatment clinic, where he was given another 16 mg of buprenorphine, with no effect. After 3 days, he was transferred to methadone and his withdrawal symptoms resolved.

In this case buprenorphine precipitated opioid withdrawal symptoms after heroin use. This highlights the importance of regular monitoring and supervision of community-dispensed buprenorphine.

Second-Generation Effects

Fetotoxicity

It is inadvisable to use buprenorphine during labor, as its effects on the fetus cannot be reversed.

Drug Administration

Drug formulations

A sublingual formulation that combines buprenorphine and naloxone is thought to be ideal for reducing parental buprenorphine abuse. In a small pilot study in nine opioid-dependent individuals already stabilized on buprenorphine 8 mg/day, naloxone 0, 4, or 8 mg was added (27). The addition of naloxone did not precipitate opiate withdrawal.

A transdermal therapeutic system (TTS) for rate-controlled delivery of buprenorphine is available in three strengths, with release rates of 35, 52.5, and 70 µg/hour for 72 hours. This is equivalent to daily doses of 0.8, 1.2, and 1.6 mg respectively. In a double-blind, randomized, controlled study using one of three dosage strengths of buprenorphine TTS in 445 patients with chronic pain the adverse effects were mild and typical of the opioid analgesics; they included nausea (17%), vomiting (9.3%), dizziness (6.8%), tiredness (5.6%), constipation (5.3%), and sweating (3.7%) (28). There was erythema in 25% and pruritus in 22%. More than half of the cases of erythema and one-third of the cases of pruritus resolved within 24 hours. In a single-blind, randomized study sublingual buprenorphine 0.2 mg provided an effective and convenient alternative in the treatment of acute renal colic compared with pethidine 50 mg intramuscularly (29). There was a slightly but non-significantly higher incidence of nausea, vomiting, and dizziness in those given buprenorphine.

Drug dosage regimens

Two doses (8 and 16 mg) of sublingual buprenorphine have been compared in a 6-week double-blind, placebo-controlled inpatient study of the reinforcing effects of intravenous diamorphine (30). Only eight diamorphine-dependent men were recruited and the authors could only postulate that doses over 16 mg might be more effective in blocking the reinforcing effects of diamorphine.

Drug administration route

Adverse effects after parenteral, sublingual, and rectal use have included hypotension, bradycardia, reduced systolic blood pressure, reduced stroke volume, nausea, sweating, vomiting, vertigo, sedation, and a reduction in respiratory rate (31). In some intravenous studies nausea and vomiting have occurred in as many as 20%. Hypotension occurs in 1–5% of patients, and hypertension, tachycardia, or bradycardia in under 1%.

Drug–Drug Interactions

Benzodiazepines

Six deaths linked to misuse of buprenorphine plus benzodiazepine combinations have been described (18). The authors emphasized that blood concentrations of buprenorphine were in the target range in three subjects, although higher in three others. Exhaustive screening detected no traces of opiates in postmortem blood, but all subjects had target range concentrations of both desmethyldiazepam and 7-aminoflunitrazepam. The risk of high-dose substitution therapy (2–8 mg), if physicians do not comply with correct practices for the prescription, and use of buprenorphine were emphasized, particularly when there is a large population of patients being treated, as there was in France in 1997 (34 000 patients).

HIV-1 protease inhibitors

The metabolism of buprenorphine is inhibited by the HIV-1 protease inhibitors (32).

Naloxone

Naloxone is of limited use in reversing the effects of buprenorphine, because of its relative inability to displace it from opioid receptors. Naloxone 1 mg had little effect on the respiratory depression caused by buprenorphine 300 µg/70 kg, although both 5 and 10 µg produced consistent reversal, which was more complete with the larger dose (33). Insignificant effects on circulation and respiration have been reported at lower doses of buprenorphine (4.5–10 µg/kg) (34).

Opioid agonists

Under some conditions the antagonist action of buprenorphine can jeopardize the effect of subsequently administered pure opioid agonists, by blocking OP_3 (μ) opioid receptors so effectively that normal doses of the opioid agonist are ineffective, necessitating the administration of a higher dose, with the attendant risk of respiratory depression, from which deaths have been reported (SEDA-13, 60). Fortunately such instances appear to be rare.

References

1. Carl P, Crawford ME, Madsen NB, Ravlo O, Bach V, Larsen AI. Pain relief after major abdominal surgery: a double-blind controlled comparison of sublingual buprenorphine, intramuscular buprenorphine, and intramuscular meperidine. Anesth Analg 1987;66(2):142–6.
2. Jakobs R, Adamek MU, von Bubnoff AC, Riemann JF. Buprenorphine or procaine for pain relief in acute pancreatitis. A prospective randomized study. Scand J Gastroenterol 2000;35(12):1319–23.
3. Gouny P, Gaitz JP, Vayssairat M. Acute hand ischemia secondary to intraarterial buprenorphine injection: treatment with iloprost and dextran-40—a case report. Angiology 1999;50(7):605–6.
4. Cracowski JL, Mallaret M, Vanzetto G. Myocardial infarction associated with buprenorphine. Ann Intern Med 1999;130(6):536–7.
5. Fincham JE. Cardiopulmonary arrest and subsequent death after administration of buprenorphine in an elderly female: a case report. J Geriatr Drug Ther 1989;3:103.
6. Schleicher G, Lechner W, Muller E. [Trophic ulcers after intraganglionic injection of buprenorphine and root canal therapy.] Aktuelle Derm 1985;11:90.
7. Lockhart SP, Baron JH. Tongue ulceration after lingual buprenorphine. BMJ (Clin Res Ed) 1984;288:1346.
8. Houdret N, Asnar V, Szostak-Talbodec N, Leteurtre E, Humbert L, Lecomte-Houcke M, Lhermitte M, Paris JC. Hépatonéphrite et ingestion massive le buprénorphines. [Hepatonephritis and massive ingestion of buprenorphine.] Acta Clin Belg Suppl 1999;1:29–31.
9. Petry NM, Bickel WK, Piasecki D, Marsch LA, Badger GJ. Elevated liver enzyme levels in opioid-dependent patients with hepatitis treated with buprenorphine. Am J Addict 2000;9(3):265–9.
10. Berson A, Gervais A, Cazals D, Boyer N, Durand F, Bernuau J, Marcellin P, Degott C, Valla D, Pessayre D. Hepatitis after intravenous buprenorphine misuse in heroin addicts. J Hepatol 2001;34(2):346–50.
11. Wisniewski B, Perlemuter G, Buffet C. Hepatite aiguë liée a l'injection intraveineuse de buprenorphine chez une toxicomane substituée. [Acute hepatitis following intravenous buprenorphine injection as a substitute drug in a drug-addict.] Gastroenterol Clin Biol 2001;25(3):328–9.
12. Woodham M. Pruritus with sublingual buprenorphine. Anaesthesia 1988;43(9):806–7.
13. Peduto VA, Di Martino M, Tani R, Toscano A, Napoleone M. Reazione anafilattoide da bupreuorfina: descrizione di un caso. [Anaphylactoid reaction to buprenorphine: a case report.] Anaesthesiol Reanim 1988;38:241.
14. Kintz P. Deaths involving buprenorphine: a compendium of French cases. Forensic Sci Int 2001;121(1–2):65–9.
15. Diamant K, Fischer G, Schneider C, Lenzinger E, Pezawas L, Schindler S, Eder H. Outpatient opiate detoxification treatment with buprenorphine. Preliminary investigation. Eur Addict Res 1998;4(4):198–202.
16. Tracqui A, Tournoud C, Flesch F, Kopferschmitt J, Kintz P, Deveaux M, Ghysel MH, Marquet P, Pepin G, Petit G, Jaeger A, Ludes B. Intoxications aiguës par traitement substitutif a base de buprénorphine haut dosage. 29 observations cliniques—20 cas mortels. [Acute poisoning during substitution therapy based on high-dosage buprenorphine. 29 clinical cases—20 fatal cases.] Presse Méd 1998;27(12):557–61.
17. Tracqui A, Kintz P, Ludes B. Buprenorphine-related deaths among drug addicts in France: a report on 20 fatalities. J Anal Toxicol 1998;22(6):430–4.
18. Reynaud M, Tracqui A, Petit G, Potard D, Courty P. Six deaths linked to misuse of buprenorphine–benzodiazepine combinations. Am J Psychiatry 1998;155(3):448–9.
19. Mendelson J, Jones RT, Welm S, Baggott M, Fernandez I, Melby AK, Nath RP. Buprenorphine and naloxone combinations: the effects of three dose ratios in

morphine-stabilized, opiate-dependent volunteers. Psychopharmacology (Berl) 1999;141(1):37–46.

20. Pani PP, Maremmani I, Pirastu R, Tagliamonte A, Gessa GL. Buprenorphine: a controlled clinical trial in the treatment of opioid dependence. Drug Alcohol Depend 2000;60(1):39–50.

21. Fischer G, Johnson RE, Eder H, Jagsch R, Peternell A, Weninger M, Langer M, Aschauer HN. Treatment of opioid-dependent pregnant women with buprenorphine. Addiction 2000;95(2):239–44.

22. Petitjean S, Stohler R, Deglon JJ, Livoti S, Waldvogel D, Uehlinger C, Ladewig D. Double-blind randomized trial of buprenorphine and methadone in opiate dependence. Drug Alcohol Depend 2001;62(1):97–104.

23. Welsh CJ, Suman M, Cohen A, Broyles L, Bennett M, Weintraub E. The use of intravenous buprenorphine for the treatment of opioid withdrawal in medically ill hospitalized patients. Am J Addict 2002;11(2):135–40.

24. Krook AL, Brors O, Dahlberg J, Grouff K, Magnus P, Roysamb E, Waal H. A placebo-controlled study of high dose buprenorphine in opiate dependents waiting for medication-assisted rehabilitation in Oslo, Norway. Addiction 2002;97(5):533–42.

25. Varescon I, Vidal-Trecan G, Nabet N, Boissonnas A. Substitution et mésusage: l'injection intraveineuse de buprénorphine haut dosage. [Buprenorphine abuse: high dose intravenous administration of buprenorphine.] Encephale 2002;28(5 Pt 1):397–402.

26. Clark NC, Lintzeris N, Muhleisen PJ. Severe opiate withdrawal in a heroin user precipitated by a massive buprenorphine dose. Med J Aust 2002;176(4):166–7.

27. Harris DS, Jones RT, Welm S, Upton RA, Lin E, Mendelson J. Buprenorphine and naloxone co-administration in opiate-dependent patients stabilized on sublingual buprenorphine. Drug Alcohol Depend 2000;61(1):85–94.

28. Bohme K. Buprenorphine in a transdermal therapeutic system—a new option. Clin Rheumatol 2002;21(Suppl 1):S13–16.

29. Chang CH, Wang CJ, Yen YC, Hsu SJ. Effectiveness of sublingual buprenorphine and intramuscular pethidine in acute renal colic. Formosan J Surg 2002;35:9–13.

30. Comer SD, Collins ED, Fischman MW. Buprenorphine sublingual tablets: effects on IV heroin self-administration by humans. Psychopharmacology (Berl) 2001;154(1):28–37.

31. Weiss P, Ritz R. Analgetische Wirkung und Nebenwirkungen von Buprenorphine bei der akuten koronaren Herzkrankheit. Ein randomisiertes Doppelblindvergleich mit Morphine. [Analgesic effect and side-effects of buprenorphine in acute coronary heart disease. A randomized double-blind comparison with morphine.] Anästh Intensivther Notfallmed 1988;23(6):309–12.

32. Iribarne C, Berthou F, Carlhant D, Dreano Y, Picart D, Lohezic F, Riche C. Inhibition of methadone and buprenorphine N-dealkylations by three HIV-1 protease inhibitors. Drug Metab Dispos 1998;26(3):257–60.

33. Gal TJ. Naloxone reversal of buprenorphine-induced respiratory depression. Clin Pharmacol Ther 1989;45(1):66–71.

34. Rifat K, Magnin C, Morel D. L'analgésie per et postopératoire à la buprénorphine: effets cardio-circulatoires et respiratoires. [Pre- and postoperative buprenorphine analgesia: cardiocirculatory and respiratory effects.] Cah Anesthesiol 1984;32(1):33–6.

Buspirone

General Information

Buspirone, an azapirone drug, similar to its analogues ipsaperone and tandospirone, is chemically and pharmacologically dissimilar to the benzodiazepines and is useful in both generalized anxiety and depression (1). In contrast to benzodiazepines, buspirone has an antidepressant-like therapeutic latency (2), and for this reason it needs to be given with considerable education and encouragement. It is effective in children with anxiety disorders (SEDA-19, 36) and as an antidepressant adjuvant in refractory depression with (3) and without (4) obsessive-compulsive symptoms. Buspirone is also effective in treating anxious alcoholics, and in patients with agitation or aggression associated with organic brain disease (5).

Originally thought to act through a dopaminergic mechanism, buspirone is now regarded as acting as a 5-HT$_{1A}$ receptor (partial) agonist (6) and produces dose-related adverse effects similar to those of the SSRIs (nausea, headache, insomnia, dizziness, and sexual dysfunction) (SEDA-22, 39) (7). Like them, it interacts with monoamine oxidase inhibitors and can produce the serotonin syndrome (8). An uncommon association with extrapyramidal movement disorders (SEDA-17, 46) (SEDA-18, 45) may reflect its structural relation to some dopamine receptor antagonists.

Compared with benzodiazepines, buspirone causes less sedation and memory impairment (9), has little interaction with alcohol (2,10), and is essentially devoid of problems of abuse, disinhibition, tolerance, and dependence.

These advantages are important in treating particular groups of patients, including patients with brain injury, elderly people, forensic populations, and the medically ill (11,12). On the other hand, over 50% of patients with cerebellar ataxia reported significant adverse effects, as described above (SEDA-21, 39).

Buspirone may also have advantages in treating individuals who are susceptible to problems with alcohol (13) or other hypnosedatives (10), although habitual users of benzodiazepines are often unwilling to persist with buspirone long enough for it to have a therapeutic effect (2).

Unlike carbamazepine or tricyclic antidepressants, buspirone is not helpful in the management of benzodiazepine withdrawal (14).

The safety results from two comparisons of buspirone 15 mg bd and buspirone 10 mg tds in patients with persistent anxiety have been subjected to meta-analysis (15). The incidences of adverse events were similar, except for a significantly higher incidence of bouts of palpitation in patients taking buspirone bd (5%) compared with tds (1%). The most frequently reported adverse events with both regimens were dizziness, headache, and nausea. There were no appreciable differences between treatments in vital signs, physical examination, electrocardiography, or clinical laboratory results. A change to twice-daily dosing with buspirone may offer convenience and possibly greater adherence to therapy in patients with persistent anxiety, without compromising the safety and tolerability profile of the drug.

The effects of hydroxyzine 50 mg/day, buspirone 20 mg/day, and placebo have been studied in 244 patients with generalized anxiety disorder in a double-blind placebo-controlled study (16). Hydroxyzine ($n = 81$) was considerably better than placebo ($n = 81$), and buspirone ($n = 82$) was intermediate. The main adverse effects were headache and migraine with buspirone (6.1 versus 4.9% with hydroxyzine and 1.2% with placebo). Somnolence occurred in 9.9% with hydroxyzine, 4.9% with buspirone, and none with placebo. Dizziness occurred in 6.1% with buspirone, none with hydroxyzine, and 2.5% with placebo.

In a 21-day, open, multicenter, dose-escalation study, 13 children and 12 adolescents with anxiety disorder and 14 healthy adults took buspirone 5–30 mg bd titrated over 3 weeks (17). Buspirone was generally safe and well-tolerated at doses up to 30 mg in adolescents and adults and in most of the children. The most common adverse events in children and adolescents were light-headedness (68%), headache (48%), and dyspepsia (20%); two children withdrew from the study at the higher doses (15 mg and 30 mg bd) owing to adverse effects. In adults, the most common adverse event was somnolence (21%); mild light-headedness, nausea, and diarrhea were also reported.

Organs and Systems

Respiratory

Because of its virtual absence of respiratory depressant effects compared with benzodiazepines (18), buspirone may be especially useful in treating anxious patients with lung disease (19).

Nervous system

The efficacy and safety of buspirone have been evaluated in the management of anxiety and irritability in 22 children with pervasive developmental disorders. One child developed abnormal involuntary movements of the mouth, cheeks, and tongue after having taken buspirone 20 mg/day for 10 months. No other drugs were prescribed. The abnormal movements disappeared completely within 2 weeks of withdrawal of buspirone. Other adverse effects in other children were minimal and included initial sedation, slight agitation, and initial nausea (20).

Long-Term Effects

Drug abuse

Despite continuing scrutiny, buspirone has shown little, if any, abuse potential (7).

Drug Administration

Drug formulations

Because of their short half-lives, buspirone and its analogues are problematic to administer (6). A single dose of

buspirone ER (extended-release) 30 mg has been compared with two doses of buspirone IR (immediate-release) 15 mg given 12 hours apart to assess differences in tolerability in an open, crossover, randomized study in 18 healthy men (21). Blood samples were obtained at 22 times. Seven subjects reported a total of 13 adverse events during the study, but none of the events recorded was unexpected. All were mild and resolved by the end of the study without medical intervention. Three adverse events (rhinitis, headache, and light-headedness) were categorized as unrelated to the study drug. The other 10 adverse events included drowsiness, dizziness, depression, tinnitus, and increased blood pressure. There were no significant differences between the two formulations.

Drug–Drug Interactions

Calcium channel blockers

In a randomized placebo-controlled trial, the possible interactions of buspirone with verapamil and diltiazem were investigated. Both verapamil and diltiazem considerably increased plasma buspirone concentrations, probably by inhibiting CYP3A4. Thus, enhanced effects and adverse effects of buspirone are possible when it is used with verapamil, diltiazem, or other inhibitors of CYP3A4 (22).

Erythromycin

Erythromycin, an inhibitor of CYP3A, can increase buspirone concentrations (SEDA-22, 39).

Fluvoxamine

The effects of fluvoxamine on the pharmacokinetics and pharmacodynamics of buspirone have been investigated in 10 healthy volunteers. Fluvoxamine moderately increased plasma buspirone concentrations and reduced the production of the active metabolite of buspirone. The mechanism of this interaction is probably inhibition of CYP3A4. However, this pharmacokinetic interaction was not associated with impaired psychomotor performance and is probably of limited clinical significance (23).

Grapefruit juice

In a randomized, two-phase crossover study, the effects of grapefruit juice on the pharmacokinetics and pharmacodynamics of oral buspirone were investigated in 10 healthy volunteers. Grapefruit juice increased the mean peak plasma concentration of buspirone 4.3-fold (24). Large amounts of grapefruit juice should be avoided in patients taking buspirone.

Haloperidol

Buspirone increases haloperidol concentrations in some patients (SEDA-21, 39).

Itraconazole

Itraconazole, an inhibitor of CYP3A, can increase buspirone concentrations (SEDA-22, 39).

Monoamine oxidase inhibitors

Buspirone interacts with monoamine inhibitors and can cause the serotonin syndrome (8).

Rifampicin

The effects of rifampicin on the pharmacokinetics and pharmacodynamics of buspirone were investigated in 10 young healthy volunteers. There was a significant reduction in the effects of buspirone in three of the six psychomotor tests used after rifampicin pretreatment. The interaction between rifampicin and buspirone is probably mostly due to increased CYP3A4 activity. Buspirone will most likely have a greatly reduced anxiolytic effect when it is used together with rifampicin or other potent inducers of CYP3A4, such as phenytoin and carbamazepine (25).

Sertraline

Serotonin syndrome has been attributed to the combination of buspirone and sertraline.

- A 49-year-old man had major adverse effects 11 days after taking a combination of sertraline, buspirone, and loxapine (26). The adverse effects were characteristic of the serotonin syndrome, which is characterized by a constellation of symptoms, including hypomania, agitation, seizures, confusion, restlessness, hyper-reflexia, tremor, myoclonus, ataxia, incoordination, anxiety, double vision, fever, shivering, variable effects on blood pressure, nausea and vomiting, sweating, and diarrhea.

St John's wort

Clinicians should inform their patients about the risks associated with taking St John's wort if they are taking psychotropic drugs that can cause the serotonin syndrome.

- A 27-year-old married woman developed symptoms of generalized anxiety disorder and was given buspirone 30 mg/day (27). During treatment she felt depressed and decided to take St John's wort. Two months later she started to have nervousness, aggressiveness, hyperactivity, insomnia, blurred vision, and very short periods of confusion and disorientation. The symptoms were consistent with serotonin syndrome. St John's wort was withdrawn and her symptoms resolved after 1 week.

Buspirone is a partial agonist at $5HT_{1A}$ receptors; St John's wort is a non-selective inhibitor of 5HT reuptake and also upregulates postsynaptic $5HT_{1A}$ and $5HT_{2A}$ receptors; it therefore causes overstimulation of $5HT_{1A}$ receptors, leading to the serotonin syndrome.

References

1. Rickels K, Amsterdam J, Clary C, Hassman J, London J, Puzzuoli G, Schweizer E. Buspirone in depressed outpatients: a controlled study. Psychopharmacol Bull 1990;26(2):163–7.
2. Lader M. Psychiatric disorders. Speight T, Holford N, editors. Avery's Drug Treatment, 4th ed. Auckland: ADIS International Press, 1997:1437.
3. Menkes DB. Buspirone augmentation of sertraline. Br J Psychiatry 1995;166(6):823–4.
4. Joffe RT, Schuller DR. An open study of buspirone augmentation of serotonin reuptake inhibitors in refractory depression. J Clin Psychiatry 1993;54(7):269–71.
5. Stanislav SW, Fabre T, Crismon ML, Childs A. Buspirone's efficacy in organic-induced aggression. J Clin Psychopharmacol 1994;14(2):126–30.
6. Blier P, Ward NM. Is there a role for $5-HT_{1A}$ agonists in the treatment of depression? Biol Psychiatry 2003;53(3):193–203.
7. Lader M. Clin pharmacology of anxiolytic drugs: past, present and future. In: Biggio G, Sanna E, Costa E, editors. GABA-A Receptors and Anxiety: From Neurobiology to Treatment. New York: Raven Press, 1995:135.
8. Napoliello MJ, Domantay AG. Buspirone: a worldwide update. Br J Psychiatry 1991;159(Suppl 12):40–4.
9. Alford C, Bhatti JZ, Curran S, McKay G, Hindmarch I. Pharmacodynamic effects of buspirone and clobazam. Br J Clin Pharmacol 1991;32(1):91–7.
10. Escande M, Frexinos M, Fabre S. Un nouvelle generation de tranquillisants. [A new generation of tranquilizing agents.] Rev Prat 1994;44(17):2316–19.
11. Steinberg JR. Anxiety in elderly patients. A comparison of azapirones and benzodiazepines. Drugs Aging 1994;5(5):335–45.
12. Weiss KJ. Management of anxiety and depression syndromes in the elderly. J Clin Psychiatry 1994;55(Suppl):5–12.
13. Cornelius JR, Bukstein O, Salloum I, Clark D. Alcohol and psychiatric comorbidity. Recent Dev Alcohol 2003;16:361–74.
14. Pelissolo A, Bisserbe JC. Dependance aux benzodiazepine. Aspects clinique et biologiques. [Dependence on benzodiazepines. Clinical and biological aspects.] Encephale 1994;20(2):147–57.
15. Sramek JJ, Hong WW, Hamid S, Nape B, Cutler NR. Meta-analysis of the safety and tolerability of two dose regimens of buspirone in patients with persistent anxiety. Depress Anxiety 1999;9(3):131–4.
16. Lader M. Anxiolytic effect of hydroxyzine: a double-blind trial versus placebo buspirone. Hum Psychopharmacol 1999;14(Suppl 1):94–102.
17. Salazar DE, Frackiewicz EJ, Dockens R, Kollia G, Fulmor IE, Tigel PD, Uderman HD, Shiovitz TM, Sramek JJ, Cutler NR. Pharmacokinetics and tolerability of buspirone during oral administration to children and adolescents with anxiety disorder and normal healthy adults. J Clin Pharmacol 2001;41(12):1351–8.
18. Rapoport DM, Greenberg HE, Goldring RM. Differing effects of the anxiolytic agents buspirone and diazepam on control of breathing. Clin Pharmacol Ther 1991;49(4):394–401.
19. Craven J, Sutherland A. Buspirone for anxiety disorders in patients with severe lung disease. Lancet 1991;338(8761):249.
20. Buitelaar JK, van der Gaag RJ, van der Hoeven J. Buspirone in the management of anxiety and irritability in children with pervasive developmental disorders: results of an open-label study. J Clin Psychiatry 1998;59(2):56–9.
21. Sakr A, Andheria M. Pharmacokinetics of buspirone extended-release tablets: a single-dose study. J Clin Pharmacol 2001;41(7):783–9.
22. Lamberg TS, Kivisto KT, Neuvonen PJ. Effects of verapamil and diltiazem on the pharmacokinetics and pharmacodynamics of buspirone. Clin Pharmacol Ther 1998;63(6):640–5.
23. Lamberg TS, Kivisto KT, Laitila J, Martensson K, Neuvonen PJ. The effect of fluvoxamine on the pharmacokinetics and pharmacodynamics of buspirone. Eur J Clin Pharmacol 1998;54(9–10):761–6.
24. Lilja JJ, Kivisto KT, Backman JT, Lamberg TS, Neuvonen PJ. Grapefruit juice substantially increases

plasma concentrations of buspirone. Clin Pharmacol Ther 1998;64(6):655–60.

25. Lamberg TS, Kivisto KT, Neuvonen PJ. Concentrations and effects of buspirone are considerably reduced by rifampicin. Br J Clin Pharmacol 1998;45(4):381–5.

26. Bonin B, Vandel P, Vandel S, Sechter D, Bizouard P. Serotonin syndrome after sertraline, buspirone and loxapine? Thérapie 1999;54(2):269–71.

27. Dannawi M. Possible serotonin syndrome after combination of buspirone and St John's wort. J Psychopharmacol 2002;16(4):401.

Busulfan

See also Cytostatic and immunosuppressant drugs

General Information

Busulfan is an alkylating agent that is used to treat myeloproliferative disorders and to produce myeloablation before bone marrow or stem cell transplantation. Busulfan is metabolized by hepatic glutathione *S*-transferase, the activity of which correlates negatively with busulfan maximum and minimum concentrations and positively with busulfan clearance (1).

General adverse effects

Leukemic patients receiving marrow from HLA-identical sibling donors were randomized to either oral busulfan 16 mg/kg ($n = 88$) or total body irradiation ($n = 79$), plus cyclophosphamide 120 mg/kg (2). Over 5–9 years the following adverse effects occurred in the two groups:

- obstructive bronchiolitis (26 versus 5%).
- cataracts (6 versus 2%).
- veno-occlusive disease of the liver (12 versus 1%).
- complete or partial alopecia (28 versus 6%).
- hemorrhagic cystitis (32 versus 10%).
- acute graft-versus-host disease (cumulative incidence at 7 years, 59 versus 47%); death from graft-versus-host disease was more common with busulfan (22 versus 3%).

Organs and Systems

Cardiovascular

Pericardial fibrosis has been reported after busulfan treatment in a man with chronic myeloid leukemia (3). Endocardial fibrosis has also been reported (4).

Respiratory

Busulfan can cause interstitial fibrosing lung disease ("busulfan lung") with an estimated incidence of 6% (5). It begins gradually, causes dyspnea and cough, and is often accompanied by skin pigmentation. It usually occurs after prolonged treatment (on average 41 months, cumulative dose 2900 mg). The respiratory function pattern is characterized by reduced lung volumes with hypoxemia and hypocapnic respiratory failure. Radiology shows interstitial and predominantly basal shadows.

Various authors have discussed the differences in busulfan-induced idiopathic pneumonia syndrome, as a result of either chronic low-dose or short-course high-dose therapy. One group found that chronic low-dose therapy (even at cumulative doses of busulfan of up to 3 g) caused different lung damage from the clinical characteristics, radiological, and pathological features of the idiopathic pneumonia syndrome (6).

Three patients with busulfan-induced interstitial pneumonitis each had circulating immune complexes and alveolitis, and histology demonstrated consistent abnormalities of type I pneumocytes and depletion of type II pneumocytes (7).

Nervous system

Busulfan can cause generalized seizures (8).

High concentrations of busulfan in the cerebrospinal fluid have been correlated with development of myoclonic epilepsy and/or other electroencephalographic changes after high-dose busulfan conditioning regimens for acute leukemia (9).

- A 21-year-old woman with acute lymphoblastic leukemia underwent bone marrow transplantation after a conditioning regimen consisting of busulfan and cyclophosphamide (10). The day after starting busulfan, she had a generalized tonic-clonic seizure and electroencephalography showed diffuse polyspikes and spike-and-wave discharges, with persistent abnormalities (slowing of background activity intermixed with diffuse slow waves and isolated delta and theta bursts) for about 20 days and complete normalization 1 month after the seizure.

Phenytoin and benzodiazepines have been successfully used to prevent seizures during busulfan therapy; benzodiazepines may be preferable, because phenytoin can induce the metabolism of busulfan, reducing its efficacy. In 29 children undergoing hemopoietic stem cell transplantation who received high-dose busulfan, intravenous or oral lorazepam (median dose 0.022 mg/kg) before each dose of busulfan and for 24 hours after the last dose was used as seizure prophylaxis; drowsiness was the only significant adverse effect and there were no seizures (11). There were no tonic-clonic or myoclonic seizures in a prospective study in 16 patients with leukemia receiving busulfan before autologous bone marrow transplantation who were given phenobarbital and clonazepam, despite electroencephalographic changes in two patients after busulfan (12).

Sensory systems

Cataract due to busulfan has been reported after long-term administration (SEDA-1, 341) (13).

- A 42-year-old Japanese woman received busulfan 212 mg/day for only 4 days and developed reduced visual acuity and blurred vision in both eyes; she had a posterior polar subcapsular opacity in the lenses in both eyes (14).

• A 49-year-old man with chronic myelogenous leukemia developed dense posterior subcapsular cataracts and punctate cortical opacities after taking busulfan for 5 years (15). Ultrastructural examination showed cortical liquefaction, with Morgagnian droplets involving primarily the region from the equator to the posterior subcapsular space, crystalloid rays, and abundant degenerate lens fiber membranes.

Hematologic

Aplastic anemia developed in 84 patients with chronic myeloid leukemia receiving busulfan; three patients died (16). The time interval until pancytopenia was detected varied considerably, ranging between 6 and 126 months. The effect did not correlate with the initial doses of busulfan.

Colony-stimulating factors have been used to treat and prevent the adverse hematological effects of busulfan (17,18).

• In a 91-year-old woman with essential thrombocythemia and marked bone marrow suppression induced by long-term busulfan, G-CSF and M-CSF increased the neutrophil and platelet counts but only transiently; there was transient eosinophilia after withdrawal of M-CSF (19).

• A 63-year-old woman with thrombocythemia was given busulfan 2 mg/day and later developed pancytopenia (20). She was given metenolone acetate 15 mg/day and G-CSF 300 µg/day, and frequent blood transfusions without effect. She was then given metenolone acetate, G-CSF 600 µg/day, and erythropoietin 24 000 units twice a week, and her pancytopenia gradually improved over several months.

One patient with busulfan-induced pancytopenia and recurrent thrombocytopenic bleeding was successfully treated prophylactically with random-donor platelet transfusions and later with HLA-matched platelets from a sibling (21).

• A patient with polycythemia vera who had undergone splenectomy received six courses of busulfan for recurrent thrombocytosis over 19 years (22). Severe pancytopenia followed and persisted for 4 months. There was marked erythroid hyperplasia in the bone marrow, with striking dyserythropoiesis, PAS-positive erythrocyte precursors, moderate numbers of circulating normoblasts, and evidence of chronic and acute hemolysis.

Of 39 patients taking busulfan 16 mg/kg/day and cyclophosphamide 120 mg/kg/day for leukemias, who received non-T cell depleted, HLA-matched sibling or unrelated donor marrow transplants 2 days after the end of chemotherapy followed by ciclosporin and methylprednisolone given to prevent graft-versus-host disease, 11 developed eosinophilia, of whom only 2 were still taking methylprednisolone (23). At the onset of eosinophilia, five of these 11 patients had graft-versus-host disease that worsened within 2 months. In the other six patients, graft-versus-host disease was not present initially but developed in all cases at a median of 4 months after the onset of eosinophilia.

Liver

In 66 patients who received busulfan in combination with cyclophosphamide, etoposide, and/or cytarabine in preparation for bone marrow transplantation, there was a higher incidence of veno-occlusive disease of the liver (sinusoidal obstruction syndrome) in those who received busulfan + cyclophosphamide (four of 10) than in those who received busulfan + cyclophosphamide + cytarabine (one of 18) or busulfan + cyclophosphamide + etoposide (seven of 38) (24). The risk of veno-occlusive disease was higher in those whose busulfan AUC was over 1500 minute.µmol/l (relative risk = 11). Other pharmacokinetic parameters, age, sex, type of bone marrow transplantation, previous therapy, or pretransplant liver function tests were not predictive of veno-occlusive disease.

In 30 patients who received oral busulfan 1 mg/kg, all six of those who developed hepatic veno-occlusive disease had a busulfan AUC greater than the mean, and five had an AUC that was greater than 1 standard deviation above the mean; veno-occlusive disease correlated with an increased AUC (25).

• Intrahepatic cholestasis has been attributed to busulfan in a 57-year-old man with chronic megakaryocytic granulocytic myelosis (26).

• Cholestatic hepatitis occurred in a 61-year-old man with chronic myelocytic leukemia who had taken busulfan for 8 years (27). He presented with fever, abdominal pain, and raised liver enzymes. A liver biopsy showed cellular cholestasis with focal liver cell necrosis accompanied by a mild inflammatory infiltrate. When busulfan was withdrawn, his liver enzymes normalized and his fever resolved.

Urinary tract

Busulfan can rarely cause hemorrhagic cystitis (28,29).

Skin

Busulfan can cause hyperpigmentation (30,31), often in combination with interstitial lung disease (5).

Hair

Of 65 patients who survived for at least 6 months after bone marrow transplantation, 31 had some degree of alopecia and 19 had extensive alopecia (32). The mean minimum busulfan concentration was 656 ng/ml in patients who developed alopecia, compared with 507 ng/ml in those who did not. Patients with more extensive alopecia had higher busulfan concentrations. In multivariate analysis, alopecia was associated with busulfan concentrations higher than the median (OR = 3.43; 95% CI = 3.04, 3.88), allogeneic transplantation (OR = 2.56; CI = 2.28, 2.88), and female sex (OR = 1.96; CI = 1.73, 2.88). There was no association between alopecia and chronic graft-versus-host disease.

Reproductive system

Busulfan can cause ovarian failure.

• A 26-year-old woman with chronic myeloid leukemia developed busulfan-induced ovarian failure, with amenorrhea, climacteric symptoms, raised plasma concentrations of luteinizing and follicle-stimulating hormones, and low 17 beta-estradiol concentrations (33). However, 1 year later she became pregnant, the busulfan was stopped, and amniocentesis showed a normal karyotype. The remainder of the pregnancy was unremarkable and ended with the normal delivery of a healthy child.

Of 21 girls aged 11–21 years who had received high-dose chemotherapy and autologous bone marrow transplantation without total body irradiation for malignant tumors 1.2–13 years before (median 7 years), 10 were given busulfan 600 mg/m^2 and melphalan (140 mg/m^2) with or without cyclophosphamide (3.6 g/m^2) (34). Eleven others did not receive busulfan. Twelve girls (57%) had clinical and hormonal evidence of ovarian failure. Among nine others who had had normal puberty, six had normal gonadotropin concentrations, one had raised gonadotropin concentrations, and two had gonadotropin concentrations at the upper limit of the reference range. All 10 girls who received busulfan developed severe persistent ovarian failure.

Second-Generation Effects

Teratogenicity

Retinal degeneration and microphthalmia have been described in the infants of women who have taken busulfan during pregnancy (35).

- Myeloschisis occurred in a 6-week-old human embryo whose 39-year-old mother had taken busulfan before and during the early stages of gestation for chronic lymphatic leukemia (36). Histology showed reduced mesenchymal elements together with somite disorganization in the affected area of the embryo.

Drug Administration

Drug overdose

A 4.6 kg infant with Wiskott–Aldrich syndrome received an accidental overdose of busulfan during preparation for allogeneic stem cell transplantation (37). Hemodialysis was immediately performed and resulted in accelerated clearance of busulfan. There were no acute neurological or hepatic adverse effects, and after cough and by rales for 2 months pulmonary symptoms resolved. There was stable partial donor chimerism after transplantation, but the patient was well 12 months later.

Drug–Drug Interactions

Cyclophosphamide

In bone marrow transplant recipients, prior administration of busulfan, which itself causes hemorrhagic cystitis, can increase the risk of cyclophosphamide-induced damage (38).

Busulfan reduces the clearance of cyclophosphamide to its active metabolite 4-hydroperoxycyclophosphamide (39). The first dose of high-dose cyclophosphamide should therefore be delayed for at least 24 hours after the last dose of busulfan.

Itraconazole

In 13 patients given bone marrow transplantation, the clearance of busulfan was reduced by an average of 20% in patients taking itraconazole compared with control patients and patients taking fluconazole (40).

Metronidazole

In 24 patients with graft-versus-host disease, metronidazole significantly increased busulfan plasma concentrations from 452 to 807 ng/ml (41). The authors concluded that metronidazole should not be administered simultaneously with busulfan, because of the risk of severe toxicity and/or mortality.

Phenytoin

In 17 patients given busulfan during conditioning before bone marrow transplantation, phenytoin increased the clearance of busulfan and shortened its half-life; diazepam did not have the same effect (42). There were reductions in the steady-state concentrations of busulfan in four of seven patients who took phenytoin and in only one of eight patients who took diazepam. This effect of phenytoin is probably due to induction of glutathione transferase.

References

1. Poonkuzhali B, Chandy M, Srivastava A, Dennison D, Krishnamoorthy R. Glutathione S-transferase activity influences busulfan pharmacokinetics in patients with beta thalassemia major undergoing bone marrow transplantation. Drug Metab Dispos 2001;29(3):264–7.
2. Ringden O, Remberger M, Ruutu T, Nikoskelainen J, Volin L, Vindelov L, Parkkali T, Lenhoff S, Sallerfors B, Mellander L, Ljungman P, Jacobsen N. Increased risk of chronic graft-versus-host disease, obstructive bronchiolitis, and alopecia with busulfan versus total body irradiation: long-term results of a randomized trial in allogeneic marrow recipients with leukemia. Nordic Bone Marrow Transplantation Group. Blood 1999;93(7):2196–201.
3. Terpstra W, de Maat CE. Pericardial fibrosis following busulfan treatment. Neth J Med 1989;35(5–6):249–52.
4. Weinberger A, Pinkhas J, Sandbank U, Shaklai M, de Vries A. Endocardial fibrosis following busulfan treatment. JAMA 1975;231(5):495.
5. Massin F, Fur A, Reybet-Degat O, Camus P, Jeannin L. La pneumopathie du busulfan. [Busulfan-induced pneumopathy.] Rev Mal Respir 1987;4(1):3–10.
6. Bilgrami SF, Metersky ML, McNally D, Naqvi BH, Kapur D, Raible D, Bona RD, Edwards RL, Feingold JM, Clive JM, Tutschka PJ. Idiopathic pneumonia syndrome following myeloablative chemotherapy and autologous transplantation. Ann Pharmacother 2001;35(2):196–201.
7. Vergnon JM, Boucheron S, Riffat J, Guy C, Blanc P, Emonot A. Pneumopathies interstitielles au busulfan: analyse histologique, évolutive et par lavage broncho-alvéolaire de trois observations. [Interstitial pneumopathies caused by busulfan. Histologic, developmental and bronchoalveolar

lavage analysis of 3 cases.] Rev Med Interne 1988; 9(4):377–83.

8. Murphy CP, Harden EA, Thompson JM. Generalized seizures secondary to high-dose busulfan therapy. Ann Pharmacother 1992;26(1):30–1.

9. Meloni G, Raucci U, Pinto RM, Spalice A, Vignetti M, Iannetti P. Pretransplant conditioning with busulfan and cyclophosphamide in acute leukemia patients: neurological and electroencephalographic prospective study. Ann Oncol 1992;3(2):145–8.

10. La Morgia C, Mondini S, Guarino M, Bonifazi F, Cirignotta F. Busulfan neurotoxicity and EEG abnormalities: a case report. Neurol Sci 2004;25(2):95–7.

11. Chan KW, Mullen CA, Worth LL, Choroszy M, Koontz S, Tran H, Slopis J. Lorazepam for seizure prophylaxis during high-dose busulfan administration. Bone Marrow Transplant 2002;29(12):963–5.

12. Meloni G, Nasta L, Pinto RM, Spalice A, Raucci U, Iannetti P. Clonazepam prophylaxis and busulfan-related myoclonic epilepsy in autografted acute leukemia patients. Haematologica 1995;80(6):532–4.

13. Honda A, Dake Y, Amemiya T. [Cataracts in a patient treated with busulfan (Mablin powder) for eight years.] Nippon Ganka Gakkai Zasshi 1993;97(10):1242–5.

14. Kaida T, Ogawa T, Amemiya T. Cataract induced by short-term administration of large doses of busulfan: a case report. Ophthalmologica 1999;213(6):397–9.

15. Hamming NA, Apple DJ, Goldberg MF. Histopathology and ultrastructure of busulfan-induced cataract. Albrecht Von Graefes Arch Klin Exp Ophthalmol 1976;200(2):139–47.

16. Krug K, Stenzel L. Verlaufsvarianten von Panzytopenien nach Busulfanbehandlung der chronischen myeloischen Leukämie (CML). [Varying course of pancytopenia after busulfan treatment of chronic myelocytic leukemia (CML).] Folia Haematol Int Mag Klin Morphol Blutforsch 1978;105(2):181–7.

17. Fiedler W, Goetz G, Weh HJ, Hossfeld DK. GM-CSF in busulfan overdosage. Eur J Haematol 1990;45(3):183–4.

18. Openshaw H, Lund BT, Kashyap A, Atkinson R, Sniecinski I, Weiner LP, Forman S. Peripheral blood stem cell transplantation in multiple sclerosis with busulfan and cyclophosphamide conditioning: report of toxicity and immunological monitoring. Biol Blood Marrow Transplant 2000;6(5A):563–75.

19. Take H, Tamura K, Kurabayashi H, Kubota K, Shirakura T. [Effect of G-CSF and M-CSF on busulfan-induced marrow failure in a 91-year old patient with essential thrombocythemia.] Nippon Ronen Igakkai Zasshi 1993;30(10):901–5.

20. Yamamoto K, Nagata K, Hamaguchi H. [Complete remission of essential thrombocythemia after recovery from severe bone marrow aplasia induced by busulfan treatment.] Gan To Kagaku Ryoho 1997;24(3):365–9.

21. Stuart JJ, Crocker DL, Roberts HR. Treatment of busulfan-induced pancytopenia. Arch Intern Med 1976;136(10):1181–3.

22. Pezzimenti JF, Kim HC, Lindenbaum J. Erythroleukemia-like syndrome due to busulfan toxicity in polycythemia vera. Cancer 1976;38(6):2242–6.

23. Kalaycioglu ME, Bolwell BJ. Eosinophilia after allogeneic bone marrow transplantation using the busulfan and cyclophosphamide preparative regimen. Bone Marrow Transplant 1994;14(1):113–15.

24. Dix SP, Wingard JR, Mullins RE, Jerkunica I, Davidson TG, Gilmore CE, York RC, Lin LS, Devine SM, Geller RB, Heffner LT, Hillyer CD, Holland HK, Winton EF, Saral R. Association of busulfan area under

the curve with veno-occlusive disease following BMT. Bone Marrow Transplant 1996;17(2):225–30.

25. Grochow LB, Jones RJ, Brundrett RB, Braine HG, Chen TL, Saral R, Santos GW, Colvin OM. Pharmacokinetics of busulfan: correlation with veno-occlusive disease in patients undergoing bone marrow transplantation. Cancer Chemother Pharmacol 1989;25(1):55–61.

26. Adang RP, Breed WP. Leverbeschadiging tijdens gebruik van busulfan. [Liver damage during use of busulfan.] Ned Tijdschr Geneeskd 1989;133(30):1515–18. Erratum in: Ned Tijdschr Geneeskd 1989;133(37):1864.

27. Morris LE, Guthrie TH Jr. Busulfan-induced hepatitis. Am J Gastroenterol 1988;83(6):682–3.

28. Millard RJ. Busulfan-induced hemorrhagic cystitis. Urology 1981;18(2):143–4.

29. Pode D, Perlberg S, Steiner D. Busulfan-induced hemorrhagic cystitis. J Urol 1983;130(2):347–8.

30. Adam BA, Ismail R, Sivanesan S. Busulfan hyperpigmentation: light and electron microscopic studies. J Dermatol 1980;7(6):405–11.

31. Simonart T, Decaux G, Gourdin JM, Peny MO, Noel JC, Leclercq-Smekens M, De Dobbeleer G. Hyperpigmentation induite par le busulfan: une observation avec étude ultrastructurale. [Hyperpigmentation induced by busulfan: a case with ultrastructure examination.] Ann Dermatol Venereol 1999;126(5):439–40.

32. Ljungman P, Hassan M, Bekassy AN, Ringden O, Oberg G. Busulfan concentration in relation to permanent alopecia in recipients of bone marrow transplants. Bone Marrow Transplant 1995;15(6):869–71.

33. Shalev O, Rahav G, Milwidsky A. Reversible busulfan-induced ovarian failure. Eur J Obstet Gynecol Reprod Biol 1987;26(3):239–42.

34. Teinturier C, Hartmann O, Valteau-Couanet D, Benhamou E, Bougneres PF. Ovarian function after autologous bone marrow transplantation in childhood: high-dose busulfan is a major cause of ovarian failure. Bone Marrow Transplant 1998;22(10):989–94.

35. Saraux H, Lefrancois A. Degenerative Netzhauterkrankungen nach Behandlung der Mutter mit Busulfan während der Schwangerschaft. [Degenerative retinal conditions after treatment with Busulfan during pregnancy.] Klin Monatsbl Augenheilkd 1977;170(6):818–20.

36. Abramovici A, Shaklai M, Pinkhas J. Myeloschisis in a six weeks embryo of a leukemic woman treated by busulfan. Teratology 1978;18(2):241–6.

37. Stein J, Davidovitz M, Yaniv I, Ben-Ari J, Gamzu Z, Hoffer E, Bentur Y, Tabak A, Krivoy N. Accidental busulfan overdose: enhanced drug clearance with hemodialysis in a child with Wiskott–Aldrich syndrome. Bone Marrow Transplant 2001;27(5):551–3.

38. Thomas AE, Patterson J, Prentice HG, Brenner MK, Ganczakowski M, Hancock JF, Pattinson JK, Blacklock HA, Hopewell JP. Haemorrhagic cystitis in bone marrow transplantation patients: possible increased risk associated with prior busulphan therapy. Bone Marrow Transplant 1987;1(4):347–55.

39. Hassan M, Ljungman P, Ringden O, Hassan Z, Oberg G, Nilsson C, Bekassy A, Bielenstein M, Abdel-Rehim M, Georen S, Astner L. The effect of busulphan on the pharmacokinetics of cyclophosphamide and its 4-hydroxy metabolite: time interval influence on therapeutic efficacy and therapy-related toxicity. Bone Marrow Transplant 2000;25(9):915–24.

40. Buggia I, Zecca M, Alessandrino EP, Locatelli F, Rosti G, Bosi A, Pession A, Rotoli B, Majolino I, Dallorso A,

Regazzi MB. Itraconazole can increase systemic exposure to busulfan in patients given bone marrow transplantation. GITMO (Gruppo Italiano Trapianto di Midollo Osseo). Anticancer Res 1996;16(4A):2083–8.

41. Nilsson C, Aschan J, Hentschke P, Ringden O, Ljungman P, Hassan M. The effect of metronidazole on busulfan pharmacokinetics in patients undergoing hematopoietic stem cell transplantation. Bone Marrow Transplant 2003;31(6):429–35.

42. Hassan M, Oberg G, Bjorkholm M, Wallin I, Lindgren M. Influence of prophylactic anticonvulsant therapy on high-dose busulphan kinetics. Cancer Chemother Pharmacol 1993;33(3):181–6.

Butibufen

See also Non-steroidal anti-inflammatory drugs

General Information

Experience with the NSAID butibufen is limited. Only gastrointestinal adverse effects have been described (1).

Reference

1. Aparicio L. Butibufen. Drugs Today 1979;15:43.

Butorphanol

See also Opioid analgesics

General Information

Butorphanol is a synthetic 14-hydroxymorphinan analogue with a low dependence potential and a low propensity to cause opioid adverse effects (1). It is a synthetic OP_2 (κ) receptor agonist and OP_3 (μ) receptor antagonist.

General adverse reactions

In some patients, effective doses cause troublesome effects. For example, in a randomized study of patients with sickle-cell crisis who received either butorphanol 2 mg intramuscularly or morphine 6 mg intramuscularly, adverse effects occurred in 23 and 13% respectively (2). On the other hand, a wide range of doses (4–48 mg/day) over 1 month failed to produce scores indicative of euphoric effects, and the withdrawal syndrome resembled a cyclazocine rather than a morphine abstinence effect (1).

Organs and Systems

Cardiovascular

Although cardiovascular toxicity with butorphanol is slight, raised pulmonary wedge pressure has occurred at cardiac catheterization (1).

Respiratory

Respiratory depression occurs minimally at doses of 2–4 mg (1).

Biliary tract

Butorphanol is generally believed to have a much smaller effect on biliary pressure than morphine, fentanyl, or pethidine, but 2 mg has caused biliary spasm (3).

Musculoskeletal

Fibrous myopathy has been reported in a 40-year-old woman who injected butorphanol intramuscularly (SEDA-17, 87).

Second-Generation Effects

Fetotoxicity

Two cases of sinusoidal fetal heart rhythm have been reported in which there was a significant temporal relation between the administration of butorphanol and the onset of the abnormal heart rhythm (4). In both instances the pattern reverted to normal after further analgesia was given.

Drug Administration

Drug administration route

Butorphanol has been used for epidural anesthesia in obstetric practice without adversely affecting the neonate, and no patients had pruritus (SEDA-16, 88).

As butorphanol is not orally active, reports of its transnasal administration are of interest. The most common adverse effects of transnasal butorphanol were dizziness, nausea and/or vomiting, headache, and drowsiness (SEDA-20, 83). Increased cardiac workload can also occur.

After cesarean section, transnasal butorphanol did not work quite as quickly as intravenous butorphanol. The effect lasted longer but the adverse effects were similar (SEDA-16, 88).

References

1. Pachter IJ, Evens RP. Butorphanol. Drug Alcohol Depend 1985;14(3–4):325–38.
2. Gonzalez ER, Ornato JP, Ware D, Bull D, Evens RP. Comparison of intramuscular analgesic activity of butorphanol and morphine in patients with sickle cell disease. Ann Emerg Med 1988;17(8):788–91.
3. Dolan PF. Butorphanol and biliary spasm. Anesthesiology 1985;63(3):340.
4. Welt SI. Sinusoidal fetal heart rate and butorphanol administration. Am J Obstet Gynecol 1985;152(3):362–3.

Butriptyline

See also Tricyclic antidepressants

General Information

Butriptyline is the isobutyl side-chain homolog of amitriptyline. Its adverse effects, reported in two open studies, were no different from those of other tricyclic antidepressants (1,2).

References

1   Madalena JC, De Matos HG. Preliminary clinical observations with butriptyline. J Med 1971;2(5):322–6.
2   Grivois H. Butriptyline. A new antidepressant compound. J Med 1971;2(5):276–89.

Butylated hydroxytoluene

General Information

Butylated hydroxytoluene is an additive used as an antioxidant in foods, such as packet cake mixes, potato crisps, salted peanuts, and dehydrated mashed potatoes. Its safety, and that of a number of other food additives, has been critically reviewed in a Danish study (1).

Organs and Systems

Immunologic

It is impossible to decide from experimental findings in animals what the result will be of prolonged human exposure to low concentrations of such substances. Butylated hydroxytoluene causes various allergies; symptoms of hay fever and asthma have been reported.

Chewing gum should be considered as a possible cause of unexplained food allergy.

- Butylated hydroxytoluene in chewing gum caused disseminated urticarial eruption in a young woman (2). An adverse drug reaction was ruled out, and the only recent dietary change had been regular use of chewing-gum containing butylated hydroxytoluene. The skin lesions showed signs of vasculitis, with a perivascular cellular infiltrate, heavy extravascular deposition of fibrinogen, and intraendothelial deposits of IgM, C'9, C3, and C9. She stopped using the gum and within a week the eruption had subsided. An oral provocation test confirmed that butylated hydroxytoluene was responsible, the cutaneous signs returning within several hours of rechallenge.

Long-Term Effects

Tumorigenicity

Although it has been suggested that butylated hydroxytoluene induces tumors in rats, others have suggested that it may protect tissues against the carcinogenic effects of many different substances.

References

1.   Zinck O, Hallas-Moller O. E-nummer Bogen. Copenhagen: Forlaget komma, 1986.
2.   Moneret-Vautrin DA, Bene MC, Faure G. She should not have chewed. Lancet 1986;1(8481):617.

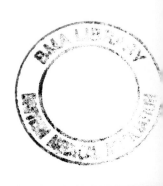